MORE LISTINGS, MORE CHOICES, MORE UP-TO-DATE INFORMATION THAN EVER BEFORE!

The latest gourmet and health foods . . . The most popular brand-name and fast-food items . . . The most exotic ethnic cuisines—including Japanese, Thai, Indian, Cajun, and Mexican . . . It's all here in the **seventh edition** of Corinne T. Netzer's *The Complete Book of Food Counts,* now completely revised and updated with all-new information on the largest possible variety of foods. Whether you're counting calories, carbs, or fat grams, boosting protein or watching your sodium intake, Corinne T. Netzer's bestselling classic gives you all the essential counts you need to make *informed and healthy* choices about the foods you eat—all in one quick and easy reference!

Thousands more listings than ever before!

THE COMPLETE BOOK OF FOOD COUNTS
SEVENTH EDITION

CORINNE T. NETZER

Books by Corinne T. Netzer

The Corinne T. Netzer Annual Calorie Counter
The Complete Book of Food Counts
Corinne T. Netzer's Big Book of Miracle Cures
The Corinne T. Netzer Carbohydrate Dieter's Diary
The Complete Book of Vitamin and Mineral Counts
The Corinne T. Netzer Carbohydrate Counter
The Corinne T. Netzer Dieter's Diary
The Corinne T. Netzer Encyclopedia of Food Values
The Corinne T. Netzer Fat Gram Counter
The Corinne T. Netzer Low-Fat Diary
The Dieter's Calorie Counter
The Corinne T. Netzer Dieter's Activity Diary

Available from Dell

Seventh Edition

THE
COMPLETE
BOOK
OF
FOOD COUNTS

Corinne T. Netzer

A DELL BOOK

THE COMPLETE BOOK OF FOOD COUNTS, SEVENTH EDITION
A Dell Book / January 2006

Published by Bantam Dell
A Division of Random House, Inc.
New York, New York

Dell is a registered trademark of Random House, Inc., and the colophon is a trademark of Random House, Inc.

ISBN-10: 0-440-24123-5
ISBN-13: 978-0-440-21423-2

Printed in the United States of America
Published simultaneously in Canada

www.bantamdell.com

OPM   10 9 8 7 6 5 4 3 2 1

For
Mary Ann and Joel Orgler

Introduction

The seventh edition of *The Complete Book of Food Counts* is the largest compilation of essential food data in this format. It contains data (calories, protein, carbohydrates, fat, cholesterol, sodium, and fiber) for basic generic foods, brand-name foods, and restaurant chains. Whether you are interested in dieting or nutrition—or both—you will find this book unique and invaluable as a reference.

Since this book is alphabetized, you should have no difficulty finding whatever you wish to look up. There are, however, times when you may have to look in more than one place. If you are searching for a particular food and cannot find it immediately, look for it under a category, such as cakes, puddings, cookies, soups. Wherever sensible, I have cross-referenced listings, but the pressure of space has made it impossible to do that for every item.

Compare only foods listed in similar measures. This rule particularly applies to the confusion between measures by capacity and measures by weight. Eight ounces is not necessarily equivalent to eight fluid ounces or one cup. Eight ounces is a measure of how much something weighs; one cup is a measure of how much space it occupies. For instance, a cup of lightweight food, such as puffed rice or popcorn, weighs about one ounce, and eight ounces of the same product would fill many cups. Naturally, you can convert a similar unit of measure into a smaller or larger amount. The following table may be useful in making such conversions.

Equivalents by Capacity
(all measures level)
1 quart = 4 cups
1 cup = 8 fluid ounces
= ½ pint
= 16 tablespoons
2 tablespoons = 1 fluid ounce
1 tablespoon = 3 teaspoons

Equivalents by Weight
1 pound = 16 ounces
3.57 ounces = 100 grams
1 ounce = 28.35 grams

All the material contained in *The Complete Book of Food Counts* is based on information from the United States government, from producers and processors of brand-name foods, and from food chains. The data contained herein is the most complete and accurate information available as this book goes to press. Please bear in mind that seasonal and regional differences can affect the nutritional value of foods. Also, the food industry often changes recipes and sizes and may discontinue products or add new ones. In the future I will revise and update this book to keep you completely informed.

Good luck and good dieting.

Corinne T. Netzer

ABBREVIATIONS AND SYMBOLS

cal.	calories
carbo.	carbohydrates
chol.	cholesterol
cont.	container
diam.	diameter
fl.	fluid
gms.	grams
"	inch
<	less than
>	more than
mgs.	milligrams
lb(s).	pound(s)
n.a.	not available
oz.	ounce
pc(s).	piece(s)
pkg.	package
pkt.	packet
prot.	protein
sod.	sodium
sq.	square
tbsp.	tablespoon
tsp.	teaspoon
tr.	trace
w/	with
*	prepared according to basic package directions, except as noted

THE
COMPLETE
BOOK
OF
FOOD COUNTS

A

Food and Measure	cal.	prot. (gms)	carbo. (gms)	fat (gms)	chol. (mgs)	sod. (mgs)	fiber (gms)
Abalone, meat only							
raw, 4 oz.	119	19.4	6.8	.9	96	341	0
Abiyuch, ½ cup, 4 oz.	79	1.7	20.1	.1	0	23	6.0
Abruzzese sausage,							
hot or sweet (*Boar's*							
Head), 1 oz.	100	8.0	<1.0	8.0	15	540	0
Acerola, fresh:							
10 fruits	15	.2	3.7	.1	0	3	.5
peeled, 1 cup	31	.4	7.5	.3	0	7	1.1
Acerola juice, fresh,							
8 fl. oz.	56	1.0	11.6	.7	0	7	.7
Achiotina, see "Lard"							
Acorn squash:							
raw:							
(*Frieda's*), ¾ cup,							
3 oz.	35	1.0	9.0	0	0	0	2.0
4" squash, 15.2 oz.	172	3.5	44.9	.4	0	13	6.6
cubed, 1 cup	56	1.1	14.6	.1	0	4	2.1
baked, cubed, ½ cup .	57	1.1	14.9	.1	0	4	4.5
boiled, mashed, ½ cup	42	.8	10.8	.1	0	4	3.2
Adobo fresco, 1 tbsp.	41	.4	3.3	3.8	0	3087	.3
Adobo sauce (*Doña*							
Maria), 2 tbsp.	230	2.0	10.0	15.0	0	370	2.0
Adobo seasoning							
(*Goya*), ¼ tsp.	0	0	0	0	0	360	0
Aduki beans, canned							
(*Eden*), ½ cup	110	7.0	19.0	0	0	10	5.0
Adzuki beans:							
dry, ¼ cup:							
(*Arrowhead Mills*) .	130	8.0	26.0	0	0	0	5.0
(*Shiloh Farms*)	160	11.0	29.0	.5	0	0	6.0
boiled, ½ cup	147	8.7	28.5	.1	0	9	8.4
Aioli, see							
"Mayonnaise"							

Food and Measure	cal.	prot. (gms)	carbo. (gms)	fat (gms)	chol. (mgs)	sod. (mgs)	fiber (gms)
Alfalfa seeds (*Shiloh Farms*), 2¼ tsp.	40	5.0	4.0	0	0	0	2.0
Alfalfa sprouts (*Jonathan's*), 1 cup	25	3.0	3.0	.5	0	5	2.0
Alfredo sauce, can or jar, ¼ cup:							
(*Classico* di Roma) ..	120	2.0	3.0	11.0	50	380	0
creamy (*Bertolli*)	110	2.0	3.0	10.0	35	420	0
creamy garlic (*Bertolli*)	100	2.0	3.0	10.0	30	360	0
garlic, roasted (*Classico* di Sorrento) ..	100	2.0	3.0	9.0	45	410	0
Parmesan (*Ragú* Classic)	110	1.0	3.0	10.0	30	400	0
tomato, sun-dried (*Classico* di Capri) .	120	2.0	4.0	10.0	50	420	2.0
Alfredo sauce, refrigerated, ¼ cup, except as noted:							
(*Buitoni* Family Size) .	140	4.0	5.0	12.0	35	430	0
(*Buitoni* Light)	80	4.0	5.0	5.0	20	370	0
(*DiGiorno*), ¼ of 10-oz. cont.	180	3.0	3.0	18.0	25	600	0
portobello mushroom (*Buitoni*)	100	2.0	5.0	8.0	20	340	0
Alfredo sauce mix, dry, creamy garlic (*McCormick*), 2 tbsp.	90	3.0	4.0	6.0	20	860	0
Allspice, 1 tsp.	5	.1	1.4	.2	0	1	.4
Almond, shelled:							
(*Beer Nuts*), 1 oz.	170	6.0	6.0	14.0	0	65	3.0
(*Fisher*), 1 oz.	170	7.0	6.0	14.0	0	0	3.0
(*Planters*), 1 oz.	170	6.0	5.0	15.0	0	0	3.0
(*Planters* Lightly Salted), .9 oz.	170	6.0	6.0	15.0	0	40	3.0
(*Planters* Salted), 1 oz.	160	6.0	6.0	15.0	0	60	3.0
raw:							
(*Shiloh Farms*), 1 oz., about 24 ..	210	7.0	7.0	18.0	0	0	4.0
(*Tree of Life*), ¼ cup	210	7.0	7.0	19.0	0	0	3.0
dried, 1 oz.	167	5.7	5.8	14.8	0	3	3.1
dry-roasted: (*New England Naturals*), ¼ cup, 1.1 oz.	180	5.0	7.0	16.0	0	220	3.0

Food and Measure	cal.	prot. (gms)	carbo. (gms)	fat (gms)	chol. (mgs)	sod. (mgs)	fiber (gms)
salted, 1 oz.	167	4.6	6.9	14.7	0	221	3.9
tamari (*Eden* Organic), 3 tbsp., 1 oz.	160	8.0	8.0	11.0	0	65	4.0
tamari (*New England Naturals*), 3 tbsp., 1 oz. . . .	160	6.0	6.0	14.0	0	100	3.0
honey-roasted, 1 oz. .	168	5.2	7.9	14.2	0	37	3.9
oil-roasted, salted, 1 oz.	176	5.8	4.5	16.4	0	221	3.2
sliced:							
(*Planters*), 1.2 oz. .	200	7.0	6.0	18.0	0	0	4.0
(*Shiloh Farms*), ¼ cup	210	7.0	7.0	18.0	0	0	4.0
slivered:							
(*Planters*), 2-oz. pkg.	340	12.0	11.0	31.0	0	0	6.0
1 cup	795	26.9	27.5	70.5	0	15	14.7
smoked:							
(*Planters*), 1 oz. . . .	170	5.0	6.0	15.0	0	200	3.0
roasted (*New England Naturals*), ¼ cup, 1.1 oz. . .	180	5.0	8.0	15.0	0	300	3.0
toasted, 1 oz.	167	5.8	6.5	14.4	0	3	3.2
Almond butter:							
(*Kettle Roaster Fresh*), 1 oz.	184	5.0	6.0	16.0	0	56	0
all varieties (*Tree of Life*), 2 tbsp.	180	5.0	7.0	16.0	0	0	4.0
Almond flour (*Shiloh Farms*), 1 oz.	170	6.0	6.0	15.0	0	0	3.0
Almond meal, 1 oz. . .	116	11.2	8.2	5.2	0	2	n.a.
Almond paste, see "Pastry filling"							
Almond syrup (*Trader Vic's* Orgeat), 2 tbsp.	100	0	25.0	0	0	15	0
Alu chole, see "Vegetarian entree, pkg."							
Amaranth, whole grain:							
(*Arrowhead Mills*), ¼ cup	180	7.0	31.0	3.0	0	10	7.0

Food and Measure	cal.	prot. (gms)	carbo. (gms)	fat (gms)	chol. (mgs)	sod. (mgs)	fiber (gms)
Amaranth *(cont.)*							
(Shiloh Farms), ¼ cup	195	7.0	36.0	3.0	0	0	6.0
1 oz.	106	4.1	18.8	1.8	0	6	4.3
Amaranth flakes, see "Cereal, ready-to-eat"							
Amaranth flour *(Arrowhead Mills)*, ⅓ cup	120	4.0	20.0	2.5	0	0	2.0
Amaranth leaves, ½ cup:							
raw, trimmed	4	.3	.6	<.1	0	3	n.a.
boiled, drained	14	1.4	2.7	.1	0	14	n.a.
Amaranth seeds *(Arrowhead Mills)*, ¼ cup	170	7.0	29.0	2.0	0	0	3.0
Amaretto syrup *(Ferrara)*, 2 oz.	130	0	32.0	0	0	12	0
Anasazi beans, dry *(Arrowhead Mills)*, ¼ cup	140	7.0	26.0	1.0	0	10	6.0
Anchovy, fresh, European, meat only, raw, 1 oz.	37	5.8	0	1.4	17	29	0
Anchovy, canned, in olive oil, drained: flat fillets:							
(Brunswick), .6 oz.	25	3.0	0	1.5	10	980	0
(Crown Prince), 9 pcs., .6 oz. . . .	35	4.0	0	2.5	15	1050	0
(Yankee Clipper), 5 pcs.	25	3.0	0	1.5	12	980	0
5 medium, .7 oz. . .	42	5.8	0	1.9	3	734	0
rolled, w/capers:							
(Crown Prince), 7 pcs., .6 oz. . . .	40	4.0	0	2.5	15	970	0
(Yankee Clipper), 6 pcs.	25	4.0	0	1.5	15	750	0
Anchovy paste *(Reese's)*, 1 tbsp. . .	30	2.0	0	2.5	55	940	0
Andouille sausage, see "Sausage"							

Food and Measure	cal.	prot. (gms)	carbo. (gms)	fat (gms)	chol. (mgs)	sod. (mgs)	fiber (gms)
Angel-hair pasta dry, see "Pasta"							
refrigerated (*Buitoni*), 1¼ cups	230	10.0	43.0	2.5	50	20	2.0
Angel-hair pasta entree, frozen, 10-oz. pkg.:							
(*Lean Cuisine Everyday Favorites*)	260	8.0	48.0	4.0	5	690	3.0
marinara (*Smart Ones*)	240	8.0	42.0	4.0	0	720	4.0
Angel-hair pasta entree mix, spicy tomato:							
(*Near East*), 2 oz.	200	8.0	39.0	2.0	0	630	3.0
(*Near East*), 1 cup* . .	240	8.0	41.0	6.0	0	630	4.0
Anise seed, 1 tsp.	7	.4	1.1	.3	0	<1	.3
Antelope, meat only, roasted, 4 oz.	170	33.4	0	3.0	143	51	0
Apple, fresh:							
(*Chiquita*), 1 medium, 5.4 oz.	80	0	22.0	0	0	0	5.0
(*Del Monte*), 5.4-oz. apple	80	0	22.0	0	0	0	5.0
(*Dole/Dole* Cameo), 5.4-oz. apple	80	0	22.0	0	0	0	5.0
(*Frieda's* Lady Apple), 5 oz.	80	0	21.0	.5	0	0	3.0
raw, w/peel:							
2¾" apple	81	.3	21.1	.5	0	1	3.7
sliced, ½ cup	32	.1	8.4	.2	0	0	3.0
raw, peeled:							
2¾" apple	72	.2	19.0	.4	0	<1	2.4
sliced, ½ cup	31	.1	8.2	.2	0	0	1.0
cooked, peeled, sliced, boiled, ½ cup	45	.2	11.7	.3	0	1	2.0
Apple, can or jar:							
baked, sliced, in syrup (*Lucky Leaf/Mussel-man's* Dutch), ½ cup	170	0	41.0	0	0	40	3.0
fried, ½ cup:							
(*Lucky Leaf*)	170	0	43.0	0	0	20	0
seasoned (*Glory*) . .	80	0	21.0	0	0	170	1.0

Food and Measure	cal.	prot. (gms)	carbo. (gms)	fat (gms)	chol. (mgs)	sod. (mgs)	fiber (gms)
Apple, can or jar *(cont.)*							
rings, spiced (*Lucky Leaf/Musselman's*),							
1 ring	35	0	9.0	0	0	5	0
sliced, ½ cup:							
(*Lucky Leaf/ Musselman's*) . . .	50	0	12.0	0	0	20	1.0
sweetened, drained	68	.2	17.0	<.1	0	3	1.7
Apple, dried (see also "Apple snack"):							
(*Shiloh Farms*), 1.4 oz., about 8 rings	120	<1.0	28.0	0	0	5	n.a.
(*Sunsweet*), ¼ cup, 1.4 oz.	110	<1.0	27.0	0	0	270	3.0
dehydrated:							
½ cup	104	.4	28.1	.2	0	74	7.4
diced (*AlpineAire*), 1 oz.	100	0	26.0	0	0	150	2.0
flakes (*AlpineAire*), 1 oz.	110	0	26.0	0	0	95	1.0
sulfured:							
1 ring	16	.1	4.2	0	0	6	4.2
2 cups	104	.4	28.3	.1	0	75	7.5
Apple, fried, see "Apple, can or jar"							
Apple, frozen:							
seasoned (*Stouffer's Harvest*), ½ of 12-oz. pkg.	190	1.0	42.0	2.5	0	130	3.0
unheated, ½ cup	42	0	10.7	0	0	3	1.6
Apple, sour, drink mixer (*Rose's* Cocktail Infusions), 1.5 fl. oz.	60	0	16.0	0	0	20	0
Apple butter, 1 tbsp.:							
(*Apple Time/Lucky Leaf/Musselman's*) .	30	0	8.0	0	0	0	0
(*Eden* Organic)	20	0	4.0	0	0	0	1.0
(*R.W. Knudsen*)	35	0	9.0	0	0	0	0
(*Shiloh Farms*)	25	0	3.0	0	0	0	0
(*Smuckers* Cider)	45	0	11.0	0	0	10	0
cherry (*Eden* Organic), 1 tbsp.	25	0	6.0	0	0	0	1.0

Food and Measure	cal.	prot. (gms)	carbo. (gms)	fat (gms)	chol. (mgs)	sod. (mgs)	fiber (gms)
Apple chips, see "Apple snack"							
Apple cider, see "Apple drink" and "Apple juice"							
Apple cider, alcoholic (*Hard Core* Crisp), 12 fl. oz.	190	1.0	19.0	0	0	15	0
Apple cinnamon glaze (*Litehouse*), 2 tbsp.	70	0	17.0	0	0	45	0
Apple dip, see "Fruit dip"							
Apple drink, 8 fl. oz.:							
(*Lincoln*)	130	0	31.0	0	0	10	0
cocktail:							
(*Langers* Diet)	60	0	14.0	0	0	10	0
(*Langers* Low Carb)	30	0	7.0	0	0	10	0
Apple dumpling, frozen (*Pepperidge Farm*), 3-oz. pc. . . .	250	3.0	33.0	11.0	0	180	1.0
Apple juice, 8 fl. oz., except as noted:							
(*After the Fall* Organic)	90	0	22.0	0	0	20	0
(*Apple Time/Lincoln/ Lucky Leaf/ Musselman's*)	120	0	31.0	0	0	25	0
(*Capri Sun Fruit Waves* Apple Splash), 6.75 fl. oz.	100	0	23.0	0	0	30	0
(*Eden* Organic)	80	0	23.0	0	0	0	0
(*Hood*)	120	0	31.0	0	0	5	0
(*Langers* Cider/Juice/ Harvest)	120	0	28.0	0	0	0	0
(*Lucky Leaf* 120% Vitamin C), 5.5-oz. can	80	0	21.0	0	0	10	0
(*Martinelli's Gold Medal* Juice/Cider) .	140	1.0	35.0	0	0	0	0
(*Minute Maid*)	110	0	28.0	0	0	20	0
(*Minute Maid*), 6.75-fl.-oz. box . . .	90	0	23.0	0	0	15	0
(*Minute Maid*), 12-fl.-oz. bottle . . .	170	0	41.0	0	0	30	0

Food and Measure	cal.	prot. (gms)	carbo. (gms)	fat (gms)	chol. (mgs)	sod. (mgs)	fiber (gms)
Apple juice *(cont.)*							
(*Musselman's* 120% Vitamin C), 5.5 oz. .	80	0	20.0	0	0	10	0
(*Nantucket Nectars* Cider/Pressed)	100	0	25.0	0	0	10	<1.0
(*Nantucket Nectars* Cloudy Organic) ...	120	0	29.0	0	0	30	0
(*Ocean Spray*)	110	0	28.0	0	0	35	0
(*R.W. Knudsen* Natural/Organic/ Cider & Spice)	120	<1.0	25.0	0	0	25	0
(*R.W. Knudsen* Organic Box)	120	0	25.0	0	0	25	0
(*Santa Cruz Organic*) .	120	<1.0	30.0	0	0	25	0
(*Santa Cruz Organic* Cider & Spice)	120	<1.0	30.0	0	0	25	0
(*S&W*)	120	0	30.0	0	0	25	0
(*Tree of Life*)	120	<1.0	30.0	0	0	25	0
(*Walnut Acres*)	110	0	29.0	0	0	0	0
frozen*:							
(*Cascadian Farm*) ..	120	0	29.0	0	0	15	0
(*Minute Maid*)	110	0	28.0	0	0	0	0
sparkling:							
(*Lucky Leaf/Mussel-man's* Cider)	150	0	36.0	0	0	20	0
(*Martinelli* Cider) ..	140	1.0	35.0	0	0	0	0
(*Martinelli* Juice), 10 fl. oz.	180	1.0	43.0	0	0	0	1.0
(*R.W. Knudsen* Crisp/Organic) ..	110	0	28.0	0	0	5	0
Apple juice blend, 8 fl. oz., except as noted:							
apricot (*R.W. Knudsen*)	120	<1.0	30.0	0	0	35	0
cherry (*Eden* Organic)	120	0	30.0	0	0	15	1.0
cranberry (*R.W. Knudsen*)	120	<1.0	25.0	0	0	25	0
grape (*Juicy Juice*) ..	120	0	29.0	0	0	10	0
sparkling, all varieties:							
(*Martinelli*)	110	0	27.0	0	0	4	0
(*Martinelli*), 10 fl. oz.	160	0	39.0	0	0	18	1.0

Food and Measure	cal.	prot. (gms)	carbo. (gms)	fat (gms)	chol. (mgs)	sod. (mgs)	fiber (gms)
Applesauce, ½ cup, except as noted:							
unsweetened/natural:							
(*Apple Time*)	50	0	13.0	0	0	10	2.0
(*Apple Time*), 4-oz. cup	50	0	12.0	0	0	10	2.0
(*Eden Organic*)	50	0	15.0	0	0	15	2.0
(*Langers*)	50	0	13.0	0	0	5	2.0
(*Lucky Leaf/Mussel-man's* Lite)	50	0	13.0	0	0	10	2.0
(*Lucky Leaf/Mussel-man's* Natural) ..	50	0	13.0	0	0	20	2.0
(*Lucky Leaf/Mussel-man's* Natural), 4-oz. cup	50	0	12.0	0	0	20	2.0
(*Mott's*)	50	0	14.0	0	0	0	1.0
(*Mott's* Single Serve), 1 cont. ..	50	0	12.0	0	0	0	1.0
(*Musselman's* Organic)	50	0	12.0	0	0	10	2.0
(*Santa Cruz Organic*)	50	0	13.0	0	0	0	2.0
(*Tree of Life*)	50	0	15.0	0	0	20	2.0
cinnamon (*Apple Time*)	50	0	12.0	0	0	10	2.0
cinnamon (*Mussel-man's Natural*) ..	50	0	13.0	0	0	10	2.0
cinnamon (*Santa Cruz Organic*) ...	80	0	19.0	0	0	10	2.0
cinnamon (*Santa Cruz Organic* Cup), 4 oz.	80	0	19.0	0	0	0	2.0
Granny Smith (*Mott's* Healthy Harvest Single Serve), 1 cont. ..	50	0	13.0	0	0	0	1.0
sweetened:							
(*Lucky Leaf/ Musselman's*) ...	90	0	22.0	0	0	10	2.0
(*Mott's* Original) ...	120	0	29.0	0	0	0	1.0
(*Musselman's* Organic), 4-oz. cup	80	0	20.0	0	0	10	2.0

Food and Measure	cal.	prot. (gms)	carbo. (gms)	fat (gms)	chol. (mgs)	sod. (mgs)	fiber (gms)
Applesauce, sweetened *(cont.)*							
chunky (*Mussel-man's Homestyle*)	100	0	25.0	0	0	25	2.0
cinnamon (*Lucky Leaf/Mussel-man's*)	100	0	25.0	0	0	10	2.0
cinnamon (*Lucky Leaf/Mussel-man's*), 4-oz. cup	80	0	20.0	0	0	10	2.0
cinnamon (*Mott's*) .	120	0	29.0	0	0	0	1.0
cinnamon (*Mott's Single Serve*), 1 cont.	100	0	25.0	0	0	0	1.0
Golden Delicious, Granny Smith, or McIntosh (*Musselman's*) . .	90	0	22.0	0	0	10	2.0
Applesauce fruit blend, ½ cup, except as noted:							
all varieties:							
(*Santa Cruz Organic*)	50	0	13.0	0	0	0	2.0
(*Santa Cruz Organic Cup*), 4 oz.	50	0	13.0	0	0	0	2.0
cherry:							
(*Eden* Organic)	70	0	17.0	0	0	10	3.0
(*Lucky Leaf/ Musselman's Lite*), 4-oz. cup . .	60	0	15.0	0	0	10	1.0
orange, raspberry, or strawberry (*Lucky Leaf/Musselman's Lite*), 4-oz. cup	60	0	14.0	0	0	10	1.0
peach (*Lucky Leaf/ Musselman's Lite*), 4-oz. cup	60	0	14.0	0	0	10	2.0
strawberry:							
(*Eden* Organic)	60	0	13.0	0	0	10	2.0
(*Mott's* Single Serve), 1 cont. . .	90	0	23.0	0	0	0	1.0
Apricot, fresh:							
(*Chiquita*), 3 medium, 4 oz.	60	0	11.0	1.0	0	0	1.0

Food and Measure	cal.	prot. (gms)	carbo. (gms)	fat (gms)	chol. (mgs)	sod. (mgs)	fiber (gms)
(*Del Monte*), 3 medium, 4 oz. . . .	60	0	11.0	1.0	0	0	1.0
(*Dole*), 3 medium, 4 oz.	60	0	11.0	1.0	0	0	1.0
3 medium, 12 per lb. .	51	1.5	11.8	.4	0	1	2.5
pitted, ½ cup:							
halves	37	1.1	8.6	.3	0	1	1.9
sliced	40	1.2	9.2	.3	0	2	2.0
Apricot, can or jar, ½ cup, halves, except as noted:							
in juice, w/liquid	59	.8	15.1	<.1	0	5	2.0
in extra light syrup (*Del Monte* Lite) . . .	60	0	16.0	0	0	10	1.0
in light syrup:							
(*Del Monte Orchard Select*)	80	<1.0	21.0	0	0	10	1.0
w/liquid	80	.7	20.9	<.1	0	5	2.0
chunks (*S&W Sun*)	90	1.0	22.0	0	0	25	1.0
almond flavor (*Del Monte*)	90	0	22.0	0	0	10	1.0
in heavy syrup:							
(*Del Monte*)	100	0	26.0	0	0	10	1.0
w/liquid	107	.7	27.7	.1	0	5	2.1
whole, peeled (*S&W*)	120	<1.0	29.0	0	0	10	1.0
Apricot, dried:							
(*Express*), 1.4 oz., about 5 pcs.	90	1.0	22.0	0	0	10	3.0
(*Shiloh Farms* California), 1.4 oz., 8 pcs.	119	2.0	31.0	0	0	5	1.0
(*Shiloh Farms* Turkish), 1.1 oz., 5 pcs.	77	1.0	20.0	.2	0	3	3.0
(*Sun•Maid Fast Fruit*), ¼ cup, 1.4 oz. . . .	100	1.0	24.0	0	0	15	3.0
(*Sunsweet* California), 5 pcs., 1.4 oz.	100	1.0	24.0	0	0	0	4.0
(*Sunsweet* Mediterranean), 6 pcs., 1.4 oz.	100	1.0	26.0	0	0	30	3.0
dehydrated, ½ cup . . .	190	2.9	49.3	.4	0	15	n.a.
sulfured, ½ cup	155	2.4	40.1	.3	0	7	5.9

Food and Measure	cal.	prot. (gms)	carbo. (gms)	fat (gms)	chol. (mgs)	sod. (mgs)	fiber (gms)
Apricot, frozen,							
sweetened, ½ cup .	119	.9	30.4	.1	0	5	2.1
Apricot juice, 8 fl. oz.:							
(*Ceres*)	120	0	30.0	0	0	10	0
(*Walnut Acres*)	130	0	32.0	0	0	15	0
Apricot nectar:							
(*Goya*), 6 fl. oz.	120	0	29.0	0	0	30	0
(*Goya*), 8 fl. oz.	130	1.0	31.0	0	0	15	0
(*Goya*), 12 fl. oz.	220	1.0	53.0	0	0	25	1.0
(*R.W. Knudsen*),							
8 fl. oz.	120	<1.0	30.0	0	0	35	0
(*Santa Cruz Organic*),							
8 fl. oz.	110	0	27.0	0	0	25	0
(*S&W*), 8 fl. oz.	140	1.0	35.0	0	0	15	1.0
(*S&W*), 12 fl. oz.	210	2.0	53.0	0	0	20	1.0
Apricot-orange drink							
(*Snapple* Snapricot),							
8 fl. oz.	120	0	30.0	0	0	10	0
Arame, see "Seaweed"							
Arby's, 1 serving:							
breakfast:							
biscuit, plain	230	5.0	26.0	12.0	0	710	<1.0
add butter	100	0	0	11.0	30	115	0
add egg	80	5.0	2.0	6.0	145	220	2.0
add Swiss cheese	40	3.0	0	3.0	10	200	0
biscuit, bacon	300	9.0	27.0	17.0	15	950	<1.0
biscuit, ham	270	12.0	27.0	13.0	20	1170	<1.0
biscuit, sausage . . .	390	10.0	26.0	27.0	30	1080	<1.0
croissant:							
bacon/egg	410	13.0	31.0	26.0	190	670	<1.0
ham/cheese	350	15.0	30.0	19.0	65	870	<1.0
sausage/egg	510	14.0	31.0	36.0	210	800	<1.0
sourdough:							
bacon/egg/cheese	500	25.0	33.0	29.0	325	1600	1.0
egg/cheese	330	15.0	31.0	16.0	165	1060	1.0
ham/egg/cheese .	450	27.0	33.0	23.0	330	1750	1.0
sandwiches:							
beef, roast:							
beef 'n cheddar .	440	22.0	44.0	21.0	50	1270	2.0
Big Montana	590	47.0	41.0	29.0	115	2080	3.0
giant	450	32.0	41.0	19.0	75	1440	2.0
junior	270	16.0	34.0	9.0	30	740	2.0
regular	320	21.0	34.0	13.0	45	950	2.0
super	440	22.0	48.0	19.0	45	1130	3.0

Food and Measure	cal.	prot. (gms)	carbo. (gms)	fat (gms)	chol. (mgs)	sod. (mgs)	fiber (gms)
chicken:							
breast fillet	500	25.0	48.0	25.0	55	1220	3.0
bacon 'n Swiss . .	550	31.0	49.0	27.0	70	1640	2.0
roast, club	470	27.0	39.0	25.0	65	1320	2.0
Market Fresh:							
BLT	780	23.0	75.0	46.0	50	1570	6.0
chicken salad . . .	770	30.0	78.0	38.0	75	1240	9.0
roast turkey,							
ranch, bacon .	830	49.0	75.0	38.0	110	2260	5.0
roast beef, Swiss	780	37.0	74.0	39.0	90	1740	6.0
roast ham, Swiss	700	36.0	74.0	31.0	85	2140	5.0
roast turkey,							
Swiss	720	45.0	74.0	27.0	90	1790	5.0
Market Fresh wraps:							
BLT	650	25.0	48.0	47.0	50	1730	31.0
chicken, Southwest	550	35.0	45.0	30.0	75	1690	30.0
chicken club	680	43.0	52.0	38.0	100	1800	31.0
roast turkey, ranch,							
bacon	710	51.0	48.0	39.0	110	2420	30.0
Market Fresh salads:							
chicken club	530	30.0	32.0	33.0	210	1120	5.0
add buttermilk							
ranch dressing	330	1.0	4.0	34.0	30	660	0
add light dressing	110	1.0	13.0	6.0	0	470	<1.0
Martha's Vineyard .	250	26.0	23.0	8.0	60	490	4.0
add almonds,							
sliced	81	4.0	2.0	7.0	0	0	1.0
add raspberry							
vinaigrette . . .	170	0	16.0	12.0	0	340	0
Santa Fe	520	27.0	40.0	29.0	60	1120	5.0
add ranch							
dressing	300	1.0	4.0	31.0	20	690	0
add tortilla strips	61	1.0	10.0	2.5	0	25	.5
sides:							
chicken fingers:							
4-pack	640	31.0	42.0	38.0	70	1590	3.0
combo	1050	37.0	89.0	60.0	70	2540	5.0
fries, curly:							
cheddar sauce . .	60	1.0	4.0	4.5	0	360	0
large	630	8.0	73.0	34.0	0	1480	7.0
medium	410	5.0	47.0	22.0	0	950	5.0
small	340	4.0	39.0	18.0	0	790	4.0
fries, home style:							
large	570	6.0	82.0	24.0	0	1030	6.0

Food and Measure	cal.	prot. (gms)	carbo. (gms)	fat (gms)	chol. (mgs)	sod. (mgs)	fiber (gms)
Arby's, sides, fries, home style *(cont.)*							
medium	380	4.0	55.0	16.0	0	690	4.0
small	300	3.0	44.0	13.0	0	550	3.0
potato cakes, 2 ...	250	2.0	26.0	15.0	0	390	2.0
Sidekickers:							
Jalapeño Bites:							
large, 10	610	11.0	58.0	37.0	55	1050	4.0
regular, 5	310	5.0	29.0	19.0	30	530	2.0
mozzarella sticks:							
large, 8	850	36.0	76.0	45.0	90	2740	4.0
regular, 4	430	18.0	38.0	23.0	45	1370	2.0
onion petals:							
large	830	10.0	88.0	48.0	0	830	5.0
regular	330	4.0	35.0	19.0	0	330	2.0
sauce/condiments:							
Arby's Sauce, pkt. ...	15	0	4.0	0	0	180	0
BBQ sauce	40	0	10.0	0	0	350	0
Bronco Berry Sauce	120	0	30.0	0	0	35.0	0
buttermilk ranch dressing	290	1.0	3.0	30.0	25	580	0
honey mustard sauce	130	0	5.0	12.0	10	170	0
Horsey Sauce, pkt. ..	60	0	3.0	5.0	5	170	0
ketchup, pkt.	20	0	4.0	0	0	170	0
mayo, pkt.	100	0	0	11.0	10	75	0
mayo, light, pkt. ...	45	0	1.0	4.5	5	115	0
marinara sauce ...	15	0	4.0	0	0	220	1.0
red ranch sauce ...	70	0	5.0	6.0	0	105	0
Tangy Southwest Sauce	330	1.0	5.0	35.0	30	370	0
three pepper sauce	20	0	3.0	1.0	0	140	0
shakes:							
chocolate, large ...	660	17.0	110.0	17.0	45	450	<1.0
chocolate, regular .	510	13.0	83.0	13.0	35	360	0
Jamocha, large ...	650	17.0	107.0	17.0	45	510	<1.0
Jamocha, regular ..	500	13.0	81.0	13.0	35	390	0
strawberry, large ..	650	16.0	107.0	17.0	45	460	<1.0
strawberry, regular .	500	13.0	81.0	13.0	35	360	0
vanilla, large	650	16.0	107.0	17.0	45	470	0
vanilla, regular	500	13.0	82.0	13.0	35	370	0
desserts:							
chocolate cookie ..	200	2.0	26.0	10.0	15	210	1.0
cinnamon roll, see *"T. J. Cinnamons"*							

Food and Measure	cal.	prot. (gms)	carbo. (gms)	fat (gms)	chol. (mgs)	sod. (mgs)	fiber (gms)
turnover, no icing:							
apple	250	4.0	35.0	10.0	0	200	2.0
cherry	250	4.0	35.0	10.0	0	200	2.0
turnover icing	130	0	29.0	1.5	0	n.a.	0
Arctic char, raw, meat only, 4 oz.	207	25.0	0	9.1	30	91	0
Arrowhead:							
raw, 1 medium corm, 2⅝"	12	.6	2.4	<.1	0	3	.<1.0
boiled, drained, 1 medium corm, .4 oz.	9	.5	1.9	<.1	0	2	<1.0
Arrowroot, raw, sliced, ½ cup	36	2.5	8.0	.1	0	16	.8
Arrowroot flour, 1 cup	457	.4	112.8	.1	0	2	4.4
Artichoke, globe, fresh:							
raw:							
(*Dole*), 1 medium, 2 oz. edible	25	2.0	6.0	0	0	70	3.0
4.5-oz. choke	60	4.2	13.5	.2	0	120	6.9
5.7-oz. choke	76	5.3	17.0	.2	0	152	8.9
boiled, drained, 1 medium, 4.2 oz. .	60	4.2	13.4	.2	0	114	6.5
hearts, boiled, drained, ½ cup	42	2.9	9.4	.1	0	80	4.5
Artichoke, canned (see also "Artichoke, marinated"), in water:							
bottoms or small (*Fanci Food*), 3 pcs., 4.6 oz.	20	2.0	3.0	0	0	490	2.0
hearts:							
(*Cento*), 2 pcs., 2.8 oz.	30	2.0	6.0	0	0	240	1.0
(*Pompeian*), 4.5 oz.	35	2.0	6.0	0	0	420	4.0
(*Progresso*), 2 pcs., 2.9 oz.	30	2.0	6.0	0	0	240	1.0
(*Vigo*), 2 pcs., 2.8 oz.	30	2.0	6.0	0	0	240	1.0
Artichoke, frozen, hearts:							
(*Birds Eye*), 12 pcs., 3 oz.	40	2.0	7.0	1.0	0	55	5.0

Food and Measure	cal.	prot. (gms)	carbo. (gms)	fat (gms)	chol. (mgs)	sod. (mgs)	fiber (gms)
Artichoke, frozen *(cont.)*							
(*C&W*), ½ cup, 3 oz. .	25	2.0	4.0	0	0	55	5.0
9-oz. pkg.	96	6.7	19.8	1.1	0	120	9.9
Artichoke, Jerusalem, see "Jerusalem artichoke"							
Artichoke, marinated:							
(*Fanci Food* Hot/Quartered/Salad), 1 oz. .	25	1.0	2.0	1.0	0	90	.5
(*Pompeian*), 1 oz.	35	.5	2.0	.5	0	90	.5
(*Progresso*), 2 pcs., 1.1 oz.	50	0	2.0	5.0	0	110	0
quarters (*S&W*), 2 pcs., 1 oz.	20	0	2.0	2.0	0	80	1.0
Artichoke dip, 2 tbsp.:							
(*Victoria*)	30	0	2.0	2.0	0	310	1.0
spinach (*Fiesta*)	60	3.0	12.0	.5	0	390	0
Artichoke paste (*Cucina Aromatica*), 1 oz.	155	.2	3.5	15.0	<5	440	2.8
Arugula, fresh:							
baby (*Ready Pac*), 3 oz.	35	3.0	5.0	1.0	0	40	3.0
10 leaves	5	.5	.7	.1	0	5	.3
½ cup	3	.3	.4	<.1	0	<1	.2
Asparagus, fresh:							
raw, spears, trimmed:							
(*Dole*), 5 medium, 3.3 oz.	25	2.0	4.0	0	0	0	2.0
4 small, 1.8 oz. . . .	14	1.3	2.6	.1	0	1	1.2
purple (*Frieda's*), 3 oz.	20	4.0	4.0	0	0	0	1.0
boiled, 4 spears, ½"-diam. base	14	1.6	2.5	.2	0	7	1.3
boiled, drained, cuts, ½ cup	22	2.3	3.8	.3	0	10	1.9
Asparagus, can or jar:							
all styles (*Del Monte*), ½ cup	20	2.0	3.0	0	0	365	1.0
spears:							
(*Green Giant*), 4.5 oz., approx. 5 spears	20	2.0	3.0	0	0	400	1.0

Food and Measure	cal.	prot. (gms)	carbo. (gms)	fat (gms)	chol. (mgs)	sod. (mgs)	fiber (gms)
white (*Fanci Food*), ½ cup	20	2.0	3.0	0	0	510	2.0
cuts, ½ cup:							
(*Green Giant*)	20	2.0	3.0	0	0	420	1.0
(*Green Giant* Low Sodium)	20	2.0	3.0	0	0	210	1.0
drained, ½ cup	23	2.6	3.0	.8	0	350	2.0
Asparagus, frozen:							
boiled, drained, 1 cup	50	5.3	8.8	.8	0	7	2.9
spears:							
(*Birds Eye*), 7 pcs., 3 oz.	20	2.0	3.0	0	0	0	0
(*C&W*), 7 pcs., 3 oz.	20	3.0	3.0	0	0	5	2.0
(*Seabrook Farms*), 7 pcs., 3 oz.	20	3.0	3.0	0	0	5	2.0
4 pcs.	14	1.9	2.4	.1	0	5	1.1
cuts:							
(*Birds Eye*), ¾ cup .	20	2.0	3.0	0	0	0	0
(*Cascadian Farm*), ⅔ cup	20	2.0	3.0	0	0	105	1.0
(*Green Giant*), ⅔ cup	20	2.0	3.0	0	0	90	2.0
Asparagus, pickled, in jars (*Tillen Farms*), 3 spears ..	10	1.0	1.0	0	0	75	0
Asparagus bean, see "Winged bean"							
Asparagus combina-tion, frozen (*Birds Eye* Stir-fry), 2 cups frozen, 1 cup*	80	3.0	15.0	0	0	35	2.0
Atemoya (*Frieda's*), 3 oz.	80	2.0	20.0	0	0	10	4.0
Au bon pain, 1 serving:							
breakfast:							
bagel:							
egg	400	25.0	63.0	4.0	120	730	3.0
egg/bacon	480	30.0	63.0	12.0	130	960	3.0
egg/cheese	480	31.0	63.0	11.0	140	870	3.0
egg/cheese/bacon	560	35.0	63.0	18.0	155	1100	3.0
yogurt, large:							
all flavors, w/fruit, granola	620	20.0	112.0	13.0	20	260	5.0

Food and Measure	cal.	prot. (gms)	carbo. (gms)	fat (gms)	chol. (mgs)	sod. (mgs)	fiber (gms)
Au bon pain, breakfast, yogurt, large *(cont.)*							
blueberry or strawberry w/fruit	380	13.0	75.0	4.5	20	190	1.0
vanilla, w/fruit	370	21.0	64.0	4.0	25	330	2.0
yogurt, small:							
plain, low fat	190	6.0	36.0	2.0	10	95	0
all flavors, w/fruit, granola	310	10.0	56.0	6.0	10	130	2.0
bakery, bagel:							
plain	300	12.0	61.0	1.0	0	470	3.0
apple, Dutch	470	13.0	98.0	3.5	0	540	5.0
asiago cheese	380	18.0	59.0	8.0	20	740	3.0
cinnamon crisp	430	11.0	96.0	6.0	0	430	3.0
cinnamon raisin	330	12.0	71.0	1.0	0	480	3.0
everything	330	13.0	63.0	3.0	0	750	3.0
French toast	420	11.0	76.0	7.0	0	440	3.0
honey 9-grain	360	14.0	75.0	2.0	0	550	6.0
jalapeño cheddar	350	18.0	56.0	6.0	15	690	2.0
sesame seed	340	13.0	62.0	4.0	0	470	3.0
bakery, cake/pastry:							
apple crumble	540	7.0	62.0	30.0	155	510	1.0
apple strudel	410	6.0	56.0	18.0	0	140	1.0
blonde w/nuts	570	6.0	57.0	36.0	65	460	2.0
butter crumb	790	9.0	96.0	42.0	50	560	2.0
cheese Danish, sweet	470	8.0	54.0	26.0	105	380	1.0
cheesecake brownie	470	5.0	55.0	26.0	95	260	1.0
cherry Danish	410	7.0	52.0	19.0	65	330	1.0
cherry strudel	390	6.0	49.0	19.0	0	135	1.0
chocolate chip brownie	480	5.0	61.0	25.0	85	220	2.0
cinnamon roll	390	9.0	67.0	12.0	45	•380	2.0
crème de fleur	550	12.0	71.0	26.0	110	540	1.0
lemon Danish	430	7.0	57.0	20.0	75	380	1.0
pecan brownie	510	5.0	55.0	31.0	80	200	3.0
pecan roll	750	14.0	112.0	29.0	15	560	4.0
raspberry crumb	770	9.0	94.0	41.0	50	550	2.0
rocky road brownie	550	13.0	49.0	33.0	115	410	2.0
bakery, cookie:							
butterscotch chip w/pecans	270	3.0	42.0	11.0	15	190	1.0
chocolate chip	260	3.0	40.0	11.0	20	240	1.0
confetti, w/*M&M's*	280	4.0	37.0	13.0	35	200	1.0

Food and Measure	cal.	prot. (gms)	carbo. (gms)	fat (gms)	chol. (mgs)	sod. (mgs)	fiber (gms)
cranberry almond macaroon, chocolate dipped	320	4.0	42.0	16.0	0	190	3.0
oatmeal raisin	250	4.0	42.0	9.0	35	170	2.0
shortbread	340	3.0	35.0	22.0	60	180	1.0
shortbread, chocolate dipped	300	6.0	52.0	10.0	20	290	1.0
shortbread, white chocolate dipped	380	8.0	46.0	21.0	40	135	2.0
toffee, English	240	2.0	26.0	14.0	20	180	1.0
bakery, croissant:							
plain	250	8.0	44.0	6.0	25	340	2.0
almond	510	13.0	63.0	25.0	95	440	3.0
apple	230	6.0	47.0	3.0	20	220	2.0
cheese, sweet	350	9.0	52.0	14.0	65	400	1.0
chocolate	380	8.0	61.0	15.0	20	300	3.0
cinnamon raisin ...	340	9.0	69.0	5.0	20	350	3.0
ham and cheese ...	340	17.0	46.0	10.0	35	720	2.0
raspberry	340	9.0	55.0	11.0	50	370	2.0
spinach and cheese	250	10.0	32.0	9.0	35	400	2.0
bakery, muffin:							
apple spice	420	7.0	65.0	15.0	20	450	3.0
banana walnut	440	9.0	60.0	19.0	20	450	3.0
berry, triple, low fat	290	5.0	61.0	2.0	25	310	2.0
blueberry	510	9.0	76.0	19.0	20	550	5.0
carrot nut	550	9.0	71.0	27.0	60	860	4.0
chocolate cake, low fat	320	4.0	74.0	2.0	20	590	4.0
chocolate chunk ...	590	10.0	83.0	20.0	25	480	5.0
corn	440	8.0	64.0	18.0	70	640	2.0
cranberry blueberry	520	9.0	76.0	20.0	20	490	5.0
cranberry walnut ..	560	1.0	69.0	26.0	20	530	5.0
raisin bran	530	14.0	100.0	13.0	35	780	12.0
bakery, scone:							
cinnamon	480	11.0	88.0	18.0	125	320	2.0
orange	410	11.0	62.0	14.0	130	350	2.0
bread, artisan:							
baguette, 2 oz.	140	5.0	30.0	0	0	360	1.0
baguette, 3.5-oz, pc.	245	8.0	53.0	0	0	630	1.0
baguette, honey multigrain, 2 oz. .	140	5.0	30.0	0	0	360	2.0
baguette, honey multigrain, 3.5-oz. pc.	245	8.0	53.0	0	0	630	3.0

Food and Measure	cal.	prot. (gms)	carbo. (gms)	fat (gms)	chol. (mgs)	sod. (mgs)	fiber (gms)
Au bon pain, bread, artisan (cont.)							
bread bowl, 9.24 oz.	640	28.0	127.0	3.0	0	1830	6.0
chocolate cherry, 2 oz.	150	4.0	31.0	2.0	0	240	2.0
cranberry raisin nut loaf, 2 oz.	150	4.0	28.0	3.0	0	220	2.0
ficelle, 2 oz.	160	5.0	34.0	0	0	400	1.0
focaccia, 4.5 oz.	310	10.0	58.0	3.5	0	640	2.0
lahvash, 3.8 oz.	250	9.0	55.0	0	0	280	4.0
multigrain, 1 slice	165	5.0	31.0	1.8	0	342	2.0
rosemary-garlic bread stick, 2.3 oz.	200	6.0	33.0	5.0	0	1430	2.0
rye, Bavarian, 1 slice	236	8.0	49.0	1.2	0	542	4.0
sun-dried tomato loaf, 2 oz.	130	5.0	27.0	0	0	370	2.0
white, French country, 2-oz. slice	130	4.0	27.0	0	0	340	1.0
white roll, soft, 4.7 oz.	400	11.0	65.0	11.0	30	700	2.0
cream cheese, 2 oz.:							
plain	120	4.0	4.0	11.0	35	180	0
honey walnut	140	3.0	12.0	9.0	30	150	0
smoked salmon	110	5.0	3.0	9.0	30	230	0
sun-dried tomato	130	4.0	5.0	10.0	35	380	0
vegetable	140	6.0	3.0	12.0	40	380	0
soup, 8 oz.:							
black bean	110	10.0	27.0	.5	0	260	14.0
black-eyed pea	190	11.0	34.0	1.0	5	400	12.0
broccoli cheddar	230	6.0	13.0	16.0	50	960	2.0
chicken chili	210	12.0	28.0	5.0	20	580	5.0
chicken Florentine	170	5.0	17.0	9.0	35	780	1.0
chicken noodle	90	7.0	11.0	2.0	15	670	0
clam chowder	240	7.0	18.0	16.0	45	670	0
corn/chili bisque	160	4.0	17.0	8.0	25	920	2.0
curried rice lentil	100	5.0	18.0	1.0	0	900	4.0
Italian wedding	100	5.0	12.0	4.0	10	960	2.0
minestrone	70	3.0	14.0	1.0	0	620	3.0
onion, French	80	3.0	11.0	3.0	10	1280	2.0
pasta e fagiole	160	7.0	24.0	4.0	5	510	5.0
pepper, Mediterranean	190	9.0	30.0	4.0	0	450	7.0

Food and Measure	cal.	prot. (gms)	carbo. (gms)	fat (gms)	chol. (mgs)	sod. (mgs)	fiber (gms)
potato, baked stuffed	240	6.0	20.0	15.0	25	720	1.0
potato leek	190	4.0	17.0	12.0	45	1020	2.0
pumpkin, harvest . .	140	2.0	15.0	7.0	15	640	4.0
red bean, rice,							
sausage	180	10.0	28.0	4.0	10	610	11.0
split pea w/ham . . .	140	10.0	23.0	1.0	5	680	8.0
tomato basil bisque	130	4.0	18.0	4.0	15	400	3.0
tomato Florentine . .	70	3.0	10.0	2.0	5	610	1.0
tomato lentil	110	6.0	19.0	1.0	0	470	6.0
tomato rice	80	3.0	15.0	.5	0	240	2.0
tortilla, Southwest .	140	3.0	17.0	6.0	10	1020	3.0
vegetable, garden . .	40	2.0	7.0	1.0	0	610	2.0
vegetable,							
Southwest	150	6.0	23.0	3.0	0	250	4.0
vegetable, Tuscan .	130	5.0	20.0	3.0	5	680	3.0
vegetable beef							
barley	80	5.0	11.0	2.0	10	810	2.0
vegetarian chili	170	9.0	30.0	1.0	0	920	15.0
wild mushroom							
bisque	110	3.0	12.0	5.0	5	920	2.0
salad, no dressing:							
Caesar	240	13.0	23.0	11.0	25	310	4.0
chef's salad	260	25.0	9.0	13.0	60	890	4.0
chicken,							
Mediterranean . .	230	19.0	13.0	12.0	50	1090	5.0
chicken, Thai	140	16.0	14.0	2.5	45	470	6.0
chicken Caesar	320	26.0	24.0	13.0	70	660	4.0
chicken pesto . . . . :	420	26.0	14.0	30.0	60	870	5.0
garden, large	110	5.0	19.0	2.0	0	300	5.0
garden, small	50	2.0	10.0	1.0	0	150	3.0
Gorgonzola walnut .	340	13.0	10.0	28.0	25	500	7.0
tuna garden	310	24.0	11.0	21.0	10	670	5.0
tuna niçoise	300	23.0	19.0	15.0	195	930	5.0
turkey Cobb	390	28.0	23.0	21.0	250	1070	6.0
salad dressing, 2.5 oz.:							
balsamic vinaigrette	150	0	9.0	12.0	0	460	0
blue cheese	370	3.0	3.0	39.0	20	690	0
Caesar	390	3.0	6.0	38.0	30	520	0
honey mustard,							
light	240	2.0	26.0	15.0	30	560	0
Mediterranean	200	1.0	4.0	20.0	5	620	0
olive oil vinaigrette,							
light	150	0	7.0	14.0	0	550	0

Food and Measure	cal.	prot. (gms)	carbo. (gms)	fat (gms)	chol. (mgs)	sod. (mgs)	fiber (gms)
Au bon pain, **salad dressing** *(cont.)*							
Parmesan peppercorn	400	3.0	5.0	38.0	20	730	0
ranch, light	200	2.0	5.0	16.0	15	800	0
raspberry vinaigrette	80	0	19.0	0	0	190	0
Thai peanut	180	2.0	24.0	8.0	0	1180	0
sandwiches:							
basil goat cheese . .	500	17.0	67.0	19.0	15	1020	6.0
beef, roast, Gorgonzola	810	49.0	86.0	31.0	120	2070	8.0
beef, roast, Swiss .	690	33.0	57.0	36.0	90	1430	2.0
chicken breast, chili Dijon w/cheddar .	530	42.0	52.0	17.0	95	1510	4.0
chicken club, grilled, chili dressing . . .	670	40.0	64.0	29.0	105	1240	4.0
chicken mozzarella .	740	55.0	73.0	24.0	85	1930	6.0
chicken salad, Asian	430	26.0	50.0	16.0	75	1390	3.0
chicken tarragon . .	800	34.0	71.0	42.0	100	1710	4.0
chicken tarragon, ficelle	330	16.0	35.0	13.0	45	760	0
honey Dijon Cordon Bleu	590	46.0	71.0	12.0	120	1560	3.0
pork, pulled, BBQ . .	610	29.0	18.0	18.0	75	1610	6.0
portobello, roasted, goat cheese	560	20.0	63.0	27.0	35	1000	6.0
steak/Gorgonzola, onion roll	780	40.0	76.0	39.0	90	1790	6.0
tomato, mozzarella ficelle	470	22.0	40.0	24.0	65	1410	0
tuna, spicy, multigrain	690	30.0	72.0	33.0	20	1170	8.0
turkey, guacamole, Swiss, baguette .	760	51.0	77.0	28.0	85	1260	6.0
turkey club, hickory smoked	710	48.0	59.0	32.0	95	2250	3.0
turkey tenderloin . .	710	34.0	67.0	35.0	85	1300	6.0
the Tuscan	710	32.0	60.0	39.0	75	1560	3.0
sandwiches, baked:							
chicken, grilled, blue cheese	672	37.0	64.0	29.0	104	1901	3.0
mozzarella, tomato, basil pesto, onion	638	23.0	66.0	30.0	52	1045	3.0

Food and Measure	cal.	prot. (gms)	carbo. (gms)	fat (gms)	chol. (mgs)	sod. (mgs)	fiber (gms)
tuna, cheddar, red pepper	553	37.0	62.0	18.0	22	1411	3.0
turkey, roasted, cranberry, cheese	554	30.0	80.0	12.1	50	1149	3.0
sandwich filling:							
beef, roast	150	26.0	1.0	5.0	70	460	0
Brie cheese	150	8.0	0	14.0	30	180	0
capicola, hot	160	15.0	1.0	10.0	55	1080	0
cheddar cheese	170	11.0	1.0	14.0	45	260	0
chicken breast	120	21.0	1.0	3.0	70	560	0
chicken tarragon	210	18.0	1.0	14.0	70	590	0
cranberry cheese	110	7.0	6.0	8.0	25	85	0
Gorgonzola cheese	210	12.0	1.0	18.0	50	780	0
ham	150	21.0	2.0	3.0	60	1140	0
hummus	100	4.0	8.0	6.0	0	210	2.0
mozzarella cheese	160	16.0	3.0	9.0	25	300	0
olive tapenade, 2 oz.	110	1.0	1.0	12.0	0	1170	1.0
provolone cheese	140	10.0	1.0	10.0	35	330	0
red peppers, roasted	45	1.0	4.0	3.5	0	190	1.0
salami, Genoa	300	18.0	0	27.0	75	1410	0
Swiss cheese	160	12.0	0	12.0	30	105	0
tarragon mayo sauce	420	0	2.0	45.0	40	420	0
tomato spread	70	1.0	4.0	6.0	0	85	0
tuna salad mix	170	25.0	3.0	8.0	0	450	0
turkey breast	120	22.0	4.0	2.0	50	950	0
wraps:							
chicken Caesar	591	33.0	63.0	24.0	80	930	5.0
chopped Cobb	561	32.0	65.0	20.0	120	1280	6.0
fields and feta	551	20.0	90.0	16.0	10	880	14.0
Mediterranean	571	19.0	80.0	22.0	5	990	9.0
tuna, Southwest	541	44.0	68.0	25.0	30	1060	7.0
Au jus gravy, canned (*Campbell's*), ¼ cup	5	1.0	0	0	0	230	0
Au jus gravy mix ¼ cup*:							
(*Lawry's*)	25	<1.0	4.0	1.0	0	320	0
(*McCormick* Natural Style)	5	0	1.0	0	0	310	0
Aubergine, see "Eggplant"							
Auntie Anne's:							
pretzel, 1 pc.:							
almond	350	9.0	72.0	1.5	0	390	2.0
w/butter	400	9.0	72.0	8.0	20	400	2.0

Food and Measure	cal.	prot. (gms)	carbo. (gms)	fat (gms)	chol. (mgs)	sod. (mgs)	fiber (gms)
Auntie Anne's, pretzel *(cont.)*							
cinnamon sugar ...	350	9.0	74.0	2.0	0	410	2.0
w/butter	450	8.0	83.0	9.0	25	430	3.0
garlic	320	9.0	66.0	1.0	0	830	2.0
w/butter	350	9.0	68.0	4.5	10	850	2.0
Glazin' Raisin	470	11.0	104.0	.5	0	460	3.0
w/butter	510	11.0	107.0	4.0	10	480	4.0
jalapeño	270	8.0	58.0	1.0	0	780	2.0
w/butter	310	8.0	59.0	4.5	10	940	2.0
maple crumb	520	10.0	112.0	3.0	0	550	3.0
w/butter	550	10.0	112.0	6.0	10	550	3.0
original	340	10.0	72.0	1.0	0	900	3.0
w/butter	370	10.0	72.0	4.0	10	930	3.0
Parmesan herb	390	11.0	74.0	5.0	10	780	4.0
w/butter	440	10.0	72.0	13.0	30	660	9.0
sesame , ...	350	11.0	63.0	6.0	0	840	3.0
w/butter	410	12.0	64.0	12.0	15	860	7.0
sour cream/onion ..	310	9.0	66.0	1.0	0	920	2.0
w/butter	340	10.0	66.0	5.0	10	930	2.0
whole wheat	350	11.0	72.0	1.5	0	1100	7.0
w/butter	370	11.0	72.0	4.5	10	1120	7.0
pretzel dips:							
caramel	235	1.0	27.0	3.0	5	110	0
cheese	100	3.0	4.0	8.0	10	510	0
chocolate flavor ...	130	1.0	24.0	4.0	2	65	1.0
cream cheese:							
light	70	3.0	1.0	6.0	25	140	0
strawberry	110	3.0	4.0	10.0	35	105	0
marinara	10	0	4.0	0	0	180	0
mustard, sweet ...	60	<1.0	8.0	1.5	40	120	0
salsa cheese, hot ..	100	2.0	4.0	8.0	10	550	0
pretzel dog	290	10.0	25.0	16.0	40	600	1.0
pretzel sticks, 4 pcs.:							
plain	227	7.0	48.0	1.0	0	600	2.0
w/butter	247	7.0	48.0	3.0	7	620	2.0
Smart Bites, 1 pc. ...	10	1.0	2.0	.5	0	30	1.0
Smart Bites, 15 pcs. .	150	15.0	30.0	7.5	0	450	15.0
Dutch Ice, 14 oz.:							
cherry, wild	210	0	48.0	0	0	25	0
grape	180	0	43.0	0	0	20	0
kiwi-banana	190	0	44.0	0	0	30	0
lemonade	315	0	77.0	0	0	0	0
mocha	400	0	74.0	10.0	0	100	0

Food and Measure	cal.	prot. (gms)	carbo. (gms)	fat (gms)	chol. (mgs)	sod. (mgs)	fiber (gms)
orange creme	280	0	64.0	0	0	35	0
piña colada	220	0	53.0	0	0	15	0
raspberry, blue	165	0	38.0	0	0	20	0
strawberry	220	0	50.0	0	0	40	0
Dutch Latte, 14 oz.:							
caramel	350	4.0	49.0	15.0	55	170	0
coffee	290	4.0	38.0	14.0	50	135	0
mocha	360	5.0	47.0	17.0	55	135	0
Dutch shake, 14 oz.:							
chocolate	580	10.0	75.0	27.0	105	380	0
coffee	240	10.0	77.0	27.0	105	304	0
strawberry	610	10.0	78.0	27.0	105	304	0
vanilla	510	10.0	58.0	27.0	105	300	0
Dutch smoothie, 14 oz.:							
cherry, wild	250	3.0	41.0	8.0	30	90	0
grape	230	3.0	36.0	8.0	30	100	0
kiwi-banana	240	3.0	38.0	8.0	30	100	0
lemonade	300	3.0	53.0	8.0	30	80	0
mocha	330	3.0	50.0	13.0	30	130	0
orange creme	280	3.0	46.0	8.0	30	100	0
piña colada	260	3.0	44.0	8.0	30	90	0
raspberry, blue	230	3.0	34.0	8.0	30	100	0
strawberry	250	3.0	40.0	8.0	30	100	0
lemonade	180	0	43.0	0	0	0	0
lemonade, strawberry	190	0	48.0	0	0	0	0
Australian blue							
squash (*Frieda's*),							
¾ cup, 3 oz.	30	1.0	7.0	0	0	0	1.0
Avocado:							
(*Chiquita*), ⅓ medium,							
1.1 oz.	55	1.0	3.0	5.0	0	0	3.0
(*Del Monte*),							
⅓ medium, 1.1 oz. . .	55	1.0	3.0	5.0	0	0	3.0
all varieties:							
cubed, 1 cup	240	3.0	12.8	22.0	0	11	10.1
pureed, ½ cup	185	2.3	9.8	16.6	0	8	7.7
California:							
pulp from							
1 medium, 6.1 oz.	289	3.4	14.9	26.7	0	14	11.8
pureed, ½ cup	192	2.3	9.9	17.7	0	9	7.8
Florida, pureed, ½ cup	138	2.6	9.0	11.6	0	2	6.4
seedless (*Frieda's*							
Cocktail), 1.4-oz. pc.	60	1.0	3.0	6.0	0	0	2.0

Food and Measure	cal.	prot. (gms)	carbo. (gms)	fat (gms)	chol. (mgs)	sod. (mgs)	fiber (gms)
Avocado dip (see also "Guacamole")							
(*Litehouse*), 2 tbsp. . . .	140	1.0	2.0	15.0	15	240	0
A&W, 1 serving:							
sandwiches:							
cheeseburger	500	29.0	43.0	24.0	90	870	3.0
cheeseburger,							
deluxe	540	29.0	43.0	28.0	95	970	4.0
double	590	32.0	47.0	31.0	110	1250	4.0
bacon	600	32.0	44.0	33.0	105	1150	4.0
bacon double . . .	670	36.0	47.0	37.0	125	1490	4.0
cheeseburger Jr. . . .	390	19.0	41.0	17.0	55	1000	3.0
chicken, crispy	580	32.0	57.0	25.0	65	1390	5.0
chicken, grilled	430	37.0	37.0	15.0	90	1080	4.0
hamburger	460	26.0	39.0	22.0	75	690	3.0
hamburger, deluxe .	500	26.0	40.0	26.0	80	800	4.0
hamburger Jr.	350	17.0	37.0	15.0	40	820	3.0
hot dogs:							
plain	280	11.0	22.0	17.0	35	710	1.0
cheese dog	320	11.0	25.0	20.0	40	910	1.0
coney (chili)	310	13.0	24.0	18.0	40	870	2.0
coney (chili) cheese	350	13.0	27.0	21.0	45	1070	2.0
chicken strips, 3 pcs. .	500	28.0	32.0	29.0	55	1050	2.0
dipping sauce, 1 oz.:							
barbecue	40	0	10.0	0	0	230	0
honey mustard	100	0	12.0	6.0	0	170	0
ranch	160	0	2.0	17.0	15	240	0
sweet and sour . . .	45	0	12.0	0	0	120	0
fries:							
cheese	380	4.0	50.0	19.0	5	870	4.0
chili	370	8.0	49.0	16.0	10	780	5.0
chili cheese	400	8.0	51.0	19.0	10	990	5.0
regular, kids	310	3.0	45.0	13.0	0	460	4.0
regular, large	430	5.0	61.0	18.0	0	640	6.0
onion rings	350	5.0	45.0	17.0	5	720	2.0

B

Food and Measure	cal.	prot. (gms)	carbo. (gms)	fat (gms)	chol. (mgs)	sod. (mgs)	fiber (gms)
Babaganoush, see "Eggplant appetizer"							
Bacon, raw, organic, hardwood smoked (*Organic Valley*), 2 strips, 2 oz.	270	5.0	1.0	27.0	35	620	0
Bacon, cooked, 2 slices, except as noted:							
(*Black Label*)	80	5.0	0	7.0	15	330	0
(*Black Label* Low Salt)	80	5.0	0	7.0	15	230	0
(*Black Label* Center Cut)	70	5.0	0	5.0	15	300	0
(*Boar's Head* Domestic)	70	4.0	0	6.0	10	190	0
(*Boar's Head* Imported)	60	4.0	0	5.0	10	190	0
(*Hatfield*), 3 slices . . .	70	5.0	0	5.0	5	280	0
(*Hatfield* Reduced Sodium), 3 slices . .	70	5.0	0	5.0	5	180	0
(*Hatfield* Thick Cut), 3 slices	80	5.0	0	6.0	10	330	0
(*Hormel* Applewood Smoked)	110	7.0	0	9.0	20	440	0
(*Hormel* Microwave) .	80	5.0	0	3.0	15	330	0
(*Hormel* Microwave Low Salt)	80	5.0	0	7.0	15	230	0
(*Oscar Mayer*)	70	4.0	0	6.0	15	290	0
(*Oscar Mayer* Center Cut)	50	4.0	0	4.0	15	270	0
(*Oscar Mayer* Lower Sodium)	70	4.0	0	6.0	10	170	0
(*Range Brand*)	110	7.0	0	9.0	20	460	0

Food and Measure	cal.	prot. (gms)	carbo. (gms)	fat (gms)	chol. (mgs)	sod. (mgs)	fiber (gms)
Bacon, cooked *(cont.)*							
hickory:							
(*Tyson*)	90	5.0	0	7.0	15	240	0
thick cut (*Tyson*) . .	140	8.0	0	11.0	25	380	0
maple flavor (*Hormel*)	80	5.0	0	7.0	15	270	0
peppered (*Hormel*) . .	110	7.0	0	9.0	20	440	0
mesquite (*Hormel*) . .	80	5.0	0	7.0	15	330	0
microwaved	143	10.9	.3	10.6	33	588	0
precooked:							
(*Hormel*), 2½ slices	70	5.0	0	5.0	20	290	0
(*Oscar Mayer*), .5 oz.	70	5.0	0	5.0	15	220	0
hickory (*Tyson*) . . .	90	5.0	0	7.0	15	240	0
spicy hot (*Boar's Head*)	60	4.0	0	5.0	10	270	0
thick cut (*Oscar Mayer*), .4-oz. slice	60	4.0	0	5.0	10	250	0
turkey, see "Turkey bacon"							
uncured (*Health is Wealth*)	70	0	0	7.0	10	380	0
Bacon, Canadian:							
(*Boar's Head*), 2 oz. . .	70	12.0	0	2.0	35	570	0
(*Hormel*), 2 oz.	70	11.0	0	2.5	30	650	0
(*Hormel Pillow Pack*), 22 slices, 2 oz.	80	10.0	2.0	3.5	30	800	0
pizza (*Hormel*), 22 slices, 2 oz.	70	10.0	1.0	3.0	30	600	0
unheated, 2 oz.	89	11.7	1.9	4.0	28	799	0
Bacon, Irish, back:							
(*Dawn Irish Gold*), 2 slices, 2 oz.	140	10.0	1.0	10.0	30	570	0
(*Shannon*), 1-oz. slice	60	4.0	0	5.0	20	220	0
Bacon, Italian, .5 oz.:							
(*Boar's Head*)	50	2.0	0	4.5	10	180	0
(*Daniele* Pancetta) . . .	50	2.0	0	4.5	10	230	0
"Bacon," vegetarian, frozen, 2 slices, except as noted:							
(*Morningstar Farms* Breakfast Strips) . .	60	2.0	2.0	4.5	0	220	<1.0
(*Worthington Stripples*)	60	2.0	2.0	4.5	0	220	<1.0
Canadian (*Yves*), 1.3 oz.	80	17.0	1.0	.5	0	480	1.0

Food and Measure	cal.	prot. (gms)	carbo. (gms)	fat (gms)	chol. (mgs)	sod. (mgs)	fiber (gms)
Bacon bits, 1 tbsp.:							
bits (*Hormel*)	30	3.0	0	1.5	5	250	0
bits (*Oscar Mayer*) . . .	25	3.0	0	1.5	5	220	0
crumbled (*Hormel*) . .	30	3.0	0	2.0	10	170	0
pieces (*Hormel*)	25	3.0	0	1.5	10	180	0
"Bacon" bits,							
imitation, 1½ tbsp.:							
(*Bac'n Pieces*)	30	3.0	2.0	1.5	0	220	0
chips/bits (*Bac-Os*) . .	30	3.0	2.0	1.5	0	120	0
Bacon dip, 2 tbsp.:							
and cheddar:							
(*Kraft* 8 oz.)	60	1.0	3.0	5.0	5	170	0
(*Kraft* 16 oz.)	60	1.0	3.0	5.0	5	180	0
horseradish (*Cabot*) . .	50	1.0	1.0	5.0	15	190	0
Bacon grease, 1 tbsp.	115	0	0	12.7	12	19	0
Bagel, 1 pc.:							
plain:							
(*Pepperidge Farm*) .	260	9.0	54.0	1.0	0	500	3.0
(*Sara Lee*), 2.2 oz. .	160	6.0	33.0	.5	0	320	1.0
(*Sara Lee*), 3.4 oz. .	250	9.0	52.0	1.0	0	490	2.0
(*Thomas'*), 3.7 oz. .	290	11.0	56.0	2.0	0	540	3.0
mini (*Pepperidge*							
Farm)	110	4.0	22.0	.5	0	200	1.0
mini (*Thomas'*),							
1.7 oz. . . . . :	130	5.0	26.0	1.0	0	260	1.0
plain, onion, poppy, or							
sesame, 2 oz.	157	6.0	30.4	.9	0	304	1.3
apple cinnamon (*Sara*							
Lee), 4 oz.	310	11.0	64.0	1.5	0	430	3.0
banana walnut (*Sara*							
Lee), 4 oz.	350	12.0	61.0	7.0	0	440	4.0
blueberry:							
(*Sara Lee* Deluxe),							
3.4 oz.	260	9.0	53.0	1.0	0	490	2.0
(*Sara Lee* Toaster							
Size), 2.2 oz. . . .	160	6.0	34.0	.5	0	310	1.0
(*Thomas'*), 3.7 oz. .	300	10.0	59.0	2.5	0	520	3.0
mini (*Sara Lee*),							
1 oz.	70	3.0	15.0	0	0	140	<1.0
swirl, mini (*Pep-*							
peridge Farm) . .	120	4.0	24.0	.5	0	190	<1.0
brown sugar							
cinnamon, mini							
(*Pepperidge Farm*) .	120	4.0	24.0	.5	0	150	2.0

Food and Measure	cal.	prot. (gms)	carbo. (gms)	fat (gms)	chol. (mgs)	sod. (mgs)	fiber (gms)
Bagel *(cont.)*							
cinnamon raisin:							
(*Pepperidge Farm*) .	270	8.0	57.0	1.0	0	450	3.0
(*Sara Lee* Deluxe),							
3.4 oz.	260	9.0	55.0	1.0	0	460	4.0
(*Sara Lee* Toaster							
Size), 2.2 oz. ...	160	6.0	33.0	.5	0	300	1.0
cranberry orange							
(*Sara Lee*), 4 oz. ..	310	11.0	64.0	1.5	0	430	3.0
egg, 2 oz.	158	6.0	30.2	1.2	14	288	1.3
everything:							
(*Pepperidge Farm*) .	270	9.0	55.0	1.5	0	550	3.0
(*Thomas'*), 3.7 oz. .	300	11.0	54.0	4.0	0	510	3.0
honey wheat (*Sara*							
Lee), 3.4 oz.	250	9.0	50.0	1.0	0	397	4.0
multigrain:							
(*Pepperidge Farm*) .	270	9.0	55.0	1.5	0	470	5.0
(*Thomas'*), 3.7 oz. .	300	11.0	57.0	2.5	0	470	4.0
oat bran, 2 oz.	145	6.1	30.4	.7	0	289	2.1
onion:							
(*Sara Lee*), 2.2 oz. .	160	6.0	33.0	1.0	0	300	1.0
(*Sara Lee* Deluxe),							
3.4 oz.	250	9.0	51.0	1.0	0	470	2.0
(*Thomas'*), 3.7 oz. .	290	11.0	56.0	2.0	0	440	3.0
sesame seed							
(*Thomas'*), 3.7 oz. .	280	11.0	53.0	3.5	0	510	3.0
sun-dried tomato/basil							
(*Sara Lee*), 4 oz. ...	300	11.0	61.0	1.5	0	480	2.0
whole wheat:							
(*Sara Lee* Heart							
Healthy), 3.3 oz..	220	11.0	47.0	1.5	0	480	6.0
(*Thomas'*), 3.7 oz. .	270	12.0	55.0	2.0	0	260	1.0
Bagel w/cream							
cheese, ½ of							
6.4-oz. pkg.:							
plain cream cheese							
(*Philadelphia* To-Go)	240	6.0	34.0	9.0	30	420	2.0
chive (*Philadelphia*							
To-Go)	240	6.0	34.0	8.0	30	440	2.0
strawberry							
(*Philadelphia* To-Go)	230	5.0	37.0	7.0	25	400	2.0
Baked beans, ½ cup,							
except as noted:							
(*Allens* Homestyle) ...	140	6.0	29.0	1.0	0	410	5.0

Food and Measure	cal.	prot. (gms)	carbo. (gms)	fat (gms)	chol. (mgs)	sod. (mgs)	fiber (gms)
(*Allens* Original)	150	6.0	29.0	1.0	0	350	8.0
(*Bush's* Bold & Spicy)	120	6.0	24.0	.5	0	550	5.0
(*Bush's* Boston)	170	6.0	32.0	1.5	0	440	6.0
(*Bush's* Country)	170	7.0	33.0	1.0	0	680	7.0
(*Bush's* Homestyle) ..	150	6.0	28.0	1.5	5	480	8.0
(*Bush's* Original)	150	7.0	29.0	1.0	0	550	7.0
(*Bush's* Original), 7.5-oz. bowl	260	11.0	51.0	1.5	0	990	11.0
bacon, maple cured :							
(*Allens*)	140	6.0	27.0	1.0	0	450	4.0
(*Bush's*)	150	7.0	28.0	1.0	0	620	7.0
(*S&W* Sweet Bacon)	140	5.0	29.0	.5	0	510	6.0
barbecue:							
(*Allens*)	150	6.0	29.0	1.0	0	410	5.0
(*Bush's*)	160	6.0	32.0	1.0	0	510	6.0
(*S&W* Country) ...	140	6.0	28.0	.5	0	510	6.0
(*S&W* Ranch Recipe)	140	6.0	25.0	1.5	0	640	8.0
brown sugar and bacon (*Campbell's*)	160	6.0	28.0	3.0	5	420	6.0
honey mustard (*S&W*)	140	6.0	28.0	.5	0	600	6.0
maple sugar (*S&W*) ..	150	7.0	29.0	0	0	640	6.0
onion:							
(*Allens*)	140	5.0	25.0	1.5	0	410	4.0
(*Bush's*)	150	7.0	26.0	1.5	0	500	6.0
w/pork:							
(*Campbell's*)	140	6.0	27.0	1.0	<5	460	7.0
(*Wagon Master*) ..	130	7.0	23.0	1.0	0	420	9.0
(*Wagon Master* 1 lb.)	130	7.0	21.0	1.0	0	330	6.0
sorghum and mustard (*Eden* Organic)	150	8.0	27.0	0	0	130	7.0
vegetarian:							
(*Allens*)	140	6.0	28.0	0	0	460	4.0
(*Amy's*)	120	5.0	24.0	.5	0	480	6.0
(*Bush's*)	130	5.0	24.0	0	0	550	6.0
(*S&W*)	120	6.0	24.0	.5	0	630	8.0
Baking mix (see also "Biscuit mix"), all purpose:							
(*Bisquick* Original), ⅓ cup	160	3.0	26.0	6.0	0	490	0
(*Bisquick* Reduced Fat), ⅓ cup	150	3.0	27.0	2.5	0	500	<1.0

Food and Measure	cal.	prot. (gms)	carbo. (gms)	fat (gms)	chol. (mgs)	sod. (mgs)	fiber (gms)
Baking mix *(cont.)*							
(*Don's Chuck Wagon*),							
¼ cup	95	3.0	21.0	0	0	665	1.0
(*"Jiffy"*), ¼ cup	130	2.0	22.0	4.5	0	320	1.0
whole wheat (*Hodgson Mill* Insta-Bake),							
⅓ cup	138	4.0	29.0	1.0	0	290	3.0
Baking powder:							
(*Calumet*), ⅛ tsp. . . .	0	0	0	0	0	60	0
(*Clabber Girl*), ¼ tsp. .	0	0	>1.0	0	0	120	0
Baking soda, ½ tsp. .	0	0	0	0	0	630	0
Baklava pastry, frozen (*Athens/Apollo*),							
2 pcs., 2 oz.	230	3.0	26.0	12.0	0	85	<1.0
Balsam pear, ½ cup, except as noted:							
(*Frieda's* Bittermelon),							
1 cup, 3 oz.	15	1.0	3.0	0	0	0	2.0
leafy-tips:							
raw	7	1.3	.8	.2	0	3	.6
boiled, drained	10	1.0	2.0	.1	0	4	.6
pods, ½" pcs.:							
raw	8	.5	1.7	.1	0	3	1.3
boiled, drained	12	.5	2.7	.1	0	4	1.2
Bamboo shoots, fresh, slices, ½ cup:							
raw	21	2.0	4.0	.2	0	3	.7
boiled, drained	8	.9	1.2	.1	0	3	<1.0
Bamboo shoots, canned, ½ cup:							
drained	13	1.1	2.1	.3	0	5	2.0
sliced (*Port Arthur*) . .	40	1.0	9.0	0	0	25	1.0
Banana (see also "Plantain"), fresh:							
(*Chiquita*), 1 medium,							
4.4 oz.	110	1.0	29.0	0	0	0	4.0
(*Del Monte*),							
1 medium	110	1.0	29.0	0	0	0	4.0
(*Dole*), 1 medium,							
4.4 oz.	110	1.0	29.0	0	0	0	4.0
(*Frieda's* Baby Nino/ Burro), 3-oz. pc. . .	80	1.0	20.0	0	0	0	1.0
1 medium, 8¾" long .	105	1.2	26.7	.6	0	1	2.7
sliced, ½ cup	69	.8	17.6	.4	0	1	1.8

Food and Measure	cal.	prot. (gms)	carbo. (gms)	fat (gms)	chol. (mgs)	sod. (mgs)	fiber (gms)
mashed, ½ cup	104	1.2	26.4	.5	0	1	2.7
red (*Frieda's*), 5 oz. . .	130	1.0	33.0	.5	0	0	2.0
red, 7¼" long	118	1.6	30.7	.3	0	1	n.a.
Banana, dried:							
(*Frieda's*), 1.2-oz. pc. .	130	1.0	33.0	.5	0	0	2.0
dehydrated:							
¼ cup	87	1.0	22.1	.5	0	1	1.9
sliced (*AlpineAire*),							
1 serving	50	1.0	12.0	0	0	0	1.0
Banana chips:							
(*Sunridge Farms*), 1 oz.	150	0	12.0	10.0	0	0	1.0
(*Tree of Life*), ¼ cup .	240	1.0	27.0	15.0	0	0	4.0
Banana drink blend,							
8 fl. oz.:							
(*After the Fall Banana*							
Casablanca)	150	1.0	37.0	0	0	20	0
(*Snapple* Go Bananas)	120	0	30.0	0	0	10	0
mango carrot							
(*Nantucket Nectars*)	120	0	30.0	0	0	30	0
Banana milk drink,							
see "Milk, flavored"							
Banana squash							
(*Frieda's*), ¾ cup,							
3 oz.	30	1.0	7.0	0	0	0	1.0
Barbecue beans, see							
"Baked beans"							
Barbecue coating mix							
see "Chicken							
coating mix"							
Barbecue rub (*D.L.*							
Jardine's 5-Star							
Ranch), 1 tbsp.	15	0	3.0	0	0	2530	0
Barbecue sauce (see							
also "Grilling							
sauce"), 2 tbsp.,							
except as noted:							
(*Annie's Natural*							
Organic Original) . .	45	0	9.0	1.0	0	240	0
(*Bilardo Brothers*							
Original)	25	1.0	5.0	0	0	240	1.0
(*Bull's-Eye* Original) . .	60	0	13.0	0	0	330	0
(*D.L. Jardine's* Chick'n							
Lik'n)	45	0	7.0	1.5	0	200	0

Food and Measure	cal.	prot. (gms)	carbo. (gms)	fat (gms)	chol. (mgs)	sod. (mgs)	fiber (gms)
Barbecue sauce *(cont.)*							
(*D.L. Jardine's* 5-Star), 1 tbsp.	45	1.0	10.0	0	0	190	<1.0
(*D.L. Jardine's* Killer)	35	1.0	6.0	1.5	0	310	<1.0
(*D.L. Jardine's* Texas Pecan)	40	0	7.0	1.0	0	250	1.0
(*Hunt's* Original)	40	0	9.0	0	0	360	<1.0
(*Hunt's* Original Bold)	50	0	13.0	0	0	280	<1.0
(*KC Masterpiece*)	60	0	15.0	0	0	240	0
(*Kraft Carb Well*)	15	0	3.0	0	0	390	0
(*Kraft* Char-Grill)	60	0	13.0	0	0	460	0
(*Kraft* Original)	40	0	9.0	0	0	420	0
(*Kraft* Original Easy Squeeze)	40	0	11.0	0	0	420	0
(*Kraft* Steakhouse)	60	0	14.0	0	0	360	0
(*Kraft* Thick 'n Spicy Original)	50	0	12.0	0	0	430	0
(*Litehouse*)	45	0	11.0	0	0	400	0
(*Lloyd's* Original)	50	1.0	11.0	0	0	300	0
(*Neera's* Southwest Sizzler), 2 tsp.	36	0	5.0	0	0	126	0
(*Silver Dollar City* Original)	40	0	11.0	0	0	400	0
(*Silver Dollar City* Ozark Recipe)	50	0	14.0	0	0	330	0
(*Woody's* Cook-in' Concentrate)	50	1.0	4.0	4.0	0	490	1.0
(*World Harbors*)	70	0	16.0	0	0	540	0
all varieties (*Maull's*)	60	0	13.0	0	0	300	0
Asian (*San-J*)	40	2.0	7.0	0	0	840	0
Cajun (*Kraft Thick 'n Spicy*)	50	0	12.0	0	0	460	0
bacon, hickory (*Kraft Thick 'n Spicy*)	60	0	13.0	0	0	460	0
brown sugar, spicy (*Kraft Thick 'n Spicy*)	60	0	15.0	0	0	350	0
chipotle:							
hot (*Annie's Naturals* Organic)	45	0	9.0	1.0	0	240	0
smokey (*Texas Longhorn*)	35	0	8.0	0	0	10	0
concentrate (*Watkins* Original), 2 tsp.	20	0	5.0	0	0	300	0

Food and Measure	cal.	prot. (gms)	carbo. (gms)	fat (gms)	chol. (mgs)	sod. (mgs)	fiber (gms)
garlic:							
(*Pain Is Good* Garlic-Que)	30	1.0	8.0	0	0	240	0
roasted (*Kraft*)	50	0	12.0	0	0	360	0
hickory:							
(*Bull's-Eye* Smokehouse) ...	60	0	13.0	0	0	340	0
(*Hunt's*)	50	0	13.0	0	0	280	<1.0
brown sugar (*Hunt's*)	70	0	16.0	0	0	360	1.0
brown sugar (*KC Masterpiece*) ...	60	0	15.0	0	0	320	0
honey (*Hunt's*)	50	0	12.0	0	0	380	<1.0
smoke (*Kraft*)	40	0	9.0	0	0	420	0
smoke (*Kraft Thick 'n Spicy*)	50	0	12.0	0	0	450	0
smoke, hot (*Kraft*) .	40	0	9.0	0	0	370	0
smoke, w/onion bits (*Kraft*)	45	0	11.0	0	0	360	0
smoke, sweet (*Bull's-Eye*)	60	1.0	15.0	0	0	370	0
sweet (*Silver Dollar City*)	45	0	11.0	0	0	260	0
honey:							
(*Kraft Thick 'n Spicy*)	60	0	13.0	0	0	340	0
concentrate (*Watkins*), 2 tsp.	20	0	5.0	0	0	280	0
mustard (*Hunt's*) ..	50	0	12.0	0	0	310	1.0
mustard (*Kraft*) ...	60	0	13.0	0	0	300	0
roasted garlic (*Kraft*)	50	0	11.0	0	0	380	0
smoke (*Bull's-Eye*) .	50	0	11.0	0	0	310	0
and spice (*Bilardo Brothers*)	30	1.0	7.0	0	0	240	1.0
spicy (*Bull's-Eye*) ..	50	0	12.0	0	0	310	0
spicy (*Kraft*)	60	0	14.0	0	0	360	0
teriyaki (*KC Masterpiece*) ...	60	0	14.0	0	0	590	0
hot:							
(*Bilardo Brothers*) .	30	1.0	8.0	0	0	240	1.0
(*Kraft*)	40	0	9.0	0	0	520	0
spicy (*Bull's-Eye*) ..	60	0	13.0	0	0	390	0
and spicy (*Hunt's*) .	45	0	11.0	0	0	440	<1.0

Food and Measure	cal.	prot. (gms)	carbo. (gms)	fat (gms)	chol. (mgs)	sod. (mgs)	fiber (gms)
Barbecue sauce *(cont.)*							
jalapeño (*Texas Longhorn* Rodeo) . .	35	0	8.0	0	0	10	0
jerk, Jamaican (*Pain Is Good*)	60	1.0	14.0	0	0	270	0
Kansas City style:							
(*Cowtown*)	45	1.0	11.0	0	0	290	0
(*Cowtown* Night of the Living)	40	0	10.0	0	0	210	0
(*Kraft*)	50	0	11.0	0	0	310	0
maple, smoky (*Annie's Naturals* Organic) . .	45	0	9.0	1.0	0	220	0
mesquite:							
(*Bull's-Eye* Texas Style)	60	0	13.0	0	0	380	0
(*D.L. Jardine's*) . . .	40	1.0	6.0	1.5	0	270	<1.0
(*Hunt's*)	40	0	9.0	0	0	360	<1.0
(*Kraft*)	40	0	9.0	0	0	420	0
concentrate (*Watkins*), 2 tsp.	20	0	5.0	0	0	290	0
smoke (*Kraft Thick 'n Spicy*)	50	0	12.0	0	0	440	0
onion, grilled, w/garlic (*Bull's-Eye*)	60	1.0	14.0	0	0	410	1.0
onion bits (*Kraft*)	45	0	11.0	0	0	360	0
Polynesian (*Sagawa's*)	60	1.0	13.0	0	0	620	0
Southern style:							
(*Pain Is Good*)	60	1.0	14.0	0	0	270	0
vinegar (*Bilardo Brothers*)	25	1.0	5.0	0	0	145	1.0
St. Louis style (*Silver Dollar City*)	35	0	9.0	0	0	370	0
sweet and mild (*Silver Dollar City*)	40	0	11.0	0	0	420	0
sweet and sour (*Woody's*)	70	0	17.0	0	0	610	1.0
tangy (*Silver Dollar City*)	30	0	7.0	0	0	390	0
teriyaki (*Kraft*)	60	0	12.0	0	0	440	0
Barbecue seasoning (*McCormick*), ¼ tsp.	0	0	0	0	0	20	0
Barley:							
dry, ¼ cup:							
(*Shiloh Farms*)	140	5.0	35.0	1.0	0	0	6.0

Food and Measure	cal.	prot. (gms)	carbo. (gms)	fat (gms)	chol. (mgs)	sod. (mgs)	fiber (gms)
pearled (*Arrowhead Mills*)	160	5.0	32.0	1.0	0	5	8.0
pearled	176	5.0	38.9	.6	0	5	7.8
cooked, pearled, ½ cup	97	1.8	22.2	.4	0	3	3.0
Barley flakes (*Arrowhead Mills*), ⅓ cup .	110	4.0	28.0	1.0	0	0	5.0
Barley flour:							
(*Arrowhead Mills*), ⅓ cup	95	3.0	19.0	1.0	0	0	4.0
(*Shiloh Farms*), ¼ cup	75	3.0	19.0	.5	0	0	3.0
Barley grits (*Shiloh Farms*), ¼ cup	140	5.0	35.0	1.0	0	0	6.0
Barley malt syrup (*Eden* Organic), 1 tbsp.	60	1.0	14.0	0	0	0	0
Barley miso, see "Miso"							
Basella, see "Vine spinach"							
Basil, fresh:							
1 oz.	8	.7	1.2	.2	0	0	.3
5 medium leaves	1	.1	.1	<.1	0	0	.1
chopped, 2 tbsp.	1	.1	.2	<.1	0	0	.2
Basil, dried, ground:							
1 tbsp.	11	.7	2.7	.2	0	2	.5
1 tsp.	4	.2	.9	.1	0	<1	.2
Baskin-Robbins, 4-oz. scoop, except as noted:							
ice cream:							
banana nut	260	5.0	27.0	16.0	45	75	1.0
black walnut	280	6.0	25.0	19.0	50	90	1.0
butter pecan	280	5.0	24.0	18.0	50	95	1.0
chocolate	260	5.0	33.0	14.0	50	130	0
chocolate *World Class*	270	5.0	33.0	15.0	45	115	0
chocolate almond ..	310	7.0	32.0	18.0	45	120	1.0
chocolate chip	270	5.0	28.0	16.0	55	95	1.0
chocolate chip cookie dough ...	290	5.0	36.0	15.0	55	130	1.0
chocolate éclair ...	300	5.0	35.0	17.0	60	130	0
chocolate fudge ...	270	4.0	35.0	15.0	50	140	0
chocolate ribbon ..	240	4.0	31.0	12.0	45	85	0
créme brûlée	280	4.0	41.0	11.0	80	115	0

Food and Measure	cal.	prot. (gms)	carbo. (gms)	fat (gms)	chol. (mgs)	sod. (mgs)	fiber (gms)
***Baskin-Robbins*, ice cream** *(cont.)*							
fudge brownie	300	5.0	35.0	19.0	45	140	1.0
German chocolate							
cake	300	5.0	36.0	16.0	45	150	1.0
gold medal ribbon .	260	5.0	34.0	13.0	45	150	0
Jamoca	240	5.0	26.0	13.0	55	90	0
Jamoca almond							
fudge	270	6.0	31.0	15.0	40	80	1.0
mint chocolate chip	270	5.0	28.0	16.0	55	95	1.0
nutty coconut	300	6.0	28.0	20.0	45	90	1.0
Oreo cookies 'n							
cream	280	5.0	32.0	15.0	50	150	1.0
peanut butter							
chocolate	320	7.0	31.0	20.0	45	180	1.0
pistachio almond ..	290	7.0	25.0	19.0	50	85	1.0
pralines 'n cream ..	270	4.0	34.0	14.0	45	170	0
Reese's peanut							
butter cup	300	6.0	31.0	18.0	50	130	0
rocky road	290	5.0	36.0	15.0	45	120	1.0
strawberry, very							
berry	220	4.0	28.0	11.0	40	70	0
strawberry							
shortcake	280	4.0	34.0	14.0	45	130	0
tiramisu	260	5.0	32.0	13.0	60	120	0
vanilla	260	4.0	26.0	16.0	65	70	0
vanilla, French	280	4.0	26.0	18.0	120	85	0
ice cream, light:							
berries 'n banana ..	110	5.0	25.0	2.0	10	125	1.0
caramel turtle	160	5.0	37.0	4.0	10	130	0
chocolate, mad							
about	160	5.0	35.0	4.0	10	125	1.0
chocolate chip	170	4.0	30.0	4.5	10	110	1.0
chocolate chocolate							
chip	150	6.0	30.0	4.5	10	140	1.0
chocolate cookie ..	160	6.0	34.0	5.0	10	190	1.0
espresso 'n cream .	180	5.0	32.0	4.0	10	120	1.0
pineapple coconut .	150	4.0	27.0	2.0	10	105	0
tin roof sundae	190	4.0	34.0	3.0	10	105	1.0
frozen yogurt, ½ cup:							
low fat:							
Maui brownie							
madness	210	6.0	39.0	4.0	10	140	1.0
perils of praline .	190	5.0	37.0	3.5	5	170	1.0
Raspberry							
Cheese Louise	190	5.0	36.0	4.0	10	150	1.0

Food and Measure	cal.	prot. (gms)	carbo. (gms)	fat (gms)	chol. (mgs)	sod. (mgs)	fiber (gms)
vanilla, nonfat	150	6.0	32.0	0	5	105	0
soft serve:							
chocolate	120	4.0	25.0	0	0	85	1.0
peppermint	110	4.0	24.0	0	0	75	0
red raspberry ...	110	4.0	25.0	0	0	75	0
Truly Free, no sugar:							
butter pecan	90	4.0	17.0	0	5	90	1.0
café mocha	90	4.0	18.0	0	5	85	1.0
chocolate	80	4.0	15.0	0	0	80	0
strawberry patch	90	4.0	17.0	0	5	85	1.0
vanilla	90	4.0	17.0	0	5	85	1.0
vanilla, nonfat ..	110	4.0	23.0	0	0	80	0
ice, daiquiri, Margarita,							
or watermelon	130	0	34.0	0	0	15	0
sherbet:							
blue raspberry,							
orange, or							
rainbow	160	1.0	34.0	2.0	10	40	0
red raspberry	160	1.0	36.0	2.0	10	40	0
sundaes, 1 serving:							
banana royale	630	9.0	91.0	27.0	85	250	5.0
banana split	1030	12.0	168.0	39.0	135	190	7.0
hot fudge, 2 scoop .	530	8.0	62.0	29.0	85	200	0
hot fudge, 3 scoop .	750	11.0	86.0	41.0	125	280	0
Bold Breeze:							
kiwi:							
16 oz.	340	1.0	87.0	0	0	30	3.0
24 oz.	470	1.0	120.0	.5	0	40	4.0
creamy, 16 oz. ..	440	4.0	107.0	.5	0	95	3.0
creamy, 24 oz. ..	620	7.0	152.0	1.0	5	150	4.0
strawberry citrus:							
16 oz.	350	1.0	89.0	1.0	0	10	2.0
24 oz.	480	2.0	122.0	1.0	0	15	4.0
creamy, 16 oz. ..	450	5.0	109.0	1.0	0	75	3.0
creamy, 24 oz. ..	630	8.0	154.0	1.5	5	120	4.0
wild mango:							
16 oz.	340	1.0	84.0	1.0	0	10	2.0
24 oz.	470	1.0	116.0	1.5	0	15	2.0
creamy, 16 oz. ..	440	4.0	104.0	1.5	0	75	2.0
creamy, 24 oz. ..	620	7.0	148.0	2.0	5	120	3.0
Cappuccino Blast,							
16 oz.:							
cappuccino	300	6.0	43.0	12.0	45	95	0
low fat	220	6.0	45.0	2.0	10	115	0

Food and Measure	cal.	prot. (gms)	carbo. (gms)	fat (gms)	chol. (mgs)	sod. (mgs)	fiber (gms)
Baskin-Robbins, Cappuccino Blast, 16 oz. *(cont.)*							
nonfat	210	7.0	45.0	0	5	120	0
w/whipped cream	480	9.0	67.0	21.0	80	160	0
chocolate	450	6.0	81.0	12.0	45	140	0
mocha	350	5.0	57.0	12.0	45	90	0
w/whipped cream	370	6.0	58.0	13.0	50	100	0
Mintopia	430	7.0	63.0	17.0	50	125	0
turtle	540	7.0	92.0	17.0	50	330	0
shakes:							
chocolate							
w/chocolate:							
16 oz.	620	15.0	81.0	30.0	105	300	1.0
24 oz.	990	20.0	149.0	39.0	135	440	1.0
chocolate w/vanilla:							
16 oz.	690	13.0	85.0	33.0	130	210	0
24 oz.	1000	19.0	133.0	45.0	175	290	0
espresso, 24 oz. . . .	790	19.0	80.0	45.0	175	300	0
vanilla, 16 oz.	680	13.0	81.0	33.0	130	380	0
vanilla, 24 oz.	980	19.0	125.0	45.0	175	640	0
Bass (see also "Sea Bass"), meat only:							
freshwater, 4 oz.:							
raw	129	21.4	0	4.2	77	79	0
baked, broiled, or microwaved	166	27.4	0	5.4	99	102	0
striped, 4 oz.:							
raw	110	20.1	0	2.7	91	78	0
baked, broiled, or microwaved	141	25.8	0	3.4	117	100	0
Batter and breading mix (see also "Tempura batter mix" and specific listings), seasoned, ¼ cup, except as noted:							
(*Old Bay Better Batter*)	110	2.0	13.0	.5	0	690	0
(*Old Bay Dip & Crisp*)	110	3.0	15.0	2.0	0	800	0
all purpose:							
batter (*Don's Chuck Wagon*)	100	4.0	20.0	0	0	580	1.0
batter (*Golden Dipt Fry Easy*)	100	2.0	20.0	0	0	770	0
breading (*Golden Dipt* Fry Easy) . .	120	2.0	20.0	1.0	0	750	0

Food and Measure	cal.	prot. (gms)	carbo. (gms)	fat (gms)	chol. (mgs)	sod. (mgs)	fiber (gms)
beer batter (*Golden Dipt* Fry Easy)	100	1.0	19.0	0	19	740	0
Cajun (*Golden Dipt Oven Easy*)	90	1.0	11.0	3.0	0	610	0
garlic and herb (*Golden Dipt Oven Easy*), 3 tbsp.	100	1.0	13.0	3.0	0	610	0
lemon and pepper (*Golden Dipt Oven Easy*)	90	1.0	12.0	3.0	0	680	0
Bay leaf, dried, crumbled, 1 tsp.	5	.1	.3	.1	0	<1	<1.0
Bean dip, 2 tbsp., except as noted:							
(*Fritos* Original)	40	2.0	5.0	1.0	0	170	1.0
(*Pace*), ½ cup	80	5.0	15.0	0	0	590	4.0
black bean:							
(*D.L. Jardine's* Texas Pate)	30	2.0	5.0	0	0	85	2.0
(*Fritos*)	30	2.0	6.0	0	0	210	2.0
(*Garden of Eatin'* Baja)	25	2.0	5.0	0	0	80	1.0
mild (*Guiltless Gourmet*)	30	2.0	5.0	0	0	115	2.0
spicy (*Guiltless Gourmet*)	30	2.0	5.0	0	0	110	2.0
jalapeño (*Fritos* Hot) .	40	2.0	5.0	1.0	0	210	1.0
jalapeño lime (*Synder's*)	25	1.0	5.0	0	0	150	n.a.
pinto bean, w/cheese, salsa (*Cedarlane* 5-Layer Mexican) ..	60	3.0	4.0	3.0	10	100	1.0
red bean, spicy chipolte (*Garden of Eatin'*)	25	1.0	5.0	0	0	90	2.0
Bean dishes, see specific bean listings							
Bean salad (see also "Beans, mixed"), ½ cup:							
dill sauce (*S&W* Provencal Recipe) .	50	6.0	14.0	0	0	560	3.0
three bean (*Green Giant*)	90	3.0	20.0	0	0	490	4.0

Food and Measure	cal.	prot. (gms)	carbo. (gms)	fat (gms)	chol. (mgs)	sod. (mgs)	fiber (gms)
Bean sauce, Asian:							
black bean, 1 tbsp.:							
(*Ka•Me*)	20	1.0	3.0	.5	0	280	0
garlic (*Lee Kum Kee*)	30	1.0	4.0	1.0	0	1270	1.0
brown bean, spicy (*House of Tsang*), 1 tsp.	15	0	3.0	0	0	130	0
Bean sprouts, fresh, see specific listings							
Beans, see specific listings							
Beans, baked, see "Baked beans"							
Beans, mixed (see also "Bean salad"), canned, ½ cup:							
(*Bush's*)	110	7.0	19.0	0	0	500	6.0
(*S&W* New York Deli Style)	90	4.0	17.0	0	0	670	6.0
(*S&W* San Antonio) ..	90	6.0	20.0	.5	0	670	6.0
(*S&W* Santa Fe)	90	6.0	21.0	.5	0	680	6.0
(*Westbrae Natural* Organic)	100	7.0	19.0	.5	0	150	5.0
(*Westbrae Natural* Organic Soup Beans)	100	6.0	19.0	0	0	140	6.0
seasoned (*Glory* Crock Pot Beans)	130	7.0	25.0	.5	0	610	7.0
Beans, snap or string, see "Green bean" and "Snap bean"							
Beans and franks, can or pkg.:							
(*Hormel*), 7.5-oz can .	280	11.0	32.0	12.0	50	1310	5.0
(*Kid's Kitchen*), 1 cup	320	13.0	37.0	13.0	35	760	7.0
Beans and rice, see "Rice dishes" and "Rice entree"							
Bear, meat only, simmered, 4 oz.	294	36.8	0	15.2	111	81	0
Béarnaise sauce, in jars (*Reese*), 2 tbsp.	110	0	1.0	11.0	30	60	0

Food and Measure	cal.	prot. (gms)	carbo. (gms)	fat (gms)	chol. (mgs)	sod. (mgs)	fiber (gms)
Béarnaise sauce mix							
(*McCormick*), 1 tsp.	10	0	1.0	0	0	180	0
Beaver, meat only,							
roasted, 4 oz.	240	39.5	0	7.9	133	67	0
Bee pollen (*Tree of*							
Life), 1 tsp.	30	.3	3.4	.8	0	30	0
Beechnuts, dried,							
shelled, 1 oz.	164	1.8	9.5	14.2	0	11	n.a.
Beef, choice grade, trimmed to ¼" fat, except as noted, meat only, 4 oz.:							
brisket, whole:							
braised, lean w/fat .	437	26.6	0	35.8	107	69	0
braised, lean only . .	274	33.7	0	14.5	105	79	0
chuck, arm pot roast:							
braised, lean w/fat .	395	30.6	0	29.2	112	67	0
braised, lean only . .	255	37.4	0	10.5	115	75	0
chuck, blade roast:							
braised, lean w/fat .	412	29.7	0	31.5	117	73	0
braised, lean only . .	298	35.2	0	16.3	120	81	0
flank steak, trimmed to 0" fat:							
braised, lean only . .	269	31.8	0	14.7	81	82	0
broiled, lean only . .	256	30.0	0	14.2	77	92	0
ground, see "Beef, ground"							
porterhouse steak:							
broiled, lean w/fat .	346	28.2	0	25.1	94	69	0
broiled, lean only . .	247	31.9	0	12.2	91	75	0
rib, whole:							
roasted, lean w/fat .	426	25.1	0	35.4	96	71	0
roasted, lean only .	276	30.9	0	15.9	91	82	0
rib, large end (ribs 6–9):							
roasted, lean w/fat .	434	25.3	0	36.2	96	71	0
roasted, lean only .	284	31.2	0	16.7	92	83	0
rib, small end (ribs 10–12):							
broiled, lean w/fat .	376	26.7	0	31.3	95	70	0
broiled, lean only . .	264	31.8	0	14.3	91	78	0
round, bottom:							
braised, lean w/fat .	322	32.5	0	20.3	109	57	0
braised, lean only . .	249	35.8	0	10.7	109	58	0

Food and Measure	cal.	prot. (gms)	carbo. (gms)	fat (gms)	chol. (mgs)	sod. (mgs)	fiber (gms)
Beef, round, bottom *(cont.)*							
round, eye of:							
roasted, lean w/fat .	273	30.2	0	16.0	82	67	0
roasted, lean only .	198	32.9	0	6.5	78	70	0
round, full cut:							
broiled, lean w/fat .	272	31.0	0	15.4	91	69	0
broiled, lean only ..	217	33.1	0	8.3	88	73	0
round, tip:							
roasted, lean w/fat .	280	30.1	0	16.9	94	70	0
roasted, lean only .	213	32.6	0	8.3	92	74	0
round, top:							
broiled, lean w/fat .	254	34.2	0	12.0	96	68	0
broiled, lean only ..	214	35.9	0	6.7	95	69	0
fried, lean w/fat ...	314	36.7	0	17.4	110	77	0
fried, lean only	257	39.8	0	9.7	110	81	0
shank, crosscuts:							
braised, lean w/fat .	298	34.8	0	16.6	91	69	0
braised, lean only ..	228	38.2	0	7.2	88	73	0
shortribs:							
braised, lean w/fat .	534	24.5	0	47.6	107	57	0
braised, lean only ..	335	34.9	0	20.6	105	66	0
sirloin, top:							
broiled, lean w/fat .	305	31.3	0	19.0	102	70	0
broiled, lean only ..	229	34.4	0	9.1	101	75	0
fried, lean w/fat ...	370	31.9	0	25.9	111	79	0
fried, lean only	270	36.8	0	12.4	112	87	0
T-bone steak:							
broiled, lean w/fat .	338	28.3	0	24.0	94	69	0
broiled, lean only ..	243	31.9	0	11.8	91	75	0
tenderloin:							
broiled, lean w/fat .	345	28.4	0	24.8	98	67	0
broiled, lean only ..	252	32.0	0	12.7	95	71	0
top loin:							
broiled, lean w/fat .	338	28.8	0	23.8	90	71	0
broiled, lean only ..	243	32.5	0	11.5	86	77	0
Beef, choice grade, trimmed to ⅛" fat, meat only, lean w/fat, 4 oz.:							
brisket, braised:							
whole	375	29.3	0	27.8	105	73	0
flat half	338	32.5	0	22.1	91	52	0
point half	396	27.7	0	30.8	104	78	0

Food and Measure	cal.	prot. (gms)	carbo. (gms)	fat (gms)	chol. (mgs)	sod. (mgs)	fiber (gms)
chuck, braised:							
arm	350	34.2	0	22.6	93	56	0
blade	407	29.9	0	30.9	117	73	0
rib, whole, broiled . . .	399	25.2	0	32.3	81	71	0
rib, whole, roasted . . .	414	25.6	0	33.8	95	73	0
rib, large end:							
broiled	420	23.7	0	35.4	82	71	0
roasted	429	25.5	0	35.5	96	71	0
rib, small end:							
broiled	345	27.8	0	25.1	132	56	0
roasted	407	25.3	0	33.1	94	71	0
round, full cut, broiled	266	31.2	0	14.7	90	70	0
round, bottom:							
braised	288	37.3	0	14.2	91	48	0
roasted	253	29.5	0	14.1	91	42	0
round, eye, roasted . .	240	32.3	0	11.4	73	42	0
round, tip, roasted . . .	259	30.9	0	14.0	93	71	0
round, top:							
braised	284	38.7	0	13.2	102	51	0
broiled	254	34.8	0	11.6	75	45	0
pan-fried	302	37.4	0	15.7	110	77	0
sirloin, top:							
broiled	291	30.4	0	17.9	94	61	0
pan-fried	355	32.6	0	23.9	111	81	0
steak, broiled:							
porterhouse	339	26.4	0	25.1	84	73	0
T-bone	324	27.3	0	20.0	74	75	0
tenderloin:							
broiled	310	30.0	0	20.2	74	59	0
roasted	375	27.1	0	28.8	96	74	0
top loin, broiled	315	29.7	0	20.9	110	59	0
Beef, canned, see "Beef entree, can or pkg." and specific listings							
Beef, corned (see also "Beef lunch meat"), cooked, 4 oz.:							
brisket	285	20.6	.5	21.5	111	1286	0
brisket, flat:							
(*Brookfield Farms*) .	230	11.0	0	20.0	55	1150	0
(*Freirich*)	210	16.0	0	17.0	110	1050	0
Beef, corned, canned:							
(*Hormel*), 2 oz.	120	15.0	0	7.0	50	490	0

Food and Measure	cal.	prot. (gms)	carbo. (gms)	fat (gms)	chol. (mgs)	sod. (mgs)	fiber (gms)
Beef, corned, canned *(cont.)*							
(*Libby's*), 2 oz.	120	15.0	0	7.0	50	490	0
hash, see "Beef hash"							
Beef, dried (see also "Beef jerky"):							
(*Hormel*), 10 slices, 1 oz.	50	8.0	1.0	1.5	25	1200	0
(*Hormel Pillow Pack*), 10 slices, 1 oz.	50	9.0	1.0	.5	25	1060	0
cured, 1 oz.	47	8.3	.4	1.1	n.a.	984	0
Beef, freeze-dried (see also "Beef entree, freeze-dried"), cooked, diced:							
(*AlpineAire*), ½ oz. . . .	60	11.0	0	2.0	35	180	0
(*Mountain House*), ⅔ cup	130	25.0	0	3.5	65	640	0
Beef, frozen or refrigerated, raw, boneless:							
ground, organic: (*Organic Valley* Chub), 4 oz.	300	20.0	0	23.0	85	75	0
(*Organic Valley* Patties), 5.25-oz. pc.	390	26.0	0	31.0	110	105	0
sirloin, marinated: peppercorn (*Always Tender*), 4 oz. . .	130	18.0	2.0	5.0	45	500	0
tequila lime (*Always Tender*), 4 oz. . .	120	17.0	3.0	5.0	45	500	0
teriyaki (*Always Tender*), 4 oz. . .	130	18.0	4.0	5.0	45	500	0
steak, frozen, 6.25-oz. pc.: center fillet (*Tyson*)	190	36.0	0	5.0	105	770	0
center fillet, peppered (*Tyson*)	190	36.0	0	5.0	105	610	0
flat iron grillers (*Tyson*)	160	31.0	0	2.0	90	340	0
steak, organic, 8 oz.: New York strip (*Organic Valley*) .	320	48.0	0	12.0	130	130	0

Food and Measure	cal.	prot. (gms)	carbo. (gms)	fat (gms)	chol. (mgs)	sod. (mgs)	fiber (gms)
rib eye (*Organic Valley*)	700	37.0	0	60.0	160	120	0
sirloin (*Organic Valley*)	490	43.0	0	34.0	150	120	0
Beef, frozen or refrigerated, cooked, 5 oz., except as noted:							
backribs, split, w/barbecue sauce (*Lloyd's*), 2 ribs w/sauce, 7.5 oz.	620	32.0	25.0	43.0	140	1730	0
barbecue, shredded:							
(*Hormel*)	90	8.0	10.0	2.0	25	530	0
original sauce w/ (*Lloyd's*), ¼ cup .	90	7.0	11.0	2.0	15	370	0
brisket, barbecued, sliced (*Hormel*) ...	290	18.0	23.0	14.0	65	1170	0
pot roast, in gravy (*Tyson*)	170	23.0	2.0	8.0	65	730	0
roast:							
(*Hormel*)	200	28.0	3.0	9.0	75	450	0
in brown gravy (*Tyson*)	130	17.0	5.0	4.0	50	980	0
shredded, Southwestern (*Hormel*), 2 oz.	70	2.0	2.0	3.0	25	260	0
steak:							
sliced, and gravy (*Hormel*)	160	22.0	3.0	4.5	60	600	0
strips, seasoned (*Tyson* Bag), 3 oz.	140	18.0	1.0	6.0	55	500	0
strips, seasoned (*Tyson* Box), 3 oz.	130	18.0	1.0	6.0	55	420	0
steak, breaded:							
fingers (*Tyson*), 2 pcs., 3.2 oz. ..	240	8.0	13.0	17.0	20	610	1.0
country fried (*Tyson*), 3.2-oz. patty	300	9.0	17.0	21.0	25	710	1.0
teriyaki (*Simply Simmered*)	100	10.0	10.0	3.0	20	940	1.0
tips:							
(*Hormel*)	160	20.0	5.0	7.0	55	760	1.0
in gravy (*Tyson*) ...	200	17.0	5.0	12.0	55	530	0

Food and Measure	cal.	prot. (gms)	carbo. (gms)	fat (gms)	chol. (mgs)	sod. (mgs)	fiber (gms)
Beef, ground, retail							
cuts, 4 oz.:							
raw:							
95% lean	155	24.3	0	6.0	70	75	0
90% lean	199	22.7	0	11.3	74	75	0
85% lean	244	21.1	0	17.0	77	75	0
80% lean	288	19.5	0	22.7	81	76	0
75% lean	332	17.9	0	28.4	85	76	0
crumbles, pan-browned:							
95% lean	219	33.1	0	8.6	101	96	0
90% lean . . . . :	261	32.3	0	13.7	101	99	0
85% lean	290	31.4	0	17.4	102	101	0
80% lean	308	30.6	0	19.7	101	103	0
75% lean	314	30.4	0	20.7	101	105	0
patty, broiled:							
95% lean	202	29.8	0	8.0	86	74	0
90% lean	246	29.6	0	13.3	96	77	0
85% lean	284	29.4	0	17.6	102	82	0
80% lean	307	29.2	0	20.2	103	85	0
75% lean	315	29.0	0	21.3	101	88	0
patty, pan-broiled:							
95% lean	186	29.3	0	7.0	86	81	0
90% lean	231	28.6	0	12.1	93	85	0
85% lean	263	27.9	0	15.9	98	90	0
80% lean	274	27.3	0	18.1	98	94	0
75% lean	281	26.6	0	18.6	94	99	0
"Beef," vegetarian							
(see also "Burger, vegetarian"):							
canned (*Worthington Prime Stakes*),							
3.2-oz. pc.	120	9.0	7.0	6.0	0	440	1.0
frozen/refrigerated:							
(*Loma Linda* Swiss Stake), 3.2-oz. pc.	130	9.0	9.0	6.0	0	430	3.0
(*Worthington Stakelets*),							
2.5-oz. pc.	150	14.0	7.0	7.0	0	480	2.0
corned (*Worthington*),							
3 slices, 2 oz. . . .	140	10.0	5.0	9.0	0	460	0
ground (*Quorn*),							
⅔ cup, 3 oz. . . .	80	13.0	5.0	2.5	0	220	4.0

Food and Measure	cal.	prot. (gms)	carbo. (gms)	fat (gms)	chol. (mgs)	sod. (mgs)	fiber (gms)
ground (*Yves* The Good Ground), 1.9 oz.	60	10.0	5.0	.5	0	260	3.0
ground, Mexican (*Yves* The Good Ground), 1.9 oz. .	90	11.0	5.0	2.5	0	300	3.0
meatballs (*Yves* The Good Ground), 2.1 oz.	110	16.0	7.0	2.4	0	420	3.0
smoked (*Worthington*), 3 slices, 2 oz. . . .	130	11.0	7.0	7.0	0	510	<1.0
strips (*Lightlife*), 3 oz.	70	11.0	6.0	0	0	460	4.0
Beef dinner, frozen, 1 pkg.:							
pot roast:							
(*Healthy Choice* Dinners), 11 oz. .	320	19.0	39.0	9.0	45	550	6.0
(*Stouffer's* Home-style), 16 oz. . . .	350	21.0	43.0	10.0	35	1610	7.0
(*Swanson Hungry-Man*), 18.5 oz. . .	430	27.0	47.0	16.0	55	1180	7.0
ribs, boneless, barbecue sauce (*Healthy Choice* Dinners), 11 oz. . . .	360	22.0	47.0	9.0	55	580	8.0
roasted:							
mushroom (*Healthy Choice* Dinners), 11 oz.	280	23.0	28.0	8.0	60	600	5.0
oven (*Healthy Choice* Dinners), 10.15 oz.	280	22.0	33.0	7.0	60	600	5.0
slow, and gravy (*Stouffer's* Home-style), 14 oz. . . .	370	21.0	41.0	14.0	35	1510	8.0
Salisbury steak:							
(*Healthy Choice* Dinners), 12.5 oz.	360	23.0	45.0	9.0	45	580	5.0
(*Lean Cuisine Dinnertime Selections*), 15.5 oz.	320	25.0	35.0	9.0	55	890	6.0

Food and Measure	cal.	prot. (gms)	carbo. (gms)	fat (gms)	chol. (mgs)	sod. (mgs)	fiber (gms)
Beef dinner, Salisbury steak *(cont.)*							
(*Stouffer's* Home-style), 16 oz. ...	470	28.0	49.0	18.0	60	1010	5.0
(*Swanson Hungry-Man*), 16.25 oz. .	410	28.0	47.0	12.0	90	1020	3.0
w/red-skin mashed potato (*Healthy Choice* Dinners), 8 oz.	210	16.0	21.0	6.0	35	600	3.0
steak:							
country fried (*Stouffer's* Home-style), 16 oz. ...	590	22.0	52.0	33.0	45	1410	4.0
Southwest, mesquite (*Stouffer's* Home-style), 14 oz. ...	440	19.0	50.0	18.0	40	1740	8.0
steak tips Dijon (*Lean Cuisine Dinnertime Selections*), 12 oz. .	310	18.0	44.0	7.0	35	820	5.0
Stroganoff (*Healthy Choice* Dinners), 11 oz.	330	22.0	40.0	9.0	60	600	7.0
tips portobello (*Healthy Choice* Dinners), 11.25 oz.	280	23.0	28.0	8.0	50	600	3.0
"Beef" dinner, vegetarian, frozen, Salisbury steak (*Amy's* Country Dinner Whole Meal), 11-oz. pkg.	390	11.0	60.0	12.0	15	570	8.0
Beef entree, can or pkg.:							
hash, see "Beef hash"							
pot roast (*Hormel* Bowl), 10 oz.	200	24.0	20.0	2.5	40	740	2.0
roast, w/gravy (*Hormel*), ½ cup ..	140	23.0	3.0	4.0	75	640	3.0
roast, w/potatoes (*Hormel* Bowl), 10 oz.	230	23.0	25.0	4.5	45	970	2.0
Salisbury steak (*Hormel* Bowl), 10 oz.	290	18.0	25.0	13.0	45	1190	3.0

Food and Measure	cal.	prot. (gms)	carbo. (gms)	fat (gms)	chol. (mgs)	sod. (mgs)	fiber (gms)
stew:							
(*Dinty Moore* Bowl), 10 oz.	250	15.0	22.0	11.0	40	1250	2.0
(*Dinty Moore* Can), 1 cup	180	10.0	17.0	8.0	30	970	2.0
(*Dinty Moore* Can), 7.5-oz. can	190	10.0	15.0	10.0	30	900	2.0
(*Dinty Moore* Cup), 1 cont.	160	10.0	14.0	7.0	30	900	2.0
(*Dinty Moore* Steak-house Can), 1 cup	170	14.0	16.0	6.0	45	1090	2.0
(*Hormel* Meal), 1 cont.	150	10.0	14.0	6.0	25	890	2.0
Beef entree, freeze-dried, 1 serving:							
patty, flame-broiled (*Mountain House*), ½ pouch	230	19.0	26.0	5.0	50	830	3.0
rotini (*AlpineAire*) ...	360	21.0	59.0	5.0	40	560	3.0
stew:							
(*Mountain House* Can/Four), 1 cup	210	13.0	24.0	8.0	20	970	3.0
(*Mountain House* Double), ½ pouch	320	14.0	37.0	13.0	20	1170	4.0
(*Mountain House* Single)	330	20.0	37.0	12.0	35	1520	4.0
Stroganoff flavor:							
(*AlpineAire*)	330	2.0	40.0	10.0	55	1010	2.0
(*Mountain House* Can/Four), 1 cup	260	11.0	31.0	11.0	20	880	2.0
(*Mountain House* Double), ½ pouch	270	16.0	30.0	9.0	25	1220	3.0
(*Mountain House* Single)	390	17.0	46.0	16.0	25	1320	2.0
w/beef and rice (*Instant Gourmet*)	440	21.0	67.0	10.0	60	1150	5.0
tamale pie (*AlpineAire* Western)	380	23.0	50.0	10.0	55	1050	7.0
teriyaki:							
(*Mountain House*), ½ pouch	330	14.0	55.0	6.0	20	1170	4.0
(*Mountain House* Can), 1 cup	260	12.0	44.0	4.0	15	910	3.0

Food and Measure	cal.	prot. (gms)	carbo. (gms)	fat (gms)	chol. (mgs)	sod. (mgs)	fiber (gms)
Beef entree, frozen (see also "beef, frozen or refrigerated, cooked"), 1 pkg., except as noted:							
chipped, creamed (*Stouffer's* 11 oz.), 4.4 oz.	140	9.0	9.0	8.0	40	610	0
chow mein (*Shanghai*), ⅓ of 24-oz. pkg. . . .	310	22.0	29.0	12.0	55	1010	3.0
and broccoli:							
garlic (*Lean Cuisine* Café Classics), 9 oz.	170	13.0	16.0	6.0	30	690	3.0
Hunan (*Lean Cuisine Everyday Favorites*), 8.5 oz.	230	12.0	36.0	4.0	15	680	1.0
spicy (*Michelina's Yu Sing* Bowls), 11 oz.	380	16.0	78.0	5.0	20	1630	2.0
spicy, w/rice (*Uncle Ben's* Rice Bowl), 12 oz.	370	21.0	62.0	4.5	25	1550	1.0
stir-fry (*Shanghai*), 1/5 of 44-oz. pkg.	220	13.0	42.0	3.0	25	890	4.0
broccoli and (*Stouffer's Skillet Sensations*), ⅓ of 25-oz. pkg.	180	10.0	29.0	10.0	35	800	2.0
fajita, see "Fajita"							
home style (*Stouffer's Skillet Sensations*), 7.1 oz.	170	10.0	19.0	6.0	25	740	2.0
Merlot (*Healthy Choice*), 10 oz.	240	16.0	26.0	8.0	40	580	7.0
Oriental:							
(*Healthy Choice*), 10.6 oz.	300	16.0	27.0	9.0	35	600	8.0
(*Lean Cuisine* Café Classics), 9.25 oz.	210	14.0	31.0	3.5	25	570	2.0
pepper steak:							
(*Smart Ones Bistro Selections*), 10 oz.	230	15.0	32.0	5.0	30	690	4.0

Food and Measure	cal.	prot. (gms)	carbo. (gms)	fat (gms)	chol. (mgs)	sod. (mgs)	fiber (gms)
green (*Stouffer's* Homestyle), 10.5 oz.	310	21.0	30.0	8.0	30	960	2.0
and rice (*Michelina's* Authentico), 8 oz.	250	11.0	43.0	4.0	20	890	1.0
and rice (*Michelina's Lean Gourmet*), 8 oz.	260	12.0	43.0	4.5	15	880	1.0
peppercorn: (*Lean Cuisine* Café Classics), 8.75 oz.	220	14.0	25.0	7.0	25	690	3.0
fillet (*Smart Ones Bistro Selections*), 9.5 oz.	230	15.0	24.0	8.0	30	790	4.0
picadillo (*Ethnic Gourmet*), 10 oz. . .	340	10.0	36.0	13.0	25	650	3.0
pie/pot pie (*Swanson*), 7 oz.	400	13.0	42.0	21.0	60	900	3.0
portobello (*Lean Cuisine* Café Classics), 9 oz.	200	14.0	25.0	5.0	30	680	2.0
pot roast: (*Lean Cuisine* Café Classics), 9 oz. . .	190	12.0	23.0	6.0	25	690	2.0
(*Smart Ones* Higher Protein), 9 oz. . .	170	25.0	9.0	9.0	60	710	2.0
(*Stouffer's* Homestyle), 8⅞ oz. . . .	260	16.0	24.0	11.0	35	960	3.0
w/potato (*Michelina's Signature*), 10 oz.	260	14.0	35.0	7.0	25	880	4.0
Yankee (*Stouffer's Skillet Sensations*), ⅓ of 24-oz. pkg.	190	10.0	24.0	6.0	25	670	4.0
roast/roasted: w/gravy (*Smart Ones Bistro Selections*), 9 oz.	220	13.0	19.0	7.0	25	830	3.0
oven (*Lean Cuisine* Café Classics), 9.25 oz.	210	16.0	18.0	8.0	35	690	2.0
portobello (*Smart Ones* Higher Protein), 9 oz. . .	200	26.0	9.0	8.0	50	660	2.0

Food and Measure	cal.	prot. (gms)	carbo. (gms)	fat (gms)	chol. (mgs)	sod. (mgs)	fiber (gms)
Beef entree, frozen *(cont.)*							
Salisbury steak:							
(*Boston Market*), 16 oz.	750	30.0	44.0	42.0	100	2420	4.0
(*Lean Cuisine* Café Classics), 9.5 oz.	280	25.0	26.0	8.0	50	670	3.0
(*Michelina's* Authentico), 8 oz.	290	12.0	22.0	16.0	40	1400	2.0
(*Michelina's Lean Gourmet*), 8.5 oz.	200	12.0	23.0	7.0	30	970	2.0
(*Michelina's Signature*), 10.5 oz. . .	410	22.0	35.0	19.0	50	1820	2.0
(*Smart Ones*), 9.5 oz.	260	22.0	25.0	6.0	30	790	4.0
(*Smart Ones* Higher Protein), 9 oz. . .	200	20.0	9.0	8.0	35	700	2.0
(*Stouffer's* Home-style), 9⅝ oz. . .	370	25.0	27.0	18.0	40	1120	1.0
(*Swanson* Angus), 13 oz.	390	25.0	24.0	20	80	750	3.0
shepherd's pie (*Ian's* Natural), ½ of 9.5-oz. pkg.	250	14.0	23.0	11.0	25	350	2.0
sirloin:							
and Asian vegetables (*Smart Ones* Higher Protein), 9 oz.	160	25.0	11.0	4.0	55	750	3.0
roasted, w/noodles (*Michelina's Lean Gourmet*/Authentico), 8 oz.	230	13.0	30.0	5.0	45	920	2.0
spicy (*Contessa* Minute Meal Bowl), 10.5 oz.	300	17.0	52.0	6.0	15	1000	4.0
steak:							
and garlic potatoes (*Birds Eye Voila!*), 1 cup*	190	9.0	22.0	7.0	15	630	5.0
grilled, roasted garlic sauce (*Healthy Choice*), 10 oz. . . .	240	17.0	46.0	7.0	40	600	6.0
grilled whiskey (*Healthy Choice*), 9.5 oz.	300	17.0	46.0	5.0	40	600	6.0

Food and Measure	cal.	prot. (gms)	carbo. (gms)	fat (gms)	chol. (mgs)	sod. (mgs)	fiber (gms)
and portobello mushrooms (*Stouffer's* Bowl Cuisine), 11 oz. .	280	16.0	33.0	9.0	35	970	4.0
strips, grilled, w/onion, peppers (*Swanson Hungry-Man* Steakhouse), 20 oz.	580	34.0	75.0	16.0	65	2370	6.0
steak w/dipping sauce:							
barbecue (*Healthy Choice*), 13 oz. . .	390	25.0	51.0	9.0	60	600	8.0
teriyaki (*Healthy Choice*), 14 oz. . .	490	26.0	74.0	10.0	60	590	6.0
zesty (*Healthy Choice*), 13 oz. . .	340	24.0	37.0	10.0	80	600	6.0
stew:							
(*Green Giant* Complete Skillet Meal), ¼ of 32-oz. pkg.	180	11.0	27.0	3.5	25	1110	4.0
(*Stouffer's* Bowl Cuisine), 11 oz. .	300	19.0	32.0	11.0	45	1070	5.0
and vegetable (*Michelina's* Homestyle Bowls), 11 oz.	230	14.0	31.0	6.0	20	1340	4.0
stir-fry (*Contessa*), 1¾ cups*	190	13.0	28.0	3.0	20	820	4.0
Stroganoff:							
(*Michelina's Lean Gourmet*), 8 oz. .	250	15.0	38.0	5.0	20	650	2.0
(*Stouffer's* Homestyle), 9¾ oz. . . .	380	22.0	34.0	17.0	70	990	2.0
(*Stouffer's Skillet Sensations* 40 oz.), 7.25 oz. .	250	17.0	24.0	10.0	35	870	3.0
teriyaki:							
(*Healthy Choice*), 9.5 oz.	310	15.0	46.0	7.0	40	600	5.0
and rice (*Lean Cuisine Skillet Sensations*), ⅓ of 24-oz. pkg.	180	9.0	31.0	2.5	15	540	2.0

Food and Measure	cal.	prot. (gms)	carbo. (gms)	fat (gms)	chol. (mgs)	sod. (mgs)	fiber (gms)
Beef entree, frozen (cont.)							
teriyaki steak:							
(*Lean Cuisine* Café Classics Bowl), 10.5 oz.	340	21.0	47.0	7.0	30	690	4.0
(*Michelina's Yu Sing* Bowls), 11 oz. ..	370	16.0	64.0	4.5	15	1160	3.0
(*Stouffer's Skillet Sensations*), ⅓ of 23.5-oz. pkg.	210	11.0	33.0	3.5	20	900	2.0
tips:							
Southern (*Lean Cuisine* Café Classics), 8.75 oz.	250	15.0	36.0	5.0	25	630	3.0
steak, portobello (*Lean Cuisine* Café Classics), 7.5 oz.	180	15.0	13.0	7.0	40	460	3.0
and vegetables:							
(*Ethnic Gourmet* Bulgogi, 10 oz. .	350	13.0	36.0	12.0	50	700	2.0
(*Smart Ones* Bowls), 11 oz.	260	12.0	40.0	7.0	20	1010	3.0
teriyaki (*Birds Eye Voila!* Reduced Carb), 1 cup* ...	160	15.0	15.0	4.0	25	950	4.0
teriyaki steak (*Green Giant* Complete Skillet Meal), ¼ of 32-oz. pkg.	300	15.0	53.0	3.5	20	1030	3.0
"Beef" entree, vegetarian, frozen, 1 pkg.:							
pepper steak (*Hain Vegetarian Classics*), 10 oz.	310	26.0	41.0	6.0	0	440	9.0
Santa Fe veggie beef (*Yves* The Good Bowl), 10.5 oz.	360	15.0	57.0	9.0	0	810	5.0
Beef entree mix, see "Hamburger entree mix"							
Beef gravy, ¼ cup:							
(*Boston Market* Classic)	30	1.0	4.0	1.0	<5	340	0

Food and Measure	cal.	prot. (gms)	carbo. (gms)	fat (gms)	chol. (mgs)	sod. (mgs)	fiber (gms)
(*Campbell's*)	25	1.0	3.0	1.0	<5	270	0
(*Campbell's* Fat Free) .	15	1.0	3.0	0	0	300	0
roast, slow:							
(*Franco-American*) .	25	1.0	3.0	.5	<5	310	0
(*Franco-American*							
Fat Free)	20	1.0	3.0	0	0	360	0
w/roasted garlic							
(*Campbell's*)	25	1.0	4.0	.5	0	280	0
savory (*Heinz* Home							
Style)	25	1.0	4.0	.5	0	210	0
Beef gravy mix, and							
herb (*McCormick*),							
¼ cup*	30	1.0	3.0	1.0	0	290	0
Beef hash, canned,							
1 cup, except as							
noted:							
corned beef:							
(*Armour*)	440	19.0	23.0	30.0	100	840	2.0
(*Castleberry*)	430	21.0	25.0	28.0	55	1070	3.0
(*Mary Kitchen*)	390	21.0	22.0	24.0	80	1000	2.0
(*Mary Kitchen*),							
7.5-oz. can	220	18.0	20.0	22.0	75	920	2.0
(*Mary Kitchen* 50%							
Less Fat)	280	19.0	25.0	12.0	65	1070	3.0
roast beef (*Mary*							
Kitchen)	390	21.0	22.0	24.0	70	790	2.0
Beef hash, freeze-							
dried, roast beef							
(*AlpineAire* All							
American), 2 oz. . . .	220	18.0	28.0	5.0	50	920	3.0
Beef jerky, 1 oz.:							
(*Pemmican* Homestyle							
Tender Original) . . .	80	12.0	3.0	2.0	35	720	1.0
(*Pemmican* Long							
Lasting Original) . .	60	12.0	5.0	.5	10	530	0
(*Pemmican* Premium							
Cut Original)	80	13.0	4.0	1.0	35	610	1.0
hot/spicy or peppered							
(*Pemmican* Long							
Lasting)	60	12.0	4.0	.5	10	340	0
kippered:							
(*Pemmican* Original)	60	10.0	2.0	1.0	25	730	0
peppered							
(*Pemmican*)	60	10.0	2.0	1.0	25	740	0

Food and Measure	cal.	prot. (gms)	carbo. (gms)	fat (gms)	chol. (mgs)	sod. (mgs)	fiber (gms)
Beef jerky, kippered *(cont.)*							
sweet/hot							
(*Pemmican*)	70	10.0	6.0	1.0	15	810	0
teriyaki (*Pemmican*) .	60	10.0	2.0	1.0	20	870	0
shredded:							
original or peppered							
(*Pemmican*)	80	12.0	3.0	2.0	35	720	1.0
teriyaki (*Pemmican*)	80	12.0	3.0	2.0	35	730	1.0
steak tips (*Pemmican*)	70	9.0	5.0	1.5	20	510	0
teriyaki (*Pemmican Long Lasting*)	70	12.0	6.0	.5	10	310	0
Beef lunch meat (see also "Bologna," "Pastrami," etc.), 2 oz., except as noted:							
corned:							
(*Black Bear* Brisket)	90	9.0	2.0	5.0	35	550	0
(*Boar's Head*)	80	14.0	0	2.5	30	490	0
(*Boar's Head* First Cut)	80	12.0	0	4.0	40	460	0
(*Dietz & Watson* Brisket)	90	4.0	0	5.0	35	550	0
(*Healthy Choice*) . .	60	10.0	0	1.5	30	430	0
(*Healthy Deli*)	80	11.0	2.0	3.0	30	480	0
(*Hormel*)	70	10.0	0	3.0	30	650	0
(*Sara Lee*)	70	11.0	0	2.5	30	530	0
(*Sara Lee* Sliced), 2 slices, 1.8 oz. .	50	8.0	1.0	2.0	25	600	0
(*Tyson* Bag), 2 slices, 2.25 oz.	70	13.0	0	2.0	20	530	0
London broil:							
(*Black Bear*)	60	12.0	0	1.5	25	390	0
(*Dietz & Watson*) . .	60	12.0	0	1.5	30	390	0
oven roasted:							
(*Boar's Head* Top Round No Salt) .	90	14.0	0	3.0	30	40	0
(*Healthy Deli* Zero Carb)	70	12.0	0	2.0	30	320	0
Italian style (*Healthy Deli*) . . .	70	11.0	1.0	1.5	30	320	0
Cajun style (*Boar's Head*)	80	14.0	0	2.0	35	260	0

Food and Measure	cal.	prot. (gms)	carbo. (gms)	fat (gms)	chol. (mgs)	sod. (mgs)	fiber (gms)
pepper seasoned (*Boar's Head* Eye Round)	90	14.0	0	3.0	40	190	0
roast/roasted:							
(*Dietz & Watson* Cap Off)	60	12.0	0	1.5	30	290	0
(*Hansel & Gretel*) . .	70	11.0	2.0	1.5	30	310	0
(*Hatfield Deli Choice*)	80	15.0	0	1.5	35	290	0
(*Sara Lee*)	60	11.0	1.0	2.0	30	420	0
(*Sara Lee* Sliced), 2 slices, 1.6 oz. . .	60	9.0	0	2.5	25	260	0
(*Tyson* Bag), 2 slices, 2.25 oz.	90	13.0	1.0	2.0	30	710	0
extra lean (*Alpine Lace* 97% Fat Free)	70	13.0	1.0	1.5	40	300	0
eye round (*Dietz & Watson*)	70	12.0	0	2.0	30	390	0
Italian style (*Boar's Head*)	80	12.0	1.0	2.0	40	370	0
Italian style (*Dietz & Watson*)	60	12.0	0	1.5	30	390	0
marinated (*Dietz & Watson* Cap Off)	60	12.0	0	1.5	30	290	0
medium (*Healthy Choice*)	70	10.0	1.0	1.5	25	480	0
peppered (*Sara Lee*)	70	11.0	1.0	2.0	30	340	0
seasoned (*Hormel*)	70	10.0	0	3.0	30	630	0
seasoned (*Williams Black Angus*) . . .	90	15.0	0	3.0	50	250	0
teriyaki, eye round (*Dietz & Watson*)	70	12.0	0	2.0	30	390	0
top round (*Boar's Head* Low Sodium)	80	15.0	<1.0	2.5	30	80	0
whole muscle (*Healthy Choice*), 2 slices, 1.6 oz. . .	50	8.0	1.0	1.0	20	450	0
Beef pie, see "Beef entree, frozen"							
Beef pocket/sandwich, frozen, 1 pc., 4.5 oz., except as noted:							
barbecue sauce w/ (*Lean Pockets*)	290	11.0	47.0	7.0	20	850	3.0

Food and Measure	cal.	prot. (gms)	carbo. (gms)	fat (gms)	chol. (mgs)	sod. (mgs)	fiber (gms)
Beef pocket/sandwich *(cont.)*							
cheeseburger:							
(*Lean Pockets*)	280	12.0	42.0	7.0	20	810	3.0
(*White Castle*),							
2 pcs., 3.7 oz. ..	310	15.0	23.0	17.0	30	480	6.0
hamburger (*White Castle*), 2 pcs.	270	12.0	23.0	14.0	20	270	5.0
Philly cheese steak:							
(*Croissant Pockets*)	360	13.0	33.0	19.0	25	810	3.0
(*Lean Pockets*)	280	13.0	40.0	7.0	25	590	3.0
sub (*Michelina's Hot Subs*), 2.1 oz.	300	14.0	36.0	12.0	20	860	1.0
steak fajita (*Lean Pockets*)	260	11.0	39.0	7.0	25	730	3.0
Beef potato puffs, frozen (*Goya*), 1 pc.	140	6.0	18.0	5.0	10	400	3.0
Beef sausage, see "Sausage" and specific listings							
Beef seasoning, and pork (*Lawry's* Perfect Blend), ¼ tsp. ..	0	0	0	0	0	200	0
Beef seasoning mix (see also specific listings):							
pot roast (*McCormick Bag 'n Season*), 1 tsp.	10	0	1.0	0	0	390	0
stew:							
(*Adolph's Meal Makers*), 1 tsp...	10	0	3.0	0	0	700	0
(*Lawry's*), 1 tsp.	10	0	2.0	0	0	500	0
(*McCormick*), 2 tsp.	15	0	2.0	0	0	410	0
(*McCormick Bag 'n Season*), 1 tsp...	15	1.0	1.0	0	0	670	0
Stroganoff:							
(*Lawry's*), 1 tbsp...	20	0	5.0	0	0	520	0
(*McCormick*), 2 tsp.	15	0	3.0	0	0	350	0
Swiss steak (*McCormick Bag 'n Season*), 1 tsp.	15	0	2.0	0	0	460	0
Beef stew, see "Beef entree"							

Food and Measure	cal.	prot. (gms)	carbo. (gms)	fat (gms)	chol. (mgs)	sod. (mgs)	fiber (gms)
Beef-tomato drink, see "Tomato-beef drink"							
Beefalo, meat only, roasted, 4 oz.	213	34.8	0	7.2	66	93	0
Beefsteak leaf, pickled, see "Shiso leaf powder"							
Beer, 12 fl. oz.:							
regular	146	.9	13.2	0	0	19	0
light	100	.7	4.8	0	0	10	0
Beerwurst, pork and beef, 2 oz.	155	7.8	2.4	12.6	35	410	.5
Beet, fresh:							
raw:							
(*Frieda's*), ½ cup, 3 oz.	35	1.0	8.0	0	0	65	2.0
2 medium, 2" diam.	70	2.6	15.6	.3	0	126	4.6
trimmed, sliced, ½ cup	29	1.1	6.5	.1	0	53	1.9
boiled, drained:							
2 medium, 2" diam.	44	1.7	10.0	.2	0	77	1.7
sliced, ½ cup	38	1.4	8.5	.2	0	65	1.4
Beet, canned, ½ cup, except as noted:							
whole:							
(*Freshlike* Small), 3 pcs., 4.4 oz. . .	40	1.0	9.0	0	0	240	2.0
whole or sliced:							
(*S&W*)	35	1.0	8.0	0	0	290	2.0
w/liquid	36	1.0	8.3	.1	0	324	1.4
sliced:							
(*Del Monte*)	35	1.0	8.0	0	0	290	2.0
(*Freshlike* Small) . .	35	1.0	9.0	0	0	230	2.0
(*Veg-All*)	40	<1.0	8.0	0	0	300	1.0
Harvard:							
(*Greenwood* Sweet & Tangy)	100	1.0	27.0	0	0	370	1.0
w/liquid	89	1.0	22.4	.1	0	199	1.0
pickled:							
(*S&W*), 1 oz.	15	0	4.0	0	0	50	1.0
whole or sliced (*Greenwood*), 1 oz.	25	0	6.0	0	0	100	0
sliced (*Del Monte*) .	80	1.0	19.0	0	0	380	2.0

Food and Measure	cal.	prot. (gms)	carbo. (gms)	fat (gms)	chol. (mgs)	sod. (mgs)	fiber (gms)
Beet, canned, pickled *(cont.)*							
sliced (*Freshlike* Selects), 4 pcs.,							
1 oz.	20	0	4.0	0	0	20	0
w/liquid	74	.9	18.5	.1	0	300	3.0
Beet greens, ½ cup:							
raw, 1" pcs.	4	.4	.8	<.1	0	38	.7
boiled, drained, 1" pcs.	20	1.9	3.9	.1	0	173	2.1
Berliner, pork and							
beef, 1 oz.	65	4.3	.7	4.9	13	368	0
Berries, mixed, frozen:							
(*Cascadian Farm* Harvest), 1 cup . . .	70	1.0	16.0	0	0	0	4.0
(*C&W* Medley), 1 cup	60	0	14.0	0	0	5	2.0
(*Tree of Life*), ¾ cup .	60	0	16.0	0	0	0	3.0
Berry drink blend, 8 fl. oz., except as noted:							
(*Bolthouse Farms* Berry Boost Smoothie)	110	1.0	30.0	0	0	0	4.0
(*Minute Maid Coolers*), 6.75-fl.-oz. pouch .	100	0	26.0	0	0	15	0
(*Sobe Black & Blue*) .	120	0	31.0	0	0	24	0
(*V8 Splash*)	110	0	27.0	0	0	35	0
(*V8 Splash* Smoothies Wild Berry Creme) .	130	3.0	30.0	0	0	70	0
kiwi:							
(*Minute Maid*)	110	0	29.0	0	0	75	0
(*Minute Maid*), 12-fl.-oz. bottle .	160	0	43.0	0	0	110	0
punch:							
(*Minute Maid*)	120	0	32.0	0	0	15	0
(*Nantucket Nectars* Maine)	110	0	27.0	0	0	30	0
frozen* (*Minute Maid*)	110	0	30.0	0	0	0	0
Berry juice, 8 fl. oz.:							
(*After the Fall* Oregon)	130	0	32.0	0	0	15	0
(*Juicy Juice*)	120	0	30.0	0	0	20	0
(*L&A*)	120	0	30.0	0	0	15	0
(*Langers*)	120	0	30.0	0	0	15	0
nectar (*Santa Cruz Organic*)	110	<1.0	30.0	0	0	25	0

Food and Measure	cal.	prot. (gms)	carbo. (gms)	fat (gms)	chol. (mgs)	sod. (mgs)	fiber (gms)
Biryani paste, see "Curry paste"							
Biscuit, plain or buttermilk, 2-oz. pc.	206	3.5	27.5	9.4	<1	596	.7
Biscuit, frozen or refrigerated, 1 pc., except as noted:							
(*Grands!* Extra Rich)	210	4.0	26.0	10.0	0	580	<1.0
(*Grands!* Original Homestyle)	190	4.0	24.0	8.0	0	590	<1.0
(*Grands! Butter Tastin'*)	190	4.0	24.0	9.0	0	590	<1.0
(*Pillsbury Butter Tastin' Golden Homestyle*)	100	2.0	14.0	4.0	0	360	0
(*Pillsbury Butter Tastin' Golden Layers*)	110	2.0	14.0	4.5	0	360	0
(*Pillsbury Butter Tastin' Microwave*)	200	4.0	24.0	10.0	0	590	<1.0
(*Pillsbury Butter Tastin' Oven Baked*)	180	4.0	22.0	9.0	0	570	<1.0
(*Pillsbury Country*)	150	4.0	29.0	2.0	0	570	<1.0
(*Pillsbury Easy Split Oven Baked Extra Large*)	280	6.0	34.0	13.0	0	870	1.0
buttermilk:							
(*Grands!*)	190	4.0	24.0	8.0	0	600	<1.0
(*Grands!* Flaky Layers)	190	4.0	23.0	9.0	0	550	<1.0
(*Grands!* Reduced Fat)	170	4.0	25.0	6.0	0	590	<1.0
(*Perfect Portions*)	200	4.0	25.0	10.0	0	520	<1.0
(*Pillsbury*)	150	4.0	29.0	2.0	0	570	<1.0
(*Pillsbury* Microwave)	200	4.0	24.0	10.0	0	610	<1.0
(*Pillsbury* Oven Baked)	180	4.0	22.0	9.0	0	580	<1.0
(*Pillsbury Golden Homestyle*)	100	2.0	14.0	4.0	0	360	0
(*Pillsbury Golden Layers*)	110	2.0	14.0	4.5	0	360	0
(*Pillsbury 1869*)	100	2.0	12.0	5.0	0	320	0
(*Rhodes*)	200	3.0	25.0	10.0	0	490	<1.0
cheddar garlic (*Pillsbury* Oven Baked)	190	5.0	20.0	10.0	10	700	<1.0

Food and Measure	cal.	prot. (gms)	carbo. (gms)	fat (gms)	chol. (mgs)	sod. (mgs)	fiber (gms)
Biscuit, frozen or refrigerated *(cont.)*							
cinnamon sugar (*Pillsbury Golden Layers*)	110	2.0	16.0	4.0	0	260	<1.0
corn, golden (*Grands!*)	190	4.0	28.0	7.0	0	620	<1.0
flaky:							
(*Grands!* Original/ Butter Tastin'*) ..	190	4.0	23.0	9.0	0	550	<1.0
(*Grands!* Original Reduced Fat) ...	170	4.0	25.0	6.0	0	590	<1.0
(*Pillsbury* Layers), 3 pcs.	160	4.0	28.0	4.0	0	550	1.0
(*Pillsbury* Oven Baked)	170	4.0	20.0	8.0	0	530	0
(*Pillsbury Golden Layers*)	110	2.0	14.0	4.5	0	360	0
honey butter (*Pillsbury Golden Layers*)	110	2.0	14.0	5.0	0	280	0
Southern style:							
(*Grands!*)	190	4.0	24.0	9.0	0	590	<1.0
(*Pillsbury* Oven Baked)	180	4.0	22.0	9.0	0	570	<1.0
wheat (*Grands!* Reduced Fat)	180	4.0	27.0	7.0	0	590	2.0
Biscuit mix (see also "Baking mix"), ⅓ cup mix, except as noted:							
(*Kentucky Kernel*) ¼ cup	171	3.0	28.0	5.0	0	659	1.0
buttermilk:							
(*Bisquick* Complete)	150	2.0	21.0	6.0	0	370	0
(*"Jiffy"*)	160	3.0	29.0	4.0	<5	380	<1.0
cheese, three (*Bisquick* Complete)	160	3.0	21.0	7.0	0	400	0
cheese garlic (*Bisquick* Complete)	160	2.0	22.0	7.0	0	350	0
cinnamon swirl (*Bisquick* Complete)	150	2.0	26.0	4.0	0	330	0
honey butter (*Bisquick* Complete)	160	2.0	24.0	6.0	0	310	0
Bison, meat only, 4 oz.:							
roasted	162	32.3	0	2.7	93	65	0
ground, pan-broiled ..	270	27.0	0	17.2	94	83	0

Food and Measure	cal.	prot. (gms)	carbo. (gms)	fat (gms)	chol. (mgs)	sod. (mgs)	fiber (gms)
Bitter melon, see "Balsam pear"							
Bitters:							
(*Angostura*), 2 tbsp...	50	0	14.0	0	0	390	0
aromatic (*Angostura*), ½ tsp.	12	0	2.0	0	0	<1	0
Black bean, dried:							
dry (*Goya*), ¼ cup ...	70	9.0	23.0	0	0	20	15.0
boiled, ½ cup	113	7.6	20.4	.5	0	1	7.5
turtle, dry, ¼ cup:							
(*Arrowhead Mills*) .	140	9.0	27.0	0	0	0	10.0
(*Shiloh Farms*)	150	10.0	28.0	.5	0	10	9.0
turtle, boiled, ½ cup .	120	7.5	22.4	.3	0	3	4.9
Black bean, canned (see also "Refried beans"), ½ cup:							
(*Allens*)	100	6.0	19.0	.5	0	400	8.0
(*Bush's*)	100	7.0	20.0	.5	0	460	7.0
(*Eden* Organic)	100	7.0	18.0	0	0	15	6.0
(*Progresso*)	110	7.0	17.0	1.0	0	400	7.0
(*S&W*)	70	5.0	17.0	0	0	480	6.0
(*S&W* 50% Less Salt)	70	5.0	17.0	0	0	240	6.0
(*Westbrae Natural* Organic)	100	6.0	19.0	0	0	140	5.0
(*Zapata*)	110	7.0	19.0	1.0	0	100	7.0
Caribbean:							
(*Eden* Organic)	90	7.0	20.0	.5	0	135	7.0
(*S&W*)	90	6.0	23.0	0	0	540	7.0
w/rice (*Glory*)	90	4.0	16.0	1.5	0	450	2.0
seasoned (*Trappey's*) .	120	7.0	20.0	1.5	0	410	7.0
Black bean, mix, instant (*Fantastic*), ⅓ cup	160	10.0	29.0	1.5	0	310	7.0
Black bean dish, frozen, seasoned, and rice (*Glory* Savory Accents), ½ cup	90	3.0	16.0	1.0	0	440	2.0
Black bean entree, frozen, and sausage (*Glory* Savory Singles), 11-oz. pkg.	400	15.0	41.0	18.0	30	1420	8.0
Black bean sauce, see "Bean sauce"							

Food and Measure	cal.	prot. (gms)	carbo. (gms)	fat (gms)	chol. (mgs)	sod. (mgs)	fiber (gms)
Blackberry, fresh, ½ cup	37	.5	9.2	.3	0	tr.	3.6
Blackberry, canned, in syrup, ½ cup	118	1.7	29.6	.2	0	3	4.4
Blackberry, dried (*Frieda's* Marion-berry), ⅓ cup, 1.4 oz.	98	0	32.0	.5	0	0	2.0
Blackberry, frozen: (*Cascadian Farm*), 1 cup	90	2.0	22.0	.5	0	0	7.0
unsweetened, ½ cup .	49	.9	11.8	.3	0	1	3.8
Blackberry syrup (*Smucker's*), ¼ cup	210	0	52.0	0	0	0	0
Black-eyed peas (see also "Cowpeas"): fresh (*Frieda's*), ⅓ cup, 3 oz.	130	8.0	21.0	1.0	0	250	11.0
dry (*Shiloh Farms*), ¼ cup	90	9.0	23.0	0	0	15	10.0
mature, boiled, ½ cup	100	6.7	17.9	.5	0	3	5.6
Black-eyed peas, canned, ½ cup: (*Allens* Dry)	110	7.0	18.0	1.0	0	275	4.0
(*Allens/East Texas Fair*)	120	7.0	21.0	1.0	0	350	6.0
(*Bush's*)	100	5.0	19.0	0	0	410	4.0
(*Eden* Organic)	90	6.0	16.0	1.0	0	25	4.0
w/bacon: (*Allens*)	120	7.0	20.0	1.5	0	390	5.0
(*Trappey's*)	120	7.0	19.0	2.0	0	470	5.0
or bacon/jalapeño (*Bush's*)	110	6.0	18.0	1.0	5	630	5.0
w/bacon/pork: (*Sunshine*)	120	7.0	20.0	1.5	0	390	5.0
(*Trappey's*)	110	6.0	19.0	2.0	0	470	5.0
w/rice (*Glory*)	90	5.0	17.0	.5	0	680	3.0
seasoned (*Glory* Southern)	140	10.0	25.0	.5	0	420	5.0
w/snaps: (*Allens/East Texas Fair*)	120	8.0	20.0	1.0	0	420	5.0
(*Bush's*)	110	7.0	17.0	.5	0	550	5.0
Black-eyed peas, frozen, ½ cup: (*McKenzie's*)	110	7.0	21.0	.5	0	10	4.0

Food and Measure	cal.	prot. (gms)	carbo. (gms)	fat (gms)	chol. (mgs)	sod. (mgs)	fiber (gms)
boiled, drained	112	7.2	20.2	.6	0	5	4.3
seasoned, and rice (*Glory* Savory Accents)	80	4.0	17.0	.5	0	360	3.0
Blackened seasoning (*Old Bay*), ½ tsp. . .	0	0	0	0	0	95	0
Blimpie, 1 serving:							
café sandwiches, 6":							
Cable Car Club	350	26.0	36.0	9.0	65	1320	2.0
Fisherman's Wharf tuna melt	350	30.0	35.0	11.0	65	1300	3.0
Golden Gate Gourmet	400	30.0	40.0	14.0	65	1470	2.0
Union Square Veggie	330	12.0	39.0	15.0	20	710	2.0
cold subs, 6":							
Blimpie Best	460	30.0	52.0	16.0	69	1690	3.3
Buffalo chicken . . .	400	32.0	50.0	8.0	60	2110	3.0
club	440	27.5	50.5	12.0	66	1437	3.3
ham and cheese . . .	436	28.0	51.5	12.5	59	1302	3.3
roast beef	468	37.0	49.0	13.5	71	1384	3.3
seafood	355	14.0	58.0	7.7	19	895	3.8
tuna	493	24.0	50.5	23.0	50	876	3.3
turkey	424	24.5	49.0	11.0	62	1597	3.3
grilled subs, 6":							
beef/turkey/cheddar	600	28.0	49.0	31.0	69	1836	2.7
Cuban	462	30.0	50.4	12.0	67	1526	2.7
pastrami special . . .	462	32.3	52.0	14.0	44	1438	3.3
Reuben	630	31.0	55.0	33.0	46	1914	2.4
ultimate club	724	33.0	51.0	42.0	81	1933	2.7
hot subs, 6":							
BLT	588	28.0	49.0	32.0	41	1596	3.3
chicken, Buffalo . . .	400	32.0	50.0	13.4	61	2108	2.7
chicken, grilled	373	29.0	50.0	9.0	35	836	3.3
ChikMax	511	29.0	71.0	13.2	0	1287	8.0
meatball	572	28.0	55.0	27.0	58	1145	1.7
pastrami	507	36.0	53.0	17.0	74	1658	3.3
steak/onion melt . .	440	29.0	49.0	15.5	68	1056	3.0
MexiMax	425	23.0	65.0	9.0	0	1012	7.3
VegiMax	395	24.0	60.0	7.0	0	982	8.3
wraps:							
BLT, ultimate	831	34.0	60.0	50.0	78	2677	3.0
chicken Caesar	646	25.0	56.0	35.0	45	1635	3.0
beef/cheddar	714	34.0	57.0	37.0	78	2183	3.0

Food and Measure	cal.	prot. (gms)	carbo. (gms)	fat (gms)	chol. (mgs)	sod. (mgs)	fiber (gms)
***Blimpie*, wraps** *(cont.)*							
Italian, zesty	638	26.0	74.0	33.0	62	2374	3.0
Southwestern	674	26.0	54.0	35.0	56	2504	3.0
steak/onion	716	30.0	64.0	37.0	78	1716	3.0
breads:							
ciabatta	230	8.0	43.0	2.5	0	620	2.0
regular, 6":							
honey oat	298	10.0	49.0	7.4	0	464	4.2
Parmesan, zesty .	267	11.0	44.0	5.4	0	552	1.8
rye, marbled	297	12.0	55.0	3.0	0	699	3.4
white	238	8.6	43.0	3.4	0	481	1.7
white, poppy . . .	245	9.0	44.0	4.0	0	481	1.8
white, sesame . .	252	9.0	43.0	4.7	0	482	1.9
wheat	297	12.0	55.0	3.0	0	699	3.4
wheat, poppy . . .	240	9.0	42.0	4.2	0	464	3.8
wheat, sesame . .	247	9.6	41.0	5.0	0	465	3.9
wrap, traditional . . .	320	8.0	51.0	8.0	0	820	2.0
wrap, spinach/herb	310	8.0	49.0	8.0	0	780	2.0
dressing/toppings:							
cheese, 1 slice:							
cheddar	52	3.0	0	4.5	10	250	0
provolone	80	6.0	0	6.0	20	200	0
Swiss	80	7.0	0	6.0	20	46	0
dressing, 1.5 oz.:							
Blimpie	180	2.0	24.0	12.0	0	860	0
blue cheese	230	2.0	2.0	24.0	25	440	0
Caesar	210	1.0	2.0	22.0	10	500	0
Dijon honey	200	1.0	8.0	18.0	20	250	0
Italian, fat free . .	25	0	5.0	0	0	380	0
Italian, light	20	0	2.0	1.0	0	760	0
Parmesan							
peppercorn . . .	240	1.0	2.0	25.0	15	390	0
ranch, light	70	1.0	8.0	4.0	0	360	0
Thousand Island	320	0	11.0	32.0	40	540	0
guacamole	194	1.8	7.4	17.5	<1	468	1.4
oil/vinegar for 6" sub	36	0	.5	4.0	0	0	0
pesto, 1 oz.	130	0	1.0	13.0	0	240	0
sides, 5 oz.:							
coleslaw	180	1.0	13.0	13.0	<5	230	1.0
macaroni salad	360	4.0	25.0	25.0	10	660	1.0
potato salad	270	2.0	19.0	19.0	10	560	1.0
potato salad,							
mustard	160	2.0	21.0	5.0	5	660	1.0

Food and Measure	cal.	prot. (gms)	carbo. (gms)	fat (gms)	chol. (mgs)	sod. (mgs)	fiber (gms)
soup, 8 oz.:							
broccoli cheese . . .	190	6.0	15.0	12.0	15	940	3.0
chicken noodle	120	7.0	18.0	2.5	20	850	1.0
chicken rice	230	10.0	21.0	12.0	30	1210	2.0
chili grande	250	18.0	30.0	7.0	40	1230	18.0
potato, cream of . .	190	5.0	24.0	9.0	<5	860	3.0
tomato basil ravioli	110	4.0	22.0	1.0	10	720	<1.0
vegetable, garden . .	80	5.0	14.0	.5	0	620	3.0
vegetable beef	80	4.0	13.0	1.5	5	1010	2.0
salad, regular:							
antipasto	244	23.0	10.0	12.6	69	1217	2.7
chef	212	20.0	9.0	9.0	66	961	3.0
Chili Olé	480	21.0	42.0	27.0	45	1240	3.0
grilled chicken, Caesar dressing .	347	18.0	8.6	27.2	45	862	2.6
Roast Beef 'n Bleu .	390	31.0	29.0	16.0	70	1550	0
seafood	122	6.0	16.0	4.4	19	418	3.2
tuna	261	16.0	8.0	19.5	50	398	2.7
turkey, Zesto Pesto	370	20.0	31.0	19.0	40	1410	0
Blintz, frozen, 2.2-oz. pc., except as noted:							
apple:							
(A&B Famous), 2.5-oz. pc.	181	3.5	28.0	4.1	8	116	1.0
raisin (Empire)	80	3.0	16.0	2.0	10	150	1.0
cheese:							
(A&B Famous), 3-oz. pc.	189	6.2	30.8	4.5	20	92	1.0
(Empire)	80	6.0	13.0	2.0	15	135	2.0
(Golden)	80	6.0	13.0	2.0	15	135	2.0
(Kineret)	65	2.0	12.0	1.0	0	120	0
potato:							
(A&B Famous), 2.5-oz. pc.	117	3.8	12.9	5.6	21	275	0
(Empire)	90	3.0	15.0	4.0	5	170	2.0
(Kineret)	70	2.0	12.0	2.0	0	110	0
Blintz, nondairy, frozen, "cheese," 1 pc.:							
(Tofutti Mintz's Blintzes)	90	3.0	15.0	4.0	0	170	0
w/apple, blueberry, or cherry (Tofutti Pillows)	70	2.0	16.0	5.0	0	290	0

Food and Measure	cal.	prot. (gms)	carbo. (gms)	fat (gms)	chol. (mgs)	sod. (mgs)	fiber (gms)
Blood sausage, 1 oz.	107	4.1	.4	9.8	34	n.a.	0
Bloody Mary drink mixer:							
(*Angostura*), 8 fl. oz. . .	80	3.0	15.0	1.0	0	940	0
(*Mr & Mrs T*), 11.5-fl.-oz. can	60	2.0	13.0	.5	0	2070	0
(*Pace*), 8 fl. oz.	50	2.0	10.0	0	0	970	2.0
(*Sacramento*), 8 fl. oz.	60	2.0	13.0	0	0	940	3.0
spicy:							
(*D.L. Jardine's* Red Snapper), 3 fl. oz.	90	1.0	5.0	0	0	680	0
(*Pain Is Good* Original/Cajun/ Jamaican), 1 fl. oz.	5	0	1.0	0	0	182	0
Bloody Mary season- ing (*Angostura*), 1 tsp.	0	0	0	0	0	300	0
Blue squash, see "Australian blue squash"							
Blueberry, fresh, ½ cup	41	.5	10.2	.3	0	5	2.0
Blueberry, canned, in heavy syrup:							
(*S&W*), ⅓ cup	70	0	16.0	0	0	0	6.0
½ cup	113	.8	28.2	.4	0	4	1.9
Blueberry, dried, ¼ cup, 1.4 oz., except as noted:							
(*Frieda's*)	140	1.0	33.0	0	0	0	4.0
wild (*Hodgson Mill*) . .	120	1.0	32.0	1.0	0	0	6.0
wild (*Shiloh Farms*), ⅓ cup	160	0	38.0	.5	0	0	2.0
Blueberry, freeze- dried (*AlpineAire*), .5 oz.	60	0	12.0	1.0	0	0	0
Blueberry, frozen:							
(*Cascadian Farm*), 1 cup	70	1.0	22.0	1.0	0	10	4.0
(*C&W*), ¾ cup	70	0	17.0	0	0	0	4.0
(*Tree of Life*), 1 cup . .	80	0	20.0	0	0	0	2.0
unsweetened, ½ cup .	40	.3	9.4	.5	0	1	2.1
sweetened, ½ cup . . .	94	.5	25.2	.2	0	2	2.4

Food and Measure	cal.	prot. (gms)	carbo. (gms)	fat (gms)	chol. (mgs)	sod. (mgs)	fiber (gms)
Blueberry glaze (*Litehouse*), 3 tbsp.	70	0	18.0	0	0	25	0
Blueberry juice, 8 fl. oz.:							
(*After the Fall* Maine Coast)	120	0	31.0	0	0	15	0
(*R.W. Knudsen* Just Blueberry)	100	0	24.0	0	0	10	0
(*Walnut Acres*)	130	0	31.0	0	0	15	<1.0
Blueberry juice concentrate (*Tree of Life*), 8 tsp.	120	0	31.0	0	0	10	0
Blueberry nectar, 8 fl. oz.:							
(*R.W. Knudsen*)	130	0	30.0	0	0	15	0
banana (*Nantucket Nectars*)	110	0	28.0	0	0	30	1.0
Blueberry syrup (*Smucker's*), ¼ cup	210	0	52.0	0	0	0	0
Blueberry-chickpea spread (*Cedar's* Mediterranean), 2 tbsp.	50	2.0	11.0	0	0	5	2.0
Blueberry-cranberry drink (*Langers*), 8 fl. oz.	135	0	34.0	0	0	10	0
Bluefish, meat only:							
raw, 4 oz.	141	22.7	0	4.8	67	68	0
baked, broiled, or microwaved, 4 oz. .	180	29.1	0	6.2	86	87	0
Boar, wild, meat only, roasted, 4 oz.	181	32.1	0	5.0	87	68	0
Bob Evans, 1 serving:							
breakfast combos:							
country biscuit	852	30.0	71.0	49.0	261	2455	4.0
eggs Benedict	418	25.0	35.0	20.0	442	1008	2.0
fruit yogurt plate ..	414	9.0	96.0	2.0	5	106	8.0
pot roast hash ..	752	45.0	37.0	46.0	529	1261	4.0
sausage, light	469	34.0	48.0	21.0	22	977	4.0
sausage gravy, bowl	403	14.0	26.0	27.0	34	1673	0
sausage gravy, cup	217	7.0	14.0	15.0	18	901	0
sunshine skillet ...	780	33.0	35.0	56.0	530	1781	4.0
breakfast omelette:							
regular, plain	285	14.0	1.0	24.0	482	142	0

Food and Measure	cal.	prot. (gms)	carbo. (gms)	fat (gms)	chol. (mgs)	sod. (mgs)	fiber (gms)
Bob Evans, breakfast omelette *(cont.)*							
cheese	477	25.0	3.0	40.0	530	428	1.0
farmer's market .	642	32.0	11.0	50.0	556	1991	1.0
ham/cheese	505	34.0	2.0	39.0	546	1278	0
sausage/cheese .	679	37.0	2.0	57.0	554	1030	0
Southwest chicken	674	45.0	5.0	51.0	590	1669	1.0
Western	522	35.0	6.0	39.0	546	1279	1.0
Egg Beaters, plain .	149	19.0	2.0	12.0	3	423	0
cheese	328	30.0	4.0	26.0	51	709	1.0
farmer's market .	493	37.0	12.0	36.0	78	2273	1.0
ham/cheese	356	39.0	3.0	25.0	67	1560	1.0
sausage/cheese .	530	42.0	3.0	43.0	76	1312	1.0
Southwest chicken	551	50.0	5.0	40.0	111	1839	2.0
Western	399	40.0	7.0	28.0	67	1449	2.0
breakfast items:							
bacon, 1 pc.	36	1.0	0	4.0	5	54	0
bacon, Canadian, 1 pc.	21	4.0	0	1.0	9	261	0
egg, hard-boiled, 1 .	60	6.0	1.0	4.0	190	55	0
eggs, scrambled . .	170	14.0	1.0	11.0	482	142	0
French toast, stuffed, 9.9 oz. . . .	566	11.0	55.0	15.0	84	659	3.0
French toast, stuffed, 6.6 oz. . . .	397	7.0	38.0	12.0	54	419	2.0
fruit cup	164	2.0	42.0	1.0	0	11	4.0
grits	187	3.0	29.0	7.0	0	186	2.0
ham, smoked, 1 pc.	66	11.0	2.0	2.0	40	857	0
home fries	193	4.0	28.0	7.0	0	577	4.0
hotcake, 1 pc.:							
blueberry	187	4.0	32.0	5.0	9	369	2.0
buttermilk	171	3.0	28.0	5.0	9	367	1.0
cinnamon	271	3.0	41.0	10.0	9	369	1.0
multigrain	208	5.0	34.0	6.0	10	505	2.0
mush, 1 slice	65	1.0	14.0	0	0	196	0
oatmeal, bowl	185	7.0	34.0	3.0	0	301	5.0
sausage, 1 link	125	5.0	0	11.0	14	184	0
sausage, lite, 1 link	100	10.0	0	7.0	19	278	0
sausage patty, 1 pc.	117	8.0	0	9.0	22	270	0
sirloin steak	423	35.0	3.0	29.0	82	680	0
strawberry yogurt .	145	6.0	28.0	1.0	5	85	1.0
waffle, Belgian, 1 pc.	342	7.0	57.0	10.0	18	735	2.0

Food and Measure	cal.	prot. (gms)	carbo. (gms)	fat (gms)	chol. (mgs)	sod. (mgs)	fiber (gms)
burgers/sandwiches:							
bacon cheeseburger	778	40.0	31.0	54.0	122	1014	1.0
big BLT	420	10.0	30.0	29.0	30	687	2.0
BLT, plain	242	7.0	26.0	13.0	15	428	2.0
Bob's BLT	751	23.0	48.0	51.0	279	1266	0
cheese, grilled	392	9.0	25.0	17.0	30	782	2.0
cheeseburger, plain	707	39.0	31.0	47.0	112	905	1.0
chicken:							
fried, club	659	42.0	40.0	36.0	110	1507	2.0
fried, plain	508	36.0	39.0	23.0	77	1032	2.0
grilled, club	594	46.0	31.0	31.0	122	1422	2.0
grilled, plain	442	41.0	30.0	17.0	90	947	2.0
chicken salad, plain	643	21.0	55.0	38.0	62	1273	3.0
haddock	520	21.0	65.0	19.0	32	889	0
hamburger, plain . .	605	34.0	30.0	38.0	82	429	1.0
pot roast	655	34.0	62.0	31.0	98	1455	1.0
turkey bacon melt .	596	40.0	56.0	24.0	120	1218	3.0
lunch savors:							
pulled pork							
sandwich	464	24.0	54.0	18.0	59	579	3.0
steak tips/noodles .	581	39.0	48.0	26.0	135	1802	3.0
stir-fry chicken	497	31.0	55.0	18.0	66	1295	5.0
stir-fry vegetable . .	278	7.0	55.0	4.0	0	855	4.0
lunch savors salad:							
Cobb, grilled							
chicken	574	48.0	9.0	39.0	319	1321	3.0
Frisco:							
fried chicken . . .	496	29.0	26.0	31.0	77	1243	4.0
grilled chicken . .	461	39.0	9.0	31.0	115	1040	3.0
spinach, country . .	545	42.0	11.0	38.0	282	1106	4.0
Wildfire:							
fried chicken . . .	646	26.0	74.0	29.0	52	1184	8.0
grilled chicken . .	610	35.0	57.0	29.0	89	981	8.0
salads, farm-fresh:							
chicken salad	781	23.0	77.0	46.0	87	1132	12.0
Cobb, grilled							
chicken	753	64.0	15.0	50.0	360	1708	6.0
Frisco salad:							
fried chicken . . .	648	38.0	40.0	38.0	91	1577	6.0
grilled chicken . .	595	52.0	1.0	38.0	148	1272	6.0
side, garden	152	6.0	26.0	4.0	0	396	2.0
side, garden, no							
croutons	23	1.0	5.0	2.0	0	10	2.0
side, specialty	174	9.0	16.0	9.0	22	449	2.0

Food and Measure	cal.	prot. (gms)	carbo. (gms)	fat (gms)	chol. (mgs)	sod. (mgs)	fiber (gms)
Bob Evans, salads, farm-fresh *(cont.)*							
side, specialty, no							
croutons	113	7.0	5.0	7.0	22	267	2.0
spinach, country . .	624	55.0	13.0	40.0	314	1350	5.0
Wildfire:							
fried chicken . . .	798	35.0	88.0	36.0	66	1518	11.0
grilled chicken . .	745	49.0	68.0	36.0	122	1213	10.0
salad dressing, 3 oz.[1]:							
bleu cheese	440	3.0	6.0	47.0	44	675	0
colonial	464	0	23.0	41.0	0	387	0
French	439	0	19.0	41.0	27	494	0
honey mustard	384	0	16.0	36.0	41	494	0
hot bacon	213	0	35.0	6.0	7	378	0
Italian, light	165	0	8.0	14.0	0	1180	0
ranch	312	3.0	3.0	31.0	28	624	0
ranch, lite	206	2.0	5.0	20.0	22	754	0
Thousand Island . .	425	0	14.0	40.0	28	709	0
vinegar and oil	51	0	0	6.0	0	1	0
Wildfire ranch	241	1.0	18.0	19.0	15	614	0
soup, hearty:							
bean, bowl	176	11.0	23.0	5.0	14	1268	7.0
bean, cup	125	8.0	16.0	3.0	10	902	5.0
cheddar potato,							
bowl	387	17.0	31.0	22.0	62	1515	2.0
cheddar potato, cup	307	14.0	25.0	18.0	49	1200	1.0
sausage chili, bowl	376	22.0	26.0	24.0	59	962	10.0
sausage chili, cup .	268	16.0	19.0	17.0	42	687	7.0
vegetable beef, bowl	219	11.0	23.0	9.0	29	962	4.0
vegetable beef, cup	127	7.0	13.0	5.0	17	556	2.0
dinner:							
catfish, grilled, 1 pc.	270	22.0	4.0	19.0	58	896	4.0
chicken, fried	291	31.0	9.0	15.0	77	666	1.0
chicken, grilled	214	33.0	0	9.0	84	544	0
w/barbecue sauce	392	34.0	27.0	16.0	84	813	2.0
w/garlic butter . .	373	34.0	15.0	20.0	85	949	2.0
chicken-n-noodles .	407	20.0	32.0	22.0	115	659	2.0
chicken pot pie	758	32.0	46.0	49.0	209	1754	2.0
chicken strip, 1 pc.	127	7.0	9.0	7.0	14	321	0
chicken tender, 1 pc.	101	10.0	0	7.0	28	191	0
cod, lemon pepper,							
1 pc.	271	17.0	15.0	16.0	56	598	0
meat loaf	630	42.0	14.0	44.0	157	1081	1.0

1. *Dinner portion; divide by 2 for the 1.5-oz. side portion.*

Food and Measure	cal.	prot. (gms)	carbo. (gms)	fat (gms)	chol. (mgs)	sod. (mgs)	fiber (gms)
noodles, buttered ..	287	7.0	35.0	13.0	47	120	2.0
pork chop	477	48.0	2.0	28.0	129	829	0
w/barbecue sauce	654	49.0	29.0	35.0	129	1099	2.0
w/garlic butter ..	635	50.0	16.0	39.0	130	1234	2.0
roast beef, open face	453	33.0	24.0	25.0	104	1042	1.0
salmon, plain	376	27.0	12.0	23.0	74	232	1.0
shrimp, fried, plain .	330	32.0	8.0	20.0	284	1499	0
spaghetti, marinara	619	34.0	104.0	7.0	15	1128	10.0
spaghetti, meatballs	1087	54.0	116.0	45.0	107	1965	13.0
seniors	617	31.0	59.0	29.0	69	1166	7.0
steak, country fried	481	20.0	26.0	33.0	60	1217	0
w/gravy	535	20.0	31.0	37.0	60	1763	0
steak Monterey ...	600	44.0	7.0	41.0	126	1671	1.0
steak tips/noodles .	1027	77.0	94.0	39.0	268	3230	7.0
seniors	573	38.0	47.0	26.0	135	1733	3.0
stir-fry chicken	727	41.0	84.0	27.0	85	1962	6.0
seniors	480	28.0	55.0	18.0	57	1236	5.0
stir-fry vegetables .	502	15.0	99.0	7.0	5	1416	12.0
strip steak	677	50.0	12.0	50.0	128	1140	1.0
w/garlic butter ..	771	50.0	15.0	59.0	129	1375	2.0
turkey and dressing	549	37.0	41.0	25.0	126	1407	4.0
side items:							
applesauce	101	0	26.0	0	0	17	2.0
baked potato, plain	207	8.0	54.0	0	0	16	6.0
loaded	433	22.0	57.0	18.0	54	612	7.0
bread dressing	362	6.0	36.0	20.0	0	1013	0
broccoli florets	44	5.0	8.0	1.0	0	41	5.0
cheddar	162	10.0	14.0	9.0	20	367	5.0
carrots, glazed	137	1.0	21.0	6.0	7	125	4.0
coleslaw	198	1.0	18.0	13.0	12	229	2.0
corn, buttered	156	3.0	18.0	9.0	12	229	2.0
cottage cheese	122	15.0	4.0	5.0	37	436	0
french fries	217	3.0	35.0	7.0	0	300	3.0
fruit dish	91	1.0	23.0	1.0	0	10	2.0
green beans w/ham	53	2.0	5.0	2.0	7	641	2.0
potatoes, mashed .	171	2.0	15.0	6.0	18	382	1.0
mushrooms, grilled	152	4.0	10.0	12.0	0	1003	5.0
onion rings	461	5.0	49.0	27.0	1	680	1.0
rice pilaf	163	3.0	32.0	3.0	0	606	1.0
vegetables, garden, grilled	283	5.0	23.0	20.0	0	203	7.0
garnish/condiments:							
cranberry relish ...	54	0	13.0	0	0	6	1.0

Food and Measure	cal.	prot. (gms)	carbo. (gms)	fat (gms)	chol. (mgs)	sod. (mgs)	fiber (gms)
Bob Evans, garnish/condiments *(cont.)*							
garlic herb butter ..	43	0	2.0	4.0	1	235	1.0
hollandaise sauce ..	52	1.0	6.0	3.0	2	219	0
onion ring garnish .	115	1.0	12.0	7.0	0	170	1.0
gravy, beef	33	1.0	5.0	2.0	2	560	0
gravy, chicken	71	0	4.0	6.0	4	460	0
gravy, country	54	0	6.0	4.0	0	546	0
bread/rolls:							
banana nut	186	3.0	30.0	7.0	7	275	1.0
biscuit	277	5.0	36.0	12.0	0	764	0
cranberry nut	170	2.0	25.0	8.0	3	307	1.0
dinner roll	201	5.0	34.0	5.0	9	268	1.0
English muffin	139	5.0	28.0	1.0	0	229	2.0
garlic bread	218	3.0	16.0	16.0	0	386	1.0
kaiser bun	167	6.0	30.0	2.0	0	310	1.0
mini bun	105	3.0	20.0	1.0	0	211	1.0
pumpkin bread	161	3.0	27.0	5.0	3	244	1.0
sourdough bread ..	130	4.0	26.0	1.0	0	253	1.0
Texas toast	120	2.0	12.0	1.0	0	125	1.0
wheat bread	69	3.0	13.0	1.0	0	148	2.0
white bread	67	2.0	12.0	1.0	0	134	1.0
desserts:							
apple dumpling ...	841	8.0	119.0	37.0	41	327	5.0
berry cobbler	631	3.0	85.0	31.0	0	546	5.0
blackberry cobbler .	671	7.0	87.0	34.0	43	435	0
hot fudge cake	785	1.0	108.0	37.0	74	672	5.0
pie, 1 slice:							
apple, no sugar .	483	3.0	52.0	28.0	0	350	2.0
caramel pecan							
silk	812	6.0	69.0	57.0	104	217	2.0
cherry supreme .	478	4.0	46.0	30.0	61	330	2.0
coconut cream ..	556	9.0	67.0	29.0	17	457	2.0
French silk	901	9.0	82.0	61.0	194	245	2.0
pecan	779	7.0	94.0	41.0	137	135	1.0
pumpkin	545	7.0	69.0	27.0	53	72	3.0
Reese's cup	597	9.0	78.0	28.0	14	510	1.0
Reese's sundae ..	769	13.0	104.0	35.0	67	352	3.0
vanilla ice cream, à la mode or							
1 serving	159	3.0	19.0	8.0	34	51	0
Bockwurst, raw, 1 oz.	87	3.8	.1	7.8	17	313	0
Bok-choy, see "Cabbage, Chinese"							

Food and Measure	cal.	prot. (gms)	carbo. (gms)	fat (gms)	chol. (mgs)	sod. (mgs)	fiber (gms)
Bologna (see also "Ham bologna," etc.), 2 oz., except as noted:							
(*Boar's Head* 28% Lower Sodium) ...	150	8.0	0	13.0	30	410	0
(*Deli Delight*)	130	8.0	4.0	8.0	25	400	0
(*Hansel & Gretel* Classic)	150	8.0	3.0	12.0	30	670	0
(*Hatfield Deli Choice*) .	160	7.0	2.0	14.0	30	550	0
(*Johnsonville* Country Style Ring)	170	7.0	1.0	15.0	35	460	0
(*Oscar Mayer* 8 oz.), 1 oz.	90	3.0	1.0	8.0	30	290	0
(*Oscar Mayer* 16 oz.), 1 oz.	90	3.0	1.0	8.0	30	300	0
(*Oscar Mayer* Light), 1 oz.	60	3.0	2.0	4.0	20	300	0
beef:							
(*Boar's Head*)	150	7.0	0	13.0	35	520	0
(*Deli Delight*)	150	8.0	4.0	11.0	30	400	0
(*Hansel & Gretel*) ..	160	7.0	4.0	13.0	30	710	0
(*Hatfield Deli Choice*)	160	7.0	2.0	13.0	30	560	0
(*Healthy Deli* Zero Carb)	120	8.0	0	10.0	30	610	0
(*Johnsonville* Hearty Ring)	170	7.0	1.0	15.0	35	460	0
(*Oscar Mayer* 8 oz.), 1 oz.	90	3.0	1.0	8.0	15	300	0
(*Oscar Mayer* 16 oz.), 1 oz.	90	3.0	1.0	8.0	20	310	0
(*Oscar Mayer* Light), 1 oz.	60	3.0	2.0	4.0	15	310	0
(*Tyson*), .9-oz. slice	80	3.0	1.0	7.0	15	330	0
lean (*Hebrew National*)	90	8.0	1.0	5.0	20	440	0
garlic (*Boar's Head*) ..	150	7.0	1.0	13.0	35	530	0
German:							
(*Hansel & Gretel*) ..	150	8.0	3.0	12.0	30	670	0
(*Hatfield Deli Choice*)	170	7.0	2.0	14.0	30	570	0
(*Healthy Deli* Zero Carb)	150	8.0	0	13.0	35	680	0

Food and Measure	cal.	prot. (gms)	carbo. (gms)	fat (gms)	chol. (mgs)	sod. (mgs)	fiber (gms)
Bologna *(cont.)*							
Lebanon (*Boar's Head*)	100	11.0	3.0	5.0	40	680	0
pork and beef (*Boar's Head*)	150	7.0	<1.0	13.0	35	530	0
"Bologna," vegetarian, frozen, slices:							
(*Worthington Bolono*), 3 slices, 2 oz.	80	11.0	3.0	3.0	0	660	2.0
(*Yves*), 2.2 oz.	80	13.0	4.0	1.0	0	430	1.0
Boniato (*Frieda's*), 3 oz.	100	1.0	24.0	0	0	10	3.0
Bonito, meat only, raw, 4 oz.	146	29.3	.5	2.3	n.a.	50	0
Bonito flakes (*Eden*), 2 tbsp.	4	1.2	0	0	1	4	0
Borage:							
raw, 1" pcs., ½ cup ..	9	.8	1.4	.3	0	35	<1.0
boiled, drained, 4 oz. .	28	2.4	4.0	.9	0	98	<2.0
Boston Market,							
1 serving:							
entree, chicken:							
crispy baked							
country w/gravy .	440	26.0	33.0	23.0	35	970	5.0
garlic, rotisserie:							
½ w/skin	590	70.0	4.0	33.0	290	1010	0
¼ dark, w/skin ..	320	30.0	2.0	21.0	155	500	0
¼ dark, no skin .	190	22.0	1.0	10.0	115	440	0
¼ white, w/skin, wing	280	40.0	2.0	12.0	135	510	0
¼ white, no skin, wing	170	33.0	2.0	4.0	85	480	0
pastry top pot pie .	750	26.0	57.0	46.0	110	1530	2.0
Tuscan, rotisserie:							
½ spicy	630	72.0	8.0	34.0	295	1370	1.0
¼ spicy, dark ...	340	31.0	4.0	22.0	160	680	1.0
¼ spicy, white ..	200	37.0	4.0	4.5	95	700	1.0
entree, other:							
cod, baked	330	37.0	11.0	16.0	130	430	0
ham, honey glazed .	210	24.0	10.0	8.0	75	1460	0
meat loaf, 2 slices .	510	32.0	22.0	34.0	140	890	2.0
w/beef gravy ...	580	33.0	27.0	39.0	140	1270	2.0
w/tomato, chunky	550	33.0	30.0	34.0	140	1270	3.0
turkey, rotisserie ..	170	36.0	3.0	1.0	100	850	0
sides, cold:							
coleslaw	310	7.0	29.0	22.0	20	230	10.0

Food and Measure	cal.	prot. (gms)	carbo. (gms)	fat (gms)	chol. (mgs)	sod. (mgs)	fiber (gms)
cranberry	120	1.0	25.0	1.5	0	0	<1.0
sides, hot:							
apples, cinnamon ..	250	0	56.0	4.5	0	45.0	3.0
butternut squash ..	150	2.0	25.0	6.0	20	560	6.0
corn, sweet	180	5.0	30.0	4.0	0	170	2.0
green bean							
casserole	80	1.0	9.0	4.5	5	670	2.0
green beans	70	1.0	6.0	4.0	0	250	2.0
macaroni and							
cheese	280	13.0	33.0	11.0	30	890	1.0
pasta, penne	240	10.0	29.0	9.0	10	680	2.0
potato, mashed ...	210	4.0	30.0	9.0	25	590	2.0
w/gravy	230	4.0	32.0	9.0	25	780	3.0
potato, new, garlic							
dill	130	3.0	25.0	2.5	0	150	2.0
poultry gravy	15	0	2.0	.5	0	180	0
spinach, sautéed ..	90	6.0	8.0	5.0	15	550	5.0
spinach, creamed ..	260	9.0	11.0	20.0	55	740	2.0
squash casserole ..	330	7.0	20.0	24.0	70	1110	3.0
sweet potato							
casserole	280	3.0	39.0	13.0	10	190	2.0
stuffing, savory ...	190	4.0	27.0	8.0	5	620	2.0
vegetables, steamed	30	2.0	6.0	0	0	135	2.0
sandwiches, w/cheese:							
chicken, w/sauce ..	670	38.0	68.0	33.0	90	420	5.0
meat loaf	1070	57.0	102.0	55.0	190	1480	7.0
turkey, w/sauce ...	690	49.0	68.0	29.0	130	690	5.0
salads:							
Caesar, entree	470	14.0	17.0	40.0	35	1070	3.0
Caesar, side	300	5.0	13.0	26.0	15	690	<1.0
chicken Caesar	640	46.0	19.0	44.0	120	1530	3.0
chicken, Asian	540	41.0	57.0	15.0	85	1880	8.0
no dressing/							
noodles	270	38.0	22.0	5.0	85	510	7.0
fruit salad	70	1.0	16.0	0	0	15.0	1.0
soup:							
chicken noodle, cup	100	6.0	8.0	4.5	30	500	0
tortilla, w/toppings .	170	8.0	18.0	8.0	25	1060	2.0
tortilla, no toppings	80	5.0	7.0	4.5	15	930	1.0
desserts:							
apple pie, 1 slice ..	550	4.0	66.0	31.0	0	240	3.0
brownie, chocolate .	580	9.0	88.0	23.0	95	350	6.0
brownie, caramel							
pecan	900	9.0	114.0	47.0	120	150	6.0

Food and Measure	cal.	prot. (gms)	carbo. (gms)	fat (gms)	chol. (mgs)	sod. (mgs)	fiber (gms)
Boston Market, desserts *(cont.)*							
cake, chocolate ...	650	6.0	86.0	32.0	60	320	2.0
cake, molten fudge	300	3.0	34.0	19.0	35	210	1.0
chocolate Mania ...	490	4.0	36.0	33.0	95	170	1.0
chocolate chip cookie	390	4.0	51.0	19.0	15	350	2.0
cornbread	120	1.0	21.0	3.5	5	220	0
oatmeal cookie	390	5.0	47.0	20.0	30	340	2.0
Bouillon (see also "Bouillon concentrate"):							
beef:							
(*Herb-Ox*), 1 cube .	5	0	0	0	0	900	0
(*Herb-Ox* Instant), 1 tsp.	5	0	0	0	0	760	0
(*Herb-Ox* Instant Broth/Seasoning), 1 pkt.	5	0	0	0	0	1020	0
(*Herb-Ox* Instant Low Sodium), 1 pkt	10	0	2.0	0	0	5	0
(*Knorr*), ½ cube ..	20	<1.0	<1.0	1.0	0	1400	0
(*Maggie* Instant), 1 tsp.	5	0	0	0	0	570	0
(*Tyson*), 1 cube or tsp.	5	1.0	0	0	0	920	0
(*Watkins*), 2 tsp. ...	15	<1.0	2.0	.5	0	710	0
chicken:							
(*Doña Maria*), 1 tsp.	10	0	0	.5	0	930	0
(*Herb-Ox*), 1 cube .	5	0	0	0	0	1100	0
(*Herb-Ox* Instant), 1 tsp.	5	0	0	0	0	880	0
(*Herb-Ox* Instant Broth/Seasoning), 1 pkt	5	0	0	0	0	1100	0
(*Herb-Ox* Instant Broth/Seasoning Low Sodium), 1 pkt.	10	0	2.0	0	0	5	0
(*Knorr*), ½ cube ..	20	<1.0	<1.0	1.5	0	1270	0
(*Maggi* Instant), 1 tsp.	5	0	1.0	0	0	640	0
(*Tyson*), 1 cube or tsp.	5	0	1.0	0	0	910	0

Food and Measure	cal.	prot. (gms)	carbo. (gms)	fat (gms)	chol. (mgs)	sod. (mgs)	fiber (gms)
(*Watkins*), 2 tsp. ...	20	<1.0	3.0	.5	0	580	0
garlic (*Herb-Ox*), 1 cube	5	0	0	0	0	1100	0
tomato (*Doña Maria*), 1 tsp.	10	0	1.0	.5	0	640	0
fish (*Knorr*), ½ cube .	10	<1.0	0	1.0	0	980	0
ham (*Knorr*), ½ cube	15	0	<1.0	1.0	0	1030	0
vegetable:							
(*Herb-Ox*), 1 cube .	5	0	0	0	0	980	0
(*Knorr* Vegetarian), ½ cube	15	<1.0	1.0	1.0	0	830	0
(*Morga*), ½ cube ..	22	.5	1.3	1.6	0	300	0
(*Maggi* Vegetarian), 1 cube	5	0	1.0	0	0	820	0
Bouillon concentrate, liquid, 1 tsp., except as noted:							
beef:							
(*Bovril*), 2 tsp.	10	<1.0	1.0	0	0	930	0
(*Home Again* Base)	10	1.0	1.0	0	0	800	0
(*Knorr*), 2 tsp.	15	2.0	1.0	0	0	850	0
beef flavor (*Savory Basics* Stock)	20	2.0	1.0	.5	0	630	0
chicken:							
(*Bovril*), 2 tsp.	15	<1.0	2.0	.5	0	880	0
(*Home Again* Base)	10	1.0	<1.0	0	0	720	0
(*Home Again* Base No MSG)	15	<1.0	2.0	.5	0	880	0
(*Knorr*), 2 tsp.	5	<1.0	<1.0	0	0	740	0
(*Savory Basics* Stock)	20	2.0	1.0	.5	0	630	0
chicken flavor (*Home Again* Stock)	20	0	2.0	1.0	0	740	0
ham (*Home Again* Base), ¾ tsp.	15	0	1.0	1.0	0	590	0
vegetable (*Savory Basics* Stock), 2 tsp.	15	1.0	3.0	0	0	650	0
Bow-tie pasta, see "Pasta, dry"							
Bow-tie pasta entree, frozen, and chicken (*Lean Cuisine Café Classics*), 9.5 oz. ...	220	15.0	31.0	4.0	40	680	3.0

Food and Measure	cal.	prot. (gms)	carbo. (gms)	fat (gms)	chol. (mgs)	sod. (mgs)	fiber (gms)
Boysenberry, fresh, see "Blackberry"							
Boysenberry, frozen, unsweetened, ½ cup	33	.7	8.1	.1	0	1	2.6
Boysenberry nectar (*R.W. Knudsen*), 8 fl. oz.	130	<1.0	35.0	0	0	35	0
Boysenberry syrup (*Smucker's*), ¼ cup	210	0	52.0	0	0	0	0
Brains, 4 oz.:							
beef, fried	222	14.3	0	18.0	2262	179	0
lamb, fried	310	19.2	0	25.2	2840	178	0
pork, braised	156	13.8	0	10.8	2894	103	0
veal, fried	242	16.4	0	19.0	2404	200	0
Bran, see "Cereal" and specific grains							
Bratwurst, cooked, 1 link, except as noted:							
(*Boar's Head*), 4 oz. . .	300	19.0	0	25.0	75	650	0
(*Johnsonville* Brat Bites Precooked), 6 links, 2 oz.	200	7.0	1.0	18.0	40	530	0
(*Johnsonville* Heat & Serve), 2.7 oz.	260	12.0	3.0	23.0	50	920	0
(*Johnsonville* Oktoberfest), 4 oz.	390	19.0	1.0	34.0	85	1060	0
(*Johnsonville* Original/ Beer 'n Bratwurst/ Savory Onion), 3 oz.	290	14.0	1.0	25.0	65	800	0
(*Johnsonville* Precooked/Stadium Style), 2.7 oz.	240	9.0	2.0	22.0	50	760	0
(*Organic Valley*), 3 oz.	255	12.0	2.0	21.0	49	465	0
beef, smoked (*Johnsonville*), 2.7 oz. . .	240	9.0	2.0	21.0	60	640	0
cheddar (*Johnsonville*), 3 oz.	300	15.0	2.0	25.0	65	800	0
chicken, w/wild rice (*Bilinski*), 2 oz. . . .	70	11.0	2.0	2.0	25	280	0
garlic and honey (*Johnsonville*), 3 oz.	280	13.0	5.0	22.0	60	700	0
hot and spicy (*Johnsonville*), 3 oz.	290	14.0	2.0	25.0	60	760	0

Food and Measure	cal.	prot. (gms)	carbo. (gms)	fat (gms)	chol. (mgs)	sod. (mgs)	fiber (gms)
smoked (*Johnsonville*), 2.7 oz.	240	9.0	2.0	21.0	60	640	0
turkey (*Shady Brook Farms*), 3 oz.	160	18.0	1.0	9.0	75	690	0
"Bratwurst," vegetar-ian, frozen (*Boca*), 2.5-oz. link	140	14.0	6.0	7.0	0	760	1.0
Bratwurst burger, grilled (*Johnson-ville*), 2.5-oz. pc. . .	240	11.0	1.0	21.0	55	660	0
Braunschweiger (see also "Liverwurst"), 2 oz.:							
(*Black Bear*)	140	9.0	2.0	15.0	55	460	0
(*Boar's Head* Lite) . . .	120	9.0	1.0	8.0	50	450	0
(*Hansel & Gretel*)	170	9.0	4.0	13.0	95	730	0
(*Oscar Mayer*)	190	8.0	1.0	17.0	90	630	0
Brazil nuts, shelled:							
(*Shiloh Farms*), ¼ cup	240	5.0	5.0	24.0	0	0	2.0
1 oz., 8 medium or 6 large	186	4.1	3.6	18.8	0	<1	1.6
Bread, 1 slice, except as noted:							
banana swirl (*Pepperidge Farm*) .	90	2.0	15.0	2.0	0	100	<1.0
buttermilk:							
(*Earth Grains*)	110	4.0	20.0	1.5	0	200	<1.0
(*Pillsbury*)	90	3.0	15.0	1.5	0	150	0
sweet (*Pepperidge Farm Farmhouse*)	110	4.0	22.0	1.0	0	210	1.0
cinnamon swirl:							
(*Pepperidge Farm*) .	90	3.0	14.0	2.5	0	115	2.0
raisin (*Pepperidge Farm*)	80	3.0	14.0	1.5	0	105	1.0
French (*Pepperidge Farm* Hot & Crusty Thin Sliced), 2 slices	150	5.0	29.0	1.5	0	320	1.0
French toast swirl:							
brown sugar cinna-mon (*Pepperidge Farm*)	140	4.0	25.0	3.5	0	170	1.0
maple syrup cinna-mon (*Pepperidge Farm*)	130	4.0	25.0	2.0	0	170	2.0

Food and Measure	cal.	prot. (gms)	carbo. (gms)	fat (gms)	chol. (mgs)	sod. (mgs)	fiber (gms)
Bread, French toast swirl *(cont.)*							
vanilla, French (*Pepperidge Farm*) ..	140	4.0	23.0	3.5	0	190	<1.0
garlic (*Pepperidge Farm* Hot & Crusty), 2 slices, ½"	170	5.0	21.0	8.0	0	310	1.0
grain, whole (*Healthy Choice*)	80	4.0	18.0	1.0	0	170	3.0
honey (*Earth Grains*) .	110	4.0	19.0	1.5	0	160	2.0
Indian flatbread, see "Chapati"							
Italian:							
(*Arnold Carb Counting*)	60	6.0	8.0	1.5	0	140	2.0
(*Pepperidge Farm*) .	90	3.0	15.0	1.5	0	180	<1.0
kamut (*Shiloh Farms* Organic)	90	6.0	18.0	1.0	0	115	3.0
multigrain:							
(*Arnold Carb Counting*)	60	5.0	9.0	1.5	0	135	3.0
(*Earth Grains*)	110	5.0	19.0	1.5	0	180	5.0
(*Pepperidge Farm* Natural Whole Grain)	90	4.0	15.0	1.0	0	140	3.0
(*Sara Lee* Heart Healthy)	100	4.0	19.0	1.0	0	180	2.0
(*Sara Lee* Heart Healthy Plus) ...	80	4.0	14.0	1.0	0	135	4.0
(*Sara Lee* Heart Healthy Plus with Honey)	110	5.0	19.0	1.5	0	180	5.0
(*Shiloh Farms* Organic Sandwich)	80	4.0	17.0	.5	0	100	3.0
crunchy (*Pepperidge Farm* Natural Whole Grain)	90	4.0	15.0	1.5	0	150	3.0
5-grain (*Shiloh Farms* Organic) .	90	5.0	19.0	.5	0	110	4.0
5-grain (*Shiloh Farms* Organic No Salt)	90	5.0	19.0	.5	0	0	4.0
7-grain (*Healthy Choice*)	80	3.0	18.0	1.0	0	170	3.0

Food and Measure	cal.	prot. (gms)	carbo. (gms)	fat (gms)	chol. (mgs)	sod. (mgs)	fiber (gms)
7-grain (*Pepperidge Farm Carb Style*)	60	5.0	8.0	1.5	0	150	3.0
7-grain (*Pepperidge Farm Farmhouse*)	110	4.0	20.0	1.5	0	190	2.0
7-grain (*Pepperidge Farm Light Style*), 3 slices	140	6.0	27.0	1.0	0	290	2.0
7-grain (*Shiloh Farms* Organic) .	90	5.0	19.0	.5	0	130	3.0
7-grain (*Shiloh Farms* Organic No Salt)	90	5.0	19.0	.5	0	0	3.0
9-grain (*Pepperidge Farm* Natural Whole Grain) ...	90	4.0	15.0	1.0	0	140	3.0
10-grain, sprouted (*Shiloh Farms* Organic), 2 slices	140	9.0	26.0	1.5	0	120	5.0
12-grain (*Pepperidge Farm Farmhouse*)	120	4.0	21.0	2.5	0	160	3.0
soft (*Healthy Choice*)	60	3.0	12.0	.5	0	120	2.0
oat:							
crunchy (*Pepperidge Farm Farmhouse*)	110	5.0	19.0	1.5	0	180	2.0
honey (*Pepperidge Farm* Natural Whole Grain) ...	90	4.0	15.0	1.5	0	135	2.0
nut (*Earth Grains*) .	120	4.0	20.0	2.5	0	210	1.0
nutty (*Pepperidge Farm Farmhouse*)	120	4.0	21.0	2.5	0	150	3.0
oatmeal:							
(*Arnold Bakery Light*), 2 slices ..	80	4.0	19.0	.5	0	170	4.0
(*Pepperidge Farm*) .	60	2.0	11.0	1.0	0	160	1.0
(*Pepperidge Farm Light Style*), 3 slices	140	7.0	27.0	.5	0	260	2.0
soft (*Pepperidge Farm Farmhouse*)	110	4.0	21.0	1.0	0	200	1.0
pita, 1 pc.:							
(*Garden of Eatin' Bible Bread*)	160	7.0	31.0	1.5	0	115	2.0

Food and Measure	cal.	prot. (gms)	carbo. (gms)	fat (gms)	chol. (mgs)	sod. (mgs)	fiber (gms)
Bread, pita *(cont.)*							
(*Garden of Eatin'* Bible Bread Very Low Salt)	160	7.0	30.0	2.0	0	30	1.0
spelt (*Shiloh Farms*)	150	6.0	29.0	1.0	0	125	4.0
white (*Sahara*)	160	5.0	32.0	1.5	0	350	2.0
whole wheat (*Sahara*)	140	6.0	27.0	1.5	0	310	5.0
whole wheat (*Shiloh Farms*)	140	6.0	31.0	0	0	130	3.0
potato:							
(*Earth Grains*)	110	4.0	20.0	1.0	0	190	<1.0
(*Pepperidge Farm Farmhouse* Golden)	110	3.0	22.0	1.0	0	220	1.0
pumpernickel:							
(*Arnold* Real Jewish)	80	2.0	16.0	1.0	0	230	1.0
(*Pepperidge Farm* Family)	80	3.0	15.0	1.0	0	230	2.0
(*Pepperidge Farm* Party), 5 slices . .	130	5.0	24.0	1.5	0	290	3.0
(*Rubschlager Rye-Ola*)	100	3.0	20.0	.5	0	200	3.0
w/whole kernels (*Mestemacher* Westphalian) . . .	80	2.0	16.0	1.0	0	160	3.0
rye:							
(*Arnold* Melba Thin), 2 slices	120	3.0	21.0	2.0	0	310	1.0
(*Arnold Carb Counting*)	60	5.0	9.0	1.5	0	210	3.0
(*Pepperidge Farm* Party), 5 slices . .	120	4.0	25.0	1.0	0	430	3.0
(*Shiloh* Rich 'n Rye), 2 slices	150	9.0	27.0	2.0	0	150	5.0
(*Wild's* Party), 3 slices	80	3.0	14.0	1.5	0	180	2.0
black (*Rubschlager Rye-Ola*)	100	3.0	20.0	.5	0	200	3.0
w/seeds (*Arnold* Real Jewish) . . .	80	2.0	15.0	1.5	0	220	1.0
w/seeds (*Levy's* Real Jewish) . . .	90	3.0	17.0	1.5	0	250	1.0

Food and Measure	cal.	prot. (gms)	carbo. (gms)	fat (gms)	chol. (mgs)	sod. (mgs)	fiber (gms)
w/seeds (*Pepperidge Farm*) ..	80	3.0	15.0	1.0	0	210	2.0
seedless (*Arnold Real Jewish*) ...	90	2.0	15.0	1.5	0	230	1.0
seedless (*Pepperidge Farm*) ..	80	3.0	15.0	1.0	0	210	1.0
rye/pumpernickel:							
(*Arnold* Deli Swirl) .	80	3.0	15.0	1.0	0	220	1.0
(*Pepperidge Farm* Deli Swirl)	80	3.0	15.0	1.0	0	220	1.0
sourdough (*Pepperidge Farm Farmhouse*)	110	4.0	20.0	1.5	0	220	1.0
spelt (*Shiloh Farms Organic*)	100	4.0	21.0	1.0	0	140	2.0
sunflower, rye (*Rubschlager Rye-Ola*) .	110	3.0	19.0	2.0	0	190	3.0
rye, soy (*Rubschlager Rye-Ola*)	100	4.0	20.0	.5	0	200	3.0
wheat:							
(*Pepperidge Farm Farmhouse Butter-topped*) ..	120	4.0	21.0	2.0	0	200	1.0
(*Pepperidge Farm Farmhouse Hearty Country*) .	110	4.0	21.0	1.5	0	190	2.0
(*Pillsbury*)	80	3.0	15.0	1.0	0	115	1.0
(*Sara Lee* Classic) .	70	3.0	13.0	1.0	0	150	2.0
(*Sara Lee* Delightful)	45	3.0	9.0	0	0	120	2.0
(*Shiloh Farms* Homestyle Organic), 2 slices	160	7.0	29.0	1.5	0	115	<1.0
buttermilk (*Pepperidge Farm Farmhouse*)	120	4.0	21.0	2.0	0	200	1.0
dark (*Pepperidge Farm* Whole Grain German)	90	4.0	15.0	1.0	0	140	3.0
honey (*Sara Lee*) ..	70	2.0	14.0	1.0	0	140	1.0
honey, soft (*Healthy Choice*)	60	3.0	12.0	.5	0	120	2.0
sesame (*Pepperidge Farm Farmhouse*)	110	4.0	19.0	2.0	0	190	2.0

Bread *(cont.)*
wheat, whole:

Food and Measure	cal.	prot. (gms)	carbo. (gms)	fat (gms)	chol. (mgs)	sod. (mgs)	fiber (gms)
(*Arnold Carb Counting*)	60	4.0	9.0	1.5	0	130	3.0
(*Earth Grains*)	110	5.0	19.0	1.5	0	190	5.0
(*Lifeworks*), 2 slices	170	9.0	27.0	2.5	0	330	3.0
(*Pepperidge Farm Thin Sliced*)	70	3.0	11.0	1.0	0	95	2.0
(*Pepperidge Farm Very Thin Sliced*), 3 slices	120	4.0	21.0	2.0	0	220	3.0
(*Pepperidge Farm Carb Style*)	60	5.0	8.0	1.5	0	170	3.0
(*Pepperidge Farm Farmhouse*)	110	5.0	19.0	2.0	0	150	3.0
(*Sara Lee* Heart Healthy)	70	4.0	19.0	1.0	0	180	2.0
(*Sara Lee* Heart Healthy Plus) ...	80	4.0	14.0	1.0	0	135	4.0
(*Sara Lee* Heart Healthy Plus with Honey)	110	5.0	19.0	1.5	0	180	5.0
(*Sara Lee* Home-style)	100	5.0	20.0	1.5	0	190	2.0
(*Sara Lee* Home-style Wide Pan) .	100	5.0	20.0	1.0	0	200	2.0
(*Shiloh Farms* Organic), 2 slices	140	7.0	26.0	1.5	0	260	4.0
(*Shiloh Farms* Organic No Salt), 2 slices	140	7.0	26.0	1.5	0	0	3.0
honey (*Earth Grains*)	110	5.0	20.0	1.5	0	180	5.0
stone ground (*Earth Grains*)	100	4.0	19.0	1.0	0	170	2.0
stone ground, whole grain (*Pepperidge Farm*)	90	4.0	16.0	1.0	0	135	2.0
wheat berry:							
(*Earth Grains*)	100	4.0	20.0	.5	0	220	1.0
(*Pepperidge Farm Farmhouse*)	110	4.0	20.0	1.5	0	200	2.0
white:							
(*Arnold* Country Classics)	110	3.0	19.0	1.5	0	210	<1.0

Food and Measure	cal.	prot. (gms)	carbo. (gms)	fat (gms)	chol. (mgs)	sod. (mgs)	fiber (gms)
(*Arnold Brick Oven*), 2 slices	140	4.0	25.0	2.5	0	260	1.0
(*Arnold Brick Oven* Big Slice)	90	3.0	17.0	1.5	0	180	<1.0
(*Lifeworks*), 2 slices	170	8.0	28.0	2.5	0	340	2.0
(*Pepperidge Farm* Canadian)	80	3.0	16.0	1.0	0	170	<1.0
(*Pepperidge Farm* Sandwich), 2 slices	130	4.0	23.0	2.5	0	260	<1.0
(*Pepperidge Farm* Sandwich Family/ Large), 2 slices .	150	4.0	27.0	3.0	0	310	0
(*Pepperidge Farm* Toasting)	90	3.0	16.0	1.0	0	200	0
(*Pepperidge Farm* Very Thin Sliced), 3 slices	120	4.0	24.0	1.0	0	250	1.0
(*Pepperidge Farm* Carb Style)	60	5.0	8.0	1.0	0	160	3.0
(*Pepperidge Farm* Farmhouse Butter-topped) . .	110	3.0	21.0	1.5	0	240	<1.0
(*Pepperidge Farm* Farmhouse Country)	110	4.0	20.0	1.0	0	200	2.0
(*Pepperidge Farm* Farmhouse Hearty)	110	3.0	22.0	1.0	0	280	1.0
(*Pillsbury*)	80	3.0	15.0	1.0	0	170	1.0
(*Sara Lee* Classic) .	80	2.0	15.0	1.5	0	140	<1.0
(*Sara Lee* Delightful)	90	5.0	18.0	1.0	0	240	4.0
honey (*Pillsbury*) . .	80	3.0	15.0	1.0	0	140	0
honey (*Sara Lee*) . .	100	3.0	22.0	.5	0	210	<1.0
Bread, brown, canned (*B&M*), ½" slice . . .	130	3.0	29.0	.5	0	390	2.0
Bread, frozen:							
challah, ready-to-bake, 2 oz., ⅛ loaf:							
(*Kineret*)	140	5.0	27.0	1.0	20	220	<1.0
round (*Kineret* Holiday)	150	5.0	25.0	4.0	20	220	<1.0
cheese, mini (*Pepperidge Farm*), 2 slices, ¼"	170	5.0	21.0	7.0	10	310	1.0

Food and Measure	cal.	prot. (gms)	carbo. (gms)	fat (gms)	chol. (mgs)	sod. (mgs)	fiber (gms)
Bread, frozen *(cont.)*							
dough, 1.8 oz.:							
wheat (*Rhodes*) . . .	130	6.0	24.0	2.0	0	280	2.0
white (*Rhodes*) . . .	140	5.0	24.0	2.0	0	280	2.0
dough, sweet, see "Dough, sweet"							
French, crusty (*Pillsbury*), 1/5 loaf	150	5.0	28.0	2.0	0	370	<1.0
garlic:							
(*Pepperidge Farm*), 2 slices, ½"	170	4.0	24.0	7.0	0	250	2.0
5 cheese (*Pepperidge Farm*), 2 slices, ½"	190	5.0	24.0	8.0	<5	300	2.0
mini (*Pepperidge Farm*), 2 slices, ½"	170	4.0	25.0	6.0	<5	280	1.0
mozzarella (*Pepperidge Farm*), 2 slices, ¼"	160	5.0	22.0	6.0	0	250	2.0
Parmesan (*Pepperidge Farm*), 2 slices, ½"	160	5.0	23.0	6.0	0	270	2.0
Italian:							
(*Pillsbury* Country), ⅛ loaf	110	4.0	21.0	1.5	0	270	<1.0
w/garlic (*Pillsbury*), 1¼" slice, ½ tsp. spread	130	4.0	21.0	3.5	0	490	<1.0
Texas toast, 1 slice:							
5 cheese (*Pepperidge Farm*) . .	150	4.0	18.0	7.0	<5	200	1.0
garlic (*Pepperidge Farm*)	150	3.0	18.0	7.0	0	190	2.0
mozzarella Monterey Jack (*Pepperidge Farm*)	160	5.0	20.0	7.0	<5	250	<1.0
Parmesan (*Pepperidge Farm*) . .	160	4.0	14.0	9.0	20	250	<1.0
Bread, mix (see also "Bread mix, sweet"), dry mix, ¼ cup, except as noted:							
barley, w/soy (*Hodgson Mill*) . . .	121	5.0	23.0	1.0	0	215	2.0

Food and Measure	cal.	prot. (gms)	carbo. (gms)	fat (gms)	chol. (mgs)	sod. (mgs)	fiber (gms)
cheese and herb							
(*Hodgson Mill*) ...	130	5.0	21.0	1.0	0	250	<1.0
focaccia, 1 serving:							
Italian herb and							
cheese (*Buitoni*)	110	3.0	21.0	2.0	0	390	0
rosemary and garlic							
(*Buitoni*)	110	3.0	21.0	2.0	0	390	0
multigrain, 9, w/soy							
(*Hodgson Mill*) ...	120	5.0	22.0	1.5	0	150	3.0
potato, w/soy							
(*Hodgson Mill*) ...	110	5.0	23.0	0	0	170	<1.0
rye, caraway, w/soy							
(*Hodgson Mill*) ...	110	5.0	22.0	1.0	0	190	3.0
white, w/soy (*Hodgson*							
Mill Wholesome) ..	120	5.0	22.0	.5	0	170	1.0
whole wheat, honey							
(*Hodgson Mill*) ...	120	5.0	22.0	.5	0	160	2.0
Bread mix, sweet:							
banana:							
(*Betty Crocker*							
Quick), 1/12 pkg.*	170	3.0	25.0	7.0	35	200	0
(*Produce Partners*),							
2 tbsp. mix	150	2.0	32.0	.5	0	250	0
carrot (*Produce Part-*							
ners), ½ cup mix ..	260	3.0	60.0	1.0	0	560	0
cinnamon streusel							
(*Betty Crocker*							
Quick), 1/14 pkg.* .	180	3.0	28.0	7.0	30	160	0
corn:							
(*Glory* Homestyle),							
1.2-oz. square* .	160	2.0	24.0	4.5	35	480	2.0
(*Hodgson Mill*),							
¼ cup mix	130	4.0	28.0	.5	0	240	3.0
(*Kentucky Kernel*),							
¼ cup	120	2.0	24.0	1.5	0	310	0
jalapeño (*Hodgson*							
Mill), ¼ cup mix	100	4.0	21.0	.5	0	310	1.0
cranberry orange							
(*Betty Crocker*							
Quick), 1/12 pkg.* .	180	3.0	29.0	6.0	35	180	0
gingerbread, whole							
wheat (*Hodgson*							
Mill), ¼ cup mix ..	110	2.0	24.0	0	0	260	2.0

Food and Measure	cal.	prot. (gms)	carbo. (gms)	fat (gms)	chol. (mgs)	sod. (mgs)	fiber (gms)
Bread mix, sweet *(cont.)*							
lemon poppy seed (*Betty Crocker* Quick), 1/12 pkg.* .	170	3.0	25.0	7.0	35	200	0
Bread crumbs (see also "Batter and breading mix"), ¼ cup or 1 oz.:							
plain:							
(*Arnold* All Purpose)	110	4.0	19.0	1.5	0	200	1.0
(*Progresso*)	110	4.0	19.0	1.5	0	210	1.0
garlic and herb (*Progresso*)	100	4.0	18.0	1.5	0	530	1.0
Italian:							
(*Contadina*)	100	3.0	19.0	1.5	0	720	1.0
(*Progresso*)	110	4.0	20.0	1.5	0	430	1.0
Parmesan (*Progresso*)	110	4.0	19.0	1.5	0	270	1.0
Bread cubes, see "Stuffing"							
Bread dough, see "Bread, frozen"							
Bread stick:							
plain:							
(*Colonna*), 2 pcs. . .	60	2.0	14.0	0	0	100	0
(*Stella D'oro*), 1 pc.	45	1.0	7.0	1.0	0	40	0
(*Stella D'oro* No Salt), 1 pc.	45	1.0	7.0	1.0	0	0	0
mini (*Stella D'oro*), 4 pcs.	70	2.0	12.0	1.5	0	65	1.0
cracked pepper, mini (*Stella D'oro*), 4 pcs.	70	2.0	11.0	2.0	0	490	0
garlic, roasted (*Stella D'oro*), 1 pc.	45	1.0	8.0	1.0	0	230	0
sesame:							
(*Stella D'oro*), 1 pc.	50	1.0	7.0	2.0	0	45	1.0
mini (*Stella D'oro*), 4 pcs.	80	2.0	11.0	3.5	0	75	1.0
Bread stick, frozen or refrigerated:							
(*Pillsbury* Soft), 2 pcs.	140	4.0	25.0	2.5	0	370	<1.0
(*Rhodes*), 1/6 pkg. . . .	180	5.0	32.0	3.0	0	250	1.0
corn bread (*Pillsbury* Twists), 1 pc.	130	3.0	17.0	6.0	0	340	1.0

Food and Measure	cal.	prot. (gms)	carbo. (gms)	fat (gms)	chol. (mgs)	sod. (mgs)	fiber (gms)
garlic:							
(*Pepperidge Farm*), 1 pc.	160	5.0	25.0	4.5	0	320	1.0
w/herbs (*Pillsbury*), 2 pcs., ½ tsp. spread	170	4.0	24.0	6.0	0	560	<1.0
Parmesan w/garlic (*Pillsbury*), 2 pcs., ½ tsp. spread	170	5.0	24.0	6.0	0	550	<1.0
Breadfruit, raw, ½ cup	113	1.2	29.8	.3	0	2	5.4
Breadfruit seeds:							
raw, 1 oz.	54	2.1	8.3	1.6	0	7	1.5
boiled, shelled, 1 oz. .	48	1.5	9.1	.7	0	7	1.4
roasted, shelled, 1 oz.	59	1.8	11.4	.8	0	8	1.7
Breading mix, see "Batter and breading mix" and specific listings							
Breadnut tree seeds, dried, 1 oz.	104	2.4	22.5	.5	0	15	4.2
Breakfast dish, see "Egg breakfast" and specific listings							
Breakfast pocket/ sandwich (see also "Burrito, breakfast" and "Taco, breakfast"), frozen, 1 pc.:							
bacon and sausage (*Toaster Scrambles*)	180	4.0	14.0	12.0	25	370	0
bagel, sausage/egg/ cheese (*Jimmy Dean*), 4.8 oz.	340	15.0	33.0	17.0	115	740	1.0
biscuit:							
bacon/egg/cheese (*Jimmy Dean*), 3.6 oz.	320	12.0	27.0	18.0	100	790	1.0
double sausage/egg/ cheese (*Swanson Hungry-Man*), 6 oz.	450	17.0	35.0	27.0	235	1180	1.0
sausage/egg/cheese (*Jimmy Dean*), 4.5 oz.	430	13.0	28.0	30.0	115	830	1.0

Food and Measure	cal.	prot. (gms)	carbo. (gms)	fat (gms)	chol. (mgs)	sod. (mgs)	fiber (gms)
Breakfast pocket/sandwich *(cont.)*							
cheese/egg, and:							
bacon (*Toaster Scrambles*)	180	4.0	14.0	12.0	25	380	0
ham or sausage (*Toaster Scrambles*)	180	4.0	14.0	12.0	25	370	0
croissant, sausage/ egg/cheese:							
(*Aunt Jemima*), 4.1 oz.	350	13.0	22.0	23.0	145	680	<1.0
(*Jimmy Dean*), 4.8 oz.	450	12.0	24.0	33.0	125	770	1.0
English muffin:							
ham and cheese (*Smart Ones*), 4 oz.	210	13.0	28.0	5.0	20	420	2.0
sausage/egg/cheese (*Jimmy Dean*), 4.6 oz.	350	13.0	28.0	21.0	110	720	1.0
veggie, w/cheese (*Morningstar Farms*)	280	28.0	35.0	3.0	10	1000	5.0
French toast:							
(*Pop-Tarts*)	220	3.0	34.0	8.0	<5	180	<1.0
sausage/egg/cheese (*Aunt Jemima*), 4.7 oz.	330	14.0	26.0	19.0	230	760	1.0
pocket, egg/cheese:							
bacon (*Hot Pockets*), 4.5 oz.	310	10.0	32.0	16.0	75	450	2.0
bacon (*Hot Pockets*), 2.25 oz.	170	6.0	20.0	7.0	45	290	1.0
bacon (*Lean Pockets*), 2.25 oz.	150	7.0	21.0	4.5	40	280	2.0
ham (*Hot Pockets*), 2.25 oz.	150	6.0	17.0	7.0	35	310	1.0
sausage (*Croissant Pockets*), 4.5 oz.	360	12.0	34.0	20.0	75	620	3.0
sausage (*Hot Pockets*), 2.25 oz.	170	6.0	19.0	7.0	45	280	1.0
sausage (*Lean Pockets*), 2.25 oz.	140	7.0	19.0	4.5	45	310	2.0

Food and Measure	cal.	prot. (gms)	carbo. (gms)	fat (gms)	chol. (mgs)	sod. (mgs)	fiber (gms)
tofu scramble (*Amy's*), 4.5 oz. . .	180	11.0	23.0	6.0	0	520	<1.0
wrap, 4.3 oz.:							
bacon/egg/cheddar (*Jimmy Dean*) . .	350	15.0	23.0	20.0	210	920	<1.0
ham/egg/cheddar (*Jimmy Dean*) . .	300	16.0	23.0	15.0	205	980	<1.0
Breakfast syrup, see "Pancake syrup"							
Brewer's yeast flakes (*Louis Labs*), 1.1 oz., 2 rounded tbsp.	116	16.0	13.0	0	0	63	6.0
Broad bean, fresh:							
raw, ½ cup	40	3.1	6.4	.4	0	28	2.3
boiled, drained, 4 oz. .	64	5.4	11.5	.6	0	47	<3.0
Broad bean, mature:							
dry:							
(*Frieda's* Fava), ¾ cup, 3 oz.	290	22.0	50.0	1.5	0	10	21.0
(*Shiloh Farms* Fava), ¼ cup	70	7.0	22.0	0	0	20	12.0
peeled (*Frieda's* Habas), ½ cup, 3 oz.	100	6.0	17.0	0	0	5	4.0
boiled, ½ cup	93	6.5	16.7	.3	0	4	4.6
Broad bean, mature, canned, ½ cup:							
(*Progresso* Fava Beans)	110	6.0	20.0	.5	0	250	5.0
w/liquid	91	7.0	15.9	.3	0	580	4.7
Broccoli, fresh:							
raw:							
(*Andy Boy*), 1 medium stalk, 5.2 oz.	45	5.0	8.0	.5	0	55	5.0
(*Dole*), 1 medium stalk, 5.2 oz. . . .	45	5.0	8.0	.5	0	55	5.0
8.7-oz. stalk	42	4.5	7.9	.5	0	40	4.5
chopped, ½ cup . . .	12	1.3	2.3	.2	0	12	1.3
boiled, drained:							
1 stalk, 6.3 oz.	51	5.4	9.1	.6	0	46	5.2
chopped, ½ cup . . .	22	2.3	3.9	.2	0	20	2.3
Broccoli, Chinese, see "Kale, Chinese"							

Food and Measure	cal.	prot. (gms)	carbo. (gms)	fat (gms)	chol. (mgs)	sod. (mgs)	fiber (gms)
Broccoli, freeze-dried							
chopped (*Alpine-Aire*), ¼ oz.	25	2.0	4.0	0	0	20	2.0
Broccoli, frozen:							
spears:							
(*Birds Eye*),							
2 spears, 3.1 oz.	30	2.0	4.0	0	0	25	2.0
(*Green Giant*),							
3.5 oz., approx.							
3 spears	25	2.0	4.0	0	0	120	2.0
(*Green Giant Select*),							
3 oz., approx.							
3 spears	25	2.0	4.0	0	0	20	2.0
baby (*Birds Eye*),							
4 spears, 3 oz. ..	30	1.0	4.0	0	0	20	2.0
10-oz. pkg.	84	8.7	15.2	1.0	0	49	8.5
spears or chopped,							
boiled, drained,							
1 cup	52	5.7	9.8	.2	0	44	5.5
florets:							
(*Cascadian Farm*							
Bag), ⅔ cup	25	2.0	4.0	0	0	15	2.0
(*Cascadian Farm*							
Box), 1⅓ cups ..	25	2.0	4.0	0	0	110	2.0
(*C&W*), 5 pcs., 3 oz.	25	2.0	4.0	0	0	20	2.0
(*Green Giant Select*),							
1⅓ cups	25	2.0	4.0	0	0	20	2.0
baby (*Birds Eye*),							
1 cup	30	1.0	4.0	0	0	20	2.0
cuts:							
(*Birds Eye* Tender),							
1 cup	30	2.0	4.0	0	0	20	2.0
(*Cascadian Farm*),							
⅔ cup	20	2.0	4.0	0	0	20	2.0
(*Green Giant*), 1 cup	25	2.0	4.0	0	0	20	2.0
(*Green Giant* Boil-in-Bag), ⅔ cup .	25	2.0	4.0	0	0	-110	2.0
(*Tree of Life*), 1 cup	25	2.0	4.0	0	0	20	2.0
chopped:							
(*Green Giant*), ¾ cup	25	2.0	4.0	0	0	20	2.0
baby (*Birds Eye*),							
¾ cup	30	1.0	4.0	0	0	20	2.0
10-oz. pkg.	75	8.0	13.6	.8	0	68	8.5

Food and Measure	cal.	prot. (gms)	carbo. (gms)	fat (gms)	chol. (mgs)	sod. (mgs)	fiber (gms)
in butter sauce, spears (*Green Giant*), 4 oz., approx. 3 spears ..	50	3.0	6.0	2.0	<5	330	2.0
in cheese sauce:							
(*Birds Eye*), ½ cup	90	3.0	8.0	5.0	5	490	1.0
(*Green Giant*), ⅔ cup	80	3.0	9.0	3.0	<5	570	2.0
cheddar (*Cascadian Farm* Bag), ½ cup	60	5.0	7.0	2.5	5	290	3.0
cheddar (*Cascadian Farm* Box), ⅔ cup	70	4.0	7.0	2.5	5	310	2.0
three cheese (*Green Giant*), ½ cup cooked	50	3.0	5.0	2.5	<5	370	2.0
creamed (*C&W*), ½ cup	120	3.0	7.0	8.0	30	320	2.0
Broccoli combinations, frozen, 1 cup, except as noted:							
carrots, water chestnuts:							
(*Birds Eye*), 1 cup .	35	1.0	6.0	0	0	35	2.0
(*Green Giant Select*), ⅔ cup	25	1.0	5.0	0	0	30	2.0
cauliflower:							
(*Birds Eye*), 1 cup .	25	1.0	4.0	0	0	25	2.0
cauliflower, carrots:							
(*Green Giant Select*), ⅔ cup	25	2.0	4.0	0	0	30	2.0
cheese sauce (*Green Giant*), ½ cup cooked ..	50	2.0	7.0	2.0	<5	320	2.0
cheese sauce (*Green Giant* Boil-in-Bag), ⅔ cup .	80	3.0	9.0	3.0	<5	560	2.0
corn, peppers (*Birds Eye*), ¾ cup	60	2.0	11.0	1.0	0	10	1.0
green beans, onion, pepper (*Birds Eye*), 1 cup	30	1.0	5.0	0	0	10	2.0
peppers, onion, mushrooms (*Birds Eye*), 1 cup	30	1.0	4.0	0	0	15	1.0

Food and Measure	cal.	prot. (gms)	carbo. (gms)	fat (gms)	chol. (mgs)	sod. (mgs)	fiber (gms)
Broccoli combinations, frozen *(cont.)*							
red peppers, sugar snap, water chestnuts (*C&W*), 1 cup	40	2.0	6.0	0	0	15	2.0
Broccoli dish, frozen:							
nuggets (*Dr. Praeger's*), 4 pcs., 1.4 oz.	45	2.0	5.0	2.0	0	135	1.0
pancake, 1.3-oz. pc.:							
(*Dr. Praeger's*)	40	1.0	5.0	2.0	0	130	<1.0
(*Dr. Praeger's* Bombay)	70	2.0	8.0	3.0	15	150	1.0
Broccoli entree, frozen pot pie (*Amy's*), 7.5 oz.	430	11.0	46.0	22.0	45	630	4.0
Broccoli rabe, fresh:							
(*Andy Boy*), 1/5 bunch, 3 oz.	30	3.0	3.0	0	0	45	2.0
(*Frieda's* Rapini), 3 oz.	25	3.0	4.0	0	0	25	0
cooked (*Ready Pac*), ½ cup	30	3.0	3.0	0	0	50	2.0
Broccoli rabe, frozen (*Seabrook Farms*), 1 cup	25	2.0	4.0	0	0	35	2.0
Broccoli snack rolls, frozen (*Health is Wealth Muchees*), 2 pcs., 1 oz.	60	2.0	10.0	1.5	0	170	1.0
Broccoli sprouts (*Jonathan's*), 1 cup	35	2.0	5.0	.5	0	25	4.0
Broccoli-cheese pocket sandwich, frozen (*Amy's*), 4.5-oz. pc.	270	8.0	37.0	10.0	15	560	3.0
Broiling sauce, see "Grilling sauce"							
Brown gravy, w/onion (*Campbell's*), 1/4 cup	25	0	4.0	1.0	0	330	<1.0
Brown gravy mix, 1/4 cup*:							
(*Lawry's*)	20	0	4.0	0	0	340	0
(*McCormick*)	20	0	3.0	.5	0	340	0
Brownie, 1 pc., except as noted:							
(*Hostess* Bites), 3 pcs., 1.3 oz.	170	2.0	21.0	9.0	30	80	1.0

Food and Measure	cal.	prot. (gms)	carbo. (gms)	fat (gms)	chol. (mgs)	sod. (mgs)	fiber (gms)
chocolate chip:							
(*Awrey's* Decadent),							
1.6 oz.	190	2.0	27.0	8.0	20	95	<1.0
(*Awrey's* Low Fat),							
1.3 oz.	130	2.0	27.0	3.0	0	115	<1.0
peanut butter							
(*Awrey's*), 1.6 oz.	200	3.0	25.0	10.0	20	100	<1.0
fudge, 1.5 oz.:							
(*Entenmann's*),							
½ pc.	180	2.0	25.0	9.0	30	85	1.0
(*Little Debbie*)	270	2.0	39.0	12.0	10	140	1.0
wheat free (*Foods by*							
George), 1/9 slice .	210	2.0	28.0	10.0	20	25	1.0
Brownie, frozen, choc-							
olate fudge, triple							
(*Sara Lee*), .7-oz. pc.	90	1.0	12.0	4.0	5	30	1.0
Brownie, mix,							
1/20 pkg.*, except							
as noted:							
(*Betty Crocker*							
Supreme Original) .	160	2.0	27.0	6.0	20	110	0
w/caramel and walnuts							
(*Betty Crocker*							
Supreme Turtle) ...	170	2.0	23.0	8.0	20	100	0
chocolate:							
dark (*Betty Crocker*							
Supreme)	170	2.0	25.0	7.0	20	110	0
fudge, dark (*Betty*							
Crocker)	170	2.0	24.0	7.0	20	110	0
fudge, dark (*Duncan*							
Hines Family),							
1/18 pkg.*	170	2.0	25.0	7.0	15	140	<1.0
German (*Betty*							
Crocker)	190	2.0	29.0	8.0	20	135	1.0
milk, chunk (*Dun-*							
can Hines Choco-							
late Lovers),							
1/16 pkg.*	170	2.0	25.0	7.0	15	110	1.0
triple (*Duncan*							
Hines Deca-							
dence), 1/16 pkg.*	180	2.0	25.0	9.0	15	110	1.0
walnut (*Duncan*							
Hines Chocolate							
Lovers),							
1/16 pkg.*	180	2.0	24.0	8.0	15	115	2.0

Food and Measure	cal.	prot. (gms)	carbo. (gms)	fat (gms)	chol. (mgs)	sod. (mgs)	fiber (gms)
Brownie, mix *(cont.)*							
chocolate chunk:							
(*Betty Crocker* Supreme)	180	2.0	25.0	9.0	20	95	1.0
triple (*Betty Crocker* Supreme)	180	2.0	25.0	9.0	20	95	1.0
walnut (*Betty Crocker* Supreme)	180	2.0	24.0	9.0	20	95	1.0
frosted (*Betty Crocker* Supreme)	200	2.0	31.0	9.0	20	130	1.0
fudge:							
(*Betty Crocker*) ...	170	2.0	23.0	7.0	20	105	0
(*Betty Crocker* Low Fat), 1/18 pkg.* .	130	2.0	27.0	2.5	0	115	1.0
(*Betty Crocker* Pouch), 1/9 pkg.*	190	2.0	27.0	8.0	25	125	1.0
(*"Jiffy"*), 1/5 cup mix	150	1.0	28.0	4.0	0	150	<1.0
chewy (*Duncan Hines* Family Style)	180	2.0	24.0	9.0	20	120	<1.0
peanut butter (*Betty Crocker* Supreme) .	180	3.0	23.0	9.0	20	105	0
pecan (*Betty Crocker* Supreme)	170	2.0	22.0	9.0	20	95	1.0
walnut (*Betty Crocker* Supreme)	180	2.0	22.0	9.0	20	95	0
w/whole wheat flour, flax seeds (*Hodgson Mill*), 3 tbsp. mix ..	120	3.0	28.0	.5	0	80	2.0
Brownie à la mode, see "Ice cream dessert"							
Browning sauce:							
(*GravyMaster*), ¼ tsp.	0	0	<1.0	0	0	30	0
(*Kitchen Bouquet*), 1 tsp.	15	0	3.0	0	0	10	0
Bruegger's:							
bagels, 1 pc.:							
plain	300	12.0	61.0	2.0	0	540	4.0
blueberry	330	11.0	68.0	2.0	0	530	4.0
chocolate chip	310	11.0	69.0	4.5	0	500	4.0
cinnamon raisin ...	320	11.0	68.0	2.0	0	510	4.0
cinnamon sugar ...	340	12.0	71.0	2.0	0	540	6.0

Food and Measure	cal.	prot. (gms)	carbo. (gms)	fat (gms)	chol. (mgs)	sod. (mgs)	fiber (gms)
cranberry orange ..	330	11.0	68.0	2.0	0	510	4.0
everything	310	12.0	62.0	2.0	0	710	4.0
garlic	310	12.0	62.0	2.0	0	540	4.0
honey grain	330	13.0	64.0	3.0	0	500	5.0
jalapeño	310	12.0	63.0	2.0	0	550	4.0
onion	310	12.0	62.0	2.0	0	540	4.0
poppy	310	12.0	61.0	2.5	0	540	4.0
pumpernickel	320	12.0	64.0	2.5	0	600	5.0
rosemary olive oil .	350	11.0	62.0	6.0	0	530	4.0
salt	300	12.0	61.0	2.0	0	1540	4.0
sesame	320	12.0	61.0	2.0	0	540	4.0
sun-dried tomato ..	320	12.0	61.0	2.0	0	540	4.0
cream cheese, 2 tbsp.:							
plain	90	2.0	4.0	8.0	25	85	0
plain, light	70	2.0	3.0	4.5	15	90	0
bacon scallion	100	2.0	4.0	8.0	30	105	0
chive	100	2.0	2.0	9.0	30	90	0
garden veggie	90	2.0	3.0	8.0	25	95	0
garden veggie, light	60	4.0	2.0	4.0	15	75	0
herb garlic, light ...	70	4.0	3.0	4.5	15	85	0
honey walnut	110	2.0	5.0	8.0	25	85	0
jalapeño	100	2.0	3.0	9.0	30	100	0
olive pimento	100	2.0	2.0	9.0	30	90	0
smoked salmon ...	100	2.0	2.0	9.0	25	105	0
strawberry, light ...	70	4.0	4.0	4.0	15	85	0
wildberry	100	2.0	4.0	9.0	25	85	0
sandwich, breakfast:							
egg/cheese	480	22.0	66.0	15.0	190	840	4.0
egg/cheese/bacon .	560	26.0	66.0	22.0	220	1070	4.0
egg/cheese/ham ...	520	28.0	66.0	17.0	205	1350	4.0
egg/cheese/sausage	680	33.0	66.0	33.0	235	1570	4.0
sandwich, deli:							
chicken breast	440	37.0	62.0	6.0	60	1230	4.0
chicken salad, mayo	460	24.0	67.0	12.0	55	820	4.0
ham, honey mustard	440	24.0	77.0	4.5	30	1440	4.0
turkey, mayo	480	25.0	65.0	14.0	35	1220	4.0
filling only:							
hummus, 2 tbsp.	60	2.0	4.0	3.5	0	85	2.0
tuna salad, 2.5 oz.	180	8.0	6.0	14.0	20	440	0
sandwich, specialty:							
chicken fajita	500	28.0	74.0	12.0	85	970	5.0
garden veggie	390	16.0	80.0	2.5	0	610	7.0
Leonardo da Veggie	460	19.0	69.0	11.0	40	740	4.0

Food and Measure	cal.	prot. (gms)	carbo. (gms)	fat (gms)	chol. (mgs)	sod. (mgs)	fiber (gms)
Bruegger's, sandwich, specialty *(cont.)*							
smoked salmon ...	470	26.0	66.0	12.0	55	590	4.0
turkey, herby	530	28.0	73.0	14.0	55	1180	4.0
turkey, Santa Fe ...	480	29.0	71.0	10.0	55	1630	4.0
desserts:							
Blondie bar	370	5.0	42.0	23.0	25	220	2.0
brownie, chocolate							
chunk	330	4.0	39.0	19.0	55	150	2.0
brownie, mint	300	3.0	34.0	17.0	40	95	0
Bruegger Bar	420	6.0	47.0	24.0	15	240	3.0
cappuccino bar ...	420	5.0	45.0	25.0	60	125	1.0
lemon bar	350	4.0	39.0	20.0	85	260	0
oatmeal cranberry							
mountain	430	7.0	49.0	24.0	60	320	3.0
pecan chocolate							
chunk bar	350	4.0	32.0	24.0	80	160	1.0
raspberry sammies	270	3.0	36.0	13.0	35	130	1.0
Bruschetta, frozen, pesto, mozzarella, tomato (*Cedarlane*), 1.25-oz. pc.	100	3.0	10.0	5.0	5	190	.5
Bruschetta topping, olive (*Delallo*), 2 tbsp.	70	0	1.0	8.0	0	140	0
Brussels sprouts, fresh:							
raw:							
(*Dole*), 4 pcs., 3 oz.	40	2.0	6.0	.5	0	25	3.0
½ cup	19	1.5	3.9	.1	0	11	1.8
boiled, .7-oz. pc.	8	.5	1.8	.1	0	4	.9
boiled, drained, ½ cup	30	2.0	6.8	.4	0	17	3.4
Brussels sprouts, frozen:							
(*Birds Eye*), 10 pcs., 3 oz.	45	3.0	8.0	0	0	15	3.0
(*Birds Eye* Tender), 6 pcs., 3 oz.	45	3.0	8.0	0	0	15	3.0
(*C&W* Petite), 3 oz., approx. 10 pcs. ...	30	3.0	5.0	0	0	25	3.0
in butter sauce (*Green Giant*), ½ cup cooked	45	3.0	6.0	1.0	<5	310	3.0
boiled, drained, ½ cup	33	2.8	6.5	.3	0	18	1.4

Food and Measure	cal.	prot. (gms)	carbo. (gms)	fat (gms)	chol. (mgs)	sod. (mgs)	fiber (gms)
Brussels sprouts com-							
binations, frozen,							
cauliflower, carrots							
(*Birds Eye*), 1 cup .	40	2.0	7.0	0	0	35	2.0
Buckwheat, grain:							
1 oz.	97	3.8	20.3	1.0	0	<1	2.8
1 cup	584	22.5	121.6	5.8	0	1	17.0
Buckwheat flour:							
(*Arrowhead Mills*),							
⅓ cup	115	5.0	20.0	1.5	0	0	6.0
(*Hodgson Mill*), ⅓ cup	160	7.0	33.0	1.0	0	10	2.0
(*Shiloh Farms*), ¼ cup	100	4.0	21.0	1.0	0	0	3.0
1 cup :	402	15.1	84.7	3.7	0	13	12.0
Buckwheat groats:							
(*Arrowhead Mills*),							
¼ cup	150	5.0	31.0	1.0	0	0	4.0
(*Shiloh Farms*), ¼ cup	140	5.0	30.0	1.0	0	0	3.0
roasted, dry:							
(*Shiloh Farms*							
Kasha), ¼ cup . .	140	5.0	30.0	1.0	0	0	3.0
(*Wolff's* Kasha),							
¼ cup	170	6.0	35.0	1.0	0	10	2.0
1 oz.	98	3.3	21.2	.8	0	3	.8
roasted, cooked, 1 cup	182	6.7	39.5	1.2	0	8	4.5
Buffalo wing sauce,							
see "Wing sauce"							
Bulgur:							
dry:							
(*Shiloh Farms*),							
¼ cup	150	5.0	33.0	.5	0	0	4.0
(*Shiloh Farms*							
Organic), ⅓ cup .	150	5.0	33.0	.5	0	0	4.0
¼ cup	120	4.3	26.6	.5	0	6	6.4
cooked, 1 cup	152	5.6	33.8	.4	0	9	8.2
Bulgur salad, see							
"Tabouli"							
Bun, see "Roll"							
Bun, sweet, frozen or							
refrigerated, 1 pc.:							
caramel (*Pillsbury*) . .	170	2.0	24.0	7.0	0	320	<1.0
cinnamon, plain:							
(*Rhodes*)	240	4.0	42.0	7.0	0	250	1.0
(*Rhodes Anytime!*)	240	4.0	39.0	6.0	0	465	1.0

Food and Measure	cal.	prot. (gms)	carbo. (gms)	fat (gms)	chol. (mgs)	sod. (mgs)	fiber (gms)
Bun, sweet, cinnamon, plain *(cont.)*							
giant *(Rhodes)*	220	4.0	37.0	6.0	0	240	1.0
cinnamon, w/frosting*							
(Rhodes Anytime!)	310	4.0	51.0	9.5	0	470	1.0
(Sara Lee Deluxe) .	320	5.0	41.0	15.0	40	300	1.0
giant *(Rhodes)*	265	4.0	44.0	8.0	5	260	1.0
cinnamon, w/icing:							
(Grands!)	330	5.0	53.0	11.0	0	650	1.0
(Grands! Reduced Fat)	310	5.0	54.0	8.0	0	660	1.0
(Pillsbury Bakery Style)	560	9.0	92.0	17.0	25	970	2.0
(Pillsbury Oven Baked)	290	6.0	46.0	10.0	15	720	1.0
(Pillsbury Reduced Fat)	140	2.0	24.0	3.5	0	340	<1.0
butter cream, extra rich *(Grands!)* . .	340	5.0	52.0	12.0	0	670	1.0
cream cheese icing *(Grands!)*	330	5.0	52.0	11.0	0	640	1.0
regular or cream cheese *(Pillsbury)*	150	2.0	23.0	5.0	0	340	<1.0
cinnamon, toaster, mini: *(Eggo Toaster Swirlz)*, 1 set, 4 pcs.	120	2.0	20.0	3.0	5	200	<1.0
cinnamon raisin, w/icing *(Pillsbury)* .	170	2.0	26.0	6.0	0	320	<1.0
orange, plain:							
(Rhodes)	240	4.0	42.0	7.0	0	250	1.0
(Rhodes Anytime!)	220	4.0	39.0	5.0	0	465	1.0
orange, w/frosting*:							
(Rhodes)	285	4.0	49.0	9.5	0	482	1.0
(Rhodes Anytime) .	300	4.0	51.0	8.5	5	500	1.0
orange, w/icing *(Pillsbury)*	170	2.0	25.0	7.0	0	340	<1.0
strawberry, toaster, mini *(Eggo Toaster Swirlz)*, 1 set, 4 pcs.	110	2.0	19.0	3.0	5	210	<1.0
Burbot, meat only:							
raw, 4 oz.	102	21.9	0	.9	68	110	0
baked, broiled, or microwaved, 4 oz. . .	130	28.1	0	1.2	87	141	0

Food and Measure	cal.	prot. (gms)	carbo. (gms)	fat (gms)	chol. (mgs)	sod. (mgs)	fiber (gms)
Burdock root:							
raw:							
(*Frieda's* Gobo Root), ¾ cup, 3 oz.	60	1.0	15.0	0	0	0	3.0
7.3-oz. pc.	112	1.3	13.6	.1	0	4	5.1
pieces, ½ cup	43	.9	10.3	.1	0	3	1.9
boiled, 1" pcs., ½ cup	55	1.3	13.2	.1	0	3	1.1
Burger, see "Beef pocket/sandwich"							
Burger, vegetarian:							
canned:							
(*Loma Linda* Redi-Burger), ⅝" slice, 3 oz.	120	18.0	7.0	2.5	0	450	4.0
(*Loma Linda* Vege-Burger), ¼ cup .	60	12.0	2.0	.5	0	130	2.0
(*Worthington* Burger), ¼ cup .	70	10.0	3.0	1.5	0	250	1.0
frozen:							
crumbles (*Morningstar Farms* Grillers), ⅔ cup	80	10.0	4.0	2.5	0	210	2.0
ground (*Boca*), 2 oz.	60	13.0	6.0	.5	0	270	3.0
mix:							
(*Fantastic* Nature's Burger), ¼ cup .	170	8.0	30.0	3.0	0	320	5.0
tofu (*Fantastic*), 3 tbsp.	80	3.0	13.0	2.5	0	400	1.0
Burger patty, vegetarian, frozen, 1 pc., 2.5 oz., except as noted:							
(*Boca* Original Vegan)	70	13.0	6.0	1.0	0	330	4.0
(*Garden Gourmet* Veggie Patties), 2.6 oz.	90	7.0	6.0	4.0	0	430	4.0
(*Morningstar Farms* Better'n Burgers) . .	100	13.0	6.0	2.0	0	310	3.0
(*Morningstar Farms* Garden Veggie Patties), 2.4 oz. . . .	100	10.0	9.0	2.5	0	350	4.0
(*Morningstar Farms* Grillers Original), 2.25 oz.	140	15.0	5.0	6.0	0	260	2.0

Food and Measure	cal.	prot. (gms)	carbo. (gms)	fat (gms)	chol. (mgs)	sod. (mgs)	fiber (gms)
Burger patty, vegetarian, frozen *(cont.)*							
(*Morningstar Farms Harvest Burgers*), 3.2 oz.	140	18.0	8.0	4.0	0	390	5.0
(*Yves* The Good Burger Original), 2.6 oz.	110	12.0	7.0	4.0	0	470	3.0
(*Yves* Veggie Authentic), 2.6 oz. . .	120	11.0	9.0	4.5	0	450	7.0
(*Yves* Veggie Chick'n), 2.6 oz.	100	15.0	5.0	2.5	0	350	2.0
all American:							
(*Amy's*)	120	10.0	15.0	3.0	0	390	3.0
(*Boca*)	150	15.0	9.0	5.0	10	500	3.0
black bean, spicy (*Morningstar Farms*), 2.75 oz. . . .	150	11.0	16.0	4.5	0	470	5.0
Bombay (*Dr. Praeger's*), 2.75 oz.	100	8.0	9.5	3.3	0	190	4.0
California:							
(*Amy's*)	130	6.0	19.0	5.0	0	430	5.0
(*Dr. Praeger's*), 2.75 oz.	100	8.0	9.5	3.3	0	190	4.0
(*Dr. Praeger's Family Pack*), 3.8 oz.	100	7.0	12.0	4.0	0	220	5.0
char-broiled (*Garden Gourmet* Veggie Patties), 2.6 oz. . . .	100	14.0	2.0	4.0	0	440	4.0
cheeseburger (*Boca*) .	100	12.0	5.0	5.0	5	360	3.0
Chicago (*Amy's*)	160	10.0	20.0	5.0	5	390	3.0
fajita (*Morningstar Farms*), 2.25 oz. . . .	130	8.0	7.0	7.0	5	290	3.0
garlic, roasted (*Boca*)	80	13.0	6.0	2.0	0	380	4.0
Italian (*Dr. Praeger's*), 2.75 oz.	100	8.0	9.5	3.3	0	190	4.0
onion, roasted (*Boca*)	130	15.0	10.0	3.0	0	500	4.0
Philly cheese steak burger (*Morningstar Farms*), 2.25 oz. . . .	120	10.0	6.0	6.0	5	400	3.0
pizza burger:							
(*Dr. Praeger's*), 3.1 oz.	120	9.0	11.5	4.0	5	240	4.0

Food and Measure	cal.	prot. (gms)	carbo. (gms)	fat (gms)	chol. (mgs)	sod. (mgs)	fiber (gms)
tomato and basil (*Morningstar Farms*), 2.4 oz...	130	11.0	7.0	6.0	10	320	7.0
portobello mushroom and peppers (*Morningstar Farms*), 2.4 oz.	120	12.0	9.0	4.0	0	470	3.0
prime (*Morningstar Farms Grillers*)	170	16.0	5.0	9.0	0	390	2.0
savory (*Yves*), 2.6 oz.	150	6.0	18.0	6.0	5	350	4.0
soy or Tex-Mex (*Dr. Praeger's*), 2.75 oz.	100	8.0	9.5	3.3	0	190	4.0
Texas (*Amy's*)	120	12.0	14.0	2.5	0	350	3.0
vegetable, grilled (*Boca*)	70	12.0	6.0	1.0	5	300	4.0
Burger King, 1 serving:							
breakfast:							
Croissan'wich:							
egg/cheese	300	12.0	26.0	17.0	195	700	<1.0
bacon/egg/cheese	340	14.0	26.0	7.0	200	920	<1.0
ham/egg/cheese .	340	17.0	26.0	18.0	210	1470	<1.0
sausage/cheese .	410	13.0	24.0	29.0	45	830	1.0
sausage/egg/ cheese	500	18.0	26.0	36.0	220	1060	1.0
Croissan'wich, double:							
double bacon ...	430	19.0	27.0	26.0	220	1360	<1.0
double ham	420	26.0	27.0	23.0	235	2450	<1.0
double, sausage .	750	28.0	26.0	60.0	260	1630	2.0
ham/bacon	420	23.0	27.0	25.0	225	1910	<1.0
ham/sausage ...	580	27.0	27.0	41.0	245	2040	1.0
sausage/bacon ..	590	24.0	27.0	43.0	240	1490	1.0
Enormous Omelet sandwich	760	35.0	44.0	50.0	420	2080	3.0
French toast sticks, 5	390	6.0	46.0	20.0	0	440	2.0
hash brown rounds:							
small	230	2.0	23.0	15.0	0	450	2.0
medium	390	3.0	38.0	25.0	0	760	4.0
jam, grape/straw- berry	30	0	7.0	0	0	0	0
syrup	80	0	21.0	0	0	20	0
burgers:							
Angus burger	570	33.0	62.0	22.0	180	1270	3.0

Food and Measure	cal.	prot. (gms)	carbo. (gms)	fat (gms)	chol. (mgs)	sod. (mgs)	fiber (gms)
Burger King, burgers *(cont.)*							
bacon/cheese ...	710	41.0	64.0	33.0	215	1990	3.0
low carb	260	24.0	2.0	18.0	180	490	<1.0
bacon cheeseburger	390	22.0	31.0	20.0	60	990	1.0
double	570	35.0	32.0	34.0	110	1250	2.0
BK Veggie Burger ..	420	23.0	46.0	16.0	10	1090	7.0
w/out mayo	340	23.0	46.0	8.0	0	1020	7.0
cheeseburger	350	19.0	31.0	17.0	50	770	1.0
cheeseburger, double	530	32.0	32.0	31.0	100	1030	2.0
Double Whopper ..	970	52.0	52.0	61.0	160	1110	4.0
w/cheese	1060	56.0	53.0	69.0	185	1540	4.0
w/cheese, no mayo	900	56.0	53.0	51.0	170	1410	4.0
w/cheese, low carb	630	48.0	5.0	47.0	170	810	<1.0
w/out mayo	810	52.0	52.0	44.0	150	980	4.0
low carb	540	43.0	3.0	40.0	150	380	<1.0
hamburger	310	17.0	30.0	13.0	40	550	1.0
hamburger double .	440	28.0	30.0	23.0	75	600	1.0
Whopper	700	31.0	52.0	42.0	85	1020	4.0
w/cheese	800	35.0	53.0	49.0	110	1450	4.0
w/cheese, no mayo	640	35.0	53.0	31.0	95	1330	4.0
w/cheese, low carb	370	27.0	5.0	28.0	95	720	<1.0
w/out mayo	540	30.0	52.0	24.0	75	900	4.0
low carb	280	22.0	3.0	20.0	75	290	<1.0
Whopper, Jr.	390	17.0	31.0	22.0	45	550	2.0
w/cheese	430	19.0	32.0	26.0	55	770	2.0
w/cheese, no mayo	350	19.0	32.0	17.0	50	700	2.0
w/cheese, low carb	190	14.0	2.0	14.0	50	360	0
w/out mayo	310	17.0	31.0	13.0	40	490	2.0
low carb	140	11.0	1.0	10.0	40	140	0
sandwiches:							
BK Big Fish	630	23.0	69.0	30.0	55	1340	4.0
spicy	630	23.0	69.0	30.0	55	1490	4.0
spicy, w/out tartar sauce	480	23.0	68.0	13.0	40	1190	4.0
chicken	560	25.0	52.0	28.0	60	1270	3.0
chicken, w/out mayo	460	25.0	52.0	17.0	55	1190	3.0
Chicken Whopper ..	570	38.0	48.0	25.0	75	1410	4.0

Food and Measure	cal.	prot. (gms)	carbo. (gms)	fat (gms)	chol. (mgs)	sod. (mgs)	fiber (gms)
w/out mayo	410	38.0	48.0	7.0	60	1280	4.0
low carb	160	30.0	3.0	3.5	60	850	1.0
Tendercrisp chicken	780	27.0	70.0	45.0	55	1730	6.0
spicy	720	26.0	71.0	37.0	50	1990	6.0
spicy, w/out							
sauce or mayo	570	26.0	70.0	21.0	40	1540	6.0
Chicken Tenders:							
4 pcs.	170	11.0	10.0	9.0	25	420	0
5 pcs.	210	14.0	13.0	12.0	30	530	<1.0
6 pcs.	250	16.0	15.0	14.0	35	630	<1.0
8 pcs.	340	22.0	20.0	19.0	50	840	<1.0
dipping sauce, 1 oz.:							
barbecue	35	0	9.0	0	0	390	0
honey flavored	90	0	23.0	0	0	0	0
honey mustard	90	0	9.0	6.0	10	150	0
onion ring sauce ..	150	0	3.0	15.0	15	210	<1.0
ranch	140	1.0	1.0	15.0	5	95	0
sweet and sour ...	40	0	10.0	0	0	65	0
sides:							
bacon, 1 strip	15.0	1.0	0	1.0	5.0	70	0
fries, salted:							
king	600	7.0	76.0	30.0	0	1070	6.0
king, no salt	600	7.0	76.0	30.0	0	620	6.0
large	500	6.0	63.0	25.0	0	880	5.0
large, no salt ...	500	6.0	63.0	25.0	0	510	5.0
medium	360	4.0	46.0	18.0	0	640	4.0
medium, no salt .	360	4.0	46.0	18.0	0	380	4.0
small	230	3.0	29.0	11.0	0	410	2.0
small, no salt ...	230	3.0	29.0	11.0	0	240	2.0
ketchup, 1 pkt.	10	0	3.0	0	0	125	0
onion rings:							
king	550	8.0	70.0	27.0	5.0	800	5.0
large	480	7.0	60.0	23.0	0	690	5.0
medium	320	4.0	40.0	16.0	0	460	3.0
small	180	2.0	22.0	9.0	0	260	2.0
salad, no dressing/							
toast:							
chicken Caesar	190	25.0	9.0	7.0	50	900	1.0
chicken Caesar,							
Tendercrisp	390	24.0	25.0	22.0	40	1160	4.0
garden	20	1.0	4.0	0	0	15.0	<1.0
garden, chicken ...	210	26.0	12.0	7.0	50	910	2.0
garden, chicken							
Tendercrisp	410	25.0	28.0	22.0	40	1170	5.0

Food and Measure	cal.	prot. (gms)	carbo. (gms)	fat (gms)	chol. (mgs)	sod. (mgs)	fiber (gms)
***Burger King,* salad, no dressing/toast** *(cont.)*							
garden, shrimp . . .	200	21.0	13.0	10.0	120	900	3.0
shrimp Caesar	180	20.0	9.0	10.0	120	880	2.0
salad dressing/toast:							
garden ranch	120	1.0	7.0	10.0	20	610	0
garlic Caesar	130	2.0	7.0	11.0	20	710	0
honey mustard	70	0	18.0	0	0	230	0
onion vinaigrette . .	100	0	8.0	8.0	0	960	0
tomato balsamic vinaigrette	110	0	9.0	9.0	0	760	0
toast, garlic Parmesan	70	2.0	9.0	2.5	0	120	0
shakes:							
vanilla, medium . . .	540	11.0	76.0	20.0	80	320	0
vanilla, large	800	16.0	113	29.0	120	480	<1.0
vanilla, small	400	8.0	57.0	15.0	60	240	0
shakes, syrup added:							
chocolate, large . . .	850	15.0	133.0	27.0	105	620	2.0
chocolate, medium	600	10.0	97.0	18.0	70	470	2.0
chocolate, small . . .	410	7.0	65.0	13.0	50	300	<1.0
strawberry, large . .	840	14.0	131.0	26.0	105	450	<1.0
strawberry, medium	590	9.0	96.0	17.0	70	300	0
strawberry, small . .	410	7.0	64.0	13.0	50	220	0
Icee, cherry or *Coca-Cola),* medium	140	0	40.0	0	0	10	0
dessert, pie:							
Dutch apple	300	2.0	45.0	13.0	0	270	1.0
Hershey's sundae . .	300	3.0	31.0	18.0	10	190	1.0
Burger sauce, see "Sandwich spread"							
Burrito (see also "Burrito, breakfast"), frozen, 1 pc.:							
bean/cheese:							
(*Amy's*), 6 oz.	280	10.0	43.0	8.0	10	540	6.0
(*El Monterey*), 4 oz.	220	7.0	24.0	6.0	5	460	4.0
(*El Monterey*), 5 oz.	280	9.0	43.0	8.0	5	580	5.0
(*El Monterey*), 8 oz.	450	14.0	69.0	12.0	10	930	8.0
(*El Monterey* XX Large!), 10 oz. . .	560	18.0	87.0	15.0	10	1160	9.0
(*Reser's*), 5 oz.	340	11.0	51.0	11.0	5	660	5.0
bean/rice (*Amy's*), 6 oz.	280	9.0	48.0	6.0	0	550	5.0
bean/rice/cheese (*Cedarlane* Low Fat), 6 oz.	260	13.0	48.0	1.0	0	490	7.0

Food and Measure	cal.	prot. (gms)	carbo. (gms)	fat (gms)	chol. (mgs)	sod. (mgs)	fiber (gms)
beef:							
grilled fajita (*El Monterey Supreme*), 5 oz. . . .	280	11.0	48.0	4.5	10	730	2.0
steak, shredded (*El Monterey* Carb Friendly), 5 oz. . .	320	20.0	26.0	15.0	60	910	14.0
taco seasoned (*El Monterey*), 4 oz.	290	9.0	32.0	14.0	15	600	2.0
beef/bean:							
(*El Monterey*), 4 oz.	300	9.0	34.0	14.0	15	580	3.0
(*El Monterey*), 5 oz.	380	11.0	42.0	18.0	20	720	4.0
(*El Monterey*), 8 oz.	600	17.0	68.0	29.0	35	1150	7.0
(*El Monterey* XX Large!), 10 oz. . .	750	21.0	86.0	36.0	40	1440	9.0
(*El Monterey* Red Hot), 5 oz.	380	11.0	42.0	18.0	20	700	4.0
(*El Monterey* Red Hot), 8 oz.	600	17.0	68.0	28.0	35	1150	7.0
(*El Monterey* Red Hot XX Large!), 10 oz.	750	21.0	86.0	36.0	40	1400	9.0
beef/bean, green chili:							
(*El Monterey*), 4 oz.	340	8.0	35.0	17.0	25	290	3.0
(*El Monterey*), 5 oz.	350	10.0	41.0	16.0	20	670	4.0
(*El Monterey* XX Large!), 10 oz. . .	700	21.0	84.0	31.0	35	1340	7.0
beef/bean, red chili:							
(*El Monterey*), 4 oz.	340	8.0	35.0	17.0	25	470	3.0
(*El Monterey*), 5 oz.	380	11.0	42.0	18.0	20	680	4.0
(*El Monterey*), 8 oz.	560	17.0	66.0	25.0	30	1030	6.0
(*El Monterey* XX Large!), 10 oz. . .	740	19.0	84.0	36.0	40	1100	8.0
beef/cheese, shredded (*El Monterey Supreme*), 5 oz.	290	13.0	37.0	10.0	30	370	1.0
black bean, 6 oz.:							
rice (*Amy's Especial*)	260	8.0	45.0	6.0	5	620	3.0
vegetable (*Amy's*) .	280	9.0	44.0	8.0	0	580	4.0
chicken:							
(*El Monterey*), 4 oz.	210	7.0	32.0	7.0	10	550	1.0
grilled (*El Monterey Supreme*), 5 oz. . .	280	10.0	44.0	7.0	20	410	2.0

Food and Measure	cal.	prot. (gms)	carbo. (gms)	fat (gms)	chol. (mgs)	sod. (mgs)	fiber (gms)
Burrito *(cont.)*							
chicken/cheese, chipotle (*El Monterey Carb Friendly*), 5 oz.	310	23.0	26.0	12.0	25	810	14.0
steak, char-broiled (*El Monterey*), 5 oz. . . .	290	15.0	39.0	9.0	25	460	1.0
vegetable/cheese (*Cedarlane*), 6 oz. . .	330	14.0	48.0	8.0	15	590	3.0
Burrito, breakfast, frozen, 1 pc.:							
(*Amy's*), 6 oz.	250	9.0	38.0	7.0	0	540	5.0
egg, cheese, salsa, bacon (*El Monterey Supreme*), 4.5 oz. .	290	13.0	36.0	11.0	120	740	1.0
egg sausage (*El Monterey Supreme*), 4.5 oz.	300	10.0	34.0	13.0	75	630	1.0
Burrito entree, frozen, ½ of 10-oz. pkg.:							
w/chili verde sauce (*Cedarlane* Grande)	230	9.0	27.0	10.0	20	540	2.0
w/salsa roja (*Cedarlane* Grande)	220	9.0	27.0	9.0	20	610	2.0
Burrito entree kit (*Old El Paso* Dinner Kit):							
as packaged, ⅛ pkg. . .	150	3.0	26.0	4.0	0	790	1.0
prepared, 1 burrito* . .	270	14.0	27.0	12.0	40	840	1.0
Burrito seasoning mix:							
(*Chi-Chi's* Fiesta), ¼ pkg.	40	1.0	6.0	1.0	0	520	1.0
(*Lawry's*), 2 tsp.	20	<1.0	4.0	0	0	390	<1.0
(*McCormick*), 1 tbsp.	25	0	5.0	.5	0	500	0
Burrito snack rolls, frozen (*Health is Wealth Munchees*), 10 pcs. 5 oz.	310	11.0	53.0	7.0	5	610	6.0
Butter, 1 tbsp., except as noted:							
(*Land O Lakes Ultra Creamy* Unsalted) .	110	0	0	12.0	30	0	0
(*Land O Lakes Ultra Creamy* Salted) . . .	110	0	0	12.0	30	85	0
regular, unsalted: (*Cabot*)	100	0	0	11.0	30	0	0

Food and Measure	cal.	prot. (gms)	carbo. (gms)	fat (gms)	chol. (mgs)	sod. (mgs)	fiber (gms)
(*Darigold*)	100	0	0	11.0	30	0	0
(*Land O Lakes*) . . .	100	0	0	11.0	30	0	0
(*Organic Valley*) . . .	100	0	0	11.0	30	0	0
1 stick or 4 oz.	813	1.0	0	92.0	248	12	0
1 tbsp.	100	.1	0	11.4	31	1	0
1 tsp.	34	<.1	0	3.8	10	<1	0
regular, salted:							
(*Cabot*)	100	0	0	11.0	30	90	0
(*Darigold*)	100	0	0	11.0	30	100	0
(*Land O Lakes*) . . .	100	0	0	11.0	30	95	0
(*Organic Valley*) . . .	100	0	0	11.0	30	75	0
1 stick or 4 oz.	813	1.0	0	92.0	248	937	0
1 tbsp.	100	.1	0	11.4	31	115	0
1 tsp.	34	<.1	0	3.8	10	39	0
whipped, unsalted:							
(*Darigold*)	70	0	0	8.0	20	0	0
(*Land O Lakes*) . . .	70	0	0	7.0	20	0	0
½ cup or 1 stick . .	542	.6	<.1	61.3	165	8	0
1 tbsp.	67	.1	tr.	7.6	20	1	0
1 tsp.	23	tr.	tr.	2.6	7	<1	0
whipped, salted:							
(*Darigold*)	70	0	0	8.0	20	65	0
(*Land O Lakes*) . . .	70	0	0	7.0	20	50	0
½ cup or 1 stick . .	542	.6	<.1	61.3	165	625	0
1 tbsp.	67	.1	tr.	7.6	20	78	0
1 tsp.	23	tr.	tr.	2.6	7	26	0
light, salted:							
(*Land O Lakes*) . . .	50	0	1.0	6.0	15	95	0
whipped (*Land O*							
Lakes)	45	0	1.0	5.0	15	80	0
w/canola oil, spread-							
able or soft baking							
(*Land O Lakes*) . . .	100	0	0	11.0	20	90	0
Butter, flavored,							
1 tbsp.:							
garlic, roasted, w/oil							
(*Land O Lakes*) . . .	100	0	0	11.0	20	110	0
honey:							
(*Downey's*)	60	0	11.0	1.0	<5	10	0
(*Land O Lakes*) . . .	90	0	4.0	8.0	15	35	0
Butter beans (see also							
"Lima beans"),							
canned, ½ cup:							
(*Bush's* Speckled) . . .	110	6.0	19.0	.5	0	420	5.0

Food and Measure	cal.	prot. (gms)	carbo. (gms)	fat (gms)	chol. (mgs)	sod. (mgs)	fiber (gms)
Butter beans *(cont.)*							
(*McKenzie's*)	100	6.0	20.0	0	0	130	4.0
(*S&W*)	80	6.0	19.0	0	0	500	5.0
baby:							
(*Allens*)	120	7.0	22.0	.5	0	460	6.0
(*Bush's*)	120	7.0	19.0	.5	0	510	5.0
green (*Sunshine*)	120	7.0	22.0	.5	0	460	6.0
large:							
(*Allens*)	120	7.0	20.0	1.0	0	290	7.0
(*Bush's*)	100	6.0	18.0	.5	0	450	5.0
white, w/sausage							
(*Trappey's*)	110	6.0	21.0	1.0	0	300	6.0
seasoned (*Glory*)	120	7.0	20.0	1.0	0	530	5.0
Butter flavor season-							
ing, 1 tsp.:							
(*Butter Buds*)	5	0	2.0	0	0	120	0
(*Molly McButter* Light							
Sodium)	5	0	2.0	0	0	90	0
(*Molly McButter*							
Natural)	5	0	1.0	0	0	180	0
cheese or roasted gar-							
lic (*Molly McButter*)	5	0	1.0	0	0	125	0
Butter oil, see "Oil"							
Butterbur, fresh:							
raw, .2-oz. stalk	1	<.1	.2	<.1	0	<1	<1.0
boiled, drained, 4 oz. .	9	.3	2.4	<.1	0	5	n.a.
Butterbur, canned,							
chopped, ½ cup . . .	2	.1	.2	.1	0	3	n.a.
Buttercup squash							
(*Frieda's*), ¾ cup,							
3 oz.	30	1.0	7.0	0	0	0	1.0
Butterfish, meat only:							
raw, 4 oz.	166	19.6	0	9.1	74	100	0
baked, broiled, or							
microwaved, 4 oz. .	212	25.1	0	11.7	94	129	0
Buttermilk, see "Milk"							
Butternut, dried:							
in shell, 1 lb.	750	30.5	14.8	69.8	0	1	5.8
shelled, 1 oz.	174	7.1	3.4	16.2	0	<1	1.3
Butternut squash:							
raw:							
(*Frieda's*), ¾ cup,							
3 oz.	30	1.0	7.0	0	0	0	1.0
cubed, ½ cup	32	.7	8.1	.1	0	3	1.1

Food and Measure	cal.	prot. (gms)	carbo. (gms)	fat (gms)	chol. (mgs)	sod. (mgs)	fiber (gms)
baked, cubed, ½ cup .	41	.9	10.7	.1	0	4	2.9
Butternut squash, frozen:							
12-oz. pkg.	192	6.0	49.0	.3	0	8	4.4
boiled, drained, mashed, ½ cup . . .	47	1.5	12.1	.1	0	2	n.a.
Butterscotch baking chips, 1 tbsp., .5 oz.:							
(*Guittard*)	80	<1.0	10.0	4.5	0	15	0
(*Hershey's Bake Shoppe*)	80	<1.0	10.0	4.0	0	10	0
Butterscotch syrup (*Smucker's Sundae Syrup*), 2 tbsp.	100	1.0	25.0	0	0	110	0
Butterscotch topping, 2 tbsp.:							
(*Hershey's*)	110	<1.0	27.0	0	0	120	0
(*Smucker's* Spoonable)	120	0	30.0	0	0	110	0
caramel (*Smucker's* Special Recipe) . . .	130	1.0	30.0	1.0	<5	70	<1.0

C

Food and Measure	cal.	prot. (gms)	carbo. (gms)	fat (gms)	chol. (mgs)	sod. (mgs)	fiber (gms)
Cabbage, fresh:							
raw:							
5¾" head, 2½ lbs. . .	228	13.1	49.3	2.4	0	164	20.9
shredded, ½ cup . .	9	.5	1.9	.1	0	6	.8
boiled, drained,							
shredded, ½ cup . .	17	.8	3.4	.3	0	6	2.1
Cabbage, can or jar:							
red, sweet and sour							
(*Greenwood*), ·							
½ cup	100	0	24.0	0	0	380	0
seasoned (*Glory*							
Country), ½ cup . .	30	1.0	6.0	0	0	300	2.0
Cabbage, Chinese,							
fresh, ½ cup, except							
as noted:							
bok-choy:							
raw (*Frieda's*),							
1 cup, 3 oz.	10	1.0	2.0	0	0	55	1.0
raw (*Frieda's Baby*),							
⅔ cup, 3 oz. . . .	10	1.0	2.0	0	0	35	1.0
raw, whole, 1 lb. . .	52	6.0	8.7	.8	0	257	4.0
raw, shredded	5	.5	.8	.1	0	23	.4
boiled, drained,							
shredded	10	1.3	1.5	.1	0	29	1.4
napa, raw (*Frieda's*),							
1 cup, 3 oz.	15	1.0	3.0	0	0	10	1.0
pe-tsai:							
raw, whole, 1 lb. . .	68	5.1	13.6	.8	0	38	4.2
raw, shredded	6	.5	1.2	.1	0	3	.4
boiled, drained,							
shredded	8	.9	1.4	.1	0	6	1.0
Cabbage, freeze-dried							
(*AlpineAire*), .9 oz. .	70	3.0	13.0	1.0	0	40	5.0

Food and Measure	cal.	prot. (gms)	carbo. (gms)	fat (gms)	chol. (mgs)	sod. (mgs)	fiber (gms)
Cabbage, frozen, seasoned (*Glory Savory Accents Country*), ½ cup ..	45	1.0	7.0	1.5	0	380	2.0
Cabbage, marinated, see "Kim chee"							
Cabbage, mustard, raw (*Frieda's* Gai Choy), 1 cup, 3 oz.	20	2.0	4.0	0	0	20	2.0
Cabbage, napa, see "Cabbage, Chinese"							
Cabbage, red, fresh:							
raw:							
whole, 1 lb.	100	5.0	22.2	.9	0	38	7.3
shredded (*Fresh Express*), 1 cup .	20	1.0	4.0	0	0	30	1.0
shredded, ½ cup ..	10	.5	2.1	.1	0	4	.7
boiled, drained,							
shredded, ½ cup ..	16	.8	3.5	.2	0	6	1.5
Cabbage, savoy, fresh:							
raw:							
whole, 1 lb.	100	7.3	22.1	.4	0	102	11.2
shredded, ½ cup ..	10	.7	2.1	<.1	0	10	1.1
boiled, drained,							
shredded, ½ cup ..	18	1.3	4.0	.1	0	17	n.a.
Cabbage, *Salad Savoy* (*Frieda's*), ⅔ cup, 3 oz.	25	2.0	5.0	0	0	25	3.0
Cabbage, stuffed, entree, frozen (*Lean Cuisine Everyday Favorites*), 9.5-oz. pkg.	200	10.0	26.0	6.0	15	700	4.0
Cabbage, Tuscan (*Frieda's*), ⅔ cup, 3 oz.	20	1.0	5.0	0	0	15	2.0
Cactus pads, fresh:							
raw:							
(*Frieda's*), ¾ cup, 3 oz.	20	1.0	4.0	0	0	5	1.0
sliced, 1 cup	14	1.1	2.9	.1	0	19	2.0
cooked:							
1 cup	22	2.0	4.9	.1	0	30	3.0
1 pad	4	.4	1.0	<.1	0	6	.6

Food and Measure	cal.	prot. (gms)	carbo. (gms)	fat (gms)	chol. (mgs)	sod. (mgs)	fiber (gms)
Cactus pads, canned:							
(*Doña Maria* Nopalitos), 2 tbsp. .	5	0	1.0	0	0	500	0
(*La Costeña* Nopalitos), 1 cup . .	20	0	4.0	0	0	2580	2.0
in escabeche (*Royal Crown* Nopalitos), ²/₃ cup	5	0	1.0	0	0	690	2.0
sliced, 2 tbsp.:							
(*Doña Maria* Nopalitos)	5	0	1.0	0	0	560	0
(*Embasa* Nopalitos)	5	0	1.0	0	0	830	2.0
Cactus pear, see "Prickly pear"							
Cajun seasoning:							
(*Luzianne*), ¼ tsp. . . .	0	0	0	0	0	260	0
(*McCormick*), ¼ tsp. .	0	0	0	0	0	135	0
(*McCormick 1 Step*), 1 tsp.	10	0	1.0	0	0	350	0
Cake, ⅛ cake, except as noted:							
banana crunch (*Entenmann's*)	230	2.0	32.0	10.0	35	290	<1.0
butter, 1/6 cake:							
(*Entenmann's* Sunshine)	310	4.0	44.0	14.0	90	380	0
loaf (*Entenmann's*) .	220	3.0	31.0	9.0	70	290	0
buttercream, French (*Awrey's* Dessert Cake), 1/9 cake . . .	230	2.0	37.0	9.0	15	280	<1.0
carrot (*Entenmann's* Deluxe), 1/9 cake . .	270	3.0	30.0	16.0	30	250	1.0
chocolate (*Bill Knapp's*)	330	3.0	54.0	12.0	20	380	1.0
chocolate chip, Swiss (*Entenmann's*), 1/9 cake	320	3.0	45.0	15.0	40	220	<1.0
chocolate fudge (*Entenmann's*)	270	3.0	40.0	12.0	15	250	2.0
crumb cake:							
(*Entenmann's* Ulti-mate), 1/10 cake	250	2.0	33.0	13.0	15	280	<1.0
chocolate chip, filled (*Entenmann's*), 1/9 cake	380	3.0	49.0	21.0	35	200	1.0

Food and Measure	cal.	prot. (gms)	carbo. (gms)	fat (gms)	chol. (mgs)	sod. (mgs)	fiber (gms)
raspberry almond (*Entenmann's* Ultimate), 1/10 cake	240	3.0	30.0	13.0	40	210	<1.0
wheat free (*Foods by George*), 1/9 cake	280	2.0	36.0	14.0	40	80	<1.0
golden, fudge iced (*Entenmann's*)	290	3.0	41.0	14.0	35	220	1.0
lemon:							
coconut (*Entenmann's*)	320	2.0	38.0	18.0	35	250	<1.0
crunch (*Entenmann's*), 1/9 cake	330	3.0	49.0	13.0	50	290	<1.0
marble loaf (*Entenmann's*)	190	2.0	27.0	8.0	40	260	<1.0
pound, wheat free (*Foods by George*), 2.7-oz. slice	290	4.0	35.0	15.0	130	190	<1.0
raisin loaf (*Entenmann's*)	220	2.0	35.0	8.0	40	210	1.0
sour cream loaf (*Entenmann's*)	220	2.0	26.0	12.0	45	160	0
Cake, frozen, 1/8 cake, except as noted:							
carrot:							
(*Mrs. Smith's*), 1/6 cake	300	3.0	37.0	16.0	30	360	1.0
(*Pepperidge Farm Dessert Classics*), 1/9 cake	280	2.0	32.0	16.0	25	230	1.0
(*Smart Ones*), 3.2-oz. pc.	220	3.0	33.0	3.5	5	260	2.0
cheese, see "Cheesecake"							
chocolate chip (*Kineret*), 2 slices, 2 oz.	200	2.0	27.0	10.0	45	170	0
chocolate:							
chunk (*Pepperidge Farm* 3 Layer) ..	260	2.0	41.0	9.0	20	115	<1.0
decadence (*Pepperidge Farm Dessert Classics*)	300	3.0	32.0	18.0	25	150	1.0

Food and Measure	cal.	prot. (gms)	carbo. (gms)	fat (gms)	chol. (mgs)	sod. (mgs)	fiber (gms)
Cake, frozen, chocolate *(cont.)*							
German (*Pepperidge Farm* 3 Layer) ..	250	2.0	31.0	13.0	25	150	<1.0
layer, double (*Sara Lee*)	260	3.0	33.0	13.0	10	230	2.0
chocolate fudge:							
(*Pepperidge Farm* 3 Layer)	250	3.0	31.0	11.0	30	160	1.0
double (*Smart Ones*), 2.7-oz. pc.	150	3.0	20.0	4.5	40	330	2.0
stripe (*Pepperidge Farm* 3 Layer) ..	250	2.0	31.0	13.0	25	140	<1.0
coffee cake:							
butter streusel (*Sara Lee*), 1/6 cake ..	190	3.0	25.0	9.0	35	190	1.0
crumb (*Sara Lee*) ..	190	2.0	30.0	8.0	20	150	1.0
pecan (*Sara Lee*), 1/6 cake	140	3.0	23.0	13.0	20	150	1.0
coconut layer:							
(*Pepperidge Farm* 3 Layer)	250	2.0	35.0	11.0	25	115	<1.0
(*Sara Lee*)	260	2.0	33.0	14.0	15	210	1.0
devil's food (*Pepperidge Farm* 3 Layer)	250	2.0	34.0	12.0	25	140	<1.0
golden layer:							
(*Pepperidge Farm* 3 Layer)	250	2.0	33.0	12.0	25	120	<1.0
fudge (*Sara Lee*) ..	260	2.0	34.0	13.0	15	200	1.0
guava (*Pepperidge Farm* 3 Layer)	190	1.0	36.0	5.0	15	100	<1.0
mango (*Pepperidge Farm* 3 Layer)	190	1.0	35.0	4.5	15	110	<1.0
marble (*Kineret*), 2 slices, 2 oz.	200	2.0	25.0	10.0	45	180	0
pineapple, golden (*Pepperidge Farm* Dessert Classics), 1/10 cake	270	2.0	34.0	14.0	15	150	1.0
pound cake:							
(*Sara Lee* Free & Light), ¼ cake ..	200	3.0	39.0	4.0	0	290	1.0
butter (*Sara Lee*), ¼ cake	240	4.0	37.0	16.0	115	160	1.0

Food and Measure	cal.	prot. (gms)	carbo. (gms)	fat (gms)	chol. (mgs)	sod. (mgs)	fiber (gms)
butter (*Sara Lee* Family Size), 1/6 cake	220	4.0	34.0	15.0	206	150	1.0
strawberry swirl (*Sara Lee*), ¼ cake	290	4.0	44.0	11.0	60	140	1.0
red, white, and blue (*Pepperidge Farm* 3 Layer)	250	2.0	35.0	11.0	25	120	<1.0
strawberry stripe (*Pepperidge Farm* 3 Layer)	250	2.0	32.0	12.0	15	110	<1.0
tiramisu (*Ritch & Famous*), 2.7-oz. pc.	360	6.0	34.0	23.0	65	50	<1.0
vanilla layer: (*Pepperidge Farm* 3-Layer)	250	2.0	35.0	11.0	25	120.	<1.0
(*Sara Lee*)	260	2.0	32.0	14.0	15	210	0
Cake, mix, 1/12 cake*, except as noted:							
angel food: (*Betty Crocker*) ...	140	3.0	32.0	0	0	320	0
(*Duncan Hines*) ...	140	3.0	31.0	0	0	310	0
confetti (*Betty Crocker*)	150	3.0	34.0	0	0	320	0
banana (*Duncan Hines*)	270	3.0	36.0	12.0	55	310	0
Boston cream pie, w/filling, frosting (*Duncan Hines Signature Dessert*), 1/6 cake*	420	6.0	59.0	19.0	85	500	1.0
butter pecan (*Super- Moist*)	240	3.0	35.0	10.0	55	290	0
carrot (*SuperMoist*), 1/10 cake*	320	4.0	42.0	15.0	65	370	0
chocolate: butter recipe (*SuperMoist*) ...	250	4.0	35.0	12.0	75	420	2.0
double swirl (*Super- Moist*)	270	4.0	35.0	13.0	55	330	1.0
German (*Super- Moist*)	270	3.0	36.0	13.0	55	330	0
milk (*SuperMoist*) .	240	4.0	34.0	11.0	55	300	1.0

Food and Measure	cal.	prot. (gms)	carbo. (gms)	fat (gms)	chol. (mgs)	sod. (mgs)	fiber (gms)
Cake, mix (cont.)							
chocolate chip (Super-Moist)	250	3.0	35.0	11.0	55	270	0
chocolate fudge:							
(SuperMoist)	270	3.0	35.0	13.0	55	340	1.0
dark (Duncan Hines)	290	4.0	36.0	15.0	55	380	1.0
chocolate silk torte w/filling and frosting (Duncan Hines Signature Dessert), 1/6 cake*	440	6.0	65.0	18.0	35	280	2.0
devil's food:							
(Duncan Hines) ...	290	4.0	35.0	15.0	55	380	1.0
("Jiffy"), 1/5 pkg...	220	3.0	40.0	5.0	0	520	1.0
(SuperMoist)	270	4.0	35.0	13.0	55	340	2.0
fudge, butter recipe (Duncan Hines), 1/10 cake*	300	4.0	43.0	16.0	85	370	1.0
fudge marble:							
(Duncan Hines) ...	270	3.0	35.0	12.0	55	300	<1.0
(SuperMoist), 1/10 cake*	290	4.0	42.0	12.0	65	340	0
funnel cake (Golden Dipt Fry Easy Batter mix), 1/4 cup	120	0	23.0	1.0	20	200	0
gingerbread (Betty Crocker), 1/8 cake* .	230	3.0	39.0	6.0	25	350	0
golden, butter recipe (Duncan Hines), 1/10 cake*	330	4.0	43.0	16.0	85	340	0
lemon:							
(Duncan Hines) ...	270	3.0	36.0	12.0	55	310	0
(SuperMoist)	240	3.0	35.0	10.0	55	290	0
orange:							
(Duncan Hines) ...	270	3.0	36.0	12.0	55	310	0
w/filling and glaze (Duncan Hines Signature Desserts Dreamsicle)	410	6.0	57.0	4.5	75	380	<1.0
pineapple:							
(Duncan Hines) ...	270	3.0	36.0	12.0	55	310	0
(SuperMoist)	250	3.0	35.0	10.0	55	290	0
upside-down (Betty Crocker), 1/6 cake*	400	3.0	64.0	14.0	35	330	0

Food and Measure	cal.	prot. (gms)	carbo. (gms)	fat (gms)	chol. (mgs)	sod. (mgs)	fiber (gms)
pound (*Betty Crocker*), ⅛ cake*	260	4.0	45.0	8.0	55	210	0
rainbow:							
chip (*SuperMoist*), 1/10 cake*	300	4.0	41.0	13.0	65	340	0
swirl (*SuperMoist*) .	250	3.0	35.0	11.0	55	290	0
sour cream white (*SuperMoist*), 1/10 cake*	280	3.0	41.0	12.0	0	380	0
strawberry:							
(*Duncan Hines*) ...	270	3.0	36.0	12.0	55	310	0
(*SuperMoist*)	250	3.0	35.0	10.0	55	290	0
spice:							
(*Duncan Hines*) ...	270	3.0	36.0	12.0	55	310	0
(*SuperMoist*)	250	3.0	35.0	10.0	55	290	0
vanilla, French (*Super-Moist*)	240	3.0	35.0	10.0	55	290	0
white:							
(*Duncan Hines*) ...	210	3.0	36.0	6.0	0	280	0
(*"Jiffy"*), 1/5 pkg. . .	210	2.0	41.0	4.5	0	320	<1.0
(*SuperMoist*)	230	3.0	34.0	10.0	0	300	0
yellow:							
(*Duncan Hines*) ...	270	3.0	36.0	12.0	55	310	0
(*SuperMoist*)	250	3.0	35.0	10.0	55	290	0
butter recipe (*SuperMoist*) ...	250	3.0	36.0	11.0	75	370	0
golden (*"Jiffy"*), 1/5 pkg.	210	2.0	41.0	4.5	0	340	<1.0
Cake, snack (see also specific listings), 1 pc., except as noted:							
caramel cookie bar (*Little Debbie*), 1.2 oz.	160	1.0	22.0	8.0	0	85	0
chocolate, w/creme:							
(*Devil Dogs*), 1.6 oz.	180	2.0	26.0	8.0	0	150	<1.0
(*Ding Dongs*), 2 pcs., 2.8 oz. ..	360	3.0	47.0	18.0	5	210	2.0
(*Drake's* Swiss Rolls), 3 oz.	340	3.0	48.0	15.0	35	320	2.0
(*Hostess Ho-Hos*), 3 oz.	380	3.0	50.0	18.0	30	220	2.0

Food and Measure	cal.	prot. (gms)	carbo. (gms)	fat (gms)	chol. (mgs)	sod. (mgs)	fiber (gms)
Cake, snack, chocolate, w/creme *(cont.)*							
(*Little Debbie* Devil Cremes), 1.7 oz.	190	1.0	29.0	8.0	0	170	0
(*Ring Dings*), 2 pcs., 2.7 oz.	340	2.0	43.0	18.0	0	220	2.0
(*Suzy Q's*), 2 oz. . . .	230	2.0	35.0	9.0	10	270	1.0
w/coconut (*Sno Balls*), 1.8 oz. . . .	180	2.0	32.0	4.5	5	210	1.0
chocolate chip creme pie (*Little Debbie*), 1.2 oz.	150	1.0	23.0	6.0	<2	95	<1.0
coffee cake:							
(*Drake's*), 1.2 oz. . .	140	1.0	20.0	6.0	5	100	0
(*Drake's* Low Fat), 1.2 oz.	110	1.0	21.0	2.0	10	110	0
(*Little Debbie*), 2 pcs., 2.2 oz. . .	240	2.0	42.0	7.0	10	190	0
crumb cake:							
(*Entenmann's*), 3 oz.	360	4.0	47.0	17.0	55	390	<1.0
apple (*Entenmann's*), 4 oz.	440	4.0	63.0	19.0	55	470	1.0
raspberry almond (*Entenmann's*), 4 oz.	250	6.0	60.0	28.0	90	470	1.0
cupcake:							
(*Hostess* Baseballs), 1.6 oz.	150	1.0	31.0	3.0	0	160	0
chocolate (*Hostess*), 1.8 oz.	180	2.0	30.0	6.0	5	290	1.0
chocolate, w/creme (*Yankee Doodles*), 2 pcs., 2 oz.	280	2.0	33.0	9.0	0	220	<1.0
golden (*Hostess*), 1.9 oz.	200	1.0	33.0	7.0	10	180	0
orange (*Hostess*), 1.9 oz.	200	1.0	35.0	7.0	15	190	0
donuts, mini, 3 pcs.:							
crumb (*Hostess Donettes*), 2 oz. .	230	3.0	31.0	10.0	10	270	0
chocolate coated (*Hostess Donettes*), 1.5 oz.	200	2.0	21.0	12.0	0	180	0
fudge cake, frosted (*Little Debbie*), 1.5 oz.	200	2.0	25.0	10.0	15	105	<1.0

Food and Measure	cal.	prot. (gms)	carbo. (gms)	fat (gms)	chol. (mgs)	sod. (mgs)	fiber (gms)
golden, w/creme:							
(*Sunny Doodles*),							
2 pcs., 2 oz.	220	2.0	33.0	9.0	15	180	0
(*Twinkies*), 1.5 oz. .	150	1.0	25.0	5.0	15	200	0
jelly creme pie (*Little*							
Debbie), 1.2 oz. . . .	160	1.0	23.0	7.0	0	100	0
maple creme pie (*Little*							
Debbie), 1.2 oz. . . .	150	1.0	23.0	6.0	<5	140	<1.0
marble cake (*Enten-*							
mann's), 2.75 oz. . .	180	2.0	25.0	9.0	30	85	1.0
oatmeal creme pie (*Lit-*							
tle Debbie), 1.2 oz.	170	1.0	26.0	7.0	0	190	<1.0
pecan swirls (*Drake's*),							
1 oz.	100	1.0	16.0	4.0	0	65	0
pound cake (*Enten-*							
mann's), 2.75 oz. . .	280	4.0	37.0	12.0	70	330	<1.0
Cake, snack, mix (see also "Cookie mix" and specific listings), 1/9 pkg., except as noted:							
banana walnut (*Betty Crocker Snackin' Cake*)	180	2.0	31.0	5.0	0	240	0
chocolate chip, golden (*Betty Crocker Snackin' Cake*)	180	2.0	32.0	5.0	0	180	1.0
chocolate chunk (*Betty Crocker Snackin' Cake*)	180	2.0	32.0	5.0	0	190	1.0
cinnamon swirl (*Betty Crocker Snackin' Cake*)	190	2.0	34.0	5.0	0	210	0
lemon (*Betty Crocker Sunkist* Supreme Dessert Bar), 1/16 pkg.*	140	2.0	24.0	4.5	40	90	0
Calabaza (*Frieda's*), ½ cup, 3 oz.	10	1.0	2.0	0	0	0	1.0
Calamari, see "Squid"							
Calamari dish, frozen, breaded, fried: (*Contessa*), 13 pcs., 2 tbsp. sauce, 2 oz.	170	5.0	16.0	9.0	65	520	0

Food and Measure	cal.	prot. (gms)	carbo. (gms)	fat (gms)	chol. (mgs)	sod. (mgs)	fiber (gms)
Calamari dish *(cont.)*							
rings (*Fisherman's Pride*), 20 pcs., 4 oz.	140	11.0	20.0	1.5	130	380	1.0
Calves liver, see "Liver"							
Camote, see "Boniato"							
Camouflage melon (*Frieda's*), 1 cup, 5 oz.	50	1.0	13.0	0	0	15	1.0
Candy:							
almond, coated:							
carob (*Tree of Life*), 1.4 oz.	220	3.0	20.0	16.0	0	45	1.0
chocolate (*Brach's Supremes*), 11 pcs., 1.4 oz. .	220	3.0	22.0	13.0	10	10	2.0
chocolate (*Planter's*), 12 pcs., 1.4 oz. .	220	4.0	19.0	15.0	<5	15	2.0
chocolate, candy (*M&M's*), 1.3-oz. pkg.	200	3.0	21.0	11.0	5	15	2.0
yogurt (*Tree of Life*), 1.4 oz.	220	3.0	20.0	15.0	0	20	2.0
almond paste, see "marzipan," below							
bridge mix (*Brach's*), 16 pcs., 1.4 oz. . . .	190	2.0	26.0	8.0	5	40	>1.0
butter rum (*Life Savers*), 2 pcs.	20	0	5.0	0	0	35	0
butter toffee creme (*Creme Savers*), .5 oz.	60	0	13.0	1.0	5	60	0
butterscotch:							
(*Brach's*), 3 pcs., .6 oz.	70	0	17.0	0	0	95	0
disks (*Star Brites*), 3 pcs., .6 oz. . . .	60	0	16.0	0	0	80	0
candy corn (*Brach's*), 26 pcs., 1.4 oz. . . .	140	0	35.0	0	0	115	0
caramel:							
(*Brach's Milk Maid*), 4 pcs., 1.4 oz. . .	160	1.0	30.0	4.5	0	80	0
(*Sugar Babies*), 30 pcs., 1.6 oz. .	180	0	41.0	1.5	0	40	0

Food and Measure	cal.	prot. (gms)	carbo. (gms)	fat (gms)	chol. (mgs)	sod. (mgs)	fiber (gms)
(*Sugar Daddy Junior*), 3 pcs., 1.3 oz.	160	1.0	35.0	2.0	0	55	0
(*Sugar Daddy Large*), 1.7 oz. ...	200	1.0	43.0	2.5	0	65	0
egg (*Cadbury*), 1.4-oz. pc.	190	2.0	24.0	10.0	<5	70	0
rolls (*Brach's Milk Maid*), 5 pcs., 1.3 oz.	140	0	28.0	3.5	0	65	0
caramel, chocolate coated:							
(*Brach's Milk Maid*), 18 pcs., 1.4 oz. .	160	1.0	28.0	6.0	5	90	0
(*Milk Duds*), 13 pcs., 1.4 oz. .	170	1.0	28.0	6.0	0	85	0
(*Mini Rolo Bites*), 19 pcs., 1.4 oz. .	190	2.0	26.0	9.0	<5	50	<1.0
(*Rolo*), 1.7-oz. pkg.	210	2.0	31.0	9.0	5	85	0
clusters (*Brach's*), 3 pcs., 1.6 oz. ...	210	4.0	23.0	13.0	5	80	1.0
clusters (*Pot of Gold*), 3 pcs., 1.6 oz.	240	4.0	24.0	14.0	5	70	1.0
cookie bar (*Twix*), 2 bars	280	3.0	37.0	14.0	5	115	1.0
dark chocolate (*Milky Way*), 5 pcs.	200	2.0	29.0	9.0	5	105	1.0
milk chocolate (*Milky Way*), 5 pcs.	200	2.0	30.0	8.0	10	115	0
peanut, nougat, white chocolate (*Zero*), 1.8-oz. bar	230	3.0	36.0	8.0	0	105	<1.0
carob chips (*Tree of Life*), 50 pcs., .5 oz.	70	1.0	9.0	4.0	0	5	1.0
cashew, chocolate coated (*Planters*), 13 pcs., 1.4 oz. ...	220	4.0	21.0	14.0	5	15	1.0
cherry, chocolate covered, 1 oz.:							
dark (*Cella's*), 2 pcs.	110	1.0	19.0	4.0	0	10	<1.0
milk (*Cella's*), 2 pcs.	120	1.0	19.0	4.5	5	20	<1.0

Food and Measure	cal.	prot. (gms)	carbo. (gms)	fat (gms)	chol. (mgs)	sod. (mgs)	fiber (gms)
Candy *(cont.)*							
cherry, dried, chocolate coated (*Harvest Sweets*), 1.25 oz. . . .	160	1.0	24.0	7.0	3	11	1.0
cherry flavor:							
(*Twizzlers* Bites), 17 pcs., 1.4 oz. .	140	1.0	32.0	.5	0	110	0
(*Twizzlers* Nibs), 2.25-oz. pkg. . . .	220	1.0	51.0	1.5	0	125	0
(*Twizzlers Pull-N Peel*), 1.2-oz. pc.	100	1.0	25.0	0	0	85	0
twists (*Twizzlers*), 4 pcs., 1.6 oz. . .	160	1.0	36.0	1.0	0	125	0
chocolate, coffee crunch (*Mauna Loa Kona*), 1.75-oz. bar	270	3.0	29.0	16.0	0	0	4.0
chocolate, cookies and cream:							
(*Hershey's*), 1.5 oz.	230	4.0	26.0	12.0	5	95	0
(*Hershey's* Limited Edition), 1.5 oz. .	230	4.0	26.0	12.0	10	70	<1.0
chocolate, dark:							
(*Cadbury Royal Dark*), 10 blocks, 1.4 oz.	220	2.0	24.0	13.0	<5	0	3.0
(*Dove*), 1.3-oz. bar	200	2.0	22.0	12.0	5	0	2.0
(*Dove Promises*), 5 pcs., 1.4 oz. . .	210	2.0	24.0	13.0	5	0	2.0
(*Hershey's Kisses* Rich), 9 pcs., 1.5 oz.	230	2.0	25.0	13.0	<5	0	3.0
(*Hershey's Special Dark*), 1.4 oz. . . .	220	2.0	25.0	12.0	<5	0	3.0
almond (*Hershey's Nuggets Special Dark*), 4 pcs., 1.3 oz.	220	3.0	20.0	14.0	<5	0	3.0
honey almond nougat (*Toblerone*), 1.2 oz.	170	1.0	20.0	9.0	5	5	2.0
mint (*Cadbury Royal Dark*), 10 blocks, 1.4 oz.	220	2.00	24.0	13.0	<5	0	3.0

Food and Measure	cal.	prot. (gms)	carbo. (gms)	fat (gms)	chol. (mgs)	sod. (mgs)	fiber (gms)
orange (*Terry's*), 1.6 oz.	240	1.0	28.0	13.0	5	5	3.0
raspberry (*Hershey's Nuggets*), 4 pcs., 1.4 oz.	220	2.0	24.0	13.0	0	0	3.0
chocolate, double (*Hershey's* Limited Edition), 1.6-oz. bar	210	3.0	29.0	9.0	5	55	<1.0
chocolate, milk:							
(*Brach's Stars*), 10 pcs., 1.3 oz. .	200	2.0	24.0	11.0	0	25	0
(*Cadbury Dairy Milk*), 10 blocks, 1.4 oz.	220	3.0	24.0	12.0	10	45	<1.0
(*Dove*), 1.3-oz. bar	200	2.0	22.0	12.0	5	25	1.0
(*Dove Promises*), 5 pcs., 1.4 oz. . .	220	2.0	24.0	13.0	5	25	1.0
(*Hershey's*), 1.5 oz.	230	3.0	25.0	13.0	10	40	1.0
(*Hershey's Hugs*), 9 pcs., 1.4 oz. . .	210	3.0	23.0	12.0	10	45	0
(*Hershey's Kisses*), 9 pcs., 1.4 oz. . .	230	3.0	24.0	13.0	10	35	1.0
(*Hershey's Nuggets*), 4 pcs., 1.4 oz. . .	230	3.0	24.0	13.0	10	35	1.0
(*Hershey's Swoops*), 1.25-oz. cup	190	3.0	20.0	11.0	10	30	<1.0
(*Milka*), ⅓ bar, 1.2 oz.	180	2.0	20.0	10.0	5	30	1.0
(*Nestlé*), ¼ of 5-oz. bar	170	1.0	23.0	10.0	<5	15	<1.0
(*Symphony*), 1.5 oz.	230	4.0	24.0	13.0	10	40	<1.0
(*Terry's*), 1.6 oz.	230	3.0	27.0	12.0	10	35	0
almond (*Cadbury Roast Almond*), 10 blocks, 1.4 oz.	220	4.0	21.0	13.0	10	80	1.0
almond (*Hershey's*), 1.4 oz.	230	5.0	20.0	14.0	5	35	1.0
almond (*Hershey's Kisses*), 9 pcs., 1.4 oz.	230	4.0	21.0	14.0	10	30	1.0
almond (*Hershey's Nuggets*), 4 pcs., 1.3 oz.	210	4.0	20.0	13.0	5	30	1.0

Food and Measure	cal.	prot. (gms)	carbo. (gms)	fat (gms)	chol. (mgs)	sod. (mgs)	fiber (gms)
Candy, chocolate, milk *(cont.)*							
almond/toffee (*Symphony*), 1.5 oz. . .	230	4.0	22.0	14.0	10	50	1.0
candy coated (*M&M's*), 1.7-oz. pkg.	240	2.0	34.0	10.0	5	30	1.0
candy coated (*M&M's* Fun Size), .7-oz. pkg.	100	1.0	15.0	4.5	5	15	1.0
candy coated, minis (*M&M's*), 1.1-oz. tube	150	1.0	21.0	7.0	5	20	1.0
caramel (*Caramello*), 6 blocks, 1.5 oz.	200	3.0	27.0	9.0	10	50	<1.0
caramel filled (*Hershey's Kisses*), 8 pcs., 1.3 oz. . .	180	2.0	24.0	8.0	10	60	0
crème egg (*Cadbury*), 1.4-oz. pc.	180	2.0	25.0	8.0	5	25	<1.0
crisps (*Crunch*), ¼ of 5-oz. bar . .	170	2.0	24.0	9.0	5	30	<1.0
crisps (*Krackel*), 1.4-oz. bar	210	2.0	28.0	10.0	<5	50	<1.0
crisps, w/caramel (*Crunch*), 1.52-oz. bar	210	2.0	29.0	11.0	5	75	<1.0
crispy, candy coated (*M&M's*), 1.5-oz. pkg.	200	2.0	31.0	8.0	5	60	1.0
fruit/nut (*Cadbury Fruit & Nut*), 10 blocks, 1.4 oz.	200	3.0	25.0	10.0	5	30	1.0
fruit/nut (*Chunky*), ¼ of 5-oz. bar . .	170	2.0	21.0	10.0	5	15	1.0
honey almond nougat (*Toblerone*), 1.4 oz.	210	2.0	26.0	11.0	10	20	1.0
honey almond nougat (*Toblerone*), 1.76-oz. bar	260	3.0	32.0	13.0	10	25	1.0
honey almond nougat (*Toblerone*), 1.23-oz. bar . . .	180	2.0	23.0	9.0	10	15	1.0

Food and Measure	cal.	prot. (gms)	carbo. (gms)	fat (gms)	chol. (mgs)	sod. (mgs)	fiber (gms)
macadamia (*Mauna Loa*), 1.75-oz. bar	280	4.0	27.0	18.0	10	45	1.0
macadamia, crisps (*Mauna Loa*), 1.75-oz. bar	270	4.0	29.0	17.0	10	55	<1.0
mint (*Hershey's Kisses*), 9 pcs., 1.4 oz.	230	3.0	24.0	13.0	10	35	1.0
orange (*Terry's*), 1.6 oz.	230	3.0	27.0	12.0	10	30	1.0
peanut butter chips (*Butterfinger*), 1/5 bar, 1.4 oz. ...	190	2.0	27.0	9.0	<5	50	<1.0
raisins/almonds, extra creamy (*Hershey's Nuggets*), 4 pcs., 1.4 oz.	200	3.0	23.0	11.0	10	30	1.0
raspberry crème (*Cadbury*), 10 blocks, 1.4 oz.	220	4.0	23.0	12.0	5	55	0
strawberry crème (*Hershey's Kisses*), 9 pcs., 1.5 oz.	220	4.0	24.0	12.0	5	60	0
toffee/almonds, extra creamy (*Hershey's Nuggets*), 4 pcs., 1.4 oz.	220	4.0	21.0	13.0	10	50	1.0
chocolate, white: w/honey almond nougat (*Toblerone*),1.2 oz. ...	180	2.0	20.0	10.0	5	30	0
chocolate assortment: (*Pot of Gold*), 1.1-oz. box	130	1.0	21.0	5.0	<5	45	<1.0
(*Pot of Gold Premium*), 1.5 oz.	220	3.0	26.0	11.0	5	45	1.0
(*Pot of Gold* Sugar Free), 1.5 oz. ...	180	2.0	22.0	16.0	10	5	1.0
caramel (*Pot of Gold*), 1.5 oz.	200	2.0	27.0	9.0	5	80	<1.0

Food and Measure	cal.	prot. (gms)	carbo. (gms)	fat (gms)	chol. (mgs)	sod. (mgs)	fiber (gms)
Candy, chocolate assortment *(cont.)*							
creme (*Pot of Gold*),							
1.4 oz.	170	1.0	32.0	4.0	0	25	<1.0
mint (*Pot of Gold*),							
1.4 oz.	200	2.0	26.0	10.0	5	35	1.0
nut (*Pot of Gold*),							
1.5 oz.	240	3.0	21.0	16.0	5	40	1.0
chocolate caramel							
creme (*Creme*							
Savers), .5 oz.	60	0	13.0	1.5	5	30	0
chocolate chews:							
(*Tootsie Roll*							
Midgees), 6 pcs.,							
1.4 oz.	140	1.0	28.0	3.0	0	15	0
(*Tootsie Roll*							
Midgees Small),							
12 pcs., 1.3 oz. .	130	0	25.0	3.0	0	15	0
chocolate thins, 1.3 oz.:							
cherry jubilee							
(*Andes*), 8 pcs. .	200	2.0	22.0	13.0	0	35	<1.0
crème de menthe							
(*Andes*), 8 pcs. .	200	2.0	22.0	13.0	0	30	1.0
mint parfait (*Andes*),							
8 pcs.	200	2.0	21.0	13.0	0	35	0
toffee crunch							
(*Andes*), 8 pcs. .	190	2.0	23.0	11.0	0	65	0
chocolate twists							
(*Twizzlers*), 4 pcs.,							
1.5 oz.	160	2.0	34.0	1.5	0	100	<1.0
cinnamon:							
(*Brach's* Imperials),							
52 pcs., .5 oz. ..	60	0	15.0	0	0	0	0
disks (*Star Brites*),							
3 pcs., .6 oz. ...	60	0	16.0	0	0	15	0
hard (*Brach's*),							
3 pcs., .6 oz. ...	70	0	17.0	0	0	10	0
hot (*Hain*), 6 pcs. ...	10	0	2.0	0	0	0	0
circus peanuts							
(*Brach's*), 6 pcs.,							
1.5 oz.	160	<1.0	39.0	0	0	0	0
coconut, w/chocolate:							
(*Almond Joy*							
Swoops),							
1.25-oz. cup	200	2.0	21.0	12.0	<5	15	<1.0

Food and Measure	cal.	prot. (gms)	carbo. (gms)	fat (gms)	chol. (mgs)	sod. (mgs)	fiber (gms)
(*Mounds*),							
1.7-oz. bar	240	2.0	29.0	13.0	0	70	2.0
almond (*Almond*							
Joy), 1.6-oz. bar	220	2.0	27.0	12.0	0	65	2.0
chocolate chocolate							
(*Amond Joy*),							
1.6-oz. bar	230	3.0	25.0	13.0	0	55	3.0
piña colada							
(*Almond Joy*),							
1.6-oz. bar	230	3.0	25.0	13.0	<5	70	2.0
coconut, Neapolitan							
(*Brach's* Sundaes),							
3 pcs., 1.3 oz.	160	1.0	28.0	5.0	0	75	1.0
cotton candy:							
(*Charms Fluffy*							
Stuff), .6-oz. bag	70	0	17.0	0	0	0	0
(*Charms Fluffy*							
Stuff), 1.1-oz. bag	120	0	30.0	0	0	0	0
(*Jays*), 2 oz.	220	3.0	56.0	0	0	0	0
cranberry, chocolate							
coated:							
dark (*Cape Cod*),							
1¼ oz.	160	1.0	23.0	8.0	0	0	2.0
milk (*SunRidge*							
Farms), 1.4 oz.. .	180	1.0	26.0	9.0	5	10	2.0
crèmes:							
assorted (*Rich &*							
Dreamy), 3 pcs.,							
1.7 oz.	170	1.0	36.0	3.0	0	5	>1.0
egg (*Cadbury*),							
1.4-oz. pc.	170	2.0	28.0	6.0	<5	25	0
dulce de leche (*Her-*							
shey's Kisses),							
8 pcs., 1.3 oz.	180	3.0	24.0	8.0	10	70	0
fruit flavor, assorted:							
(*Brach's* Jube Jels),							
12 pcs., 1.4 oz. .	140	0	34.0	0	0	40	0
(*Jolly Rancher Stix*),							
.6-oz. pkg.	70	0	17.0	0	0	10	0
(*Life Savers* Fruit							
Slices), 1.4 oz. . .	140	2.0	36.0	0	0	10	0
(*Mason Dots*),							
12 pcs., 1.5 oz. .	140	0	35.0	0	0	10	0

Food and Measure	cal.	prot. (gms)	carbo. (gms)	fat (gms)	chol. (mgs)	sod. (mgs)	fiber (gms)
Candy, fruit flavor, assorted *(cont.)*							
(*Wild 'n Fruity* Rainbow Bears), 4 pcs., 1.6 oz. ..	150	0	38.0	0	0	15	0
all varieties, except sours (*Skittles*), 2.2-oz. bag	240	0	54.0	2.5	0	10	0
chews (*Jolly Rancher*), 6 pcs., 1.14 oz.	150	0	33.0	2.0	0	0	0
chews (*Starburst*), 2.1-oz. pkg.	240	0	48.0	5.0	0	0	0
chews (*Tootsie Frooties*), 12 pcs., 1.3 oz.	140	0	29.0	3.0	0	20	0
chews (*Tootsie Roll*), 6 pcs., 1.4 oz. ..	140	0	28.0	3.0	0	15	0
chews, sour (*Twizzlers Sourz*), 1.8-oz. pkg.	180	1.0	41.0	1.5	0	300	<1.0
chews, tangy (*Wild 'n Fruity*), 12 pcs., 1.4 oz.	160	0	32.0	3.5	0	20	0
gummy (*Brach's*), 13 pcs., 1.4 oz. .	110	2.0	25.0	0	0	10	0
gummy (*Jolly Rancher*), 10 pcs., 1.4 oz.	120	2.0	29.0	0	0	15	0
gummy (*Life Savers*), 1.4 oz. .	130	2.0	30.0	0	0	0	0
gummy (*Wild 'n Fruity* Bears/ Worms), 5 pcs., 1.4 oz.	140	2.0	32.0	0	0	15	0
gummy, sour (*Wild 'n Fruity* Fish), 8 pcs., 1.4 oz. ..	110	2.0	26.0	0	0	10	0
gummy, sour (*Wild 'n Fruity* Worms), 5 pcs., 1.6 oz. ..	150	2.0	36.0	0	0	15	0
slices (*Brach's*), 3 pcs., 1.6 oz. ..	150	0	38.0	0	0	10	0
sours (*Jolly Rancher Screaming Sours*), 16 pcs., 1.4 oz. .	140	0	34.0	0	0	60	0

Food and Measure	cal.	prot. (gms)	carbo. (gms)	fat (gms)	chol. (mgs)	sod. (mgs)	fiber (gms)
sours (*Skittles*), 1.8-oz. bag	200	0	44.0	2.0	0	5	0
fruit flavor, hard:							
(*Jolly Rancher*), 3 pcs., .6 oz. . . .	70	0	17.0	0	0	0	0
(*Jolly Rancher* Sugar Free), 4 pcs., .6 oz. . . .	35	0	13.0	0	0	0	0
(*Life Savers*), 2 pcs.	20	0	5.0	0	0	0	0
(*Life Savers* Sours), .5 oz.	60	0	15.0	0	0	0	0
(*Life Savers* Fusions), .5 oz. .	60	0	15.0	0	0	10	0
(*Wild 'n Fruity*), 3 pcs., .6 oz. . . .	70	0	18.0	0	0	5	0
(*Jolly Rancher* Rocks), 1.1 oz. . .	120	0	30.0	0	0	15	0
(*Starburst*), 3 pcs., .5 oz.	50	0	13.0	0	0	25	0
and crème, .5 oz.:							
orange (*Creme Savers*)	70	0	13.0	1.5	0	35	0
raspberries (*Creme Savers*)	60	0	13.0	1.5	0	35	0
strawberries (*Creme Savers*)	70	0	13.0	1.5	0	30	0
sour balls (*Charms*), 1 pc.	20	0	5.0	0	0	0	0
squares (*Charms*), 2 pcs., .2 oz. . . .	20	0	6.0	0	0	0	0
fudge:							
double (*Hershey's Kisses*), 9 pcs., 1.5 oz.	230	3.0	25.0	13.0	10	35	1.0
ginger, chocolate (*Sun-Ridge Farms*), ¼ cup, 1.8 oz.	240	8.0	25.0	13.0	5	15	6.0
ginger, hard (*Gin-Gins*), 3 pcs., .3 oz.	35	0	8.0	0	0	0	0
gum, chewing, 1 pc., except as noted:							
(*Abra Cabubble*) . . .	45	0	10.0	0	0	0	0
(*Bubble Yum*)	25	0	6.0	0	0	0	0

Food and Measure	cal.	prot. (gms)	carbo. (gms)	fat (gms)	chol. (mgs)	sod. (mgs)	fiber (gms)
Candy, gum, chewing *(cont.)*							
(*Bubble Yum* Sugarless)	10	0	3.0	0	0	0	0
(*Big Red/Juicy Fruit/ Wrigley's Spearmint/Doublemint/ Winterfresh*)	10	0	2.0	0	0	0	0
(*Skittles*), 2 pcs. . . .	10	0	2.0	0	0	0	0
all varieties:							
(*Freedent*)	10	0	2.0	0	0	0	0
(*Orbit/Elipse* Sugar Free), 2 pcs.	5	0	2.0	0	0	0	0
except bubble (*Extra* Sugar Free)	5	0	2.0	0	0	0	0
bubble (*Extra* Sugar Free)	5	0	1.0	0	0	0	0
jelly beans:							
(*Brach's*), 14 pcs., 1.4 oz.	150	0	37.0	0	0	5	0
(*Jelly Belly*), 35 pcs., 1.4 oz.	140	0	37.0	0	0	10	0
(*Jolly Rancher* Assorted), 1.4 oz. .	140	0	34.0	0	0	25	0
(*Jolly Rancher* Bold Smoothie), 1.4 oz.	140	0	35.0	0	0	25	0
(*Smucker's*), 25 pcs., 1.4 oz.	150	0	37.0	0	0	10	0
(*Starburst*), ¼ cup, 1.5 oz.	150	0	38.0	0	0	15	0
licorice:							
(*Crows*), 12 pcs., 1.5 oz.	140	0	35.0	0	0	10	0
(*Kookaburra*), 4 pcs., 1.4 oz.	130	1.0	31.0	.5	0	65	0
(*Twizzlers*), 4 pcs., 1.6 oz.	150	2.0	34.0	.5	0	200	0
(*Twizzlers* Bites), 18 pcs., 1.4 oz. .	130	1.0	30.0	.5	0	180	0
(*Twizzlers* Nibs), 2.25-oz. pkg. . . .	210	2.0	48.0	1.5	0	315	0
candy coated (*Good & Plenty*), 1.75-oz. pkg. . . .	170	<1.0	43.0	0	0	120	0

Food and Measure	cal.	prot. (gms)	carbo. (gms)	fat (gms)	chol. (mgs)	sod. (mgs)	fiber (gms)
chews (*SunRidge Farms*), ¼ cup, 1.4 oz.	140	3.0	27.0	2.0	0	30	<1.0
lollipop, 1 pop, except as noted:							
(*Charms* Sweet/ Sour), .6 oz.	70	0	17.0	0	0	0	0
(*Charms Blow Pop*), .6 oz.	60	0	16.0	0	0	0	0
(*Charms Blow Pop* Junior), .5 oz. . .	50	0	14.0	0	0	0	0
(*Charms Blow Pop* Super), 1.3 oz. . .	130	0	35.0	0	0	0	0
(*Jolly Rancher* As- sorted), .6 oz. . .	60	0	16.0	0	0	10	0
(*Jolly Rancher* Filled), .6 oz. . . .	60	0	15.0	0	0	30	0
(*Life Savers*), .4 oz.	40	0	10.0	0	0	0	0
(*Starburst* Fruit Chew), .5 oz.	50	0	13.0	0	0	5	0
(*Tootsie Roll* Pop), .6 oz.	60	0	15.0	0	0	0	0
(*Tootsie Roll* Pop Miniature), 3 pcs., .5 oz.	50	0	13.0	0	0	0	0
(*Tootsie Roll* Pop Small), .45 oz. . .	45	0	11.0	0	0	0	0
macadamias, coated:							
butter candy glaze (*Mauna Loa*), 1 oz.	190	2.0	10.0	15	<5	55	1.0
butter corn crunch (*Mauna Loa*), 1 oz.	150	1.0	18.0	8.0	1	140	1.0
chocolate, dark (*Mauna Loa*), 9 pcs., 1.3 oz. . .	200	2.0	18.0	16.0	0	0	3.0
chocolate, milk (*Mauna Loa*), 1 oz., ¼ cup	150	2.0	15.0	10.0	5	10	1.0
chocolate, milk (*Mauna Loa* Deluxe), 4 pcs., 1.3 oz.	210	2.0	19.0	16.0	5	15	1.0

Food and Measure	cal.	prot. (gms)	carbo. (gms)	fat (gms)	chol. (mgs)	sod. (mgs)	fiber (gms)
Candy, macadamias, coated *(cont.)*							
chocolate, milk (*Mauna Loa Mountains*), 4 pcs., 1.3 oz. ..	200	2.0	21.0	14.0	5	15	1.0
chocolate, milk, candy (*Mauna Loa*), 1.4 oz.	200	2.0	25.0	12.0	5	10	1.0
chocolate, milk, toffee (*Mauna Loa*), 7 pcs., 1.4 oz. ..	210	2.0	23.0	13.0	5	70	1.0
malt balls, coated:							
carob (*SunRidge Farms*). ¼ cup, 1.9 oz.	210	1.0	34.0	2.5	0	50	0
carob (*Tree of Life*), 1.4 oz.	200	0	28.0	10.0	0	80	0
chocolate (*Brach's Malts*), 15 pcs., 1.4 oz.	190	2.0	30.0	7.0	10	25	1.0
chocolate (*Whoppers*), ¾-oz. pkg.	100	1.0	16.0	3.5	0	70	0
chocolate, candy (*Whoppers Robin Eggs*), 24 pcs., 1.4 oz.	170	<1.0	31.0	5.0	0	95	0
marshmallows:							
(*Kraft Jet-Puffed*), 1 oz.	90	1.0	23.0	0	0	30	0
all flavors, 1.1 oz.:							
(*Kraft Fun-Mallows*)	100	1.0	24.0	0	0	30	0
mini (*Kraft Fun-Mallows*)	100	1.0	24.0	0	0	15	0
crème (*Kraft*), .4 oz.	40	00	10.0	0	0	10	0
toasted coconut (*Kraft*), 1 oz. ...	100	1.0	21.0	2.5	0	20	0
marzipan (*Biermann*), .42-oz. pc.	50	1.0	10.0	1.0	0	5	1.0
mint:							
(*Brach's* Kentucky), 7 pcs., .6 oz. ...	60	0	16.0	0	0	0	0
(*Brach's Ice Blue Mint Coolers*), 3 pcs., .6 oz. ...	70	0	17.0	0	0	10	0

Food and Measure	cal.	prot. (gms)	carbo. (gms)	fat (gms)	chol. (mgs)	sod. (mgs)	fiber (gms)
(*BreathSavers*), 1 pc.	5	0	2.0	0	0	0	0
(*Life Savers Cryst-O-Mint/Pep-O-Mint/Wint-O-Green*), 2 pcs. . . .	20	0	5.0	0	0	0	0
dessert (*Brach's*), 14 pcs., .5 oz. . . .	60	0	15.0	0	0	0	0
peppermint, cool (*Hain*), 6 pcs.	10	0	2.0	0	0	0	0
peppermint or spearmint (*Star Brites* Starlight), 3 pcs., .5 oz. . . .	60	0	15.0	0	0	10	0
mint, chocolate coated (see also "peppermint," below) (*Junior Mints*), 16 pcs., 1.4 oz.	170	1.0	30.0	3.0	0	30	<1.0
nonpareils:							
(*Brach's Sprinkles*), 17 pcs., 1.4 oz. . .	200	2.0	29.0	9.0	15	35	1.0
(*Snow-Caps*), ¼ cup, 1.4 oz. . . .	180	1.0	30.0	8.0	<5	0	2.0
nougat, jelly (*Brach's*), 5 pcs., 1.4 oz.	160	0	34.0	2.5	0	50	0
nougat, w/chocolate:							
(*Milky Way*), 2-oz. bar	270	2.0	41.0	10.0	5	95	1.0
(*Milky Way* Fun Size), 2 bars, 1.4 oz. . .	180	2.0	28.0	7.0	5	65	0
(*Milky Way* Miniature), 5 pcs., 1.5 oz.	190	2.0	30.0	7.0	5	70	0
(*Milky Way* Pop'ables), 13 pcs., 1.4 oz. . .	180	1.0	28.0	7.0	5	55	0
(*3 Musketeers*), 2.13-oz. bar	260	2.0	46.0	8.0	5	110	1.0
(*3 Musketeers* Fun Size), 2 bars, 1.2 oz.	140	1.0	25.0	4.5	5	60	1.0
(*3 Musketeers* Miniature), 7 pcs., 1.5 oz.	180	1.0	31.0	5.0	5	75	1.0

Food and Measure	cal.	prot. (gms)	carbo. (gms)	fat (gms)	chol. (mgs)	sod. (mgs)	fiber (gms)
Candy, nougat, w/chocolate *(cont.)*							
chocolate (*Charleston Chew*), 1.9-oz. bar	230	2.0	43.0	6.0	0	35	<1.0
chocolate chews (*3 Musketeers Chewlicious*), .8-oz. bar	100	0	18.0	2.5	5	30	0
dark (*Milky Way Midnight*), 1.76-oz. bar	220	1.0	36.0	8.0	5	85	1.0
dark (*Milky Way Midnight* Fun Size), 2 bars, 1.4 oz.	170	1.0	28.0	7.0	5	65	1.0
dark (*Milky Way Midnight* Miniature), 5 pcs., 1.4 oz.	180	1.0	29.0	7.0	5	70	1.0
strawberry (*Charleston Chew*), 1.9-oz. bar	230	2.0	43.0	6.0	0	35	0
vanilla (*Charleston Chew*), 1.9-oz. bar	230	2.0	44.0	6.0	0	35	0
vanilla (*Charleston Chew* Mini), 13 pcs., 1.4 oz. .	170	2.0	29.0	6.0	0	30	0
orange slices (*Brach's*), 2 pcs., 1.3 oz.	130	0	32.0	0	0	10	0
peanut bar:							
(*Planters*), 1.6 oz. .	230	6.0	22.0	14.0	0	70	2.0
(*Planters* Carb Well), 1.23 oz.	160	6.0	16.0	12.0	0	140	2.0
chocolate (*Chew-ets/ Peanut Chews*), 3 pcs., 1 oz.	140	3.0	17.0	6.0	0	30	<1.0
peanut butter, w/chocolate:							
(*Brach's* Meltaways), 3 pcs., 1.3 oz. . .	200	3.0	19.0	13.0	0	90	1.0
(*Butterfinger*), 2.1-oz. bar	270	4.0	43.0	11.0	0	135	1.0
(*Butterfinger* King), ⅓ bar, 1.25 oz. . .	160	2.0	25.0	6.0	0	80	<1.0

Food and Measure	cal.	prot. (gms)	carbo. (gms)	fat (gms)	chol. (mgs)	sod. (mgs)	fiber (gms)
(*Butterfinger* Minis), 4 bars, 1.4 oz.	180	2.0	29.0	7.0	0	90	<1.0
(*Butterfinger Crisp*), 1.76-oz. bar	250	3.0	33.0	13.0	0	140	1.0
(*Butterfinger Crisp* Minis), 4 bars, 1.6 oz.	220	2.0	29.0	11.0	0	120	1.0
(*5th Avenue*), 2-oz. bar	290	5.0	35.0	14.0	0	125	2.0
(*Reese's Bites*), 16 pcs., 1.4 oz.	220	4.0	23.0	12.0	<5	70	1.0
(*Reese's Peanut Butter Cups*), 1.5 oz.	230	4.0	23.0	13.0	<5	130	1.0
(*Reese's Peanut Butter Cups Big Cup*), 1.5-oz. pc.	230	4.0	23.0	13.0	<5	140	1.0
(*Reese's Pieces*), 1.5-oz. pkg.	220	5.0	26.0	11.0	0	80	1.0
(*Reese's Swoops*), 1.25-oz. cup	190	6.0	17.0	11.0	0	130	2.0
candy coated (*M&M's*), 1.6-oz. pkg.	240	5.0	26.0	14.0	5	100	2.0
coconut (*Zagnut*), 1.75-oz. bar	230	3.0	31.0	10.0	0	85	2.0
cookie bar (*Twix*), 2 bars	280	4.0	28.0	17.0	5	120	2.0
dark (*Reese's Peanut Butter Cups*), 1.5 oz.	230	4.0	22.0	14.0	0	120	2.0
fudge (*Reese's Peanut Butter Cups*), 1.5 oz.	230	5.0	22.0	13.0	<5	140	2.0
nougat (*Reese's Fast Break*), 2-oz. bar	280	5.0	34.0	14.0	<5	200	2.0
nuts (*Reese's NutRageous*), 1.8-oz. bar	280	6.0	27.0	16.0	0	70	2.0
white chocolate (*Reese's Peanut Butter Cups*), 1.5 oz.	230	5.0	22.0	13.0	<5	150	1.0

Food and Measure	cal.	prot. (gms)	carbo. (gms)	fat (gms)	chol. (mgs)	sod. (mgs)	fiber (gms)
Candy *(cont.)*							
peanut caramel bar:							
(*Baby Ruth*),							
2.1-oz. bar	280	4.0	37.0	13.0	0	130	2.0
(*PayDay*),							
1.8-oz. bar	260	6.0	28.0	14.0	0	140	2.0
(*Snickers*)							
2.1-oz. bar	280	4.0	35.0	14.0	5	140	1.0
(*Snickers* Fun Size),							
2 bars, 1.4 oz. . .	190	3.0	24.0	10.0	5	100	1.0
(*Snickers* Miniature),							
4 pcs., 1.3 oz. . .	170	3.0	22.0	9.0	5	90	1.0
(*Snickers Crunchier*)							
1.55-oz. bar	230	4.0	25.0	13.0	5	140	1.0
(*Snickers Pop'ables*),							
13 pcs., 1.4 oz. .	190	3.0	24.0	9.0	5	85	1.0
(*Whatchamacallit*),							
1.6-oz. bar	230	3.0	29.0	11.0	<5	125	<1.0
honey roasted (*Pay-Day*), 1.8-oz. bar	240	6.0	30.0	11.0	0	130	2.0
peanuts, coated:							
butter toffee (*Fisher*),							
¼ cup, 1 oz.	130	3.0	17.0	6.0	0	150	1.0
butter toffee (*Old Dominion*), 1 oz.	140	4.0	16.0	7.0	0	20	2.0
butter toffee, maple (*Brach's* Maple Nut Goodies),							
7 pcs., 1.5 oz. . .	200	3.0	30.0	8.0	0	70	1.0
candy (*M&M's*),							
1.7-oz. pkg.	250	5.0	30.0	13.0	5	25	2.0
candy (*M&M's* Fun Size), .7-oz. pkg.	110	2.0	13.0	5.0	0	10	1.0
carob (*Tree of Life*),							
1.4 oz.	220	3.0	20.0	16.0	0	45	<1.0
chocolate (*Brach's* Double Dippers),							
15 pcs., 1.4 oz. .	210	4.0	23.0	12.0	10	65	2.0
chocolate (*Goober's*),							
¼ cup, 1.4 oz. . .	210	4.0	22.0	14.0	5	15	2.0
chocolate (*Mr. Goodbar*), 1.7-oz. bar	270	5.0	27.0	16.0	5	20	2.0
chocolate (*Mr. Goodbar Bites*), 25 pcs.,							
1.4 oz.	230	4.0	21.0	14.0	<5	120	1.0

Food and Measure	cal.	prot. (gms)	carbo. (gms)	fat (gms)	chol. (mgs)	sod. (mgs)	fiber (gms)
chocolate clusters (*Brach's*), 3 pcs., 1.4 oz.	210	4.0	21.0	13.0	5	65	2.0
French burnt (*Brach's*), 31 pcs., 1.4 oz.	170	3.0	29.0	6.0	0	0	1.0
yogurt (*Tree of Life*), 1.4 oz.	220	4.0	19.0	15.0	0	20	<1.0
pecan caramel clusters, chocolate:							
(*Nestlé* Turtles), 4 pcs., 1.5 oz. . .	210	2.0	25.0	12.0	5	45	1.0
(*Pot of Gold*), 3 pcs., 1.6 oz. . .	250	3.0	24.0	16.0	5	65	1.0
(*Russell Stover* Pecan Delights Sugar-Free), 2 pcs., 1.2 oz. . .	150	2.0	17.0	11.0	0	30	3.0
peppermint, w/chocolate:							
(*Brach's* Mint Patties), 3 pcs., 1.3 oz.	140	0	29.0	3.0	0	0	0
(*York* Pattie), 1.4-oz. pc.	160	<1.0	32.0	3.0	0	10	<1.0
(*York Bites*), 15 pcs., 1.4 oz.	160	<1.0	33.0	3.0	0	25	<1.0
(*York Swoops*), 1.25-oz. cup	190	2.0	21.0	11.0	<5	0	2.0
pretzel, caramel, peanut chocolate (*Take 5*), 1.5-oz. bar	220	4.0	25.0	11.0	<5	180	1.0
pretzel, coated:							
chocolate, milk (*Synders* Dips), 1 oz.	130	2.0	18.0	6.0	<5	110	n.a.
chocolate, white (*Synders* Dips), 1 oz.	140	3.0	19.0	6.0	<5	110	n.a.
chocolate, white (*Hershey's Bites*), 23 pcs., 1.4 oz. . .	200	4.0	25.0	9.0	<5	290	1.0
yogurt (*SunRidge Farms*), 8 pcs., 1.4 oz.	210	2.0	27.0	10.0	0	190	0

Food and Measure	cal.	prot. (gms)	carbo. (gms)	fat (gms)	chol. (mgs)	sod. (mgs)	fiber (gms)
Candy, pretzel, coated *(cont.)*							
yogurt (*Tree of Life*), 1.4 oz.	190	2.0	28.0	9.0	0	75	0
raisins, coated:							
carob (*SunRidge Farms*), ¼ cup, 2.1 oz.	290	1.0	41.0	14.0	0	40	1.0
carob (*Tree of Life*), 1.4 oz.	180	1.0	28.0	9.0	0	45	<1.0
chocolate (*Brach's California*), 35 pcs., 1.4 oz. .	170	1.0	28.0	6.0	10	10	1.0
chocolate (*Raisinets*), ¼ cup, 1.4 oz.	190	2.0	32.0	8.0	5	15	1.0
yogurt (*SunRidge Farms*), 1.4 oz. . .	170	1.0	29.0	7.0	0	20	<1.0
yogurt (*Tree of Life*), 1.4 oz.	180	1.0	27.0	8.0	0	20	<1.0
root beer (*Brach's Barrels*), 3 pcs., .6 oz. .	70	0	17.0	0	0	5	0
soy nuts, coated, 1oz.:							
chocolate (*GeniSoy*)	140	4.0	15.0	7.5	<5	25	2.0
praline (*GeniSoy*) . .	120	6.0	18.0	2.5	0	110	2.0
spearmint (*Brach's Leaves*), 5 pcs., 1.4 oz.	130	0	34.0	0	0	15	0
spice drops (*Brach's*), 12 pcs., 1.4 oz. ...	130	0	33.0	0	0	15	0
strawberry twists (*Twizzlers*), 4 pcs., 1.6 oz.	160	1.0	36.0	1.0	0	130	0
toffee, 3 pcs., .6 oz.:							
coffee (*Brach's Special Treasures*)	70	0	14.0	1.0	0	70	0
fruit and cream (*Brach's Special Treasures*)	60	0	13.0	.5	0	50	0
golden (*Brach's Special Treasures*)	80	0	15.0	2.0	10	95	0
toffee, w/chocolate:							
(*Heath*), 1.4-oz. bar	210	1.0	24.0	12.0	10	125	<1.0
(*Heath Bites*), 15 pcs., 1.4 oz. .	210	1.0	25.0	12.0	5	95	<1.0

Food and Measure	cal.	prot. (gms)	carbo. (gms)	fat (gms)	chol. (mgs)	sod. (mgs)	fiber (gms)
(*Skor*), 1.4-oz. bar .	210	1.0	24.0	12.0	15	120	<1.0
truffles:							
(*Truffelettes*), 4 pcs., 1.1 oz.	189	1.6	14.0	14.0	0	18	1.4
assorted (*Pot of Gold*), 1.5 oz. . . .	200	2.0	27.0	9.0	5	20	1.0
chocolate, dark (*Harry and David*), 2 pcs., 1.3 oz. . .	200	2.0	19.0	16.0	0	10	2.0
cookies and cream bar (*Milka*),⅓ bar, 1.2 oz.	180	2.0	19.0	11.0	5	25	1.0
wafer, w/chocolate:							
(*KitKat*), 1.5-oz. bar	220	3.0	27.0	11.0	<5	25	<1.0
(*KitKat Bites*), 15 pcs., 1.4 oz. .	200	3.0	25.0	10.0	<5	25	<1.0
mint (*KitKat*), 1.5-oz. bar	220	3.0	27.0	11.0	<5	25	<1.0
peanut butter (*ReeseSticks*), 1.5 oz.	230	4.0	23.0	13.0	<5	115	1.0
triple chocolate (*Kit-Kat*), 1.5-oz. bar	220	3.0	26.0	12.0	<5	35	1.0
white chocolate (*Kit-Kat*), 1.5-oz. bar	220	3.0	26.0	12.0	5	45	0
walnuts, glazed (*Emerald* Original), 1 oz.	140	2.0	12.0	10.0	0	125	1.0
Cane juice, dehydrated (*Tree of Life* Organic), 1 level tsp.	15	0	3.0	1.5	0	10	0
Cane syrup, 1 tbsp. . . .	52	0	13.4	0	0	<1	0
Cannellini beans, see "Kidney beans"							
Cannelloni entree, frozen, cheese (*Lean Cuisine Everyday Favorites*), 9⅛-oz. pkg.	260	18.0	30.0	7.0	20	690	3.0
Cannoli shell (*Ferrara*), .5 -oz. shell	80	1.0	8.0	4.0	0	0	0
Cantaloupe:							
(*Chiquita*), ¼ medium	50	1.0	12.0	0	0	25	1.0
(*Del Monte*), ¼ medium	50	1.0	12.0	0	0	25	1.0

Food and Measure	cal.	prot. (gms)	carbo. (gms)	fat (gms)	chol. (mgs)	sod. (mgs)	fiber (gms)
Cantaloupe *(cont.)*							
(*Dole*), ¼ medium . . .	50	1.0	12.0	0	0	25	1.0
½ of 5" melon	94	2.3	22.3	.7	0	23	2.1
cubed, 1 cup	56	1.4	13.4	.5	0	14	1.3
Cantaloupe, dried (*SunRidge Farms*),							
¼ cup, 1.4 oz.	140	0	34.0	0	0	30	1.0
Caper berries (*Haddon House*), ½ oz.	0	0	1.0	0	0	410	0
Capers, 1 tbsp., except as noted:							
(*Bellino*), 2 tbsp.	5	5	1.0	0	0	350	0
(*Crosse & Blackwell*) .	5	0	1.0	0	0	350	0
(*Goya*)	5	0	1.0	0	0	380	0
(*Roland*)	0	0	1.0	0	0	315	0
Capicola, see "Ham lunch meat"							
Capon, see "Chicken"							
Caponata, see "Egg-plant appetizer"							
Cappuccino, see "Coffee, flavored, mix" and "Coffee, iced"							
Carambola, fresh: (*Frieda's* Starfruit),							
5 oz.	45	1.0	11.0	0	0	0	4.0
1 medium, 4.7 oz. . . .	42	.7	9.9	.4	0	2	3.4
sliced, ½ cup	18	.3	1.0	.2	0	1	1.5
Carambola, dried (*Frieda's* Starfruit),							
⅓ cup, 1.4 oz.	120	2.0	29.0	0	0	5	1.0
Caramel dip, see "Fruit dip"							
Caramel syrup, 2 tbsp.:							
(*Hershey's Classic Caramel* Sundae) . .	100	0	25.0	0	0	95	0
(*Smucker's Sundae Syrup*)	100	1.0	25.0	0	0	110	0
Caramel topping, 2 tbsp.:							
(*Hershey's Classic Caramel*)	110	<1.0	27.0	0	0	140	0
(*Smucker's*)	130	1.0	31.0	0	0	110	0

Food and Measure	cal.	prot. (gms)	carbo. (gms)	fat (gms)	chol. (mgs)	sod. (mgs)	fiber (gms)
(*Smucker's Magic Shell*)	220	2.0	14.0	18.0	5	30	0
(*Smucker's Plate-Scapers*)	100	1.0	25.0	0	0	105	0
butterscotch, see "Butterscotch topping"							
dulce de leche:							
(*Smucker's*)	110	2.0	23.0	1.5	10	45	0
(*Smucker's* Spoonable)	140	1.0	25.0	4.0	5	40	0
hot (*Smucker's* Spoonable)	140	1.0	29.0	2.5	0	75	0
Caraway seed, 1 tsp.	7	.4	1.1	.3	0	<1	<1.0
Cardamom, ground:							
1 tsp.	6	.2	1.4	.1	0	<1	.5
1 tbsp.	18	.6	4.0	.4	0	1	1.6
Cardoon:							
raw:							
(*Frieda's*), 1 cup, 3 oz.	15	1.0	4.0	0	0	140	1.0
shredded, ½ cup	18	.6	4.4	.1	0	151	1.4
boiled, drained, 4 oz.	25	.9	6.0	.1	0	200	n.a.
Caribou, meat only, roasted, 4 oz.	189	33.8	0	5.0	123	68	0
Carissa:							
1 medium, .8 oz.	12	.1	2.7	.3	0	1	n.a.
sliced, ½ cup	46	.4	10.2	1.0	0	2	n.a.
Carl's Jr., 1 serving:							
breakfast items:							
burrito	560	29.0	37.0	32.0	495	990	1.0
Croissant Sunrise Sandwich	360	13.0	29.0	21.0	245	470	0
w/bacon	410	16.0	29.0	25.0	255	610	0
w/sausage	550	21.0	31.0	40.0	285	970	0
eggs, scrambled:							
w/bacon	760	23.0	69.0	42.0	500	1140	5.0
w/sausage	900	27.0	72.0	56.0	525	1480	5.0
French Toast Dips:							
6 pcs., no syrup	450	10.0	59.0	20.0	5	570	0
9 pcs., no syrup	670	15.0	88.0	30.0	5	850	1.0
French toast syrup.	90	0	21.0	0	0	0	0
jelly or jam	40	0	9.0	0	0	15	0
quesadilla	390	17.0	38.0	18.0	285	920	2.0
sourdough sandwich	410	21.0	39.0	19.0	255	510	2.0
w/bacon	470	25.0	39.0	24.0	305	680	2.0

Food and Measure	cal.	prot. (gms)	carbo. (gms)	fat (gms)	chol. (mgs)	sod. (mgs)	fiber (gms)
***Carl's Jr.*, breakfast items, sourdough sandwich** *(cont.)*							
w/ham	450	26.0	40.0	20.0	270	850	2.0
w/sausage	610	28.0	39.0	37.0	290	1040	2.0
sandwiches:							
Carl's bacon Swiss							
crispy chicken ..	750	31.0	91.0	28.0	80	1900	3.0
Carl's Catch Fish ..	560	19.0	58.0	27.0	80	990	2.0
Carl's ranch crispy							
chicken	660	24.0	72.0	31.0	70	1180	3.0
Carl's western							
bacon crispy							
chicken	760	31.0	72.0	38.0	90	1550	3.0
Charbroiled BBQ							
Chicken	370	35.0	47.0	4.0	60	1070	4.0
Charbroiled Chicken							
Club	550	42.0	43.0	23.0	95	1330	4.0
Charbroiled Santa							
Fe Chicken	610	38.0	43.0	32.0	100	1440	4.0
chicken, spicy	460	14.0	48.0	26.0	40	1220	2.0
chili burger	690	39.0	57.0	35.0	110	1400	5.0
double sourdough							
bacon cheese-							
burger	920	52.0	45.0	59.0	170	1020	2.0
Double Western							
Bacon Cheese-							
burger	920	51.0	65.0	50.0	155	1730	2.0
Famous Star burger	590	24.0	50.0	32.0	70	910	3.0
w/cheese	650	28.0	51.0	37.0	85	1170	3.0
hamburger	260	14.0	36.0	9.0	35	480	1.0
sourdough bacon							
cheeseburger ...	550	31.0	41.0	29.0	85	500	2.0
Super Star burger .	790	41.0	52.0	47.0	130	980	3.0
w/double cheese	920	48.0	53.0	57.0	160	1490	3.0
The Six Dollar							
Burger	1000	39.0	72.0	62.0	135	1690	6.0
The Western Bacon							
Six Dollar Burger	1060	45.0	79.0	61.0	135	2180	2.0
Western Bacon							
Cheeseburger ...	660	32.0	64.0	30.0	85	1410	2.0
side dishes:							
chicken breast strips:							
3 pcs.	380	22.0	27.0	21.0	55	1360	1.0
5 pcs.	630	37.0	45.0	34.0	90	2269	2.0

Food and Measure	cal.	prot. (gms)	carbo. (gms)	fat (gms)	chol. (mgs)	sod. (mgs)	fiber (gms)
chicken stars:							
6 pcs.	270	14.0	15.0	17.0	40	500	0
9 pcs.	410	21.0	23.0	26.0	60	760	1.0
chili cheese fries . .	920	20.0	89.0	16.0	65	1030	9.0
CrissCut Fries	410	5.0	43.0	24.0	0	950	4.0
fries:							
kids	250	4.0	32.0	12.0	0	150	3.0
large	620	10.0	80.0	8.0	0	380	7.0
medium	460	7.0	59.0	22.0	0	280	5.0
small	290	5.0	37.0	14.0	0	170	3.0
hash brown nuggets	330	3.0	32.0	21.0	0	470	3.0
onion rings	440	7.0	53.0	5.0	0	700	3.0
zucchini	320	6.0	31.0	19.0	0	860	2.0
potato, baked:							
plain	280	7.0	63.0	0	0	30	7.0
plain, w/margarine .	380	7.0	63.0	12.0	0	140	7.0
bacon/cheese	620	22.0	71.0	29.0	40	1160	7.0
broccoli/cheese . . .	510	12.0	71.0	21.0	15	940	7.0
sour cream/chive . .	410	9.0	65.0	14.0	10	190	7.0
salad:							
Buffalo ranch							
chicken	380	19.0	42.0	16.0	35	1180	6.0
Charbroiled Chicken							
Salad-To-Go	330	34.0	17.0	7.0	75	880	5.0
Garden Salad-To-Go	120	3.0	5.0	3.0	5	230	2.0
salad croutons, .5 oz.	70	1.0	8.0	3.0	0	170	0
salad dressing, 2 oz.:							
blue cheese	320	2.0	1.0	35.0	25	370	0
Buffalo ranch	330	1.0	2.0	35.0	25	720	0
French, fat free	60	0	16.0	0	0	660	0
house	220	1.0	3.0	22.0	20	440	0
Italian, fat free	15	0	4.0	0	0	770	0
Thousand Island . .	250	1.0	7.0	24.0	25	450	0
sauce, dipping:							
barbecue	50	1.0	11.0	0	0	270	0
buffalo wing	0	0	0	0	0	30.0	0
honey	90	0	22.0	0	0	0	0
house	110	0	2.0	11.0	10	220	0
mustard	50	0	11.0	0	0	210	0
sweet and sour .	50	0	12.0	0	0	80	0
desserts:							
chocolate chip							
cookie	350	3.0	46.0	18.0	20	330	1.0
chocolate cake	300	3.0	48.0	12.0	30	350	1.0

Food and Measure	cal.	prot. (gms)	carbo. (gms)	fat (gms)	chol. (mgs)	sod. (mgs)	fiber (gms)
Carl's Jr., desserts *(cont.)*							
strawberry swirl cheesecake	290	6.0	30.0	17.0	55	230	0
shakes:							
chocolate, medium	820	22.0	148.0	16.0	70	550	0
chocolate, small . . .	540	15.0	98.0	11.0	45	360	0
strawberry, medium	750	20.0	133.0	15.0	65	490	0
strawberry, small . .	520	14.0	93.0	11.0	45	340	0
vanilla, medium . . .	700	22.0	115.0	16.0	70	520	0
vanilla, small	470	15.0	77.0	45.0	11	350	0
Carnival squash *(Frieda's)*, ¾ cup, 3 oz.	30	1.0	7.0	0	0	0	1.0
Carob drink mix, powder, 3 tsp.	45	.2	11.2	tr.	0	12	<1.0
Carob flour, 1 cup . . .	395	4.8	91.6	.7	0	36	41.0
Carob powder *(Shiloh Farms)*, 1 tbsp. . . .	45	0	11.0	0	0	12	1.0
Carp, meat only:							
raw, 4 oz.	144	20.2	0	6.4	75	58	0
baked, broiled, or microwaved, 4 oz. .	184	25.9	0	8.1	95	71	0
Carrot, fresh:							
raw:							
(Dole), 7" long, 1¼" diam.	35	1.0	8.0	0	0	40	2.0
(Frieda's Gold*)*, ⅔ cup, 3 oz. . . .	35	1.0	9.0	0	0	30	3.0
(Grimmway), 7" long, 1¼" diam.	35	1.0	8.0	0	0	40	2.0
whole, 7½" long, 2.8 oz.	31	.7	7.3	.1	0	25	2.2
shredded *(Fresh Express)*, 1 cup, 3 oz.	45	1.0	10.0	0	0	55	3.0
shredded, ½ cup . .	24	.6	5.6	.1	0	19	1.7
raw, baby:							
(Grimmway), 3 oz. .	38	1.0	9.0	0	0	30	2.0
(Mann's), 3 oz.	38	1.0	9.0	0	0	44	2.0
1 medium, 2¾" long	4	.1	.8	.1	0	3	.2
peeled mini *(Dole)*, 3 oz., ¾ cup	40	1.0	9.0	0	0	45	2.0

Food and Measure	cal.	prot. (gms)	carbo. (gms)	fat (gms)	chol. (mgs)	sod. (mgs)	fiber (gms)
boiled, drained, sliced, ½ cup	35	.9	8.2	.1	0	52	2.6
Carrot, can or jar, ½ cup, except as noted:							
baby (*Reese*)	15	<1.0	3.0	0	0	410	1.0
crinkle sliced (*Fresh-like*)	45	1.0	11.0	0	0	180	3.0
shredded (*Hengsten-berg* Salad), ¼ cup	10	0	3.0	0	0	85	1.0
sliced:							
(*Allens* Tiny)	35	0	8.0	0	0	40	3.0
(*Del Monte*)	35	0	8.0	0	0	300	3.0
(*S&W*)	35	0	8.0	0	0	300	1.0
(*Veg-All* Tender) ...	30	0	5.0	0	0	320	2.0
w/liquid	28	.8	6.2	.2	0	297	1.1
drained	17	.5	4.0	.1	0	176	1.1
honey:							
(*Glory*)	50	1.0	13.0	0	0	220	2.0
glazed (*Del Monte Savory Sides*) ..	70	1.0	18.0	0	0	440	1.0
Carrot, dehydrated, diced (*AlpineAire*), ¾ oz.	80	2.0	17.0	0	0	55	2.0
Carrot, frozen, ⅔ cup, except as noted:							
baby (*Birds Eye*)	35	0	7.0	0	0	60	2.0
crinkle cut (*Dr. Praeger's*)	35	1.0	7.0	0	0	60	2.0
round (*C&W* Parisienne)	40	0	10.0	0	0	50	3.0
sliced:							
(*Birds Eye*)	35	0	7.0	0	0	55	2.0
boiled, drained, ½ cup	26	.9	6.0	.1	0	43	2.6
Carrot, glazed, frozen: (*Green Giant*), ½ cup cooked	70	<1.0	7.0	4.0	0	260	2.0
honey (*Green Giant* Boil-in-Bag), 1 cup .	90	1.0	13.0	3.5	0	180	2.0
Carrot, pickled, in jars (*Hogue Farms*), 5 pcs., 1.1 oz.	30	0	7.0	0	0	5	1.0

Food and Measure	cal.	prot. (gms)	carbo. (gms)	fat (gms)	chol. (mgs)	sod. (mgs)	fiber (gms)
Carrot drink blend, 8 fl. oz.:							
w/fruit juices (*AriZona* Crazy Cocktail)	150	.5	38.0	0	0	35	.8
orange mango (*Nantucket Nectars*)	130	0	30.0	0	0	5	0
Carrot juice, 8 fl. oz.:							
(*Bolthouse Farms*) ...	70	2.0	14.0	0	0	150	>1.0
(*Hain*)	80	2.0	16.0	.5	0	65	0
(*Hollywood*)	120	2.0	27.0	1.0	0	250	1.0
Carvel, 1 serving:							
ice cream, ½ cup:							
chocolate	190	4.0	22.0	10.0	25	100	0
chocolate, nonfat ..	120	2.0	28.0	0	0	40	0
vanilla	200	5.0	21.0	10.0	40	110	0
vanilla, nonfat	120	2.0	25.0	0	0	55	0
vanilla, no sugar ..	130	5.0	25.0	3.0	15	85	0
sherbet, ½ cup	140	2.0	31.0	1.0	5	45	0
sundaes:							
caramel	590	10.0	73.0	27.0	95	390	0
caramel apple	810	14.0	88.0	46.0	90	330	2.0
cherries, Bordeaux .	550	11.0	69.0	26.0	95	250	1.0
banana barge	1050	20.0	132.0	53.0	110	300	7.0
fudge, bittersweet .	600	11.0	69.0	31.0	95	310	1.0
fudge, hot	590	11.0	65.0	31.0	95	310	1.0
fudge, nonfat	380	7.0	84.0	0	5	190	0
fudge brownie	1020	16.0	109.0	58.0	135	480	5.0
strawberry	500	10.0	58.0	26.0	95	250	1.0
strawberry, nonfat .	290	8.0	63.0	0	5	100	1.0
strawberry shortcake	760	14.0	96.0	35.0	90	240	2.0
turtle	1110	13.0	95.0	78.0	90	460	3.0
coladas, 16 fl. oz.:							
banana or strawberry	370	1.0	68.0	10.0	0	150	0
peach or raspberry	370	1.0	69.0	10.0	0	150	0
piña colada	400	1.0	61.0	17.0	0	230	0
Creammachino, 16 fl. oz.:							
caramel cream	590	14.0	74.0	26.0	90	450	0
classic	410	13.0	36.0	24.0	90	260	0
mocha fudge	610	14.0	61.0	35.0	90	310	1.0
drinks, fountain:							
Carvelanche:							
w/topping	600	12.0	71.0	30.0	95	280	<1.0

Food and Measure	cal.	prot. (gms)	carbo. (gms)	fat (gms)	chol. (mgs)	sod. (mgs)	fiber (gms)
nonfat, fruit	390	12.0	82.0	0	0	160	0
Fizzlers, regular ...	340	2.0	75.0	4.5	10	105	1.0
ice cream soda	400	7.0	63.0	15.0	55	200	0
chocolate	440	8.0	68.0	16.0	55	230	1.0
nonfat	290	2.0	68.0	0	0	115	8.0
shake, nonfat:							
chocolate	440	5.0	104.0	0	0	n.a.	0
mocha	440	10.0	97.0	0	0	230	0
vanilla	300	9.0	62.0	0	0	135	0
shake, thick:							
chocolate	720	18.0	96.0	31.0	115	420	0
chocolate, re-duced fat	520	17.0	100.0	8.0	35	350	<1.0
vanilla	660	17.0	79.0	30.0	115	350	0
vanilla, reduced fat	460	16.0	84.0	7.0	35	280	<1.0
smoothies, 16 fl. oz.:							
banana or raspberry	310	1.0	79.0	.5	0	40	0
berry, Staten Island	310	1.0	80.0	.5	0	40	0
berry, Times Square cooler, Grand	310	1.0	75.0	.5	0	40	0
Central	290	1.0	73.0	.5	0	40	0
Casaba melon:							
1/10 of 7¾" melon ...	43	1.5	10.2	.2	0	20	1.3
cubed, 1 cup	44	1.5	10.5	.2	0	10	1.4
Cashew, 1 oz., except as noted:							
(*Beer Nuts*)	170	5.0	8.0	13.0	0	80	1.0
(*Fisher* Jumbo)	170	5.0	8.0	15.0	0	140	1.0
(*Frito Lay* Salted)	160	4.0	8.0	13.0	0	115	1.0
(*Kettle* Lightly Salted)	160	5.0	8.0	14.0	0	180	1.0
(*Kettle* Unsalted)	160	5.0	8.0	14.0	0	0	1.0
(*Planters* Fancy 6 oz.)	170	5.0	8.0	14.0	0	120	1.0
(*Planters* Fancy 10 oz.)	170	5.0	8.0	14.0	0	115	1.0
(*Planters* Whole)	170	5.0	8.0	14.0	0	120	1.0
(*Planters* Whole Lightly Salted)	170	5.0	8.0	14.0	0	60	1.0.
raw, whole, ¼ cup:							
(*Shiloh Farms*)	190	5.0	11.0	15.0	0	5	1.0
dry-roasted:							
18 medium, 1 oz. ...	163	4.4	9.3	13.2	0	4	.9
whole or halves, 1 cup	787	21.0	44.8	63.5	0	21	4.1

Food and Measure	cal.	prot. (gms)	carbo. (gms)	fat (gms)	chol. (mgs)	sod. (mgs)	fiber (gms)
Cashew *(cont.)*							
halves and pieces:							
(*Planters*)	170	6.0	7.0	14.0	0	120	1.0
(*Planters* Lightly							
Salted	170	6.0	7.0	14.0	0	55	1.0
honey-roasted							
(*Planters*)	150	4.0	11.0	12.0	0	85	1.0
oil-roasted:							
18 medium, 1 oz. ...	163	4.6	8.1	13.7	0	5	1.1
whole or halves,							
1 cup	748	21.0	37.1	62.7	0	22	4.9
Cashew butter:							
(*Kettle Roaster Fresh*),							
1 oz.............	165	4.0	9.0	14.0	0	4	0
(*Tree of Life*), 2 tbsp. .	180	4.0	9.0	15.0	0	0	1.0
Cashew sesame mix,							
w/peanuts (*Planters*),							
1 oz.	160	5.0	9.0	13.0	0	240	2.0
Cassava (see also							
"Yuca root"), raw:							
14.4-oz. root	653	5.6	155.2	1.1	0	57	7.3
1 cup	330	2.8	78.4	.6	0	29	3.7
Catfish, channel, meat							
only:							
farmed, 4 oz.:							
raw	153	17.7	0	8.6	15	60	0
baked, broiled, or							
microwaved	172	21.2	0	9.1	73	91	0
wild, 4 oz.:							
raw	108	18.6	0	3.2	66	49	0
baked, broiled, or							
microwaved	119	20.9	0	3.2	82	57	0
Catfish, frozen or re-							
frigerated, 4 oz.:							
fillets (*Delta Pride*) ...	90	16.0	0	3.5	40	160	0
nuggets (*Delta Pride*) .	170	17.0	0	11.0	80	100	0
steaks (*Delta Pride*) ..	160	17.0	0	10.0	60	70	0
strips (*Delta Pride*) ..	120	16.0	0	6.0	50	170	0
whole (*Delta Pride*) ..	130	17.0	0	6.0	50	85	0
Catfish entree, frozen,							
strips, fried (*Delta*							
Pride Country Crisp),							
4 oz.	240	10.0	20.0	12.0	25	450	0

Food and Measure	cal.	prot. (gms)	carbo. (gms)	fat (gms)	chol. (mgs)	sod. (mgs)	fiber (gms)
Catjang, boiled, ½ cup	100	7.0	17.5	.6	0	16	3.1
Cauliflower, fresh:							
raw:							
(*Andy Boy*), 1/6 medium head, 3.5 oz.	25	2.0	5.0	0	0	30	2.0
(*Dole*), 1/6 medium head, 3.5 oz. ...	25	2.0	5.0	0	0	30	2.0
florets, 3 pcs.	14	1.1	2.9	.1	0	17	1.4
1" pcs., ½ cup	13	1.0	2.6	.1	0	15	1.3
boiled, drained, 1" pcs., ½ cup	14	1.1	2.6	.3	0	9	1.7
green:							
raw, 1/5 head	28	2.7	5.7	.3	0	22	3.0
raw, 1" pcs., ½ cup	16	1.5	3.0	.2	0	12	1.6
boiled, drained, 1" pcs., ½ cup ..	20	1.9	3.9	.2	0	14	2.0
Cauliflower, frozen:							
florets:							
(*Birds Eye*), 4 pcs., 3 oz.	25	1.0	4.0	0	0	25	1.0
(*Green Giant*), 1 cup	20	2.0	3.0	0	0	25	2.0
boiled, drained, 1" pcs., ½ cup	17	1.5	3.4	.2	0	16	2.0
in cheese sauce (*Green Giant*), ½ cup	60	2.0	7.0	2.5	<5	510	1.0
in garlic sauce (*Birds Eye*), 1¼ cups	60	2.0	6.0	4.0	0	460	2.0
Cauliflower combinations, frozen, w/carrots, snow pea pods (*Birds Eye*), 1 cup .	30	1.0	6.0	0	0	35	2.0
Caviar (see also "Roe"), 1 tbsp., except as noted:							
black or red	40	3.9	.6	2.9	94	240	0
lumpfish, black, red or gold (*Romanoff*) ..	15	1.0	0	1.0	50	380	0
salmon (*Romanoff*) ..	35	3.0	0	1.5	55	310	0
sturgeon, granular (*Romanoff* Beluga/ Osetra/Sevruga), 1 oz.	74	9.5	.9	4.3	n.a.	624	0

Food and Measure	cal.	prot. (gms)	carbo. (gms)	fat (gms)	chol. (mgs)	sod. (mgs)	fiber (gms)
Caviar *(cont.)*							
whitefish, black or gold (*Romanoff*) ..	25	1.0	1.0	1.5	45	300	0
Caviar spread, see "Taramosalata"							
Cayenne, see "Pepper"							
Ceci bean, see "Garbanzo bean"							
Celeriac, fresh, raw:							
(*Frieda's* Celery Root), ¾ cup, 3 oz.	35	1.0	8.0	0	0	85	2.0
trimmed, 4 oz.	44	1.7	10.4	.3	0	113	2.0
trimmed, ½ cup	31	1.2	7.2	.2	0	78	1.4
Celery:							
raw:							
(*Dole*) 2 stalks	20	1.0	2.0	0	0	100	2.0
7½"-stalk, 1.6 oz. ..	6	.3	1.5	.1	0	35	.7
diced, ½ cup	10	.5	2.2	.1	0	52	1.0
boiled, drained, diced, ½ cup	13	.6	3.0	.1	0	68	1.2
Celery, Chinese (*Frieda's* Kahn Choy), 1 cup, 3 oz.	15	1.0	3.0	0	0	75	1.0
Celery, dehydrated (*AlpineAire*), .3 oz. ..	25	1.0	5.0	0	0	125	1.0
Celery, dried, flake or seed (*Tone's*), 1 tsp.	9	.4	.9	.5	0	4	.3
Celery root, see "Celeriac"							
Celery salt:							
(*McCormick*), ¼ tsp. .	0	0	0	0	0	250	0
(*Tone's*), 1 tsp.	6	.3	.6	.4	0	1584	.2
Cellophane noodles, see "Noodle, Asian"							
Celtus, raw, trimmed:							
1 oz.	6	.2	1.0	.1	0	3	.3
.3-oz. leaf	1	<.1	.3	0	0	1	.1
Cereal, ready-to-eat (see also specific grains), 1 cup, except as noted:							
amaranth flakes (*Arrowhead Mills*) .	140	4.0	26.0	2.0	0	0	3.0

Food and Measure	cal.	prot. (gms)	carbo. (gms)	fat (gms)	chol. (mgs)	sod. (mgs)	fiber (gms)
bran:							
(*All-Bran* Original), ½ cup	80	4.0	23.0	1.0	0	80	10.0
(*All-Bran Bran Buds*), ⅓ cup	70	2.0	24.0	1.0	0	200	13.0
(*Fiber One*), ½ cup	60	2.0	25.0	1.0	0	105	14.0
(*Post* 100%), ⅓ cup	80	4.0	22.0	1.0	0	125	9.0
flakes (*Arrowhead Mills*)	110	4.0	22.0	1.0	0	85	5.0
flakes (*Kellogg's Complete*), ¾ cup	90	3.0	23.0	.5	0	210	5.0
flakes (*Malt-O-Meal Balance*), ¾ cup	90	3.0	23.0	.5	0	210	3.0
flakes (*Post*), ¾ cup	100	3.0	24.0	.5	0	220	5.0
bran, raisin:							
(*Cascadian Farm*)	180	5.0	43.0	1.5	0	340	6.0
(*Erewhon*)	170	5.0	40.0	1.0	0	100	6.0
(*General Mills* Para su Familia), 1⅓ cups	170	4.0	42.0	1.0	0	300	7.0
(*Kellogg's*)	190	5.0	45.0	1.5	0	350	7.0
(*Kellogg's Raisin Bran Crunch*)	190	3.0	45.0	1.0	0	210	4.0
(*Malt-O-Meal*)	190	6.0	45.0	1.5	0	350	8.0
(*Post*)	190	4.0	46.0	1.0	0	300	8.0
(*Total*)	170	3.0	42.0	1.0	0	240	5.0
nut (*General Mills*), 1¼ cups	200	4.0	44.0	2.5	0	270	5.0
buckwheat flakes, maple (*Arrowhead Mills*)	170	4.0	35.0	1.0	0	190	1.0
corn:							
(*Barbara's Puffins*), ¾ cup	90	2.0	23.0	1.0	0	190	5.0
(*Boo Berries*)	120	1.0	26.0	1.0	0	190	0
(*Chex Corn*)	110	2.0	25.0	.5	0	280	1.0
(*Cocomotion*), ¾ cup	100	2.0	22.0	.5	0	95	<1.0
(*Franken Berry*)	120	1.0	26.0	1.0	0	190	0
(*French Toast Crunch*), ¾ cup	120	1.0	26.0	1.5	0	150	1.0
(*Kaboom*), 1¼ cups	120	1.0	25.0	1.0	0	190	1.0
(*Kellogg's Corn Pops*)	120	1.0	28.0	0	0	120	<1.0

Food and Measure	cal.	prot. (gms)	carbo. (gms)	fat (gms)	chol. (mgs)	sod. (mgs)	fiber (gms)
Cereal, ready-to-eat, corn *(cont.)*							
(*Kellogg's Smorz*) .	120	1.0	25.0	2.0	0	140	<1.0
(*Kix*), 1⅓ cups	120	2.0	25.0	1.0	0	220	1.0
(*Malt-O-Meal Corn*							
Bursts)	120	1.0	28.0	0	0	120	0
(*Trix*)	120	1.0	26.0	1.5	0	190	1.0
(*Trix* Reduced							
Sugar)	120	1.0	26.0	1.5	0	180	1.0
berry berry (*Kix*) . .	120	1.0	26.0	1.5	0	160	1.0
berry (*Malt-O-Meal*							
Berry Colossal							
Crunch), ¾ cup .	120	1.0	26.0	1.5	0	210	1.0
caramel (*Barbara's*							
Organic Wild							
Puffs)	110	2.0	25.0	1.0	0	160	<1.0
cinnamon (*Barbara's*							
Puffins), ¾ cup .	100	2.0	26.0	1.0	0	150	6.0
cinnamon bun							
(*Kellogg's Mini*							
Swirlz)	120	2.0	25.0	2.0	0	115	1.0
cocoa (*Barbara's*							
Organic Wild							
Puffs)	110	2.0	25.0	1.0	0	190	1.0
cocoa (*Malt-O-Meal*							
Coco-Roos),							
¾ cup	120	1.0	27.0	1.0	0	190	0
fruity punch							
(*Barbara's* Organic							
Wild Puffs)	110	2.0	26.0	1.0	0	55	1.0
peanut butter							
(*Barbara's Puf-*							
fins), ¾ cup	110	3.0	23.0	2.0	0	230	2.0
puffed (*Arrowhead*							
Mills)	60	2.0	12.0	1.0	0	5	2.0
corn flakes:							
(*Arrowhead Mills*) .	120	2.0	27.0	0	0	70	2.0
(*Barbara's*)	110	2.0	26.0	0	0	130	2.0
(*Erewhon*), 1¼ cups	210	5.0	45.0	2.5	0	100	3.0
(*General Mills*							
Country)	110	2.0	25.0	.5	0	270	1.0
(*Kellogg's Corn*							
Flakes Original) .	100	2.0	24.0	0	0	200	1.0
(*Malt-O-Meal*)	110	2.0	26.0	0	0	320	1.0

Food and Measure	cal.	prot. (gms)	carbo. (gms)	fat (gms)	chol. (mgs)	sod. (mgs)	fiber (gms)
(*New Morning*)	120	2.0	26.0	1.0	0	180	2.0
(*Organic Promise Cranberry Sunshine*)	110	2.0	26.0	1.0	0	100	2.0
(*Post Toasties*)	100	2.0	24.0	0	0	260	1.0
(*Total*), 1⅓ cups ..	110	2.0	23.0	.5	0	210	1.0
frosted (*Malt-O-Meal*), ¾ cup ...	120	1.0	28.0	0	0	200	1.0
frosted (*New Morning*)	120	2.0	27.0	1.0	0	150	2.0
frosted, w/strawberries (*New Morning*)	120	1.0	27.0	1.0	0	150	2.0
honey crunch (*Kellogg's Corn Flakes*), ¾ cup ..	110	2.0	26.0	.5	0	220	1.0
corn and amaranth (*Erewhon Aztec*) ...	110	2.0	26.0	0	0	70	1.0
corn and rice:							
(*Cinnamon Crunch Crispix*), ¾ cup ..	120	1.0	26.0	1.0	0	180	<1.0
(*Crispix*)	110	2.0	25.0	0	0	210	<1.0
corn and wheat (*Malt-O-Meal Honey Graham Squares*), ¾ cup	120	1.0	25.0	1.0	0	270	1.0
granola:							
(*Almond Raisin Crisp Granola*), ½ cup	220	7.0	36.0	9.0	0	50	6.0
(*Apple Raisin Walnut Granola Organic*), ½ cup .	230	6.0	33.0	8.0	0	0	4.0
(*Apple Sunrise Granola*), ⅓ cup .	190	5.0	30.0	6.0	0	40	3.0
(*Banana Crunch Granola Organic*), ⅔ cup	230	6.0	47.0	2.5	0	0	4.0
(*Berry Good Granola*), ⅔ cup ...	250	6.0	44.0	6.0	0	40	4.0
(*Cascadian Farm Oats & Honey*), ⅔ cup	230	5.0	42.0	6.0	0	110	3.0

Food and Measure	cal.	prot. (gms)	carbo. (gms)	fat (gms)	chol. (mgs)	sod. (mgs)	fiber (gms)
Cereal, ready-to-eat, granola *(cont.)*							
(*Cape Cod Cranberry Granola*), ½ cup	200	5.0	41.0	2.5	0	35	3.0
(*Cinnamon Spice & Everything Nice Granola*), ½ cup .	240	6.0	37.0	8.0	0	0	4.0
(*Grateful Date Granola*), ½ cup .	240	6.0	37.0	8.0	0	45	4.0
(*Honey Crunch Granola*), ½ cup .	280	8.0	37.0	13.0	0	20	4.0
(*Magical Maple Granola*), ½ cup .	220	6.0	34.0	8.0	0	20	3.0
(*Maple Almond Date Granola*), ½ cup .	280	8.0	39.0	11.0	0	0	5.0
(*Outrageous Raspberry Granola*), ½ cup	200	6.0	37.0	3.0	0	40	4.0
(*Peachy Keen Granola*), ½ cup .	220	5.0	33.0	7.0	0	70	3.0
(*Pecan Splendor Granola*), ½ cup .	290	8.0	37.0	13.0	0	45	5.0
(*Save the Forest Absolutely Nuts Organic*), ⅔ cup	220	6.0	30.0	9.0	0	5	4.0
(*Save the Forest Raspberry Razzmataz Organic*), ¾ cup	250	6.0	37.0	9.0	0	0	4.0
(*Shiloh Farms Apple Pie*), ½ cup	250	7.0	39.0	8.0	0	5	5.0
(*Shiloh Farms Festive Flavors*), ½ cup	240	7.0	39.0	7.0	0	60	5.0
(*Shiloh Farms Maple Morning*), ½ cup	250	7.0	37.0	9.0	0	20	5.0
(*Shiloh Farms Sunny Honey Oat*), ½ cup	210	6.0	36.0	5.0	0	45	4.0
(*Shiloh Farms Sunrise Almond*), ½ cup	230	7.0	35.0	7.0	0	0	4.0
cinnamon raisin (*Cascadian Farm*), ⅔ cup	210	5.0	42.0	3.0	0	200	3.0

Food and Measure	cal.	prot. (gms)	carbo. (gms)	fat (gms)	chol. (mgs)	sod. (mgs)	fiber (gms)
nut (*Save the Forest*), ½ cup ..	270	7.0	35.0	12.0	0	45	4.0
w/raisins (*Kellogg's Crunchy Blends*) ⅔ cup	220	5.0	48.0	3.0	0	150	3.0
w/out raisins (*Kellogg's Crunchy Blends*), ½ cup	190	4.0	39.0	3.0	0	120	3.0
spelt and kamut (*Shiloh* Flaky), ½ cup	220	7.0	45.0	1.5	0	0	4.0
kamut:							
flakes (*Arrowhead Mills*)	120	4.0	25.0	1.0	0	70	2.0
flakes (*Erewhon*), ⅔ cup	110	5.0	25.0	0	0	75	4.0
flakes (*Shiloh Farms*), ½ cup ..	140	6.0	28.0	.5	0	0	4.0
puffed (*Arrowhead Mills Puffed Kamut*)	50	3.0	11.0	0	0	0	2.0
millet, puffed (*Arrowhead Mills*)	60	2.0	11.0	.5	0	0	1.0
multigrain (see also "granola," above):							
(*Alpen* No Sugar), ⅔ cup	200	7.0	40.0	3.0	0	30	4.0
(*Alpen* Original), ⅔ cup	200	6.0	41.0	3.0	0	30	4.0
(*Apple Jacks*)	130	1.0	30.0	.5	0	150	1.0
(*Arrowhead Mills Perfect Harvest*)	140	5.0	25.0	2.0	0	60	5.0
(*Barbara's* Grain Shop), ½ cup ...	90	3.0	24.0	1.0	0	125	8.0
(*Barbara's* Honey Crunch'n Oats), ¾ cup	120	2.0	24.0	1.0	0	135	2.0
(*Basic 4*)	200	4.0	42.0	3.0	0	320	3.0
(*Blueberry Muesli* Fat Free), ½ cup	170	3.0	39.0	0	0	5	3.0
(*Cascadian Farm* Squares), ¾ cup	110	3.0	25.0	.5	0	115	2.0

Food and Measure	cal.	prot. (gms)	carbo. (gms)	fat (gms)	chol. (mgs)	sod. (mgs)	fiber (gms)
Cereal, ready-to-eat, multigrain *(cont.)*							
(*Cascadian Farm Hearty Morning*), ¾ cup	200	5.0	43.0	2.5	0	360	8.0
(*Cheerios*)	110	3.0	24.0	1.0	0	200	3.0
(*Chex* Multi-Bran)	190	4.0	46.0	1.5	0	360	7.0
(*Cocoa Puffs*)	120	1.0	26.0	1.5	0	160	1.0
(*Cocoa Puff* Reduced Sugar)	120	1.0	25.0	1.5	0	220	1.0
(*Cookie Crisp*)	120	1.0	26.0	1.5	0	170	1.0
(*Count Chocula*)	120	1.0	26.0	1.0	0	170	1.0
(*Cranberry Muesli Fat Free*), ½ cup	170	3.0	39.0	0	0	0	3.0
(*Froot Loops*)	120	1.0	28.0	1.0	0	150	1.0
(*GoLean*)	140	9.0	36.0	1.0	0	85	8.0
(*GoLean Crunch*)	190	9.0	36.0	3.0	0	95	8.0
(*Good Friends*)	170	5.0	43.0	2.0	0	130	12.0
(*Good Friends Cinna-Raisin Crunch*)	170	4.0	41.0	1.5	0	105	8.0
(*Grape-Nuts*), ½ cup	200	7.0	47.0	1.0	0	310	6.0
(*Grape-Nuts O's*)	120	2.0	28.0	0	0	140	2.0
(*Heart to Heart*), ¾ cup	110	4.0	25.0	1.5	0	90	5.0
(*Honey Comb*)	110	2.0	26.0	.5	0	220	1.0
(*Kashi Medley*), ¾ cup	120	3.0	26.0	1.0	0	75	3.0
(*Kellogg's Crunchy Blends Just Right*), ¾ cup	200	4.0	43.0	2.0	0	240	3.0
(*Kellogg's Crunchy Blends Müeslix*), ⅔ cup	200	5.0	40.0	3.0	0	170	4.0
(*Kellogg's Smart Start* Antioxidants)	190	3.0	43.0	.5	0	280	3.0
(*Kellogg's Smart Start* Healthy Heart), 1¼ cups	230	6.0	49.0	2.0	0	140	5.0
(*Kellogg's Smart Start* Soy Protein)	200	10.0	40.0	1.5	0	260	4.0
(*Malt-O-Meal Honey Buzzers*), 1⅓ cups	110	1.0	26.0	.5	0	220	<1.0
(*Malt-O-Meal Tootie Fruities*)	120	2.0	28.0	1.0	0	150	1.0

Food and Measure	cal.	prot. (gms)	carbo. (gms)	fat (gms)	chol. (mgs)	sod. (mgs)	fiber (gms)
(New England Natural Muesli Organic), ½ cup .	220	8.0	40.0	5.0	0	40	8.0
(Product 19)	100	2.0	25.0	0	0	210	1.0
(Reese's Puffs), ¾ cup	130	2.0	23.0	3.5	0	200	1.0
(Seven in the Morning), ½ cup	210	7.0	47.0	1.5	0	260	7.0
(Team Cheerios) ...	110	2.0	25.0	1.0	0	200	2.0
(Total), ¾ cup	100	2.0	23.0	1.0	0	190	3.0
(Waffle Crisp)	120	2.0	25.0	2.5	0	115	1.0
almond (Honey Bunches of Oats), ¾ cup	130	3.0	25.0	2.5	0	170	2.0
banana (Honey Bunches of Oats), ¾ cup	120	2.0	26.0	2.0	0	120	2.0
banana (Post Selects Banana Nut Crunch)	240	5.0	44.0	6.0	0	250	5.0
blueberry (Post Selects Blueberry Morning), 1¼ cups	230	15.0	48.0	3.5	0	240	2.0
brown sugar and oat (Total), ¾ cup ..	110	2.0	23.0	.5	0	200	1.0
cranberry almond (Post Selects Cranberry Almond Crunch) ..	210	4.0	43.0	3.0	0	190	3.0
dates, raisins, walnuts (Post Fruit & Bran)	200	4.0	42.0	3.0	0	260	6.0
flakes (Arrowhead Mills)	170	5.0	33.0	2.0	0	180	3.0
flakes (Fiber One Honey Clusters) .	170	3.0	47.0	1.0	0	170	14.0
flakes (Grape-Nuts), ¾ cup	110	3.0	24.0	1.0	0	120	3.0
honey nut (Clusters)	210	4.0	46.0	2.5	0	280	3.0
honey roasted (Honey Bunches of Oats), ¾ cup .	120	2.0	25.0	1.5	0	170	2.0

Food and Measure	cal.	prot. (gms)	carbo. (gms)	fat (gms)	chol. (mgs)	sod. (mgs)	fiber (gms)
Cereal, ready-to-eat, multigrain *(cont.)*							
maple pecan (*Post Selects Maple Pecan Crunch*), ½ cup	220	4.0	39.0	6.0	0	135	3.0
marshmallow bits (*Oreo O's*)	110	1.0	22.0	2.0	0	90	1.0
peaches (*Honey Bunches of Oats*), ¾ cup	120	2.0	26.0	2.0	0	125	1.0
peaches, raisins, almonds (*Post Fruit & Bran*) ...	190	4.0	42.0	3.0	0	260	6.0
pecans, crunchy (*Post Selects Great Grains*), ½ cup	220	5.0	38.0	6.0	0	200	4.0
puffed (*Kashi*)	70	2.0	15.0	.5	0	0	1.0
puffed, honey (*Kashi*)	120	3.0	25.0	1.0	0	6	2.0
raisins, dates, pecans (*Post Selects Great Grains*), ½ cup ..	210	4.0	40.0	4.5	0	130	4.0
strawberry (*Honey Comb*), 1⅓ cups	120	2.0	26.0	1.0	0	150	10
strawberry (*Honey Bunches of Oats*), ¾ cup	120	2.0	26.0	2.0	0	150	1.0
oat/oats:							
(*Alpha-Bits*)	130	3.0	27.0	1.5	0	210	1.0
(*Arrowhead Mills Organic Nature O's*)	130	4.0	25.0	2.0	0	0	2.0
(*Barbara's Breakfast O's*), 1¼ cups ..	130	4.0	22.0	2.0	0	115	3.0
(*Cascadian Farm Purely O's*)	110	3.0	29.0	2.0	0	280	3.0
(*Cheerios*)	110	3.0	22.0	2.0	0	210	3.0
(*Fruit-E-O's*)	120	3.0	25.0	1.5	0	85	2.0
(*Lucky Charms*) ...	120	2.0	25.0	1.0	0	200	1.0
(*Malt-O-Meal Marshmallow Mateys*)	110	2.0	25.0	1.0	0	210	2.0

Food and Measure	cal.	prot. (gms)	carbo. (gms)	fat (gms)	chol. (mgs)	sod. (mgs)	fiber (gms)
(*Malt-O-Meal Toasty O's*)	110	4.0	22.0	2.0	0	280	3.0
(*Oatios* Original)	110	3.0	22.0	2.0	0	125	3.0
almond (*Oatmeal Crisp*)	220	5.0	42.0	4.5	0	250	4.0
apple (*Malt-O-Meal Apple Zings*)	130	1.0	30.0	1.0	0	150	1.0
apple cinnamon (*Barbara's* Toasted O's), ¾ cup	110	3.0	24.0	1.0	0	80	2.0
apple cinnamon (*Malt-O-Meal Toasty O's*), ¾ cup	120	2.0	25.0	1.5	0	160	1.0
apple cinnamon (*Oatios*)	120	3.0	18.0	1.0	0	60	2.0
apple cinnamon (*Oatmeal Crisp*) .	210	4.0	45.0	2.0	0	270	4.0
berry, triple (*Cheerios* Berry Bursts)	110	3.0	24.0	1.5	0	180	2.0
berry, triple (*Oatmeal Crisp*)	210	5.0	45.0	2.5	0	260	5.0
chocolate (*Lucky Charms*)	120	1.0	26.0	1.0	0	160	1.0
cocoa (*Oatios*)	110	3.0	17.0	1.0	0	40	2.0
honey almond (*Cascadian Farm*)	120	3.0	24.0	1.5	0	250	2.0
honey almond (*Oatios*)	120	3.0	17.0	1.0	0	50	2.0
honey nut (*Barbara's* Toasted O's), ¾ cup	120	3.0	23.0	2.0	0	75	2.0
honey nut (*Cheerios*)	120	3.0	23.0	1.5	0	210	2.0
honey nut (*Malt-O-Meal Toasty O's*)	110	3.0	24.0	1.0	0	270	2.0
w/marshmallows (*Alpha-Bits*)	120	2.0	26.0	1.0	0	230	1.0
raisin (*Oatmeal Crisp*)	210	5.0	44.0	2.0	0	220	3.0
shredded (*Barbara's* Shredded Spoonfuls), ¾ cup	120	4.0	24.0	1.5	0	200	4.0

Food and Measure	cal.	prot. (gms)	carbo. (gms)	fat (gms)	chol. (mgs)	sod. (mgs)	fiber (gms)
Cereal, ready-to-eat, oat/oats *(cont.)*							
shredded, vanilla almond (*Barbara's*)	220	7.0	42.0	3.0	0	210	4.0
strawberry (*Cheerios Berry Bursts*) ...	110	3.0	24.0	1.5	0	180	2.0
strawberry banana (*Cheerios* Berry Bursts)	110	3.0	24.0	1.5	0	180	3.0
oat bran:							
(*Hodgson Mill*), ¼ cup	120	6.0	23.0	3.0	0	3	6.0
(*Kellogg's Cracklin' Oat Bran*), ¾ cup	200	4.0	35.0	7.0	0	150	6.0
(*Ultimate Oat Bran*), ⅔ cup	110	5.0	22.0	2.0	0	55	3.0
flakes (*Kellogg's Complete*), ¾ cup	110	3.0	23.0	1.0	0	210	4.0
oat bran flakes:							
(*Arrowhead Mills*) .	140	5.0	24.0	2.5	0	80	4.0
oat and corn:							
(*Apple Stroodles*), ¾ cup	110	3.0	25.0	.5	0	15	1.0
apple cinnamon (*Cheerios*), ¾ cup	120	2.0	25.0	1.5	0	120	1.0
frosted (*Cheerios*) .	120	2.0	25.0	1.0	0	210	1.0
rice:							
(*Chex* Rice), 1¼ cups	120	2.0	26.0	.5	0	270	<1.0
(*Fruity Pebbles*), ¾ cup	110	1.0	24.0	1.0	0	160	0
(*Rice Krispies*), 1¼ cups	120	2.0	29.0	0	0	320	0
(*Rice Krispies Treats*), ¾ cup ..	120	1.0	26.0	1.5	0	170	0
(*Rice Twice*), ¾ cup	120	2.0	26.0	0	0	60	0
(*Tony's Cinnamon Crunchers*), ¾ cup	130	1.0	23.0	3.5	0	160	<1.0
brown, crisps (*Barbara's*)	110	2.0	25.0	<1.0	0	125	1.0
brown, crispy (*Erewhon*)	110	2.0	25.0	0	0	180	1.0
brown, crispy, w/berries (*Erewhon*)	120	2.0	27.0	.5	0	100	1.0

Food and Measure	cal.	prot. (gms)	carbo. (gms)	fat (gms)	chol. (mgs)	sod. (mgs)	fiber (gms)
brown, crispy (*Erewhon* Gluten Free)	110	2.0	25.0	.5	0	160	0
brown, crispy (*Erewhon* No Salt)	110	2.0	25.0	0	0	10	1.0
cocoa (*Cocoa Pebbles*), ¾ cup .	120	1.0	25.0	1.5	0	180	0
cocoa (*Kellogg's Rice Krispies*), ¾ cup	120	1.0	27.0	1.0	0	190	1.0
cocoa (*Malt-O-Meal Cocoa Dyno-Bites*), ¾ cup ...	120	1.0	27.0	1.0	0	160	1.0
cocoa, crispy (*New Morning*), ¾ cup	120	2.0	26.0	.5	0	100	1.0
crispy (*Malt-O-Meal*), 1¼ cups	130	2.0	29.0	0	0	320	0
flakes (*Arrowhead Mills* Sweetened)	180	3.0	40.0	1.0	0	190	1.0
fruit (*Malt-O-Meal Fruity Dyno-Bites*), ¾ cup	100	<1.0	24.0	.5	0	160	0
honey (*Barbara's Puffins*), ¾ cup .	120	2.0	25.0	1.5	0	125	2.0
puffed (*Arrowhead Mills*)	60	1.0	14.0	0	0	50	<1.0
puffed (*Malt-O-Meal*)	60	1.0	13.0	0	0	0	0
rice and corn:							
frosted (*Chex*)	110	1.0	26.0	.5	0	180	0
honey nut (*Chex*) ..	120	2.0	26.0	.5	0	220	0
rice and wheat:							
(*Organic Promise Strawberry Fields*)	120	2.0	28.0	0	0	200	1.0
banana berry (*Fruit Harvest*), ¾ cup .	120	2.0	25.0	2.0	0	140	1.0
peach strawberry (*Fruit Harvest*), ¾ cup	110	2.0	26.0	0	0	170	1.0
red berries (*Kellogg's Special K*)	110	3.0	25.0	0	0	220	1.0
strawberry blueberry (*Fruit Harvest*), ¾ cup	110	2.0	25.0	0	0	140	1.0

Food and Measure	cal.	prot. (gms)	carbo. (gms)	fat (gms)	chol. (mgs)	sod. (mgs)	fiber (gms)
Cereal, ready-to-eat, rice and wheat *(cont.)*							
vanilla almond (*Kellogg's Special K*), ¾ cup	110	2.0	25.0	1.5	0	160	1.0
spelt flakes (*Arrowhead Mills*)	120	4.0	24.0	1.0	0	100	3.0
wheat:							
(*Barbara's* Organic Crispy Wheats), ¾ cup	110	3.0	25.0	.5	0	190	3.0
(*Barbara's* Organic Wild Puffs)	100	2.0	23.0	.5	0	40	<1.0
(*Barbara's* Soy-Essence), ¾ cup	110	3.5	25.0	.5	0	115	5.0
(*Chex* Wheat)	180	5.0	40.0	1.0	0	420	5.0
(*Cinnamon Toast Crunch*), ¾ cup .	120	1.0	24.0	3.0	0	190	2.0
(*Golden Crisp*), ¾ cup	110	2.0	25.0	0	0	25	1.0
(*Golden Grahams*), ¾ cup	120	1.0	25.0	1.0	0	270	1.0
(*Honey Smacks*), ¾ cup	100	2.0	24.0	.5	0	50	1.0
(*Kellogg's Tiger Power*)	110	6.0	21.0	.5	0	250	2.0
(*Malt-O-Meal Golden Puffs*), ¾ cup ...	100	2.0	25.0	0	0	40	<1.0
(*Total* Protein), ¾ cup	120	13.0	11.0	3.5	0	270	3.0
(*Weetabix*), 2 pcs. .	120	4.0	28.0	1.0	0	130	4.0
(*Wheaties*)	110	3.0	24.0	1.0	0	220	3.0
berries (*Malt-O-Meal Balance*) ..	110	3.0	26.0	.5	0	170	5.0
cinnamon (*Malt-O-Meal Cinnamon Toasters*), ¾ cup	130	1.0	24.0	3.5	0	210	1.0
flakes (*Cascadian Farm* Wheat Crunch), ¾ cup .	110	2.0	25.0	.5	0	190	2.0
peanut butter (*Toast Crunch*), ¾ cup .	130	2.0	23.0	3.5	0	210	1.0
whole, flakes (*Erewhon*)	180	6.0	42.0	1.0	0	135	6.0

Food and Measure	cal.	prot. (gms)	carbo. (gms)	fat (gms)	chol. (mgs)	sod. (mgs)	fiber (gms)
whole, w/flaxseed (*Uncle Sam*)	190	7.0	38.0	5.0	0	135	10.0
whole, w/flaxseed, berries (*Uncle Sam*)	220	8.0	39.0	4.5	0	120	10.0
wheat, puffed:							
(*Arrowhead Mills*) .	60	3.0	12.0	0	0	0	2.0
(*Malt-O-Meal*)	50	2.0	11.0	0	0	0	1.0
wheat, shredded:							
(*Arrowhead Mills*) .	190	6.0	38.0	1.0	0	5	6.0
(*Arrowhead Mills Sweetened*)	200	5.0	42.0	1.0	0	5	5.0
(*Barbara's*), 2 pcs. .	140	4.0	31.0	1.0	0	0	5.0
(*Malt-O-Meal Frosted Mini Spooners*)	190	5.0	45.0	1.0	0	0	6.0
(*Organic Promise Autumn Wheat*) .	190	5.0	45.0	1.0	0	0	6.0
(*Post Shredded Wheat 'N Bran Spoon Size*), 1¼ cups	200	7.0	48.0	1.5	0	0	8.0
(*Post Shredded Wheat Original*), 1/6 of 10-oz. pkg.	160	5.0	37.0	1.0	0	0	6.0
(*Post Shredded Wheat Original Spoon Size*)	170	6.0	40.0	1.0	0	0	6.0
frosted (*Kellogg's Mini-Wheats*), approx. 24 pcs., 1.8 oz.	190	4.0	44.0	1.0	0	0	5.0
frosted (*Kellogg's Mini-Wheats Big Bite*), approx. 5 pcs., 1.8 oz. ..	180	5.0	41.0	1.0	0	5	5.0
frosted (*Kellogg's Mini-Wheats Bite Size*), approx. 24 pcs., 2.1 oz. .	200	6.0	48.0	1.0	0	5	6.0
frosted (*Post Shredded Wheat Spoon Size*)	180	4.0	43.0	1.0	0	0	5.0

Food and Measure	cal.	prot. (gms)	carbo. (gms)	fat (gms)	chol. (mgs)	sod. (mgs)	fiber (gms)
Cereal, ready-to-eat, wheat, shredded *(cont.)*							
honey nut (*Post Shredded Wheat Spoon Size*)	200	5.0	43.0	1.5	0	70	4.0
raisin (*Kellogg's Mini-Wheats*), approx. 23 pcs., ¾ cup	180	5.0	42.0	1.0	0	5	5.0
strawberry (*Kellogg's Mini-Wheats*), approx. 23 pcs., ¾ cup ..	170	4.0	40.0	1.0	0	15	5.0
vanilla crème, frosted (*Kellogg's Mini-Wheats*), approx. 24 pcs., ¾ cup.	180	4.0	43.0	1.0	0	0	5.0
wheat and rice (*Cinnamon Toast Crunch*), ¾ cup	130	1.0	24.0	3.5	0	210	1.0
wheat, soy, rice flakes (*Kellogg's Special K Low Carb Lifestyle*), ¾ cup	100	10.0	14.0	3.0	0	110	5.0
wheat bran, see "bran," above							
Cereal, cooking/hot (see also specific grains), uncooked, except as noted:							
barley, ¼ cup:							
(*Arrowhead Mills Bits O Barley*)	160	4.0	34.0	1.0	0	0	6.0
(*Erewhon* Plus) ...	170	5.0	37.0	1.0	0	0	4.0
buckwheat, cream of (*Wolff's*), ⅓ cup ...	90	1.0	21.0	0	0	0	0
bulgur, w/soy (*Hodgson Mill*), ¼ cup ..	115	10.0	22.0	1.0	0	0	3.0
farina, see "wheat," below							
grits, see "Corn grits"							
multigrain:							
(*Country Choice Naturals*), ½ cup	130	6.0	29.0	1.5	0	0	5.0

Food and Measure	cal.	prot. (gms)	carbo. (gms)	fat (gms)	chol. (mgs)	sod. (mgs)	fiber (gms)
(*Kashi* Pilaf), ½ cup*	170	6.0	30.0	3.0	0	15	6.0
4 grain (*Arrowhead Mills* Plus Flax), ¼ cup	140	5.0	28.0	1.5	0	0	9.0
7 grain (*Arrowhead Mills*), ⅓ cup	140	8.0	28.0	1.0	0	0	6.0
7 grain (*Arrowhead Mills* Wheat Free), ¼ cup	150	5.0	30.0	2.5	0	0	3.0
w/flax seeds and soy (*Hodgson Mill*), ⅓ cup	160	7.0	25.0	3.0	0	0	6.0
oat bran:							
(*Arrowhead Mills*), ⅓ cup	130	6.0	21.0	2.5	0	0	4.0
(*Shiloh Farms* 12 oz.), ⅓ cup	130	7.0	25.0	3.0	0	0	6.0
w/wheat germ (*Erewhon*), ⅓ cup	170	10.0	31.0	2.5	0	0	5.0
oat:							
(*Country Choice Naturals* Old Fashioned/Quick), ½ cup	150	5.0	27.0	3.0	0	0	4.0
(*Quaker* Old Fashioned/Quick), ½ cup	150	5.0	27.0	3.0	0	0	4.0
flakes (*Arrowhead Mills*), ⅓ cup	130	5.0	23.0	2.0	0	0	4.0
steel cut (*Arrowhead Mills*), ¼ cup	160	6.0	27.0	3.0	0	0	8.0
oatmeal, 1 pkt., except as noted:							
(*Arrowhead Mills* Instant Original)	110	4.0	19.0	2.0	0	0	2.0
(*Arrowhead Mills* Old Fashioned), ⅓ cup	130	5.0	23.0	2.0	0	0	4.0
(*Country Choice Naturals* Instant)	110	4.0	19.0	2.0	0	0	3.0
(*Malt-O-Meal Big Bowl*)	150	5.0	28.0	3.0	0	150	4.0
(*Uncle Sam* Instant)	130	5.0	24.0	3.0	0	20	5.0

Food and Measure	cal.	prot. (gms)	carbo. (gms)	fat (gms)	chol. (mgs)	sod. (mgs)	fiber (gms)
Cereal, cooking/hot, oatmeal *(cont.)*							
w/added oat bran (*Erewhon* Instant)	130	6.0	25.0	2.5	0	0	4.0
apple cinnamon (*Country Choice Naturals* Instant)	140	4.0	27.0	1.5	0	85	3.0
apple cinnamon (*Erewhon* Instant)	130	5.0	24.0	2.0	0	100	3.0
apple cinnamon (*Heart to Heart* Instant)	160	4.0	33.0	2.0	0	130	5.0
apple cinnamon (*Malt-O-Meal Big Bowl*)	190	4.0	41.0	2.0	0	260	5.0
apple cinnamon (*Fantastic Big Cereal*)	270	8.0	54.0	3.5	0	320	6.0
banana nut barley (*Fantastic Big Cereal*)	270	6.0	55.0	3.5	0	320	8.0
brown sugar or French vanilla (*Country Choice Naturals* Organic Plus)	180	7.0	32.0	3.0	0	140	3.0
cinnamon raisin almond (*Arrowhead Mills*)	140	5.0	24.0	3.0	0	0	3.0
cinnamon spice (*Malt-O-Meal Big Bowl*)	250	6.0	54.0	3.0	0	360	5.0
cranberry orange (*Fantastic Big Cereal*)	300	9.0	56.0	4.0	0	290	7.0
maple, golden brown (*Heart to Heart* Instant) . . .	160	4.0	33.0	2.0	0	95	5.0
maple apple spice (*Arrowhead Mills*)	140	4.0	26.0	2.0	0	45	3.0
maple brown sugar (*Malt-O-Meal Big Bowl*)	230	6.0	49.0	3.0	0	360	5.0
maple raisin 3-grain (*Fantastic Big Cereal*)	270	7.0	60.0	2.0	0	310	8.0

Food and Measure	cal.	prot. (gms)	carbo. (gms)	fat (gms)	chol. (mgs)	sod. (mgs)	fiber (gms)
maple spice (*Erewhon* Instant)	130	5.0	25.0	2.0	0	100	3.0
maple syrup (*Country Choice Naturals* Instant)	170	6.0	32.0	2.0	0	80	4.0
raisin, dates, walnuts (*Erewhon* Instant)	130	4.0	24.0	2.5	0	40	3.0
raisin spice (*Heart to Heart* Instant) .	150	3.0	33.0	2.0	0	100	4.0
steel cut (*Country Choice Naturals*), 1.4 oz.	150	5.0	27.0	3.0	0	0	4.0
wheat 'n berries (*Fantastic Big Cereal*)	260	7.0	56.0	2.0	0	310	8.0
rice:							
(*Arrowhead Mills* Rice and Shine), ¼ cup	150	3.0	32.0	1.0	0	0	2.0
(*Cream of Rice*), 1 pkt.	170	3.0	38.0	0	0	0	0
(*Lundberg* Organic Hot'n Creamy), ⅓ cup	190	4.0	43.0	2.0	0	0	3.0
almond, sweet (*Lundberg* Hot'n Creamy), ⅓ cup .	200	3.0	40.0	3.5	0	0	4.0
brown, cream (*Erewhon*), ¼ cup .	170	5.0	36.0	1.0	0	30	1.0
cinnamon raisin (*Lundberg* Hot'n Creamy), ⅓ cup .	190	3.0	42.0	1.5	0	0	4.0
wheat:							
(*Arrowhead Mills* Bear Mush), ¼ cup	150	5.0	32.0	1.0	0	0	2.0
(*Cream of Wheat* 1, 2½, or 10 Minute), 1 pkt.	120	3.0	25.0	0	0	0	1.0
(*Cream of Wheat* Instant), 1 pkt. . .	90	3.0	17.0	0	0	170	1.0
(*Farina*), 3 tbsp. . . .	120	3.0	22.0	0	0	0	<1.0
(*Malt-O-Meal* Original), 3 tbsp.	120	5.0	26.0	.5	0	0	1.0

Food and Measure	cal.	prot. (gms)	carbo. (gms)	fat (gms)	chol. (mgs)	sod. (mgs)	fiber (gms)
Cereal, cooking/hot, wheat *(cont.)*							
(*Malt-O-Meal* Perfect Balance), ⅓ cup .	160	7.0	32.0	1.5	0	0	3.0
apple cinnamon (*Cream of Wheat* Instant), 1 pkt. . . .	130	2.0	29.0	0	0	160	1.0
chocolate (*Malt-O-Meal*), 3 tbsp. . . .	120	4.0	27.0	.5	0	0	1.0
cinnamon swirl (*Cream of Wheat* Instant), 1 pkt. . . .	130	2.0	28.0	0	0	170	1.0
cracked (*Hodgson Mill*), ¼ cup	110	5.0	25.0	1.0	0	0	5.0
maple brown sugar (*Cream of Wheat* Instant), 1 pkt. . . .	120	2.0	27.0	0	0	140	1.0
maple brown sugar (*Malt-O-Meal*), ¼ cup	170	4.0	37.0	0	0	0	1.0
peaches or strawberries and cream (*Cream of Wheat* Instant), 1 pkt. . . .	130	2.0	28.0	0	0	270	1.0
wheat, rye, and flax: (*Red River* Original), ¼ cup	154	5.5	27.0	2.5	0	4	5.7
(*Red River* Ready-to-Serve), 1 pkt. .	136	4.9	24.0	2.2	0	0	5.3
maple brown sugar (*Red River* Ready-to-Serve), 1 pkt. .	153	4.6	29.0	1.8	0	0	4.5
Cereal crumbs, see "Corn flake crumbs"							
Cereal bar, see "Granola/cereal bar"							
Cervelat, see "Summer sausage"							
Challah, see "Bread, frozen"							
Chapati (*Garden of Eatin'*), 1.3-oz. pc. .	120	3.0	20.0	2.5	0	110	2.0
Chayote:							
raw:							
1 medium, 7.2 oz. .	49	1.8	11.0	.6	0	8	6.1

Food and Measure	cal.	prot. (gms)	carbo. (gms)	fat (gms)	chol. (mgs)	sod. (mgs)	fiber (gms)
1" pcs., ½ cup	16	.6	3.6	.2	0	3	2.0
boiled, drained, 1" pcs., ½ cup	19	.5	4.1	.4	0	1	2.3
Cheese (see also "Cheese food/ product" and "Cheese spread"), 1 oz., except as noted:							
all varieties, except Monterey Jack (*Land O Lakes Snack 'n Cheese To-Go*), ¾ oz.	80	5.0	0	7.0	20	140	0
American, processed:							
(*Boar's Head* Loaf) .	100	6.0	1.0	9.0	25	380	0
(*Cabot*), ¾-oz. slice	80	4.0	1.0	7.0	20	270	0
(*Kraft* Singles), ⅔ oz.	60	3.0	1.0	4.5	15	250	0
(*Kraft* Singles), ¾ oz.	70	4.0	2.0	5.0	20	270	0
(*Kraft* Singles Extra Thick), 1.2 oz. ..	110	6.0	3.0	8.0	30	440	0
(*Kraft* Singles Fat Free), ⅔ oz.	30	4.0	2.0	0	5	250	0
(*Kraft* Singles Fat Free), ¾ oz.	30	5.0	2.0	0	5	270	0
(*Kraft Deli Deluxe* Slices)	100	5.0	1.0	9.0	30	460	0
(*Kraft Deli Deluxe* Slices), ⅔ oz. ..	70	4.0	0	6.0	20	310	0
(*Kraft Deli Deluxe* Slices), ¾ oz.	80	4.0	0	7.0	20	340	0
(*Land O Lakes*) ...	110	6.0	1.0	9.0	25	400	0
(*Land O Lakes* Less Salt)	110	6.0	1.0	9.0	30	260	0
(*Land O Lakes* Light)	70	7.0	1.0	4.0	15	370	0
(*Land O Lake* Slices), ¾ oz.	70	4.0	2.0	5.0	15	350	0
(*Land O Lakes Naturally Slender*)	90	6.0	1.0	7.0	20	360	0
(*Sara Lee*)	100	7.0	1.0	8.0	25	260	0
(*Sara Lee* Slices), .8 oz.	80	5.0	0	7.0	25	340	0

Food and Measure	cal.	prot. (gms)	carbo. (gms)	fat (gms)	chol. (mgs)	sod. (mgs)	fiber (gms)
Cheese, American, processed (cont.)							
(Sargento Burger-Cheese), ⅔-oz. slice	70	4.0	<1.0	6.0	20	240	0
sharp (Land O Lakes Slices)	110	6.0	1.0	9.0	25	390	0
white (Hatfield Deli Choice)	110	6.0	0	9.0	25	180	0
white or yellow (Alpine Lace Reduced Fat)	90	6.0	1.0	6.0	20	300	0
yellow (Alpine Lace Reduced Fat Loaf)	90	6.0	1.0	7.0	20	300	0
asiago:							
(BelGioioso)	100	7.0	0	8.0	25	340	0
(Sara Lee)	110	8.0	0	9.0	20	310	0
shredded (Sara Lee)	110	8.0	0	9.0	20	310	0
shredded (Sargento Extra Fine), 2 tsp.	20	1.0	0	1.5	5	55	0
(BelGioioso Auribella)	110	7.0	0	9.0	30	265	0
(BelGioioso Italico)	100	6.0	0	8.0	30	280	0
blend, shredded, ¼ cup:							
(Cabot Fancy)	100	7.0	1.0	7.0	20	180	0
4 cheese (Kraft Classic Melts)	120	7.0	1.0	10.0	30	310	0
blue/bleu:							
(Athenos)	100	6.0	<1.0	8.0	30	390	0
(Point Reyes Original)	100	6.0	0	8.0	25	390	0
creamy (Boar's Head)	90	6.0	0	8.0	30	310	0
blue, crumbled:							
(Athenos), 3 tbsp.	110	7.0	2.0	9.0	30	430	<1.0
(Litehouse Idaho), ¼ cup, 1.1 oz.	100	5.0	2.0	8.0	35	400	0
(Sargento), ¼ cup	100	6.0	1.0	8.0	25	380	0
brick (Land O Lakes)	110	7.0	1.0	8.0	25	170	0
Brie	95	5.9	.1	7.9	20	229	0
butterkäse, plain or smoked (Boar's Head)	100	6.0	0	9.0	30	180	0
Camembert	85	5.6	.1	6.9	20	239	0
caraway	107	7.1	.9	8.3	2.6	196	0

Food and Measure	cal.	prot. (gms)	carbo. (gms)	fat (gms)	chol. (mgs)	sod. (mgs)	fiber (gms)
Chedarella (Land O Lakes)	110	7.0	0	9.0	25	190	0
cheddar:							
(*Alpine Lace Reduced Fat*) ...	90	7.0	0	7.0	20	200	0
(*Cabot*)	110	7.0	<1.0	9.0	30	180	0
(*Boar's Head Canadian/Vermont*)	110	7.0	0	10.0	30	170	0
(*Cabot Light 75% Reduced Fat*) ...	60	9.0	<1.0	2.5	10	200	0
(*Cabot Light 50% Reduced Fat*) ...	70	8.0	1.0	4.5	15	170	0
(*Kraft 2% Fat*)	90	7.0	1.0	6.0	20	240	0
(*Land O Lakes*) ...	110	7.0	0	9.0	30	190	0
(*Organic Valley*) ...	110	7.0	<1.0	9.0	30	180	0
(*Organic Valley*), ¾-oz. slice	90	5.0	0	7.0	20	140	0
(*Sargento Slices*) ..	80	5.0	0	6.0	20	140	0
(*Tree of Life Low Sodium*)	110	7.0	0	9.0	25	110	0
(*Tree of Life Organic 33% Less Fat*) ..	90	8.0	1.0	6.0	15	135	0
medium (*Kraft*) ...	110	7.0	1.0	9.0	30	180	0
mild (*Cracker Barrel Cracker Cuts*) ...	120	6.0	0	10.0	25	180	0
mild (*Kraft Longhorn*)	110	7.0	0	9.0	30	180	0
mild (*Kraft Deli Deluxe* Slices), .8 oz.	90	5.0	0	7.0	25	160	0
mild (*Sara Lee*) ...	110	7.0	1.0	9.0	30	180	0
mild (*Sara Lee* Slices), .8 oz. ...	90	5.0	0	7.0	20	140	0
mild (*Sargento* Snack Single) ...	110	7.0	1.0	9.0	30	180	0
mild (*Sargento* Snack 6-Pack), .8 oz.	100	6.0	0	8.0	25	150	0
mild (*Sargento* Cubes), 7 pcs., 1.1 oz.	120	7.0	<1.0	10.0	30	190	0
mild (*Tree of Life* Organic)	110	7.0	1.0	9.0	30	180	0
mild or sharp (*Tree of Life*)	110	7.0	0	9.0	25	180	0

Food and Measure	cal.	prot. (gms)	carbo. (gms)	fat (gms)	chol. (mgs)	sod. (mgs)	fiber (gms)
Cheese, cheddar *(cont.)*							
mild or smoked							
(*Cabot*)	110	7.0	<1.0	9.0	30	180	0
raw or sharp							
(*Organic Valley*) .	110	7.0	0	9.0	30	170	0
sharp (*Boar's Head*)	110	7.0	<1.0	9.0	30	190	0
sharp (*Cracker*							
Barrel Reduced							
Fat)	90	7.0	1.0	6.0	20	240	0
sharp (*Cracker*							
Barrel Slices),							
¾ oz.	90	5.0	0	8.0	25	150	0
sharp (*Kraft*)	120	6.0	0	10.0	30	180	0
sharp (*Kraft* Singles),							
¾ oz.	60	4.0	2.0	4.5	15	270	0
sharp (*Kraft* Singles							
Fat Free), ¾ oz. .	30	5.0	2.0	0	5	280	0
sharp (*Kraft* Singles							
2% Fat), ¾ oz. . .	50	4.0	1.0	3.0	10	290	0
sharp (*Kraft Deli*							
Deluxe Slices),							
.8 oz.	90	5.0	0	8.0	25	150	0
sharp, extra							
(*Cracker* Barrel							
Reduced Fat) . . .	90	7.0	1.0	9.0	20	240	0
sharp, extra							
(*Cracker Barrel*							
Cracker Cuts) . . .	120	6.0	0	10.0	30	180	0
sharp, extra (*Land O*							
Lakes Processed)	110	6.0	1.0	9.0	25	350	0
sharp or extra sharp							
(*Cracker Barrel*) .	120	6.0	0	10.0	30	180	0
sharp or extra sharp							
(*Sara Lee*)	110	7.0	1.0	9.0	30	180	0
sharp, white							
(*Cracker Barrel*							
Vermont)	110	7.0	1.0	9.0	30	180	0
sharp, white							
(*Cracker Barrel*							
Reduced Fat) . . .	90	7.0	1.0	6.0	20	240	0
cheddar, shredded,							
¼ cup:							
(*Organic Valley*) . . .	110	7.0	1.0	9.0	30	180	0

Food and Measure	cal.	prot. (gms)	carbo. (gms)	fat (gms)	chol. (mgs)	sod. (mgs)	fiber (gms)
(*Sargento* Thick & Hearty)	110	6.0	1.0	9.0	25	200	0
all styles (*Sargento* ChefStyle)	110	7.0	1.0	9.0	30	190	0
fine (*Kraft* Free) ...	45	9.0	1.0	0	5	280	0
mild (*Kraft* 2% Fat)	80	7.0	1.0	6.0	20	230	0
mild (*Sargento*) ...	110	7.0	1.0	9.0	30	190	0
mild (*Sargento* 4 oz.)	110	7.0	1.0	9.0	30	180	0
mild (*Sargento* Reduced Fat) ...	80	7.0	1.0	6.0	20	180	0
mild, fine (*Kraft*) ..	110	6.0	1.0	9.0	25	180	0
sharp (*Cabot*)	110	7.0	1.0	9.0	30	180	0
sharp (*Kraft*)	110	6.0	1.0	9.0	25	180	0
sharp, fine (*Kraft*) .	120	7.0	1.0	10.0	30	190	0
sharp, fine (*Kraft* 2% Fat)	80	7.0	1.0	6.0	20	230	0
w/tomato, jalapeño, salsa (*Sargento* Bistro)	110	7.0	2.0	9.0	25	190	0
cheddar, flavored:							
bacon (*Kraft*)	90	5.0	2.0	7.0	20	480	0
chipotle, Parmesan, pepperoni pizza, or smoky bacon (*Cabot*)	110	7.0	1.0	9.0	30	180	0
garlic, roasted (*Kraft*)	80	5.0	1.0	2.0	25	380	0
garlic herb, roasted garlic, habanero, Mediterranean, peppercorn, or tomato basil (*Cabot*)	110	7.0	<1.0	9.0	30	180	0
horseradish (*Boar's Head*)	110	6.0	0	9.0	30	190	0
horseradish (*Cabot*)	110	6.0	1.0	9.0	30	270	0
horseradish (*Williams*)	110	6.0	0	9.0	30	460	0
jalapeño (*Cabot* Light 50% Reduced Fat)	70	8.0	1.0	4.5	15	170	0
cheddar blend, shredded ¼ cup:							
American (*Kraft* Classic Melts) ..	120	7.0	1.0	10.0	30	310	0

Food and Measure	cal.	prot. (gms)	carbo. (gms)	fat (gms)	chol. (mgs)	sod. (mgs)	fiber (gms)
Cheese, cheddar blend *(cont.)*							
Jack (*Kraft* Mexican)	110	6.0	1.0	9.0	25	190	0
Jack (*Sargento*) . . .	110	7.0	1.0	9.0	30	180	0
Jack, w/jalapeño							
(*Sargento*)	110	6.0	1.0	9.0	25	180	0
Monterey Jack							
(*Kraft*)	100	6.0	1.0	8.0	25	170	0
cheddar Monterey Jack,							
marbled (*Kraft*) . . .	110	7.0	1.0	9.0	30	200	0
Cheshire	110	6.6	1.4	8.7	29	198	0
Colby:							
(*Boar's Head*							
Longhorn)	110	7.0	<1.0	9.0	30	170	0
(*Kraft*)	110	6.0	1.0	9.0	30	180	0
(*Kraft* Longhorn) . .	110	7.0	0	9.0	30	180	0
(*Kraft* 2% Fat)	80	7.0	0	6.0	20	220	0
(*Land O Lakes*) . . .	110	7.0	1.0	9.0	25	190	0
(*Organic Valley*) . . .	110	7.0	<1.0	9.0	25	170	0
(*Sara Lee*)	110	7.0	1.0	9.0	30	170	0
(*Sara Lee* Longhorn							
Slices)	110	7.0	0	9.0	30	170	0
(*Sargento* Slices),							
¾ oz.	80	5.0	<1.0	7.0	20	140	0
(*Tree of Life*)	110	7.0	1.0	9.0	30	170	0
Colby Jack:							
(*Alpine Lace Co-Jack*							
Reduced Fat) . . .	90	6.0	1.0	7.0	20	135	0
(*Boar's Head*)	110	6.0	0	9.0	25	180	0
(*Cabot*)	110	7.0	1.0	9.0	30	170	0
(*Cracker Barrel*							
Cracker Cuts) . . .	110	7.0	1.0	9.0	30	180	0
(*Kraft Deli Deluxe*							
Slices), .8 oz. . . .	90	5.0	0	7.0	25	150	0
(*Land O Lakes Co-*							
Jack)	110	7.0	0	9.0	25	190	0
(*Sara Lee*)	100	7.0	0	8.0	30	170	0
(*Sargento* Slices),							
⅔ oz.	70	4.0	0	6.0	15	125	0
(*Sargento* Snacks) .	110	6.0	<1.0	9.0	25	190	0
(*Sargento* Snacks),							
¾-oz. pc.	80	5.0	<1.0	7.0	20	140	0
(*Sargento* Cubes),							
7 pcs., 1.1 oz. . .	110	6.0	<1.0	9.0	25	200	0

Food and Measure	cal.	prot. (gms)	carbo. (gms)	fat (gms)	chol. (mgs)	sod. (mgs)	fiber (gms)
(*Sargento Cubes 8 oz.*), 7 pcs., 1.1 oz.	110	6.0	<1.0	9.0	25	190	0
marbled (*Kraft*) ...	110	7.0	0	9.0	30	180	0
Colby Jack, shredded, ¼ cup or 1 oz.:							
(*Sargento*)	110	7.0	1.0	9.0	30	190	0
fine (*Kraft*)	100	6.0	1.0	8.0	25	190	0
cottage, 4%, ½ cup:							
(*Darigold* Large Curd)	130	14.0	5.0	5.0	25	490	0
(*Darigold* Small Curd)	120	14.0	5.0	5.0	25	470	0
(*Friendship*)	110	15.0	3.0	5.0	20	380	0
(*Hood* Country/ Large Curd)	110	13.0	5.0	4.5	25	380	0
(*Organic Valley*) ...	110	14.0	3.0	5.0	15	450	0
chive (*Darigold*) ...	120	14.0	5.0	5.0	25	470	0
chive (*Hood*)	110	13.0	5.0	4.5	25	380	0
pineapple (*Darigold*)	150	11.0	17.0	4.0	20	410	0
pineapple (*Friend-ship*)	140	12.0	14.0	4.0	15	300	0
pineapple (*Hood*) ..	130	10.0	15.0	3.5	20	290	0
cottage, 2%, ½ cup:							
(*Breakstone's* Large Curd	90	11.0	6.0	2.5	15	410	0
(*Breakstone's* Small Curd	90	12.0	6.0	2.5	15	400	0
(*Cabot*)	100	13.0	4.0	4.5	15	400	0
(*Darigold*)	100	14.0	5.0	2.5	15	470	0
(*Friendship* Pot Style)	90	15.0	3.0	2.5	10	400	0
(*Knudsen* Low Fat) .	100	13.0	6.0	2.5	15	440	0
(*Organic Valley*) ...	100	15.0	4.0	2.0	10	450	0
cottage, 1%, ½ cup:							
(*Friendship*)	90	16.0	3.0	1.0	5	360	0
(*Friendship* No Salt)	90	16.0	4.0	1.0	5	50	0
(*Hood*)	80	13.0	6.0	1.0	10	380	0
(*Hood* No Salt)	80	13.0	6.0	1.0	10	60	0
black pepper and herbs (*Hood*) ...	80	13.0	6.0	1.0	10	430	0
chive and toasted onion (*Hood*) ...	110	13.0	5.0	4.5	25	380	0
peaches (*Hood*) ...	110	9.0	18.0	1.0	5	270	0
pineapple (*Friend-ship*)	120	12.0	16.0	1.0	5	290	0

Food and Measure	cal.	prot. (gms)	carbo. (gms)	fat (gms)	chol. (mgs)	sod. (mgs)	fiber (gms)
Cheese, cottage, 1% *(cont.)*							
pineapple and cherry							
(*Hood*)	80	13.0	6.0	1.0	10	380	0
strawberries (*Hood*)	120	9.0	19.0	1.0	5	270	0
cottage, nonfat, ½ cup:							
(*Breakstone's*)	90	12.0	8.0	0	10	450	0
(*Cabot*)	70	13.0	5.0	0	5	410	0
(*Darigold*)	90	15.0	6.0	0	5	460	0
(*Friendship*)	80	15.0	4.0	0	<5	350	0
(*Hood*)	80	13.0	7.0	0	5	320	0
(*Knudsen Free*) . . .	80	13.0	7.0	0	5	430	0
peach (*Friendship*) .	110	12.0	15.0	0	<5	300	0
pineapple (*Friend-							
ship*)	110	12.0	16.0	0	<5	300	0
pineapple (*Hood*) . .	100	10.0	16.0	0	5	240	0
cream cheese, 2 tbsp.:							
(*Boar's Head*)	100	2.0	2.0	10.0	30	100	0
(*Organic Valley* Bar),							
1 oz.	100	.5	1.0	10.0	35	95	0
(*Organic Valley* Tub)	90	2.0	2.0	9.0	30	140	0
(*Philadelphia* Bar) .	100	2.0	1.0	10.0	30	90	0
(*Philadelphia* Bar Fat							
Free)	30	4.0	2.0	0	5	200	0
(*Philadelphia* Light)	60	3.0	2.0	4.5	15	150	0
(*Philadelphia* ⅓ Less							
Fat)	80	3.0	1.0	6.0	20	120	0
(*Philadelphia* Tub) .	100	2.0	1.0	9.0	35	120	0
(*Philadelphia* Tub Fat							
Free)	30	5.0	1.0	0	5	200	0
berries or brown							
sugar cinnamon							
(*Philadelphia*							
Swirls)	90	1.0	4.0	8.0	30	115	0
chive and onion							
(*Philadelphia*) . . .	90	2.0	2.0	9.0	35	160	0
garlic herb (*Philadel-							
phia* Swirls)	90	1.0	3.0	8.0	35	140	0
honey nut (*Philadel-							
phia*)	100	1.0	4.0	8.0	30	100	0
pineapple (*Philadel-							
phia*)	90	1.0	4.0	8.0	30	100	0
salmon (*Philadelphia*)	90	2.0	1.0	8.0	35	210	0
strawberry (*Philadel-							
phia*)	90	1.0	4.0	8.0	30	100	0

Food and Measure	cal.	prot. (gms)	carbo. (gms)	fat (gms)	chol. (mgs)	sod. (mgs)	fiber (gms)
strawberry (*Philadelphia* Light)	70	2.0	6.0	4.0	15	120	0
vegetable, garden (*Philadelphia*) ...	90	1.0	2.0	9.0	35	150	0
cream cheese, whipped, 2 tbsp.:							
(*Philadelphia*)	60	1.0	1.0	6.0	20	90	0
berry, mixed (*Philadelphia*)	70	1.0	3.0	6.0	20	50	0
chive (*Philadelphia*)	60	1.0	<1.0	6.0	15	130	0
cinnamon brown sugar (*Philadelphia*)	70	1.0	3.0	6.0	20	55	0
garlic and herb (*Philadelphia*) ...	60	1.0	1.0	6.0	20	100	0
ranch (*Philadelphia*)	60	1.0	1.0	6.0	15	150	0
Edam:							
(*Boar's Head*)	90	7.0	0	7.0	20	280	0
(*Sara Lee*)	100	8.0	0	8.0	25	280	0
1 oz.	90	7.0	0	7.0	25	280	0
farmer:							
(*Friendship*)	50	5.0	0	2.5	10	120	0
(*Friendship* No Salt)	50	5.0	0	2.5	10	10	0
farmer, kefir, 2 tbsp.:							
(*Lifeway*)	40	3.0	4.0	1.5	6	10	0
(*Lifeway* Lite)	25	3.0	2.0	1.0	<5	10	0
feta:							
(*Alpine Lace* Reduced Fat) ...	50	6.0	1.0	3.0	10	370	0
(*Athenos* Mild)	80	5.0	<1.0	6.0	20	190	0
(*Athenos* Traditional)	70	5.0	<1.0	6.0	20	320	0
(*Athenos* Traditional Reduced Fat) ...	60	6.0	<1.0	4.0	10	390	0
(*Boar's Head*)	60	5.0	1.0	4.0	10	360	0
(*Organic Valley*) ...	70	4.0	1.0	6.0	10	430	0
(*Shiloh Farms* Goat)	110	6.0	0	9.0	15	150	0
basil tomato (*Athenos*)	80	5.0	<1.0	6.0	20	320	<1.0
garlic herb (*Athenos*)	80	5.0	0	7.0	20	340	0
peppercorn (*Athenos*)	80	5.0	<1.0	6.0	20	330	<1.0
feta, crumbled, ¼ cup:							
(*Athenos* Mild)	90	6.0	1.0	7.0	20	220	<1.0
(*Athenos* Traditional)	90	5.0	2.0	7.0	20	380	<1.0

Food and Measure	cal.	prot. (gms)	carbo. (gms)	fat (gms)	chol. (mgs)	sod. (mgs)	fiber (gms)
Cheese, feta, crumbled *(cont.)*							
(*Athenos* Traditional Reduced Fat) ...	70	7.0	1.0	4.5	10	470	<1.0
basil tomato (*Athenos*)	100	6.0	2.0	8.0	25	380	<1.0
basil tomato (*Athenos* Reduced Fat)	70	7.0	2.0	4.5	10	460	<1.0
garlic herb (*Athenos*)	100	6.0	1.0	8.0	20	400	1.0
peppercorn (*Athenos*)	100	6.0	2.0	7.0	25	400	<1.0
(*Finlandia Lappi*)	100	7.0	<1.0	8.0	25	160	0
fontina:							
(*BelGioioso*)	100	6.0	0	8.0	25	170	0
(*Denmark's Finest*)	90	7.0	0	7.0	15	160	0
(*Gjetost*)	130	3.0	11.0	9.0	30	90	0
Gloucester, double (*Boar's Head*)	110	7.0	0	10.0	35	200	0
goat:							
(*Shiloh Farms* Just Jack)	110	7.0	<1.0	9.0	20	130	0
hard type	128	8.7	.6	10.1	30	98	0
semisoft type	103	6.1	.7	8.5	22	146	0
soft type	76	5.3	.3	6.0	13	104	0
chive (*Shiloh Farms* Chive 'n Jack) ..	100	7.0	0	8.0	20	110	0
garlic and herbs (*Maitre D'*)	80	5.0	0	6.0	20	130	0
tomato basil (*Shiloh Farms*)	100	7.0	0	8.0	20	110	0
gorgonzola:							
(*Athenos*)	100	6.0	<1.0	8.0	25	380	0
(*BelGioioso Creamy-Gorg*)	100	6.0	0	8.0	30	280	0
crumbled (*Athenos*), 3 tbsp.	110	7.0	2.0	9.0	30	400	<1.0
Gouda:							
(*Boar's Head*)	110	6.0	0	9.0	30	280	0
(*Finlandia Naturals*)	100	7.0	<1.0	8.0	25	160	0
(*Finlandia Sandwich Naturals*)	100	7.0	<1.0	8.0	25	160	0
(*Sara Lee*)	110	7.0	0	9.0	30	260	0
aged (*Rembrandt*) .	120	7.0	0	9.0	27	264	0

Food and Measure	cal.	prot. (gms)	carbo. (gms)	fat (gms)	chol. (mgs)	sod. (mgs)	fiber (gms)
smoked (*Sara Lee*)	110	7.0	0	9.0	30	260	0
Gruyère	117	8.5	.1	9.2	31	95	0
havarti:							
(*Finlandia Naturals*)	110	8.0	<1.0	9.0	25	160	0
(*Finlandia Sandwich*							
Naturals)	110	7.0	<1.0	9.0	25	160	0
(*Land O Lakes*) . . .	110	7.0	0	9.0	25	170	0
(*Sara Lee*)	120	5.0	0	10.0	25	150	0
cream, all varieties							
(*Boar's Head*) . . .	110	6.0	0	10.0	35	210	0
dill (*Sara Lee*)	110	6.0	0	9.0	25	170	0
Italian, shredded,							
¼ cup:							
(*Maggio*)	90	7.0	<1.0	6.0	20	190	0
4 cheese (*Organic*							
Valley)	90	8.0	1.0	7.0	20	220	0
4 cheese (*Sargento*							
Reduced Fat) . . .	80	8.0	1.0	4.5	15	220	0
5 cheese (*Kraft*) . . .	90	7.0	1.0	6.0	20	240	0
6 cheese (*Sargento*)	90	7.0	1.0	7.0	20	200	0
w/garlic (*Sargento*)	100	7.0	1.0	7.0	20	170	0
jalapeño Jack (*Tree of*							
Life Organic)	110	6.0	1.0	9.0	20	160	0
(*Jarlsberg*):							
regular	100	7.0	0	8.0	20	180	0
(*Jarlsberg Lite*) . . .	70	9.0	0	3.5	10	130	0
(*Sargento Jarlsberg*							
Slices), .8 oz. . . .	80	6.0	<1.0	6.0	15	110	0
kasseri (*BelGioioso*) . .	110	7.0	0	9.0	30	270	0
limburger	93	5.7	.1	7.7	26	227	0
mascarpone:							
(*BelGioioso*)	120	2.0	0	13.0	35	15	0
(*BelGioioso* Tiramisu)	130	2.0	0	13.0	35	15	0
Mexican, mild, jalapeño							
(*Kraft* Singles), ¾ oz.	60	4.0	2.0	4.5	15	270	0
Mexican, shredded,							
¼ cup:							
(*Maggio*)	110	6.0	1.0	9.0	25	200	0
(*Sargento*)	110	6.0	1.0	9.0	25	200	0
(*Sargento* Reduced							
Fat)	80	8.0	1.0	6.0	20	200	0
(*Sargento* Thick &							
Hearty)	80	7.0	1.0	6.0	15	190	0

Food and Measure	cal.	prot. (gms)	carbo. (gms)	fat (gms)	chol. (mgs)	sod. (mgs)	fiber (gms)
Cheese, Mexican, shredded *(cont.)*							
4 cheese (*Kraft*) . . .	100	6.0	1.0	9.0	25	190	0
4 cheese (*Kraft* 2% Fat)	80	7.0	1.0	5.0	15	240	0
Monterey Jack:							
(*Boar's Head*)	100	6.0	0	9.0	25	180	0
(*Cabot*)	110	7.0	<1.0	9.0	30	170	0
(*Kraft* 8 oz.)	100	6.0	0	9.0	30	190	0
(*Kraft* 16 oz.)	110	6.0	0	9.0	30	190	0
(*Kraft* 2% Fat)	80	7.0	1.0	6.0	20	240	0
(*Kraft* Singles), ¾ oz.	70	4.0	1.0	5.0	20	280	0
(*Land O Lakes*) . . .	110	7.0	0	9.0	25	190	0
(*Land O Lakes* Snack 'n Cheese To-Go), ¾ oz. . . .	80	5.0	0	7.0	20	125	0
(*Organic Valley*) . . .	100	7.0	0	9.0	30	170	0
(*Sara Lee*)	100	7.0	0	8.0	30	170	0
(*Sara Lee* Slices) .8 oz.	80	5.0	0	7.0	20	135	0
(*Sargento* Slices), ¾ oz.	80	5.0	0	6.0	20	135	0
(*Tree of Life* Organic)	100	6.0	1.0	8.0	20	170	0
hot pepper (*Land O Lakes*)	110	6.0	0	9.0	25	190	0
jalapeño (*Boar's Head*)	100	6.0	0	9.0	25	170	0
jalapeño (*Land O Lakes*)	110	6.0	1.0	9.0	25	190	0
jalapeño (*Sara Lee*)	100	6.0	1.0	8.0	20	190	0
jalapeño (*Sara Lee* Slices), .8 oz. . . .	80	5.0	0	6.0	20	125	0
semisoft (*Tree of Life*)	110	7.0	0	9.0	25	150	0
Monterey Jack, shredded, ¼ cup:							
(*Colby*)	110	7.0	1.0	9.0	30	170	0
(*Kraft*)	100	6.0	1.0	8.0	25	190	0
(*Sargento*)	110	7.0	1.0	9.0	30	190	0
Monterey Jack and Colby, see "Colby Jack," above							
mozzarella:							
(*Alpine Lace* Reduced Fat) . . .	70	8.0	1.0	3.0	10	200	0

Food and Measure	cal.	prot. (gms)	carbo. (gms)	fat (gms)	chol. (mgs)	sod. (mgs)	fiber (gms)
(*Alpine Lace* Reduced Fat Low Moisture)	70	6.0	1.0	5.0	20	250	0
(*BelGioioso* Fresh) .	80	5.0	1.0	6.0	25	170	0
(*Boar's Head* Low Moisture)	90	6.0	1.0	7.0	20	150	0
(*Kraft* Low Moisture)	80	7.0	1.0	5.0	20	220	0
(*Kraft* Singles), ¾ oz.	50	4.0	1.0	3.0	10	290	0
(*Kraft Deli Deluxe* Slices), ¾ oz. . . .	60	6.0	0	5.0	10	150	0
(*Land O Lakes*) . . .	90	7.0	1.0	6.0	15	190	0
(*Organic Valley*) . . .	80	5.0	<1.0	6.0	20	105	0
(*Polly-O* Fresh)	80	5.0	0	7.0	20	15	0
(*Sara Lee* Slices), .8 oz.	60	6.0	1.0	4.0	10	130	0
(*Sargento* Slices 8 oz.), ¾ oz.	60	5.0	0	4.0	10	140	0
(*Sargento* Slices 12 oz.), ¾ oz. . . .	60	5.0	1.0	4.0	15	140	0
(*Sargento Twirls*), .8-oz. pc.	70	6.0	<1.0	4.5	15	200	0
(*Tree of Life*)	80	8.0	1.0	5.0	15	150	0
(*Tree of Life* Organic)	80	8.0	1.0	5.0	15	170	0
whole (*Maggio*) . . .	80	6.0	1.0	6.0	25	180	0
whole (*Polly-O*) . . .	80	6.0	1.0	6.0	20	200	0
part skim (*Maggio*)	80	7.0	1.0	5.0	20	180	0
part skim (*Polly-O*)	70	6.0	1.0	5.0	15	200	0
nonfat (*Kraft* Singles), ¾ oz.	30	5.0	2.0	0	5	270	0
nonfat (*Polly-O*) . . .	35	7.0	1.0	0	5	220	0
mozzarella, shredded, ¼ cup:							
(*Cabot*)	80	8.0	1.0	6.0	15	170	0
(*Kraft*)	80	6.0	1.0	5.0	20	220	0
(*Maggio*)	80	8.0	1.0	5.0	15	170	0
(*Organic Valley*) . . .	80	8.0	1.0	5.0	15	170	0
(*Polly-O*)	90	6.0	1.0	7.0	20	190	0
(*Polly-O* Lite)	60	7.0	1.0	2.5	10	230	0
(*Polly-O* Nonfat) . . .	40	8.0	1.0	0	5	240	0
(*Polly-O* Part Skim)	80	7.0	1.0	5.0	15	200	0
(*Sargento* ChefStyle Whole)	90	7.0	1.0	7.0	25	190	0
(*Sargento* ChefStyle/ Fancy)	80	7.0	1.0	6.0	15	190	0

Food and Measure	cal.	prot. (gms)	carbo. (gms)	fat (gms)	chol. (mgs)	sod. (mgs)	fiber (gms)
Cheese, mozzarella, shredded *(cont.)*							
(*Sargento* Reduced Fat) . . . . :	80	8.0	<1.0	4.5	10	200	0
(*Sargento* Thick & Hearty)	110	7.0	1.0	9.0	30	190	0
asiago, w/roasted garlic (*Sargento Bistro*)	80	7.0	2.0	6.0	15	270	0
Parmesan, fine (*Polly-O*)	90	6.0	1.0	7.0	20	210	0
provolone (*Sargento*)	90	6.0	0	7.0	20	170	0
provolone, Romano, Parmesan (*Polly-O*)	90	0	1.0	7.0	20	230	0
w/sun-dried tomato and basil (*Sargento Bistro*)	90	7.0	1.0	6.0	20	220	0
Muenster:							
(*Alpine Lace* Reduced Fat) . . .	100	7.0	1.0	9.0	25	85	0
(*Boar's Head*)	100	6.0	0	8.0	25	180	0
(*Boar's Head* Low Sodium)	100	6.0	0	8.0	20	75	0
(*Finlandia*)	115	7.0	<1.0	10.0	13	170	0
(*Finlandia Naturals*)	110	7.0	<1.0	9.0	25	180	0
(*Finlandia Sandwich Naturals*)	110	7.0	<1.0	9.0	25	180	0
(*Land O Lakes*) . . .	100	7.0	0	8.0	25	180	0
(*Organic Valley*) . . .	100	7.0	1.0	8.0	25	180	0
(*Sara Lee*)	100	6.0	0	8.0	25	190	0
(*Sara Lee* Slices), .8 oz.	80	5.0	0	7.0	20	150	0
(*Sargento* Slices), ¾ oz.	80	5.0	0	6.0	20	135	0
nacho, shredded, ¼ cup:							
(*Sargento*)	110	7.0	1.0	9.0	30	200	0
(*Sargento* 4 oz.) . . .	110	7.0	1.0	9.0	25	220	0
Neufchâtel (*Philadelphia*)	70	3.0	1.0	6.0	20	120	0
Parmesan:							
(*BelGioioso/BelGioioso* Vegetarian)	110	10.0	0	7.0	25	260	0

Food and Measure	cal.	prot. (gms)	carbo. (gms)	fat (gms)	chol. (mgs)	sod. (mgs)	fiber (gms)
(*BelGioioso American Grana*)	110	10.0	0	7.0	25	260	0
(*Sara Lee*)	110	10.0	1.0	7.0	20	350	0
Parmesan, grated, 2 tsp.:							
(*Kraft*)	20	2.0	0	1.5	5	85	0
(*Kraft* Reduced Fat)	20	1.0	2.0	1.0	5	75	0
(*Polly-O*)	20	2.0	0	1.5	5	85	0
(*Rienzi*)	20	2.0	0	1.5	5	75	0
(*Sara Lee*)	20	2.0	0	1.5	5	70	0
(*Sargento*)	25	2.0	0	1.5	5	80	0
(*Tree of Life*)	20	2.0	0	1.0	5	30	0
Romano (*Kraft*) ...	20	2.0	0	1.0	5	85	0
Romano (*Polly-O*) .	20	2.0	0	1.5	5	85	0
Romano (*Sargento*)	25	2.0	0	1.5	5	80	0
Parmesan, shredded, ¼ cup:							
(*Kraft*)	110	9.0	1.0	8.0	25	410	0
(*Organic Valley*) ...	110	10.0	0	7.0	20	350	0
(*Sara Lee*)	110	10.0	1.0	7.0	20	350	0
(*Tree of Life*)	100	9.0	1.0	7.0	20	180	0
mozzarella and Romano (*Sargento Angel Hair*)	100	8.0	1.0	7.0	20	280	0
Romano and asiago (*Kraft*)	110	8.0	1.0	8.0	25	400	0
pepato (*BelGioioso*) ..	100	7.0	0	8.0	25	340	0
pepper, hot:							
(*Alpine Lace* Reduced Fat American) ...	90	6.0	1.0	7.0	20	300	0
(*BelGioioso Peperoncino*) ...	100	7.0	0	8.0	25	340	0
pepper Jack:							
(*Cabot*)	110	7.0	<1.0	9.0	30	170	0
(*Kraft*)	110	6.0	1.0	9.0	30	170	0
(*Kraft* Singles), ¾ oz.	50	4.0	2.0	2.5	10	360	0
(*Kraft Deli Deluxe* Slices), .8 oz. ...	90	5.0	0	7.0	25	150	0
(*Land O Lakes C-Jack*)	110	7.0	0	9.0	25	190	0
(*Organic Valley*) ...	100	6.0	0	8.0	20	190	0
shredded, w/habanero (*Sargento*), ¼ cup	100	6.0	<1.0	9.0	25	190	0

Food and Measure	cal.	prot. (gms)	carbo. (gms)	fat (gms)	chol. (mgs)	sod. (mgs)	fiber (gms)
Cheese *(cont.)*							
pimento (*Kraft* Singles), ¾ oz.	60	4.0	2.0	4.5	20	270	0
pizza, shredded, ¼ cup:							
(*Maggio*)	100	7.0	1.0	7.0	20	180	0
(*Sargento Double Cheese*)	90	7.0	1.0	6.0	20	190	0
4 cheese (*Kraft*)	90	6.0	1.0	7.0	20	220	0
mozzarella/cheddar (*Kraft*)	90	6.0	1.0	7.0	20	200	0
mozzarella/provolone (*Kraft*)	90	6.0	1.0	7.0	20	210	0
Port du Salut	100	6.7	.2	8.0	35	151	0
provolone:							
(*Alpine Lace Reduced Fat*)	90	7.0	1.0	6.0	15	180	0
(*Boar's Head 42% Lower Sodium*)	100	7.0	1.0	8.0	20	140	0
(*Hatfield Deli Choice*)	100	7.0	1.0	8.0	20	240	0
(*Kraft Deli Deluxe Slices*)	100	7.0	0	8.0	25	230	0
(*Organic Valley*)	100	7.0	1.0	5.0	15	150	0
(*Sara Lee*)	100	7.0	1.0	8.0	25	260	0
(*Sargento* Slices 8 oz.), ⅔ oz.	70	5.0	0	5.0	15	125	0
(*Sargento* Slices 12 oz.), ⅔ oz.	70	5.0	0	5.0	15	140	0
(*Sargento* Slices Reduced Fat), ⅔ oz.	50	5.0	0	3.5	10	140	0
(*Tree of Life*)	100	7.0	1.0	8.0	20	250	0
medium (*BelGioioso*)	100	7.0	0	8.0	30	320	0
mild (*BelGioioso*)	100	7.0	0	8.0	25	120	0
sharp (*BelGioioso*)	110	7.0	0	9.0	30	320	0
sharp, picante (*Boar's Head*)	100	7.0	1.0	8.0	25	250	0
smoke (*Land O Lakes*)	100	7.0	1.0	8.0	20	250	0
smoked (*Sara Lee* Slices), .8 oz.	80	6.0	0	6.0	15	190	0
ricotta, ¼ cup:							
(*Polly-O* Lite)	70	8.0	3.0	3.0	10	80	0
(*Polly-O* Original)	110	7.0	2.0	8.0	25	65	0
(*Sargento* Light)	60	5.0	3.0	2.5	15	55	0

Food and Measure	cal.	prot. (gms)	carbo. (gms)	fat (gms)	chol. (mgs)	sod. (mgs)	fiber (gms)
whole (*BelGioioso Ricotta con Latte*)	100	8.0	0	7.0	25	100	0
whole (*Maggio*) . . .	100	6.0	3.0	7.0	25	150	0
whole (*Sargento*) ..	90	7.0	3.0	6.0	25	75	0
part skim (*Maggio*)	80	4.0	3.0	5.0	20	150	0
part skim (*Polly-O*)	90	8.0	2.0	6.0	20	65	0
part skim (*Sargento*)	70	6.0	3.0	4.5	25	85	0
nonfat (*Maggio*) . . .	50	7.0	3.0	0	5	170	0
nonfat (*Polly-O*) . . .	45	8.0	3.0	0	5	80	0
nonfat (*Sargento*) ..	50	5.0	5.0	0	10	65	0
Romano:							
(*BelGioioso*)	100	9.0	0	7.0	25	330	0
shredded (*Sara Lee*)	100	8.0	1.0	7.0	20	330	0
shredded (*Maggio*), 1 tbsp.	20	1.0	0	2.0	0	100	0
Romano, grated:							
(*Kraft*), 2 tsp.	20	2.0	0	1.5	5	85	0
(*Maggio*), 1 tbsp. . .	25	1.0	2.0	1.5	0	85	0
(*Sara Lee*), 2 tsp. .	20	1.0	0	1.5	5	60	0
(*Tree of Life*), 2 tsp.	15	1.0	0	1.0	5	55	0
Roquefort	105	6.1	.6	8.7	26	513	0
string:							
(*Maggio*)	80	8.0	<1.0	5.0	15	170	0
(*Organic Valley*) . . .	80	8.0	<1.0	5.0	15	150	0
(*Organic Valley* Stringles)	90	7.0	1.0	6.0	20	190	1.0
(*Polly-O String-Ums*)	80	7.0	1.0	6.0	20	220	0
(*Polly-O String-Ums* Reduced Fat) . . .	80	8.0	1.0	4.5	15	220	0
(*Sargento* Snacks Single)	80	8.0	<1.0	6.0	15	240	0
(*Sargento* Snacks), .8-oz. pc.	70	6.0	<1.0	4.5	15	200	0
(*Sargento* Snacks Light), ¾-oz. slice	50	6.0	<1.0	2.5	10	180	0
Swiss:							
(*Alpine Lace* Reduced Fat) . . .	90	7.0	1.0	6.0	15	180	0
(*Alpine Lace* Reduced Fat), 1.2-oz. slice	110	10.0	0	7.0	25	75	0
(*Boar's Head* Gold Label Imported) .	110	8.0	<1.0	8.0	20	65	0

Food and Measure	cal.	prot. (gms)	carbo. (gms)	fat (gms)	chol. (mgs)	sod. (mgs)	fiber (gms)
Cheese, Swiss *(cont.)*							
(*Boar's Head* Lacey)	90	9.0	0	6.0	15	35	0
(*Boar's Head* Natural No Salt)	110	8.0	<1.0	8.0	25	10	0
(*Cabot* Slices)	110	9.0	1.0	8.0	30	60	0
(*Finlandia*)	110	8.0	<1.0	8.0	25	60	0
(*Finlandia Heavenly Light*)	80	8.0	<1.0	4.0	15	130	0
(*Finlandia Naturals*)	110	8.0	<1.0	8.0	25	60	0
(*Finlandia Sandwich Naturals*)	110	8.0	<1.0	8.0	25	60	0
(*Hatfield Deli Choice*), 1.2-oz. slice	130	10.0	1.0	9.0	30	570	0
(*Kraft* Singles), ¾ oz.	60	4.0	2.0	4.5	20	280	0
(*Kraft* Singles Deli Deluxe Aged) ...	110	8.0	0	9.0	30	50	0
(*Kraft* Singles Deli Thin)	110	8.0	0	9.0	30	50	0
(*Kraft* Singles Fat Free), ¾ oz.	30	5.0	2.0	0	20	280	0
(*Kraft* Singles 2% Milk), ¾ oz.	50	4.0	2.0	2.5	10	310	0
(*Kraft* Singles 2% Milk Deli Deluxe), ¾ oz.	70	6.0	0	4.5	15	50	0
(*Kraft Deli Deluxe* Slices)	90	6.0	1.0	7.0	25	340	0
(*Kraft Deli Deluxe* Slices 8 oz.), ⅔ oz.	80	6.0	0	7.0	20	35	0
(*Kraft Deli Deluxe* Slices 12 oz.), ⅔ oz.	70	6.0	0	5.0	20	260	0
(*Land O Lakes*) ...	110	8.0	1.0	8.0	25	115	0
(*Sara Lee* Slices), .8 oz.	80	6.0	0	6.0	20	45	0
(*Sara Lee* Specialty)	100	8.0	1.0	8.0	25	60	0
(*Sargento* Aged/Thin Slices), ⅔ oz. ..	70	5.0	0	5.0	20	40	0
(*Sargento* Reduced Fat Slices), ¾ oz.	60	7.0	1.0	4.0	10	30	0
(*Sargento* Thick Sliced)	110	8.0	1.0	8.0	25	60	0
(*Tree of Life*)	110	8.0	1.0	8.0	25	75	0

Food and Measure	cal.	prot. (gms)	carbo. (gms)	fat (gms)	chol. (mgs)	sod. (mgs)	fiber (gms)
smoked (*Williams*) .	90	5.0	0	7.0	20	390	0
Swiss, baby:							
(*Boar's Head*)	110	7.0	<1.0	9.0	25	135	0
(*Cracker Barrel*) ...	110	7.0	0	9.0	25	110	0
(*Land O Lakes*) ...	110	8.0	1.0	8.0	25	115	0
(*Organic Valley*) ...	110	7.0	0	9.0	25	125	0
(*Sara Lee*)	100	7.0	1.0	9.0	20	190	0
(*Sara Lee* Slices), .8 oz.	90	6.0	0	6.0	15	160	0
(*Sara Lee* Specialty)	110	7.0	0	9.0	25	125	0
(*Sargento* Slices), ⅔ oz.	70	5.0	0	5.0	15	40	0
Swiss, shredded, ¼ cup:							
(*Kraft*)	110	7.0	1.0	8.0	25	60	0
(*Sargento*)	110	8.0	<1.0	8.0	25	60	0
Swiss and American, processed (*Land O Lakes*)	100	6.0	1.0	9.0	25	410	0
Swiss and cheddar, smokey (*Kraft*)	100	5.0	1.0	8.0	25	380	0
Cheese, freeze-dried:							
cheddar, powder (*AlpineAire*), 1 oz. .	170	11.0	0	14.0	n.a.	560	0
cottage (*Mountain House*), ½ cup	110	14.0	3.0	4.5	25	400	0
"Cheese," substitute and nondairy:							
American:							
(*Tofutti*), .7-oz. slice	70	2.0	2.0	5.0	0	290	0
(*Yves* Good Slice), .7-oz. slice	35	4.0	0	2.0	0	290	0
cheddar style:							
(*Yves* Good Slice), .7-oz. slice	35	4.0	1.0	2.0	0	320	0
shredded (*Yves* Good Shreds), 1 oz.	60	7.0	0	3.0	0	330	0
cream "cheese," 2 tbsp.:							
plain, except non-hydrogenated (*Tofutti Better Than Cream Cheese*)	80	1.0	1.0	8.0	0	135	0

Food and Measure	cal.	prot. (gms)	carbo. (gms)	fat (gms)	chol. (mgs)	sod. (mgs)	fiber (gms)
"Cheese," substitute and nondairy, cream "cheese" *(cont.)*							
plain, nonhydrogenated (*Tofutti Better Than Cream Cheese*) .	120	1.0	13.0	7.0	0	150	0
flavored, all varieties (*Tofutti Better Than Cream Cheese*)	80	1.0	1.0	8.0	0	135	0
garlic, roasted (*Tofutti*), .7-oz. slice	70	2.0	2.0	5.0	0	290	0
mozzarella style:							
(*Tofutti*), .7-oz. slice	70	2.0	2.0	5.0	0	290	0
(*Yves* Good Slice), .7-oz. slice	35	4.0	0	2.0	0	280	0
shredded (*Yves* Good Shreds), 1 oz.	60	7.0	1.0	3.0	0	300	0
Cheese appetizer/ snack, frozen:							
jalapeño (*Health is Wealth Munchees*), 2 pcs., 1 oz.	60	2.0	10.0	1.5	0	220	1.0
sticks, mozzarella, breaded:							
(*Health is Wealth*), 2 pcs., 1.3 oz. . .	120	5.0	14.0	5.0	15	250	0
(*Ian's* Natural), 2 pcs., 1.3 oz. . .	120	4.0	10.0	7.0	15	300	0
three cheese (*Athens* Tyropita), 2 pcs., 2 oz.	180	6.0	9.0	13.0	30	290	0
Cheese dip, 2 tbsp.:							
(*Cheez Whiz* Light) . . .	80	6.0	6.0	3.5	20	500	0
(*Cheez Whiz* Original)	90	3.0	4.0	7.0	30	490	0
(*D.L. Jardine's* Queso Caliente/Loco)	40	0	4.0	2.0	0	190	0
beef or chicken and cheese (*Chi-Chi's*) .	40	0	2.0	3.0	10	160	0
cheddar:							
jalapeño (*Fritos*) . . .	50	1.0	4.0	4.0	5	200	0
jalapeño (*Litehouse*)	150	1.0	1.0	16.0	20	170	0
mild (*Fritos*)	60	1.0	3.0	4.0	5	330	0

Food and Measure	cal.	prot. (gms)	carbo. (gms)	fat (gms)	chol. (mgs)	sod. (mgs)	fiber (gms)
mild (*Snyder's*) ...	100	2.0	3.0	9.0	5	450	0
cheese (*Snyder's*) ...	90	3.0	3.0	7.0	10	470	0
chili (*Fritos*)	45	1.0	3.0	3.0	<5	310	0
Monterey Jack (*Tostitos* Party Bowl)	40	1.0	4.0	2.5	<5	210	0
nacho: (*Kaukauna*)	90	3.0	4.0	7.0	10	330	0
nondairy, mild or spicy (*Road's End Organics Chreese*)	20	2.0	3.0	0	0	110	<1.0
onion, French (*Kaukauna*)	50	1.0	4.0	3.0	10	150	0
salsa con queso: (*Cheez Whiz*)	90	3.0	4.0	7.0	30	500	0
(*Chi-Chi's*)	45	0	3.0	3.0	0	280	0
(*Pace*)	45	1.0	4.0	3.0	5	230	1.0
(*Tostitos*)	40	<1.0	5.0	2.5	<5	280	<1.0
flame roasted (*Snyder's*)	35	0	4.0	2.0	0	160	0
medium (*Taco Bell*)	40	1.0	2.0	3.0	5	300	0
mild (*Taco Bell*) ...	40	1.0	3.0	3.0	5	330	0
veggie ranch (*Kaukauna*)	50	1.0	3.0	3.0	10	240	0
Cheese dip kit:							
cheddar (*Sargento Cheese Dips!*), 3.75-oz. pkg.:							
w/bagel chips, ranch	280	9.0	24.0	17.0	15	1130	<1.0
w/butter pretzels ..	360	9.0	47.0	16.0	15	1430	2.0
w/tortilla chips	320	7.0	26.0	21.0	15	860	1.0
cheese (*Handi-Snacks*):							
w/breadsticks (*Premium*), 1.1 oz.	110	3.0	13.0	4.5	10	340	0
w/crackers (*Ritz*), 1 oz.	100	2.0	10.0	6.0	10	330	0
w/pretzel sticks (*Mr. Salty*), 1 oz.	100	3.0	12.0	3.5	10	380	0
Cheese entree, frozen (see also "Spinach entree" and specific listings), 1 pkg.:							
matter paneer (*Amy's* Whole Meal), 10 oz.	320	11.0	54.0	8.0	5	780	6.0

Food and Measure	cal.	prot. (gms)	carbo. (gms)	fat (gms)	chol. (mgs)	sod. (mgs)	fiber (gms)
Cheese entree *(cont.)*							
shahi paneer (*Ethnic Gourmet*), 12 oz. ...	510	20.0	52.0	25.0	30	500	4.0
Cheese food/product (see also "Cheese" and "Cheese spread"), 1 oz., except as noted:							
(*Velveeta*)	80	5.0	3.0	6.0	25	410	0
(*Velveeta* Light)	60	5.0	4.0	3.0	15	420	0
(*Velveeta* Slices), ¾ oz.	60	4.0	1.0	4.5	15	260	0
(*Velveeta* Slices Extra Thick), 1.2 oz.	100	5.0	2.0	7.0	30	430	0
Jack, w/jalapeño (*Land O Lakes*)	90	5.0	1.0	8.0	20	420	0
w/jalapeño (*Land O Lakes*)	90	6.0	2.0	7.0	20	450	0
Mexican:							
(*Velveeta*)	90	5.0	3.0	6.0	25	430	0
mild (*Velveeta*)	90	5.0	3.0	6.0	25	420	0
w/onion (*Land O Lakes*)	90	5.0	2.0	7.0	20	420	0
w/pepperoni (*Land O Lakes*)	90	5.0	2.0	7.0	20	430	0
shredded (*Velveeta*), ¼ cup, 1.3 oz.	130	8.0	3.0	9.0	30	500	0
Cheese salt (*Watkins*), ¼ tsp.	0	0	0	0	0	310	0
Cheese sandwich, frozen, grilled (*Smucker's Uncrustables*), 1.75-oz. pc.	150	6.0	17.0	6.0	15	500	<1.0
Cheese sauce, ¼ cup:							
jalapeño (*Zapata*)	50	2.0	4.0	3.5	15	260	0
mild (*Zapata*)	60	2.0	7.0	2.5	10	490	0
Cheese sauce, cooking, in jars, ¼ cup:							
Alfredo (*Ragú Cheese Creations* Classic) .	110	1.0	3.0	10.0	30	480	0
cheddar, double:							
(*Ragú Carb Options*)	90	2.0	2.0	8.0	25	480	0
(*Ragú Cheese Creations*)	100	2.0	3.0	9.0	25	510	0

Food and Measure	cal.	prot. (gms)	carbo. (gms)	fat (gms)	chol. (mgs)	sod. (mgs)	fiber (gms)
Cheese sauce base (*Watkins* Soup and Sauce Base), 2½ tbsp.	80	1.0	14.0	2.0	5	440	0
Cheese sauce mix, four, Italian (*Mc-Cormick*), 1⅓ tbsp.	40	1.0	5.0	1.5	5	600	0
"Cheese" sauce mix, nondairy, dry, ⅓ pkt.:							
Alfredo or cheddar style, gluten free (*Road's End Organics Chreese*)	35	3.0	5.0	0	0	240	1.0
cheddar or mozzarella style (*Road's End Organics Chreese*) .	35	2.0	6.0	0	0	260	1.0
Cheese spread (see also "Cheese," and "Cheese food product"), 2 tbsp., except as noted:							
(*Kraft* Manchego Singles), ¾-oz. slice	70	4.0	1.0	5.0	15	290	0
(*Viola*), 1 oz.	90	4.0	<1.0	8.0	20	220	0
all varieties (*Kaukauna* Log)	90	6.0	4.0	6.0	15	230	1.0
bacon:							
(*Kraft*)	90	5.0	1.0	8.0	25	570	0
smokey (*Kaukauna/ WisPride* Ball) ..	90	6.0	4.0	6.0	15	230	1.0
beef and onion (*Kaukauna* Ball) ...	120	2.0	5.0	10.0	30	180	0
blue cheese (*Kraft Roka*)	80	3.0	2.0	7.0	20	340	0
cheddar, sharp:							
(*Kaukauna* Ball) ...	90	6.0	4.0	6.0	15	230	1.0
(*WisPride* Lite)	70	5.0	5.0	3.5	15	190	0
double (*WisPride* Cup/Log)	90	6.0	4.0	6.0	15	230	1.0
extra (*KauKauna/ WisPride*)	90	5.0	3.0	7.0	20	190	0
extra (*Kaukauna/ WisPride* Ball) ..	100	6.0	4.0	7.0	15	230	0

Food and Measure	cal.	prot. (gms)	carbo. (gms)	fat (gms)	chol. (mgs)	sod. (mgs)	fiber (gms)
Cheese spread, cheddar, sharp *(cont.)*							
or smokey (*Kaukauna/Wis-Pride*)	90	5.0	3.0	7.0	20	210	0
or smokey (*Kaukauna/Wis-Pride* Lite)	70	5.0	5.0	3.5	15	190	0
or smokey (*WisPride* Log)	90	6.0	4.0	6.0	15	230	1.0
cheddar cream cheese (*Kaukauna/WisPride* Ball)	100	6.0	3.0	7.0	20	190	1.0
feta, original or sun-dried tomato (*Athenos*)	80	3.0	<1.0	7.0	20	190	0
garlic herb:							
(*Kaukauna/WisPride*)	90	2.0	2.0	8.0	25	190	0
(*Kaukauna/WisPride* Ball)	120	2.0	5.0	10.0	30	180	1.0
horseradish:							
(*Kaukauna/WisPride*)	90	5.0	3.0	7.0	20	210	0
(*Kaukauna/WisPride* Ball)	90	6.0	4.0	6.0	15	230	1.0
nacho (*Easy Cheese*)	90	5.0	3.0	7.0	25	480	0
olive and pimiento (*Kraft*)	70	2.0	3.0	6.0	20	220	0
onion, Vidalia (*Kaukauna* Ball)	100	5.0	3.0	7.0	20	190	0
pimiento (*Kraft*)	80	2.0	3.0	6.0	20	170	0
pineapple (*Kraft*)	70	2.0	4.0	5.0	15	120	0
port wine:							
(*Kaukauna/WisPride*)	90	5.0	3.0	7.0	20	210	0
(*Kaukauna/WisPride* Lite)	70	5.0	5.0	3.5	15	190	0
(*Kaukauna/WisPride* Ball)	90	6.0	4.0	6.0	15	230	1.0
ranch cream cheese (*Kaukauna/WisPride* Ball)	120	2.0	6.0	10.0	30	180	1.0
sharp (*Kraft Old English*)	90	5.0	1.0	8.0	25	520	0
Swiss:							
(*Kaukauna* Ball)	80	6.0	2.0	6.0	20	420	0
(*WisPride* Ball/Log)	80	5.0	2.0	6.0	20	220	1.0

Food and Measure	cal.	prot. (gms)	carbo. (gms)	fat (gms)	chol. (mgs)	sod. (mgs)	fiber (gms)
almond (*Kaukauna*)	90	5.0	3.0	7.0	20	140	0
sharp, double (*Wis-Pride* Log)	90	6.0	4.0	6.0	15	230	1.0
vegetable, garden:							
(*Kaukauna/WisPride*)	90	2.0	2.0	8.0	25	190	0
(*WisPride* Ball)	120	2.0	5.0	10.0	30	180	1.0
Cheese sticks, see "Cheese appetizer/ snack"							
Cheeseburger, see "Beef pocket/ sandwich"							
Cheesecake, fresh, French style (*Entenmann's* Deluxe), 1/5 cake	470	7.0	46.0	29.0	45	470	<1.0
Cheesecake, freezedried, see "Dessert, freeze-dried"							
Cheesecake, frozen or refrigerated:							
(*Baby Watson*), 1/6 of 18-oz. cake	240	4.0	19.0	16.0	55	170	0
(*Mother's Kitchen*), 1/6 of 60-oz. cake .	330	5.0	29.0	21.0	75	210	<1.0
(*Sara Lee* Original), 1/4 of 17-oz. cake ..	340	7.0	38.0	18.0	60	320	1.0
amaretto (*Impromptu Gourmet*), 1 slice ..	380	7.0	30.0	26.0	120	350	1.0
caramel fudge (*Impromptu Gourmet*), 1 slice	380	6.0	38.0	22.0	80	230	1.0
cherry (*Sara Lee* Original), 1/4 of 19-oz. cake	350	6.0	55.0	12.0	35	310	2.0
chocolate swirl (*Atkins*), 1/8 of 24-oz. cake ..	250	6.0	19.0	20.0	110	170	0
dulce de leche (*Impromptu Gourmet*), 1 slice	370	6.0	36.0	22.0	110	250	1.0
French style: (*Sara Lee* Classic), 1/5 of 23.5-oz. cake	410	6.0	41.0	25.0	25	330	1.0

Food and Measure	cal.	prot. (gms)	carbo. (gms)	fat (gms)	chol. (mgs)	sod. (mgs)	fiber (gms)
Cheesecake, frozen or refrigerated, French style *(cont.)*							
(Smart Ones), 3.9-oz. pc.	170	7.0	28.0	4.0	15	230	2.0
chocolate *(Sara Lee)*, 1/5 of 21-oz. cake	430	5.0	52.0	22.0	15	340	2.0
strawberry *(Sara Lee)*, 1/6 of 26-oz. cake	320	4.0	43.0	14.0	20	230	1.0
New York style:							
(Impromptu Gourmet), 1 slice	350	6.0	33.0	22.0	110	240	1.0
(Sara Lee), 1/6 of 30-oz. cake	350	6.0	35.0	21.0	65	360	1.0
(Smart Ones), 2.5-oz. pc.	150	6.0	21.0	5.0	15	140	1.0
chocolate swirl *(Sara Lee)*, 1/6 of 28-oz. cake	470	7.0	45.0	29.0	125	460	1.0
pumpkin *(Atkins)*, 1/8 of 24-oz. cake	240	6.0	18.0	19.0	95	135	1.0
raspberry swirl *(Atkins)*, 1/8 of 24-oz. cake	240	6.0	19.0	19.0	105	170	0
strawberry *(Sara Lee Original)*, 1/4 of 19-oz. cake	330	6.0	49.0	12.0	40	310	2.0
vanilla *(Atkins)*, 1/8 of 24-oz. cake	250	6.0	19.0	20.0	110	170	0
Cheesecake mix, dry:							
(Jell-O No Bake Homestyle), 1/6 pkg.	220	2.0	44.0	4.5	0	400	1.0
(Jell-O No Bake Real), 1/6 pkg.	220	2.0	42.0	5.0	0	380	1.0
cherry or strawberry *(Jell-O No Bake)*, 1/9 pkg.	200	2.0	42.0	3.5	0	270	1.0
strawberry swirl *(Jell-O No Bake Reduced Fat)*, 1/8 pkg.	180	4.0	39.0	1.5	0	290	1.0
Cheesecake snack:							
bars, 1 pc.:							
marble brownie *(Philadelphia Snack Bars 9 oz.)*, 1.5 oz.	170	3.0	20.0	9.0	25	110	1.0

Food and Measure	cal.	prot. (gms)	carbo. (gms)	fat (gms)	chol. (mgs)	sod. (mgs)	fiber (gms)
marble brownie (*Philadelphia* Snack Bars 9.5 oz.), 1.6 oz.	190	3.0	20.0	11.0	35	105	1.0
strawberry (*Philadelphia* Snack Bars), 1.5 oz.	180	2.0	22.0	9.0	10	80	0
bites, 1-oz. pc.:							
strawberry, chocolate covered (*Philadelphia* Snack Bites)	130	1.0	15.0	7.0	10	55	0
turtle (*Philadelphia* Snack Bites)	130	2.0	15.0	7.0	10	55	0
bites, chocolate dipped, ½ of 7.75-oz. pkg.:							
(*Sara Lee* Original)	100	1.0	8.0	7.0	15	55	0
praline pecan (*Sara Lee*)	90	1.0	8.0	6.0	15	55	1.0
Cherimoya (see also "Custard apple"):							
(*Frieda's*), 5 oz.	120	2.0	34.0	.5	0	0	3.0
1 medium, 1.9 lb.	515	7.1	131.3	2.2	0	n.a.	13.1
Cherries jubilee topping (*Lucky Leaf/ Musselman's*), ¼ cup	80	0	20.0	0	0	10	1.0
Cherry, fresh:							
(*Chiquita*), 1 cup, approx. 21 pcs.	90	2.0	22.0	.5	0	0	3.0
(*Del Monte*), 1 cup, 4.9 oz.	90	2.0	22.0	0	0	0	3.0
(*Dole*), 1 cup, approx. 21 pcs.	90	2.0	22.0	.5	0	0	3.0
sour, red, ½ cup:							
w/pits	26	.5	6.3	.2	0	2	.6
red, pitted	39	.8	9.4	.2	0	3	.9
sweet, w/pits, ½ cup	52	.9	12.0	.7	0	1	1.7
sweet, 10 medium	49	.8	11.3	.7	0	<1	1.6
Cherry, canned, ½ cup:							
dark, pitted:							
in extra heavy syrup (*S&W*)	140	1.0	34.0	0	0	10	1.0
in heavy syrup (*Del Monte*)	100	<1.0	24.0	0	0	10	<1.0

Food and Measure	cal.	prot. (gms)	carbo. (gms)	fat (gms)	chol. (mgs)	sod. (mgs)	fiber (gms)
Cherry, canned *(cont.)*							
red, tart, pitted, in water *(Lucky Leaf/ Musselman's)*	50	0	12.0	0	0	10	1.0
sour, pitted:							
in water	44	1.0	10.9	.1	0	9	1.3
in light syrup	95	.9	24.3	.1	0	9	1.0
in heavy syrup	116	.9	29.8	.1	0	9	1.0
sweet, w/liquid:							
in water	57	1.0	14.6	.2	0	1	1.9
in juice	68	1.1	17.3	<.1	0	4	1.9
in light syrup	84	.8	21.8	.2	0	4	1.9
Cherry, dried:							
bing:							
(Frieda's), ¼ cup, 1.4 oz.	120	2.0	26.0	0	0	5	3.0
(Shiloh Farms), ⅓ cup, 1.6 oz. . .	150	2.0	35.0	0	0	7	9.0
sour/tart:							
(Eden Montmorency), ¼ cup, 1.6 oz. . .	140	0	36.0	0	0	15	3.0
(Frieda's), ⅓ cup, 1.4 oz.	150	2.0	33.0	0	0	0	2.0
(Shiloh Farms), ⅓ cup, 1.4 oz. . .	135	3.0	31.0	0	0	7	4.0
Cherry, frozen:							
unsweetened:							
sweet *(Cascadian Farm)*, 1 cup . . .	90	2.0	24.0	.5	0	0	3.0
½ cup	36	7.1	8.5	.3	0	1	1.2
sweetened, ½ cup . . .	116	1.5	29.0	.2	0	1	2.7
Cherry, maraschino, 1 pc.:							
red or green mint *(S&W)*	10	0	3.0	0	0	0	0
w/stems *(Great Expectations)*	10	0	2.0	0	0	5	0
Cherry, West Indian, see "Acerola"							
Cherry butter *(Eden Organic)*, 1 tbsp. . . .	35	0	9.0	0	0	0	1.0
Cherry drink:							
(Minute Maid Coolers), 6.75-fl.-oz. pouch . .	100	0	28.0	0	0	15	0

Food and Measure	cal.	prot. (gms)	carbo. (gms)	fat (gms)	chol. (mgs)	sod. (mgs)	fiber (gms)
black, 8 fl. oz.:							
(*Ocean Spray*)	140	0	33.0	0	0	35	0
(*R.W. Knudsen*							
Concentrate) ...	130	1.0	31.0	0	0	15	0
Cherry juice, 8 fl. oz.:							
(*Juicy Juice*)	130	0	30.0	0	0	10	0
(*Walnut Acres*)	140	0	34.0	0	0	15	0
black:							
(*L&A*)	180	0	45.0	0	0	10	0
(*R.W. Knudsen*) ...	180	2.0	43.0	0	0	40	0
(*R.W. Knudsen* Just							
Cherry)	180	2.0	44.0	0	0	40	0
cider (*R.W. Knudsen*) .	130	1.0	31.0	0	0	15	0
tart:							
(*Eden* Organic							
Montmorency) ..	140	1.0	33.0	1.0	0	30	0
(*R.W. Knudsen* Just							
Cherry)	130	1.0	32.0	0	0	20	0
Cherry juice blend, berries (*Ceres* Secrets of the Valley), 8 fl. oz.	120	0	30.0	0	0	10	0
Cherry juice concentrate:							
(*Eden* Organic), 2 tbsp.	110	1.0	26.0	0	0	20	0
black (*Tree of Life*), 8 tsp.	110	0	28.0	0	0	0	0
Cherry syrup, maraschino (*Trader Vic's*), 1 fl. oz.	90	0	23.0	0	0	15	0
Chervil, dried, 1 tsp. .	1	.1	.3	<.1	0	<1	.1
Chestnut, Chinese, shelled, 1 oz.:							
dried	103	1.9	22.7	.5	0	2	<1.0
boiled or steamed ...	44	.8	9.6	.2	0	1	<1.0
roasted	68	1.3	14.9	.3	0	1	<1.0
Chestnut, European: raw:							
in shell, 1 lb.	714	8.1	152.8	7.6	0	9	27.2
shelled, w/peel, 1 cup, 13 pcs. ...	308	3.5	66.0	3.3	0	4	11.7
dried, peeled, 1 oz. ..	105	1.4	23.3	1.1	0	11	<2.0
boiled, 1 oz.	37	.8	7.9	.4	0	8	<1.0

Food and Measure	cal.	prot. (gms)	carbo. (gms)	fat (gms)	chol. (mgs)	sod. (mgs)	fiber (gms)
Chestnut, European *(cont.)*							
roasted, peeled:							
1 oz.	70	.9	15.0	.6	0	1	3.3
1 cup, 17 kernels . .	350	4.3	75.7	3.2	0	3	16.7
Chestnuts, European, in jars *(Minerve)*,							
4 whole, 1.1 oz. . . .	50	1.0	12.0	0	0	0	2.0
Chestnut spread							
(Faugier), 2 tbsp. . . .	80	0	20.0	0	0	0	0
Chia seeds, dried:							
(Shiloh Farms), 3 tbsp.	140	5.0	13.0	7.0	0	15	10.0
1 oz.	139	4.4	12.4	10.8	8	5	10.7
Chicken, fresh, 4 oz., except as noted:							
broiler-fryer, roasted:							
w/skin, ½ chicken, 10.5 oz. (15.8 oz. w/bone)	715	81.6	0	40.7	263	244	0
w/skin	271	31.0	0	15.4	100	93	0
meat only	215	32.8	0	8.4	101	98	0
meat only, chopped or diced, 1 cup . .	266	40.5	0	10.4	125	120	0
skin only, 1 oz.	129	5.8	0	11.5	24	18	0
dark meat only	232	31.0	0	11.0	105	105	0
light meat only	196	35.1	0	5.1	96	87	0
breast, w/skin, ½ breast, 3½ oz. (8½ oz. w/bone)	193	29.2	0	7.6	83	69	0
drumstick, w/skin, 1.8 oz. (2.9 oz. w/bone)	112	14.1	0	5.8	48	47	0
leg, w/skin (5.7 oz. w/bone)	265	29.6	0	15.4	105	99	0
thigh, w/skin, 2.2 oz. (2.9 oz. w/bone) .	153	15.5	0	9.6	58	52	0
wing, w/skin, 1.2 oz. (2.3 oz. w/bone) .	99	9.1	0	6.6	29	28	0
capon, roasted, w/skin:							
½ capon, 1.4 lbs. (2 lbs. w/bone) .	1457	184.5	0	74.2	549	313	0
w/skin	260	32.8	0	13.2	98	56	0
ground, see "Chicken, ground"							

Food and Measure	cal.	prot. (gms)	carbo. (gms)	fat (gms)	chol. (mgs)	sod. (mgs)	fiber (gms)
roaster, roasted:							
w/skin, ½ chicken, 1 lb. (1½ lbs. w/bone)	1071	115.0	0	64.3	365	349	0
meat w/skin	253	27.2	0	15.2	86	83	0
stewing, stewed:							
w/skin, ½ chicken, 9.2 oz. (13½ oz. w/bone)	744	70.2	0	49.2	205	190	0
meat w/skin	323	30.5	0	21.4	90	83	0
meat only	269	34.5	0	13.5	94	88	0
meat only, chopped or diced, 1 cup ..	332	42.6	0	16.6	117	109	0
Chicken, canned, chunk, 2 oz.:							
(*Hormel*)	60	9.0	0	2.5	25	250	0
(*Tyson*)	60	10.0	0	2.5	30	200	0
(*Tyson* Pouch)	70	14.0	0	1.5	45	210	0
breast:							
(*Hormel*)	50	9.0	0	1.0	20	250	0
(*Hormel* No Salt) ..	50	9.0	0	1.0	20	50	0
(*Swanson*)	50	10.0	1.0	1.0	20	270	0
(*Tyson*)	60	13.0	0	.5	30	200	0
white and dark (*Swanson*)	60	10.0	0	2.0	30	250	0
Chicken, freeze-dried, cooked, diced:							
(*AlpineAire*), ½ oz. ...	60	13.0	0	1.0	35	15	0
(*Mountain House*), ¾ cup	170	24.0	0	8.0	105	380	0
Chicken, frozen or refrigerated, raw, 4 oz., except as noted:							
whole, edible portion:							
(*Organic Valley*) ...	240	21.0	0	17.0	85	80	0
cut up (*Tyson*)	220	19.0	0	16.0	80	170	0
whole, fryer, rotisserie: dark, all seasonings (*Perdue*)	240	15.0	1.0	20.0	75	260	0
white, all seasonings (*Perdue*)	170	19.0	1.0	10.0	80	370	0
whole, roasting: garlic, toasted, dark (*Perdue*)	260	16.0	1.0	21.0	100	440	0

Food and Measure	cal.	prot. (gms)	carbo. (gms)	fat (gms)	chol. (mgs)	sod. (mgs)	fiber (gms)
Chicken, frozen or refrigerated, raw, whole, roasting *(cont.)*							
garlic, toasted, white (*Perdue*)	180	20.0	1.0	10.0	90	440	0
honey, dark (*Perdue*)	260	16.0	4.0	20.0	100	820	0
honey, white (*Perdue*)	190	20.0	4.0	10.0	85	810	0
breast, bone-in:							
split (*Tyson*)	180	22.0	0	10.0	65	160	0
split (*Tyson Individually Fresh Frozen*), 5.25-oz. pc.	230	29.0	0	12.0	100	440	0
split, skinless (*Tyson*)	110	24.0	0	1.5	60	160	0
breast, boneless, marinated:							
(*Always Tender*) . . .	150	29.0	2.0	3.0	80	790	0
Italian (*Always Tender*)	170	29.0	3.0	4.5	85	770	0
lemon pepper (*Always Tender*) .	180	28.0	5.0	5.0	80	770	0
teriyaki (*Always Tender*)	180	29.0	8.0	3.0	80	820	0
breast, boneless, skinless:							
(*Organic Valley*) . . .	120	26.0	0	1.5	65	75	0
(*Perdue* Individually Frozen), 5.9-oz. pc.	160	35.0	0	1.5	100	310	0
(*Perdue Fit & Easy*)	110	26.0	0	1.0	75	45	0
(*Perdue Oven Stuffer*)	130	27.0	0	2.0	75	45	0
(*Tyson*)	100	23.0	0	1.5	60	230	0
(*Tyson Individually Fresh Frozen*), 7-oz. pc.	170	34.0	0	3.5	85	290	0
sandwich steaks (*Bell & Evans*), 2 oz.	60	14.0	<.1	.5	40	25	0
thin sliced (*Perdue*), 2.8 oz.	80	18.0	0	1.5	50	35	0
breast, breaded:							
broccoli and cheese stuffed (*Tyson*), 6-oz. pc.	340	20.0	22.0	19.0	75	710	1.0
Cordon Bleu (*Tyson*), 6-oz., pc.	390	25.0	19.0	24.0	95	990	0

Food and Measure	cal.	prot. (gms)	carbo. (gms)	fat (gms)	chol. (mgs)	sod. (mgs)	fiber (gms)
garlic Pramesan (*Bell & Evans*) ..	190	29.0	12.0	2.0	65	640	<2.0
Kiev (*Tyson*), 6-oz. pc.	500	20.0	20.0	38.0	125	660	0
breast tenders (*Tyson*)	100	22.0	0	.5	45	220	0
breast tenders, breaded: (*Bell & Evans*)	190	20.0	13.0	6.0	45	440	1.0
coconut (*Bell & Evans*)	180	18.0	16.0	5.0	45	370	<1.0
drumsticks (*Tyson Individually Fresh Frozen*), 2 pcs., 4 oz.	140	17.0	0	7.0	90	290	0
leg quarters (*Tyson*) ..	190	19.0	0	13.0	85	180	0
nuggets (*Bell & Evans*)	190	20.0	13.0	6.0	45	440	1.0
patties. breaded: (*Bell & Evans*)	170	20.0	13.0	4.0	60	370	<1.0
w/mozzarella (*Bell & Evans*)	190	22.0	11.0	6.0	60	520	0
tenderloin, breast: (*Perdue* Individually Frozen)	110	24.0	0	1.5	65	160	0
(*Perdue Fit & Easy*)	120	27.0	0	1.0	70	45	0
tenders, see "breast tenders," above							
thigh: (*Organic Valley*) ...	240	19.0	0	17.0	95	85	0
(*Perdue* Individually Frozen), 6.2-oz. pc.	260	29.0	0	16.0	140	270	0
(*Tyson*)	220	18.0	0	16.0	90	170	0
(*Tyson Individually Fresh Frozen*), 5-oz. pc.	380	17.0	1.0	34.0	110	350	0
thigh, bone/skinless: (*Tyson Individually Fresh Frozen*), 4-oz. pc.	170	17.0	0	11.0	70	270	0
cutlets (*Tyson*)	110	20.0	0	4.0	85	250	0
thigh, skinless (*Tyson*)	210	19.0	0	15.0	95	75	0
wing: (*Tyson*)	230	19.0	0	17.0	80	170	0

Food and Measure	cal.	prot. (gms)	carbo. (gms)	fat (gms)	chol. (mgs)	sod. (mgs)	fiber (gms)
Chicken, frozen or refrigerated, raw, wing *(cont.)*							
(*Tyson Individually Fresh Frozen*), 4 pcs., 4 oz. . . . . :	240	20.0	0	18.0	95	340	0
Chicken, frozen or refrigerated, cooked (see also "Chicken entree, frozen"):							
whole, 3 oz.:							
dark (*Perdue*)	210	17.0	0	16.0	110	55	0
dark (*Perdue* Soup/ Stew Baking) . . .	210	18.0	0	15.0	100	60	0
. dark, cut up or split (*Perdue*)	210	17.0	0	16.0	110	55	0
white (*Perdue*)	170	21.0	0	10.0	85	45	0
white (*Perdue* Soup/ Stew Baking) . . .	170	21.0	0	9.0	80	50	0
white, cut up or split (*Perdue*)	170	21.0	0	10.0	85	45	0
whole, roasted, 3 oz.:							
(*Tyson*)	160	16.0	1.0	11.0	75	490	1.0
dark (*Perdue Oven Stuffer*)	210	18.0	0	15.0	100	60	0
white (*Perdue Oven Stuffer*)	170	21.0	0	9.0	80	50	0
whole, roasted, seasoned, 3 oz.:							
garlic, toasted, dark (*Perdue*)	190	16.0	1.0	14.0	100	330	0
garlic, toasted, light (*Perdue*)	160	19.0	1.0	9.0	75	320	0
honey, dark (*Perdue*)	220	13.0	3.0	17.0	85	690	0
honey, white (*Perdue*)	160	17.0	3.0	9.0	75	690	0
lemon pepper (*Tyson*)	160	16.0	1.0	11.0	75	560	1.0
whole, rotisserie, 3 oz.							
dark, seasoned (*Perdue*)	180	15.0	0	13.0	100	260	0
white, seasoned (*Perdue*)	140	17.0	0	7.0	75	260	0
barbecue sauce w/, shredded, ¼ cup:							
honey hickory sauce (*Lloyd's*)	90	6.0	12.0	2.0	20	490	0

Food and Measure	cal.	prot. (gms)	carbo. (gms)	fat (gms)	chol. (mgs)	sod. (mgs)	fiber (gms)
original sauce (*Lloyd's*)	90	6.0	11.0	2.0	15	420	0
bites, breaded (*Tyson*), 13 pcs., 3 oz.	270	13.0	15.0	18.0	40	400	1.0
breast, bone-in, roasted:							
whole (*Perdue Oven Stuffer*), 3 oz. . .	150	21.0	0	2.5	70	40	0
half (*Tyson*), 5.1-oz. pc.	260	34.0	1.0	13.0	110	670	0
split (*Perdue*), 6.8-oz. pc.	370	48.0	0	20.0	180	100	0
split, skinless (*Perdue*), 5.8-oz. pc.	250	46.0	0	7.0	150	95	0
breast, bone-in, skin-less:							
(*Perdue* Individually Frozen), 4.2 oz. pc.	140	32.0	0	1.5	90	280	0
(*Perdue Fit & Easy*), 3 oz.	110	25.0	0	1.0	70	30	0
(*Perdue Oven Stuffer*), 3 oz. . .	120	25.0	0	1.5	70	30	0
roasted (*Tyson*), 3.75-oz. pc.	120	25.0	1.0	2.0	65	550	0
breast, carved, ½ cup, 2.5 oz.:							
grilled, Italian (*Per-due Short Cuts*) .	90	17.0	3.0	1.5	50	580	0
grilled, lemon pepper (*Perdue Short Cuts*)	100	17.0	2.0	2.0	45	580	0
grilled, Southwest (*Perdue Short Cuts*)	100	18.0	2.0	2.0	55	580	0
honey roasted (*Per-due Short Cuts*) .	90	17.0	3.0	1.5	50	580	0
roasted (*Perdue Short Cuts Original*)	90	17.0	2.0	1.5	55	580	0
breast, diced, 3 oz.:							
(*Tyson*)	90	20.0	0	1.0	45	250	0
roasted (*Tyson*) . . .	110	19.0	2.0	2.5	60	370	1.0

Food and Measure	cal.	prot. (gms)	carbo. (gms)	fat (gms)	chol. (mgs)	sod. (mgs)	fiber (gms)
Chicken, frozen or refrigerated, cooked *(cont.)*							
breast cutlet, breaded, white, 3 oz.:							
(*Perdue*)	200	13.0	14.0	10.0	40	530	0
(*Perdue* Homestyle Low Fat)	140	14.0	14.0	3.0	35	510	0
Italian (*Perdue*) . . .	140	13.0	15.0	3.0	35	540	<1.0
breast cuts, 3 oz.:							
(*Louis Rich*)	130	22.0	1.0	2.5	60	790	0
honey roasted (*Louis Rich*)	130	22.0	3.0	2.5	60	780	0
breast fillets:							
breaded (*Tyson*), 4.6-oz. pc.	240	19.0	20.0	9.0	30	680	0
char grilled (*Perdue Short Cuts*), 2.4-oz. pc.	70	14.0	2.0	1.0	40	450	0
w/gravy (*Hormel*), 6 oz.	130	21.0	4.0	3.0	50	1070	0
honey roasted (*Perdue Short Cuts*), 2.4-oz pc.	80	14.0	5.0	1.0	40	450	0
mesquite (*Tyson*), 3 oz.	130	17.0	1.0	7.0	45	540	0
teriyaki (*Hormel*), 5.7 oz.	230	28.0	30.0	2.5	50	1400	0
teriyaki (*Hormel* Family Pack), 6 oz.	240	21.0	35.0	2.5	45	1521	0
teriyaki (*Tyson*), 3.1 oz.	170	20.0	7.0	7.0	55	620	0
breast medallions:							
in Marsala sauce (*Tyson*), 5 oz. . . .	130	17.0	4.0	4.5	50	700	0
in sesame sauce (*Tyson*), 5 oz. . . .	190	18.0	22.0	3.0	50	840	0
chunks, w/sauce:							
Alfredo (*Simply Simmered*), 1 cup	200	27.0	8.0	7.0	35	310	<1.0
garlic (*Simply Simmered*), 5 oz. . . .	140	16.0	10.0	4.0	15	750	3.0
marinara (*Simply Simmered*), 5 oz.	150	8.0	9.0	5.0	20	810	3.0
sesame (*Simply Simmered*), 5 oz.	180	15.0	26.0	2.5	10	750	5.0

Food and Measure	cal.	prot. (gms)	carbo. (gms)	fat (gms)	chol. (mgs)	sod. (mgs)	fiber (gms)
sweet and sour (*Simply Simmered*), 5 oz. ...	180	15.0	26.0	2.5	10	750	5.0
Szechuan (*Simply Simmered*), 5 oz.	180	19.0	16.0	4.5	10	810	5.0
teriyaki (*Simply Simmered*), 5 oz.	190	16.0	23.0	3.5	20	950	1.0
drumstick, roasted:							
(*Perdue*), 2.2-oz. pc.	110	14.0	0	6.0	80	65	0
(*Perdue Oven Stuffer*), 3.6-oz. pc. .	190	22.0	0	11.0	120	100	0
(*Tyson*), 3 pcs., 5.8 oz.	320	44.0	2.0	15.0	230	1200	0
fillet, breaded, Italian style (*Barber Foods*), 3.5-oz. pc.	240	15.0	14.0	14.0	40	820	<1.0
fingers, breaded:							
(*Barber Foods* All American), 3.3-oz. pc.	190	16.0	15.0	8.0	35	460	<1.0
(*Ian's* Natural), 3 oz., approx. 3 pcs. ..	100	15.0	14.0	8.0	40	450	0
Buffalo (*Barber Foods*), 3.3-oz. pc.	160	15.0	18.0	3.5	35	380	<1.0
Italian (*Barber Foods*), 3.3-oz. pc.	190	15.0	15.0	8.0	35	560	<1.0
ground, see "Chicken, ground"							
leg, roasted (*Perdue*), 5.6-oz. pc.	370	33.0	0	27.0	200	105	0
meatballs, Italian style, (*Tyson*), 6 pcs., 3 oz.	180	13.0	6.0	11.0	45	610	2.0
nuggets:							
(*Barber Foods* All American), 4 pcs., 3 oz. ....:.	150	14.0	12.0	12.0	35	340	0
(*Health is Wealth*), 4 pcs., 3 oz.	150	14.0	9.0	6.0	40	180	0
(*Ian's* Natural Allergen Free), 3 oz., approx. 5 pcs. ..	100	15.0	14.0	8.0	40	250	0
(*Tyson* Bag), 5 pcs., 3.25 oz.	280	14.0	16.0	18.0	40	480	0

Food and Measure	cal.	prot. (gms)	carbo. (gms)	fat (gms)	chol. (mgs)	sod. (mgs)	fiber (gms)
Chicken, frozen or refrigerated, cooked, nuggets *(cont.)*							
(*Tyson* Box), 5 pcs., 3.2 oz.	280	13.0	16.0	18.0	50	430	0
breast (*Perdue* Individually Frozen), 5 pcs., 3.4oz.	250	11.0	15.0	16.0	40	720	1.0
cheddar and bacon (*Barber Foods*), 3 pcs., 2.8 oz. ..	190	12.0	8.0	12.0	35	350	0
golden brown (*Perdue*), 5 pcs., 3.4 oz.	240	11.0	14.0	15.0	35	530	0
ham and cheese (*Barber Foods*), 3 pcs., 2.8 oz. ..	180	12.0	8.0	12.0	35	390	0
pizza stuffed (*Barber Foods*), 3 pcs., 2.8 oz.	180	11.0	7.0	11.0	30	410	0
Southern style (*Tyson*), 6 pcs., 3 oz.	270	10.0	11.0	21.0	45	570	1.0
white (*Perdue*), 3 oz.	200	13.0	14.0	10.0	40	530	0
white (*Perdue Fun Shapes*), 4 pcs., 2.7 oz.	180	12.0	12.0	9.0	40	490	0
white, and cheese (*Perdue*), 5 pcs., 3 oz.	210	13.0	14.0	11.0	50	560	0
patties, breaded:							
(*Health is Wealth*), 3-oz. pc.	150	13.0	9.0	6.0	40	180	0
(*Ian's* Natural), 3.5-oz. pc.	220	18.0	16.0	9.0	40	300	0
breast (*Tyson*), 2.6-oz. pc.	180	10.0	12.0	11.0	25	300	1.0
breast, Southern style (*Tyson*), 2.6-oz. pc.	240	9.0	10.0	18.0	40	490	1.0
popcorn:							
(*Tyson*), 9 pcs., 3 oz.	230	13.0	21.0	11.0	30	710	1.0
(*Tyson Popcorn Chicken Bites*), 6 pcs., 3.1 oz. ..	250	14.0	22.0	12.0	30	760	2.0

Food and Measure	cal.	prot. (gms)	carbo. (gms)	fat (gms)	chol. (mgs)	sod. (mgs)	fiber (gms)
white (*Perdue*), 3 oz.	140	16.0	11.0	4.0	40	560	0
sticks, 3 pcs., 2.8 oz.:							
barbecue (*Barber Foods*)	230	13.0	15.0	13.0	40	600	<1.0
honey crunch (*Barber Foods*) . .	240	13.0	15.0	15.0	40	330	<1.0
potato chip (*Barber Foods*)	230	13.0	15.0	13.0	40	790	<1.0
strips:							
Buffalo (*Tyson*), 2 pcs., 3.5 oz. . . .	230	14.0	21.0	10.0	45	1250	1.0
crispy (*Tyson*), 2 pcs., 3.3 oz. . . .	200	16.0	13.0	10.0	30	520	1.0
fajita (*Tyson* Bag), 3 oz.	110	17.0	1.0	4.0	55	540	1.0
fajita (*Tyson* Box), 3 oz.	120	18.0	1.0	5.0	60	450	0
Southwest (*Hormel*), 2 oz.	50	7.0	3.0	1.5	20	430	0
strips, breast, 3 oz.:							
(*Perdue*)	140	16.0	12.0	4.0	40	570	0
(*Perdue Kick'n Chicken* Original)	120	14.0	14.0	1.0	35	750	0
(*Tyson*) . . . . :	120	21.0	1.0	3.5	60	500	0
barbecue (*Perdue Kick'n Chicken*) .	120	12.0	16.0	1.0	30	720	- 0
Buffalo (*Perdue*) . .	140	15.0	12.0	4.0	40	580	0
fajita (*Tyson*)	110	19.0	3.0	2.0	60	450	0
grilled (*Louis Rich*)	110	19.0	1.0	3.0	55	770	0
grilled (*Tyson*)	110	19.0	2.0	3.0	50	480	0
hot and spicy (*Perdue Kick'n Chicken*)	110	12.0	13.0	1.0	30	930	0
Italian (*Louis Rich*)	110	19.0	1.0	3.0	55	770	0
Southwest (*Louis Rich*)	110	19.0	1.0	3.0	55	770	0
Southwest (*Tyson*) .	110	18.0	2.0	3.0	40	400	0
Southwest (*Tyson* Refrigerated) . . .	120	22.0	2.0	2.5	60	250	0
tenderloin, 3 oz.:							
(*Perdue* Individually Frozen)	100	23.0	0	1.0	55	100	0
(*Perdue Fit & Easy*)	100	24.0	0	.5	60	30	0

Food and Measure	cal.	prot. (gms)	carbo. (gms)	fat (gms)	chol. (mgs)	sod. (mgs)	fiber (gms)
Chicken, frozen or refrigerated, cooked *(cont.)*							
tenderloin, breaded:							
(*Perdue*), 3 oz.	170	13.0	13.0	7.0	25	360	0
(*Perdue* Individually							
Frozen), 3 oz.	200	15.0	15.0	10.0	30	510	0
(*Tyson*), 2.4-oz. pc.	150	10.0	12.0	7.0	20	370	1.0
Southern (*Tyson*),							
2.4-oz. pc.	150	10.0	9.0	7.0	20	360	1.0
spicy (*Tyson*),							
2.4-oz. pc.	160	11.0	13.0	7.0	20	620	0
white (*Perdue* Low							
Fat), 3 oz.	140	15.0	15.0	2.5	35	500	0
tenders, breast:							
(*Health is Wealth*),							
3 pcs., 3 oz.	130	14.0	11.0	3.0	35	230	0
(*Tyson* Bag), 5 pcs.,							
3 oz.	240	12.0	15.0	14.0	35	330	0
(*Tyson* Box), 5 pcs.,							
3 oz.	220	14.0	15.0	11.0	35	330	0
honey battered							
(*Tyson*), 5 pcs.,							
3 oz.	220	13.0	13.0	13.0	35	250	2.0
w/rib meat (*Tyson*							
Box), 5 pcs., 3 oz.	220	13.0	13.0	13.0	35	250	2.0
thigh, roasted:							
(*Perdue*), 3.2-oz. pc.	240	17.0	0	19.0	115	65	0
(*Tyson*), 3.6-oz. pc.	270	19.0	1.0	21.0	120	650	1.0
wingettes:							
roasted (*Perdue*),							
3 pcs., 3.1 oz. . .	210	10.0	0	15.0	110	70	0
roasted (*Perdue*							
Oven Stuffers*),							
3 pcs., 3.4 oz. . .	220	21.0	0	15.0	120	80	0
wings:							
barbecue (*Tyson*),							
3 pcs., 3.2 oz. . .	200	15.0	7.0	13.0	110	380	0
Buffalo, hot (*Tyson*),							
4 pcs., 3.4 oz. . .	220	20.0	1.0	15.0	110	560	1.0
honey (*Tyson* Bag),							
4 pcs., 3.4 oz. . .	220	15.0	9.0	14.0	95	450	0
honey (*Tyson* Box),							
3 pcs., 3.5 oz. . .	250	15.0	13.0	15.0	90	410	1.0
hot (*Tyson* Wings of							
Fire), 3 pcs., 3.5 oz.	260	15.0	14.0	16.0	90	1130	2.0

Food and Measure	cal.	prot. (gms)	carbo. (gms)	fat (gms)	chol. (mgs)	sod. (mgs)	fiber (gms)
hot and spicy (*Perdue* Individually Frozen)	180	16.0	1.0	12.0	95	430	0
hot and spicy (*Tyson*), 3 pcs., 3 oz.	180	16.0	1.0	12.0	80	780	1.0
hot and spicy (*Tyson* Box), 3 pcs., 3.4 oz.	220	20.0	1.0	15.0	110	560	0
roasted (*Perdue*), 2 pcs., 3.2 oz. ..	210	19.0	0	15.0	115	75	0
split, Buffalo (*Perdue Wingsters*), 3 oz.	170	14.0	3.0	10.0	75	440	0
Chicken, ground:							
raw, 4 oz.:							
(*Organic Valley*) ...	210	19.0	0	14.0	125	70	0
(*Perdue*)	180	19.0	0	12.0	135	75	0
(*Wampler*)	220	22.0	0	14.0	90	65	0
breast (*Perdue*) ...	100	24.0	0	.5	65	75	0
burgers (*Bell & Evans*)	160	22.0	0	7.0	90	240	0
burgers (*Perdue*) ..	170	19.0	0	11.0	130	75	0
cooked, 3 oz.:							
(*Perdue*)	170	18.0	0	11.0	125	50	0
breast (*Perdue*) ...	80	19.0	0	.5	55	60	0
burgers (*Perdue*) ..	160	17.0	0	10.0	110	55	0
"Chicken," vegetarian:							
canned:							
(*Worthington FriChik* Original), 2 pcs., 3.2 oz.	140	12.0	3.0	8.0	0	40	1.0
diced, drained (*Worthington Chik*), ¼ cup ...	50	9.0	2.0	0	0	220	1.0
sliced (*Worthington Chik*), 3 slices, 3.2 oz.	80	15.0	3.0	.5	0	360	2.0
frozen/refrigerated:							
cutlets (*Quorn*), 2.4-oz. pc.	80	11.0	5.0	2.5	5	420	2.0
cutlet, garlic and herb (*Quorn*), 3.5-oz,. pc.	200	10.0	20.0	8.0	0	610	4.0

Food and Measure	cal.	prot. (gms)	carbo. (gms)	fat (gms)	chol. (mgs)	sod. (mgs)	fiber (gms)
"Chicken," vegetarian, frozen/refrigerated (cont.)							
drumsticks (*Garden Gourmet*), 1.8-oz. pc.	90	7.0	10.0	4.0	0	400	2.0
fingers (*Health is Wealth*), 2 oz. . . .	70	10.0	5.0	1.5	0	320	1.0
fried, w/gravy (*Loma Linda*), 2 pcs., 2.9 oz. . .	150	12.0	5.0	10.0	0	430	2.0
Italian marinara (*Morningstar Farms*), 1 pc. and 1 pkt. sauce, 5 oz.	250	12.0	29.0	9.0	0	890	2.0
nuggets (*Boca* Chik'n Original), 3 oz. . .	170	14.0	18.0	6.0	0	670	2.0
nuggets (*Dr. Praeger's*) 2 pcs., 1.3 oz.	70	4.0	9.0	2.0	0	150	1.0
nuggets (*Health is Wealth*), 3 pcs., 2.2 oz.	140	14.0	13.0	4.5	0	450	2.0
nuggets (*Loma Linda*), 5 pcs., 3 oz.	250	13.0	14.0	15.0	0	490	2.0
nuggets (*Morningstar Farms* Chik'n), 4 pcs., 3 oz.	190	12.0	18.0	7.0	0	490	2.0
nuggets (*Quorn*), 3-4 pcs., 3 oz. . .	180	8.0	18.0	8.0	0	650	3.0
patties (*Boca* Chik'n), 2.5-oz. pc.	150	11.0	14.0	6.0	0	480	1.0
patties (*Health is Wealth*), 3-oz. pc.	120	14.0	15.0	1.5	0	440	2.0
patties (*Morningstar Farms Chik Patties*), 2.5-oz. pc. .	150	9.0	16.0	6.0	0	540	2.0
patties (*Worthington Crispy Chik Patties*), 2.5-oz. pc. .	150	9.0	16.0	6.0	0	540	2.0
patties (*Quorn*), 2.6-oz. pc.	160	8.0	12.0	7.0	0	525	3.0
patties, Parmesan ranch (*Morningstar Farms Chik Patties*), 2.5-oz. pc.	170	10.0	17.0	7.0	0	680	2.0

Food and Measure	cal.	prot. (gms)	carbo. (gms)	fat (gms)	chol. (mgs)	sod. (mgs)	fiber (gms)
patties, spicy (*Boca Chik'n*), 2.5-oz. pc.	160	11.0	14.0	6.0	0	600	2.0
roll (*Worthington Meatless Chicken*), ⅜" slice, 2 oz. ..	90	9.0	2.0	4.5	0	240	1.0
slices (*Worthington Meatless Chicken*), 3 slices, 2 oz.	90	9.0	2.0	4.5	0	250	<1.0
sticks (*Worthington ChikStiks*), 1.7-oz. pc.	100	10.0	4.0	6.0	0	300	2.0
strips (*Lightlife*), 3 oz.	70	11.0	6.0	0	0	460	4.0
tenders (*Quorn*), 1 cup, 3 oz.	90	12.0	8.0	2.0	0	350	3.0
tenders, honey mustard (*Morningstar Farms Chik'n*), 2 pcs., 2.9 oz. ..	190	13.0	20.0	7.0	0	480	4.0
wings, Buffalo (*Boca Chik'n Hot & Spicy*), 3 oz.	160	14.0	14.0	7.0	0	700	3.0
wings, Buffalo (*Health is Wealth*), 3 pcs., 2.2 oz. ..	100	10.0	11.0	1.5	0	490	3.0
wings, Buffalo (*Morningstar Farms*), 5 pcs., 3 oz.	200	12.0	18.0	9.0	0	630	3.0
Chicken coating mix (see also "Batter and breading mix"), seasoned:							
(*Don's Chuck Wagon Baking Mix*), ¼ cup	95	3.0	21.0	0	0	665	1.0
(*McCormick Bag 'n Season*), 1 tbsp....	20	0	3.0	0	0	460	0
(*Oven Fry Extra Crispy*), ⅛ pkg.	60	2.0	10.0	1.0	0	420	0
(*Oven Fry Homestyle Flour*), ⅛ pkg.	40	1.0	7.0	1.0	0	470	0
(*Shake 'n Bake Original*), 1/16 of 5.5-oz. pkg.	40	1.0	7.0	1.0	0	220	0

Food and Measure	cal.	prot. (gms)	carbo. (gms)	fat (gms)	chol. (mgs)	sod. (mgs)	fiber (gms)
Chicken coating mix *(cont.)*							
barbecue glaze (*Shake 'n Bake*), 1/16 pkg.	45	0	9.0	1.0	0	410	0
Buffalo wings:							
(*McCormick Bag 'n Season*), 1 tbsp.	30	0	5.0	0	0	710	0
(*Shake 'n Bake*), 1/16 pkg.	40	3.0	8.0	1.0	0	300	0
Cajun (*Luzianne*), 2 tbsp.	100	3.0	20.0	1.0	0	1260	1.0
country style (*McCormick Bag 'n Season*), 1 tbsp.	25	0	3.0	1.0	0	880	0
fry mix:							
(*Golden Dipt* Fry Easy Extra Crispy), 1½ tbsp.	60	1.0	9.0	0	0	310	0
(*Golden Dipt* Fry Easy Original Homestyle), 2 tbsp.	50	0	9.0	0	0	660	0
(*McCormick Season 'n Fry*), 1 tbsp.	35	0	6.0	0	0	760	0
herb and spice (*Golden Dipt* Fry Easy), 2 tbsp.	70	0	13.0	0	0	490	0
hot and spicy (*Golden Dipt* Fry Easy), 2 tbsp.	50	0	9.0	0	0	430	0
garlic herb (*Shake 'n Bake*), 1/16 pkg.	35	1.0	7.0	.5	0	180	0
honey glaze:							
(*Shake 'n Bake Tangy*), 1/16 pkg.	45	0	9.0	1.0	0	300	0
mustard (*Shake 'n Bake*), 1/16 pkg.	45	6.0	9.0	1.0	0	300	0
hot and spicy (*Shake 'n Bake*), 1/16 pkg.	40	1.0	7.0	1.0	0	170	0
Italian:							
(*Shake 'n Bake*), 1/16 pkg.	40	1.0	7.0	.5	0	280	0
herb (*McCormick Bag 'n Season*), 1 tbsp.	15	0	2.0	0	0	480	0

Food and Measure	cal.	prot. (gms)	carbo. (gms)	fat (gms)	chol. (mgs)	sod. (mgs)	fiber (gms)
nuggets, crispy (*Shake 'n Bake*), 1/16 pkg.	50	1.0	9.0	1.0	0	360	0
Oriental (*McCormick Bag 'n Season*), 1 tbsp.	25	0	4.0	0	0	550	0
Santa Fe (*McCormick*), 2 tsp.	20	0	2.0	1.0	0	300	0
Southwestern (*McCormick Bag 'n Season*), 1 tbsp.	25	0	3.0	.5	0	490	0
Chicken dinner, frozen, 1 pkg.:							
asiago portobello (*Healthy Choice Dinners*), 12.5 oz. . .	330	20.0	47.0	6.0	30	600	6.0
blackened (*Healthy Choice Dinners*), 11 oz.	300	20.0	36.0	6.0	35	600	5.0
breaded, country (*Healthy Choice Dinners*), 10.6 oz. .	370	17.0	55.0	9.0	45	600	5.0
broccoli Alfredo (*Healthy Choice Dinners*), 11.5 oz. . .	300	25.0	34.0	7.0	50	530	2.0
fettuccine:							
(*Lean Cuisine Dinnertime Selections*), 13⅝ oz. .	380	26.0	51.0	8.0	45	870	5.0
(*Stouffer's* Home-style), 16.75 oz. .	500	30.0	55.0	18.0	40	1330	6.0
Florentine (*Lean Cuisine Dinnertime Selections*), 13.25 oz.	330	25.0	44.0	6.0	40	840	6.0
fried (*Swanson Hungry-Man Classic*), 16.5 oz.	790	33.0	75.0	40.0	80	1940	6.0
glazed:							
(*Lean Cuisine Dinnertime Selections*), 13 oz. . . .	310	24.0	39.0	6.0	50	610	4.0
honey (*Healthy Choice Dinners*), 11 oz.	320	18.0	46.0	6.0	40	580	6.0

Food and Measure	cal.	prot. (gms)	carbo. (gms)	fat (gms)	chol. (mgs)	sod. (mgs)	fiber (gms)
Chicken dinner, frozen, glazed *(cont.)*							
Oriental (*Lean Cuisine Dinnertime Selections*), 14 oz.	330	21.0	58.0	2.0	30	850	2.0
grilled:							
w/barbecue sauce, smokey (*Healthy Choice* Dinners), 12 oz.	370	18.0	59.0	6.0	25	600	6.0
lime, Southwestern (*Stouffer's* Homestyle), 14 oz. . . .	490	25.0	67.0	13.0	40	1780	9.0
and penne (*Lean Cuisine Dinnertime Selections*), 14 oz.	340	25.0	46.0	6.0	35	680	5.0
Tuscan (*Lean Cuisine Dinnertime Selections*), 12.5 oz.	270	20.0	34.0	6.0	35	610	3.0
herb, country (*Healthy Choice* Dinners), 11.35 oz.	280	18.0	37.0	6.0	40	600	5.0
mesquite barbecue (*Healthy Choice* Dinners), 10.5 oz. .	300	18.0	44.0	5.0	45	480	5.0
parmigiana (*Healthy Choice* Dinners), 11 oz.	320	19.0	40.0	9.0	20	600	6.0
roasted:							
(*Lean Cuisine Dinnertime Selections*), 12.5 oz. . .	320	21.0	48.0	4.5	35	730	4.0
breast (*Healthy Choice* Dinners), 11 oz.	280	18.0	32.0	8.0	45	600	7.0
sesame (*Healthy Choice* Dinners), 10.8 oz.	330	24.0	38.0	8.0	50	600	5.0
Southwestern:							
Monterey (*Stouffer's* Homestyle), 14.25 oz.	530	26.0	58.0	21.0	60	1330	4.0

Food and Measure	cal.	prot. (gms)	carbo. (gms)	fat (gms)	chol. (mgs)	sod. (mgs)	fiber (gms)
smothered (*Stouffer's* Home-style), 14 oz. ...	490	26.0	61.0	16.0	55	1470	6.0
sweet and sour (*Healthy Choice* Dinners), 11 oz. ...	340	15.0	54.0	7.0	25	580	3.0
teriyaki (*Healthy Choice* Dinners), 11 oz.	270	16.0	37.0	6.0	40	600	6.0
Chicken entree, can or pkg.:							
à la king (*Swanson*), 10.5-oz. can	320	18.0	20.0	19.0	45	1370	2.0
and dumplings:							
(*Dinty Moore* Can), 1 cup	230	12.0	28.0	8.0	35	860	1.0
(*Dinty Moore* Can), 7.5-oz. can	190	11.0	24.0	6.0	25	890	1.0
(*Dinty Moore* Cup), 1 cont.	190	11.0	24.0	6.0	25	890	1.0
(*Hormel* Bowl), 10 oz.	280	15.0	33.0	10.0	40	1010	2.0
(*Swanson*), 1 cup .	230	11.0	26.0	9.0	35	1220	2.0
and noodles:							
(*Dinty Moore* Can), 1 cup	230	14.0	24.0	9.0	65	910	1.0
(*Hormel* Bowl), 10 oz.	250	17.0	28.0	8.0	65	1260	2.0
noodles and (*Dinty Moore* Cup), 1 cont.	190	7.0	20.0	9.0	35	1200	1.0
w/potatoes (*Hormel* Bowl), 10 oz.	230	20.0	27.0	5.0	40	1020	2.0
and rice (*Hormel* Bowl), 10 oz.	260	13.0	30.0	10.0	40	1500	3.0
rice and:							
(*Dinty Moore* Cup), 1 cont.	190	7.0	23.0	8.0	20	1200	1.0
(*Hormel* Cup Fiesta), 7.5 oz.	360	11.0	32.0	21.0	70	1090	2.0
stew (*Dinty Moore* Can), 1 cup	220	12.0	17.0	11.0	35	1020	2.0
Chicken entree, freeze-dried, 1 serving:							
(*AlpineAire* Kung Fu) .	360	16.0	68.0	3.0	25	890	4.0

Food and Measure	cal.	prot. (gms)	carbo. (gms)	fat (gms)	chol. (mgs)	sod. (mgs)	fiber (gms)
Chicken entree, freeze-dried *(cont.)*							
(*AlpineAire* Sierra) . . .	330	21.0	54.0	4.0	25	670	3.0
(*AlpineAire* Summer) .	340	23.0	38.0	10.0	50	650	2.0
à la king and noodles:							
(*Mountain House*),							
½ pouch	390	25.0	42.0	14.0	85	990	3.0
(*Mountain House*							
Can), 1 cup	280	18.0	31.0	10.0	60	720	2.0
almond (*AlpineAire*) . .	380	24.0	53.0	8.0	20	780	5.0
barbecue, Texas:							
(*AlpineAire*)	305	18.0	53.0	2.0	n.a.	922	7.0
(*Instant Gourmet*) .	470	25.0	85.0	3.5	20	730	11.0
breast, grilled							
(*Mountain House*),							
½ pouch	230	26.0	22.0	4.5	75	840	<1.0
gumbo:							
(*AlpineAire*)	520	21.0	102.0	3.0	35	1420	17.0
(*Instant Gourmet*							
New Orleans) . . .	270	15.0	48.0	2.0	20	1370	5.0
noodles and:							
(*Mountain House*							
Can), 1 cup	220	10.0	34.0	5.0	40	970	1.0
(*Mountain House*),							
½ pouch	270	12.0	42.0	6.0	50	1200	2.0
Oriental, w/vegetables:							
(*Mountain House*							
Can), 1 cup	230	12.0	33.0	5.0	25	930	2.0
(*Mountain House*),							
½ pouch	300	16.0	44.0	7.0	30	1240	3.0
Polynesian (*Mountain*							
House), ½ pouch . .	270	12.0	44.0	5.0	30	1020	1.0
primavera (*AlpineAire*)	280	17.0	45.0	3.0	25	670	3.0
rice and:							
(*Mountain House*							
Can/Four), 1 cup . .	310	9.0	46.0	11.0	20	1140	2.0
(*Mountain House*							
Double), ½ pouch	410	11.0	59.0	14.0	25	1480	2.0
(*Mountain House*							
Single)	510	14.0	74.0	17.0	35	1840	3.0
Mexican (*Mountain*							
House), ½ pouch	320	18.0	46.0	7.0	30	1290	9.0
w/vegetables							
(*AlpineAire*)	330	20.0	55.0	3.0	30	1300	8.0

Food and Measure	cal.	prot. (gms)	carbo. (gms)	fat (gms)	chol. (mgs)	sod. (mgs)	fiber (gms)
rotelle (*AlpineAire*) ...	360	23.0	44.0	10.0	50	870	2.0
Santa Fe (*Instant Gourmet*)	440	21.0	81.0	3.0	15	910	13.0
stew:							
(*Mountain House*), ½ pouch	300	16.0	34.0	12.0	50	1180	4.0
(*Mountain House* Can), 1 cup	250	13.0	26.0	10.0	40	1040	3.0
teriyaki:							
(*Mountain House*), ½ pouch	280	12.0	49.0	3.5	30	1020	3.0
(*Mountain House* Can), 1 cup	240	11.0	42.0	2.5	20	870	2.0
Chicken entree, frozen (see also "Chicken, frozen or refrigerated, cooked"), 1 pkg., except as noted:							
à la king (*Stouffer's*), 11.5 oz.	370	20.0	45.0	12.0	50	620	2.0
Alfredo:							
(*Birds Eye Voila!*), 1 cup*	320	14.0	26.0	17.0	60	480	2.0
(*Contessa*), 8 oz. ..	330	16.0	26.0	18.0	80	680	2.0
(*Green Giant* Complete Skillet Meal), ¼ of 32-oz. pkg.	270	19.0	35.0	6.0	35	900	2.0
(*Green Giant* Complete Skillet Meal), ¼ of 32-oz. pkg. w/2% milk*	290	20.0	37.0	7.0	*40	920	2.0
(*Lean Cuisine Skillet Sensations* 24 oz.), 6.9 oz.	180	13.0	23.0	4.0	25	480	2.0
(*Stouffer's* Family Style Recipes), 1/7 of 57-oz. pkg.	380	17.0	33.0	20.0	30	950	3.0
(*Stouffer's Skillet Sensations* 25 oz.), 7.1 oz.	240	15.0	25.0	9.0	25	630	2.0
Florentine (*Michelina's Lean Gourmet*), 8.5 oz.	270	15.0	38.0	6.0	40	610	2.0

Food and Measure	cal.	prot. (gms)	carbo. (gms)	fat (gms)	chol. (mgs)	sod. (mgs)	fiber (gms)
Chicken entree, frozen, Alfredo *(cont.)*							
grilled, w/broccoli (*Michelina's* Homestyle Bowls), 11 oz.	490	24.0	48.0	21.0	90	920	3.0
grilled, w/broccoli (*Michelina's Signature*), 10 oz.	400	21.0	36.0	19.0	80	850	3.0
w/almonds (*Lean Cuisine* Café Classics), 8.5 oz. . .	260	18.0	38.0	4.0	30	620	3.0
arroz con pollo (*Jeff Nathan Creations*), 10 oz.	340	26.0	40.0	26.0	65	1220	4.0
baked:							
(*Lean Cuisine* Café Classics), 8⅝ oz. .	230	16.0	32.0	4.5	30	650	2.0
(*Stouffer's* Homestyle), 8 oz.	270	21.0	21.0	11.0	55	770	2.0
basil (*Smart Ones Bistro Selections*), 9.5 oz.	270	20.0	34.0	6.0	25	700	2.0
w/basil cream sauce:							
(*Lean Cuisine* Café Classics), 8.5 oz.	270	19.0	32.0	7.0	30	490	2.0
(*Lean Cuisine* Café Classics Bowl), 10.5 oz.	310	17.0	39.0	9.0	35	690	3.0
biryani (*Ethnic Gourmet*), 11 oz. . .	410	19.0	57.0	12.0	25	930	3.0
w/black beans, vegetables (*Smart Ones* Santa Fe Higher Protein), 9 oz.	140	33.0	10.0	2.5	60	850	3.0
breast:							
strips, w/mac and cheese (*Healthy Choice*), 8 oz.	290	34.0	35.0	5.0	40	600	3.0
tenders, barbecue sauce (*Stouffer's* Homestyle), 10 oz.	430	26.0	37.0	20.0	70	1230	3.0
and vegetables (*Healthy Choice*), 10.5 oz.	230	18.0	29.0	5.0	25	550	6.0

Food and Measure	cal.	prot. (gms)	carbo. (gms)	fat (gms)	chol. (mgs)	sod. (mgs)	fiber (gms)
breast, stuffed:							
asparagus and cheese (*Barber Foods*), 6-oz. pc.	350	25.0	19.0	19.0	80	690	<1.0
broccoli and cheese (*Barber Foods*), 6-oz. pc.	330	23.0	20.0	20.0	65	750	<2.0
broccoli and cheese (*Barber Foods* Light), 5.5-oz. pc.	220	25.0	15.0	7.0	50	560	<1.0
Cordon Bleu (*Barber Foods*), 6-oz. pc.	360	30.0	14.0	20.0	95	1060	<1.0
Cordon Bleu (*Barber Foods* Light), 5.5-oz. pc.	240	28.0	14.0	8.0	65	730	0
créme brie and apple (*Barber Foods*), 6-oz. pc.	320	23.0	12.0	20.0	95	800	<1.0
Kiev (*Barber Foods*), 6-oz. pc.	420	26.0	16.0	28.0	110	780	<1.0
mashed potato (*Barber Foods*), 6-oz. pc.	340	21.0	21.0	18.0	85	630	<1.0
rice and vegetables, skinless (*Barber Foods* Homestyle), 6-oz. pc.	270	22.0	26.0	9.0	50	790	<1.0
scallop and lobster (*Barber Foods*), 6-oz. pc.	380	25.0	25.0	20.0	70	790	<1.0
Caesar, grilled (*Lean Cuisine* Café Classics Bowl), 9 oz.	270	19.0	32.0	7.0	35	690	3.0
cacciatore (*Organic Classics*), 10 oz. . . .	350	25.0	38.0	10.0	80	580	3.0
Cajun style, and shrimp (*Healthy Choice*), 10.4 oz.	240	18.0	32.0	3.5	70	600	5.0
carbonara:							
(*Healthy Choice*), 9 oz.	310	23.0	39.0	7.0	40	600	2.0
(*Lean Cuisine* Café Classics), 9 oz. . . .	270	18.0	33.0	7.0	30	690	2.0
(*Smart Ones Bistro Selections*), 9.5 oz.	260	23.0	33.0	5.0	40	760	3.0

Food and Measure	cal.	prot. (gms)	carbo. (gms)	fat (gms)	chol. (mgs)	sod. (mgs)	fiber (gms)
Chicken entree, frozen *(cont.)*							
cheese, three:							
(*Birds Eye Voila!*), 1 cup*	210	13.0	21.0	8.0	30	940	2.0
(*Lean Cuisine Café Classics*), 8 oz.	230	21.0	14.0	10.0	45	520	2.0
(*Lean Cuisine Skillet Sensations 24 oz.*), 6.9 oz.	210	13.0	28.0	5.0	20	460	2.0
chow mein:							
(*Contessa*), 1¾ cups*	190	13.0	28.0	3.0	20	820	4.0
(*Lean Cuisine Everyday Favorites*), 9 oz.	200	14.0	31.0	2.5	25	620	2.0
curry, Thai style (*Organic Classics*), 10 oz.	390	20.0	42.0	17.0	55	330	2.0
w/dipping sauce:							
barbecue (*Healthy Choice*), 13 oz.	390	31.0	46.0	9.0	60	580	5.0
honey mustard (*Healthy Choice*), 13.5 oz.	360	28.0	49.0	5.0	60	600	6.0
roasted garlic tomato (*Healthy Choice*), 13 oz.	410	34.0	47.0	9.0	65	600	5.0
roasted red pepper (*Healthy Choice*), 13 oz.	390	36.0	39.0	10.0	60	570	7.0
teriyaki (*Healthy Choice*), 14 oz.	450	31.0	59.0	9.0	45	600	5.0
dumplings:							
(*C&W Ultimate Stir Fry Feast*), 1½ cups w/sauce	190	11.0	25.0	5.0	30	1350	3.0
(*C&W Ultimate Stir Fry Feast*), 1½ cups w/out sauce	160	10.0	20.0	5.0	30	410	2.0
and dumplings:							
(*Glory Savory Singles*), 11 oz.	290	16.0	40.0	8.0	75.0	1400	6.0
(*Glory Savory Singles Family Size*), 1 cup	250	14.0	34.0	7.0	65	1200	5.0

Food and Measure	cal.	prot. (gms)	carbo. (gms)	fat (gms)	chol. (mgs)	sod. (mgs)	fiber (gms)
(*Stouffer's Skillet Sensations* 24 oz.), 6.9 oz.	200	13.0	22.0	7.0	40	640	2.0
enchilada, see "Enchilada entree"							
escalloped, and noodles:							
(*Stouffer's*), 10 oz. . .	360	17.0	29.0	19.0	60	1020	4.0
(*Stouffer's* Family Style Recipes), 1/5 of 40-oz. pkg.	370	14.0	26.0	23.0	35	1080	2.0
fajita, see "Fajita"							
fettuccine:							
(*Lean Cuisine Every-day Favorites*), 9.25 oz.	280	22.0	33.0	7.0	35	690	2.0
(*Smart Ones Bistro Selections*), 10 oz.	300	21.0	39.0	8.0	70	630	4.0
(*Stouffer's* Home-style), 10.5 oz. . .	380	25.0	37.0	15.0	40	1090	3.0
primavera (*Michelina's* Authentico), 8 oz. . . .	270	12.0	37.0	9.0	25	540	3.0
fettuccine w/, see "Fettuccine entree"							
fettuccine Alfredo:							
(*Healthy Choice*), 8.5 oz.	280	25.0	28.0	7.0	55	570	3.0
(*Uncle Ben's* Pasta Bowl), 12 oz. . . .	350	27.0	47.0	7.0	140	1160	2.0
chicken and broccoli (*Michelina's* Authentico), 8.5 oz.	300	14.0	37.0	11.0	40	600	2.0
Florentine, baked (*Lean Cuisine* Café Classics), 8 oz.	200	18.0	14.0	8.0	40	660	3.0
fried:							
(*Swanson* Classic), 11.5 oz.	590	35.0	45.0	30.0	150	2030	4.0
breast (*Stouffer's* Homestyle), 8⅞ oz.	390	19.0	37.0	18.0	50	1040	2.0
w/mashed potato, gravy (*Michelina's* Authentico), 8 oz.	310	11.0	27.0	18.0	40	960	2.0

Food and Measure	cal.	prot. (gms)	carbo. (gms)	fat (gms)	chol. (mgs)	sod. (mgs)	fiber (gms)
Chicken entree, frozen *(cont.)*							
fritters, w/mashed potato (*Michelina's* Authentico Pop'n), 5.5 oz.	350	10.0	38.0	17.0	20	790	3.0
garlic:							
(*Lean Cuisine Skillet Sensations*), ⅓ of 24-oz. pkg.	240	14.0	36.0	4.5	30	580	2.0
(*Stouffer's Skillet Sensations*), ¼ of 23-oz. pkg.	190	13.0	25.0	4.0	20	680	2.0
golden baked (*Smart Ones Bistro Selections*), 10 oz.	270	17.0	42.0	5.0	25	670	2.0
roasted (*Lean Cuisine* Café Classics), 8⅞ oz.	200	17.0	14.0	8.0	40	690	2.0
garlic, and vegetables:							
(*Birds Eye Voila!*), 1 cup*	240	11.0	21.0	8.0	30	940	3.0
and pasta (*Green Giant* Complete Skillet Meal), ¼ of 32-oz. pkg.	260	17.0	31.0	7.0	35	990	2.0
roasted (*Birds Eye Voila!* Reduced Carb), 1 cup* ...	120	12.0	13.0	2.5	30	520	3.0
glazed:							
(*Lean Cuisine* Café Classics), 8.5 oz.	220	20.0	27.0	3.5	35	610	2.0
(*Michelina's Lean Gourmet*), 8 oz.	260	11.0	45.0	3.5	30	920	2.0
(*Smart Ones Bistro Selections*), 8.5 oz.	260	14.0	45.0	2.5	35	770	5.0
country (*Healthy Choice*), 8.5 oz.	230	17.0	29.0	5.0	40	600	3.0
w/green beans, rice (*Michelina's* Authentico), 8 oz.	250	11.0	45.0	3.5	20	850	2.0
white (*Boston Market*), 10 oz.	290	20.0	29.0	10.0	55	1220	2.0

Food and Measure	cal.	prot. (gms)	carbo. (gms)	fat (gms)	chol. (mgs)	sod. (mgs)	fiber (gms)
grilled:							
(*Lean Cuisine* Café Classics), 9⅜ oz.	160	14.0	15.0	5.0	35	690	4.0
(*Lean Cuisine* Café Classics Fiesta), 8.5 oz.	250	19.0	31.0	6.0	40	580	3.0
Baja (*Healthy Choice*), 10 oz. ...	270	22.0	33.0	5.0	30	600	7.0
basil (*Healthy Choice*), 10.6 oz.	290	23.0	33.0	7.0	40	580	5.0
Caesar (*Healthy Choice*), 10 oz. ...	290	17.0	42.0	7.0	25	580	7.0
Caesar (*Michelina's* Homestyle Bowls), 11 oz.	310	20.0	45.0	4.5	35	820	3.0
garlic herb sauce (*Smart Ones* Higher Protein), 9 oz.	190	23.0	9.0	8.0	45	540	2.0
marinara (*Healthy Choice*), 10 oz. ...	280	17.0	37.0	4.5	35	580	5.0
and mashed potato (*Healthy Choice*), 8.5 oz.	230	19.0	22.0	7.0	50	580	4.0
herb:							
garden (*Birds Eye Voila!*), 1 cup* ..	280	13.0	40.0	11.0	35	600	3.0
grilled (*Stouffer's*), 9 oz.	250	20.0	33.0	4.5	35	510	3.0
and roasted potatoes (*Lean Cuisine Skillet Sensations*), ⅓ of 24-oz. pkg.	170	12.0	24.0	3.0	25	510	2.0
w/honey barbecue sauce (*Organic Classics*), 9 oz.	220	21.0	26.0	5.0	45	570	4.0
honey Dijon:							
(*Smart Ones*), 8.5 oz.	210	11.0	38.0	3.5	30	620	2.0
grilled (*Lean Cuisine* Café Classics), 8 oz.	220	17.0	22.0	7.0	50	640	2.0
honey ginger (*Michelina's Yu Sing* Bowls), 11 oz.	350	16.0	60.0	6.0	30	990	3.0

Food and Measure	cal.	prot. (gms)	carbo. (gms)	fat (gms)	chol. (mgs)	sod. (mgs)	fiber (gms)
Chicken entree, frozen *(cont.)*							
honey mustard (*Lean Cuisine Café Classics*), 8 oz.	250	17.0	37.0	4.0	30	650	1.0
korma (*Ethnic Gourmet*), 11 oz. ..	360	21.0	34.0	10.0	70	750	3.0
kung pao (*Ethnic Gourmet*), 12 oz. ..	420	20.0	61.0	10.0	30	850	3.0
lemon (*Lean Cuisine Spa Cuisine*), 9 oz. ..	270	12.0	38.0	8.0	25	650	2.0
lemongrass:							
(*Lean Cuisine Spa Cuisine*), 9⅝ oz.	240	18.0	29.0	6.0	30	660	4.0
and basil (*Ethnic Gourmet*), 11 oz.	400	22.0	53.0	12.0	40	540	4.0
lemon pepper, grilled (*Stouffer's*), 9 oz. ..	240	20.0	27.0	6.0	45	630	5.0
lo mein (*Green Giant Complete Skillet Meal*), ¼ of 32-oz. pkg.	200	15.0	30.0	2.5	25	760	3.0
mandarin:							
(*Healthy Choice*), 10 oz.	280	20.0	43.0	3.5	35	520	4.0
(*Lean Cuisine Everyday Favorites*), 9 oz.	270	14.0	46.0	3.5	30	690	2.0
Margherita (*Healthy Choice*), 10 oz.	340	16.0	25.0	8.0	40	600	6.0
Marsala:							
(*Lean Cuisine Café Classics*), 8⅛ oz.	140	14.0	12.0	4.0	35	620	3.0
(*Organic Classics*), 9.5 oz.	440	18.0	41.0	22.0	70	980	3.0
w/broccoli (*Smart Ones Higher Protein*), 9 oz. ..	180	19.0	12.0	7.0	50	660	3.0
w/garlic potatoes (*Michelina's Signature*), 8.5 oz.	270	13.0	22.0	13.0	50	1010	2.0
roasted (*Healthy Choice*), 10.4 oz.	240	22.0	23.0	6.0	50	600	4.0
Massaman (*Ethnic Gourmet*), 11 oz. ..	330	18.0	44.0	9.0	35	780	4.0

Food and Measure	cal.	prot. (gms)	carbo. (gms)	fat (gms)	chol. (mgs)	sod. (mgs)	fiber (gms)
Mediterranean:							
(*Lean Cuisine* Café Classics), 10.5 oz.	260	17.0	38.0	4.0	20	690	4.0
(*Lean Cuisine Spa Cuisine*), 10.5 oz.	240	16.0	35.0	3.5	20	690	5.0
noodle, creamy:							
(*Green Giant* Complete Skillet Meal), ¼ of 32-oz. pkg.	290	19.0	42.0	5.0	30	1280	3.0
(*Green Giant* Complete Skillet Meal), ¼ of 32-oz. pkg. w/2% milk*	320	21.0	45.0	6.0	35	1310	3.0
and noodles:							
(*Michelina's* Homestyle Bowls), 11 oz.	300	20.0	43.0	6.0	70	880	4.0
(*Stouffer's* Bowl Cuisine Homestyle), 12 oz.	350	13.0	45.0	13.0	60	1160	5.0
(*Stouffer's Skillet Sensations* 25 oz.), 7.1 oz.	260	18.0	28.0	8.0	50	640	3.0
rice noodles, Thai (*Smart Ones Bistro Selections*), 9 oz.	290	13.0	39.0	4.0	25	830	2.0
noodles and (*Michelina's* Zap'ems), 8 oz.	280	12.0	36.0	10.0	70	770	2.0
nuggets entree:							
w/dessert (*Ian's* Natural Kids Meal), 8 oz.	440	18.0	60.0	14.0	50	320	2.0
w/mac and cheese (*Stouffer's Maxaroni*), 8 oz.	370	17.0	33.0	19.0	40	790	1.0
orange:							
(*Contessa* Minute Meal Bowl), 10.5 oz.	300	14.0	51.0	3.5	25	880	2.0
à l'orange (*Lean Cuisine* Café Classics), 9 oz. . .	230	18.0	35.0	15.0	35	340	2.0
Oriental:							
(*Healthy Choice*), 8.5 oz.	240	21.0	28.0	5.0	35	600	7.0

Food and Measure	cal.	prot. (gms)	carbo. (gms)	fat (gms)	chol. (mgs)	sod. (mgs)	fiber (gms)
Chicken entree, frozen, Oriental *(cont.)*							
(*Lean Cuisine Skillet Sensations* 24 oz.), 6.9 oz.	170	12.0	23.0	3.0	20	610	2.0
(*Smart Ones*), 9 oz.	230	15.0	34.0	4.5	35	790	3.0
Parmesan:							
(*Lean Cuisine* Café Classics), 10⅞ oz.	280	22.0	36.0	5.0	40	510	3.0
(*Smart Ones Bistro Selections*), 11 oz. ...	300	20.0	32.0	5.0	30	670	3.0
creamy, w/garden vegetables (*Smart Ones* Higher Protein), 9 oz. ..	210	28.0	12.0	8.0	90	790	4.0
parmigiana:							
(*Stouffer's* Family Style Recipes), ¼ of 52.5-oz. pkg.	160	22.0	59.0	18.0	40	1570	4.0
(*Stouffer's* Homestyle), 12 oz. ...	460	24.0	53.0	17.0	40	750	5.0
w/linguine (*Michelina's Signature*), 10 oz.	410	20.0	49.0	15.0	35	890	4.0
and pasta:							
(*Healthy Choice* Homestyle), 9 oz.	270	21.0	32.0	6.0	35	570	5.0
bake, and broccoli (*Stouffer's* Family Style Recipes), 1/5 of 40-oz. pkg.	340	19.0	27.0	17.0	50	1060	2.0
Cordon Bleu (*Stouffer's* Family Style Recipes), ¼ of 37-oz. pkg.	330	18.0	34.0	13.0	30	890	1.0
Italiano (*Contessa*), 1¾ cups*	300	17.0	29.0	12.0	65	710	2.0
and vegetables (*Smart Ones* Mirabella), 9.2 oz.	180	11.0	30.0	2.0	20	480	4.0
pasta, cheese sauce:							
(*Green Giant* Complete Skillet Meal), ¼ of 32-oz. pkg.	270	18.0	37.0	6.0	40	950	3.0

Food and Measure	cal.	prot. (gms)	carbo. (gms)	fat (gms)	chol. (mgs)	sod. (mgs)	fiber (gms)
(*Green Giant* Complete Skillet Meal), ¼ of 32-oz. pkg. w/2% milk*	300	19.0	39.0	7.0	40	970	3.0
patties, breaded, w/fries (*Michelina's* Authentico Chicken Littles), 5.5 oz.	300	13.0	31.0	14.0	30	660	2.0
peanut satay (*Ethnic Gourmet*), 11 oz. ..	410	25.0	51.0	12.0	35	940	3.0
in peanut sauce (*Lean Cuisine* Café Classics/ Spa Cuisine), 9 oz. .	280	21.0	32.0	7.0	25	690	2.0
pecan (*Lean Cuisine* Spa Cuisine), 9 oz. .	260	18.0	34.0	6.0	30	570	4.0
penne w/:							
(*Michelina's* Authentico), 8.5 oz.	330	16.0	48.0	9.0	40	610	2.0
(*Smart Ones* Bistro Selections Penne Pollo), 10 oz. ...	290	22.0	38.0	6.0	55	590	3.0
pesto primavera (*Birds Eye Voila!*), 1 cup*	210	12.0	24.0	7.0	20	590	2.0
piccata:							
(*Healthy Choice*), 9 oz.	270	17.0	40.0	5.0	30	600	2.0
(*Jeff Nathan Creations*), 12 oz. ...	290	27.0	24.0	6.0	65	1240	6.0
(*Lean Cuisine* Café Classics), 9 oz. ...	270	13.0	41.0	6.0	25	670	1.0
lemon herb (*Smart Ones*), 9 oz.	250	15.0	36.0	5.0	45	510	2.0
pie/pot pie:							
(*Boston Market*), 1 cup	600	15.0	35.0	39.0	65	1110	2.0
(*Ian's Natural*), 9 oz.	554	20.0	82.0	16.0	38	724	3.5
(*Stouffer's*) 10 oz. .	740	23.0	56.0	47.0	65	1170	4.0
(*Stouffer's*), ½ of 16-oz. pkg......	600	19.0	45.0	38.0	50	950	3.0
(*Swanson*), 7 oz. ...	410	11.0	40.0	23.0	55	690	2.0
Alfredo, creamy, and broccoli (*Pepperidge Farm*), 1 cup	600	16.0	46.0	40.0	40	1180	4.0

Food and Measure	cal.	prot. (gms)	carbo. (gms)	fat (gms)	chol. (mgs)	sod. (mgs)	fiber (gms)
Chicken entree, frozen, pie/pot pie *(cont.)*							
broccoli and (*Pepperidge Farm*), 1 cup	490	12.0	42.0	30.0	30	1020	2.0
Parmesan, chunky (*Pepperidge Farm*), 1 cup	520	15.0	57.0	26.0	20	1180	2.0
primavera, w/garlic, herbs (*Pepperidge Farm*), 1 cup	530	14.0	49.0	31.0	10	1080	2.0
roasted (*Pepperidge Farm*), 1 cup . . .	510	13.0	43.0	32.0	30	870	3.0
portobello, grilled (*Stouffer's*), 9 oz. . .	230	19.0	26.0	6.0	35	900	4.0
pot stickers:							
(*C&W Pot Sticker Stir Fry Feast*), 2 cups w/sauce .	200	10.0	30.0	4.0	15	1200	4.0
(*C&W Pot Sticker Stir Fry Feast*), 2 cups w/out sauce	160	9.0	23.0	4.0	15	230	4.0
Oriental style (*Lean Cuisine Everyday Favorites*), 9 oz. .	320	11.0	55.0	6.0	20	610	3.0
primavera:							
(*Lean Cuisine Skillet Sensations 24 oz.*), 6.9 oz.	180	11.0	28.0	2.5	20	430	1.0
w/spirals (*Michelina's* Authentico), 8 oz.	250	13.0	37.0	6.0	30	750	3.0
ranchero sauce, spicy (*Smart Ones* Fiesta), 8.5 oz.	210	13.0	35.0	2.0	25	570	5.0
w/rice:							
beans and vegetables (*Smart Ones* Southwestern Bowl), 11 oz.	230	16.0	32.0	3.5	25	710	5.0
cheesy (*Healthy Choice*), 9 oz. . . .	230	14.0	33.0	4.0	30	580	5.0

Food and Measure	cal.	prot. (gms)	carbo. (gms)	fat (gms)	chol. (mgs)	sod. (mgs)	fiber (gms)
savory (*Stouffer's Skillet Sensations*), 1/5 of 40-oz. pkg.	230	14.0	36.0	3.0	35	870	5.0
vegetable rice bake (*Stouffer's* Family Recipes Grand- ma's), ¼ of 36-oz. pkg.	320	19.0	31.0	13.0	50	990	1.0
rice, fried, see "Rice entree, frozen"							
roast/roasted:							
(*Lean Cuisine Every- day Favorites*), 8⅛ oz.	250	16.0	32.0	6.0	30	670	2.0
Chardonnay (*Healthy Choice*), 10.6 oz.	280	22.0	32.0	7.0	40	600	4.0
herb (*Lean Cuisine Café Classics*), 8 oz.	190	17.0	23.0	3.5	30	610	3.0
herb, creamy (*Healthy Choice*), 10 oz.	220	20.0	35.0	5.0	35	600	7.0
oven (*Smart Ones Bistro Selections*), 9 oz.	260	17.0	37.0	6.0	30	770	2.0
w/sour cream (*Smart Ones Bistro Selections*), 9.5 oz.	190	14.0	19.0	3.5	40	990	2.0
w/stuffing (*Stouffer's* Homestyle), 9⅝ oz.	460	26.0	34.0	24.0	80	990	5.0
and vegetables, w/rice (*Uncle Ben's* Rice Bowl), 12 oz.	360	21.0	25.0	4.5	25	1020	3.0
rosemary (*Lean Cuisine Spa Cuisine*), 8.25 oz.	230	17.0	29.0	5.0	35	720	3.0
and sausage (*Birds Eye Voila!* Tuscan Reduced Carb), 1 cup*	170	14.0	10.0	8.0	35	620	4.0

Food and Measure	cal.	prot. (gms)	carbo. (gms)	fat (gms)	chol. (mgs)	sod. (mgs)	fiber (gms)
Chicken entree, frozen *(cont.)*							
sesame:							
(*Healthy Choice*),							
9 oz.	260	17.0	34.0	6.0	35	580	4.0
(*Lean Cuisine* Café							
Classics), 9 oz. . . .	330	15.0	49.0	8.0	20	690	2.0
(*Michelina's Yu Sing*							
Bowls), 11 oz. . .	390	13.0	67.0	6.0	35	1450	2.0
smoked sausage, rice:							
(*Glory* Savory							
Singles Casserole),							
11 oz.	440	18.0	49.0	18.0	60	1390	1.0
(*Glory* Savory							
Singles Casserole							
Family Size),							
1 cup	320	14.0	36.0	13.0	45	1030	1.0
stir-fry:							
(*Birds Eye Voila!*),							
1 cup*	160	10.0	22.0	3.0	15	1030	2.0
(*Contessa*), 1¾ cups*	140	15.0	15.0	2.0	35	360	4.0
(*Tyson* Meal Kit),							
2¾ cups*	430	24.0	73.0	4.5	45	1700	5.0
w/rice (*Uncle Ben's*							
Rice Bowl), 12 oz.	360	23.0	35.0	4.0	35	1430	3.0
sweet and sour:							
(*Green Giant* Com-							
plete Skillet Meal),							
¼ of 32-oz. pkg.	320	14.0	62.0	1.5	25	550	3.0
(*Lean Cuisine* Café							
Classics), 10 oz. .	290	14.0	52.0	2.5	25	680	1.0
(*Smart Ones* Higher							
Protein), 9 oz. . .	150	21.0	13.0	3.0	45	740	1.0
w/rice (*Michelina's*							
Yu Sing Bowls),							
11 oz.	420	13.0	82.0	4./0	30	830	2.0
w/rice (*Uncle Ben's*							
Rice Bowl), 12 oz.	360	17.0	65.0	3.0	30	620	2.0
tandoori w/spinach							
(*Ethnic Gourmet*),							
11 oz.	330	17.0	39.0	10.0	35	870	5.0
tenderloins, w/barbe-							
cue sauce (*Smart*							
Ones Bistro Selec-							
tions), 9 oz.	300	17.0	30.0	8.0	45	780	3.0

Food and Measure	cal.	prot. (gms)	carbo. (gms)	fat (gms)	chol. (mgs)	sod. (mgs)	fiber (gms)
teriyaki:							
(*Birds Eye Voila!*), 1 cup*	250	12.0	44.0	2.5	20	980	2.0
(*Ethnic Gourmet*), 11 oz.	340	17.0	63.0	3.0	30	870	2.0
(*Green Giant* Complete Skillet Meal), ¼ of 32-oz. pkg.	250	15.0	45.0	1.5	25	810	3.0
(*Jeff Nathan Creations*), 12 oz.	350	28.0	48.0	5.5	65	1450	4.0
(*Lean Cuisine* Café Classics), 10 oz.	280	19.0	42.0	3.5	40	660	0
(*Lean Cuisine* Café Classics Bowl), 11 oz.	320	16.0	58.0	3.0	30	690	3.0
(*Lean Cuisine* Skillet Sensations 24 oz.), 9.6 oz.	230	14.0	37.0	3.0	25	620	4.0
(*Michelina's Yu Sing*), 11 oz.	400	15.0	77.0	3.0	30	1390	2.0
(*Stouffer's Skillet Sensations* 25 oz.), 7.1 oz.	160	11.0	24.0	2.0	30	640	2.0
grilled (*Stouffer's*), 9⅜ oz.	300	21.0	45.0	3.5	40	880	4.0
w/rice (*Michelina's Authentico*), 8.5 oz.	280	11.0	64.0	2.5	15	1160	1.0
w/rice (*Uncle Ben's* Rice Bowl), 12 oz.	400	20.0	66.0	3.5	25	1450	3.0
stir-fry (*Lean Cuisine* Everyday Favorites), 10 oz.	300	17.0	49.0	4.5	30	690	3.0
tetrazzini, Cajun style (*Organic Classics*), 10 oz.	370	23.0	46.0	4.5	45	850	2.0
Thai:							
pad (*Ethnic Gourmet*), 10 oz.	430	20.0	71.0	8.0	30	880	3.0
style (*Lean Cuisine* Café Classics), 9 oz.	230	18.0	30.0	4.0	30	620	2.0
style (*Uncle Ben's* Pasta Bowl), 12 oz.	400	21.0	60.0	8.0	80	980	6.0

Food and Measure	cal.	prot. (gms)	carbo. (gms)	fat (gms)	chol. (mgs)	sod. (mgs)	fiber (gms)
Chicken entree, frozen *(cont.)*							
tikka masala (*Ethnic Gourmet*), 11 oz. . .	350	25.0	37.0	11.0	95	700	7.0
Tuscany (*Healthy Choice*), 10.6 oz. . .	330	25.0	42.0	9.0	50	600	6.0
vegetable stir-fry (*Michelina's* Authentico), 8 oz.	200	10.0	29.0	5.0	10	910	3.0
vegetables and:							
(*Michelina's Yu Sing* Bowls), 11 oz. . .	360	14.0	59.0	9.0	40	970	3.0
spicy Szechuan (*Smart Ones*), 9 oz.	220	11.0	34.0	5.0	10	890	4.0
and vegetables:							
(*Birds Eye Voila!* Down Home Reduced Carb), 1 cup*	180	16.0	17.0	5.0	40	840	4.0
(*Ethnic Gourmet* Thit Ga Kho Tieu), 10 oz.	330	18.0	43.0	2.5	30	840	1.0
(*Glory* Savory Singles Casserole), 11 oz.	330	17.0	27.0	17.0	55	943	2.0
(*Lean Cuisine* Café Classics), 10.5 oz.	240	19.0	30.0	5.0	30	630	2.0
(*Smart Ones* Homestyle Higher Protein), 9 oz. . .	220	27.0	8.0	9.0	70	600	2.0
fire-grilled (*Smart Ones Bistro Selections*), 10 oz. . . .	280	18.0	45.0	3.5	55	700	2.0
grilled (*Stouffer's Skillet Sensations*), ⅓ of 25-oz. pkg.	260	16.0	28.0	9.0	30	760	2.0
hearty (*Stouffer's Bowl Cuisine*), 12 oz.	330	19.0	30.0	15.0	90	1150	4.0
and potato (*Michelina's Lean Gourmet* French Recipe), 8.5 oz. .	180	10.0	23.0	4.5	30	830	4.0
and rice (*Healthy Choice* Princess), 10.75 oz.	310	18.0	41.0	7.0	55	580	5.0

Food and Measure	cal.	prot. (gms)	carbo. (gms)	fat (gms)	chol. (mgs)	sod. (mgs)	fiber (gms)
stew, hearty (*Organic Classics*), 9.5 oz.	420	20.0	39.0	19.0	70	970	3.0
teriyaki (*Birds Eye Voila!* Reduced Carb), 1 cup* . . .	150	17.0	15.0	2.5	25	990	4.0
teriyaki (*Smart Ones* Bowls), 10.5 oz. .	280	16.0	48.0	3.0	20	700	3.0
vegetarian, see "Vegetarian entree, frozen"							
vindaloo (*Ethnic Gourmet*), 11 oz.	320	19.0	46.0	7.0	35	910	3.0
w/zucchini, creamy (*Smart Ones* Tuscan Higher Protein), 9 oz.	180	22.0	9.0	8.0	55	700	2.0
"Chicken" entree, vegetarian, frozen (see also "Vegetarian entree, frozen"), 1 pkg., except as noted:							
fire-grilled, and vegetables (*Linda Mc-Cartney*), 10 oz. . . .	340	12.0	35.0	11.0	<5	950	4.0
w/lemongrass and basil (*Ethnic Gourmet*), 11 oz.	390	12.0	58.0	13.0	0	950	7.0
Szechuan (*Ethnic Gourmet*), 12 oz. . . .	380	13.0	69.0	6.0	0	840	6.0
tenders, w/noodles, Thai (*Quorn* Simply Saute), ½ of 18-oz. pkg.	240	14.0	34.0	9.0	15	660	8.0
tenders, w/rice:							
Indian (*Quorn* Simply Saute), ½ of 18-oz. pkg.	240	14.0	47.0	4.0	15	800	9.0
Mexican (*Quorn* Simply Saute), ½ of 18-oz. pkg.	340	15.0	61.0	7.0	15	850	7.0
teriyaki stir-fry, w/chick'n (*Cedarlane*), 10 oz.	460	14.0	86.0	6.0	0	680	4.0

Food and Measure	cal.	prot. (gms)	carbo. (gms)	fat (gms)	chol. (mgs)	sod. (mgs)	fiber (gms)
"Chicken" entree, vegetarian, frozen *(cont.)*							
Thai lemongrass chick'n (*Yves* The Good Bowl), 10.5 oz.	320	16.0	49.0	8.0	0	930	4.0
Chicken entree mix, 1 cup*, except as noted:							
Alfredo (*Annie's* Organic Skillet Meal) .	330	34.0	30	8.0	80	430	1.0
basil Parmesan, creamy (*Betty Crocker Cookbook Favorites*)	340	27.0	29.0	14.0	75	880	1.0
and biscuits, buttermilk (*Betty Crocker Complete Meals*), 1/5 pkg.*	320	10.0	41.0	13.0	25	1070	2.0
cheddar:							
and broccoli (*Chicken Helper*)	310	29.0	26.0	10.0	65	790	1.0
herb (*Annie's* Organic Skillet Meals)	310	31.0	30.0	7.0	75	460	1.0
cheese, four (*Chicken Helper*)	310	25.0	26.0	12.0	60	740	1.0
cheesy:							
enchilada (*Chicken Helper*)	340	26.0	40.0	9.0	60	770	<1.0
w/pasta (*Campbell's Supper Bakes*), 1/6 pkg.	180	7.0	28.0	4.0	10	860	1.0
con queso, and Mexican rice (*Betty Crocker Cookbook Favorites*), 1/5 pkg.*	340	23.0	24.0	17.0	65	610	1.0
and dumplings (*Chicken Helper*) . .	280	22.0	27.0	10.0	50	1010	1.0
dumplings and (*Betty Crocker Complete Meals*), 1/5 pkg.* . .	250	9.0	33.0	9.0	20	1150	2.0
fettuccine Alfredo: (*Betty Crocker Complete Meals*), 1/5 pkg.*	310	14.0	38.0	11.0	40	940	2.0

Food and Measure	cal.	prot. (gms)	carbo. (gms)	fat (gms)	chol. (mgs)	sod. (mgs)	fiber (gms)
(Betty Crocker Cookbook Favorites) .	340	26.0	27.0	15.0	60	870	1.0
(Chicken Helper) . .	270	26.0	25.0	7.0	65	800	1.0
fried rice (Chicken Helper)	260	23.0	22.0	8.0	120	660	1.0
garlic, w/pasta (Campbell's Supper Bakes), 1/6 pkg.	230	11.0	44.0	1.0	<5	780	2.0
herb, rice: (Campbell's Supper Bakes), 1/6 pkg. .	190	5.0	40.0	1.0	<5	790	1.0
(Chicken Helper) . .	260	24.0	24.0	7.0	56	440	1.0
lemon, w/herb rice (Campbell's Supper Bakes), 1/6 pkg. . . .	200	4.0	43.0	1.0	<5	790	2.0
Parmesan pasta (Chicken Helper) . .	290	25.0	30.0	8.0	55	850	1.0
penne, garlic and herb (Betty Crocker Cookbook Favorites), 1/5 pkg.*	240	23.0	21.0	7.0	50	420	2.0
and potatoes, au gratin (Chicken Helper) . .	270	26.0	25.0	7.0	65	800	1.0
roast, w/stuffing (Campbell's Supper Bakes Traditional), 1/6 pkg.	160	5.0	29.0	3.0	<5	760	2.0
Southwestern, w/rice (Campbell's Supper Bakes), 16 pkg. . . .	150	4.0	32.0	1.0	5	590	2.0
and stuffing (Chicken Helper)	290	27.0	27.0	9.0	65	820	1.0
teriyaki (Chicken Helper)	300	26.0	36.0	6.0	60	880	<1.0
Chicken fat:							
1 tbsp.	115	0	0	12.8	11	0	0
rendered (Empire Kosher), 1 tbsp. . . .	120	0	<1.0	13.0	10	0	0
Chicken frankfurter, see "Frankfurter"							
Chicken giblets:							
simmered, 4 oz.	178	29.3	1.1	5.4	446	66	0
simmered, chopped, 1 cup	228	37.5	1.4	6.9	570	85	0

Food and Measure	cal.	prot. (gms)	carbo. (gms)	fat (gms)	chol. (mgs)	sod. (mgs)	fiber (gms)
Chicken gravy, can or jar, ¼ cup:							
(*Campbell's*)	40	0	3.0	3.0	5	260	0
(*Campbell's* Fat Free) .	15	<1.0	3.0	0	<5	310	0
(*Heinz* Home Style) . .	25	0	4.0	1.0	0	340	0
giblet (*Campbell's*) . . .	30	1.0	2.0	1.5	15	310	0
roast, slow:							
(*Franco-American*) .	20	1.0	3.0	.5	<5	240	0
(*Franco-American* Fat Free)	15	<1.0	3.0	0	<5	240	0
roasted (*Boston Market*)	30	1.0	4.0	1.5	<5	300	0
w/roasted garlic (*Campbell's*)	35	<1.0	4.0	2.0	5	270	0
Chicken gravy mix, ¼ cup*:							
(*McCormick*)	20	0	4.0	0	0	330	0
roasted, and herb (*McCormick*)	25	0	3.0	1.0	0	260	0
Chicken lunch meat, breast, 2 oz., except as noted:							
(*Dietz & Watson* Gourmet)	70	11.0	1.0	2.0	30	400	0
barbecue (*Boar's Head Bar BQ Sauce Basted*)	60	11.0	3.0	.5	30	490	0
browned (*Healthy Choice*)	60	11.0	1.0	1.0	25	400	0
Buffalo style (*Boar's Head Blazing Buffalo*)	60	13.0	0	1.0	35	390	0
golden roasted (*Tyson* Bag), 3 slices, 2.25 oz.	60	12.0	1.0	1.0	30	620	0
honey roasted:							
(*Tyson* Bag), 2 slices, 1.6 oz.	50	8.0	3.0	1.0	15	530	0
(*Tyson* Box), 2 slices, 1.8 oz.	60	9.0	3.0	1.0	20	590	0
oven roasted:							
(*Boar's Head Golden Classic*)	60	13.0	0	1.0	35	350	0

Food and Measure	cal.	prot. (gms)	carbo. (gms)	fat (gms)	chol. (mgs)	sod. (mgs)	fiber (gms)
(*Healthy Choice* Hearty Slices 6 oz.), 1 oz.	30	5.0	2.0	1.0	15	240	0
(*Healthy Choice* Hearty Slices 10 oz.), 1 oz. ...	35	5.0	2.0	1.0	15	240	0
(*Healthy Choice Deli Thin*), 4 slices, 1.8 oz.	60	10.0	3.0	1.5	25	450	0
(*Sara Lee*)	45	10.0	1.0	0	20	420	0
(*Sara Lee* Sliced), 2 slices, 1.6 oz. . .	45	9.0	1.0	.5	15	380	0
(*Tyson* Bag), 2 slices, 1.6 oz.	40	8.0	1.0	1.0	20	530	0
(*Tyson* Box), 5 slices, 1.8 oz.	50	9.0	2.0	1.0	20	590	0
(*Tyson* Reseal Bag), 3 slices, 2 oz. ...	60	10.0	2.0	1.0	25	640	0
oil-braised (*Williams*)	60	9.0	1.0	2.0	25	350	0
rotisserie style/flavor:							
(*Dietz & Watson*) ..	70	11.0	1.0	2.0	30	400	0
(*Sara Lee*)	50	10.0	2.0	0	20	450	0
(*Tyson* Box), 2 slices, 1.8 oz. .	50	9.0	2.0	1.0	20	590	0
seasoned (*Boar's Head Aroastica*)	60	13.0	0	1.0	35	400	0
skinless (*Healthy Choice*)	50	9.0	1.0	1.0	20	470	0
smoked:							
(*Tyson* Bag), 2 slices, 1.6 oz.	45	9.0	1.0	.5	20	530	0
(*Tyson* Box), 5 slices, 1.8 oz.	50	10.0	1.0	1.0	25	590	0
(*Tyson* Reseal Bag), 3 slices, 2.25 oz.	60	12.0	1.0	1.0	30	620	0
hickory (*Boar's Head*)	60	13.0	0	.5	35	360	0
honey (*Healthy Choice Deli Thin*), 4 slices, 1.8 oz. .	70	9.0	4.0	1.5	25	450	0
mesquite (*Healthy Choice*)	60	11.0	1.0	1.0	30	440	0
Chicken pie, frozen, see "Chicken entree, frozen"							

Food and Measure	cal.	prot. (gms)	carbo. (gms)	fat (gms)	chol. (mgs)	sod. (mgs)	fiber (gms)
Chicken pocket/ sandwich, frozen, 1 pc., 4.5 oz., except as noted:							
(*Pot Pie Express*)	350	8.0	40.0	17.0	15	860	3.0
(*Pot Pie Express* Value 5 Pack)	340	9.0	36.0	18.0	15.0	860	3.0
Alfredo (*Croissant Pockets*)	320	11.0	35.0	15.0	20	690	3.0
and broccoli:							
(*Pot Pie Express*) ..	350	10.0	40.0	17.0	15	870	3.0
cheddar (*Croissant Pockets*)	310	11.0	34.0	15.0	15	540	3.0
cheese, three, and (*Lean Pockets Quesadilla*)	280	14.0	41.0	7.0	25	630	3.0
cheddar and broccoli (*Lean Pockets*)	260	11.0	39.0	7.0	20	590	3.0
fajita (*Lean Pockets*) .	260	11.0	38.0	7.0	25	730	3.0
grilled Casear (*Michelina's Hot Subs*), 2.1 oz.	300	12.0	38.0	12.0	20	740	2.0
Parmesan:							
(*Croissant Pockets*)	370	11.0	36.0	20.0	15	760	3.0
(*Lean Pockets*)	280	13.0	43.0	7.0	30	620	3.0
Chicken salad, ⅓ cup:							
(*Wampler*)	200	9.0	9.0	14.0	30	420	1.0
(*Wampler* Low Fat) ..	90	8.0	9.0	1.5	20	440	0
Chicken salad, freeze-dried, 1 serving:							
almond (*AlpineAire*) ..	210	22.0	10.0	9.0	n.a.	570	2.0
Oriental (*AlpineAire*) .	210	19.0	16.0	8.0	n.a.	580	2.0
Chicken salad kit, w/crackers:							
(*Bumble Bee*):							
2.9-oz can salad ...	140	8.0	10.0	8.0	25	410	0
6 crackers, .6 oz. ..	90	2.0	12.0	4.5	0	180	0
(*Hormel*), 1 pkg.	220	17.0	16.0	9.0	65	710	0
(*Tyson* Salad Kit), 1 pkg.	210	18.0	15.0	9.0	50	640	1.0
Chicken sandwich, see "Chicken pocket/ sandwich"							

Food and Measure	cal.	prot. (gms)	carbo. (gms)	fat (gms)	chol. (mgs)	sod. (mgs)	fiber (gms)
Chicken sauce, see specific listings							
Chicken sauce mix (see also specific listings), dry:							
cheese, three (*Mc-Cormick*), 1 tbsp. . . .	45	1.0	2.0	3.0	10	470	0
Dijon (*McCormick*), 1⅔ tbsp.	40	0	5.0	1.5	0	420	0
Italian (*McCormick*), 2 tsp.	15	0	3.0	0	0	320	0
herb, country (*Mc-Cormick*), 1 tbsp. . . .	40	1.0	4.0	2.0	10	470	0
lemon herb (*Mc-Cormick*), 1 tbsp. . . .	30	0	5.0	0	0	410	0
Parmesan (*McCormick*), 2 tsp.	25	0	3.0	1.0	0	190	0
rice, fried (*McCormick*), 1 tbsp.	35	1.0	6.0	0	0	780	0
and rice dinner (*A Taste of Thai*), ¼ pkg.	15	0	3.0	0	0	740	0
stir fry (*McCormick*), 2 tsp.	20	0	4.0	0	0	520	0
teriyaki (*McCormick*), 1⅓ tbsp.	40	1.0	5.0	1.0	0	520	0
Chicken sausage, see "Sausage"							
Chicken seasoning, ¼ tsp.:							
(*McCormick*)	0	0	0	0	0	130	0
herb (*McCormick*) . . .	0	0	0	0	0	85	0
mesquite (*McCormick*)	0	0	0	0	0	70	0
and poultry (*Lawry's* Perfect Blend)	0	0	0	0	0	125	0
rotisserie (*McCormick*)	0	0	0	0	0	130	0
Chicken seasoning mix, see "Chicken coating mix," "Chicken sauce mix" and specific listings							
Chicken snacks, see "Chicken, frozen and refrigerated, cooked"							

Food and Measure	cal.	prot. (gms)	carbo. (gms)	fat (gms)	chol. (mgs)	sod. (mgs)	fiber (gms)
Chicken spread (*Underwood*), ¼ cup . .	110	8.0	3.0	7.0	30	410	0
Chick-fil-A, 1 serving:							
breakfast:							
bagel, wheat	220	7.0	41.0	3.0	0	350	2.0
bagel w/chicken/ egg/cheese	500	31.0	49.0	20.0	290	1260	3.0
biscuit, buttered . . .	270	4.0	38.0	12.0	0	660	1.0
biscuit w/:							
bacon	330	8.0	38.0	16.0	15	890	1.0
bacon/egg	420	15.0	38.0	22.0	255	960	1.0
bacon/egg/cheese	470	18.0	39.0	26.0	270	1190	1.0
egg	350	11.0	38.0	16.0	240	740	1.0
egg/cheese	400	14.0	38.0	21.0	35	970	1.0
sausage	490	11.0	45.0	29.0	35	780	1.0
sausage/egg	580	18.0	45.0	35.0	275	850	1.0
sausage/egg/ cheese	630	21.0	46.0	40.0	290	1080	1.0
biscuit w/gravy	330	5.0	44.0	15.0	5	930	1.0
Chick-fil-A burrito:							
chicken	420	23.0	39.0	19.0	270	960	2.0
sausage	460	20.0	40.0	24.0	270	750	2.0
Chick-fil-A Chick-N-Minis:							
3 pcs.	270	14.0	28.0	11.0	50	640	1.0
4 pcs.	360	19.0	37.0	15.0	65	860	2.0
Chick-fil-A chicken biscuit	420	18.0	44.0	19.0	35	1270	2.0
Chick-fil-A chicken biscuit w/cheese . . .	470	21.0	45.0	23.0	50	1500	2.0
hash browns	260	2.0	25.0	17.0	5	380	3.0
chicken sandwiches:							
char-grilled	270	28.0	33.0	3.5	65	940	3.0
char-grilled club, no sauce	380	35.0	33.0	11.0	90	1240	3.0
Chick-fil-A	410	28.0	38.0	16.0	60	1300	1.0
no butter	380	28.0	37.0	13.0	60	1290	1.0
chicken salad	350	20.0	32.0	15.0	65	880	5.0
chicken deluxe	420	28.0	39.0	16.0	60	1300	2.0
Cool Wraps:							
char-grilled chicken	390	29.0	54.0	7.0	65	1020	3.0
chicken Caesar	460	36.0	52.0	10.0	80	1350	3.0
spicy chicken	380	30.0	52.0	6.0	60	1090	3.0

Food and Measure	cal.	prot. (gms)	carbo. (gms)	fat (gms)	chol. (mgs)	sod. (mgs)	fiber (gms)
chicken dishes:							
chicken fillet	230	23.0	10.0	11.0	60	990	0
chicken fillet, char-grilled	100	21.0	1.0	1.5	65	610	0
Chick-N-Strips, 4-pack	290	29.0	14.0	13.0	65	730	1.0
Chick-fil-A nuggets, 8-pack	260	26.0	12.0	12.0	70	1090	<1.0
dipping sauce, 1 pkt.:							
barbeque	45	0	11.0	0	0	180	0
Chick-fil-A Buffalo .	15	0	1.0	1.5	0	410	0
honey roasted barbecue	60	0	2.0	0	5	90	0
honey mustard	45	0	10.0	0	0	150	0
ranch, buttermilk . .	110	0	1.0	12.0	5	200	0
Polynesian	110	0	13.0	6.0	0	210	0
sides:							
carrot raisin salad .	170	1.0	28.0	6.0	10	110	2.0
chicken soup, hearty 1 cup	140	8.0	18.0	3.5	25	900	1.0
coleslaw, small	260	2.0	17.0	21.0	25	220	2.0
fruit cup, medium .	60	1.0	16.0	0	0	0	2.0
Waffle Potato Fries .	270	3.0	34.0	13.0	0	115	4.0
salad:							
Chick-N Strips	390	34.0	22.0	18.0	80	860	4.0
garden	180	22.0	9.0	6.0	65	620	3.0
side salad	60	3.0	4.0	3.0	10	75	2.0
Southwest	240	25.0	17.0	8.0	60	770	5.0
salad dressing, 2 tbsp.:							
blue cheese	150	1.0	1.0	16.0	20	300	0
buttermilk ranch . . .	150	1.0	1.0	16.0	5	270	0
Caesar	160	1.0	1.0	17.0	30	240	0
honey mustard, fat free	60	0	14.0	0	0	200	0
Italian, light	15	0	2.0	.5	0	570	0
raspberry vinaigrette	80	0	15.0	2.0	0	190	0
spicy	140	0	2.0	14.0	5	130	0
Thousand Island . .	150	0	5.0	14.0	10	250	0
salad sides, 1 pkt.:							
croutons	50	<1.0	6.0	3.0	0	90	0
sunflower kernels . .	80	2.5	3.0	7.0	0	38	1.0
tortilla strips	70	2.0	9.0	3.5	0	53	1.0
desserts:							
brownie, fudge nut .	330	4.0	45.0	15.0	20	210	2.0

Food and Measure	cal.	prot. (gms)	carbo. (gms)	fat (gms)	chol. (mgs)	sod. (mgs)	fiber (gms)
Chick-fil-A, desserts (cont.)							
cheesecake, slice . .	340	6.0	30.0	21.0	90	270	2.0
IceDream, small cup	240	6.0	41.0	6.0	25	105	0
IceDream, small cone	160	4.0	28.0	4.0	15	80	0
lemon pie, slice . . .	320	7.0	51.0	10.0	110	220	3.0
Chickpeas, see "Garbanzo beans"							
Chicory, witloof:							
(*Frieda's* Endive), 2 cups, 3 oz.	15	1.0	3.0	0	0	20	3.0
5–7" head, 1.9 oz. . . .	9	.5	2.1	.1	0	1	1.6
½ cup	8	.4	1.8	<.1	0	1	1.4
Chicory greens:							
trimmed, 1 oz.	7	.5	1.3	.1	0	13	1.1
chopped, ½ cup	21	1.5	4.2	.3	0	41	3.6
Chicory root:							
1 medium, 2.6 oz. . . .	44	.8	10.5	.1	0	30	n.a.
1" pcs., ½ cup	33	.6	7.9	.1	0	23	n.a.
Chili (see also "Chili starter"), 1 cup, except as noted: w/beans:							
(*Bush's* Original) . .	250	14.0	26.0	10.0	15	1250	7.0
(*Campbell's Chunky* Roadhouse)	220	13.0	25.0	8.0	25	790	7.0
(*Campbell's Chunky* Sizzlin' Steak) . . .	190	15.0	26.0	3.0	20	880	7.0
(*Castleberry's*)	350	14.0	26.0	21.0	45	1090	8.0
(*Hormel*)	270	16.0	34.0	7.0	30	1220	7.0
(*Hormel* Homestyle)	350	16.0	28.0	20.0	45	1060	5.0
(*Hormel* Less Salt) .	270	16.0	34.0	7.0	30	910	7.0
(*Hormel* Meal), 1 cont.	220	15.0	27.0	6.0	30	1050	6.0
(*Hormel/Hormel* Hot), 7.5-oz. can	230	14.0	29.0	6.0	30	1070	6.0
(*Stagg Chunkero*) . .	310	16.0	27.0	17.0	45	820	5.0
(*Stagg Classic*)	330	17.0	28.0	17.0	45	820	5.0
(*Stagg Country*) . . .	330	16.0	30.0	17.0	40	1120	5.0
(*Stagg Fiesta Grill*) .	240	15.0	25.0	9.0	40	850	5.0
(*Stagg Laredo*)	320	18.0	27.0	15.0	45	1150	6.0
(*Stagg Quick Draw*)	270	19.0	28.0	9.0	40	1380	6.0
(*Stagg Ranch House*)	270	17.0	26.0	11.0	50	840	6.0
(*Stagg Rio Blanco*) .	250	17.0	20.0	12.0	60	1000	5.0

Food and Measure	cal.	prot. (gms)	carbo. (gms)	fat (gms)	chol. (mgs)	sod. (mgs)	fiber (gms)
(*Stagg Silverado*) ..	230	18.0	33.0	3.0	45	880	6.0
chunky (*Bush's*) ...	260	15.0	28.0	10.0	15	1250	8.0
chunky (*Hormel*) ..	270	18.0	34.0	7.0	35	1240	7.0
hot (*Bush's*)	250	14.0	26.0	10.0	15	1260	7.0
hot (*Hormel*)	270	16.0	34.0	7.0	30	1220	7.0
hot (*Hormel* Meal), 1 cont.	220	15.0	27.0	6.0	30	1050	6.0
hot (*Stagg Dynamite Hot*)	340	17.0	31.0	17.0	45	870	6.0
hot/spicy (*Hormel*)	270	15.0	33.0	7.0	30	1250	7.0
w/out beans:							
(*Bush's* Original) ..	240	13.0	16.0	14.0	25	1380	3.0
(*Hormel*)	210	16.0	17.0	9.0	40	970	3.0
(*Hormel* Less Salt) .	210	16.0	17.0	9.0	35	710	3.0
(*Hormel* Meal), 1 cont.	190	14.0	15.0	8.0	30	800	2.0
(*Stagg Steak House*)	340	17.0	16.0	22.0	70	1060	2.0
chunky (*Hormel*) ..	210	18.0	22.0	6.0	40	1040	5.0
hot (*Hormel*)	210	16.0	17.0	9.0	40	970	3.0
hot/spicy (*Hormel*)	230	16.0	19.0	10.0	40	1050	3.0
turkey, w/beans:							
(*Campbell's Chunky*)	190	15.0	27.0	2.0	20	880	6.0
(*Health Valley* 99% Fat Free)	220	16.0	34.0	3.0	30	480	8.0
(*Hormel*)	210	17.0	26.0	3.0	45	1200	5.0
(*Stagg Ranchero*) ..	240	21.0	31.0	3.0	35	850	6.0
turkey, w/out beans (*Hormel*)	190	24.0	17.0	3.0	75	1250	3.0
vegetable/vegetarian:							
(*Hormel*)	200	12.0	38.0	1.0	0	780	7.0
(*Morningstar Farms* Vegan)	180	16.0	25.0	1.5	0	900	10.0
(*Stagg Vegetable Garden*)	200	10.0	37.0	1.0	0	870	7.0
(*Worthington*)	280	24.0	25.0	10.0	0	1130	8.0
bean, four (*Walnut Acres*)	140	6.0	28.0	1.5	0	640	4.0
black bean (*Amy's*)	200	11.0	31.0	2.0	0	680	15.0
black bean or 3-bean (*Health Valley* 99% Fat Free)	160	13.0	28.0	1.0	0	320	12.0
burrito flavor (*Health Valley*)	160	14.0	30.0	1.0	0	390	11.0

Food and Measure	cal.	prot. (gms)	carbo. (gms)	fat (gms)	chol. (mgs)	sod. (mgs)	fiber (gms)
Chili, vegetable/vegetarian *(cont.)*							
lentil (*Health Valley*)	160	15.0	28.0	1.0	0	390	11.0
medium, w/vegetables (*Amy's*) ..	190	7.0	29.0	6.0	0	590	8.0
medium or spicy (*Amy's*)	190	8.0	26.0	6.0	0	590	7.0
mild or spicy (*Health Valley*)	160	14.0	30.0	1.0	0	390	11.0
mild or spicy (*Health Valley* No Salt) ..	160	14.0	30.0	1.0	0	65	11.0
Chili, frozen or refrigerated (see also "Chili entree, frozen"), 1 cup:							
(*Organic Classics* Our Favorite)	220	14.0	31.0	5.0	15	450	9.0
(*P.J.'s Beantown*)	350	20.0	32.0	16.0	60	1080	4.0
two-bean vegetable (*Moosewood* Texas)	200	9.0	34.0	4.0	0	840	8.0
Chili, mix, vegetarian:							
(*Fantastic*), ¼ cup ...	100	8.0	17.0	1.0	0	480	4.0
black bean or Texas (*Health Valley* Low Fat), ⅓ cup	120	10.0	21.0	1.0	0	290	6.0
Chili beans (see also "Chili starter" and "Mexican beans"), canned, ½ cup:							
(*Bush's*)	120	6.0	20.0	1.0	0	480	6.0
(*Westbrae Natural* Organic)	100	7.0	19.0	0	0	150	5.0
w/chipotle (*S&W* Santa Fe)	90	7.0	21.0	0	0	570	6.0
w/jalapeño/red pepper (*Eden* Organic)	130	9.0	21.0	0	0	250	7.0
tomato sauce, zesty (*S&W*)	110	7.0	23.0	1.0	0	580	6.0
Chili dip (see also "Salsa"), chunky (*La Victoria*), 2 tbsp.	10	0	2.0	0	0	140	0
Chili entree, freeze-dried, 1 serving:							
(*AlpineAire* Mountain)	300	23.0	48.0	3.0	n.a.	1280	13.0

Food and Measure	cal.	prot. (gms)	carbo. (gms)	fat (gms)	chol. (mgs)	sod. (mgs)	fiber (gms)
(*Instant Gourmet* Hearty Mountain) ..	330	25.0	52.0	3.0	0	1390	14.0
w/beans (*AlpineAire* Black Bart)	330	30.0	41.0	5.0	65	1640	10.0
mac, w/beef:							
(*Mountain House* Can), 1 cup	20	14.0	30.0	3.5	35	840	5.0
(*Mountain House* Double), ½ pouch	290	15.0	40.0	8.0	25	1130	6.0
Chili entree, frozen, 1 pkg., except as noted:							
bean:							
black (*Michelina's* Authentico), 10 oz.	400	13.0	76.0	5.0	0	520	10.0
three (*Lean Cuisine Everyday Favorites*), 10 oz.	260	9.0	40.0	7.0	10	600	8.0
beef and bean, chunky (*Stouffer's* Bowl Cuisine), 11 oz. . . .	330	24.0	32.0	12.0	55	1300	6.0
cheese pie (*Cedarlane Carb Buster* Relleno Pie), 9.5 oz.	520	32.0	9.0	40.0	105	990	1.0
and cornbread (*Amy's* Whole Meal), 10.5 oz.	340	11.0	59.0	6.0	10	680	10.0
mac (*Michelina's* Zap'ems), 8 oz. . . .	280	14.0	37.0	9.0	25	830	3.0
vegetarian (*Yves Veggie*), 10.5 oz. . .	230	21.0	37.0	1.0	0	850	14.0
Chili entree, pkg., 8 oz.:							
mac (*Fantastic Carb 'Tastic*)	290	21.0	19.0	18.0	10	760	14.0
three-bean (*Fantastic Fast Naturals*)	180	1.0	28.0	4.0	0	680	5.0
Chili pepper, see "Pepper, chili"							
Chili pepper paste, see "Thai sauce"							
Chili powder:							
(*McCormick*), ¼ tsp. . .	0	0	0	0	0	20	0
1 tbsp.	24	.9	4.1	1.3	0	76	2.6
1 tsp.	8	.3	1.4	.4	0	26	.9

Food and Measure	cal.	prot. (gms)	carbo. (gms)	fat (gms)	chol. (mgs)	sod. (mgs)	fiber (gms)
Chili relish, hot, Indian (*Patak's* Chile), 1 tbsp.	50	<1.0	0	5.0	0	510	0
Chili sauce, red (*Las Palmas*), ¼ cup ...	20	0	2.0	.5	0	310	1.0
Chili sauce, black bean, see "Black bean sauce"							
Chili sauce, hot, see "Hot sauce" and "Thai sauce"							
Chili sauce, tomato, 1 tbsp.:							
(*Del Monte*)	20	0	5.0	0	0	480	0
(*Heinz*)	20	0	4.0	0	0	230	0
(*Red Gold*)	20	0	5.0	0	0	180	0
(*Texas Pete*)	10	1.0	<1.0	0	0	70	0
Chili seasoning mix, dry:							
(*Adolph's Meal Makers*), 1 tbsp.	30	<1.0	5.0	0	0	270	<1.0
(*Carroll Shelby's* Original Texas Mix), 2 tbsp.	60	2.0	12.0	1.0	0	1320	0
(*D.L. Jardine's* Texas Bag O' Fixins/Chili Works), 3 tbsp. ...	60	2.0	9.0	1.5	0	15	0
(*Ducks Unlimited*), 1⅓ tbsp.	30	1.0	5.0	1.0	0	530	0
(*Lawry's*). 1 tsp.	10	0	2.0	0	0	500	0
(*McCormick*), 1⅓ tbsp.	30	1.0	5.0	.5	0	310	0
hot:							
(*McCormick*), 1⅓ tbsp.	35	1.0	4.0	1.0	0	340	0
(*Wick Fowler's* 2-Alarm Kit), 3 tbsp.	60	2.0	10.0	2.0	0	980	0
mild:							
(*McCormick*), 1⅓ tbsp.	30	1.0	5.0	0	0	400	0
(*Wick Fowler's* False-Alarm Kit), 2 tbsp.	50	2.0	9.0	2.0	0	980	0
Tex-Mex (*McCormick*), 1⅓ tbsp.	35	0	4.0	1.0	0	360	0

Food and Measure	cal.	prot. (gms)	carbo. (gms)	fat (gms)	chol. (mgs)	sod. (mgs)	fiber (gms)
white, chicken (*Mc-Cormick*), 1⅓ tbsp.	30	0	5.0	.5	0	450	0
Chili starter, canned, ½ cup, except as noted:							
(*S&W* Chili Makin's Home Style)	80	7.0	19.0	0	0	630	6.0
(*S&W* Chili Makin's Original)	80	5.0	20.0	.5	0	820	5.0
(*S&W* Chili Makin's Santa Fe)	80	6.0	18.0	0	0	870	5.0
black bean (*S&W* Chili Makin's)	80	6.0	19.0	0	0	750	6.0
Louisiana:							
(*Bush's Chili Magic*)	110	4.0	21.0	1.5	0	1070	5.0
(*Bush's Chili Magic*), 1 cup*	220	22.0	16.0	7.0	60	820	3.0
Texas:							
(*Bush's Chili Magic*)	120	5.0	20.0	2.0	0	1130	5.0
(*Bush's Chili Magic*), 1 cup*	230	22.0	15.0	9.0	55	880	4.0
traditional:							
(*Bush's Chili Magic*)	110	5.0	19.0	1.0	0	890	5.0
(*Bush's Chili Magic*), 1 cup*	220	22.0	15.0	8.0	55	770	3.0
Chili-garlic sauce, Vietnamese (*Huy Fong*), 1 tsp.	0	0	<1.0	0	0	70	0
Chili-ginger sauce, sweet (*The Ginger People*), 2 tbsp. . . .	60	0	15.0	0	0	0	0
Chimichanga, frozen, 1 pc., except as noted:							
bean, taco picante (*El Monterey XX Large!*), ½ of 10-oz. pc. . . .	360	10.0	42.0	16.0	15	670	3.0
beef, shredded (*José Olé*), 5 oz.	380	13.0	42.0	17.0	25	810	2.0
beef/bean:							
(*El Monterey*), 4 oz.	350	8.0	32.0	21.0	15	540	3.0
(*El Monterey* Red Hot XX Large!), 10 oz.	800	21.0	86.0	41.0	40	1400	9.0

Food and Measure	cal.	prot. (gms)	carbo. (gms)	fat (gms)	chol. (mgs)	sod. (mgs)	fiber (gms)
Chimichanga *(cont.)*							
beef/cheese:							
mini (*El Monterey Fiesta Pack*), 3 pcs., 4.5 oz. ..	370	12.0	33.0	21.0	35	530	1.0
shredded (*El Monterey Supreme*), 5 oz.	330	12.0	35.0	15.0	30	350	1.0
chicken (*José Olé*), 5 oz.	380	13.0	42.0	17.0	25	810	2.0
chicken/cheese:							
mini (*El Monterey Fiesta Pack*), 3 pcs., 4.5 oz.	300	11.0	33.0	14.0	20	960	2.0
Monterey Jack (*El Monterey Supreme*), 5 oz. ...	350	12.0	36.0	18.0	25	340	2.0
cream cheese/jalapeño (*El Monterey* Fiesta Minis), 4.5 oz.	370	7.0	32.0	24.0	45	560	1.0
nacho cheese/beef, mini, fried (*El Monterey Cruncheros*), 3 pcs., 4.5 oz.	330	10.0	35.0	16.0	20	560	2.0
Chimichurri sauce, see "Marinade"							
Chipotle oil (*Watkins* Liquid Spice), 1 tsp.	40	0	0	4.5	0	0	0
Chipotle sauce (*La Morena*), 2 tbsp. ..	25	<1.0	6.0	0	0	680	0
Chitterlings, pork, simmered, 4 oz.	344	11.6	0	32.6	162	44	0
Chives:							
fresh:							
1 oz.	9	.9	1.2	.2	0	1	.9
chopped, 1 tbsp. ...	1	.1	.1	<.1	0	<1	.1
freeze-dried:							
¼ cup	2	.2	.5	<.1	0	24	<1.0
1 tbsp.	1	<.1	.1	<.1	0	6	<1.0
Chocolate, see "Candy"							
Chocolate, baking, ½ oz. or 1 tbsp., except as noted:							
(*Nestlé Choco Bake*) ..	80	1.0	4.0	8.0	0	0	2.0

Food and Measure	cal.	prot. (gms)	carbo. (gms)	fat (gms)	chol. (mgs)	sod. (mgs)	fiber (gms)
bars:							
bittersweet (*Baker's*)	70	1.0	7.0	6.0	0	0	1.0
semisweet (*Baker's*)	70	1.0	7.0	6.0	0	0	1.0
semisweet (*Hershey's Bake Shoppe*)	70	<1.0	9.0	4.0	0	0	<1.0
semisweet (*Nestlé Toll House*)	70	<1.0	9.0	4.0	0	0	<1.0
sweet (*German's*)	60	1.0	8.0	3.5	0	0	1.0
unsweetened (*Baker's*)	70	2.0	4.0	7.0	0	0	2.0
unsweetened (*Hershey's Bake Shoppe*)	90	2.0	4.0	7.0	0	0	2.0
unsweetened (*Nestlé Toll House*)	80	2.0	5.0	7.0	0	0	3.0
white (*Baker's Premium*)	80	1.0	8.0	4.5	5	15	0
white (*Nestlé Toll House*)	80	1.0	8.0	5.0	<5	15	0
chips or morsels:							
(*Guittard* Super Cookie Chip)	70	<1.0	9.0	4.5	0	0	1.0
dark (*Hershey's Bake Shoppe Special Dark*)	80	<1.0	9.0	4.5	0	0	<1.0
milk (*Hershey's Bake Shoppe*)	80	1.0	9.0	4.5	<5	10	0
milk (*Hershey's Bake Shoppe Kisses* Unwrapped), 9 pcs., 1.4 oz.	230	3.0	24.0	13.0	10	35	1.0
milk (*Hershey's Bake Shoppe Mini Kisses*), 11 pcs., .5oz.	80	1.0	9.0	4.5	<5	15	0
milk (*M&M's* Mini)	70	1.0	10.0	3.5	5	10	0
milk (*Nestlé Toll House*)	70	<1.0	9.0	4.0	<5	0	0
mint (*Hershey's Bake Shoppe*)	80	<1.0	10.0	4.0	0	30	0
raspberry (*Hershey's Bake Shoppe*)	80	<1.0	10.0	4.0	0	0	0

Food and Measure	cal.	prot. (gms)	carbo. (gms)	fat (gms)	chol. (mgs)	sod. (mgs)	fiber (gms)
Chocolate, baking, chips or morsels *(cont.)*							
semisweet (*Guittard*)	70	<1.0	10.0	4.0	0	10	<1.0
semisweet (*Hershey's Bake Shoppe*)	80	<1.0	10.0	4.5	0	0	<1.0
semisweet (*Hershey's Bake Shoppe Minichips*)	80	1.0	9.0	4.5	<5	15	0
semisweet (*M&M's Mini*)	70	1.0	9.0	3.5	0	0	1.0
semisweet (*Nestlé Toll House*)	70	<1.0	9.0	4.0	0	0	<1.0
vanilla (*Guitard ChocAu-Lait*) ...	80	1.0	9.0	5.0	<5	20	0
white (*Hershey's Bake Shoppe Premier*)	80	1.0	9.0	4.0	0	30	0
white (*Nestlé Toll House*)	70	0	9.0	4.0	0	15	0
chunks:							
(*Nestlé Toll House*)	70	1.0	8.0	4.0	0	0	1.0
milk (*Baker's*)	80	1.0	9.0	5.0	5	25	0
semisweet (*Baker's Real*)	60	1.0	9.0	3.5	0	0	1.0
white (*Baker's*)	80	1.0	9.0	5.0	5	15	0
wafers, 27 pcs., 1.4 oz.:							
dark, bittersweet (*Guittard* Coucher du Soleil)	210	3.0	18.0	17.0	0	0	4.0
dark, semisweet (*Guittard* Lever du Soleil)	200	2.0	21.0	15.0	0	0	3.0
milk (*Guittard* Soleil d'Or)	220	3.0	20.0	15.0	10	35	1.0
white (*Guittard* Creme Francaise)	230	3.0	21.0	15.0	10	40	0
Chocolate dip, see "Fruit dip"							
Chocolate drink:							
(*Yoo-hoo*), 8 fl. oz.	130	2.0	29.0	1.0	0	180	0
(*Yoo-hoo* Lite), 9 fl. oz.	70	2.0	15.0	1.0	0	150	0
fudge, double (*Yoo-hoo*), 8 fl. oz.	140	2.0	33.0	1.0	0	180	0

Food and Measure	cal.	prot. (gms)	carbo. (gms)	fat (gms)	chol. (mgs)	sod. (mgs)	fiber (gms)
Chocolate drink mix (see also "Cocoa mix"), 2 tbsp., except as noted:							
(*Hershey's* Milk Mix), 3 tbsp.	90	0	23.0	0	0	60	<1.0
(*Nesquik*)	90	<1.0	19.0	.5	0	30	1.0
(*Nesquik* No Sugar) . .	40	1.0	7.0	1.0	0	85	1.0
double (*Nesquik*)	90	1.0	17.0	.5	0	80	1.0
Chocolate milk, see "Milk, flavored"							
Chocolate mousse, frozen (*Smart Ones*), 2.7-oz. pc.	180	6.0	24.0	4.0	<5	125	4.0
Chocolate sprinkles (*Hershey's* Triple Dessert), 2 tbsp. . .	90	<1.0	12.0	4.0	0	35	<1.0
Chocolate syrup, 2 tbsp., except as noted:							
(*Fox's U-Bet*)	120	1.0	29.0	0	0	35	0
(*Hershey's*)	100	<1.0	25.0	0	0	25	<1.0
(*Hershey's Lite*)	50	0	12.0	0	0	35	<1.0
(*Nesquik*)	100	0	24.0	0	0	50	<1.0
(*Santa Cruz Organic*) .	120	1.0	22.0	3.5	0	0	2.0
(*Smucker's Sunday Syrup*)	110	1.0	26.0	0	0	20	1.0
dark (*Hershey's Special Dark*)	110	<1.0	26.0	0	0	35	0
double (*Hershey's* Sundae)	100	<1.0	24.0	0	0	20	1.0
malt (*Hershey's Whoppers*)	100	<1.0	25.0	0	0	55	<1.0
Chocolate topping, 2 tbsp.:							
(*Hershey's* Shell)	230	1.0	16.0	18.0	0	15	1.0
(*Smucker's Magic Shell*)	210	1.0	16.0	17.0	0	20	1.0
(*Smuckers Plate-Scapers*)	100	1.0	23.0	1.0	0	20	1.0
crisps (*Krackel* Shell) .	190	<1.0	14.0	14.0	0	25	<1.0
dark (*Smucker's Dove*)	140	<1.0	22.0	5.0	0	80	1.0
fudge:							
(*Smucker's* Micro) .	130	0	28.0	1.5	0	60	1.0

Food and Measure	cal.	prot. (gms)	carbo. (gms)	fat (gms)	chol. (mgs)	sod. (mgs)	fiber (gms)
Chocolate topping, fudge *(cont.)*							
(*Smucker's* Spoonable)	130	0	28.0	1.5	0	60	1.0
(*Smucker's Magic Shell*)	200	1.0	19.0	14.0	0	50	1.0
fudge, hot:							
(*Hershey's* Fat Free)	100	1.0	23.0	0	0	135	1.0
(*Smucker's* Micro)	140	2.0	24.0	4.0	0	60	1.0
(*Smucker's* Special Recipe)	140	2.0	22.0	4.0	0	70	<1.0
(*Smucker's* Spoonable)	140	2.0	24.0	4.0	0	60	1.0
(*Smucker's* Spoonable Light)	90	2.0	23.0	0	0	90	2.0
(*Smucker's* Spoonable Sugar Free)	90	1.0	23.0	0	0	30	1.0
milk (*Smucker's Dove*)	130	2.0	21.0	4.0	0	75	1.0
mocha (*Smucker's* Spoonable)	110	1.0	28.0	0	0	100	<1.0
Chocolate-raspberry spread (*Cedar's* Meditarranean), 2 tbsp.	80	1.0	10.0	3.5	0	15	1.0
Chorizo:							
(*Fiorucci* Cantimpalo), 1 oz.	110	5.0	1.0	10.0	25	490	0
pork, spicy (*Battisoni*), 1 oz.	80	4.0	0	7.0	20	180	0
pork and beef, 2-oz. link	255	13.5	1.0	21.4	49	692	0
Chorizo, vegetarian (*Soyrizo*), 4 tbsp., 1.9 oz.	120	7.0	5.0	9.0	0	440	12.0
Chow chow pickle:							
(*Crosse & Blackwell*), 1 tbsp.	10	0	1.0	0	0	105	<1.0
sweet, w/cauliflower, ¼ cup	74	.9	16.5	.5	0	321	.9
Chrysanthemum garland, 1" pcs.:							
raw, ½ cup	2	.2	.5	<.1	0	7	.4
boiled, drained, ½ cup	10	.8	2.2	.1	0	27	1.2
Chubs, smoked, see "Whitefish, smoked"							

Food and Measure	cal.	prot. (gms)	carbo. (gms)	fat (gms)	chol. (mgs)	sod. (mgs)	fiber (gms)
Church's Chicken:							
chicken, 1 pc.:							
breast	200	19.0	4.0	12.0	65	510	0
leg	140	13.0	2.0	9.0	45	160	0
thigh	230	16.0	5.0	16.0	80	520	0
wing	250	19.0	8.0	16.0	60	540	0
chicken, batter and skin removed, 1 pc.:							
breast	145	21.0	1.0	5.5	60	480	0
leg	118	14.0	1.3	6.2	40	145	0
thigh	180	17.0	3.0	11.0	70	470	0
wing	160	20.5	2.0	7.5	56	475	0
Crunchy Tenders, 1 pc.	137	11.0	11.0	5.0	25	431	.4
Tender Crunchers, 6-8 pcs.	411	34.0	32.0	15.0	64	1294	1.0
sauces, 1 pkt.:							
barbecue	29	0	7.0	0	0	181	0
honey mustard :	111	0	4.0	11.0	10	130	0
jalapeño, creamy . .	102	0	1.0	11.0	10	137	0
Purple Pepper Sauce	46	0	12.0	0	0	26	0
sweet and sour . . .	31	0	8.0	0	0	116	0
sides, regular:							
coleslaw	92	4.0	8.0	6.0	0	230	2.0
collard greens	25	2.0	5.0	0	0	170	2.0
corn on cob	139	4.0	24.0	3.0	0	15	9.0
corn nuggets	250	3.0	30.0	12.0	0	530	2.0
fries	210	3.0	29.0	11.0	0	60	2.0
Honey Butter Biscuit	250	2.0	26.0	16.0	<5	640	1.0
Jalapeño Cheese Bombers, 4 pcs. .	240	8.0	29.0	10.0	28	968	3.0
jalapeños, 2 whole .	10	0	2.0	0	0	390	1.0
macaroni and cheese	210	8.0	23.0	11.0	15	690	1.0
mashed potato/gravy	90	1.0	14.0	3.0	0	520	1.0
okra, fried	210	3.0	19.0	16.0	0	520	4.0
rice, Cajun	130	1.0	16.0	7.0	5	260	<1.0
dessert pie:							
apple	280	2.0	41.0	12.0	<5	340	1.0
lemon, double	300	5.0	39.0	14.0	25	160	0
strawberry cream cheese	280	4.0	32.0	15.0	15	130	2.0
Churro, cinnamon:							
(*Bearitos*), ½ cup	150	1.0	20.0	7.0	0	<1	0
waffle sticks, crispy (*Tio Pepe's Churros*), 1-oz. pc.	110	1.0	14.0	5.0	15	100	2.0

Food and Measure	cal.	prot. (gms)	carbo. (gms)	fat (gms)	chol. (mgs)	sod. (mgs)	fiber (gms)
Chutney, 1 tbsp., except as noted: (*Trader Vic's* Calcutta), 2 tbsp.	44	.5	11.0	0	0	270	0
ginger pineapple (*Neera's*)	31	0	7.0	0	0	54	0
mango: (*Bombay Brand* Major Grey's), 2 tbsp.	110	0	25.0	0	0	210	0
(*Crosse & Blackwell* Major Grey's) ...	60	0	14.0	0	0	170	0
(*Neera's*) ...:....	20	0	5.0	0	0	26	0
(*Patak's*)	50	<1.0	12.0	.5	0	240	0
ginger (*Bombay Brand*), 2 tbsp. .	90	0	23.0	0	0	25	1.0
ginger (*Patak's* Major Grey)	50	0	12.0	.5	0	90	0
hot (*Crosse & Blackwell*)	60	0	14.0	0	0	170	0
hot (*Patak's*)	60	0	12.0	.5	0	70	0
lime (*Patak's*)	50	0	12.0	0	0	240	0
sweet, mild (*Patak's*)	60	0	13.0	0	0	70	0
peach (*Neera's*)	22	0	6.0	0	0	30	0
pear cardamom (*Neera's*)	30	0	7.0	0	0	23	1.0
tomato (*Neera's*)	30	1.0	5.0	2.0	0	54	1.0
vegetable, hot (*Neera's*)	21	0	2.0	2.0	0	43	0
Cilantro, see "Coriander"							
Cinnamon, ground, 1 tsp.	6	.1	2.1	.1	0	1	1.4
Cinnamon baking chips (*Hershey's Bake Shoppe*), 1 tbsp.	80	1.0	9.0	4.0	0	35	0
Cinnamon raisin spread (*Cedar's* Meditarranean), 2 tbsp.	60	1.0	8.0	2.5	0	5	2.0
Cinnamon sugar (*Mc-Cormick*), ¼ tsp. ...	15	0	3.0	0	0	0	0
Cisco, meat only: raw, 4 oz.	112	21.5	0	2.2	57	62	0

Food and Measure	cal.	prot. (gms)	carbo. (gms)	fat (gms)	chol. (mgs)	sod. (mgs)	fiber (gms)
smoked, 4 oz.	201	18.6	0	13.5	36	545	0
Citron, candied, diced (*Seneca* Glacé), 2 tbsp.	70	0	18.0	0	0	25	<1.0
Citronella root, see "Lemongrass"							
Citrus drink blend, 8 fl. oz., except as noted:							
(*AriZona Extreme Energy Shot*), 8.3-oz. can	130	0	34.0	0	0	25	0
(*Five Alive*)	120	0	30.0	0	0	15	0
(*V8 Splash*)	110	0	28.0	0	0	45	0
frozen* (*Five Alive*) . .	110	0	29.0	0	0	0	0
frozen*	114	.7	28.5	0	0	7	0
punch (*Minute Maid*) .	120	0	32.0	0	0	15	0
tropical (*Minute Maid*), 12-fl.-oz. bottle . . .	160	0	44.0	0	0	120	0
Citrus fruit salad, see "Fruit, mixed, can or jar"							
Clam, meat only:							
raw:							
4 oz.	84	14.5	2.9	1.1	39	64	0
9 large or 20 small, 6.3 oz.	133	23.0	4.6	1.8	60	100	0
boiled, poached or steamed, 4 oz.	168	29.0	5.8	2.2	76	127	0
Clam, canned, 2 oz. or ¼ cup, except as noted:							
baby, whole:							
(*Brunswick*)	50	8.0	0	1.0	25	360	0
(*Bumble Bee/ Orleans*)	50	9.0	2.0	1.0	40	270	0
(*Yankee Clipper*) . .	50	9.0	2.0	1.0	50	250	0
boiled (*Crown Prince*), ⅓ cup . .	50	8.0	1.0	1.0	25	70	0
chopped or minced:							
(*Bumble Bee/ Orleans*)	25	4.0	2.0	0	10	320	0
(*Yankee Clipper*) . .	30	5.0	3.0	0	20	280	0
arctic (*Chincoteague*)	15	2.0	1.0	0	5	240	0

Food and Measure	cal.	prot. (gms)	carbo. (gms)	fat (gms)	chol. (mgs)	sod. (mgs)	fiber (gms)
Clam, canned, chopped or minced *(cont.)*							
ocean (*Chincoteague*)	30	6.0	1.0	0	10	290	0
sea (*Chincoteague*)	25	6.0	0	0	15	260	0
Clam, smoked, canned, in oil, drained:							
(*Bumble Bee/Orleans*), 2 oz.	130	11.0	1.0	9.0	40	460	0
baby (*Yankee Clipper*), 1 can drained, 2.3 oz.	140	14.0	2.0	1.5	45	330	2.0
Clam chowder, see "Soup"							
Clam dip (*Cabot*), 2 tbsp.	50	1.0	1.0	5.0	15	120	0
Clam dish, frozen:							
fried, breaded (*Mrs. Paul's*), 18 pcs., 3 oz.	230	9.0	26.0	12.0	20	560	1.0
stuffed, in shell, 2 pcs.:							
casino (*Matlaw's*), 1.3 oz.	60	3.0	7.0	3.0	0	230	<1.0
oreganata (*Matlaw's*), 1.2 oz.	80	3.0	6.0	5.0	0	125	0
New England style (*Matlaw's*), 3.1 oz.	180	8.0	20.0	8.0	0	640	2.0
Clam juice:							
(*Orleans*), 1 tbsp.	0	1.0	0	0	0	100	0
(*Yankee Clipper*), 1 tbsp.	0	0	0	0	0	100	0
ocean (*Chincoteague*), ½ cup	10	2.0	1.0	0	0	1490	0
sea (*Chincoteague*), ½ cup	15	1.0	0	0	0	590	0
and tomato, see "Tomato-clam drink"							
Clam sauce, canned:							
red, ½ cup:							
(*Chincoteague*) ...	100	5.0	8.0	5.0	10	550	<1.0
(*Progresso*)	60	4.0	8.0	1.0	10	350	1.0
(*Snow's*)	70	4.0	6.0	3.0	10	530	0
white, ½ cup:							
(*Chincoteague*) ...	120	4.0	9.0	8.0	10	490	0
(*Progresso*)	140	7.0	5.0	10.0	15	510	0

Food and Measure	cal.	prot. (gms)	carbo. (gms)	fat (gms)	chol. (mgs)	sod. (mgs)	fiber (gms)
(*Snow's*)	90	6.0	4.0	6.0	15	720	0
creamy (*Progresso*)	110	5.0	8.0	6.0	10	440	0
Clover sprouts							
(*Jonathan's*), 1 cup	25	3.0	3.0	.5	0	5	2.0
Cloves, ground:							
1 tbsp.	21	.4	4.0	1.3	0	16	<1.0
1 tsp.	7	.1	1.3	.4	0	5	.2
Cobbler, frozen:							
apple:							
(*Sara Lee* Anytime),							
½ of 8-oz. pkg. .	350	3.0	47.0	17.0	10	240	1.0
w/raisins (*Jeff*							
Nathan Creations),							
½ of 8.5-oz. pkg.	310	3.0	47.0	13.0	0	25	2.0
blackberry (*Sara Lee*							
Anytime), ½ of							
8-oz. pkg.	350	3.0	48.0	17.0	5	240	2.0
peach:							
(*Mrs. Smith's*), ⅛ of							
32-oz. pkg.	230	3.0	34.0	10.0	0	230	1.0
(*Sara Lee* Anytime),							
½ of 8-oz. pkg. .	340	3.0	43.0	17.0	5	240	1.0
Cocktail mixers, see							
specific listings							
Cocktail sauce, see							
"Seafood sauce"							
Cocoa, 1 tbsp.:							
(*Shiloh Farms*)	15	0	2.0	1.0	0	0	1.0
Dutch or unsweetened							
(*Hershey's*)	20	1.0	3.0	.5	0	0	1.0
Cocoa mix, 1 pkt.,							
except as noted:							
(*Hershey's Goodnight*							
Hugs)	150	3.0	27.0	3.5	<5	180	0
(*Hershey's Goodnight*							
Kisses)	150	3.0	28.0	3.0	<5	150	<1.0
chocolate:							
Dutch (*Hershey's*) .	220	2.0	28.0	7.0	0	260	2.0
raspberry (*Hershey's*)	140	2.0	29.0	2.0	0	200	<1.0
rich (*Hershey's*) . . .	110	1.0	23.0	2.0	0	140	1.0
rich, w/marsh-							
mallows							
(*Hershey's*)	110	1.0	23.0	2.0	0	130	1.0

Food and Measure	cal.	prot. (gms)	carbo. (gms)	fat (gms)	chol. (mgs)	sod. (mgs)	fiber (gms)
Cocoa mix, chocolate *(cont.)*							
Royal or Irish mint (*Country Choice Naturals*), 1 oz.	100	3.0	23.0	0	0	160	<1.0
Royal or Irish mint (*Country Choice Naturals* Soy), 1 oz.	100	2.0	23.0	1.0	0	130	1.0
vanilla, French (*Hershey's*)	140	4.0	28.0	1.5	<5	135	0
Cocoa-coffee mix (*Trader Vic's Kafe-La-Te*), 2 rounded tsp., ½ oz.	50	0	13.0	0	0	30	0
Coconut, fresh, shelled:							
(*Frieda's* White/Young), ¼ cup, 1.4 oz.	140	1.0	6.0	13.0	0	10	4.0
1 oz.	100	.9	4.3	9.5	0	6	2.6
shredded or grated, 1 cup not packed	283	2.7	12.2	26.8	0	16	7.2
Coconut, cream of:							
(*Goya* Coco Cream of Coconut), 2 tbsp.	140	0	22.0	5.0	0	15	0
(*Vigo*), 2 tbsp.	110	0	17.0	10.0	0	15	0
1 tbsp.	36	.5	1.6	3.4	0	10	.4
Coconut, dried:							
flaked, sweetened:							
(*Baker's Angel Flake*), 2 tbsp.	70	1.0	6.0	5.0	0	40	1.0
(*Mounds*), 2 tbsp.	70	<1.0	6.0	4.5	0	35	1.0
⅓ cup	117	.8	11.8	7.9	0	63	1.1
shredded:							
(*Shiloh Farms*), 3 tbsp.	100	1.0	4.0	9.0	0	5	2.0
(*Tree of Life/Tree of Life* Macaroon), 1 oz.	180	2.0	7.0	18.0	0	10	5.0
toasted, 1 oz.	168	1.5	12.6	13.4	0	11	1.0
Coconut juice drink (*Foco*), 11.8-fl.-oz. can	120	0	29.0	1.0	0	130	1.0
Coconut milk:							
(*Goya*), 1 tbsp.	50	1.0	1.0	5.0	0	5	0

Food and Measure	cal.	prot. (gms)	carbo. (gms)	fat (gms)	chol. (mgs)	sod. (mgs)	fiber (gms)
(*Port Arthur* Lite), ¼ cup	35	<1.0	2.0	4.0	0	10	0
(*A Taste of Thai*), ⅓ cup	140	1.0	3.0	15.0	0	20	0
(*A Taste of Thai* Lite), ⅓ cup	45	1.0	3.0	4.0	0	20	0
(*Thai Kitchen*), ¼ cup	115	1.0	4.0	10.0	0	31	0
(*Thai Kitchen* Lite), ¼ cup	45	0	1.0	4.0	0	12	0
Coconut nectar (*R.W. Knudsen*), 8 fl. oz.	140	1.0	26.0	5.0	0	55	2.0
Coconut water (*Goya*), 12 fl. oz.	150	2.0	31.0	2.5	0	85	n.a.
Cod, meat only:							
Atlantic, 4 oz.:							
raw	93	20.2	0	.8	49	62	0
baked, broiled, or microwaved	119	25.9	0	1.0	62	88	0
Pacific, 4 oz.:							
raw	93	20.3	0	.7	42	81	0
baked, broiled, or microwaved	119	26.0	0	.9	53	103	0
Cod, canned:							
Atlantic, w/liquid, 4 oz.	119	25.8	0	1.0	62	247	0
in Biscayan sauce (*Goya*), ¼ cup	100	7.0	1.0	8.0	30	450	0
Cod, dried, Atlantic, salted, 1 oz.	81	17.6	0	.7	42	1968	0
Cod entree, frozen, 5-oz. pc.:							
au gratin (*Oven Poppers*)	220	24.0	5.0	11.0	75	450	1.0
stuffed w/broccoli and cheese (*Oven Poppers*)	150	20.0	4.0	6.0	55	330	1.0
Cod liver oil, see "Oil"							
Coffee:							
brewed, 6 fl. oz.	4	.1	.8	0	0	4	0
instant, regular, 1 rounded tsp.	4	.2	.7	tr.	0	1	0
Coffee, flavored, mix (*General Foods International Coffees*), 1⅓ tbsp.:							
café Vienna	70	<1.0	12.0	2.5	0	110	0

Food and Measure	cal.	prot. (gms)	carbo. (gms)	fat (gms)	chol. (mgs)	sod. (mgs)	fiber (gms)
Coffee, flavored, mix *(cont.)*							
cappuccino, Italian ...	60	<1.0	10.0	2.0	0	50	0
chocolate, white, Swiss	70	1.0	12.0	3.0	0	30	0
chocolate café,							
Viennese	50	1.0	10.0	1.5	0	30	0
crème caramel	70	0	12.0	2.0	0	55	0
hazelnut Belgian café .	70	<1.0	12.0	2.0	0	60	0
Suisse mocha	60	0	10.0	2.0	0	40	0
vanilla or vanilla nut,							
French	60	0	10.0	2.5	0	55	0
Coffee, iced, cappuc-cino, 10.5 fl. oz.:							
(*AriZona* Shake Double Roast/Rich							
Cholocaty)	180	4.0	36.0	3.5	9	150	.5
(*AriZona Kahlúa*)	130	5.0	24.0	2.0	7	130	.5
Coffee, iced, mix (*General Foods International Coffees Cappuccino Coolers*), 1 pkt.:							
chocolate	60	0	16.0	0	0	0	1.0
vanilla, French	60	0	15.0	0	0	0	0
Coffee creamer, see "Creamer"							
Coffee liqueur, 1 fl. oz.:							
53 proof	117	<.1	16.3	.1	0	3	0
w/cream, 34 proof ...	102	.9	6.5	4.9	0	29	0
Coffee substitute, cereal grain (*Postum*),							
1 tsp.	10	0	3.0	0	0	0	0
Cold cuts, see "Lunch meat" and specific listings							
Coleslaw, refrigerated:							
(*Blue Ridge Farm*),							
4 oz.	200	1.0	19.0	14.0	10	120	2.0
(*Reser's* Homestyle),							
½ cup	150	1.0	19.0	8.0	5	230	2.0
Coleslaw blend, see "Salad blend" and "Salad kit"							
Coleslaw dressing, see "Salad dressing"							

Food and Measure	cal.	prot. (gms)	carbo. (gms)	fat (gms)	chol. (mgs)	sod. (mgs)	fiber (gms)
Coleslaw seasoning:							
(*Produce Partners*							
Super Slaw), 1 tsp.	10	0	2.0	0	0	340	0
(*Watkins*), ½ tsp.	5	0	1.0	0	0	190	0
Collard greens, fresh:							
raw:							
(*Glory*), 2 cups	25	2.0	5.0	0	0	15	3.0
chopped (*Del Monte*),							
2 cups	25	1.0	5.0	0	0	30	1.0
chopped, ½ cup	6	.3	1.3	<.1	0	4	.7
trimmed, 1 oz.	9	.4	2.0	.1	0	6	1.0
boiled, drained,							
chopped, ½ cup	17	.9	3.9	.1	0	10	1.3
Collard greens,							
canned, ½ cup:							
(*Allens* No Salt)	30	1.0	5.0	.5	0	20	3.0
(*Bush's*)	30	2.0	4.0	0	0	410	2.0
seasoned:							
(*Allens/Sunshine*)	35	3.0	5.0	.5	0	830	1.0
Southern (*Glory*)	50	3.0	7.0	1.0	0	470	3.0
turkey flavor (*Glory*)	40	4.0	6.0	.5	0	510	2.0
Collard greens,							
frozen, chopped,							
½ cup:							
(*Seabrook Farms*)	30	2.0	2.0	0	0	20	2.0
boiled, drained	31	2.5	6.1	.4	0	42	n.a.
seasoned (*Glory*							
Savory Accents)	60	2.0	10.0	0	0	630	2.0
Conch, baked or							
broiled, 4 oz.	147	29.8	1.9	1.4	74	174	0
Cookie (see also "Cake,							
snack" and specific							
listings):							
(*Gamesa Marias*),							
8 pcs., 1 oz.	120	2.0	24.0	1.5	0	160	<1.0
(*Stella D'oro* Breakfast							
Treats), .8 oz.	90	1.0	15.0	3.0	15	70	0
(*Stella D'oro* Breakfast							
Treats Mini), 1 oz.	120	2.0	21.0	3.5	0	95	0
(*Stella D'oro* Angel							
Wings), 2 pcs.,							
1.1 oz.	170	2.0	14.0	12.0	0	105	0
(*Stella D'oro* Anginetti),							
4 pcs., 1.1 oz.	130	2.0	22.0	3.5	30	10	0

Food and Measure	cal.	prot. (gms)	carbo. (gms)	fat (gms)	chol. (mgs)	sod. (mgs)	fiber (gms)
Cookie *(cont.)*							
(Stella D'oro Marghe-							
rite), 2 pcs., 1 oz. . .	130	2.0	20.0	4.5	20	85	0
all varieties, except							
oatmeal raisin							
(*Health Valley* Fat							
Free), 3 pcs., 1.2 oz.	100	2.0	24.0	0	0	90	3.0
almond:							
(*Frieda's*), 2 pcs.,							
1 oz.	170	2.0	19.0	10.0	0	75	0
(*Stella D'oro* Delight),							
1.1 oz.	160	2.0	18.0	8.0	10	85	1.0
(*Stella D'oro* Toast),							
2 pcs., 1 oz.	110	2.0	19.0	2.5	25	85	1.0
butter, toasted (*Tree*							
of Life Fat Free),							
.8-oz. pc.	70	2.0	16.0	0	0	35	1.0
animal:							
(*Animalitos*), 14 pcs.,							
1.1 oz.	110	2.0	25.0	.5	0	160	<1.0
(*Austin* Zoo), 16 pcs.,							
1.1 oz.	130	2.0	25.0	2.0	0	90	<1.0
chocolate chip							
(*Barbara's Snack-*							
imals), 10 pcs.,							
1.1 oz.	120	1.0	19.0	4.0	0	75	0
frosted (*Keebler*),							
8 pcs., 1.1 oz. . .	150	1.0	21.0	7.0	0	75	0
iced (*Keebler*), 6 pcs.,							
1.1 oz.	140	2.0	23.0	5.0	0	100	<1.0
oatmeal (*Barbara's*							
Snackimals),							
10 pcs., 1.1 oz. .	110	1.0	18.0	4.0	0	90	1.0
vanilla (*Barbara's*),							
8 pcs., 1.1 oz. . .	120	2.0	18.0	4.5	0	85	<1.0
vanilla (*Barbara's*							
Snackimals),							
10 pcs., 1.1 oz. .	110	2.0	17.0	4.0	0	50	0
apricot raspberry							
(*Pepperidge Farm*							
Verona), 3 pcs.,							
.9 oz.	140	2.0	22.0	6.0	5	110	<1.0
anisette:							
(*Stella D'oro* Sponge),							
2 pcs., .9 oz.	90	2.0	18.0	1.0	40	75	0

Food and Measure	cal.	prot. (gms)	carbo. (gms)	fat (gms)	chol. (mgs)	sod. (mgs)	fiber (gms)
(*Stella D'oro* Toast), 3 pcs., 1.2 oz.	130	2.0	27.0	1.0	35	105	0
mini (*Stella D'oro* Toast), 1.2 oz.	130	2.0	27.0	1.0	30	105	0
arrowroot (*Nabisco*), .2-oz. pc.	20	0	4.0	.5	0	15	0
assortment (*Stella D'oro Lady Stella*), 1 oz.	130	1.0	20.0	4.5	5	55	1.0
banana walnut (*Stella D'oro* Toast), 2 pcs., .9 oz.	100	2.0	19.0	2.0	30	90	0
biscotti:							
(*Nonnis* Original), 1-oz. pc.	100	2.0	15.0	4.0	25	65	1.0
almond (*Stella D'oro*), .7-oz. pc.	100	2.0	13.0	4.5	5	45	1.0
amaretto or chocolate (*Health Valley*), 2 pcs., 1.1 oz.	120	3.0	23.0	3.0	0	50	3.0
chocolate, chocolate dipped (*Nonnis* Decadence), 1.2-oz. pc.	130	2.0	19.0	5.0	25	65	1.0
chocolate almond (*Stella D'oro*), .7-oz. pc.	90	2.0	13.0	4.0	5	40	1.0
chocolate chunk (*Stella D'oro*), .7-oz. pc.	90	1.0	14.0	4.0	5	35	0
vanilla, French (*Stella D'oro*), .7-oz. pc.	90	1.0	15.0	3.5	10	55	0
blueberry (*Stella D'oro* Toast), 2 pcs., .9 oz.	100	2.0	20.0	1.0	30	95	0
brownie, fudge:							
(*SnackWell's*), .8 oz.	90	1.0	17.0	3.5	0	130	0
double (*Country Choice*), .8-oz. pc.	90	1.0	16.0	3.0	5	85	<1.0
butter:							
(*Pepperidge Farm Chessmen*), 3 pcs., .9 oz.	120	2.0	18.0	5.0	20	80	<1.0

Food and Measure	cal.	prot. (gms)	carbo. (gms)	fat (gms)	chol. (mgs)	sod. (mgs)	fiber (gms)
Cookie, butter *(cont.)*							
(*Pepperidge Farm Chessmen* Mini), 9 pcs., 1 oz.	140	2.0	21.0	6.0	25	95	<1.0
Danish, 4 pcs., 1.1 oz.	160	2.0	19.0	8.0	20	80	1.0
butter pecan (*Pepperidge Farm Chessmen*), 3 pcs., .9 oz.	130	1.0	18.0	6.0	10	120	<1.0
caramel apple bar (*Newtons*), 2 pcs., 1.3 oz.	130	1.0	26.0	2.5	0	85	0
carob:							
(*Tree of Life* Wheat Free California), .8-oz. pc.	110	1.0	14.0	5.0	0	75	6.0
chip (*Tree of Life* Monster), 1/5 pc.	140	2.0	19.0	7.0	2	75	1.0
carrot cake:							
(*Tree of Life* Fat Free), .8-oz. pc.	60	1.0	13.0	0	0	50	1.0
(*Tree of Life* Monster Fat Free), ¼ pc. . .	90	2.0	20.0	0	0	40	2.0
cherries and cheese-cake bar (*Newtons*), 2 pcs., 1.3 oz.	120	1.0	25.0	2.5	0	125	0
chocolate:							
(*Stella D'oro* Breakfast Treats), .8-oz. pc.	90	1.0	15.0	3.0	15	55	1.0
almond (*Hershey's*), 2 pcs., 1 oz.	150	2.0	16.0	9.0	<5	65	<1.0
double Dutch (*Barbara's*), .6-oz. pc.	80	1.0	9.0	4.0	5	45	<1.0
top (*Carr's Imperials*), 2 pcs., 1 oz.	140	2.0	18.0	7.0	<5	50	1.0
top (*Pepperidge Farm Geneva*), 3 pcs., 1.1 oz. . .	160	2.0	19.0	9.0	0	95	1.0
top, dark (*Carr's Imperials*), 2 pcs., 1 oz.	150	2.0	19.0	7.0	0	40	2.0

Food and Measure	cal.	prot. (gms)	carbo. (gms)	fat (gms)	chol. (mgs)	sod. (mgs)	fiber (gms)
wafer (*Famous*),							
5 pcs., 1.1 oz. . .	140	2.0	24.0	4.0	5	230	1.0
chocolate chip/chunk:							
(*Barbara's*), .6-oz. pc.	80	1.0	9.0	4.0	5	40	<1.0
(*Chips Ahoy!*),							
3 pcs., 1.1 oz. . .	160	2.0	21.0	8.0	0	105	1.0
(*Chips Ahoy!* Candy							
Blasts), .5-oz. pc.	80	1.0	10.0	4.0	0	50	0
(*Chips Ahoy!* Chewy),							
.9-oz. pc.	120	1.0	17.0	5.0	0	100	1.0
(*Chips Ahoy!* Chewy							
Real), .9-oz. pc. .	120	1.0	17.0	6.0	0	80	1.0
(*Chips Ahoy!* Mini),							
5 pcs., 1.1 oz. . .	150	2.0	21.0	8.0	0	100	1.0
(*Chips Ahoy!* Mini							
Bite-Size Go-Pack),							
1.1 oz.	150	2.0	20.0	7.0	0	105	1.0
(*Chips Ahoy!* Re-							
duced Fat), 3 pcs.,							
1.1 oz.	140	2.0	22.0	5.0	0	140	1.0
(*Famous Amos*),							
4 pcs., 1 oz.	150	2.0	20.0	7.0	<5	100	<1.0
(*Grandma's* Home-							
style), 1.4-oz. pc.	200	2.0	28.0	9.0	15	125	1.0
(*Grandma's* Mini							
Bites), 1 pkg. . . .	210	2.0	29.0	9.0	10	150	1.0
(*Grandma's* Rich 'n							
Chewy), 1 pkg. . .	270	2.0	39.0	12.0	10	130	1.0
(*Health Valley* Chunk),							
.9-oz. pc.	120	1.0	15.0	7.0	10	150	1.0
(*Health Valley* Mini),							
4 pcs., 1 oz.	120	1.0	16.0	6.0	5	125	1.0
(*Health Valley Café*							
Creations),							
.8-oz. pc.	100	1.0	13.0	5.0	5	50	2.0
(*Keebler Chips*							
Deluxe Chocolate							
Lovers), .6-oz. pc.	80	1.0	10.0	4.5	<5	65	0
(*Keebler Chips*							
Deluxe Soft &							
Chewy), .6-oz. pc.	70	1.0	10.0	3.0	0	35	0
(*Keebler Soft Batch*),							
.6-oz. pc.	80	<1.0	10.0	3.5	0	70	<1.0

Food and Measure	cal.	prot. (gms)	carbo. (gms)	fat (gms)	chol. (mgs)	sod. (mgs)	fiber (gms)
Cookie, chocolate chip/chunk *(cont.)*							
(*Murray* Sugar Free), 3 pcs., 1.1 oz. . .	150	2.0	20.0	8.0	<5	135	<1.0
(*SnackWell's*), 13 pcs., 1 oz. . . .	130	2.0	22.0	4.0	0	160	1.0
(*Tofutti*), 1.1-oz. pc.	139	2.0	19.0	6.0	0	79	0
almond (*Pepperidge Farm Sanibel*), .9-oz. pc.	140	2.0	16.0	8.0	5	85	<1.0
caramel (*Pepperidge Farm Soft*), 1-oz. pc.	140	1.0	21.0	6.0	5	75	<1.0
chocolate (*Health Valley* Mini), 4 pcs., 1 oz.	130	1.0	16.0	7.0	5	110	1.0
chocolate (*Health Valley Café Creations*), .8-oz. pc. .	100	1.0	13.0	5.0	5	50	2.0
coconut (*Keebler Chips Deluxe Tropical Coconut*), .5-oz. pc.	80	<1.0	9.0	4.5	0	40	0
dark chocolate (*Pepperidge Farm Soft*), 1.1-oz. pc.	150	2.0	20.0	8.0	10	95	0
double (*Health Valley* Chunk), .9-oz. pc.	120	1.0	15.0	7.0	5	140	1.0
double (*Pepperidge Farm Nantucket*), .9-oz. pc.	140	2.0	18.0	7.0	10	80	1.0
fudge (*Grandma's* Homestyle), 1.4-oz. pc.	190	2.0	28.0	7.0	10	80	1.0
macadamia (*Mauna Loa*), 2 pcs., .9 oz.	130	2.0	18.0	6.0	5	55	1.0
macadamia (*Pepperidge Farm Sausalito*), .9-oz. pc.	140	2.0	16.0	8.0	10	80	0
macadamia (*Pepperidge Farm Sausalito* Mini), 4 pcs., 1 oz.	150	2.0	17.0	8.0	10	90	0

Food and Measure	cal.	prot. (gms)	carbo. (gms)	fat (gms)	chol. (mgs)	sod. (mgs)	fiber (gms)
oatmeal (*Country Choice*), .8-oz. pc.	100	2.0	15.0	4.0	5	70	1.0
oatmeal (*Health Valley*), .8-oz. pc.	100	2.0	14.0	4.0	0	50	1.0
oatmeal and walnuts (*Famous Amos*), 4 pcs., 1 oz.	150	2.0	19.0	7.0	<5	105	1.0
pecan (*Famous Amos*), 4 pcs., 1 oz.	150	2.0	19.0	8.0	0	85	<1.0
pecan (*Murray Sugar Free*), 3 pcs., 1.1 oz. ..	160	2.0	19.0	10.0	<5	135	<1.0
pecan (*Pepperidge Farm Chesapeake*), .9-oz. pc.	140	2.0	15.0	8.0	10	80	0
powdered sugar (*Keebler* Danish Wedding), 4 pcs., .9 oz.	130	1.0	18.0	6.0	0	70	<1.0
rainbow (*Keebler Chips Deluxe*), .6-oz. pc.	80	0	10.0	4.0	0	50	<1.0
rainbow, mini (*Keebler Chips Deluxe*), 4 pcs., 1.1 oz.	150	2.0	20.0	8.0	0	70	0
toffee pecan (*Pepperidge Farm Sedona*), .9-oz. pc.	130	1.0	17.0	7.0	5	100	1.0
walnut (*Country Choice*), .8-oz. pc.	100	1.0	16.0	4.0	5	65	<1.0
wheat free (*Foods by George*), 3.25-oz. pc.	380	4.0	57.0	16.0	75	135	2.0
white chocolate (*Health Valley* Chunk), .9-oz. pc.	140	1.0	17.0	7.0	5	140	1.0
white chocolate, macadamia (*Mauna Loa*), 2 pcs., .9 oz. ...	130	2.0	18.0	6.0	6	55	1.0

Food and Measure	cal.	prot. (gms)	carbo. (gms)	fat (gms)	chol. (mgs)	sod. (mgs)	fiber (gms)
Cookie, chocolate chip/chunk *(cont.)*							
white chocolate, macadamia (*Pepperidge Farm Tahoe*), .9-oz. pc.	130	1.0	17.0	6.0	<5	85	<1.0
white fudge, chunky (*Chips Ahoy!*), .6-oz. pc.	80	1.0	10.0	4.0	0	50	0
chocolate chip sandwich, vanilla creme (*Chips Ahoy! Cremewiches*), 1.1 oz. ...	150	1.0	22.0	7.0	0	65	1.0
chocolate sandwich:							
(*Austin Choco Cremes*), 1 pkg. ..	240	3.0	37.0	10.0	0	220	2.0
(*Country Choice Cremes*), 2 pcs., 1 oz.	130	1.0	19.0	5.0	0	100	0
(*Emperador*), 2 pcs., .9 oz.	120	1.0	19.0	4.0	0	105	<1.0
(*Famous Amos Cremes*), 3 pcs., 1.2 oz.	150	2.0	24.0	6.0	0	140	<1.0
(*Murray* Sugar Free Cremes), 3 pcs., 1 oz.	120	2.0	18.0	7.0	0	110	<1.0
(*Oreo*), 3 pcs., 1.2 oz.	160	2.0	24.0	7.0	0	210	1.0
(*Oreo*), 1.5-oz. pkg.	210	2.0	29.0	10.0	0	200	1.0
(*Oreo* Mini Bite Size), 9 pcs., 1 oz.	140	1.0	21.0	6.0	0	160	1.0
(*Oreo* Reduced Fat), 3 pcs., 1.2 oz. ..	150	2.0	26.0	4.5	0	190	1.0
(*Oreo Carb Well*), .8 oz.	100	2.0	16.0	5.0	0	105	3.0
(*Oreo Double Stuf*), 2 pcs., 1 oz.	140	1.0	20.0	7.0	0	135	1.0
(*Pepperidge Farm Bordeaux*), 4 pcs., .9 oz.	130	2.0	19.0	5.0	10	95	<1.0
(*Pepperidge Farm Bordeaux* Mini), 13 pcs., 1 oz.	140	2.0	21.0	6.0	10	100	<1.0
(*Pepperidge Farm Brussels*), 3 pcs., 1.1 oz.	150	2.0	20.0	7.0	5	65	1.0

Food and Measure	cal.	prot. (gms)	carbo. (gms)	fat (gms)	chol. (mgs)	sod. (mgs)	fiber (gms)
(*Pepperidge Farm Brussels* Mini), 8 pcs., 1 oz.	150	2.0	19.0	7.0	5	65	1.0
(*Pepperidge Farm Milano*), 3 pcs., 1.2 oz.	180	2.0	21.0	10.0	10	80	<1.0
(*Pepperidge Farm Milano* Mini), 6 pcs., 1 oz.	160	2.0	18.0	8.0	10	70	<1.0
chocolate crème (*Oreo*), 3 pcs., 1.1 oz.	150	1.0	21.0	7.0	0	135	1.0
chocolate crème, mini (*Oreo*), 9 pcs., 1 oz.	140	1.0	21.0	6.0	0	160	1.0
chocolate crème, mini (*Oreo*), 1.25-oz. pkg. . . .	170	2.0	25.0	7.0	0	200	1.0
double (*Health Valley Cookie Cremes*), 2 pcs., .9 oz.	120	1.0	19.0	5.0	0	100	0
double (*Pepperidge Farm Milano*), 2 pcs., 1 oz.	140	2.0	17.0	8.0	10	70	<1.0
fudge coated, white (*Oreo*), .75-oz. pc.	110	1.0	14.0	6.0	0	70	0
fudge coated (*Oreo*), .7-oz. pc.	90	1.0	13.0	5.0	0	70	1.0
fudge mint coated (*Oreo*), .6-oz. pc.	90	1.0	12.0	4.5	0	70	1.0
golden, w/chocolate creme (*Oreo Uh-Oh!*), 1.2 oz. . . .	170	2.0	24.0	7.0	0	130	1.0
mint (*Health Valley Cookie Cremes*), 2 pcs., .9 oz. . . .	120	1.0	19.0	5.0	0	100	0
mint/creme (*Oreo Double Delight*), 1 oz.	140	1.0	20.0	7.0	0	120	1.0
mint or orange (*Pepperidge Farm Milano*), 2 pcs., .9 oz.	130	1.0	16.0	7.0	<5	50	<1.0

Food and Measure	cal.	prot. (gms)	carbo. (gms)	fat (gms)	chol. (mgs)	sod. (mgs)	fiber (gms)
Cookie, chocolate sandwich *(cont.)*							
rainbow crème (*Austin Snackerz*), 7 pcs., 1 oz.	130	1.0	20.0	5.0	0	70	<1.0
raspberry (*Pepperidge Farm Milano*), 2 pcs., .9 oz.	130	1.0	16.0	7.0	<5	40	<1.0
vanilla creme (*Health Valley Bars*), 1.7-oz. pc.	200	2.0	32.0	8.0	20	90	1.0
cinnamon:							
(*Roscas*), 3 pcs., 1 oz.	130	2.0	22.0	4.0	0	130	1.0
(*Stella D'oro* Viennese Breakfast Treats), .8-oz. pc.	90	1.0	16.0	2.5	15	60	0
raisin (*Stella D'oro* Toast), 2 pcs., .9 oz.	100	2.0	20.0	1.0	40	90	0
coconut:							
(*Arcoiris*), 1 pkg., 6 pcs.	220	3.0	44.0	3.5	0	130	1.0
(*Gamesa* Barras de Coco), 5 pcs., 1 oz.	120	2.0	21.0	3.5	0	130	<1.0
(*Hawaianas*), 3 pcs., 1 oz.	130	2.0	22.0	3.5	0	115	<1.0
filled (*Almond Joy*), 2 pcs., 1 oz.	150	1.0	17.0	9.0	0	55	<1.0
cream sandwich (*Country Choice* Organic Duplex), 2 pcs. 1 oz.	130	1.0	19.0	5.0	0	115	0
crème filled stick:							
chocolate hazelnut (*Pepperidge Farm Pirouette*), 2 pcs., .9 oz.	130	1.0	10.0	6.0	10	60	<1.0
mint chocolate (*Pepperidge Farm Pirouette*), 2 pcs., .9 oz.	130	1.0	19.0	6.0	<5	50	0

Food and Measure	cal.	prot. (gms)	carbo. (gms)	fat (gms)	chol. (mgs)	sod. (mgs)	fiber (gms)
vanilla (*Pepperidge Farm Pirouette*), 2 pcs., .9 oz. . . .	140	1.0	18.0	6.0	<5	50	0
devil's food:							
(*Tree of Life* Monster Fat Free), ¼ pc. .	80	2.0	20.0	0	0	45	2.0
cake (*SnackWell's*), .6-oz. pc.	50	1.0	12.0	0	0	30	0
chocolate (*Tree of Life* Fat Free), .8-oz. pc.	70	2.0	15.0	0	0	80	1.0
egg biscuits:							
(*Stella D'oro* Jumbo), 2 pcs., 1.2 oz.	120	2.0	26.0	1.5	45	85	0
(*Stella D'oro* Roman), 1.2-oz. pc.	130	2.0	21.0	4.0	10	120	0
fig filled/bar:							
(*Barbara's*), .7-oz. pc.	60	0	14.0	.5	0	20	0
(*Barbara's* Wheat Free/Whole Wheat), .7-oz. pc.	60	1.0	13.0	0	0	25	1.0
(*Newtons*), 2 pcs., 1.1 oz. . . . . :	110	1.0	22.0	2.5	0	115	1.0
(*Newtons*), 2-oz. pkg.	200	2.0	40.0	4.0	0	230	3.0
(*Tofutti Tofiggy*), 1.1-oz. pc.	100	2.0	21.0	2.0	0	35	0
apple cinnamon or raspberry (*Barbara's*), .7-oz. pc.	60	1.0	14.0	0	0	25	1.0
blueberry (*Barbara's*), .7-oz. pc.	70	0	15.0	.5	0	20	0
fortune (*Port Arthur*), 3 pcs.	110	2.0	23.0	1.0	0	0	0
fruit slices (*Stella D'oro*), 1.2 oz.	130	2.0	20.0	5.0	5	90	1.0
fudge:							
(*Stella D'oro* Swiss), 2 pcs., 1.2 oz. . .	170	1.0	22.0	9.0	5	65	1.0
double (*Murray* Sugar Free), 3 pcs., 1.2 oz. . .	140	2.0	23.0	7.0	0	85	2.0

Food and Measure	cal.	prot. (gms)	carbo. (gms)	fat (gms)	chol. (mgs)	sod. (mgs)	fiber (gms)
Cookie, fudge *(cont.)*							
sticks (*Keebler Fudge Shoppe*), 3 pcs., 1 oz.	150	1.0	19.0	8.0	0	50	0
sticks (*Keebler Fudge Shoppe* Fudge Lovers'), 3 pcs., 1 oz.	160	1.0	17.0	10.0	0	20	<1.0
stripe (*Keebler Fudge Shoppe*), 3 pcs., 1.1 oz.	150	1.0	20.0	7.0	0	105	<1.0
stripe (*Keebler Fudge Shoppe* Sugar Free*), 3 pcs., 1 oz.	130	2.0	18.0	7.0	0	75	1.0
stripe, mini (*Keebler Fudge Shoppe*), 14 pcs., 1.1 oz. .	150	2.0	20.0	7.0	0	110	<1.0
fudge sandwich:							
(*Keebler E. L. Fudge Butterfinger Blasted*), 2 pcs., 1.2 oz.	180	2.0	23.0	9.0	<5	105	<1.0
(*Keebler E. L. Fudge S'mores Blasted*), 2 pcs., 1.2 oz. . .	170	1.0	23.0	9.0	<5	115	0
double stuffed (*Keebler E. L. Fudge*), 2 pcs., 1.2 oz.	180	2.0	23.0	9.0	<5	90	0
fudge cookies (*Keebler E. L. Fudge*), 2 pcs., .9 oz.	120	2.0	18.0	5.0	0	105	<1.0
mini (*Keebler E. L. Fudge*), 7 pcs., 1 oz.	130	1.0	21.0	6.0	0	75	0
ginger:							
(*Country Choice*), .8-oz. pc.	90	1.0	17.0	2.0	5	75	<1.0
(*Pepperidge Farm* Gingerman), 4 pcs., .9 oz.	130	2.0	21.0	4.0	10	100	<1.0
snaps (*Country Choice*), 5 pcs. . . .	120	1.0	19.0	5.0	0	85	2.0

Food and Measure	cal.	prot. (gms)	carbo. (gms)	fat (gms)	chol. (mgs)	sod. (mgs)	fiber (gms)
snaps (*Murray* Sugar Free), 7 pcs., 1.1 oz.	130	2.0	23.0	4.5	0	120	0
snaps (*Nabisco*), 4 pcs., 1 oz.	120	1.0	22.0	2.5	0	230	0
ginger-lemon sandwich:							
(*Carr's*), 2 pcs., 1 oz.	140	1.0	19.0	7.0	<5	105	<1.0
(*Country Choice* Cremes), 2 pcs., 1 oz.	130	1.0	19.0	5.0	0	130	0
graham cracker:							
amaranth or oat bran (*Health Valley Graham Crackers*), 6 pcs., 1 oz.	120	3.0	22.0	3.0	0	80	3.0
cinnamon (*Barbara's* Organic Go Go), 8 pcs., 1.1 oz. ...	130	2.0	23.0	3.5	0	130	<1.0
cinnamon (*Honey Maid*), 1.1 oz. ..	130	2.0	25.0	2.5	0	150	1.0
cinnamon (*Honey Maid* Low Fat), 1.1 oz.	120	2.0	26.0	1.5	0	170	1.0
cinnamon (*New Morning*), 2 pcs., 1.1 oz.	130	3.0	24.0	3.0	0	170	<1.0
cinnamon (*Ricanelas*), 8 pcs., 1.1 oz. ..	140	2.0	24.0	4.0	0	180	2.0
cinnamon (*Teddy Grahams*), 1.25-oz. pkg.	160	2.0	27.0	5.0	0	170	1.0
cinnamon, sticks (*Honey Maid*), 1-oz. pkg.	120	2.0	23.0	2.5	0	160	1.0
cinnamon or honey (*Teddy Grahams*), 24 pcs., 1.1 oz. .	130	2.0	23.0	4.0	0	150	1.0
honey (*Barbara's* Organic Go Go), 8 pcs., 1.1 oz. ..	130	2.0	22.0	4.0	0	150	<1.0
honey (*Honey Maid*), 1.1 oz.	140	2.0	24.0	3.0	0	190	1.0
honey (*Honey Maid* Low Fat), 1.1 oz.	120	2.0	25.0	1.5	0	190	1.0

Food and Measure	cal.	prot. (gms)	carbo. (gms)	fat (gms)	chol. (mgs)	sod. (mgs)	fiber (gms)
Cookie, graham cracker *(cont.)*							
honey (*New Morning*), 2 pcs., 1.1 oz.	130	3.0	24.0	3.0	0	180	1.0
honey (*New Morning* Bites), 22 pcs., 1 oz.	110	2.0	18.0	3.0	0	160	0
honey (*Teddy Grahams*), 1.25-oz. pkg.	150	2.0	26.0	4.5	0	170	1.0
honey, sticks (*Honey Maid*), 1.1 oz.	130	2.0	25.0	3.0	0	170	1.0
lemon ginger (*Barbara's* Organic Go Go), 8 pcs., 1.1 oz.	130	2.0	22.0	4.0	0	140	<1.0
graham, chocolate:							
(*Barbara's* Organic Go Go), 8 pcs., 1.1 oz.	130	2.0	23.0	3.5	0	125	1.0
(*Honey Maid*), 1.1 oz.	130	2.0	24.0	3.0	0	190	1.0
(*New Morning* Bites), 22 pcs., 1 oz.	110	2.0	19.0	3.0	0	110	0
(*Teddy Grahams*), 24 pcs., 1.1 oz. .	130	2.0	22.0	4.5	0	170	1.0
(*Teddy Grahams*), 1.25-oz. pkg.	150	2.0	26.0	5.0	0	200	1.0
chip (*Teddy Grahams*), 24 pcs., 1.1 oz.	130	1.0	22.0	4.0	0	170	1.0
chip, mini (*Teddy Grahams*), 1.1 oz.	140	2.0	22.0	4.5	0	170	1.0
sticks (*Honey Maid*), 1.1 oz.	130	2.0	24.0	3.0	0	170	1.0
graham, fudge coated:							
(*Keebler Fudge Shoppe*), 3 pcs., 1 oz.	140	1.0	19.0	7.0	0	105	<1.0
mini (*Keebler Fudge Shoppe*), 10 pcs., 1.2 oz.	160	2.0	22.0	8.0	0	120	<1.0

Food and Measure	cal.	prot. (gms)	carbo. (gms)	fat (gms)	chol. (mgs)	sod. (mgs)	fiber (gms)
graham sandwich:							
chocolate, crème (*Teddy Grahams Bearwiches*), 1.1-oz. pc.	150	1.0	21.0	7.0	0	105	1.0
chocolate, peanut butter (*New Morning*), 2 pcs., 1 oz.	120	2.0	18.0	5.0	0	95	0
honey, crème (*Teddy Grahams Bearwiches*), 1-oz. pc.	150	1.0	21.0	7.0	0	90	0
honey, peanut butter (*New Morning*), 2 pcs., 1 oz.	130	2.0	18.0	5.0	0	120	0
honey, vanilla (*New Morning*), 2 pcs., 1 oz.	130.	1.0	19.0	5.0	0	95	0
S'mores (*Austin*), 7 pcs., 1 oz.	140	1.0	21.0	5.0	0	90	0
S'mores (*Ritz Bits*), 1.1 oz.	150	1.0	22.0	6.0	0	130	1.0
granola (*Tree of Life Monster*), 1/5 pc. . . .	140	2.0	19.0	6.0	2	95	1.0
hazelnut cream sandwich (*Bahlsen*), 3 pcs., 1.1 oz.	170	2.0	19.0	10.0	5	40	0
lemon:							
nut (*Pepperidge Farm*), 3 pcs., 1.1 oz.	170	2.0	19.0	9.0	15	60	2.0
wafers (*Murray Sugar Free*), 4 pcs., 1 oz.	130	<1.0	19.0	10.0	0	15	0
lemon sandwich:							
(*Austin Lemon Ohs!*), 1 pkg.	250	2.0	37.0	11.0	0	140	<1.0
(*Emperador*), 1 pkg., 6 pcs.	270	3.0	45.0	8.0	0	260	1.0
(*Murray* Sugar Free), 3 pcs., 1 oz.	120	1.0	19.0	6.0	0	55	<1.0
(*SnackWell's* Sugar Free), 3 pcs., 1.1 oz.	130	2.0	24.0	6.0	0	135	0

Food and Measure	cal.	prot. (gms)	carbo. (gms)	fat (gms)	chol. (mgs)	sod. (mgs)	fiber (gms)
Cookie *(cont.)*							
lemon tartlets (*Bonne Maman*), .6-oz. pc. .	80	<1.0	11.0	3.5	15	25	0
macadamia nut crunch (*Mauna Loa*), 2 pcs., .9 oz.	150	2.0	15.0	8.0	10	30	1.0
macaroon:							
coconut (*Streit's*), 2 pcs., 1 oz.	100	1.0	12.0	6.0	0	70	2.0
honey (*Tree of Life* Monster), 1/5 pc.	150	1.0	17.0	9.0	2	75	1.0
oatmeal (*Famous Amos*), 3 pcs., 1.2 oz.	160	2.0	23.0	7.0	0	65	<1.0
maple pecan (*Tree of Life* Monster Fat Free), ¼ pc.	90	2.0	21.0	0	0	50	2.0
marshmallow, chocolate:							
(*Arcoiris*), 2 pcs., 1 oz.	120	1.0	18.0	5.0	0	50	<1.0
(*Mallomars*), 2 pcs., .9 oz.	120	1.0	17.0	5.0	0	35	1.0
fudge (*Twirls*), 1.1 oz.	130	1.0	20.0	6.0	0	75	0
marshmallow sandwich (*Arcoiris*), 1 pkg., 6 pcs.	200	3.0	43.0	2.5	0	170	1.0
mint, chocolate coated:							
(*Keebler Fudge Shoppe Grass-hopper*), 4 pc., 1 oz.	150	2.0	19.0	7.0	0	85	<1.0
(*York*), 2 pcs., 1 oz.	160	2.0	17.0	9.0	0	55	1.0
mint sandwich (*Country Choice* Cremes), 2 pcs., 1 oz.	130	1.0	19.0	5.0	0	100	0
oatmeal:							
(*Barbara's*), .6-oz. pc.	60	<1.0	8.0	3.0	5	90	<1.0
(*Country Choice* Old Fashioned), .8-oz. pc.	100	2.0	16.0	3.0	5	90	1.0
(*Murray* Sugar Free), 3 pcs., 1.1 oz. . .	150	2.0	21.0	7.0	0	160	1.0

Food and Measure	cal.	prot. (gms)	carbo. (gms)	fat (gms)	chol. (mgs)	sod. (mgs)	fiber (gms)
(*SnackWell's* Sugar Free), .8 oz.	90	1.0	17.0	2.5	0	80	1.0
(*Tree of Life* Wheat Free Americana), .8-oz. pc.	90	1.0	11.0	5.0	0	25	1.0
peanut crunch (*Health Valley*), .8-oz. pc.	100	2.0	14.0	4.0	0	60	1.0
oatmeal raisin:							
(*Country Choice*), .8-oz. pc.	100	1.0	16.0	3.0	5	70	1.0
(*Famous Amos*), 4 pcs., 1 oz.	140	2.0	21.0	5.0	<5	125	<1.0
(*Grandma's* Home-style), 1.4-oz. pc.	180	2.0	30.0	6.0	10	240	1.0
(*Health Valley*), .8-oz. pc.	90	2.0	14.0	3.5	0	50	1.0
(*Health Valley* Fat Free), 3 pcs., 1.2 oz.	100	2.0	24.0	0	0	80	3.0
(*Health Valley Café Creations*), .8-oz. pc.	90	1.0	15.0	3.5	5	50	1.0
(*Pepperidge Farm Santa Cruz*), .9-oz. pc.	130	2.0	23.0	4.5	<5	90	2.0
golden (*Tree of Life* Fat Free), .8-oz. pc.	70	2.0	16.0	0	0	40	1.0
orange (*Morelianas*), .9 oz.	130	1.0	19.0	5.0	0	80	0
peanut butter:							
(*Chips Ahoy!*), .5-oz. pc.	80	1.0	9.0	4.0	0	75	0
(*Country Choice*), .8-oz. pc.	100	2.0	13.0	5.0	5	75	<1.0
(*Grandma's* Home-style), 1.4-oz. pc.	200	4.0	24.0	10.0	10	200	1.0
(*Health Valley* Mini), 4 pcs., 1 oz.	120	3.0	16.0	5.0	10	180	0
(*Murray* Sugar Free), 3 pcs., 1.1 oz. ..	150	3.0	17.0	9.0	<5	135	1.0
(*Tofutt*), 1.1-oz. pc.	137	3.0	18.0	7.0	0	108	0

Food and Measure	cal.	prot. (gms)	carbo. (gms)	fat (gms)	chol. (mgs)	sod. (mgs)	fiber (gms)
Cookie, peanut butter *(cont.)*							
(*Tree of Life* Monster), 1/5 pc.	140	3.0	17.0	7.0	4	105	1.0
(*Tree of Life* Wheat Free Georgia), .8-oz. pc.	100	2.0	8.0	6.0	0	110	1.0
cup (*Keebler Chips Deluxe*), .6-oz. pc.	90	1.0	10.0	4.5	0	50	0
filled (*Reese's*), 2 pcs., 1 oz.	150	2.0	17.0	8.0	0	90	<1.0
fudge sticks (*Keebler Fudge Shoppe*), 3 pcs., 1 oz.	150	2.0	18.0	8.0	0	70	<1.0
swirl (*Health Valley* Bars), 1.7-oz. pc.	190	3.0	33.0	6.0	20	200	1.0
peanut butter sandwich:							
(*Nutter Butter*), 1 oz.	130	2.0	18.0	6.0	5	110	1.0
(*Nutter Butter* Bites), 10 pcs., 1.1 oz. .	140	2.0	20.0	6.0	0	115	1.0
(*Nutter Butter* Bites), 1.25-oz. pkg. . . .	170	3.0	23.0	7.0	5	135	1.0
crèmes (*Grandma's*), 5 pcs., 1.2 oz. . .	210	3.0	28.0	10.0	0	200	1.0
double stuffed (*Keebler E. L. Fudge*), 2 pcs., 1.2 oz.	180	3.0	21.0	9.0	0	170	<1.0
pecan, wheat free (*Foods by George*), 3.25-oz. pc.	410	4.0	50.0	22.0	75	135	1.0
rainbow chips sandwich crèmes (*Keebler Chips Deluxe*), .6-oz. pc. .	90	<1.0	11.0	4.5	0	35	0
raspberry:							
(*Pepperidge Farm Chantilly*), 2 pcs., .9 oz.	120	1.0	23.0	3.0	0	115	<1.0
bar (*Newtons*), 2 pcs., 1 oz.	100	1.0	21.0	1.5	0	100	1.0
shortbread:							
(*Barbara's*), .6-oz. pc.	80	1.0	9.0	4.0	5	50	<1.0
(*Lorna Doone*), 4 pcs., 1 oz.	150	1.0	19.0	7.0	0	140	0

Food and Measure	cal.	prot. (gms)	carbo. (gms)	fat (gms)	chol. (mgs)	sod. (mgs)	fiber (gms)
(*Murray* Sugar Free), 8 pcs., 1.1 oz. ..	120	2.0	22.0	6.0	0	150	1.0
(*Pepperidge Farm*), 2 pcs., .9 oz. . . .	140	2.0	16.0	7.0	10	105	<1.0
(*Sandies* Simply Shortbread), .6-oz. pc.	80	<1.0	10.0	4.5	5	65	0
(*SnackWell's* Sugar Free), 3 pcs., 1.1 oz.	130	2.0	22.0	5.0	5	150	1.0
caramel pecan or cinnamon swirl (*Sandies*), .6-oz. pc.	80	<1.0	9.0	5.0	<5	55	0
chocolate chip pecan (*Sandies*), .6-oz. pc.	80	<1.0	9.0	5.0	0	45	0
fudge dipped (*Murray* Sugar Free), 5 pcs., 1 oz.	130	2.0	20.0	7.0	0	85	<1.0
fudge stripe (*Snack-Wells*), .8 oz. . . .	110	1.0	16.0	6.0	0	80	1.0
pecan (*Sandies*), .6-oz. pc.	90	<1.0	9.0	5.0	<5	50	0
pecan (*Murray* Sugar Free), 3 pcs., 1.1 oz.	170	2.0	18.0	11.0	<5	115	<1.0
strawberry filled (*Health Valley Bars*), 1.7-oz. pc.	200	2.0	33.0	7.0	15	80	1.0
spice (*Stella D'oro* Pfeffernusse), .9 oz.	100	1.0	18.0	3.0	15	50	0
strawberry:							
(*Newtons*), 2 pcs., 1 oz.	100	1.0	20.0	1.5	0	100	1.0
(*Pepperidge Farm Verona*), 3 pcs., .9 oz.	140	2.0	22.0	5.0	10	105	<1.0
cheesecake (*Sandies* Fruit Delights), .6-oz. pc.	80	0	11.0	3.5	<5	55	<1.0
yogurt bar (*Newtons*), 2 pcs., 1.3 oz. ..	130	1.0	26.0	3.0	0	100	1.0

Food and Measure	cal.	prot. (gms)	carbo. (gms)	fat (gms)	chol. (mgs)	sod. (mgs)	fiber (gms)
Cookie *(cont.)*							
strawberry sandwich (*Emperador*), 2 pcs., .9 oz.	120	2.0	19.0	4.0	<5	65	<1.0
sugar (*Pepperidge Farm*), 3 pcs., 1.1 oz.	140	2.0	20.0	6.0	15	90	<1.0
sugar wafer:							
(*Biscos*), 8 pcs., 1 oz.	140	1.0	21.0	6.0	0	40	0
(*Gamesa*), 3 pcs., 1.2 oz.	160	1.0	23.0	7.0	0	30	0
strawberry (*Gamesa*), 3 pcs., 1.2 oz.	160	1.0	24.0	6.0	0	25	0
vanilla (*Gamesa*), 3 pcs., 1.2 oz. . .	160	1.0	25.0	7.0	0	25	0
vanilla (*Murray Sugar Free*), 4 pcs., 1 oz.	130	<1.0	19.0	10.0	0	15	0
vanilla sandwich:							
(*Austin* Cremes), 1 pkg.	250	2.0	37.0	11.0	0	130	<1.0
(*Country Choice* Cremes), 2 pcs., 1 oz.	130	1.0	19.0	5.0	0	125	0
(*Emperador*), 2 pcs., .9 oz.	120	2.0	19.0	3.5	<5	75	0
(*Grandma's* Mini Bites), 9 pcs., 1.1 oz.	150	2.0	22.0	7.0	<5	85	<1.0
(*Grandma's* Sandwich Cremes), 5 pcs., 1.5 oz. . .	210	2.0	30.0	10.0	5	125	<1.0
(*Health Valley Cookie Cremes*), 2 pcs., .9 oz. . . .	120	1.0	19.0	5.0	0	125	0
(*Murray* Sugar Free Cremes), 3 pcs., 1 oz.	120	1.0	19.0	6.0	0	55	<1.0
(*SnackWell's*), 2 pcs., .9 oz.	110	1.0	20.0	3.0	0	130	0
(*SnackWell's*), 1.7-oz. pkg.	210	2.0	38.0	5.0	0	240	1.0
(*Vienna Fingers*), 2 pcs., 1.1 oz. . .	150	1.0	21.0	6.0	0	85	0

Food and Measure	cal.	prot. (gms)	carbo. (gms)	fat (gms)	chol. (mgs)	sod. (mgs)	fiber (gms)
rainbow crème (*Austin Snackerz*), 7 pcs., 1 oz.	130	1.0	21.0	5.0	0	90	0
vanilla wafer:							
(*Country Choice*), 7 pcs.	120	1.0	19.0	5.0	5	100	2.0
(*Keebler* Reduced Fat), 8 pcs., 1.1 oz.	130	2.0	25.0	3.5	0	140	<1.0
(*Murray* Sugar Free), 9 pcs., 1 oz.	120	2.0	22.0	4.5	0	100	<1.0
(*Murray* Sugar Free Reduced Fat), 8 pcs., 1.1 oz. . .	130	2.0	25.0	3.5	0	140	<1.0
(*Nilla*), 8 pcs., 1.1 oz. 140	1.0	21.0	6.0	5	115	0	
(*Nilla* Reduced Fat), 8 pcs., 1 oz.	120	1.0	24.0	2.0	0	110	0
fudge dipped (*Murray* Sugar Free), 4 pcs., 1.1 oz.	140	1.0	19.0	10.0	0	35	<1.0
mini, golden (*Murray* Sugar Free), 18 pcs., 1.1 oz. . .	140	1.0	21.0	6.0	0	120	<1.0
Cookie, frozen or re-frigerated, ready-to-bake, 1 pc., except as noted:							
chocolate candy, w/chips (*Pillsbury*)	120	1.0	16.0	5.0	5	70	0
chocolate chip:							
(*Kineret*)	130	1.0	17.0	7.0	10	85	0
(*Pillsbury* Family Size), 1 oz., 1½" ball	130	1.0	17.0	7.0	5	85	<1.0
(*Pillsbury* Reduced Fat), 1 oz., 1½" ball	110	1.0	19.0	3.0	<5	85	<1.0
(*Pillsbury* Big Deluxe Classics) .	200	2.0	25.0	10.0	5	105	<1.0
(*Pillsbury* Ready to Bake*)	120	1.0	15.0	6.0	<5	65	<1.0
(*Pillsbury* Ready to Bake* Sugar Free)	90	1.0	16.0	4.0	<5	85	3.0

Food and Measure	cal.	prot. (gms)	carbo. (gms)	fat (gms)	chol. (mgs)	sod. (mgs)	fiber (gms)
Cookie, frozen or refrigerated, chocolate chip *(cont.)*							
w/caramel, pecans (*Pillsbury Big Deluxe Classics Turtle Supreme*) .	200	2.0	25.0	10.0	5	120	<1.0
chips and chunks (*Pillsbury Ready to Bake*)	120	1.0	15.0	6.0	<5	60	<1.0
chips and chunks, double (*Pillsbury*), 1 oz., 1½" ball . .	130	1.0	17.0	7.0	5	85	<1.0
mini (*Pillsbury Ready to Bake Bites*), 4 pcs. . . .	120	1.0	15.0	6.0	5	80	1.0
walnut (*Pillsbury*), 1 oz., 1½" ball . .	130	1.0	16.0	7.0	5	90	<1.0
walnut (*Pillsbury Ready to Bake*) .	120	1.0	14.0	7.0	<5	75	0
chocolate chunk (*Pillsbury*), 1 oz., 1½" ball	130	1.0	17.0	7.0	5	85	<1.0
gingerbread (*Pillsbury*), 1 cutout pc.	90	1.0	12.0	5.0	10	70	0
oatmeal:							
chocolate chip (*Pillsbury*), 1 oz., 1½" ball	130	1.0	17.0	6.0	5	95	<1.0
raisin (*Pillsbury Big Deluxe Classics*) .	180	2.0	26.0	7.0	10	115	1.0
peanut butter:							
(*Pillsbury*), 1 oz., 1½" ball	120	2.0	17.0	5.0	5	135	0
(*Pillsbury Ready to Bake Reese's Pieces*)	120	2.0	15.0	5.0	<5	90	0
cup (*Pillsbury Big Deluxe Classics*) .	190	3.0	24.0	9.0	5	160	<1.0
sugar:							
(*Pillsbury*), 2 slices, ¼"	140	1.0	19.0	6.0	10	85	0
(*Pillsbury Ready to Bake*)	120	1.0	15.0	6.0	5	70	0
Christmas, w/images (*Pillsbury*)	140	1.0	18.0	7.0	5	75	0

Food and Measure	cal.	prot. (gms)	carbo. (gms)	fat (gms)	chol. (mgs)	sod. (mgs)	fiber (gms)
Easter, w/images (*Pillsbury*)	140	1.0	18.0	7.0	5	80	0
shapes, all varieties (*Pillsbury*), 2 pcs.	140	1.0	17.0	7.0	5	100	0
white chunk macadamia (*Pillsbury Big Deluxe Classics*)	200	2.0	24.0	11.0	10	110	<1.0
Cookie, mix, 2 pcs.*:							
chocolate chip (*Betty Crocker*)	160	2.0	21.0	8.0	10	105	0
chocolate chunk, double (*Betty Crocker*)	150	2.0	21.0	6.0	10	105	0
chocolate peanut butter chip (*Betty Crocker*)	150	3.0	30.0	7.0	10	120	0
oatmeal chocolate chip (*Betty Crocker*)	150	2.0	21.0	7.0	10	135	0
peanut butter (*Betty Crocker*)	160	3.0	20.0	8.0	10	150	0
rainbow chocolate candy (*Betty Crocker*)	150	2.0	22.0	7.0	10	110	0
sugar (*Betty Crocker*)	160	2.0	22.0	8.0	10	115	0
Cookie crumbs:							
(*Oreo*), 2 tbsp.	90	1.0	13.0	4.0	0	95	1.0
(*Oreo* Crunchies), 2 tbsp.	50	1.0	8.0	2.5	0	60	0
Cookie pie crust, see "Pie crust"							
Coquito nut (*Frieda's*), 11 pcs., 1 oz.	110	1.0	5.0	10.0	0	5	3.0
Coriander, fresh, ¼ cup	1	.1	.1	<.1	0	1	.1
Coriander, dried:							
leaf, 1 tsp.	2	.1	.3	<.1	0	1	.1
seed, 1 tsp.	5	.2	1.0	.3	0	1	.5
Corn, fresh:							
baby, .28-oz. ear	9	.3	2.0	.1	0	1	.2
golden or white:							
raw, 5-oz. ear	123	4.6	27.2	1.7	0	21	3.9
kernels, boiled, drained, ½ cup	89	2.7	20.6	1.1	0	14	2.3
white, boiled, drained, 2.72-oz. ear	83	2.6	19.3	1.0	0	13	2.1

Food and Measure	cal.	prot. (gms)	carbo. (gms)	fat (gms)	chol. (mgs)	sod. (mgs)	fiber (gms)
Corn, canned, ½ cup, except as noted:							
whole, baby, stir-fry (*Port Arthur*)	30	1.0	3.0	1.5	0	30	4.0
kernel, golden:							
(*Del Monte*)	90	2.0	18.0	1.0	0	360	3.0
(*Del Monte* Super-sweet)	60	2.0	11.0	1.0	0	360	3.0
(*Del Monte* Super-sweet No Salt) ..	60	2.0	11.0	1.0	0	10	3.0
(*Del Monte* Super-sweet Vac Pac) .	70	2.0	13.0	1.0	0	270	3.0
(*Del Monte* Super-sweet Vac Pac No Salt)	70	2.0	13.0	1.0	0	10	3.0
(*Freshlike*)	80	3.0	17.0	1.5	0	310	2.0
(*Green Giant*)	80	2.0	18.0	.5	0	360	2.0
(*Green Giant* 50% Less Sodium) ...	80	2.0	17.0	.5	0	180	2.0
(*Green Giant Niblets* Extra Sweet), ⅓ cup	50	2.0	10.0	.5	0	200	2.0
(*Green Giant Niblets* No Salt), ⅓ cup .	60	2.0	13.0	0	0	0	2.0
(*Green Giant Niblets* Vac Pac), ⅓ cup	80	2.0	16.0	.5	0	230	<1.0
(*S&W*)	60	2.0	11.0	0	0	360	3.0
(*S&W* Vac Pac)	70	2.0	13.0	0	0	270	3.0
(*Veg-All*)	80	2.0	16.0	1.0	0	340	2.0
(*Westbrae Natural Organic*)	90	2.0	14.0	1.0	0	340	2.0
kernel, golden/white:							
(*Del Monte* Super-sweet)	80	2.0	18.0	.5	0	360	2.0
(*Green Giant* Vac Pac), ⅓ cup	50	1.0	11.0	0	0	200	1.0
kernel, white:							
(*Del Monte*)	60	2.0	11.0	1.0	0	360	3.0
(*Green Giant* Shoe-peg Vac Pac), ⅓ cup	80	2.0	16.0	.5	0	220	1.0
(*Westbrae Natural Organic*)	100	2.0	20.0	1.0	0	340	1.0

Food and Measure	cal.	prot. (gms)	carbo. (gms)	fat (gms)	chol. (mgs)	sod. (mgs)	fiber (gms)
cream style:							
(*Del Monte*)	90	2.0	20.0	.5	0	360	2.0
(*Del Monte* No Salt)	90	2.0	20.0	.5	0	10	2.0
(*Del Monte* Super-							
sweet)	60	1.0	14.0	.5	0	360	2.0
(*Del Monte* Super-							
sweet No Salt) ..	60	1.0	14.0	.5	0	10	2.0
(*Freshlike/Veg-All*),							
⅓ cup	100	2.0	21.0	1.0	0	280	2.0
(*Green Giant*)	90	2.0	19.0	.5	0	400	1.0
(*S&W*)	60	1.0	14.0	.5	0	360	2.0
seasoned (*Glory*							
Skillet Corn)	90	2.0	22.0	.5	0	580	2.0
white (*Del Monte*) .	100	2.0	21.0	1.0	0	360	2.0
in butter sauce (*Del*							
Monte Savory Sides)	90	2.0	14.0	2.5	5	530	<1.0
w/diced pepper:							
(*Freshlike* Selects) .	80	2.0	16.0	1.0	0	240	1.0
(*Green Giant* Mexi-							
corn), ⅓ cup ...	60	2.0	14.0	0	0	250	1.0
seasoned (*Del Monte*							
Fiesta Supersweet) .	50	2.0	12.0	1.0	0	310	2.0
w/tomato, black beans							
(*Del Monte Savory*							
Sides Santa Fe) ...	70	3.0	16.0	1.0	0	510	1.0
Corn, dried (*John*							
Cope's), ¼ cup	130	2.0	15.0	1.0	0	0	1.0
Corn, freeze-dried,							
½ cup:							
(*AlpineAire*)	90	3.0	16.0	2.0	0	0	3.0
(*Mountain House*) ...	90	3.0	16.0	1.5	0	0	2.0
Corn, frozen:							
on cob:							
(*Green Giant*),							
4.4-oz. ear	120	4.0	22.0	2.0	0	0	3.0
(*Green Giant* Nibbers							
Halves), ½ ear,							
2.2 oz.	70	2.0	14.0	.5	0	5	1.0
kernel, golden:							
(*Birds Eye* Sweet),							
⅔ cup	100	3.0	21.0	1.0	0	0	1.0
(*Birds Eye* Super							
Sweet), ⅔ cup ..	70	3.0	14.0	1.0	0	0	2.0

Food and Measure	cal.	prot. (gms)	carbo. (gms)	fat (gms)	chol. (mgs)	sod. (mgs)	fiber (gms)
Corn, frozen, kernel, golden *(cont.)*							
(*Cascadian Farm Super Sweet*), ¾ cup	70	2.0	16.0	1.0	0	90	2.0
(*Cascadian Farm Sweet*), ¾ cup ..	70	3.0	18.0	.5	0	0	2.0
(*C&W/C&W Early Harvest*/Organic/ Petite), ⅔ cup ..	80	3.0	19.0	1.0	0	10	1.0
(*Green Giant*), ½ cup cooked	50	2.0	4.0	3.0	0	100	2.0
(*Green Giant Niblets*), ⅓ cup cooked ..	80	2.0	17.0	.5	0	5	2.0
(*Green Giant Niblets Extra Sweet*), ⅓ cup cooked ..	70	2.0	13.0	1.0	0	0	2.0
(*McKenzie's Southern*), ½ cup	80	3.0	19.0	1.0	0	10	1.0
(*Dr. Praeger's*), ⅔ cup	100	3.0	21.0	1.0	0	0	1.0
(*Tree of Life*), ⅔ cup	80	3.0	19.0	1.0	0	10	1.0
kernel, golden/white:							
(*C&W Petite*), ⅔ cup	80	3.0	19.0	1.0	0	10	1.0
(*Green Giant Select*), ¾ cup	70	2.0	14.0	1.0	0	0	2.0
baby (*Birds Eye*), ⅔ cup	100	3.0	20.0	1.0	0	0	2.0
kernel, white:							
(*C&W Petite*), ⅔ cup	80	3.0	19.0	1.0	0	10	1.0
(*Green Giant Shoe-peg*), ½ cup	70	2.0	14.0	.5	0	45	2.0
(*Green Giant Select Shoepeg*), ¾ cup	100	3.0	20.0	1.0	0	0	3.0
baby (*Birds Eye*), ⅔ cup	90	3.0	18.0	1.0	0	0	3.0
in butter sauce:							
(*Birds Eye* 9 oz.), ½ cup	150	3.0	28.0	3.0	0	260	2.0
(*Birds Eye* 24 oz.), ¾ cup	140	3.0	22.0	5.0	5	370	1.0
(*Cascadian Farm*), ½ cup	100	3.0	19.0	3.0	5	310	2.0
(*Green Giant Niblets*), ½ cup cooked ..	100	3.0	19.0	1.5	<5	300	2.0

Food and Measure	cal.	prot. (gms)	carbo. (gms)	fat (gms)	chol. (mgs)	sod. (mgs)	fiber (gms)
(*Green Giant Niblets* Boil-in-Bag), ⅔ cup	110	3.0	22.0	1.5	<5	340	2.0
white (*Green Giant* Shoepeg), ¾ cup	110	3.0	21.0	2.0	<5	310	3.0
cream style (*Green Giant*), ½ cup	110	2.0	23.0	1.0	0	330	2.0
fried (*Glory* Savory Accents), ½ cup ..	110	3.0	24.0	1.5	0	470	2.0
Corn, whole-grain:							
1 oz.	103	2.7	21.1	1.3	0	10	2.1
1 cup	605	15.6	123.3	7.9	0	58	12.2
Corn bran, crude, 1 cup	170	6.4	65.1	.7	0	5	64.3
Corn bread, see "Bread mix, sweet"							
Corn bread and bean entree, frozen, red beans (*Moosewood*), 10-oz. pkg.	350	12.0	62.0	7.0	20	570	9.0
Corn cake mix, sweet, dry, ½ cup:							
(*Chi Chi's*)	100	1.0	22.0	.5	0	120	0
(*El Torito*)	100	1.0	22.0	.5	0	120	0
Corn combinations, frozen:							
baby carrots, sugar snap peas (*C&W*), ⅔ cup	60	2.0	10.0	.5	0	45	2.0
baby corn and:							
green beans, peas (*Birds Eye*), ¾ cup	70	2.0	13.0	0	0	0	2.0
vegetable blend (*Birds Eye*), ⅔ cup	50	2.0	9.0	1.0	0	10	3.0
black beans, tomatoes (*C&W Corn Salsa*), 1 cup	100	3.0	18.0	2.0	0	320	3.0
broccoli florets, red peppers (*C&W*), ⅔ cup	60	2.0	14.0	.5	0	10	1.0
and peas, herb butter sauce (*Green Giant*), ¾ cup	90	4.0	14.0	1.5	<5	390	3.0

Food and Measure	cal.	prot. (gms)	carbo. (gms)	fat (gms)	chol. (mgs)	sod. (mgs)	fiber (gms)
Corn combinations *(cont.)*							
red peppers, roasted, Southwestern (*Green Giant*), ¾ cup	80	2.0	17.0	.5	0	125	2.0
Corn crisps/chips (see also "Snack chips"), 1 oz., except as noted:							
(*Corn Nuts* Original) ..	120	3.0	20.0	4.5	0	180	2.0
(*Dipsy Doodles*)	160	1.0	16.0	10.0	0	180	1.0
(*Fritos*)	160	2.0	15.0	10.0	0	170	1.0
(*Fritos* King Size)	160	2.0	16.0	10.0	0	150	1.0
(*Fritos Scoops!*)	160	2.0	16.0	10.0	0	110	1.0
(*O-Ke-Doke* Puffs), 2½ cups	170	2.0	18.0	11.0	0	180	<1.0
(*Sun Chips* Original) .	140	2.0	19.0	6.0	0	115	2.0
(*Wise/Moore's*)	160	1.0	16.0	10.0	0	180	1.0
barbecue:							
(*Bugles* Smokin'), 1.1 oz.	150	1.0	18.0	8.0	0	360	0
(*Corn Nuts*)	130	2.0	20.0	4.5	0	170	2.0
(*Dipsy Doodles/ Moore's*)	160	1.0	16.0	10.0	0	250	1.0
(*Fritos*)	150	2.0	16.0	10.0	0	280	1.0
honey (*Fritos Flavor Twists*)	160	2.0	16.0	10.0	0	210	1.0
butter flavor:							
(*Chester's* Puffcorn)	160	1.0	12.0	11.0	0	300	<1.0
(*Hain PureSnax* Zoinks), 1.1 oz. ..	140	2.0	23.0	4.5	0	270	<1.0
cheese:							
(*Barbara's* Puff Bakes)	160	2.0	13.0	11.0	0	190	0
(*Barbara's* Puffs) ..	150	2.0	16.0	10.0	0	130	0
(*Bugles*), 1.1 oz. ..	160	1.0	18.0	9.0	0	310	<1.0
(*Cheese Doodles* Crunchy)	190	2.0	20.0	11.0	0	240	0
(*Cheese Doodles* Puffed)	110	1.0	13.0	6.0	0	270	0
(*Cheetos* Crunchy) .	160	2.0	15.0	10.0	0	290	<1.0
(*Cheetos* Crunchy Baked!)	130	2.0	19.0	5.0	0	240	0
(*Cheetos* Puffs/ Twisted)	160	2.0	13.0	10.0	0	350	0

Food and Measure	cal.	prot. (gms)	carbo. (gms)	fat (gms)	chol. (mgs)	sod. (mgs)	fiber (gms)
(*Cheetos Asteroids*)	160	2.0	15.0	10.0	0	320	1.0
(*Cheetos Edge* Puffs)	160	8.0	7.0	11.0	0	440	<1.0
(*Chester's* Puffcorn)	160	2.0	12.0	11.0	0	310	0
(*Snyder's* Twist) . . .	170	2.0	15.0	12.0	<5	230	<1.0
chili (*Bugles*), 1.1 oz.	160	2.0	18.0	9.0	0	310	0
hot (*Cheetos Asteroids Flamin' Hot*)	160	0	13.0	11.0	0	340	<1.0
hot (*Cheetos Flamin' Hot*)	170	2.0	14.0	11.0	0	250	<1.0
hot (*Cheetos Flamin' Hot* Limón)	160	1.0	15.0	11.0	0	190	<1.0
hot (*Chester's Flamin' Hot* Fries)	150	2.0	17.0	8.0	0	270	<1.0
jalapeño (*Barbara's* Puffs)	150	2.0	16.0	10.0	0	130	0
nacho (*Corn Nuts*) .	130	3.0	19.0	5.0	0	240	2.0
nacho (*Bugles*), 1.1 oz.	160	1.0	18.0	9.0	0	310	<1.0
nacho (*Doodle Twisters*)	210	2.0	16.0	14.0	0	310	1.0
cheese, cheddar:							
(*Shiloh Farms* Curls)	160	2.0	13.0	7.0	<5	110	0
(*Sun Chips* Harvest)	140	2.0	19.0	6.0	0	170	2.0
ranch (*Fritos Flavor Twists*)	150	2.0	17.0	9.0	0	230	1.0
w/rice (*Snyder's CheddAirs* Puffs)	135	3.0	20.0	5.0	0	90	n.a.
white (*Barbara's* Puff Bakes)	160	2.0	13.0	11.0	0	190	0
white (*Cheetos* Puffs)	150	2.0	16.0	8.0	<5	290	<1.0
white (*Hain Pure-Snax Zoinks*), 1.1 oz.	140	3.0	22.0	4.5	0	340	1.0
chili cheese (*Fritos*) . .	160	2.0	15.0	10.0	0	260	1.0
chili lime (*Sabritones*)	150	2.0	13.0	10.0	0	690	1.0
chili picante (*Corn Nuts*)	130	2.0	19.0	4.5	0	290	2.0
hot (*Fritos Flamin' Hot*)	160	2.0	15.0	10.0	0	160	1.0
mac and cheese (*Cheese Doodles*) . .	120	1.0	12.0	7.0	0	180	0
onion:							
(*Funyuns* Rings) . .	140	2.0	18.0	7.0	0	270	<1.0
(*Funyuns* Rings Mini), 1 pkg. . . .	260	3.0	30.0	14.0	0	400	1.0
French (*Sun Chips*)	140	2.0	18.0	6.0	0	160	2.0

Food and Measure	cal.	prot. (gms)	carbo. (gms)	fat (gms)	chol. (mgs)	sod. (mgs)	fiber (gms)
Corn crisps/chips, onion *(cont.)*							
rings (*Wise*), .5 oz.	70	0	10.0	3.0	0	210	1.0
ranch (*Corn Nuts*) ...	130	3.0	19.0	5.0	0	240	2.0
salsa (*Corn Nuts* Jalisco)	130	3.0	20.0	4.5	0	150	2.0
tortilla:							
(*Cape Cod* Whole Earth)	140	2.0	19.0	6.0	0	110	2.0
(*Cape Cod* Whole Earth Reduced Carb)	140	9.0	11.0	6.0	0	110	2.0
(*Doritos* Ranchero!)	150	2.0	17.0	8.0	0	290	1.0
(*Doritos* Toasted Corn)	140	2.0	18.0	7.0	0	120	1.0
(*D.L. Jardine's* Texaditas)	140	2.0	19.0	7.0	0	25	2.0
(*Garden of Eatin'* White Chips) ...	140	2.0	19.0	6.0	0	70	2.0
(*Guiltless Gourmet* White Corn)	110	3.0	22.0	2.0	0	160	2.0
(*Snyder's*)	140	2.0	23.0	4.5	0	110	1.0
(*Santitas*)	130	2.0	19.0	6.0	0	110	1.0
(*Tostitos* Bite Size) .	140	2.0	17.0	8.0	0	110	1.0
(*Tostitos* Bite Size Baked!)	110	3.0	24.0	1.0	0	200	2.0
(*Tostitos* Light) ...	90	2.0	20.0	1.0	0	105	1.0
(*Tostitos* Restaurant Style)	130	2.0	19.0	6.0	0	80	1.0
(*Tostitos* Rounds) .	140	2.0	18.0	7.0	0	120	1.0
(*Tostitos* Edge) ...	140	10.0	9.0	8.0	0	220	3.0
(*Tostitos* Gold)	140	2.0	19.0	7.0	0	110	1.0
(*Tostitos* Scoops!) .	140	2.0	18.0	7.0	0	120	1.0
black pepper Jack (*Doritos*)	150	2.0	18.0	7.0	0	240	1.0
cheese (*Doritos* Spicier Nacho!) .	140	2.0	18.0	7.0	0	210	1.0
cheese (*Doritos* Nacho Cheesier*)	140	2.0	17.0	7.0	0	200	1.0
cheese (*Doritos* Nacho Cheesier Baked!)	120	2.0	21.0	3.5	0	220	2.0
cheese (*Doritos* Nacho Cheesier Light)	90	2.0	18.0	1.0	0	240	1.0

Food and Measure	cal.	prot. (gms)	carbo. (gms)	fat (gms)	chol. (mgs)	sod. (mgs)	fiber (gms)
cheese (*Doritos Rollitos Nacho Cheesier*)	150	2.0	17.0	8.0	0	200	1.0
cheese (*Guiltless Gourmet Mucho Nacho*)	100	2.0	20.0	2.0	0	200	3.0
cheese, four (*Doritos*)	140	2.0	17.0	8.0	0	240	1.0
cheese, nacho (*Snyder's*)	160	2.0	16.0	9.0	0	170	1.0
cheese, nacho (*Wise Bravos!*)	150	2.0	17.0	8.0	0	180	1.0
cheese, white nacho (*Doritos* Natural)	150	2.0	17.0	8.0	0	190	1.0
chili (*Kettle Fire Roasted Chili* Organic)	140	3.0	18.0	7.0	0	150	2.0
chili lime (*Garden of Eatin'*)	140	2.0	18.0	7.0	0	125	2.0
chili lime (*Guiltless Gourmet*)	110	2.0	22.0	2.0	0	200	2.0
garlic herb (*Cape Cod* Whole Earth)	140	2.0	19.0	6.0	0	110	2.0
guacamole (*Doritos*)	150	4.0	16.0	8.0	0	230	1.0
guacamole (*Garden of Eatin'*)	140	2.0	19.0	6.0	0	170	2.0
multigrain, black bean, w/garlic, onion (*Kettle* Organic)	120	3.0	16.0	6.0	0	85	2.0
multigrain, 5 grain (*Kettle* Organic) .	140	2.0	18.0	6.0	0	80	2.0
mini strips or rounds (*Garden of Eatin'*)	140	2.0	19.0	6.0	0	60	2.0
w/mixed grains (*Garden of Eatin' Garden Grains*) ..	140	2.0	18.0	7.0	0	70	2.0
lime, hint of (*Tostitos*)	140	2.0	19.0	6.0	0	160	1.0
pico de gallo (*Garden of Eatin'*)	140	2.0	18.0	7.0	0	150	3.0
ranch (*Doritos* Cool Natural)	140	2.0	18.0	7.0	0	200	1.0
ranch (*Doritos Cooler Ranch*) ..	140	2.0	18.0	7.0	0	170	1.0

Food and Measure	cal.	prot. (gms)	carbo. (gms)	fat (gms)	chol. (mgs)	sod. (mgs)	fiber (gms)
Corn crisps/chips, tortilla *(cont.)*							
ranch (*Doritos Cooler Ranch Baked!*)	120	2.0	21.0	3.5	0	200	2.0
ranch (*Doritos Edge*)	150	9.0	9.0	9.0	0	240	3.0
ranch (*Doritos Rollitos Cooler Ranch*)	140	2.0	17.0	8.0	0	250	1.0
salsa (*Doritos*)	140	3.0	17.0	7.0	0	170	1.0
salsa verde (*Doritos*)	140	2.0	19.0	7.0	0	210	1.0
sesame rye, w/caraway (*Kettle* Organic) .	140	3.0	17.0	6.0	0	80	2.0
taco (*Doritos*)	140	2.0	18.0	7.0	0	170	1.0
taco (*Doritos Rollitos* Zesty) ..	150	2.0	17.0	8.0	0	140	1.0
tamari (*Garden of Eatin'*)	140	2.0	18.0	7.0	0	160	3.0
veggie (*Cape Cod Whole Earth*) ...	140	2.0	18.0	6.0	0	110	1.0
tortilla, blue corn:							
(*Garden of Eatin'*) .	140	2.0	18.0	7.0	0	60	2.0
(*Garden of Eatin'* No Salt)	140	2.0	18.0	7.0	0	10	2.0
(*Garden of Eatin' Little Soy Blues*) .	140	3.0	17.0	7.0	0	70	2.0
(*Garden of Eatin' Red Hot Blues*) ..	140	2.0	18.0	7.0	0	150	2.0
(*Garden of Eatin' Sesame Blues*) ..	150	3.0	16.0	8.0	0	90	2.0
(*Garden of Eatin' Sunny Blues*) ...	150	2.0	17.0	8.0	0	70	2.0
(*Guiltless Gourmet*)	110	3.0	22.0	2.0	0	160	2.0
(*Kettle* Organic) ...	140	3.0	18.0	6.0	0	80	2.0
(*Snyder's* Organic) .	140	2.0	17.0	7.0	0	120	n.a.
(*Tostitos* Natural) ..	140	2.0	19.0	6.0	0	80	1.0
black bean, spicy (*Guiltless Gourmet*)	110	3.0	22.0	2.0	0	200	2.0
sesame (*Cape Cod Whole Earth*) ...	150	2.0	19.0	7.0	0	110	2.0
sesame (*Kettle* Blue Moons Organic) .	150	3.0	19.0	8.0	0	80	2.0

Food and Measure	cal.	prot. (gms)	carbo. (gms)	fat (gms)	chol. (mgs)	sod. (mgs)	fiber (gms)
sesame (*Snyder's* Organic)	140	2.0	17.0	7.0	0	115	n.a.
tortilla, red corn:							
(*Garden of Eatin'*) .	140	2.0	18.0	7.0	0	70	1.0
(*Guiltless Gourmet*)	110	3.0	22.0	2.0	0	160	2.0
salsa (*Garden of Eatin'*)	140	2.0	18.0	7.0	0	170	3.0
tortilla, yellow corn:							
(*Garden of Eatin'*) .	140	2.0	18.0	7.0	0	70	2.0
(*Garden of Eatin'* Mini Rounds) ...	140	2.0	18.0	7.0	0	60	2.0
(*Guiltless Gourmet*)	110	3.0	22.0	2.0	0	160	2.0
(*Guiltless Gourmet* Unsalted)	110	2.0	22.0	1.0	0	26	2.0
(*Kettle Little Dippers* Organic)	140	2.0	19.0	6.0	0	80	2.0
(*Santitas*)	130	2.0	19.0	6.0	0	110	1.0
(*Snyder's*)	140	2.0	23.0	4.5	0	135	1.0
(*Tostitos* Natural) ..	140	2.0	19.0	6.0	0	80	1.0
(*Tostitos* Santa Fe) .	140	1.0	20.0	6.0	0	80	1.0
black bean (*Garden of Eatin'*)	140	3.0	18.0	7.0	0	70	4.0
black bean chili (*Garden of Eatin'*)	140	3.0	17.0	7.0	0	130	4.0
cheese, nacho (*Garden of Eatin'*)	140	2.0	18.0	6.0	0	140	2.0
chili verde (*Guiltless Gourmet*)	120	2.0	22.0	2.0	0	200	2.0
chipotle (*Guiltless Gourmet*)	120	2.0	22.0	2.0	0	200	2.0
Corn dogs, see "Frankfurter, wrapped"							
Corn flake crumbs (*Kellogg's*), 2 tbsp. .	40	1.0	9.0	0	0	80	0
Corn flour:							
(*Shiloh Farms*), ¼ cup	130	2.4	27.0	1.4	0	0	5.0
whole-grain, 1 oz. ...	102	2.0	21.8	1.1	0	1	3.8
whole-grain, 1 cup ...	422	8.1	89.9	4.5	0	6	15.7
masa, 1 oz.	103	2.6	21.6	1.1	0	1	2.7
masa, 1 cup	416	10.7	87.0	4.3	0	6	10.9
Corn fritters, frozen (*Delta Pride*), 3 pcs.	160	2.0	19.0	9.0	0	85	0
Corn grits, ¼ cup:							
(*Quaker* Quick)	130	3.0	29.0	.5	0	0	2.0

Food and Measure	cal.	prot. (gms)	carbo. (gms)	fat (gms)	chol. (mgs)	sod. (mgs)	fiber (gms)
Corn grits *(cont.)*							
white (*Arrowhead Mills*)	150	3.0	33.0	0	0	0	1.0
yellow (*Arrowhead Mills*)	130	3.0	30.0	0	0	0	1.0
Corn relish (*Mrs. Renfro's*), 1 tbsp.	15	0	4.0	0	0	45	0
Corn soufflé, frozen (*Stouffer's*), ½ cup	170	5.0	21.0	7.0	55	480	1.0
Corn syrup, 2 tbsp.:							
dark (*Karo*)	120	0	31.0	0	0	45	0
light (*Karo*)	120	0	31.0	0	0	35	0
Cornichon, see "Pickle"							
Cornish hen, roasted:							
meat w/skin, 4 oz.	295	25.3	0	20.7	149	73	0
meat only, 4 oz.	152	26.4	0	4.4	120	71	0
Cornish hen, frozen or refrigerated, whole:							
raw, w/out giblets (*Tyson*), 4 oz.	200	19.0	0	14.0	130	65	0
cooked, 3 oz.:							
dark (*Perdue*)	200	17.0	0	14.0	125	55	0
light (*Perdue*)	160	21.0	0	8.0	100	40	0
Cornmeal (see also "Corn flour" and "Polenta"):							
(*Goya* Fine), 3 tbsp.	100	2.0	23.0	0	0	0	1.0
blue (*Arrowhead Mills*), ⅓ cup	130	3.0	25.0	1.5	0	0	5.0
white, stone ground (*Hodgson Mill*), <¼ cup	100	3.0	22.0	1.0	0	0	3.0
yellow:							
(*Arrowhead Mills*), ⅓ cup	120	3.0	27.0	1.0	0	0	3.0
(*Hodgson Mill*), <¼ cup	100	3.0	22.0	1.0	0	0	3.0
(*Shiloh Farms*), ¼ cup	120	3.0	27.0	1.0	0	0	3.0
self-rising (*Hodgson Mill*), <¼ cup	90	3.0	21.0	1.0	0	260	3.0
whole grain, ½ cup	221	5.0	46.9	2.2	0	21	4.5
Cornstarch:							
(*Argo*), 1 tbsp.	30	0	7.0	0	0	0	0
(*Hodgson Mill*), 2 tsp.	35	0	9.0	0	0	0	1.0

Food and Measure	cal.	prot. (gms)	carbo. (gms)	fat (gms)	chol. (mgs)	sod. (mgs)	fiber (gms)
Cottonseed flour, partially defatted, 1 cup	337	38.5	38.1	5.8	8	33	2.8
Cottonseed kernels, roasted, 1 tbsp. . . .	51	3.3	2.2	3.6	0	3	.6
Cottonseed meal, partially defatted, 1 oz.	104	13.9	10.9	1.4	0	10	<1.0
Couscous, dry, ¼ cup, except as noted:							
(*Fantastic*)	190	8.0	43.0	1.0	0	0	2.0
(*Hodgson Mills*), ⅓ cup	210	8.0	47.0	1.0	0	0	5.0
(*Marrakesh Express*), 1 cup*	220	8.0	45.0	0	0	10	1.0
(*Near East*), ⅓ cup . .	220	8.0	46.0	1.0	0	5	2.0
(*Near East*), 1 cup* . .	230	8.0	46.0	2.0	0	5	2.0
(*Shiloh Farms*)	210	7.0	43.0	0	0	5	7.0
whole wheat:							
(*Fantastic*)	210	8.0	45.0	1.0	0	0	7.0
(*Shiloh Farms*)	150	6.0	34.0	.5	0	10	8.0
whole wheat, w/flax seed/soy, ⅓ cup:							
(*Hodgson Mill*) . . .	230	10.0	48.0	2.0	0	0	6.0
garlic basil (*Hodgson Mill*) .	235	10.0	50.0	2.0	0	625	6.0
Parmesan cheese (*Hodgson Mill*) .	240	10.0	50.0	2.5	10	482	6.0
Couscous, freeze-dried, precooked (*AlpineAire*), 1 oz. .	100	3.0	20.0	0	0	0	1.0
Couscous dish, mix: basil pesto (*Fantastic*), ⅓ cup	220	7.0	41.0	2.5	0	660	3.0
broccoli and cheese:							
(*Near East*), 2 oz. . .	190	7.0	41.0	.5	0	670	3.0
(*Near East*), 1 cup*	230	8.0	42.0	3.5	10	710	3.0
chicken:							
herb (*Near East*), 2 oz.	190	7.0	42.0	.5	0	510	3.0
herb (*Near East*), 1 cup*	220	7.0	42.0	3.5	0	510	3.0
w/vegetables (*Marrakesh Express*), 1 cup* . .	190	8.0	39.0	0	0	700	2.0

Food and Measure	cal.	prot. (gms)	carbo. (gms)	fat (gms)	chol. (mgs)	sod. (mgs)	fiber (gms)
Couscous dish, mix *(cont.)*							
curry:							
(*Marrakesh Express*),							
1 cup*	190	8.0	39.0	0	0	530	2.0
(*Near East* Mediter-							
ranean), 2 oz. . . .	190	7.0	42.0	.5	0	550	3.0
(*Near East* Mediter-							
ranean), 1 cup* .	220	7.0	42.0	3.5	0	550	3.0
garlic, roasted:							
olive oil (*Fantastic*),							
⅓ cup	220	7.0	43.0	.5	0	540	3.0
olive oil (*Near East*),							
2 oz.	200	7.0	41.0	1.5	0	570	2.0
olive oil (*Near East*),							
1 cup*	230	7.0	41.0	4.5	0	570	2.0
red pepper (*Fan-*							
tastic), ⅓ cup . .	200	7.0	41.0	1.0	0	440	3.0
mango salsa (*Marra-*							
kesh Express),							
1 cup*	190	6.0	38.0	0	0	380	1.0
Moroccan pasta (*Mar-*							
rakesh Express),							
1 cup*	220	8.0	45.0	0	0	10	1.0
mushroom, wild:							
(*Marrakesh Express*),							
1 cup*	190	8.0	39.0	.5	0	510	1.0
herb (*Near East*),							
2 oz.	190	8.0	42.0	.5	0	590	3.0
herb (*Near East*),							
1 cup*	230	8.0	42.0	4.0	10	630	3.0
Parmesan:							
(*Marrakesh Express*),							
1 cup*	200	8.0	38.0	1.0	0	830	2.0
(*Near East*), 2 oz. . .	200	8.0	41.0	1.5	5	580	2.0
(*Near East*), 1 cup*	220	8.0	41.0	4.0	10	600	2.0
pine nut:							
Parmesan (*Fantastic*),							
⅓ cup	220	8.0	41.0	2.5	5	530	3.0
toasted (*Near East*),							
2 oz.	200	7.0	40.0	2.5	0	510	2.0
toasted (*Near East*),							
1 cup*	230	7.0	40.0	6.0	0	510	2.0
sun-dried tomato							
(*Marrakesh Express*),							
1 cup*	190	8.0	39.0	0	0	600	2.0

Food and Measure	cal.	prot. (gms)	carbo. (gms)	fat (gms)	chol. (mgs)	sod. (mgs)	fiber (gms)
tomato lentil:							
(*Near East*), 2 oz. . . .	190	8.0	42.0	.5	0	670	3.0
(*Near East*), 1 cup*	220	8.0	42.0	3.5	0	.670	3.0
Couscous entree,							
frozen, stew,							
w/vegetables							
(*Moosewood* Moroc-							
can), 10-oz. pkg. . . .	170	5.0	32.0	3.0	0	670	5.0
Cousins Subs:							
subs, 7½":							
BLT	613	17.0	45.0	42.0	35	917	1.0
cappacola/cheese .	637	28.0	48.0	39.0	60	1420	1.0
cappacola/Genoa . .	630	23.0	48.0	40.0	64	1680	1.0
cheese steak	540	36.0	46.0	24.0	80	1126	1.0
cheese steak, double	851	61.0	46.0	46.0	160	1593	1.0
cheese steak, Philly	680	42.0	49.0	36.0	100	1250	1.0
chicken breast	618	35.0	46.0	34.0	73	1172	1.0
chicken cheddar							
deluxe	928	48.0	46.0	61.0	148	1887	1.0
club	744	43.0	48.0	43.0	107	2004	2.0
Genoa/provolone . .	730	29.0	48.0	49.0	83	1678	1.0
gyro	680	31.0	55.0	40.0	58	1539	2.0
ham/provolone	644	28.0	47.0	39.0	67	1333	2.0
Italian, regular	683	28.0	48.0	44.0	75	1722	1.0
Italian, special	797	36.0	48.0	53.0	107	2168	1.0
meatball/provolone	586	36.0	50.0	27.0	80	1386	2.0
pepperoni melt	784	33.0	47.0	52.0	102	1803	2.0
pizza sub	771	35.0	50.0	49.0	120	2008	2.0
pork, barbecue	420	30.0	63.0	6.0	57	1809	1.0
provolone	686	25.0	46.0	45.0	63	957	2.0
roast beef	618	33.0	46.0	36.0	75	883	1.0
seafood w/crab . . .	554	15.0	53.0	32.0	20	957	1.0
tuna	832	28.0	46.0	60.0	67	939	2.0
turkey breast	559	25.0	48.0	32.0	50	1493	1.0
veggie, garden	365	20.0	49.0	11.0	30	661	2.0
veggie, hot	491	25.0	49.0	23.0	50	1100	2.0
sub, lower fat, 7½":							
BLT	358	17.0	45.0	14.0	23	802	1.0
chicken breast	363	35.0	46.0	6.0	60	1057	1.0
club	369	34.0	48.0	6.0	65	1604	2.0
ham	309	22.0	47.0	5.0	35	1028	2.0
roast beef	363	33.0	46.0	6.0	62	478	1.0
steak	420	27.0	46.0	15.0	50	550	1.0
turkey breast	304	25.0	48.0	3.0	38	1087	1.0

Food and Measure	cal.	prot. (gms)	carbo. (gms)	fat (gms)	chol. (mgs)	sod. (mgs)	fiber (gms)
Cousins Subs,* sub, lower fat, 7½" *(cont.)							
veggie, garden	245	11.0	49.0	2.0	0	376	2.0
veggie, hot	289	10.0	49.0	7.0	0	593	1.0
sub, mini, 4":							
ham, lower fat	189	12.0	30.0	3.0	17	574	1.0
ham/provolone	382	15.0	30.0	23.0	35	738	1.0
Italian, special	431	18.0	31.0	27.0	49	1089	1.0
meatballs/provolone	329	22.0	32.0	14.0	40	756	1.0
provolone	422	15.0	30.0	27.0	38	597	1.0
seafood w/crab ...	311	9.0	33.0	16.0	10	583	1.0
tuna	476	15.0	30.0	33.0	35	541	1.0
turkey breast	347	15.0	31.0	19.0	30	890	1.0
turkey breast, lower fat............	194	15.0	31.0	2.0	23	676	1.0
ciabatta sandwich:							
chicken, Sedona ...	480	35.0	36.0	23.0	87	1579	4.0
club, Tuscan	438	28.0	33.0	23.0	66	1698	2.0
pork, Cubano	592	31.0	38.0	34.0	93	1628	1.0
fries:							
large	525	7.0	72.0	24.0	21	460	1.0
medium	400	5.0	55.0	19.0	16	350	1.0
small	275	4.0	38.0	13.0	11	240	1.0
salad:							
chef	280	25.0	15.0	15.0	65	1185	3.0
chicken, Oriental sesame	263	30.0	20.0	8.0	60	828	4.0
chicken Sedona ...	312	33.0	14.0	14.0	90	1580	5.0
garden	195	10.0	14.0	13.0	25	424	3.0
garden, w/chicken .	335	35.0	15.0	17.0	85	1114	3.0
Italian	359	20.0	15.0	25.0	11	1411	3.0
seafood	440	14.0	19.0	35.0	40	865	3.0
side	103	5.0	7.0	7.0	n.a.	308	1.0
tuna	369	19.0	14.0	28.0	52	652	3.0
soup, 8 oz. regular:							
broccoli cheese ...	190	6.0	15.0	12.0	15	940	3.0
cheese	240	7.0	18.0	16.0	20	1350	2.0
chicken dumpling ..	170	11.0	19.0	5.0	50	970	3.0
chicken noodle	120	7.0	18.0	3.0	20	850	1.0
chicken rice	230	10.0	21.0	12.0	30	1210	2.0
chili	250	18.0	26.0	9.0	35	1220	14.0
clam chowder	150	8.0	19.0	5.0	10	1060	3.0
potato, cream of ..	190	5.0	24.0	9.0	5	860	3.0
tomato basil ravioli	110	4.0	22.0	1.0	10	720	1.0
vegetable beef	80	4.0	13.0	2.0	5	1010	2.0

Food and Measure	cal.	prot. (gms)	carbo. (gms)	fat (gms)	chol. (mgs)	sod. (mgs)	fiber (gms)
soup, 12 oz. large:							
broccoli cheese ...	285	9.0	23.0	18.0	23	1410	5.0
cheese	360	11.0	27.0	24.0	30	2025	3.0
chicken dumpling ..	255	17.0	29.0	8.0	75	1455	5.0
chicken noodle	180	11.0	27.0	4.0	3	1275	2.0
chicken rice	345	15.0	32.0	180	45	1815	3.0
chili	375	27.0	39.0	14.0	53	1830	21.0
clam chowder	225	12.0	29.0	8.0	15	1590	5.0
potato, cream of ..	285	8.0	36.0	14.0	8	1290	5.0
tomato basil ravioli	165	6.0	33.0	2.0	15	1080	2.0
vegetable beef	120	6.0	20.0	2.0	8	1515	3.0
breads:							
ciabatta	230	9.0	47.0	1.0	0	557	1.0
Italian, 15"	420	18.0	84.0	3.0	0	720	0
Parmesan-asiago, 15"	620	34.0	84.0	18.0	50	1196	0
wheat, 15"	420	18.0	84.0	3.0	0	900	6.0
wrap, low-carb	188	10.0	19.0	8.0	0	619	12.0
chocolate chip cookie	210	2.0	25.0	11.0	10	115	1.0
Cowpeas (see also "Black-eyed peas"), fresh, ½ cup:							
raw:							
immature seeds ...	65	2.1	13.7	.3	0	3	3.6
leafy tips, chopped .	5	.7	.9	<.1	0	1	n.a.
pods, w/seeds	21	1.6	4.5	.1	0	2	n.a.
boiled, drained:							
immature seeds ...	80	2.6	16.8	.3	0	3	4.1
leafy tips, chopped .	6	1.2	.7	0	0	2	n.a.
pods, w/seeds	16	1.2	3.3	.1	0	1	n.a.
Cowpeas, canned or frozen, see "Black-eyed peas"							
Cowpeas, catjang, see "Catjang"							
Crab, meat only, 4 oz.:							
Alaska king:							
raw	95	20.8	0	.7	47	948	0
boiled, poached, or steamed	110	21.9	0	1.7	60	1216	0
blue:							
raw	99	20.5	.1	1.2	89	332	0
boiled, poached, or steamed	116	22.9	0	2.0	113	316	0

Food and Measure	cal.	prot. (gms)	carbo. (gms)	fat (gms)	chol. (mgs)	sod. (mgs)	fiber (gms)
Crab *(cont.)*							
Dungeness:							
raw	98	19.8	.8	1.1	67	335	0
boiled, poached, or							
steamed	125	25.3	1.1	1.4	86	429	0
queen:							
raw	102	21.0	0	1.4	62	611	0
boiled, poached, or							
steamed	130	26.9	0	1.7	81	784	0
Crab, canned, 2 oz.,							
except as noted:							
w/leg meat (*Brunswick*)	40	9.0	1.0	1.0	50	240	0
lump (*Brunswick*) . . .	45	9.0	1.0	.5	50	350	0
lump, regular, or leg							
meat (*Yankee*							
Clipper)	40	7.0	2.0	0	40	400	0
lump, jumbo, or claw							
(*Orleans*)	40	8.0	0	1.0	50	300	0
pink (*Bumble Bee*) . . .	35	7.0	0	.5	50	300	0
white lump:							
(*Bumble Bee/Orleans*)	40	8.0	0	1.0	50	300	0
(*Crown Prince*) . . .	45	10.0	1.0	0	50	210	0
"Crab," imitation,							
frozen, ½ cup, 3 oz.,							
except as noted:							
chunk, flake, or leg							
style (*Louis Kemp*							
Crab Delights)	80	8.0	11.0	0	10	470	0
shredded (*Louis Kemp*							
Crab Delights Easy							
Shreds)	80	7.0	13.0	0	5	620	0
from surimi, 1 oz. . . .	29	3.4	3.0	.4	6	238	0
Crab apple, fresh:							
(*Frieda's*), 5 oz.	110	1.0	28.0	0	0	0	1.0
1 oz.	22	.1	5.7	.1	0	<1	.3
sliced, ½ cup	42	.2	11.0	.2	0	1	.6
Crab apple, spiced, in							
jars (*Lucky Leaf/*							
Musselman's), 1 pc.	35	0	8.0	0	0	15	1.0
Crab cake, frozen:							
(*Nancy's* Seafood),							
6 pcs., 3 oz.	180	18.0	16.0	10.0	75	600	1.0
deviled, breaded (*Mrs.*							
Paul's), 2.9-oz. pc. .	220	20.0	12.0	12.0	60	390	3.0

Food and Measure	cal.	prot. (gms)	carbo. (gms)	fat (gms)	chol. (mgs)	sod. (mgs)	fiber (gms)
Maryland style:							
(*Mrs. Friday's*), 2.25-oz. pc.	140	7.0	7.0	10.0	15	570	0
(*Phillips*), 3-oz. pc.	160	12.0	7.0	10.0	85	560	<1.0
mini (*Yankee Trader*), 6 pcs., 2.5 oz. ..	150	7.0	8.0	9.0	23	429	1.0
Crab cake seasoning (*Old Bay* Classic), 1/6 pkg.	30	0	2.0	1.0	30	290	0
Crab spread, w/jalapeños (*Sau-Sea*), 2 tbsp. .	70	1.0	1.0	8.0	15	85	0
Cracker (see also "Snack chips):							
(*Barbara's* Rite Lite Rounds Original), 5 pcs., .5 oz.	60	1.0	11.0	2.0	0	200	0
(*Bremner* Cracker), 7 pcs., .5 oz.	60	1.0	10.0	1.5	0	120	0
(*Bremner* Wafer), 7 pcs. .5 oz.	70	2.0	11.0	1.5	0	105	0
(*Bremner* Wafer Low Sodium), 7 pcs., .5 oz.	70	2.0	12.0	1.5	0	10	0
(*Goldfish* Original), 55 pcs., 1.1 oz. ...	150	3.0	20.0	6.0	0	230	<1.0
(*Lavosh-Hawaii* Classic/ Bite Size), 1 oz. ...	120	3.0	19.0	3.0	21	290	1.0
(*Munch'ems* Original), 41 pcs., 1.1 oz. ...	140	2.0	21.0	5.0	0	220	1.0
(*Sabrosas*), 11 pcs., 1.1 oz.	150	2.0	20.0	6.0	0	190	0
bacon (*Nabisco* Baked), 1.1 oz.	160	2.0	19.0	8.0	0	430	2.0
bruschetta vegetable:							
(*Health Valley*), 6 pcs., .5 oz. ...	60	2.0	10.0	1.5	0	140	1.0
(*Health Valley* No Salt), 6 pcs., .5 oz.	60	2.0	10.0	1.5	0	40	1.0
butter/butter flavor:							
(*Keebler Club* Low Salt), 4 pcs., .5 oz.	70	1.0	9.0	3.0	0	80	0
(*Keebler Club* Original), 4 pcs., .5 oz.	70	1.0	9.0	3.0	0	140	0

Food and Measure	cal.	prot. (gms)	carbo. (gms)	fat (gms)	chol. (mgs)	sod. (mgs)	fiber (gms)
Cracker, butter/butter flavor *(cont.)*							
(*Keebler Club* Reduced Fat), 5 pcs., .6 oz.	70	1.0	12.0	2.0	0	200	0
(*Ritz* Low Sodium), 5 pcs., .6 oz. . . .	80	1.0	10.0	4.0	0	35	0
(*Ritz* Original), 5 pcs., .6 oz.	80	1.0	10.0	4.0	0	135	0
(*Ritz* Reduced Fat), 5 pcs., .5 oz. . . .	70	1.0	11.0	2.0	0	150	0
(*Ritz* Sticks), 1.1 oz.	150	2.0	19.0	7.0	0	280	1.0
(*Ritz* Top'ems), .5 oz.	70	1.0	10.0	3.0	0	150	0
(*Sara Lee* Country), 7 pcs., 1.1 oz. . .	140	2.0	20.0	6.0	0	340	<1.0
(*Toasteds* Buttercrisp), 5 pcs., .6 oz. . . .	80	1.0	10.0	3.5	0	150	0
(*Town House* Low Salt), 5 pcs., .6 oz.	80	1.0	10.0	4.5	0	75	<1.0
(*Town House* Original), 5 pcs., .6 oz.	80	1.0	9.0	4.5	0	150	<1.0
(*Town House* Reduced Fat), 6 pcs., .5 oz.	70	1.0	11.0	2.0	0	180	<1.0
(*Tree of Life* Golden Classic), 5 pcs., .5 oz.	60	1.0	12.0	<1.0	0	220	0
garlic (*Ritz*), .6 oz. .	80	1.0	10.0	4.0	0	150	0
thins (*Pepperidge Farm*), 4 pcs., .5 oz.	70	1.0	10.0	3.0	10	95	0
wheat (*Town House*), 5 pcs., .6 oz. . . .	80	1.0	9.0	4.5	0	230	<1.0
caraway (*Bremner* Wafer), 7 pcs., .5 oz	70	2.0	11.0	1.5	0	105	0
cheese:							
(*Barbara's* Cheese Bites), 22 pcs., 1 oz.	120	3.0	20.0	3.0	<5	380	<1.0
(*Cheese Nips* Big), 1 oz.	140	3.0	18.0	7.0	0	320	1.0
(*Cheez-It* Big), 13 pcs., 1.1 oz. .	160	4.0	18.0	8.0	0	250	<1.0
(*Cheez-It* Original), 27 pcs., 1.1 oz. .	160	4.0	18.0	8.0	0	250	<1.0

Food and Measure	cal.	prot. (gms)	carbo. (gms)	fat (gms)	chol. (mgs)	sod. (mgs)	fiber (gms)
(*Cheez-It* Reduced Fat), 29 pcs., 1.1 oz.	130	4.0	20.0	4.5	0	360	<1.0
(*Cheez-It Twisterz* Hot Wings Cheesy Blue), 17 pcs., 1.1 oz.	140	2.0	19.0	6.0	0	280	<1.0
(*Doritos Nacho Cheesier Golden Toast*), 1 pkg. . .	240	4.0	25.0	14.0	<5	390	1.0
(*Pepperidge Farm* Snack Sticks), 25 pcs., 1.1 oz. .	150	3.0	20.0	6.0	<5	380	<1.0
colors (*Goldfish*), 55 pcs., 1.1 oz. .	140	4.0	20.0	5.0	5	260	<1.0
four (*Cheese Nips*), 1.1 oz.	150	3.0	19.0	7.0	5	300	1.0
four (*Goldfish* Crisps), 37 pcs., 1.1 oz. . .	150	3.0	18.0	7.0	<5	320	<1.0
hot and spicy (*Cheez-It*), 26 pcs., 1.1 oz.	150	4.0	17.0	8.0	0	300	<1.0
hot and spicy (*Goldfish* Explosive), 51 pcs., 1.1 oz. .	150	3.0	17.0	7.0	<5	310	1.0
jalapeño (*Doritos Golden Toast*), 1 pkg.	230	3.0	26.0	13.0	<5	450	1.0
sour cream and onion (*Cheez-It*), 25 pcs., 1.1 oz. .	150	3.0	19.0	7.0	0	250	0
cheese, cheddar:							
(*Annie's* Bunnies), 1.1 oz., 50 pcs. .	150	3.0	19.0	7.0	<5	250	1.0
(*Austin Dolphins & Friends*), 60 pcs., 1.1 oz.	140	3.0	20.0	6.0	<5	270	<1.0
(*Better Cheddars*), 22 pcs., 1.1 oz. .	150	3.0	18.0	7.0	5	350	1.0
(*Better Cheddars* Reduced Fat), 24 pcs., 1.1 oz. .	140	3.0	20.0	5.0	5	320	3.0
(*Cheese Nips* Mini Go Pack), 1.1 oz.	150	3.0	19.0	6.0	0	340	1.0

Food and Measure	cal.	prot. (gms)	carbo. (gms)	fat (gms)	chol. (mgs)	sod. (mgs)	fiber (gms)
Cracker, cheese, cheddar *(cont.)*							
(*Cheese Nips* Reduced Fat),							
31 pcs., 1.1 oz. .	130	3.0	21.0	3.5	0	310	1.0
(*Cheetos Golden Toast*), 1 pkg. . .	240	4.0	25.0	14.0	5	440	1.0
(*Cheez-It Twisterz*),							
17 pcs.,. 1.1 oz. .	140	2.0	19.0	6.0	0	270	<1.0
(*Goldfish*), 55 pcs.,							
1.1 oz.	140	4.0	20.0	5.0	<5	250	<1.0
(*Goldfish* Baby),							
89 pcs., 1.1 oz. .	150	3.0	19.0	6.0	<5	250	<1.0
(*Goldfish* Giant),							
14 pcs., 1.1 oz. .	140	3.0	19.0	6.0	<5	230	1.0
(*Munch'ems*),							
39 pcs., 1.1 oz. .	140	3.0	19.0	6.0	0	380	1.0
(*TLC* Country),							
18 pcs., 1.1 oz. .	130	3.0	20.0	4.5	0	220	<1.0
(*Triscuit*), 1 oz. . . .	120	3.0	19.0	4.5	0	220	3.0
barbecue (*Annie's* Bunnies), 1.1 oz.,							
50 pcs.	130	3.0	18.0	6.0	0	250	2.0
barbecue (*Cheez-It*),							
25 pcs., 1.1 oz. .	150	3.0	17.0	8.0	0	300	<1.0
extra (*Goldfish*),							
51 pc., 1.1 oz. . .	140	3.0	18.0	6.0	<5	250	1.0
Jack (*Cheez-It*),							
26 pcs., 1.1 oz. .	160	3.0	18.0	8.0	0	260	0
jalapeño (*Cheese Nips*), 1.1 oz.	150	3.0	19.0	7.0	0	300	1.0
ranch (*Annie's* Bunnies), 1.1 oz.,							
50 pcs.	130	3.0	17.0	6.0	0	250	2.0
salsa (*Cheese Nips*),							
1.1 oz.	150	2.0	19.0	7.0	0	270	1.0
white (*Cheez-It*),							
26 pcs., 1.1 oz. .	150	3.0	18.0	7.0	<5	280	<1.0
whole wheat (*Annie's* Bunnies), 1.1 oz.,							
50 pcs.	130	3.0	17.0	6.0	0	250	3.0
cheese sandwich:							
(*Austin* Bite Size),							
14 pcs., 1.1 oz. .	160	2.0	17.0	9.0	<5	280	0

Food and Measure	cal.	prot. (gms)	carbo. (gms)	fat (gms)	chol. (mgs)	sod. (mgs)	fiber (gms)
(*Pepperidge Farm Mini*), 1-oz. pkg.	150	3.0	18.0	7.0	<5	270	<1.0
(*Ritz Bits*), 1.1 oz.	160	2.0	18.0	9.0	5	280	0
(*Ritz Bits*), 1.5-oz. pkg.	230	3.0	25.0	13.0	5	390	1.0
American/mozzarella (*Ritz Bits*), 1.1 oz.	150	2.0	17.0	9.0	5	300	0
cheddar on wheat (*Austin*), 1.4-oz. pkg.	200	3.0	24.0	10.0	<5	330	<1.0
w/cheddar Jack (*Austin*), 1.4-oz. pkg.	200	3.0	23.0	10.0	<5	330	<1.0
grilled cheese (*Austin*), 1.4-oz. pkg.	200	3.0	23.0	10.0	<5	400	<1.0
jalapeño cheddar (*Ritz Bits*), 1.1 oz.	160	2.0	17.0	10.0	5	340	0
chicken flavor (*Chicken in a Bisket*), 12 pcs., 1.1 oz.	170	2.0	18.0	10.0	0	280	1.0
corn bread:							
(*Town House Bistro*), 2 pcs., .6 oz. ...	80	1.0	11.0	3.0	0	105	<1.0
bell pepper (*Health Valley*), 4 pcs., .5 oz.	60	1.0	11.0	1.5	0	150	1.0
butter (*Health Valley*), 4 pcs., .5 oz. ...	60	1.0	11.0	1.5	0	160	1.0
honey (*Health Valley*), 4 pcs., .5 oz. ...	60	1.0	11.0	1.5	0	140	1.0
cream cheese and chive wafer sandwich (*Austin*), 1 pkg. ...	190	3.0	24.0	10.0	<5	370	<1.0
croissant (*Carr's*), 3 pcs., .5 oz.	70	1.0	10.0	3.0	<5	115	0
flatbread:							
chive garlic (*Margaret's Artisan*), .9-oz. pc.	110	3.0	18.0	3.0	0	75	<1.0
garlic and herb, bite size (*Tree of Life* Fat Free), 12 pcs., .5 oz.	50	1.0	12.0	0	0	80	0

Food and Measure	cal.	prot. (gms)	carbo. (gms)	fat (gms)	chol. (mgs)	sod. (mgs)	fiber (gms)
Cracker *(cont.)*							
graham cracker, see "Cookie"							
herb:							
garden (*Health Valley*), 6 pcs., .5 oz.	60	2.0	10.0	1.5	0	140	1.0
and garlic (*Tree of Life*), 10 pcs., 1.1 oz. ...,...	120	2.0	22.0	2.5	0	220	1.0
matzo, 1.1-oz. pc.:							
(*Manischewitz*)	120	3.0	27.0	0	0	0	1.0
(*Streit's*)	110	3.0	25.0	0	0	0	1.0
multigrain:							
(*Town House Bistro*), 2 pcs., .6 oz. ...	80	1.0	11.0	3.0	0	180	<1.0
(*Wheat Thins*), 17 pcs., 1.1 oz. .	130	3.0	21.0	4.5	0	230	2.0
5 grain (*Harvest Crisps*), 1.1 oz. .	140	3.0	23.0	3.5	0	240	1.0
7 grain (*TLC*), 15 pcs., 1.1 oz. .	130	3.0	22.0	3.0	0	160	2.0
7 grain (*Wheatables*), 17 pcs., 1.1 oz. .	140	2.0	20.0	6.0	0	320	1.0
10 grain (*Lavosh-Hawaii*), 1 oz.	110	1.0	19.0	3.0	0	300	3.0
onion:							
(*Toasteds*), 5 pcs., .6 oz.	80	1.0	10.0	3.0	0	150	0
French (*Health Valley*), 10 pcs., .5 oz.	60	2.0	10.0	1.5	0	140	1.0
slightly (*Lavosh-Hawaii*), 1 oz.	120	3.0	19.0	3.0	21	300	1.0
toasted (*Tree of Life*), 10 pcs., 1.1 oz. .	120	2.0	22.0	2.5	0	210	1.0
Parmesan:							
(*Goldfish*), 60 pcs., 1.1 oz.	140	4.0	19.0	6.0	<5	300	<1.0
and garlic (*Cheez-It*), 26 pcs., 1.1 oz. .	150	3.0	19.0	7.0	0	240	0
peanut butter sandwich:							
(*Austin* PB & J), 1.4-oz. pkg.	200	3.0	24.0	10.0	0	300	<1.0

Food and Measure	cal.	prot. (gms)	carbo. (gms)	fat (gms)	chol. (mgs)	sod. (mgs)	fiber (gms)
(*Pepperidge Farm* Mini), 1-oz. pkg.	130	3.0	18.0	5.0	0	270	<1.0
(*Ritz Bits*), 1.25-oz. pkg.	180	3.0	21.0	9.0	0	270	1.0
(*Ritz Bits* 9.5 oz.), 1 oz.	140	3.0	16.0	8.0	0	240	1.0
cheese (*Cheese Nips*), 1.4-oz. pkg.	190	4.0	23.0	8.0	0	350	1.0
cheese (*Frito Lay*), 1 pkg.	210	5.0	23.0	10.0	0	350	1.0
toast (*Austin* Toasty), 1.4-oz. pkg.	200	4.0	23.0	10.0	0	370	1.0
toast (*Frito Lay*), 1 pkg.	210	5.0	23.0	11.0	0	280	1.0
pepper, cracked: (*Health Valley*), 5 pcs., .5 oz. ...	60	2.0	10.0	1.5	0	140	1.0
(*Tree of Life*), 10 pcs., 1.1 oz.	120	3.0	23.0	2.0	0	135	<1.0
bite size (*Tree of Life* Fat Free), 12 pcs., .5 oz.	50	1.0	12.0	0	0	80	0
peppercorn (*Lavosh-Hawaii*), 1 oz.	115	3.0	20.0	3.0	21	300	1.0
pizza: (*Goldfish*), 55 pcs., 1.1 oz.	150	3.0	19.0	7.0	0	180	2.0
(*Goldfish* Explosive), 51 pcs., 1.1 oz. .	140	3.0	19.0	6.0	0	240	1.0
poppy seed, savory (*Barbara's* Rite Lite Rounds), 5 pcs., .5 oz.	60	1.0	11.0	0	0	200	0
pumpernickel (*Pepperidge Farm* Snack Sticks), 15 pcs., 1 oz.	120	4.0	22.0	1.5	0	380	2.0
ranch: (*Munch'ems*), 39 pcs., 1.1 oz.	140	3.0	20.0	5.0	0	240	1.0
(*TLC* Natural), 15 pcs., 1.1 oz.	130	3.0	22.0	3.0	0	200	2.0
rice, brown: (*Eden*), 1.1 oz.	120	3.0	22.0	2.0	0	230	2.0

Food and Measure	cal.	prot. (gms)	carbo. (gms)	fat (gms)	chol. (mgs)	sod. (mgs)	fiber (gms)
Cracker, rice, brown *(cont.)*							
(*Westbrae Natural Wafers No Salt*), 7 pcs., .5 oz. . . .	50	1.0	11.0	.5	0	0	0
nori maki (*Eden*), 15 pcs., 1.1 oz. . .	110	3.0	24.0	0	0	160	2.0
sesame (*San-J*), 5 pcs., 1 oz.	130	3.0	19.0	5.0	0	170	1.0
sesame (*Westbrae Natural* Wafers), 7 pcs., .5 oz. . . .	50	1.0	11.0	0	0	70	0
sesame, black (*San-J*), 5 pcs., 1 oz.	140	4.0	17.0	6.0	0	180	1.0
tamari (*San-J*), 6 pcs., 1.1 oz.	120	3.0	26.0	1.0	0	170	1.0
tamari or 5-spice (*Westbrae Natural* Wafers), 7 pcs., .5 oz.	50	1.0	11.0	0	0	65	0
rice bran (*Health Valley*), 6 pcs., 1 oz.	110	3.0	19.0	3.0	0	70	3.0
rosemary:							
(*Carr's*), 7 pcs., 1 oz.	130	2.0	19.0	5.0	0	230	<1.0
garlic (*Lavosh-Hawaii*), 1 oz. . . .	125	3.0	19.0	3.0	21	230	1.0
rye:							
(*Town House Bistro*), 2 pcs., .6 oz. . . .	80	1.0	10.0	3.5	0	160	<1.0
(*Triscuit* Deli Style), 1 oz.	120	3.0	19.0	4.5	0	150	3.0
caraway (*Lavosh-Hawaii*), 1 oz. . . .	115	3.0	20.0	3.0	21	300	1.0
saltines, 5 pcs., .5 oz.:							
(*Krispy* Original) . . .	60	1.0	11.0	1.5	0	190	<1.0
(*Premium* Fat Free)	60	1.0	12.0	0	0	170	0
(*Premium* Gold) . . .	70	1.0	10.0	3.0	0	160	0
(*Premium* Low Sodium)	60	1.0	10.0	1.5	0	35	0
(*Premium* Original)	70	1.0	11.0	2.0	0	220	0
(*Premium* Original 4 oz.)	60	1.0	10.0	1.5	0	180	0
(*Premium* Unsalted Top)	70	1.0	11.0	2.0	0	115	0
(*Zesta* Fat Free) . . .	60	1.0	13.0	0	0	250	0

Food and Measure	cal.	prot. (gms)	carbo. (gms)	fat (gms)	chol. (mgs)	sod. (mgs)	fiber (gms)
(*Zesta* Original) ...	60	1.0	11.0	1.5	0	170	0
(*Zesta* Reduced Sodium)	60	1.0	11.0	1.5	0	75	0
(*Zesta* Unsalted Top)	60	1.0	11.0	1.5	0	60	0
w/multigrain (*Premium*)	60	1.0	10.0	1.5	0	150	0
whole wheat (*Krispy*)	60	1.0	11.0	1.5	0	230	<1.0
whole wheat (*Zesta*)	60	1.0	11.0	1.5	0	230	<1.0
savory (*Sociables*), 7 pcs., .5 oz.	70	1.0	9.0	3.5	0	140	1.0
sesame:							
(*Bremner* Wafer), 7 pcs., .5 oz. ...	70	2.0	11.0	2.0	0	105	0
(*Health Valley*), 5 pcs., .5 oz. ...	60	2.0	10.0	1.5	0	140	1.0
(*Pepperidge Farm* Snack Sticks), 12 pcs., 1.1 oz. .	140	3.0	20.0	6.0	0	380	1.0
(*Toasteds*), 5 pcs., .6 oz.	80	1.0	10.0	4.0	0	135	<1.0
cheese sticks (*Twigs*), 1.1 oz.	150	3.0	18.0	7.0	0	270	3.0
and flax seed (*Tree of Life*), 10 pcs., 1.1 oz.	140	3.0	23.0	4.0	0	230	1.0
honey (*TLC*), 15 pcs., 1.1 oz.	130	3.0	22.0	3.0	0	160	2.0
tamari (*Barbara's* Rite Lite Rounds), 5 pcs., .5 oz. ...	70	1.0	10.0	2.0	0	200	0
soda/water:							
(*Carr's Table Water*), 5 pcs., .6 oz. ...	70	2.0	13.0	1.5	0	100	<1.0
(*Wellington* Traditional), 4 pcs., .5 oz.	60	2.0	12.0	1.0	0	75	0
assorted (*Carr's* Biscuits for Cheese), 2 pcs., .4 oz. ...	50	1.0	8.0	2.0	<5	85	<1.0
cracked pepper (*Carr's Table Water*), 5 pcs., .6 oz.	70	2.0	13.0	1.5	0	100	<1.0

Food and Measure	cal.	prot. (gms)	carbo. (gms)	fat (gms)	chol. (mgs)	sod. (mgs)	fiber (gms)
Cracker, soda/water *(cont.)*							
cracked pepper trio (*Sara Lee*), 7 pcs., 1.1 oz.	130	3.0	22.0	4.0	0	270	<1.0
garlic, roasted (*Carr's Table Water*), 5 pcs., .6 oz. . . .	70	2.0	12.0	1.5	0	140	<1.0
poppy and sesame (*Carr's*), 4 pcs., .6 oz.	80	2.0	9.0	5.0	<5	135	<1.0
soup/oyster, .5 oz.:							
(*Bremner* Oyster Cracker), 50 pcs.	60	1.0	10.0	1.0	0	130	0
(*Bremner* Soup/Chili Cracker), 50 pcs.	60	2.0	11.0	1.5	0	110	0
(*Krispy*), 17 pcs. . .	70	2.0	12.0	1.5	0	240	0
(*Premium*), 23 pcs.	60	1.0	11.0	1.5	0	170	0
(*Zesta*), 45 pcs. . . .	70	1.0	10.0	3.0	0	140	0
sour cream and onion:							
(*Goldfish* Crisps), 37 pcs., 1.1 oz. .	150	3.0	17.0	7.0	<5	360	<1.0
(*Munch'ems*), 39 pcs., 1.1 oz. .	140	3.0	20.0	5.0	0	270	1.0
Swiss cheese (*Nabisco* Baked), 1 oz.	140	2.0	18.0	7.0	0	360	2.0
tomato (*Garden* Savory), 4 pcs., .5 oz.	70	1.0	9.0	3.5	0	170	0
vegetable:							
(*Sara Lee* Harvest), 6 pcs., 1 oz.	140	2.0	19.0	6.0	0	350	<1.0
(*Vegetable Thins* Baked), 14 pcs., 1.1 oz.	160	2.0	19.0	9.0	0	360	2.0
garden (*Harvest Crisps*), 1.1 oz. .	130	2.0	22.0	3.5	0	230	1.0
garden (*Tree of Life*), 10 pcs., 1.1 oz. . .	120	3.0	22.0	2.5	0	250	<1.0
garden, bite size (*Tree of Life* Fat Free), 12 pcs., .5 oz.	50	1.0	12.0	0	0	80	0
wheat:							
(*Pepperidge Farm* Hearty), 3 pcs., .5 oz.	80	2.0	10.0	3.5	0	100	1.0

Food and Measure	cal.	prot. (gms)	carbo. (gms)	fat (gms)	chol. (mgs)	sod. (mgs)	fiber (gms)
(*Pepperidge Farm* Snack Sticks), 30 pcs., 1.1 oz. .	130	3.0	22.0	3.5	0	370	1.0
(*Toasteds*), 5 pcs., .6 oz.	80	1.0	10.0	3.5	0	150	<1.0
(*Wheat Thins* Big), 11 pcs., 1.1 oz. .	150	2.0	21.0	6.0	0	260	1.0
(*Wheat Thins* Low Sodium), 16 pcs., 1.1 oz.	150	3.0	21.0	6.0	0	80	1.0
(*Wheat Thins* Original), 16 pcs., 1.1 oz.	150	3.0	21.0	6.0	0	270	1.0
(*Wheatables* Original), 19 pcs., 1.1 oz. .	140	2.0	20.0	6.0	0	300	1.0
(*Wheatables* Reduced Fat), 19 pcs., 1.1 oz.	140	3.0	22.0	4.0	0	220	2.0
(*Wheatsworth*), 5 pcs., .6 oz. . . .	80	2.0	10.0	3.5	0	170	1.0
cracked (*Bremner* Wafer), 7 pcs., .5 oz.	70	2.0	11.0	1.5	0	100	0
golden (*Sara Lee*), 6 pcs., 1 oz.	140	3.0	18.0	6.0	0	210	1.0
honey (*Wheat Thins*), 1.1 oz.	150	2.0	21.0	6.0	0	260	1.0
honey (*Wheatables*), 17 pcs., 1.1 oz. .	140	2.0	20.0	6.0	0	290	1.0
ranch (*Wheat Thins*), 1 oz.	140	2.0	19.0	6.0	0	220	1.0
stoned (*Health Valley* Low Fat), 5 pcs., .5 oz.	60	1.0	10.0	1.0	0	140	1.0
stoned (*Red Oval Farms*), 2 pcs., .5 oz.	60	2.0	10.0	1.5	0	140	1.0
stoned (*Red Oval Farms* Lower Sodium), 2 pcs., .5 oz.	60	2.0	10.0	1.5	0	70	1.0
wheat, whole: (*Barbara's Wheatines*), 4 pcs., .5 oz. . . .	60	1.0	11.0	1.0	0	80	<1.0

Food and Measure	cal.	prot. (gms)	carbo. (gms)	fat (gms)	chol. (mgs)	sod. (mgs)	fiber (gms)
Cracker, wheat, whole *(cont.)*							
(*Carr's*), 2 pcs., .6 oz.	80	1.0	11.0	3.5	0	100	1.0
(*Health Valley*), 6 pcs., .5 oz. ...	60	2.0	10.0	1.5	0	140	2.0
(*Ritz*), 5 pcs., .5 oz.	70	1.0	11.0	2.5	0	125	1.0
(*Triscuit* Low Sodium), 1 oz.	130	3.0	19.0	5.0	0	50	3.0
(*Triscuit* Original), 1 oz.	120	3.0	19.0	4.5	0	180	3.0
(*Triscuit* Reduced Fat), 1 oz.	120	3.0	21.0	3.0	0	160	3.0
(*Triscuit Thin Crisps*), 15 pcs., 1.1 oz. .	130	3.0	21.0	5.0	0	180	3.0
cracked pepper (*Barbara's Wheatines*), 4 pcs., .5 oz.	50	1.0	11.0	1.0	0	120	1.0
garlic, roasted (*Triscuit*), 1 oz. .	120	3.0	20.0	4.5	0	140	3.0
herb, garden (*Triscuit*), 1 oz. .	120	3.0	20.0	4.0	0	125	3.0
zwieback (*Nabisco*), .3-oz. pc.	35	1.0	6.0	1.0	0	10	0
Cracker meal, ¼ cup:							
(*Golden Dipt* Fry Easy)	130	2.0	23.0	1.0	0	10	0
(*Nabisco*)	110	3.0	22.0	0	0	15	1.0
matzo meal:							
(*Manischewitz*) ...	130	3.0	23.0	0	0	0	1.0
(*Streit's*)	110	3.0	24.0	.5	0	0	1.0
Cranberry, fresh, ½ cup:							
(*Dole*)	30	0	7.0	0	0	0	2.0
(*Ocean Spray*)	30	0	7.0	0	0	35	2.0
whole	23	.2	6.0	.1	0	1	2.0
chopped	27	.2	7.0	.1	0	1	2.3
Cranberry, canned, see "Cranberry fruit blend" and "Cranberry sauce"							
Cranberry, dried, ⅓ cup, 1.4 oz.:							
(*Craisins*)	130	0	33.0	0	0	0	2.0
(*Frieda's*)	119	0	28.0	1.0	0	3	2.0
(*Shiloh Farms*)	140	0	33.0	0	0	0	1.0
(*Tree of Life*)	129	0	35.0	0	0	0	3.5

Food and Measure	cal.	prot. (gms)	carbo. (gms)	fat (gms)	chol. (mgs)	sod. (mgs)	fiber (gms)
cherry flavor (*Craisins*)	130	0	33.0	0	0	0	2.0
orange flavor (*Craisins*)	130	0	34.0	0	0	0	2.0
Cranberry bean:							
boiled, ½ cup	120	8.2	21.5	.4	0	1	3.0
canned, ½ cup	108	7.2	19.7	.4	0	431	n.a.
Cranberry drink,							
8 fl. oz.:							
(*Langers* Caribbean) .	135	0	34.0	0	0	10	0
(*Langers* Diet)	30	0	8.0	0	0	10	0
(*Ocean Spray*)	130	0	32.0	0	0	35	0
(*R.W. Knudsen* Con-							
centrate)	45	0	13.0	0	0	10	0
(*Walnut Acres*)	110	0	26.0	0	0	15	0
cocktail:							
(*Langers*)	140	0	35.0	0	0	10	0
(*Nantucket Nectars*)	140	0	34.0	0	0	5	0
(*Ocean Spray*)	130	0	33.0	0	0	35	0
(*Ocean Spray*							
Calcium)	150	0	37.0	0	0	35	0
(*Ocean Spray* Light)	40	0	10.0	0	0	75	0
(*Ocean Spray* Re-							
duced Calorie) . .	50	0	13.0	0	0	35	0
diet (*Langers*)	30	0	8.0	0	0	10	0
nectar (*Santa Cruz*							
Organic)	110	<1.0	27.0	0	0	25	0
white:							
(*Langers*)	120	0	28.0	0	0	10	0
(*Ocean Spray*)	120	0	29.0	0	0	35	0
(*Ocean Spray* Light)	40	0	10.0	0	0	75	0
Cranberry drink blend,							
8 fl. oz., except as noted:							
all varieties (*Langers*							
Diet/Low Carb) . . .	30	0	8.0	0	0	10	0
apple:							
(*Langers* Fuji)	160	0	39.0	0	0	10	0
(*Minute Maid*),							
11.5-fl.-oz. can . .	220	0	60.0	0	0	30	0
(*Cranapple*)	160	0	40.0	0	0	35	0
white cranberry							
(*Ocean Spray*) . .	120	0	30.0	0	0	35	0
apple raspberry:							
(*Minute Maid*)	120	0	33.0	0	0	20	0
(*Minute Maid*),							
11.5-fl.-oz. can . .	170	0	46.0	0	0	25	0

Food and Measure	cal.	prot. (gms)	carbo. (gms)	fat (gms)	chol. (mgs)	sod. (mgs)	fiber (gms)
Cranberry drink blend *(cont.)*							
berry (*Langers*)	135	0	34.0	0	0	10	0
cherry:							
(*Cran•Cherry*)	150	0	39.0	0	0	35	0
(*Cran•Grape Light*) .	40	0	10.0	0	0	75	0
grape:							
(*Cran•Grape*)	160	0	40.0	0	0	35	0
(*Langers*)	165	0	41.0	0	0	10	0
(*Minute Maid*),							
11.5-fl.-oz. can ..	150	0	39.0	0	0	20	0
(*Ocean Spray*)	170	0	41.0	0	0	35	0
grapefruit (*Sobe*							
Elixer 3C)	100	0	28.0	0	0	10	0
mango (*Cran•Mango*)	130	0	35.0	0	0	35	0
orange:							
(*Langers*)	130	0	33.0	0	0	10	0
(*Nantucket Nectars*							
Organic)	130	0	31.0	0	0	30	0
peach, white cranberry							
(*Ocean Spray*)	120	0	30.0	0	0	35	0
raspberry:							
(*Cran•Raspberry*) .	140	0	34.0	0	0	35	0
(*Cran•Raspberry*							
Light)	40	0	10.0	0	0	75	0
(*Langers*)	150	0	36.0	0	0	10	0
(*R.W. Knudsen*) ...	130	0	31.0	0	0	15	0
(*Snapple*)	120	0	29.0	0	0	10	0
white cranberry							
(*Langers*)	120	0	28.0	0	0	10	0
strawberry:							
(*Cran•Strawberry*) .	140	0	37.0	0	0	35	0
white cranberry							
(*Ocean Spray*) ..	120	0	31.0	0	0	35	0
tangerine (*Cran•*							
Tangerine)	130	0	35.0	0	0	35	0
wildberry (*Ocean Spray*							
Cravin' Less Sugar)	80	0	20.0	0	0	100	0
Cranberry fruit blend,							
orange or raspberry							
(*Cran•Fruit*), ¼ cup	120	0	29.0	0	0	35	1.0
Cranberry juice,							
8 fl. oz.:							
(*After the Fall* Cape							
Cod)	120	0	30.0	0	0	15	0

Food and Measure	cal.	prot. (gms)	carbo. (gms)	fat (gms)	chol. (mgs)	sod. (mgs)	fiber (gms)
(L&A Delight)	140	0	34.0	0	0	10	0
(L&A 100)	140	0	35.0	0	0	15	0
(Langers)	140	0	35.0	0	0	15	0
(Northland)	140	0	35.0	0	0	35	0
(R.W. Knudsen Just							
Cranberry)	60	<1.0	14.0	0	0	25	0
(R.W. Knudsen Nectar)	140	1.0	34.0	0	0	40	0
frozen* (Cascadian							
Farm)	120	0	29.0	0	0	0	0
white cranberry:							
(L&A 100)	160	0	40.0	0	0	15	0
(Langers)	160	0	40.0	0	0	15	0
Cranberry juice blend,							
8 fl. oz.:							
(Ocean Spray)	140	0	35.0	0	0	35	0
apple, red delicious							
(Ocean Spray)	130	0	32.0	0	0	35	0
berry, mixed:							
(Langers)	135	0	34.0	0	0	10	0
(Ocean Spray)	150	0	38.0	0	0	35	0
blueberry (Walnut							
Acres)	110	0	29.0	0	0	10	0
grape:							
(Langers)	150	0	38.0	0	0	15	0
(Ocean Spray							
Concord)	150	0	37.0	0	0	35	0
kiwi (Ceres)	110	0	28.0	0	0	14	0
peach (Ocean Spray							
Georgia)	140	0	34.0	0	0	35	0
raspberry:							
(After the Fall)	130	0	32.0	0	0	10	0
(Langers)	145	0	36.0	0	0	15	0
(Ocean Spray							
Pacific)	140	0	34.0	0	0	35	0
(Walnut Acres)	110	0	27.0	0	0	10	<1.0
raspberry grape (Nan-							
tucket Nectars)	150	0	38.0	0	0	45	0
Cranberry juice cock-							
tail, see "Cranberry							
drink"							
Cranberry juice con-							
centrate (Tree of							
Life), 8 tsp.	110	0	28.0	0	0	0	0

Food and Measure	cal.	prot. (gms)	carbo. (gms)	fat (gms)	chol. (mgs)	sod. (mgs)	fiber (gms)
Cranberry sauce, can or jar, ¼ cup, except as noted:							
(*R.W. Knudsen*), 1 tbsp.	25	0	6.0	0	0	0	0
whole (*Ocean Spray*) .	110	0	27.0	0	0	10	1.0
whole or jellied							
(*Harvest Moon*) ...	100	0	26.0	0	0	35	1.0
(*S&W*)	100	0	26.0	0	0	35	1.0
jellied (*Ocean Spray*) .	110	0	25.0	0	0	10	1.0
Cranberry twist drink mixer (*Rose's* Cocktail Infusions), 1.5 fl. oz.	60	0	15.0	0	0	15	0
Crayfish, mixed species:							
farmed, meat only:							
raw, 4 oz.	82	16.8	0	1.1	122	70	0
raw, 8 pcs., .95 oz.	19	4.0	0	.3	29	17	0
boiled or steamed, 4 oz.	99	19.9	0	1.5	155	110	0
wild, meat only:							
raw, 4 oz.	87	18.1	0	1.1	129	66	0
raw, 8 pcs., .95 oz.	21	4.3	0	.3	31	16	0
boiled or steamed, 4 oz.	93	19.0	0	1.4	151	107	0
Cream:							
half-and-half:							
(*Darigold*), 2 tbsp. .	40	1.0	1.0	3.0	15	15	0
(*Hood*), 2 tbsp. ...	40	1.0	1.0	3.5	15	20	0
(*Organic Valley*) ...	40	<1.0	1.0	3.5	10	10	0
(*Simply Smart* Fat Free), 2 tbsp.	15	1.0	2.0	0	0	30	0
1 cup	315	7.2	10.4	27.8	89	98	0
1 tbsp.	20	.4	.6	1.7	6	6	0
light, coffee or table:							
(*Hood*), 1 tbsp. ...	30	0	<1.0	3.0	10	10	0
1 cup	469	6.5	8.8	46.3	159	95	0
1 tbsp.	29	.4	.6	2.9	10	6	0
medium (25% fat):							
1 cup	583	5.9	8.3	59.8	209	88	0
1 tbsp.	37	.4	.5	3.8	13	6	0
sour, see "Cream, sour"							
whipped topping, see "Cream topping"							

Food and Measure	cal.	prot. (gms)	carbo. (gms)	fat (gms)	chol. (mgs)	sod. (mgs)	fiber (gms)
whipping[1], light:							
(*Darigold*), 1 tbsp. .	45	0	1.0	4.5	20	0	0
(*Hood*), 1 tbsp. . . .	45	0	<1.0	4.5	20	5	0
1 cup	699	5.2	7.1	73.9	265	82	0
1 tbsp.	44	.3	.4	4.6	17	5	0
whipping[1], heavy:							
(*Darigold*), 1 tbsp. .	50	0	1.0	5.0	20	0	0
(*Hood*), 1 tbsp. . . .	50	0	0	5.0	20	0	0
(*Organic Valley*) . . .	50	0	0	6.0	20	5	0
1 cup	821	4.9	6.6	88.1	326	89	0
1 tbsp.	52	.3	.4	5.6	21	6	0
Cream, clotted (*The Devon Cream Company*), 2 tbsp. . .	150	0	<1.0	17.0	50	5	0
Cream, sour, 2 tbsp., except as noted:							
(*Breakstone's*)	60	1.0	1.0	5.0	20	10	0
(*Cabot*)	50	1.0	1.0	5.0	15	35	0
(*Darigold*)	60	1.0	2.0	5.0	20	45	0
(*Hood*)	60	1.0	2.0	5.0	20	20	0
(*Hood* Squeezable) . .	60	<1.0	2.0	5.0	20	50	0
(*Knudsen Hampshire*)	60	1.0	1.0	6.0	25	15	0
(*Organic Valley*)	60	0	1.0	5.0	15	15	0
1 cup	493	7.3	9.8	48.2	102	123	0
light (low fat):							
(*Breakstone's*)	40	1.0	2.0	3.0	15	20	0
(*Cabot*)	35	1.0	2.0	2.5	10	25	0
(*Darigold*)	40	1.0	3.0	2.5	10	65	0
(*Hood*)	35	1.0	3.0	1.5	5	20	0
(*Knudsen* Light) . . .	30	2.0	2.0	2.0	10	20	0
(*Knudsen* Light 16 oz.)	40	2.0	2.0	2.5	10	20	0
(*Organic Valley*) . . .	40	1.0	1.0	2.5	10	15	0
nonfat:							
(*Breakstone's* 8 oz.)	30	1.0	5.0	0	5	25	0
(*Breakstone's* 16 oz.)	35	2.0	6.0	0	5	25	0
(*Cabot*)	20	1.0	3.0	0	0	40	0
(*Darigold*)	25	2.0	4.0	0	5	50	0
(*Hood*)	25	1.0	4.0	0	0	25	0
(*Knudsen Free*) . . .	30	2.0	5.0	0	5	25	0
Cream, sour, powder (*AlpineAire*), 2 oz. .	310	13.0	20.0	20.0	80	200	0

1. *Unwhipped; volume approximately doubled when whipped.*

Food and Measure	cal.	prot. (gms)	carbo. (gms)	fat (gms)	chol. (mgs)	sod. (mgs)	fiber (gms)
"Cream," sour, non-dairy, 2 tbsp.:							
(*Tofutti Sour Supreme*)	85	2.0	9.0	7.0	0	160	0
nonhydrogenated (*Tofutti Better Than Sour Cream*)	85	2.0	9.0	5.0	0	160	0
Cream puffs, frozen:							
chocolate, mini:							
(*Delizza*), 7 pcs., 3.5 oz.	375	4.9	33.5	25.4	130	68	.1
(*Ritch & Famous Dreamy*), 4 pcs., 1.7 oz.	100	2.0	13.0	11.0	60	80	1.0
vanilla, French, mini (*Ritch & Famous*), .4-oz. pc.	35	<1.0	3.0	2.5	15	20	0
Cream of tartar, 1 tsp.	7	0	1.9	0	0	2	0
Cream topping, 2 tbsp.:							
(*Cabot* Whipped Cream)	30	0	2.0	2.0	10	0	0
(*Cool Whip*)	25	0	2.0	1.5	0	0	0
(*Cool Whip* Extra Creme)	25	0	2.0	0	5	0	0
(*Cool Whip* Free)	15	0	3.0	0	0	5	0
(*Cool Whip* Lite)	20	0	3.0	1.0	0	0	0
(*Hood* Instant)	20	0	<1.0	1.5	5	0	0
(*Hood* Instant Light) .	15	0	1.0	.5	<5	0	0
(*Reddi Wip* Extra Creamy)	15	0	<1.0	1.5	5	0	0
(*Reddi Wip* Fat Free) .	5	0	1.0	0	0	0	0
(*Reddi Wip* Original) .	15	0	<1.0	1.0	<5	0	0
chocolate (*Reddi Wip*)	15	0	1.0	1.0	<5	0	0
Creamer, 2 tbsp.:							
half-and-half:							
(*Coffee-mate*)	40	<1.0	1.0	3.5	15	70	0
hazelnut (*Coffee-mate*)	70	<1.0	8.0	4.0	15	60	0
vanilla (*Coffee-mate*)	60	<1.0	4.0	4.0	15	60	0
powder:							
(*Coffee-mate* Latte Creations Classic)	100	1.0	12.0	6.0	0	125	0
mocha or vanilla (*Coffee-mate* Latte Creations)	90	<1.0	14.0	4.0	0	125	0

Food and Measure	cal.	prot. (gms)	carbo. (gms)	fat (gms)	chol. (mgs)	sod. (mgs)	fiber (gms)
Creamer, nondairy:							
fluid, 1 tbsp.:							
(*Coffee-mate*)	20	0	2.0	1.0	0	0	0
(*Coffee-mate* Fat Free)	10	0	2.0	0	0	0	0
(*Coffee-mate* Low Fat)	10	0	1.0	.5	0	5	0
(*Country Creamer*) .	20	0	2.0	1.5	0	0	0
(*Silk*)	15	0	1.0	1.0	0	10	0
powder, 1 tsp.:							
(*Coffee-mate*)	10	0	1.0	.5	0	0	0
(*Coffee-mate* Lite) .	10	0	2.0	0	0	0	0
(*Cremora*)	10	0	<1.0	1.0	0	10	0
(*Cremora* Fat Free) .	10	0	2.0	0	0	5	0
(*Cremora* Lite & Creamy)	10	0	1.0	0	0	5	0
(*Cremora* No Carb) .	15	0	0	1.5	0	0	0
(*Cremora* Royale) . .	15	0	1.0	1.0	0	10	0
Creamer, nondairy, flavored:							
fluid, 1 tbsp.:							
almond, toasted, or amaretto (*Coffee-mate*)	40	0	5.0	2.0	0	5	0
café mocha (*Coffee-mate*)	40	0	5.0	2.0	0	5	0
café mocha or Irish creme (*Coffee-mate* Fat Free) . .	25	0	5.0	0	0	0	0
chocolate raspberry (*Coffee-mate*) . . .	40	0	5.0	2.0	0	10	0
cinnamon vanilla creme (*Coffee-mate*)	40	0	5.0	2.0	0	5	0
hazelnut (*Coffee-mate*)	40	0	5.0	2.0	0	5	0
hazelnut or French vanilla (*Silk*)	20	0	3.0	1.0	0	10	0
hazelnut or Irish crème (*Coffee-mate*)	40	0	5.0	2.0	0	5	0
vanilla, French (*Coffee-mate*) . . .	40	0	5.0	2.0	0	0	0

Food and Measure	cal.	prot. (gms)	carbo. (gms)	fat (gms)	chol. (mgs)	sod. (mgs)	fiber (gms)
Creamer, nondairy, flavored, fluid *(cont.)*							
vanilla, French (*Coffee-Mate Fat Free*)	10	0	2.0	0	0	0	0
vanilla caramel (*Coffee-mate*) . . .	40	0	5.0	2.0	0	15	0
vanilla nut (*Coffee-mate*) . . .	40	0	5.0	2.0	0	5	0
powder, 4 tsp.:							
chocolate, creamy (*Coffee-mate*) . . .	60	0	9.0	2.5	0	30	0
chocolate, creamy (*Coffee-mate Fat Free*)	50	0	11.0	0	0	30	0
cinnamon vanilla creme (*Coffee-mate*)	60	0	9.0	3.0	0	15	0
dulce de leche (*Cremora*)	60	0	9.0	2.5	0	25	0
hazelnut (*Coffee-mate*)	60	0	9.0	3.0	0	15	0
hazelnut (*Coffee-mate Fat Free*) . .	50	0	11.0	0	0	15	0
hazelnut (*Cremora Nutty for Hazelnut*)	25	0	<1.0	2.5	0	0	0
Irish creme (*Coffee-mate*)	60	0	9.0	3.0	0	15	0
peppermint mocha (*Coffee-mate*) . . .	60	0	9.0	3.0	0	15	0
vanilla (*Cremora Ooh-la-la*)	25	0	<1.0	2.5	0	0	0
vanilla, French (*Coffee-mate*) . . .	60	0	9.0	3.0	0	15	0
vanilla, French (*Coffee-mate Fat Free*)	50	0	11.0	0	0	15	0
vanilla caramel (*Coffee-mate*) . . .	60	0	9.0	3.0	0	15	0
vanilla nut (*Coffee-mate*) . . .	60	0	8.0	2.5	0	15	0
Crème fraîche:							
(*Santè*), 2 tbsp.	100	<1.0	<1.0	11.0	40	10	0
(*Vermont Butter & Cheese*), 1 oz.	110	1.0	1.0	11.0	25	20	0

Food and Measure	cal.	prot. (gms)	carbo. (gms)	fat (gms)	chol. (mgs)	sod. (mgs)	fiber (gms)
Crepe, 1 pc.:							
(*A&B Famous*), 1.4 oz	86	2.0	9.0	3.8	27	89	0
(*Frieda's*), .4 oz.	30	1.0	5.0	.5	5	50	0
Cress, garden, ½ cup:							
raw	8	.7	1.4	.2	0	4	.3
boiled, drained	16	1.3	2.6	.4	0	5	.5
Cress, water, see "Watercress"							
Croaker, meat only, raw, Atlantic, 4 oz. .	119	20.2	0	3.6	69	63	0
Croissant:							
butter, 1-oz. pc.	115	2.3	13.0	6.0	19	211	.7
apple, 2-oz. pc.	144	4.2	21.0	4.9	18	155	1.4
cheese, 1.5-oz. pc. ...	174	3.9	19.7	8.8	24	233	1.1
Croissant, frozen, French style:							
(*Sara Lee* Original), 1.5-oz. pc.	170	4.0	20.0	8.0	5	200	1.0
petite (*Sara Lee*), 2 pcs., 2 oz.	230	6.0	26.0	11.0	5	260	1.0
Crookneck squash:							
(*Frieda's* Baby), ⅔ cup, 3 oz.	15	1.0	3.0	0	0	0	1.0
sliced, ½ cup:							
raw, ends trimmed .	12	.6	2.6	.2	0	1	.7
boiled, drained	18	.8	3.9	.3	0	1	1.3
Crookneck squash, canned, cut, drained, no salt, ½ cup	14	.7	3.2	.1	0	5	1.1
Crookneck squash, frozen, boiled, sliced, ½ cup	24	1.2	5.3	.2	0	6	1.2
Croutons (see also "Salad toppers"):							
Caesar salad:							
(*Mrs. Cubbison's*), 5 pcs.	30	1.0	4.0	1.0	0	110	0
(*Pepperidge Farm* Generous Cut Classic), 6 pcs. .	35	1.0	4.0	1.5	0	90	0
(*Pepperidge Farm* Generous Cut Fat Free), 6 pcs.	30	<1.0	5.0	0	0	80	0

Food and Measure	cal.	prot. (gms)	carbo. (gms)	fat (gms)	chol. (mgs)	sod. (mgs)	fiber (gms)
Croutons *(cont.)*							
cheese, sourdough (*Pepperidge Farm Generous Cut*), 6 pcs.	30	1.0	4.0	1.0	0	80	0
cheese and garlic:							
(*Mrs. Cubbison's*), 5 pcs.	30	1.0	4.0	1.0	0	90	0
(*Pepperidge Farm Classic Cut*), 11 pcs.	35	<1.0	5.0	1.0	0	70	0
garlic and butter (*Mrs. Cubbison's* Zesty), 5 pcs.	30	0	5.0	1.0	0	100	0
herb (*Mrs. Cubbison's* Fat Free), 5 pcs.	30	1.0	5.0	0	0	80	0
Italian, zesty (*Pepperidge Farm Generous Cut*), 6 pcs.	35	<1.0	4.0	1.5	0	85	0
onion and garlic:							
(*Mrs. Cubbison's*), 5 pcs.	30	1.0	5.0	1.0	0	120	0
(*Pepperidge Farm Classic Cut*), 11 pcs.	30	<1.0	5.0	1.0	0	60	0
pepper, cracked, and Parmesan (*Pepperidge Farm Generous Cut*), 6 pcs.	35	1.0	4.0	1.0	0	70	0
ranch:							
buttermilk (*Pepperidge Farm Generous Cut*), 6 pcs.	30	<1.0	5.0	1.0	0	80	0
cool herb (*Mrs. Cubbison's*), 5 pcs.	30	1.0	5.0	1.0	0	70	0
seasoned:							
(*Mrs. Cubbison's*), 5 pcs.	30	1.0	4.0	1.0	0	80	0
(*Pepperidge Farm Classic Cut*), 11 pcs.	30	<1.0	5.0	1.0	0	65	0

Food and Measure	cal.	prot. (gms)	carbo. (gms)	fat (gms)	chol. (mgs)	sod. (mgs)	fiber (gms)
Crowder peas, see "Peas, crowder"							
Cucumber, w/peel:							
(*Chiquita*), ⅓ medium, 3.5 oz.	15	1.0	3.0	0	0	0	1.0
(*Frieda's* Hothouse/ Japanese), ⅔ cup, 3 oz.	10	1.0	2.0	0	0	0	1.0
1 medium, 8¼" long .	38	2.1	8.3	.4	0	6	2.4
sliced, ½ cup	7	.4	1.4	.1	0	1	.4
Cucumber, pickled, see "Pickles"							
Cucuzza squash (*Frieda's*), ¾ cup, 3 oz.	10	1.0	3.0	0	0	0	0
Cumin seed, ground:							
1 tsp.	8	.4	.9	.5	0	4	.2
Cupcake, see "Cake, snack"							
Curaçao, blue (*Angostura*), 1 fl. oz.	80	0	19.0	0	0	0	0
Currants:							
fresh, ½ cup:							
black, Europe	36	.8	8.6	.2	0	1	3.0
red or white	31	.8	7.7	.1	0	1	2.4
dried, Zante:							
½ cup	204	2.9	53.3	.2	0	6	4.9
Curry, vegetable, see "Vegetable entree, pkg."							
Curry paste (see also "Curry sauce base"):							
green (*Thai Kitchen*), 1 tbsp.	10	0	2.0	0	0	270	0
hot:							
(*Patak's*), 2 tbsp. . . .	160	1.0	4.0	16.0	0	1130	0
(*Patak's* Garam Masala), 2 tsp. . . .	130	1.0	4.0	12.0	0	1080	0
(*Patak's* Kashmiri Masala), 1 tsp. . . .	15	<1.0	<1.0	1.0	0	270	0
(*Patak's* Madras), 2 tbsp.	160	1.0	4.0	16.0	0	1010	0
hot, vindaloo:							
(*Neera's*), 2 tsp.	48	0	3.0	4.0	0	118	1.0

Food and Measure	cal.	prot. (gms)	carbo. (gms)	fat (gms)	chol. (mgs)	sod. (mgs)	fiber (gms)
Curry paste, hot, vindaloo *(cont.)*							
(*Patak's* Vindaloo), 2 tbsp.	160	1.0	4.0	16.0	0	1020	0
medium, 2 tbsp.:							
(*Patak's* Balti)	115	2.0	6.0	10.0	0	640	<1.0
(*Patak's* Biryani Paste)	170	1.0	3.0	17.0	0	920	0
(*Patak's* Tikka Masala)	110	1.0	5.0	9.0	0	700	<1.0
mild (*Patak's*), 2 tbsp.	180	1.0	8.0	16.0	0	910	4.0
red (*Thai Kitchen*), 1 tbsp.	10	0	2.0	0	0	140	0
tandoori:							
(*Neera's* Grilling), 2 tsp.	19	0	3.0	2.0	0	156	1.0
(*Patak's*), 2 tbsp. . . .	30	<1.0	3.0	1.0	0	1440	2.0
Curry powder:							
1 tbsp.	20	.8	3.7	.9	0	3	1.0
1 tsp.	6	.3	1.2	.3	0	1	.3
Masala:							
(*Neera's*), 2 tsp.	13	1.0	3.0	1.0	0	167	1.0
(*Neera's* Garam), ¼ tsp.	2	0	0	0	0	0	0
Curry sauce, cooking (see also "Thai sauce"), ½ cup:							
chile, hot:							
w/coriander (*Patak's* Vindaloo)	320	3.0	15.0	28.0	0	790	1.0
w/cumin (*Patak's* Madras 10 oz.) . .	280	3.0	15.0	23.0	0	770	1.0
w/cumin (*Patak's* Madras 15 oz.) . .	140	2.0	13.0	9.0	0	550	1.0
coconut, rich creamy:							
mild (*Patak's* Korma 10 oz.)	210	4.0	11.0	17.0	0	670	2.0
mild (*Patak's* Korma 15 oz.)	110	2.0	11.0	6.0	0	520	1.0
coriander and lemon, tangy, medium:							
(*Patak's* Tikka Masala 10 oz.) . .	210	3.0	13.0	16.0	0	1030	2.0
(*Patak's* Tikka Masala 15 oz.) . .	110	2.0	13.0	6.0	0	760	1.0

Food and Measure	cal.	prot. (gms)	carbo. (gms)	fat (gms)	chol. (mgs)	sod. (mgs)	fiber (gms)
sweet peppers and coconut, hot (*Patak's* Jalfrezi) ...	140	2.0	12.0	9.0	0	340	2.0
tomato:							
rich, mild (*Patak's* Dopiaza)	110	2.0	13.0	5.0	0	800	1.0
spicy, and cardamom (*Patak's* Rogan Josh 10 oz.)	180	2.0	12.0	13.0	0	840	1.0
spicy, and cardamon (*Patrak's* Rogan Josh 15 oz.)	110	2.0	12.0	6.0	0	600	1.0
Curry sauce base (see also "Curry paste"), 1 tsp.:							
green (*A Taste of Thai*)	15	0	1.0	1.5	0	200	1.0
Panang (*A Taste of Thai*)	25	0	2.0	2.0	0	170	0
red (*A Taste of Thai*) .	20	0	1.0	1.5	0	260	0
yellow (*A Taste of Thai*)	30	0	1.0	3.0	0	135	1.0
Cusk, meat only:							
raw, 4 oz.	99	21.6	0	.8	47	36	0
baked, broiled, or microwaved, 4 oz. .	127	27.6	0	1.0	60	45	0
Custard apple, trimmed, 1 oz.	29	.5	7.1	.2	0	1	1.0
Custard marrow, see "Chayote"							
Cuttlefish, meat only, 4 oz.:							
raw	90	18.4	.9	.8	127	422	0
boiled or steamed ...	179	36.8	1.9	1.6	254	844	0
Cuttlefish, canned, in ink (*Goya*), ¼ cup .	120	8.0	2.0	9.0	15	350	0

D

Food and Measure	cal.	prot. (gms)	carbo. (gms)	fat (gms)	chol. (mgs)	sod. (mgs)	fiber (gms)
Dal/Dahl, see "Lentil dish, mix"							
Daikon, fresh/dried, see "Radish, Oriental"							
Daikon, pickled (*Eden*), 2 slices, .5 oz.	5	0	1.0	0	0	250	0
Daiquiri drink mixer:							
(*Trader Vic's* Hawaiian), 4 fl. oz.	170	0	42.0	0	0	20	0
banana, frozen (*Bacardi*), 2 fl. oz.	140	0	36.0	0	0	0	0
peach, frozen (*Bacardi*), 2 fl. oz.	120	0	32.0	0	0	0	0
strawberry:							
(*Bacardi*), 4 fl. oz. .	160	0	46.0	0	0	30	0
(*Mr & Mrs T*), 3.5 fl. oz.	150	0	34.0	0	0	20	0
frozen (*Bacardi*), 2 fl. oz.	120	0	32.0	0	0	0	0
Daiquiri/Margarita drink mixer, 4 fl. oz.:							
lime (*Daiq-or-Rita*) ...	210	0	55.0	0	0	85	1.0
mango (*Daiq-or-Rita*) .	270	0	55.0	0	0	85	1.0
peach (*Daiq-or-Rita*) .	270	1.0	41.0	0	0	45	1.0
strawberry:							
(*Daiq-or-Rita*)	260	1.0	55.0	0	0	85	1.0
(*Holland House*) ...	180	0	46.0	0	0	25	0
Dairy Queen/Brazier, 1 serving:							
burgers:							
DQ Homestyle:							
burger	290	17.0	29.0	12.0	45	630	2.0
cheeseburger ...	340	20.0	29.0	17.0	55	850	2.0

Food and Measure	cal.	prot. (gms)	carbo. (gms)	fat (gms)	chol. (mgs)	sod. (mgs)	fiber (gms)
double cheese-burger	540	35.0	30.0	31.0	115	1130	2.0
double cheese-burger w/bacon	610	41.0	31.0	36.0	130	1380	2.0
DQ Ultimate	670	40.0	29.0	43.0	135	1210	2.0
Flame Thrower	810	43.0	27.0	60.0	160	1390	2.0
Grillburger:							
bacon cheese	710	36.0	40.0	45.0	105	1430	1.0
California	630	26.0	37.0	42.0	75	820	1.0
classic	540	27.0	41.0	30.0	65	990	2.0
classic w/cheese	610	31.0	41.0	36.0	85	1110	2.0
½ lb.	800	47.0	41.0	50.0	130	1230	2.0
½ lb. w/cheese	930	56.0	41.0	60.0	160	1380	2.0
mushroom Swiss	700	30.0	37.0	47.0	90	890	1.0
Chicken Strip Basket:							
4-pc.	920	32.0	92.0	49.0	40	2090	7.0
6-pc.	1120	45.0	102.0	60.0	60	2450	9.0
hot dog, regular	240	9.0	19.0	14.0	25	730	1.0
hot dog, chili 'n cheese	330	14.0	22.0	21.0	45	1090	2.0
popcorn shrimp basket	730	19.0	88.0	35.0	115	2420	7.0
sandwich, chicken:							
crispy	590	21.0	50.0	34.0	40	1100	4.5
grilled	340	22.0	26.0	16.0	55	1000	2.0
fries/onion rings:							
fries, large	480	5.0	72.0	19.0	0	1140	5.0
fries, medium	380	4.0	56.0	15.0	0	880	4.0
fries, small	300	3.0	45.0	12.0	0	700	3.0
onion rings	470	6.0	45.0	30.0	0	740	3.0
salad, no dressing:							
crispy chicken	350	21.0	21.0	20.0	40	620	6.0
grilled chicken	240	26.0	12.0	10.0	65	950	4.0
side salad	60	3.0	6.0	2.5	5	60	2.0
salad dressing:							
DQ blue cheese	210	2.0	4.0	20.0	5	700	0
DQ honey mustard	260	1.0	18.0	21.0	20	370	0
DQ ranch	310	1.0	3.0	33.0	25	390	0
honey mustard, nonfat	50	0	13.0	0	0	160	0
Italian, nonfat	10	0	3.0	0	0	390	0
ranch, nonfat	60	0	13.0	0	0	410	0
ranch, buttermilk, nonfat	30	1.0	6.0	0	0	440	0
red French, nonfat	40	0	10.0	0	0	330	0

Food and Measure	cal.	prot. (gms)	carbo. (gms)	fat (gms)	chol. (mgs)	sod. (mgs)	fiber (gms)
Dairy Queen/Brazier, salad dressing (cont.)							
Thousand Island, nonfat	60	0	16.0	0	0	400	0
Blizzard:							
banana split:							
large	810	17.0	134.0	23.0	70	134	2.0
medium	580	12.0	97.0	17.0	50	97	1.0
small	460	10.0	73.0	14.0	40	73	<1.0
chocolate chip cookie:							
large	1320	21.0	193.0	52.0	90	193	0
medium	1030	17.0	150.0	40.0	70	150	0
small	720	12.0	105.0	28.0	50	105	0
Oreo cookie:							
large	1010	19.0	148.0	37.0	70	148	2.0
medium	700	13.0	103.0	26.0	45	103	1.0
small	570	11.0	83.0	21.0	40	83	<1.0
Reese's Cup:							
large	1050	25.0	152.0	38.0	70	370	0
medium	790	18.0	114.0	28.0	50	280	0
small	600	14.0	87.0	21.0	40	220	0
Blizzard CheeseQuake:							
blueberry, large . . .	1030	20.0	148.0	41.0	160	600	1.0
blueberry, medium .	760	15.0	108.0	30.0	120	450	1.0
blueberry, small . . .	560	11.0	78.0	22.0	85	330	0
raspberry, large . . .	1100	20.0	165.0	41.0	160	600	1.0
raspberry, medium .	810	15.0	119.0	30.0	120	450	1.0
raspberry, small . . .	580	11.0	84.0	22.0	85	330	1.0
strawberry, large . .	980	20.0	136.0	41.0	160	610	1.0
strawberry, medium	710	14.0	97.0	30.0	115	440	1.0
strawberry, small . .	520	11.0	71.0	22.0	85	320	0
cones:							
DQ soft serve:							
chocolate, ½ cup	150	4.0	22.0	5.0	15	75	0
vanilla, ½ cup . .	140	3.0	22.0	4.5	15	70	0
chocolate, medium	340	8.0	53.0	11.0	30	160	0
chocolate, small . . .	240	6.0	37.0	8.0	20	115	0
dipped, large	710	12.0	85.0	36.0	45	250	0
dipped, medium . . .	490	8.0	59.0	24.0	30	190	1.0
dipped, small	340	6.0	42.0	17.0	20	130	1.0
vanilla, large	480	11.0	76.0	15.0	45	230	0
vanilla, medium . . .	330	8.0	53.0	9.0	30	160	0
vanilla, small	230	6.0	38.0	7.0	20	115	0
DQ round cake, ⅛ cake	370	7.0	56.0	13.0	25	289	<1.0
malt, chocolate:							
large	1320	29.0	222.0	35.0	110	670	2.0

Food and Measure	cal.	prot. (gms)	carbo. (gms)	fat (gms)	chol. (mgs)	sod. (mgs)	fiber (gms)
medium	870	20.0	153.0	22.0	70	450	2.0
small	640	15.0	111.0	16.0	55	340	1.0
Misty slush, medium .	290	0	74.0	0	0	30	0
Misty slush, small ...	220	0	56.0	0	0	20	0
MooLatte:							
caramel, 16 oz. ...	630	9.0	96.0	20.0	35	250	0
caramel, 24 oz. ...	870	13.0	139.0	26.0	55	360	0
cappuccino, 16 oz. .	490	7.0	68.0	18.0	30	170	0
cappuccino, 24 oz. .	690	11.0	102.0	23.0	50	260	0
mocha, 16 oz.	590	8.0	80.0	23.0	30	210	1.0
mocha, 24 oz.	830	12.0	118.0	31.0	50	310	1.0
vanilla, 16 oz.	570	7.0	87.0	18.0	30	170	0
vanilla, 24 oz.	790	11.0	127.0	23.0	50	260	0
novelties:							
Buster Bar	500	11.0	45.0	28.0	15	230	2.0
Chocolate Dilly bar .	220	3.0	25.0	13.0	15	85	0
DQ fudge bar	50	4.0	13.0	0	0	70	0
DQ sandwich	200	4.0	31.0	6.0	10	140	1.0
DQ vanilla orange bar	60	2.0	17.0	0	0	40	0
lemon *DQ Freez'r* ..	80	0	20.0	0	0	10	0
Starkiss	80	0	21.0	0	0	10	0
Royal Treats:							
banana split	510	8.0	96.0	12.0	30	180	3.0
Brownie Earthquake	740	10.0	112.0	27.0	50	350	0
Peanut Buster parfait	730	16.0	99.0	31.0	35	400	2.0
Triple Chocolate							
Utopia	770	12.0	96.0	39.0	55	390	5.0
strawberry shortcake	430	7.0	70.0	14.0	60	360	1.0
shake, chocolate:							
large	1140	26.0	186.0	33.0	105	550	2.0
medium	760	17.0	129.0	20.0	70	370	2.0
small	560	13.0	93.0	15.0	50	280	1.0
sundae, chocolate:							
large	580	11.0	100.0	15.0	45	260	1.0
medium	400	8.0	71.0	10.0	30	210	0
small	280	5.0	49.0	7.0	20	140	0
sundae, strawberry:							
large	500	10.0	83.0	15.0	45	230	<1.0
medium	340	7.0	58.0	9.0	30	160	<1.0
small	240	5.0	40.0	7.0	20	110	0
Dandelion greens:							
raw:							
(*Frieda's*), 2 cups,							
3 oz.	40	2.0	8.0	0	0	65	3.0
½ cup chopped, 1 oz.	13	.8	2.6	.2	0	22	1.0

Food and Measure	cal.	prot. (gms)	carbo. (gms)	fat (gms)	chol. (mgs)	sod. (mgs)	fiber (gms)
Dandelion greens *(cont.)*							
boiled, drained, chopped, ½ cup	17	1.0	3.3	.3	0	23	1.5
Danish, 1 pc.:							
cheese *(Entenmann's)*, 3.5 oz.	330	6.0	60.0	8.0	10	330	<1.0
pineapple cheese *(Entenmann's)*, 4 oz.	460	6.0	45	28.0	<5	500	1.0
Dasheen, see "Taro"							
Date, dried:							
(Dole), 1.4 oz.	120	1.0	33.0	0	0	10	3.0
(Frieda's Medjool), 2-3 pcs., 1.4 oz.	120	1.0	31.0	0	0	0	3.0
(Shiloh Farms Deglet Noor), 5-6 pcs., 1.4 oz.	120	1.0	31.0	0	0	0	3.0
(Sunsweet), 5-6 pcs. or ¼ cup chopped, 1.4 oz.	120	1.0	32.0	0	0	0	3.0
(Tree of Life Deglet Noor), 5 pcs., 1.5 oz.	120	1.0	31.0	0	0	0	3.0
10 pcs. , 2.9 oz.	228	1.6	61.0	.4	0	2	6.2
pitted, ½ cup	245	1.8	65.4	.5	0	3	6.7
Date, Indian, see "Tamarindo"							
Date-nut rolls, w/coconut and almonds *(Shiloh Farms)*, 1.4 oz., 1½ pcs.	80	1.0	30.0	0	0	20	4.0
Del Taco, 1 serving:							
breakfast:							
burrito:							
breakfast	250	10.0	24.0	11.0	160	520	1.0
egg/cheese	450	23.0	39.0	24.0	530	740	3.0
steak/egg	580	33.0	41.0	34.0	560	1270	3.0
hash brown sticks:							
5 pcs.	250	0	20.0	19.0	0	200	0
8 pcs.	410	0	32.0	30.0	0	320	0
Macho Bacon & Egg Burrito	1030	40.0	82.0	60.0	790	1760	6.0
quesadilla, bacon/ egg	450	21.0	40.0	23.0	260	920	2.0

Food and Measure	cal.	prot. (gms)	carbo. (gms)	fat (gms)	chol. (mgs)	sod: (mgs)	fiber (gms)
burgers:							
Bacon Double Del Cheeseburger ...	610	29.0	35.0	39.0	95	1130	4.0
bun taco	440	24.0	37.0	21.0	65	830	4.0
cheeseburger	330	16.0	37.0	13.0	35	870	3.0
Del Cheeseburger ..	430	16.0	35.0	25.0	45	710	4.0
Double Del Cheese-burger	560	26.0	35.0	35.0	85	960	4.0
hamburger	280	13.0	37.0	9.0	25	640	3.0
burrito:							
bean/cheese green .	280	11.0	38.0	8.0	15	1030	6.0
bean/cheese red	270	11.0	38.0	8.0	15	1020	6.0
carnitas	440	25.0	41.0	21.0	70	1050	3.0
chicken, spicy	480	23.0	66.0	16.0	40	1850	8.0
chicken works	520	26.0	57.0	23.0	65	1620	4.0
Del Beef	550	31.0	42.0	30.0	90	1090	3.0
Del Classic Chicken	560	24.0	41.0	36.0	70	1100	3.0
Del Combo	530	28.0	61.0	22.0	55	1680	11.0
Deluxe Combo	570	29.0	64.0	25.0	60	1700	12.0
Deluxe Del Beef ...	590	32.0	45.0	33.0	95	1110	4.0
half pound green ..	430	20.0	59.0	12.0	20	1690	13.0
half pound red	430	20.0	65.0	12.0	20	1670	13.0
Macho Beef	1170	60.0	89.0	62.0	190	2190	7.0
Macho Chicken ...	930	47.0	111.0	33.0	100	2990	16.0
Macho Combo	1050	49.0	113.0	44.0	115	2760	17.0
steak works	590	27.0	58.0	31.0	70	1820	5.0
veggie works	490	18.0	69.0	18.0	25	1660	9.0
quesadilla:							
cheddar	500	23.0	39.0	27.0	75	860	2.0
chicken cheddar ...	580	33.0	41.0	31.0	104	1240	2.0
chicken spicy Jack .	570	32.0	40.0	30.0	105	1300	2.0
spicy Jack	490	23.0	38.0	26.0	75	920	2.0
taco :							
Big Fat	320	16.0	39.0	11.0	35	680	3.0
Big Fat Chicken ...	340	18.0	38.0	13.0	45	840	3.0
Big Fat Steak	390	18.0	38.0	19.0	45	960	3.0
carnitas	170	9.0	18.0	6.0	25	370	2.0
chicken, soft	210	11.0	16.0	12.0	30	520	1.0
chicken del carbon .	170	12.0	19.0	5.0	30	530	2.0
fish, crispy	290	7.0	30.0	16.0	20	460	2.0
steak del carbon ...	170	12.0	19.0	11.0	30	680	2.0
taco	160	7.0	11.0	10.0	20	150	1.0
taco, soft	160	8.0	16.0	8.0	20	330	1.0
ultimate	260	14.0	13.0	17.0	50	470	2.0

Food and Measure	cal.	prot. (gms)	carbo. (gms)	fat (gms)	chol. (mgs)	*sod. (mgs)	fiber (gms)
Del Taco (cont.)							
salad:							
chicken, deluxe ...	740	33.0	77.0	34.0	70	2610	15.0
Deluxe Taco Salad .	780	33.0	76.0	40.0	80	2250	14.0
taco salad	350	10.0	10.0	30.0	45	390	2.0
nachos/sides:							
beans/cheese cup .	260	16.0	44.0	3.0	5	1810	16.0
chips/salsa, medium	310	5.0	43.0	14.0	0	580	3.0
fries:							
chili cheese	670	17.0	51.0	46.0	45	880	5.0
Deluxe Chili							
Cheese	710	17.0	53.0	49.0	50	880	6.0
macho	690	7.0	68.0	46.0	0	550	6.0
medium	490	5.0	47.0	32.0	0	380	5.0
small	350	3.0	34.0	23.0	0	270	3.0
Macho Nachos	1100	31.0	113.0	63.0	55	2640	15.0
nachos	380	5.0	40.0	24.0	5	630	2.0
rice cup	140	3.0	27.0	2.0	2	910	1.0
shakes:							
chocolate	680	16.0	117.0	16.0	45	350	1.0
strawberry	540	14.0	100.0	8.0	40	280	1.0
vanilla	550	16.0	97.0	10.0	50	320	0
Delicata squash							
(*Frieda's*), ¾ cup,							
3 oz.	30	1.0	7.0	0	0	0	1.0
Denny's, 1 serving:							
breakfast menu, no							
bread or syrup:							
All American Slam .	816	46.0	3.0	67.0	828	1826	1.0
Belgian waffle platter	619	22.0	28.0	45.0	274	1683	0
corned beef hash							
slam	668	32.0	11.0	55.0	535	816	1.0
country-fried steak							
and eggs	464	29.0	13.0	34.0	527	828	6.0
country scramble ..	1038	42.0	79.0	62.0	481	3935	4.0
Denver scramble ..	940	48.0	75.0	51.0	551	3331	4.0
French Slam	1196	48.0	74.0	83.0	789	2302	3.0
French toast platter	1261	44.0	110.0	79.0	422	2495	3.0
Grand Slam	665	26.0	33.0	49.0	515	1106	2.0
Grand Slam Slugger	927	34.0	74.0	55.0	476	2399	3.0
grits, 4 oz.	80	2.0	18.0	0	0	520	0
ham-cheddar							
omelette	595	41.0	5.0	47.0	783	*1200	0

Food and Measure	cal.	prot. (gms)	carbo. (gms)	fat (gms)	chol. (mgs)	sod. (mgs)	fiber (gms)
hash browns	197	2.0	20.0	12.0	0	446	2.0
w/cheddar cheese	280	7.0	21.0	19.0	23	583	2.0
w/onion, cheese,							
gravy	493	14.0	54.0	25.0	29	3534	3.0
heartland scramble	1111	42.0	79.0	66.0	550	3197	8.0
Lumberjack Slam,							
w/hash browns .	1035	51.0	73.0	58.0	589	4462	3.0
meat lover's	1027	44.0	72.0	60.0	497	3462	3.0
meat lover's							
scramble	1241	51.0	82.0	76.0	561	4563	8.0
meat lover's skillet .	1031	39.0	27.0	74.0	528	2374	10.0
Moons Over My							
Hammy	841	54.0	42.0	51.0	580	2699	2.0
pancakes, 3	223	6.0	47.0	4.0	0	901	2.0
pancake platter	466	20.0	47.0	23.0	47	2077	2.0
potatoes, country							
fried	394	3.0	23.0	20.0	9	938	10.0
sirloin steak/eggs ..	675	62.0	1.0	45.0	643	368	1.0
Slim Slam	421	31.0	39.0	13.0	50	2625	1.0
T-bone steak/eggs ..	991	73.0	1.0	77.0	657	1003	1.0
Ultimate Omelette ..	619	36.0	8.0	50.0	770	1214	1.0
veggie-cheese							
omelette	484	30.0	11.0	39.0	747	719	2.0
breakfast items:							
bacon, 4 strips	162	12.0	1.0	18.0	36	640	0
bagel, dry	235	9.0	46.0	1.0	0	495	0
biscuit, dry	192	3.0	22.0	10.0	<1	519	0
cinnamon apple							
filling	90	0	21.0	2.0	0	70	1.0
cream cheese	100	2.0	1.0	10.0	31	90	0
egg, 1	120	6.0	>1.0	10.0	210	120	0
eggs, 2, hash browns	678	26.0	20.0	55.0	506	898	2.0
English muffin, dry	125	5.0	24.0	1.0	0	198	1.0
ham, grilled slice ..	85	15.0	6.0	3.0	49	1700	0
margarine, whipped	87	0	0	10.0	0	117	0
oatmeal, *Quaker* ...	100	5.0	18.0	2.0	0	175	3.0
sausage, 4 links ...	354	16.0	0	32.0	64	944	0
syrup, maple	143	0	36.0	0	0	26	0
syrup, maple, sugar							
free	23	0	9.0	0	0	71	0
toast, 1, dry	90	3.0	17.0	1.0	0	166	1.0
topping, 3 oz.:							
blueberry	106	0	26.0	0	0	15	0
cherry	86	0	21.0	0	0	5	0

Denny's, breakfast items, topping *(cont.)*

Food and Measure	cal.	prot. (gms)	carbo. (gms)	fat (gms)	chol. (mgs)	sod. (mgs)	fiber (gms)
strawberry	115	1.0	26.0	1.0	0	12	1.0
whipped cream .	23	0	2.0	2.0	7	1	0
sandwiches, no fries:							
bacon, lettuce and							
tomato	610	15.0	50.0	38.0	35	862	2.0
Boca Burger	452	32.0	64.0	11.0	14	1290	9.0
burger, classic	694	40.0	56.0	35.0	100	785	4.0
w/cheese	852	49.0	57.0	48.0	140	1385	4.0
burger, mushroom							
Swiss	880	51.0	63.0	49.0	137	1619	5.0
chicken, barbecued	1089	48.0	86.0	62.0	103	1872	5.0
chicken, grilled, no							
dressing	476	36.0	56.0	14.0	77	1494	4.0
chicken melt, Italian	1134	51.0	68.0	62.0	115	3735	7.0
chicken melt hoagie	751	46.0	43.0	44.0	93	1834	2.0
chicken ranch melt .	838	47.0	57.0	47.0	109	2481	3.0
club	602	31.0	45.0	38.0	41	2450	2.0
fish	589	22.0	30.0	30.0	30	1557	3.0
Philly melt hoagie .	874	47.0	58.0	50.0	114	2444	5.0
The Super Bird	479	24.0	32.0	29.0	47	1764	2.0
soup, 8 oz.:							
broccoli cheddar ..	574	6.0	41.0	43.0	0	1174	2.0
chicken noodle	118	1.0	14.0	5.0	30	1130	1.0
clam chowder	624	7.0	55.0	42.0	5	1474	4.0
vegetable beef	79	6.0	11.0	1.0	5	820	2.0
appetizers, w/out							
condiments:							
Buffalo strips	734	48.0	43.0	42.0	96	1673	0
Buffalo wings	974	67.0	11.0	72.0	267	4049	2.0
chicken strips	635	47.0	55.0	25.0	95	1510	0
mozzarella sticks ..	710	36.0	49.0	41.0	48	5220	6.0
nacho	1276	54.0	117.0	64.0	181	1654	11.0
Sampler	1405	47.0	124.0	80.0	75	5305	4.0
smothered cheese							
fries	767	27.0	69.0	48.0	78	875	0
entrees, no sides:							
burgers, mini, 6,							
w/onion rings ...	2044	61.0	179.0	122.0	145	3834	10.0
chicken, grilled	200	25.0	15.0	5.0	67	824	1.0
chicken strips	635	47.0	55.0	25.0	95	1510	0
country fried steak .	644	28.0	30.0	46.0	89	2149	11.0
fish and chips	958	34.0	83.0	54.0	88	1390	6.0
shrimp, fried	219	17.0	18.0	10.0	133	774	1.0

Food and Measure	cal.	prot. (gms)	carbo. (gms)	fat (gms)	chol. (mgs)	sod. (mgs)	fiber (gms)
shrimp, fried and							
scampi	346	27.0	15.0	20.0	241	1104	1.0
shrimp scampi skillet	289	25.0	3.0	19.0	192	766	.3
sirloin steak	337	18.0	1.0	28.0	687	344	1.0
steak and shrimp . .	645	36.0	31.0	42.0	150	1143	2.0
T-bone steak	860	65.0	0	65.0	196	867	0
turkey, roast,							
w/stuffing, gravy	435	42.0	62.0	10.0	100	4620	2.0
sides/condiments:							
applesauce	60	0	15.0	0	0	13	1.0
barbecue sauce .	47	0	11.0	1.0	0	595	0
bread stuffing . . .	100	3.0	19.0	1.0	0	405	1.0
brown gravy	13	0	2.0	0	0	184	0
coleslaw	274	2.0	14.0	24.0	37	588	2.0
corn	105	3.0	23.0	2.0	0	184	3.0
cottage cheese . .	72	9.0	2.0	3.0	10	281	0
country gravy . . .	17	0	2.0	1.0	0	93	0
fries, no salt	423	6.0	57.0	7.0	0	144	1.0
fries, seasoned . .	261	5.0	35.0	12.0	0	556	
garlic dinner bread,							
2 pcs.	170	2.0	15.0	11.0	<1	325	1.0
green beans	40	2.0	8.0	1.0	0	47	3.0
marinara sauce .	48	1.0	7.0	2.0	0	206	1.0
onion rings	381	5.0	38.0	23.0	6	1003	1.0
pico de gallo . . .	21	1.0	5.0	0	0	125	1.0
potato, baked . . .	220	5.0	51.0	0	0	16	5.0
potato, mashed .	168	3.0	23.0	7.0	8	498	2.0
sour cream	91	1.0	2.0	9.0	19	23	0
tartar sauce	225	0	3.0	23.0	15	157	0
tomato, 3 slices .	13	1.0	3.0	0	0	6	1.0
turkey gravy	125	4.0	29.0	9.0	69	3323	0
salad, no dressing,							
except as noted:							
Caesar, side							
w/dressing	362	11.0	20.0	26.0	23	913	2.0
chef's	365	41.0	14.0	16.0	289	1376	4.0
chicken breast,							
grilled	259	32.0	10.0	11.0	90	724	4.0
chicken strip, fried .	438	33.0	26.0	26.0	78	1030	4.0
garden, side	113	7.0	6.0	7.0	0	144	2.0
taco	505	18.0	57.0	22.0	54	553	8.0
salad croutons	112	2.0	12.0	6.0	0	195	1.0
salad dressing:							
blue cheese	163	1.0	1.0	18.0	20	205	0

Food and Measure	cal.	prot. (gms)	carbo. (gms)	fat (gms)	chol. (mgs)	sod. (mgs)	fiber (gms)
Denny's, salad dressing *(cont.)*							
Caesar	133	1.0	1.0	14.0	2	380	0
French	106	0	3.0	10.0	7	274	0
honey mustard	160	0	20.0	15.0	20	123	0
Italian, low cal	15	0	3.0	.5	0	390	0
ranch	129	0	1.0	14.0	8	189	0
ranch, fat free	25	.1	6.0	.2	0	300	0
Thousand Island ..	118	0	5.0	11.0	15	170	0
dessert/shakes:							
apple crisp à la mode	723	6.0	133.0	21.0	32	394	6.0
banana split	894	15.0	121.0	43.0	78	177	6.0
carrot cake	799	9.0	99.0	45.0	125	630	2.0
cheesecake	580	8.0	51.0	38.0	174	380	0
float, cola/root beer	280	3.0	47.0	10.0	39	109	0
hot fudge brownie à la mode	997	12.0	147.0	42.0	14	82	6.0
milkshake	560	11.0	76.0	26.0	100	272	<1.0
milkshake, malted .	583	12.0	82.0	26.0	100	278	<1.0
Oreo Blender Blaster	895	16.0	112.0	46.0	135	280	2.0
pie, no topping:							
apple	470	3.0	64.0	24.0	0	470	1.0
blueberry	681	5.0	90.0	22.0	0	299	5.0
chocolate peanut butter	653	15.0	64.0	39.0	27	319	3.0
coconut cream ..	582	5.0	63.0	33.0	0	482	3.0
French silk	690	7.0	54.0	49.0	80	225	4.0
sundae:							
single scoop	188	3.0	14.0	14.0	37	43	0
double scoop ...	375	6.0	29.0	27.0	74	86	0
topping, 2 oz.:							
blueberry	71	0	17.0	0	0	10	0
cherry	57	0	14.0	0	0	3	0
chocolate	133	2.0	34.0	.5	0	109	1.0
fudge	201	1.0	30.0	10.0	3	96	1.0
strawberry	77	1.0	17.0	1.0	0	8	1.0
whipped cream ...	23	0	2.0	2.0	7	3	0
Dessert, see specific listings							
Dessert, freeze-dried, 1 serving:							
apple almond crisp (*AlpineAire*)	260	5.0	57.0	1.0	0	25	4.0
apple blueberry cobbler (*AlpineAire*)	210	6.0	38.0	4.0	n.a.	550	4.0

Food and Measure	cal.	prot. (gms)	carbo. (gms)	fat (gms)	chol. (mgs)	sod. (mgs)	fiber (gms)
bananas Foster (*Alpine-Aire*)	250	2.0	47.0	5.0	n.a.	75	2.0
cheesecake:							
blackberry (*Alpine-Aire* Mountain) ..	670	6.0	134.0	13.0	n.a.	490	1.0
blueberry (*Mountain House*), ¼ pouch, ½ cup	210	7.0	37.0	4.0	5	330	<1.0
chocolate hazelnut Bavarian cream (*AlpineAire*)	300	7.0	36.0	14.0	n.a.	60	4.0
ice cream, 1 pkg.:							
Neapolitan (*Mountain House*)	120	2.0	15.0	6.0	25	50	0
sandwich (*Mountain House*)	170	2.0	25.0	7.0	15	169	1.0
peach crumble, deep dish (*AlpineAire*) ..	220	2.0	48.0	3.0	0	35	1.0
raspberry crumble (*Mountain House*), ¼ pouch, ½ cup ..	160	1.0	31.0	3.0	0	85	3.0
Dill dip (*Litehouse* Dilly), 2 tbsp.	150	1.0	2.0	16.0	15	200	0
Dill seed, 1 tsp.	6 —	.3	1.2	.3	0	<1	.4
Dill weed, fresh:							
5 sprigs	<1	<1.0	.1	<.1	0	1	<.1
1 cup	4	.3	.6	.1	0	5	.2
Dill weed, dried, 1 tsp.	3	.2	.6	<.1	0	2	.1
Dip, see specific listings							
Dipping sauce, see specific listings							
Dock:							
raw, chopped, 1 cup .	29	2.6	4.3	.9	9	5	3.9
boiled, drained, 4 oz. .	23	2.1	3.3	.7	0	3	<1.0
Dolphin fish, meat only:							
raw, 4 oz.	97	21.0	0	.8	83	99	0
baked, broiled or microwaved, 4 oz. ..	124	26.9	0	1.0	107	128	0
Domino's Pizza, ⅛ pizza, except as noted:							
deep dish, 12":							
America's Favorite Feast	309	12.0	29.0	17.0	25	797	2.0

Food and Measure	cal.	prot. (gms)	carbo. (gms)	fat (gms)	chol. (mgs)	sod. (mgs)	fiber (gms)
Domino's Pizza, deep dish, 12" *(cont.)*							
Bacon Cheeseburger							
Feast	325	14.0	28.0	18.5	30	805	2.0
Barbecue Feast	304	12.0	32.0	15.0	23	771	2.0
beef	277	11.0	28.0	14.5	19	664	2.0
cheese	238	9.0	28.0	11.0	11	556	2.0
Deluxe Feast	287	11.0	29.0	15.0	20	712	2.0
ExtravaganZZa Feast	341	14.0	30.0	19.5	31	935	2.0
green pepper/onion/							
mushroom	244	9.0	30.0	11.0	11	556	2.0
ham	250	11.0	28.0	11.5	16	663	2.0
ham/pineapple	252	10.0	30.0	11.5	15	637	2.0
Hawaiian Feast	275	12.0	30.0	13.0	19	717	2.0
MeatZZa Feast	333	14.0	29.0	19.0	31	911	2.0
pepperoni	275	11.0	28.0	14.0	19	692	2.0
Pepperoni Feast ...	317	13.0	29.0	17.5	27	841	2.0
pepperoni/sausage .	307	12.0	29.0	17.0	25	796	2.0
sausage	283	11.0	29.0	15.0	19	701	2.0
Vegi Feast	270	11.0	30.0	13.5	15	397	2.0
deep dish, 14":							
America's Favorite							
Feast	433	17.0	42.0	23.5	34	1110	3.0
Bacon Cheeseburger							
Feast	459	20.0	41.0	25.5	42	1146	3.0
Barbecue Feast	424	17.0	46.0	20.5	31	1078	2.0
beef	392	15.0	41.0	20.0	26	937	2.0
cheese	336	13.0	41.0	15.0	16	782	2.0
Deluxe Feast	396	15.0	42.0	20.0	26	975	3.0
ExtravaganZZa Feast	468	20.0	43.0	25.5	40	1260	3.0
green pepper/onion/							
mushroom	343	13.0	42.0	15.0	16	783	3.0
ham	352	15.0	41.0	15.5	22	929	2.0
ham/pineapple	355	14.0	42.0	15.5	21	900	2.0
Hawaiian Feast	389	17.0	43.0	18.0	26	1011	3.0
MeatZZa Feast	458	19.0	40.0	25.0	40	1230	3.0
pepperoni	385	15.0	41.0	19.5	26	964	2.0
Pepperoni Feast ...	443	18.0	42.0	24.0	37	1166	3.0
pepperoni/sausage .	430	17.0	41.0	23.0	34	1109	3.0
sausage	400	15.0	42.0	20.5	27	990	3.0
Vegi Feast	380	15.0	43.0	18.0	21	924	3.0
hand-tossed, 12":							
America's Favorite							
Feast	257	10.0	29.0	11.5	22	626	2.0

Food and Measure	cal.	prot. (gms)	carbo. (gms)	fat (gms)	chol. (mgs)	sod. (mgs)	fiber (gms)
Bacon Cheeseburger Feast	273	12.0	28.0	13.0	27	634	2.0
Barbecue Feast	252	11.0	31.0	10.0	20	600	1.0
beef	225	9.0	28.0	9.0	16	493	2.0
cheese	186	7.0	28.0	5.5	9	385	1.0
Deluxe Feast	234	9.0	29.0	9.5	17	542	2.0
ExtravaganZZa Feast	289	13.0	30.0	14.0	28	764	2.0
green pepper/onion/ mushroom	191	8.0	29.0	5.5	9	386	2.0
ham	198	9.0	28.0	6.0	13	492	1.0
ham/pineapple	200	9.0	29.0	6.0	12	467	2.0
Hawaiian Feast	223	10.0	30.0	8.0	16	547	2.0
MeatZZa Feast	281	13.0	29.0	13.5	28	740	2.0
pepperoni	223	9.0	28.0	9.0	16	522	2.0
Pepperoni Feast ...	265	11.0	28.0	12.5	24	670	2.0
pepperoni/sausage .	255	10.0	28.0	11.5	22	626	2.0
sausage	231	9.0	28.0	9.5	17	530	2.0
Vegi Feast	218	9.0	29.0	8.0	13	489	2.0
hand-tossed, 14":							
America's Favorite Feast	353	14.0	39.0	16.0	31	864	2.0
Bacon Cheeseburger Feast	379	17.0	38.0	18.0	38	900	2.0
Barbecue Feast	344	14.0	43.0	13.5	27	832	2.0
beef	312	13.0	38.0	12.5	23	690	2.0
cheese	256	10.0	38.0	8.0	12	536	2.0
Deluxe Feast	316	13.0	39.0	12.5	23	729	2.0
ExtravaganZZa Feast	388	17.0	40.0	18.5	37	1014	3.0
green pepper/onion/ mushroom	263	11.0	39.0	8.0	12	537	2.0
ham	272	12.0	38.0	8.5	18	682	2.0
ham/pineapple	275	12.0	40.0	8.5	17	653	2.0
Hawaiian Feast	309	14.0	41.0	11.0	23	765	2.0
MeatZZa Feast	378	17.0	39.0	18.0	37	984	2.0
pepperoni	305	12.0	38.0	12.0	22	718	2.0
Pepperoni Feast ...	363	16.0	39.0	17.0	33	920	2.0
pepperoni/sausage .	350	14.0	39.0	16.0	31	863	2.0
sausage	320	13.0	39.0	13.5	24	744	2.0
Vegi Feast	300	13.0	40.0	11.0	18	678	3.0
thin crust, 12":							
America's Favorite Feast	208	8.0	15.0	13.5	23	533	1.0
Bacon Cheeseburger Feast	224	10.0	14.0	14.5	29	542	1.0

Food and Measure	cal.	prot. (gms)	carbo. (gms)	fat (gms)	chol. (mgs)	sod. (mgs)	fiber (gms)
Domino's Pizza, thin crust, 12" (cont.)							
Barbecue Feast	203	8.0	17.0	11.5	22	508	1.0
beef	175	7.0	14.0	10.5	17	400	1.0
cheese	137	5.0	14.0	7.0	10	293	1.0
Deluxe Feast	185	7.0	15.0	11.5	19	449	1.0
ExtravaganZZa Feast	240	11.0	16.0	15.5	29	672	1.0
green pepper/onion/ mushroom	142	6.0	15.0	7.5	10	293	1.0
ham	148	7.0	14.0	7.5	14	400	1.0
ham/pineapple	150	7.0	15.0	7.5	13	374	1.0
Hawaiian Feast	174	8.0	16.0	9.5	17	454	1.0
MeatZZa Feast	232	11.0	15.0	15.0	29	647	1.0
pepperoni	174	7.0	14.0	10.5	17	429	1.0
Pepperoni Feast . . .	216	9.0	14.0	14.0	26	577	1.0
pepperoni/sausage .	206	8.0	14.0	13.5	23	533	1.0
sausage	181	7.0	14.0	11.0	18	438	1.0
Vegi Feast	168	7.0	15.0	9.5	14	397	1.0
thin crust, 14":							
America's Favorite Feast	285	11.0	20.0	18.5	32	737	2.0
Bacon Cheeseburger Feast	311	14.0	19.0	20.5	40	773	1.0
Barbecue Feast	276	11.0	24.0	15.5	29	704	1.0
beef	243	10.0	19.0	15.0	24	563	1.0
cheese	188	7.0	19.0	10.0	13	409	1.0
Deluxe Feast	248	10.0	20.0	15.0	24	601	2.0
ExtravaganZZa Feast	320	14.0	21.0	20.5	38	887	2.0
green pepper/onion/ mushroom	201	8.0	21.0	10.0	13	410	2.0
ham	204	9.0	19.0	10.5	20	555	1.0
ham/pineapple	207	9.0	21.0	10.5	18	526	1.0
Hawaiian Feast	240	11.0	21.0	13.0	24	638	2.0
MeatZZa Feast	310	14.0	20.0	20.0	38	857	2.0
pepperoni	237	10.0	19.0	14.5	24	591	1.0
Pepperoni Feast . . .	295	13.0	20.0	19.0	35	793	1.0
pepperoni/sausage .	282	11.0	19.0	18.5	32	736	2.0
sausage	252	10.0	20.0	15.5	25	616	2.0
Vegi Feast	231	10.0	21.0	13.5	19	551	2.0
salad, Amazin' Greens, ½ cont.:							
garden fresh	63	3.8	4.5	3.7	11	81	1.6
grilled chicken Caesar	98	11.8	4.2	3.9	26	316	1.3

Food and Measure	cal.	prot. (gms)	carbo. (gms)	fat (gms)	chol. (mgs)	sod. (mgs)	fiber (gms)
sides, 1 pc. or cont.:							
bread stick	115	2.0	12.0	6.3	0	122	0
Buffalo Chicken							
Kickers	47	4.0	3.0	2.0	9	163	0
Buffalo wings:							
barbecue	50	6.0	2.0	2.5	26	176	0
hot	45	5.0	1.0	2.5	26	255	0
cheesy bread	123	4.0	13.0	6.5	6	162	0
Cinna Stix	123	2.0	15.0	6.1	0	111	1.0
icing, sweet	250	0	57.0	2.5	0	0	0
sauce, dipping:							
blue cheese	223	1.0	2.0	23.5	20	417	0
garlic	440	0	0	49.0	0	380	0
hot	15	0	4.0	0	0	1820	0
marinara	25	1.0	5.0	.2	0	263	0
ranch	197	1.0	2.0	20.5	9	380	0
Donuts, 1 pc., except as noted:							
plain:							
(*Awrey's*), 2 pcs., 2.8 oz.	330	5.0	38.0	18.0	15	380	0
(*Entenmann's Softee*), 1.7 oz.	200	3.0	24.0	12.0	20	240	<1.0
chocolate frosted (*Entenmann's*), 2 oz.	280	2.0	28.0	19.0	10	190	1.0
crumb topped (*Entenmann's*), 2.1 oz. ...	260	2.0	35.0	12.0	10	220	<1.0
glazed (*Entenmann's*), 1.8 oz.	210	3.0	25.0	11.0	5	190	<1.0
Dough, bread, see "Bread, frozen"							
Dough, sweet (*Rhodes*), 1.8 oz.	145	5.0	24.0	3.0	10	260	1.0
Dow gok, see "Yard-long bean"							
Drum, freshwater, meat only:							
raw, 4 oz.	135	19.9	0	5.6	73	85	0
baked, broiled, or microwaved, 4 oz. .	173	25.5	0	7.2	93	109	0
Duck, domesticated, roasted, 4 oz.:							
meat w/skin	382	21.5	0	32.1	95	67	0
meat only	228	26.6	0	12.7	101	74	0

Food and Measure	cal.	prot. (gms)	carbo. (gms)	fat (gms)	chol. (mgs)	sod. (mgs)	fiber (gms)
Duck *(cont.)*							
young, Pekin:							
breast, meat w/skin	229	27.8	0	12.3	154	95	0
leg, meat w/skin . . .	246	30.3	0	12.9	129	125	0
Duck, wild, raw:							
meat w/skin, 4 oz. . . .	239	19.8	0	17.2	91	64	0
breast meat, 4 oz. . . .	139	22.5	0	4.8	87	65	0
Duck fat, 1 tbsp.	115	0	0	12.8	13	0	0
Duck sauce, see "Sweet and sour sauce"							
Dulce de leche topping, see "Caramel topping"							
Dulse flakes, see "Seaweed"							
Dumpling squash, see "Sweet dumpling squash"							
Dumplings, frozen:							
chicken, see "Chicken entree, frozen"							
meatless, 2 pcs.:							
(*Health is Wealth* Potstickers), 1.6 oz.	80	4.0	11.0	4.0	0	300	1.0
steamed (*Health is Wealth*), 1.6 oz. .	50	4.0	12.0	1.5	0	310	1.0
Dunkin Donuts,							
1 serving:							
breakfast sandwich:							
bacon/egg/cheese:							
bagel	480	17.0	69.0	14.0	150	1300	2.0
croissant	480	17.0	39.0	28.0	140	880	0
English muffin . .	330	19.0	34.0	12.0	155	1210	1.0
egg/cheese:							
bagel	470	23.0	71.0	10.0	140	1190	2.0
biscuit	370	15.0	32.0	20.0	140	1190	1.0
croissant	440	14.0	39.0	26.0	125	640	0
English muffin . .	280	15.0	34.0	9.0	140	1010	1.0
ham/egg/cheese:							
bagel	510	30.0	71.0	11.0	160	1460	2.0
croissant	470	20.0	38.0	27.0	150	940	0
English muffin . .	310	21.0	34.0	10.0	160	1270	1.0
sausage/egg/cheese:							
bagel	680	33.0	72.0	29.0	185	1700	2.0
biscuit	570	24.0	32.0	39.0	185	1700	1.0

Food and Measure	cal.	prot. (gms)	carbo. (gms)	fat (gms)	chol. (mgs)	sod. (mgs)	fiber (gms)
croissant	650	22.0	39.0	45.0	165	1010	0
English muffin ..	480	24.0	35.0	27.0	185	1520	1.0
steak/egg/cheese, bagel	590	30.0	66.0	24.0	235	1420	2.0
steak/mushroom/ Swiss, bagel	660	34.0	67.0	29.0	255	1570	2.0
bagel:							
plain	320	12.0	62.0	2.5	0	650	2.0
blueberry	330	10.0	66.0	2.5	0	600	2.0
cinnamon raisin ...	330	10.0	65.0	3.0	0	430	3.0
everything	370	14.0	67.0	6.0	0	650	3.0
harvest	350	13.0	61.0	6.0	0	500	7.0
multigrain	380	14.0	68.0	6.0	0	650	5.0
onion	320	12.0	61.0	3.5	0	610	3.0
poppy seed	370	14.0	65.0	7.0	0	650	3.0
reduced carb	380	25.0	45.0	12.0	20	780	14.0
salsa	310	13.0	60.0	2.5	0	790	2.0
salt	320	12.0	62.0	2.5	0	4520	2.0
sesame	380	14.0	64.0	8.0	0	650	3.0
sourdough	370	15.0	71.0	3.0	0	760	2.0
wheat	330	12.0	62.0	4.0	0	610	4.0
biscuit	250	5.0	29.0	13.0	0	780	1.0
croissant:							
plain	330	5.0	37.0	18.0	5	270	0
reduced carb	370	18.0	19.0	24.0	5	300	2.0
cream cheese, 2 oz.:							
plain	190	4.0	4.0	17.0	55	190	0
plain, light	110	4.0	6.0	9.0	30	230	0
chive	170	4.0	4.0	17.0	45	230	2.0
salmon	170	4.0	2.0	17.0	45	180	0
strawberry	190	4.0	9.0	17.0	45	150	0
vegetable, garden ..	170	2.0	4.0	15.0	45	340	0
Shedd's buttermatch, 1 tbsp.	80	0	0	9.0	0	100	0
cookies, 2 pcs.:							
chocolate chunk ...	220	3.0	28.0	11.0	35	105	1.0
w/walnuts	230	3.0	27.0	12.0	35	110	1.0
white chocolate .	230	3.0	28.0	12.0	35	120	1.0
oatmeal raisin pecan	220	3.0	29.0	10.0	30	110	1.0
donuts:							
apple crumb	230	3.0	34.0	10.0	0	270	1.0
apple crumb cake ..	290	3.0	41.0	15.0	15	320	1.0
apple 'n spice	200	3.0	29.0	8.0	0	270	1.0
Bavarian kreme ...	210	3.0	30.0	9.0	0	270	1.0

Food and Measure	cal.	prot. (gms)	carbo. (gms)	fat (gms)	chol. (mgs)	sod. (mgs)	fiber (gms)
Dunkin Donuts, donuts *(cont.)*							
black raspberry ...	210	3.0	32.0	8.0	0	280	1.0
blueberry cake	290	3.0	35.0	16.0	10	400	1.0
blueberry crumb ..	240	3.0	36.0	10.0	0	260	1.0
Boston kreme	240	3.0	36.0	9.0	0	280	1.0
chocolate coconut .	300	4.0	31.0	19.0	0	370	1.0
chocolate frosted ..	200	3.0	29.0	9.0	0	260	1.0
chocolate frosted cake	360	4.0	40.0	20.0	25	350	1.0
chocolate glazed cake	290	3.0	33.0	16.0	0	370	1.0
chocolate kreme filled	270	3.0	35.0	13.0	0	260	1.0
cinnamon cake	330	4.0	34.0	20.0	25	340	1.0
crueller, French ...	150	2.0	17.0	8.0	20	105	1.0
double chocolate cake	310	2.0	37.0	17.0	0	370	2.0
gingerbread, glazed	260	3.0	35.0	11.0	20	320	1.0
glazed	180	3.0	25.0	8.0	0	250	1.0
glazed cake	350	4.0	41.0	19.0	25	340	1.0
jelly filled	210	3.0	32.0	8.0	0	280	1.0
lemon burst	300	3.0	35.0	14.0	0	300	3.0
lemon cake	240	2.0	28.0	14.0	0	150	0
maple frosted	200	3.0	29.0	9.0	0	260	1.0
old-fashioned cake .	300	4.0	28.0	19.0	25	330	1.0
powdered cake	330	4.0	36.0	19.0	25	330	1.0
strawberry	210	3.0	32.0	8.0	0	260	1.0
strawberry frosted .	210	3.0	30.0	9.0	0	260	1.0
sugar raised	170	3.0	22.0	8.0	0	250	1.0
vanilla kreme filled .	270	3.0	36.0	13.0	0	250	1.0
whole wheat glazed	310	4.0	32.0	19.0	0	380	2.0
donut fancies:							
apple fritter	300	4.0	41.0	14.0	0	360	1.0
chocolate iced Bismark	340	3.0	50.0	15.0	0	290	1.0
bow tie donut	300	4.0	34.0	17.0	0	340	1.0
coffee roll	270	4.0	33.0	14.0	0	340	1.0
coffee roll, frosted .	290	4.0	36.0	14.0	0	340	1.0
éclair	270	3.0	39.0	11.0	0	290	1.0
glazed fritter	260	4.0	31.0	14.0	0	330	1.0
donut *Munchkins:*							
cinnamon, 4 pcs. ...	270	3.0	31.0	15.0	25	210	1.0
cake, 4 pcs.	270	3.0	27.0	16.0	25	240	1.0
cake, glazed, 3 pcs.	280	3.0	38.0	13.0	20	190	1.0

Food and Measure	cal.	prot. (gms)	carbo. (gms)	fat (gms)	chol. (mgs)	sod. (mgs)	fiber (gms)
cake, powdered, 4 pcs.	270	3.0	31.0	14.0	25	210	1.0
chocolate cake, glazed, 3 pcs.	200	2.0	26.0	10.0	0	250	1.0
glazed, 5 pcs.	200	3.0	27.0	9.0	0	220	1.0
jelly filled, 5 pcs. ..	210	3.0	30.0	9.0	0	240	1.0
lemon filled, 4 pcs.	170	2.0	23.0	8.0	0	190	0
sugar raised, 7 pcs.	220	4.0	26.0	12.0	0	290	1.0
donut sticks, cake:							
plain	420	4.0	35.0	29.0	35	310	1.0
cinnamon	450	4.0	42.0	30.0	35	310	1.0
chocolate, glazed ..	470	4.0	49.0	29.0	0	490	2.0
glazed	490	4.0	51.0	29.0	35	310	1.0
jelly	530	4.0	61.0	29.0	35	320	1.0
powdered	450	4.0	42.0	29.0	35	310	1.0
muffins:							
banana walnut	540	10.0	69.0	25.0	65	520	3.0
blueberry	470	8.0	73.0	17.0	60	500	2.0
blueberry, reduced fat	440	8.0	75.0	12.0	55	650	2.0
chocolate chip	630	10.0	89.0	26.0	70	560	2.0
cranberry orange ..	440	8.0	66.0	17.0	65	480	3.0
coffee cake muffin .	580	9.0	78.0	19.0	65	520	1.0
corn	510	8.0	77.0	18.0	75	860	1.0
English	160	6.0	32.0	1.5	0	590	1.0
honey bran	480	8.0	79.0	15.0	60	480	5.0
pumpkin	610	10.0	83.0	18.0	15	690	3.0
panini:							
chicken fajita	390	23.0	57.0	9.0	40	990	3.0
meatball	480	22.0	56.0	19.0	40	1180	3.0
steak	450	30.0	56.0	12.0	45	1630	3.0
pastry/pie:							
apple Danish	250	4.0	36./0	10.0	5	220	0
apple pie	610	9.0	82.0	28.0	0	610	4.0
apple pie à la mode	810	12.0	107.0	38.0	40	610	4.0
cheese Danish	270	11.0	32.0	14.0	15	210	1.0
cinnamon stick	460	7.0	60.0	21.0	15	300	2.0
S'mores	140	2.0	20.0	6.0	0	135	1.0
strawberry cheese danish	250	4.0	33.0	12.0	10	200	0
Coolatta:							
coffee, w/cream ...	350	3.0	40.0	22.0	75	65	0
coffee, w/milk	210	4.0	42.0	4.0	15	80	0
coffee, w/milk, 2% .	190	4.0	41.0	2.0	10	80	0

Food and Measure	cal.	prot. (gms)	carbo. (gms)	fat (gms)	chol. (mgs)	sod. (mgs)	fiber (gms)
Dunkin Donuts, Coolatta (cont.)							
coffee, w/milk, skim	170	4.0	41.0	0	0	80	0
lemonade	240	0	49.0	0	0	35	0
orange mango	270	1.0	66.0	0	0	25	2.0
strawberry fruit ...	290	0	72.0	0	0	30	1.0
vanilla bean	440	1.0	70.0	17.0	0	95	1.0
espresso drinks, hot:							
cappuccino, w/milk	80	4.0	7.0	4.5	20	70	0
w/milk, sugar ...	130	4.0	21.0	4.5	20	65	0
w/soy milk	70	4.0	6.0	2.5	0	80	1.0
w/soy milk, sugar	120	4.0	20.0	2.5	0	80	1.0
latte, w/milk	120	6.0	10.0	6.0	25	95	0
w/milk, sugar ...	160	6.0	22.0	6.0	25	95	0
w/soy milk	90	6.0	8.0	3.5	0	110	1.0
w/soy milk, sugar	150	6.0	22.0	3.5	0	110	1.0
caramel swirl ...	230	8.0	36.0	6.0	25	140	0
caramel swirl, soy	210	8.0	34.0	3.5	0	160	1.0
mocha swirl	230	6.0	37.0	7.0	25	110	1.0
mocha swirl, soy	210	7.0	35.0	2.5	0	80	1.0
peppermint mocha	290	6.0	51.0	9.0	25	110	1.0
white chocolate							
raspberry	270	6.0	42.0	9.0	25	115	0
latte, iced:							
w/milk	120	6.0	11.0	7.0	25	105	0
w/milk, sugar	170	6.0	23.0	7.0	25	110	0
w/soy milk	90	6.0	8.0	3.5	0	115	1.0
w/soy milk, sugar .	140	6.0	20.0	3.5	0	115	1.0
caramel swirl	240	8.0	37.0	7.0	25	150	0
caramel swirl, soy .	210	8.0	34.0	3.5	0	160	1.0
mocha swirl	240	7.0	38.0	8.0	25	125	1.0
mocha swirl, soy ..	210	7.0	35.0	4.5	0	130	2.0
drinks, other:							
Dunkaccino	230	2.0	35.0	10.0	5	210	0
hot chocolate	220	2.0	38.0	8.0	0	280	2.0
vanilla chai	230	1.0	40.0	8.0	5	50	0
Durian, fresh:							
½ of 1.3-lb. fruit	442	4.4	81.5	16.0	0	3	11.4
chopped, ½ cup	179	1.8	32.9	6.5	0	2	4.6
Dutch brand loaf, see "Lunch meat"							

E

Food and Measure	cal.	prot. (gms)	carbo. (gms)	fat (gms)	chol. (mgs)	sod. (mgs)	fiber (gms)
Éclair, chocolate, frozen:							
(*Smart Ones*),							
2.1-oz. pc.	150	2.0	25.0	4.0	30	170	1.0
mini:							
(*Delizza* Belgian),							
7 pcs., 3.5 oz. . .	333	5.1	32.2	20.8	63	128	.9
(*Ritch & Famous*),							
.6-oz. pc.	50	<1.0	5.0	3.5	15	25	0
Edamame (see also "Soybean"), fresh (*Frieda's*), 2.6 oz., ½ cup in pod, 1 cup shelled	100	8.0	10.0	3.0	0	10	3.0
Edamame, frozen:							
in pod, ½ cup:							
(*C&W*)	60	5.0	8.0	.5	0	0	5.0
(*Dr. Praeger's*)	74	8.0	6.0	2.0	0	4	7.5
shelled:							
(*Cascadian Farm*),							
⅔ cup	120	10.0	9.0	5.0	0	10	4.0
(*Dr. Praeger's*),							
½ cup	95	9.0	8.0	3.0	0	4	5.0
Eel, meat only:							
raw, 4 oz.	209	20.9	0	3.2	143	58	0
baked, broiled, or microwaved, 4 oz. . .	268	26.8	0	17.0	183	74	0
Egg, chicken:							
raw, 1 large:							
whole	75	6.3	.6	5.0	213	63	0
white only (*Egg Beaters*), 3 tbsp.	25	5.0	0	0	0	75	0
white only	17	3.5	.3	0	0	55	0
yolk only[1]	59	2.8	.3	5.1	213	7	0

1. Includes a small portion of white.

Food and Measure	cal.	prot. (gms)	carbo. (gms)	fat (gms)	chol. (mgs)	sod. (mgs)	fiber (gms)
Egg, chicken *(cont.)*							
raw, brown:							
extra large (*Organic Valley*)	80	7.0	<1.0	6.0	240	70	0
extra large (*Organic Valley* Omega-3)	80	8.0	1.0	4.5	250	95	0
jumbo (*Organic Valley*)	90	8.0	<1.0	6.0	270	80	0
large (*Organic Valley*)	70	6.0	<1.0	5.0	215	65	0
medium (*Organic Valley*)	70	5.0	1.0	4.5	185	55	0
cooked:							
hard-boiled, chopped, 1 cup	210	17.1	1.5	14.4	578	169	0
poached, 1 large ..	74	6.2	.6	5.0	212	140	0
Egg, chicken, dried:							
whole:							
1 oz.	168	13.0	1.4	11.9	544	148	0
stabilized, 1 oz. ...	174	13.7	.7	12.5	572	155	0
white, flakes, 1 oz. ...	100	21.8	1.2	<.1	0	328	0
yolk, 1 oz.	195	8.7	.1	17.4	830	26	0
Egg, duck, 1 egg	130	9.0	1.0	9.6	619	102	0
Egg, goose, 1 egg ...	267	20.0	1.9	19.1	1227	199	0
Egg, quail, 1 egg	14	1.2	<.1	1.0	76	13	0
Egg, substitute, ¼ cup:							
(*Egg Beaters*)	30	6.0	1.0	0	0	115	0
(*Kineret* Light 'n Tasty)	30	6.0	1.0	0	0	80	0
(*Morningstar Farms Better'n Eggs*)	20	5.0	0	0	0	90	0
(*Morningstar Farms Scramblers*)	35	6.0	2.0	0	0	95	0
(*Tofutti Egg Watchers*)	30	6.0	1.0	0	0	80	0
cheese and chive (*Egg Beaters*)	35	6.0	1.0	1.0	<5	210	0
garden vegetable (*Egg Beaters*)	30	6.0	1.0	0	0	160	0
Southwestern (*Egg Beaters*)	30	6.0	1.0	0	0	180	0
Egg, turkey, 1 egg ...	135	10.8	.9	9.4	737	119	0
Egg breakfast, freeze-dried, 1 serving:							
w/bacon:							
(*Mountain House* Can), ⅔ cup	180	14.0	7.0	10.0	410	700	0

Food and Measure	cal.	prot. (gms)	carbo. (gms)	fat (gms)	chol. (mgs)	sod. (mgs)	fiber (gms)
(*Mountain House Pouch*)	320	26.0	12.0	18.0	730	1250	<1.0
w/ham and peppers:							
(*Mountain House Can*), ⅔ cup	160	12.0	6.0	9.0	350	530	<1.0
(*Mountain House Pouch*)	350	27.0	14.0	21.0	790	1200	1.0
omelette, ranch w/beef (*AlpineAire*)	390	28.0	17.0	24.0	n.a.	580	1.0
scrambled:							
(*AlpineAire*)	170	11.0	2.0	13.0	n.a.	180	0
(*Mountain House*) .	310	23.0	14.0	18.0	570	1040	0
scrambling/omelette mix (*AlpineAire*) ...	339	27.0	3.0	23.0	n.a.	300	0
Egg breakfast, frozen (see also "Breakfast pocket/sandwich" and specific listings):							
omelette:							
cheese, three (*Jimmy Dean*), 4.3 oz. ..	290	16.0	5.0	23.0	305	830	<1.0
ham/cheese, w/home fries (*Aunt Jemima Great Starts*), 5.2-oz. pkg.	250	13.0	19.0	14.0	265	810	1.0
Western style (*Jimmy Dean*), 4.3 oz.	210	13.0	6.0	15.0	280	590	<1.0
scrambled, w/hash browns:							
w/bacon (*Aunt Jemima Great Starts*), 5.25-oz. pkg.	320	13.0	16.0	22.0	300	740	<1.0
w/sausage (*Aunt Jemima Great Starts*), 6.25-oz. pkg.	370	14.0	18.0	27.0	335	750	2.0
Egg roll (see also "Spring roll"), frozen or refrigerated:							
broccoli (*Health is Wealth*), 3 oz.	150	6.0	23.0	4.5	5	560	2.0

Food and Measure	cal.	prot. (gms)	carbo. (gms)	fat (gms)	chol. (mgs)	sod. (mgs)	fiber (gms)
Egg roll *(cont.)*							
pizza *(Health is Wealth)*, 3 oz.	200	7.0	23.0	9.0	0	470	3.0
w/sauce, 3.1-oz. pc:							
seafood *(Chung's)*	170	6.0	24.0	5.0	5	470	2.0
shrimp *(Chung's)*	160	6.0	24.0	5.0	15	450	2.0
vegetable *(Chung's)*	160	4.0	25.0	6.0	0	470	2.0
spinach *(Health is Wealth)*, 3 oz.	180	7.0	20.0	8.0	0	300	3.0
vegetable:							
(Empire), 3 oz.	130	3.0	15.0	6.0	15	390	3.0
(Health is Wealth Oriental), 3 oz.	160	4.0	23.0	4.0	0	390	2.0
(Health is Wealth Veggie), 3 oz.	130	4.0	21.0	4.0	0	550	3.0
(Kahiki), 3 oz.	120	4.0	23.0	2.0	5	730	2.0
mini *(Barney's)*, 3 pcs., 2.4 oz.	160	5.0	22.0	16.0	0	300	1.0
vegetarian, chicken-free *(Health is Wealth)*, 3 oz.	120	8.0	21.0	4.0	0	390	2.0
Egg roll entree, frozen, vegetable *(Lean Cuisine Everyday Favorites)*, 9-oz. pkg.	310	7.0	60.0	5.0	5	640	3.0
Egg roll sauce (see also "Sweet and sour sauce"), orange *(Port Arthur)*, 2 tbsp.	50	0	13.0	0	0	140	0
Egg roll wrapper (see also "Wrappers") *(Frieda's)*, 2 pcs.	130	5.0	28.0	.5	0	250	1.0
Eggnog, dairy, ½ cup:							
(Darigold)	180	3.0	22.0	9.0	65	85	0
(Darigold Light)	140	6.0	20.0	4.5	50	85	0
(Hood Fat Free)	110	8.0	18.0	0	<5	100	0
(Hood Golden)	180	4.0	22.0	9.0	65	100	0
(Hood Light)	140	4.0	22.0	4.0	45	100	0
(Hood Carb Countdown Reduced Sugar)	120	4.0	9.0	8.0	60	125	0
(Organic Valley)	140	4.0	15.0	7.0	65	65	0
(Turkey Hill)	190	5.0	23.0	9.0	65	105	0
(Turkey Hill CarbIQ)	140	5.0	11.0	9.0	60	110	2.0
vanilla *(Hood)*	180	4.0	22.0	9.0	65	100	0

Food and Measure	cal.	prot. (gms)	carbo. (gms)	fat (gms)	chol. (mgs)	sod. (mgs)	fiber (gms)
Eggnog, canned							
(*Borden*), ½ cup ..	160	4.0	17.0	9.0	75	80	0
"Eggnog," nondairy							
(*Silk* Nog), ½ cup .	90	3.0	15.0	2.0	0	75	0
Eggplant, fresh:							
raw:							
(*Frieda's* Chinese/							
Japanese), ⅔ cup,							
3 oz.	20	1.0	5.0	0	0	0	2.0
1" pcs., ½ cup	11	.4	2.5	.1	0	1	1.0
boiled, drained,							
1" cubes, ½ cup . . .	13	.4	3.2	.1	0	2	1.2
Eggplant appetizer:							
baba ghanoush, 2 tbsp.:							
(*Cedar's*)	50	2.0	5.0	2.0	0	80	3.0
roasted (*Cedar's*) ..	50	3.0	5.0	2.0	0	120	3.0
caponata (*Alessi*),							
⅓ cup	140	2.0	7.0	7.0	0	310	4.0
spread (*Peloponnese*),							
2 tbsp.	20	0	3.0	1.0	0	240	0
Eggplant dip (*Victoria*),							
2 tbsp.	30	0	2.0	2.0	0	310	1.0
Eggplant entree,							
frozen, 1 pkg.,							
except as noted:							
bhartha (*Ethnic*							
Gourmet), 12 oz. . . .	290	8.0	46.0	9.0	0	770	8.0
cutlets, breaded							
(*Dominex*), 3-oz. pc. .	180	2.0	18.0	11.0	0	150	1.0
Parmesan:							
(*Cedarlane*), 5 oz. .	160	7.0	16.0	8.0	15	390	3.0
(*Cedarlane Carb*							
Buster), 9.5 oz. . .	220	12.0	15.0	15.0	40	620	4.0
parmigiana, w/sauce							
(*Celentano*), ½ of							
14-oz. pkg.	260	7.0	13.0	20.0	50	430	3.0
rollettes (*Celentano*),							
10 oz.	340	8.0	20.0	26.0	35	700	4.0
Eggplant entree, pkg.							
(*Tasty Bite* Punjab),							
½ of 10-oz. pkg. . .	112	4.0	13.0	9.0	0	515	2.0
Eggplant relish, Indian							
(*Patak's* Brinjal),							
1 tbsp.	50	<1.0	5.0	4.0	0	240	0

Food and Measure	cal.	prot. (gms)	carbo. (gms)	fat (gms)	chol. (mgs)	sod. (mgs)	fiber (gms)
Eggplant spread, see "Eggplant appetizer"							
Eight ball squash (*Frieda's*), 1 cup, 4.4 oz.	18	2.0	4.0	0	0	4	1.0
El Pollo Loco, 1 serving:							
chicken, flame-grilled:							
breast, w/skin	187	30.0	0	7.0	128	540	0
breast, w/out skin .	153	29.0	0	4.0	95	540	0
leg	86	14.0	0	3.0	80	206	0
thigh	120	14.0	0	7.0	82	225	0
wing	83	13.0	0	3.0	58	334	0
tortilla, 3 pcs.:							
corn, 6"	210	3.0	42.0	3.0	0	105	3.0
flour, 6.5"	330	9.0	48.0	12.0	0	630	3.0
burritos:							
BRC	528	17.0	79.0	15.0	15	1394	6.0
chicken, spicy	555	29.0	64.0	19.0	72	1962	6.0
Chicken Lover's Burrito	526	34.0	55.0	18.0	101	1808	2.0
Classic Chicken Burrito	636	32.0	81.0	19.0	63	1749	6.0
Grilled Fiesta Burrito	1068	55.0	91.0	54.0	124	3006	5.0
Twice Grilled Burrito	853	59.0	62.0	41.0	151	2936	2.0
Ultimate Chicken Burrito	701	35.0	84.0	24.0	65	2281	6.0
favorites:							
chicken nachos . . .	1299	65.0	90.0	77.0	202	2340	12.0
chicken quesadilla .	654	38.0	53.0	30.0	108	1530	2.0
cheese quesadilla . .	543	22.0	51.0	26.0	60	1177	2.0
chicken taquito, 2 . .	370	15.0	43.0	17.0	25	690	3.0
chicken soft taco . .	237	17.0	18.0	11.0	45	526	1.0
taco al carbon	134	9.0	18.0	3.0	29	224	1.0
bowls:							
chicken Caesar	535	25.0	47.0	29.0	51	1451	5.0
Pollo	543	31.0	84.0	10.0	42	2159	12.0
salad:							
Caesar	535	23.0	17.0	42.0	59	1242	4.0
w/out dressing . .	221	22.0	15.0	9.0	44	908	4.0
fiesta	747	31.0	29.0	57.0	97	1654	5.0
w/out dressing . .	439	30.0	26.0	26.0	82	1249	4.0
Monterray Pollo Salad	258	22.0	17.0	13.0	52	1266	3.0
w/out dressing . .	176	22.0	12.0	6.0	44	836	3.0

Food and Measure	cal.	prot. (gms)	carbo. (gms)	fat (gms)	chol. (mgs)	sod. (mgs)	fiber (gms)
tostada	740	34.0	83.0	33.0	65	1823	11.0
w/out shell	414	29.0	42.0	16.0	65	1479	7.0
salad dressing:							
chipotle	269	1.0	3.0	28.0	13	354	1.0
cilantro	275	1.0	1.0	29.0	13	292	0
cilantro, lite	83	0	5.0	7.0	8	430	0
Italian, lite	20	0	2.0	1.0	0	780	0
ranch, buttermilk . .	220	1.0	2.0	24.0	10	420	0
Thousand Island . . .	220	0	7.0	21.0	30	360	0
sides:							
black beans	306	7.0	35.0	16.0	13	731	5.0
coleslaw	206	2.0	12.0	16.0	11	358	2.0
corn cobbette	42	1.0	10.0	0	0	7.0	1.0
fries	444	6.0	61.0	19.0	0	605	0
garden salad	111	5.0	8.0	7.0	15	271	2.0
gravy	12	0	2.0	0	1	151	0
macaroni/cheese . .	381	11.0	25.0	26.0	65	891	2.0
pinto beans	154	7.0	24.0	4.0	0	674	9.0
mashed potatoes . .	110	2.0	23.0	1.0	0	406	2.0
Spanish rice	161	3.0	33.0	1.0	0	421	1.0
vegetables, fresh . .	68	3.0	6.0	4.0	0	78	4.0
condiments:							
guacamole	51	0	5.0	3.0	0	272	0
jalapeño hot sauce .	3	0	0	0	0	112	0
salsa, avocado	18	0	1.0	1.0	0	226	0
salsa, house	6	0	1.0	0	0	87	0
salsa, pico de gallo	10	0	1.0	0	0	136	0
salsa, spicy chipotle	7	0	1.0	0	0	180	0
tortilla chips	304	4.0	34.0	17.0	0	430	3.0
sour cream	104	2.0	2.0	10.0	22	26	0
Serrano pepper, fried	23	0	3.0	1.0	0	2.0	0
dessert:							
churro	181	3.0	24.0	11.0	5	221	1.0
caramel flan	303	4.0	43.0	12.0	54	160	0
Foster's Freeze, w/out							
cone	180	4.0	30.0	5.0	20	100	0
Elderberries, ½ cup .	53	.5	13.3	.4	0	4	5.1
Elderberry nectar (*R.W.*							
Knudsen), 8 fl. oz. .	120	<1.0	29.0	0	0	20	0
Elk, meat only, roasted,							
4 oz.	166	34.2	0	2.2	83	69	0
Empanada, frozen,							
2 pcs., 4.75 oz.:							
beef (*Goya*)	380	11.0	58.0	12.0	15	800	2.0

Food and Measure	cal.	prot. (gms)	carbo. (gms)	fat (gms)	chol. (mgs)	sod. (mgs)	fiber (gms)
Empanada *(cont.)*							
cheese (*Goya*)	350	10.0	44.0	15.0	20	990	2.0
pizza (*Goya*)	370	11.0	56.0	12.0	15	930	40
Emu, ground,							
panbroiled, 4 oz. ..	185	32.2	0	5.3	99	74	0
Enchilada, frozen, 1 pc.:							
beef, w/sauce:							
(*El Monterey*), 4 oz.	150	6.0	16.0	7.0	15	450	2.0
(*El Monterey*), 5 oz.	180	8.0	18.0	9.0	25	680	2.0
cheese (*Cedarlane*),							
4.8 oz.	270	14.0	19.0	17.0	45	390	2.0
cheese, w/sauce:							
(*El Monterey*), 4 oz.	170	7.0	15.0	10.0	25	600	1.0
(*El Monterey*), 5 oz.	220	10.0	16.0	13.0	35	610	1.0
chicken, suiza sauce							
(*El Monterey*), 5 oz.	210	11.0	19.0	11.0	35	530	1.0
Enchilada dinner,							
frozen, 1 pkg.:							
black bean (*Amy's*							
Whole Meal), 10 oz.	320	7.0	55.0	8.0	0	740	9.0
cheese (*Amy's* Whole							
Meal), 9 oz.	330	15.0	38.0	14.0	30	680	6.0
Enchilada entree,							
frozen, 1 pkg.,							
except as noted:							
(*Amy's* Bowls Santa Fe),							
10 oz.	340	17.0	47.0	9.0	5	780	10.0
black bean vegetable:							
(*Amy's*), ½ of 9							
.5-oz. pkg.	170	5.0	26.0	5.0	0	390	3.0
(*Amy's* Family Size),							
1/7 of 35-oz. pkg.	170	5.0	26.0	5.0	0	390	3.0
cheese:							
(*Amy's*), ½ of							
9-oz. pkg.......	220	10.0	18.0	12.0	35	460	2.0
(*Amy's* Family Size),							
1/7 of 35-oz. pkg.	240	11.0	19.0	13.0	35	460	2.0
(*Linda McCartney*),							
5-oz. pc.	250	8.0	23.0	11.0	30	570	2.0
chicken:							
(*Healthy Choice*),							
9 oz............	310	16.0	46.0	7.0	40	600	6.0
(*Healthy Choice*),							
11.3 oz.	360	13.0	59.0	7.0	30	580	8.0

Food and Measure	cal.	prot. (gms)	carbo. (gms)	fat (gms)	chol. (mgs)	sod. (mgs)	fiber (gms)
(*Lean Cuisine Everyday Favorites*), 9 oz.	280	10.0	49.0	5.0	20	540	3.0
(*Stouffer's* Family Style Recipes), ⅛ of 57-oz. pkg.	310	11.0	33.0	15.0	40	650	2.0
Suiza (*Smart Ones*), 9 oz.	340	12.0	38.0	10.0	40	800	3.0
pie, 3-layer (*Cedarlane*), ½ of 11-oz. pkg.	215	13.0	27.0	7.0	15	595	3.0
spinach feta (*Cedarlane Carb Buster*), 9 oz.	490	32.0	11.0	37.0	105	1219	4.0
vegetable, garden (*Cedarlane*), ½ of 9-oz. pkg.	140	9.0	20.0	3.0	10	310	3.0
Enchilada sauce, ¼ cup:							
(*La Victoria* Traditional)	10	0	2.0	1.5	0	330	0
(*Pace*)	25	1.0	5.0	0	0	550	1.0
green chili:							
(*La Victoria*)	15	0	3.0	0	0	270	1.0
(*Las Palmas*)	25	0	3.0	1.5	0	340	0
(*Old El Paso*)	30	<1.0	3.0	1.5	0	330	0
hot (*Las Palmas*)	15	0	2.0	.5	0	330	0
hot, medium, or mild (*Old El Paso*)	20	0	3.0	1.0	0	220	0
medium (*Las Palmas*)	15	0	2.0	.5	0	310	1.0
mild (*Las Palmas*)	20	0	2.0	.5	0	310	1.0
red chili (*La Victoria*)	15	0	2.0	.5	0	270	0
tomato (*Las Palmas*)	20	<1.0	5.0	0	0	290	<1.0
Enchilada sauce mix:							
(*Lawry's*), 2 tsp.	20	0	4.0	0	0	260	<1.0
(*McCormick*), 2 tsp.	15	0	3.0	0	0	280	0
Endive, chopped, ½ cup	4	.3	.8	.1	0	6	.8
Endive, Belgian, see "Chicory, witloof"							
Epazote, raw, 2 sprigs	1	0	.3	0	0	172	.2
Eppaw, raw, ½ cup	75	2.3	15.8	.9	0	6	n.a.
Escarole, see "Endive"							
European soldier bean, canned (*Westbrae Natural* Organic Heirloom Beans), ½ cup	90	6.0	16.0	0	0	140	5.0

F

Food and Measure	cal.	prot. (gms)	carbo. (gms)	fat (gms)	chol. (mgs)	sod. (mgs)	fiber (gms)
Fajita, frozen or refrigerated:							
beef (*Tyson* Meal Kit),							
3.8-oz. pc.*	140	9.0	17.0	4.0	15	310	2.0
chicken:							
(*Birds Eye Voila!*),							
1 cup*	150	10.0	13.0	6.0	25	730	3.0
(*Smart Ones Bistro Selections* Su-							
preme), 9.25 oz.	260	18.0	33.0	7.0	35	650	3.0
(*Tyson* Meal Kit),							
3.8-oz. pc.*	130	8.0	17.0	3.5	15	350	2.0
Fajita kit (*Old El Paso* No-Fuss Dinner Kit):							
1/5 pkg. mix	190	4.0	33.0	4.5	0	1020	1.0
2 fajitas*	300	24.0	36.0	7.0	55	1070	2.0
(*Taco Bell* Dinner Home Originals),							
1/5 pkg. mix	230	5.0	38.0	5.0	0	1080	3.0
Fajita marinade/sauce, see "Marinade"							
Fajita seasoning (*McCormick*), 1/4 tsp.	0	0	0	0	0	130	0
Fajita seasoning mix:							
(*Chi-Chi's*), 1/4 pkg.	35	0	7.0	1.0	0	510	0
(*D.L. Jardine's*), 1 tsp.	10	0	1.0	0	0	38	0
(*Lawry's*), 2 tsp.	10	0	3.0	0	0	400	0
marinade (*McCormick*), 2 tsp.	15	0	2.0	0	0	290	0
Falafel mix:							
(*Fantastic*), 1/4 cup ...	120	7.0	21.0	2.0	0	370	6.0
(*Near East*), 1/4 cup ..	100	10.0	18.0	1.0	0	560	5.0
(*Near East*), about 2½ patties*	230	10.0	18.0	15.0	0	560	5.0

Food and Measure	cal.	prot. (gms)	carbo. (gms)	fat (gms)	chol. (mgs)	sod. (mgs)	fiber (gms)
Farfalle pasta entree, frozen, spinach pesto sauce (*Moosewood*), 10-oz. pkg.	410	13.0	57.0	16.0	20	590	6.0
Farina, whole grain:							
dry, 1 oz.	105	3.0	22.1	.1	0	1	.8
cooked, 1 cup	116	3.4	24.6	.2	0	1	3.3
Farro, see "Spelt"							
Fava bean, see "Broad bean, mature"							
Feijoa, raw:							
(*Frieda's*), 5 oz.	70	2.0	15.0	1.0	0	0	0
w/skin, 1 medium, 2.3 oz.	25	.6	5.3	.4	0	2	0
pureed, ½ cup	60	1.5	12.9	1.0	0	4	0
Fennel, bulb:							
(*Andy Boy*), 1 medium bulb	73	5.8	17.0	.5	0	122	7.3
(*Frieda's*), ¾ cup, 3 oz.	25	1.0	6.0	0	0	45	0
8.3-oz. bulb	72	2.9	17.1	.5	0	122	7.3
sliced, 1 cup	27	1.1	6.3	.2	0	45	2.7
Fennel seed, 1 tsp. . . .	7	.3	1.1	.3	0	2	<1.0
Fenugreek seed, 1 tsp.	12	.9	2.2	.2	0	2	<1.0
Fettuccine:							
dry, see "Pasta"							
refrigerated:							
(*Buitoni*), 1¼ cups	240	10.0	45.0	2.5	55	20	2.0
(*DiGiorno*), 2.5 oz. .	200	8.0	39.0	1.5	0	140	2.0
(*Monterey Carb Smart* Egg Recipe), 3.5 oz.	200	12.0	27.0	5.0	140	70	5.0
spinach (*Buitoni*), 1¼ cups	260	12.0	45.0	3.0	75	110	2.0
Fettuccine dish, freeze-dried (*AlpineAire* Leonardo da Fettuc-cine), 1 serving . . .	330	16.0	44.0	10.0	30	740	1.0
Fettuccine dish, mix:							
Alfredo (*Annie's Organic*), 1 cup* . .	270	11.0	43.0	8.0	20	580	2.0
curly, cheddar, broccoli sauce (*Annie's Natural*), 1 cup* . . .	350	11.0	51.0	12.0	30	560	1.0

Food and Measure	cal.	prot. (gms)	carbo. (gms)	fat (gms)	chol. (mgs)	sod. (mgs)	fiber (gms)
Fettuccine entree, frozen, 1 pkg.:							
Alfredo:							
(*Healthy Choice*), 8 oz.	240	10.0	36.0	6.0	15	600	4.0
(*Lean Cuisine Everyday Favorites*), 9.25 oz.	290	12.0	44.0	7.0	15	660	2.0
(*Linda McCartney*), 10 oz.	360	14.0	35.0	13.0	35	950	4.0
(*Michelina's* Authentico), 9 oz.	370	14.0	46.0	16.0	40	670	3.0
(*Michelina's Lean Gourmet*), 9 oz. . .	250	12.0	41.0	5.0	10	570	2.0
(*Smart Ones*), 9.25 oz.	270	14.0	39.0	6.0	15	650	3.0
(*Stouffer's*), 11.5 oz.	530	17.0	49.0	30.0	105	1100	3.0
w/chicken, see "Chicken entree, frozen"							
Fettuccine entree, pkg., Alfredo (*Kraft It's Pasta Anytime*), 11.5-oz. pkg.	580	21.0	74.0	22.0	50	1800	4.0
Fiddlehead fern, fresh, 4 oz.	39	5.2	6.3	.5	0	1	n.a.
Fig, fresh:							
1 large, 2.3 oz.	47	.5	12.3	.2	0	1	2.1
1 medium, 1.8 oz. . . .	37	.4	9.6	.2	0	1	1.7
Fig, can or jar, ½ cup:							
in light syrup	87	.5	22.6	.1	0	1	2.3
in heavy syrup	114	.5	29.7	.1	0	2	2.8
Fig, dried:							
(*Shiloh Farms* Adriatic/ Black Mission), ⅓ cup	113	3.0	26.0	0	0	5	5.0
(*Shiloh Farms* Calimyrna), 2 figs, 1.6 oz.	120	1.0	30.0	.5	0	5	4.0
10 figs, 6.6 oz.	477	5.7	122.2	2.2	0	20	17.4
Filberts, see "Hazelnuts"							
Fillo dough, frozen:							
(*Athens* Twin Pack), 5 sheets, 9" x 14", 2 oz.	180	4.0	37.0	1.5	0	230	1.0

Food and Measure	cal.	prot. (gms)	carbo. (gms)	fat (gms)	chol. (mgs)	sod. (mgs)	fiber (gms)
(*Athens/Apollo*), 2 oz., about 2½ sheets, 14" x 18"	180	4.0	37.0	1.5	0	230	1.0
extra thick (*Apollo* Country Style), 2-oz. sheet	200	5.0	33.0	5.0	0	430	<1.0
shells, mini (*Athens*), 2 shells	35	0	4.0	2.0	0	25	0
shredded (*Athens/ Apollo*), ⅛ of 12-oz. pkg.	120	3.0	22.0	1.5	0	115	<1.0
Fireweed, leaves, fresh, 1 cup	24	1.1	4.4	.7	0	8	2.4
Fish, see specific listings							
Fish cake, see "Fish entree" and specific fish listings							
Fish coating mix (see also "Batter and breading mix" and "Seafood coating mix"), seasoned:							
(*Don's Chuck Wagon*), ¼ cup	95	4.0	21.0	0	0	710	1.0
(*Golden Dipt* Fish Fry), 1⅓ tbsp.	35	0	6.0	0	0	230	0
(*Oven Fry*), ⅛ pkg. . .	45	1.0	9.0	.5	0	290	0
Cajun (*Golden Dipt* Fry Easy), 1⅓ tbsp. . . .	35	0	6.0	0	0	250	0
fish and chips mix: (*Don's Chuck Wagon*), ¼ cup	100	3.0	21.0	0	0	740	1.0
batter (*Golden Dipt* Fry Easy), ¼ cup	100	0	20.0	0	0	840	0
Fish dinner, frozen, 1 pkg.:							
herb baked (*Healthy Choice* Dinners), 10.9 oz.	360	16.0	55.0	8.0	40	590	5.0
lemon pepper (*Healthy Choice* Dinners), 10.7 oz.	280	11.0	49.0	5.0	30	580	5.0

Food and Measure	cal.	prot. (gms)	carbo. (gms)	fat (gms)	chol. (mgs)	sod. (mgs)	fiber (gms)
Fish entree, frozen (see also specific fish listings):							
cake, breaded:							
(*Kineret*), 2 pcs., 4 oz.	160	4.0	23.0	6.0	5	310	1.0
(*Dr. Praeger's*), 2.9-oz. pc.	158	12.0	14.0	6.0	30	190	<1.0
fillet, baked, lemon pepper (*Lean Cuisine* Café Classics), 9-oz. pkg.	220	22.0	20.0	6.0	65	630	7.0
fillet, beer batter:							
(*Gorton's*), 2 pcs., 3.6 oz.	230	9.0	18.0	14.0	20	640	0
(*Mrs. Paul's* Tenders), 4 pcs., 4 oz.	230	11.0	22.0	11.0	25	710	1.0
fillet, breaded:							
(*Dr. Praeger's*), 2.1-oz. pc.	113	6.5	11.0	4.0	24	211	<1.0
(*Ian's* Natural), 3.5-oz. pc.	260	14.0	32.0	8.0	20	410	2.0
crunchy (*Mrs. Paul's*), 2 pcs., 3.7 oz. . .	260	6.0	22.0	15.0	25	430	0
sandwich (*Dr. Praeger's*), 4 oz. . .	210	12.0	19.0	9.0	60	230	<1.0
fillet, grilled:							
Alfredo, w/broccoli (*Gorton's* Meal), 10-oz. pkg.	160	19.0	14.0	3.0	40	990	5.0
Caesar Parmesan (*Gorton's*), 3.8-oz. pc.	100	17.0	1.0	3.0	60	250	0
Cajun blackened (*Gorton's*), 3.8-oz. pc.	100	17.0	1.0	3.0	60	330	0
char-grilled (*Gorton's*), 3.8-oz. pc.	100	17.0	1.0	3.0	60	250	0
garlic butter (*Gorton's*), 3.8-oz. pc.	100	17.0	1.0	3.0	60	370	0
garlic butter (*Mrs. Paul's* Meals), 11-oz. pkg.	270	21.0	34.0	3.0	70	730	3.0
herb, Italian (*Gorton's*), 3.8-oz. pc.	100	17.0	1.0	3.0	60	280	0

Food and Measure	cal.	prot. (gms)	carbo. (gms)	fat (gms)	chol. (mgs)	sod. (mgs)	fiber (gms)
lemon butter (*Gorton's*), 3.8-oz. pc.	100	17.0	1.0	3.0	60	250	0
lemon pepper (*Gorton's*), 3.8-oz. pc.	100	17.0	1.0	3.0	60	380	0
lemon pepper, w/rice, vegetables (*Gorton's* Meal), 10-oz. pkg.	240	17.0	34.0	3.5	40	890	3.0
fillet, w/macaroni and cheese (*Stouffer's* Homestyle), 9-oz. pkg.	430	20.0	47.0	18.0	55	1040	2.0
nuggets, fish shaped (*Dr. Praeger's* Fishies), 4 pcs., 1.6 oz.	90	7.0	9.0	3.5	18	127	<1.0
portions, breaded: crunchy (*Kineret* 11.4 oz.), 2 pcs., 3.8 oz.	250	13.0	27.0	10.0	35	260	<1.0
crunchy (*Kineret* 20 oz.), 2 pcs., 4 oz.	260	14.0	29.0	10.0	35	270	<1.0
w/shrimp, crab, vegetables (*Oven Poppers*), 4.5-oz. pc.	200	13.0	13.0	11.0	85	380	0
w/spinach and cheese (*Oven Poppers*), 4.5-oz. pc.	160	15.0	8.0	8.0	70	310	0
sticks, breaded: (*Dr. Praeger's*), 3 pcs., 2.8 oz. ..	138	7.0	14.0	6.0	24	185	<1.0
(*Dr. Praeger's* Family Pack), 3 pcs., 2.8 oz.	145	7.0	14.0	6.0	24	185	<1.0
(*Ian's* Natural), 5 pcs., 3.3 oz.	190	11.0	24.0	6.0	15	310	1.0
(*Kineret*), 5 pcs., 3.8 oz.	250	11.0	30.0	9.0	30	690	<1.0
(*Mrs. Paul's*), 6 pcs., 3.4 oz.	230	10.0	21.0	12.0	20	380	1.0
(*Van de Kamp's*), 6 pcs., 4 oz.	260	3.0	23.0	13.0	30	370	0

Food and Measure	cal.	prot. (gms)	carbo. (gms)	fat (gms)	chol. (mgs)	sod. (mgs)	fiber (gms)
Fish entree, sticks, breaded *(cont.)*							
crunchy (*Kineret* 10.8 oz.), 6 pcs., 3.6 oz.	230	12.0	28.0	8.0	30	300	<1.0
crunchy (*Kineret* 25 oz.), 6 pcs., 3.1 oz.	230	9.0	29.0	9.0	15	290	1.0
w/mac and cheese (*Stouffer's Maxaroni*), 7.75-oz. pkg.	330	16.0	35.0	14.0	35	670	1.0
Fish oil, see "Oil"							
Fish sauce, Thai, see "Thai sauce"							
Fish seasoning, see specific listings							
Fish seasoning mix, see "Fish coating mix"							
Flatfish, meat only:							
raw, 4 oz.	104	21.4	0	1.4	54	92	0
baked, broiled, or microwaved, 4 oz. .	133	27.4	0	1.7	77	119	0
Flavor enhancer, see "Monosodium glutamate"							
Flax seeds, 3 tbsp., except as noted:							
(*Arrowhead Mills*) . . .	140	6.0	9.0	9.0	0	0	7.0
(*Hodgson Mill*), 2 tbsp.	60	3.0	4.0	5.0	0	0	4.0
(*Tree of Life/Tree of Life Organic Golden*) . . .	140	5.0	11.0	10.0	0	0	6.0
brown (*Shiloh Farms*)	140	5.0	11.0	10.0	0	0	6.0
golden:							
(*Arrowhead Mills*) .	160	8.0	10.0	10.0	0	10	9.0
(*Shiloh Farms*), 1 tbsp.	61	2.0	3.0	4.0	0	0	3.0
Flounder, fresh, see "Flatfish"							
Flounder entree, frozen, 5-oz. pc.:							
au gratin (*Oven Poppers*)	220	24.0	5.0	11.0	75	450	1.0
stuffed:							
w/broccoli, cheese (*Oven Poppers*) .	150	20.0	4.0	6.0	55	330	1.0

Food and Measure	cal.	prot. (gms)	carbo. (gms)	fat (gms)	chol. (mgs)	sod. (mgs)	fiber (gms)
w/crab (*Oven Poppers*)	240	17.0	15.0	13.0	35	400	0
w/garlic, shrimp, almonds (*Oven Poppers*)	260	16.0	16.0	14.0	40	380	0
Flour, see "Wheat flour" and specific listings							
Flour, mixed grains (*Arrowhead Mills Perfect Harvest*), ¼ cup	130	5.0	24.0	1.5	0	0	4.0
Focaccia, mix, see "Bread, mix"							
Foo qua, see "Balsam pear"							
Frankfurter, 1 link, except as noted:							
(*Ball Park* Bun Size/ Franks), 2 oz.	180	6.0	3.0	16.0	40	610	0
(*Ball Park* Fat Free), 1.8 oz.	50	6.0	6.0	0	10	490	0
(*Ball Park* Lite), 1.8 oz.	100	6.0	3.0	7.0	25	540	0
(*Ball Park* Single), 1.6 oz.	150	5.0	3.0	13.0	30	490	0
(*Hatfield*), 2 oz.	180	7.0	1.0	16.0	35	510	0
(*Hatfield* Original), 1.6 oz.	130	5.0	0	12.0	25	350	0
(*Hatfield* Reduced Sodium), 2 oz.	170	7.0	1.0	15.0	35	300	0
(*Hatfield* Phillies), 2 oz.	170	7.0	1.0	15.0	30	540	0
(*Healthy Choice*), 1.75 oz.	70	6.0	6.0	2.5	20	440	0
(*Hormel* Fat Free), 1.8 oz.	45	5.0	5.0	0	15	580	0
(*Dietz & Watson* Gourmet Lite), 2 oz.	60	8.0	3.0	1.5	15	390	0
(*Oscar Mayer* Wieners Light), 1.6 oz.	90	5.0	1.0	7.0	30	460	0
beef:							
(*Ball Park* Bun Size/ Franks), 2 oz. ...	180	6.0	3.0	16.0	35	620	0
(*Ball Park* Fat Free), 1.8 oz.	55	6.0	7.0	0	10	490	0

Food and Measure	cal.	prot. (gms)	carbo. (gms)	fat (gms)	chol. (mgs)	sod. (mgs)	fiber (gms)
Frankfurter, beef *(cont.)*							
(Ball Park Grillmaster), 2.9 oz.	250	9.0	3.0	23.0	50	780	0
(Ball Park Grillmaster Deli Style), 2.9 oz.	250	8.0	3.0	23.0	50	830	0
(Ball Park Lite), 1.8 oz.	100	6.0	3.0	7.0	20	510	0
(Ball Park Single), 1.6 oz.	150	5.0	2.0	13.0	30	500	0
(Boar's Head Lite), 1.6 oz.	90	7.0	0	6.0	25	270	0
(Boar's Head Natural Casing), 2 oz.	160	7.0	1.0	14.0	30	440	0
(Boar's Head Skinless), 1.6 oz.	120	6.0	0	11.0	20	350	0
(Dietz & Watson Fat Free), 2 oz.	40	6.0	4.0	0	15	390	0
(Dietz & Watson Gourmet Lite), 2 oz.	60	8.0	3.0	1.5	15	390	0
(Hatfield), 2 oz. ...	170	7.0	1.0	15.0	30	540	0
(Healthy Choice), 1.75 oz.	70	6.0	7.0	2.5	15	440	0
(Hebrew National), 1.7 oz.	150	6.0	1.0	14.0	30	370	0
(Hebrew National Family Pack), 2 oz.	180	7.0	1.0	16.0	40	450	0
(Hebrew National 97% Fat Free), 1.7 oz.	45	6.0	3.0	1.5	15	400	0
(Hebrew National Party Pack), 2 oz.	180	7.0	1.0	16.0	40	450	0
(Hebrew National Reduced Fat), 1.7 oz.	120	6.0	0	10.0	25	360	0
(Hormel), 2 oz. ...	170	6.0	0	15.0	35	490	0
(Hormel Fat Free), 1.8 oz.	45	6.0	5.0	0	10	590	0
(Nathan's Casing), 2 oz.	180	7.0	1.0	15.0	35	400	1.0
(Nathan's Skinless), 2 oz.	170	7.0	1.0	15.0	35	470	0
(Oscar Mayer XXL Deli Style), 2.7 oz.	230	9.0	1.0	22.0	50	740	0

Food and Measure	cal.	prot. (gms)	carbo. (gms)	fat (gms)	chol. (mgs)	sod. (mgs)	fiber (gms)
(*Oscar Mayer XXL* Premium), 2.7 oz.	240	9.0	1.0	23.0	45	680	0
(*Shiloh Farms*) 2 oz.	110	8.0	0	9.0	30	470	0
(*Wranglers*), 2 oz. .	170	7.0	1.0	15.0	35	560	0
dinner (*Hebrew National*), 4 oz. .	350	13.0	1.0	32.0	70	990	0
uncured (*Organic Valley*), 2 oz. . . .	120	8.0	1.0	9.0	30	330	0
cheese:							
(*Ball Park* Single), 1.6 oz.	150	6.0	2.0	13.0	35	450	0
(*Hatfield*), 2 oz. . . .	170	7.0	1.0	15.0	35	550	0
(*Wranglers*), 2 oz. .	170	7.0	1.0	15.0	35	610	0
chicken (*Organic Valley*), 2 oz.	90	7.0	1.0	7.0	45	330	0
cocktail:							
(*Hormel* Smokies), 6 pcs., 2 oz.	170	8.0	1.0	15.0	35	550	0
beef (*Boar's Head*), 5 pcs., 2 oz.	170	8.0	0	15.0	30	430	0
beef (*Hormel* Smokies), 6 pcs., 2 oz.	180	8.0	2.0	16.0	35	530	0
w/cheese (*Hormel* Smokies), 6 pcs., 2 oz.	170	9.0	1.0	14.0	40	620	0
hot and spicy:							
(*Ball Park* Grillmaster), 2.9 oz.	260	9.0	4.0	24.0	50	780	0
(*Oscar Mayer XXL*), 2.7 oz.	210	10.0	1.0	19.0	45	750	0
jalapeño (*Wranglers*), 2 oz.	170	1.0	7.0	15.0	35	610	0
pork and beef (*Boar's Head*), 2 oz.	150	7.0	0	14.0	25	460	0
salmon (*A&B Famous*), 2 pcs., 2.6 oz.	190	10.0	4.0	15.0	30	680	0
smoked:							
(*Ball Park* Bun Size Smokies), 2 oz. .	180	6.0	2.0	17.0	35	580	0
(*Ball Park* Grillmaster Smokehouse), 2.9 oz.	260	9.0	3.0	24.0	50	790	0

Food and Measure	cal.	prot. (gms)	carbo. (gms)	fat (gms)	chol. (mgs)	sod. (mgs)	fiber (gms)
Frankfurter, smoked *(cont.)*							
(*Hormel* Smokies), 1 oz.	80	4.0	0	7.0	20	290	0
(*Johnsonville* Natural Casing Wieners), 1.75 oz.	150	6.0	1.0	14.0	40	410	0
(*Oscar Mayer XXL* Original), 2.7 oz.	240	9.0	1.0	23.0	45	680	0
(*Wranglers*), 2 oz. .	170	7.0	1.0	15.0	35	560	0
w/cheese (*Hormel* Smokies), 1 oz. . .	80	4.0	0	7.0	20	310	0
turkey:							
(*Louis Rich/Oscar Mayer*), 1.6 oz. .	100	5.0	2.0	8.0	30	510	0
(*Louis Rich/Oscar Mayer Bun Length*), 2 oz.	120	1.0	3.0	10.0	35	640	0
(*Oscar Mayer*), 1.6 oz.	100	5.0	2.0	8.0	30	510	0
cheese (*Louis Rich/ Oscar Mayer*), 1.6 oz.	100	6.0	2.0	8.0	30	490	0
smoked, white (*Ball Park* Bun Size), 1.8 oz.	45	6.0	5.0	0	10	420	0
uncured (*Health is Wealth*), 1.5 oz. . . .	80	6.0	1.0	6.0	20	340	0
"Frankfurter," vegeta- rian, 1 link or pc., except as noted:							
canned, 1.8 oz.:							
(*Loma Linda* Big Franks)	110	11.0	3.0	6.0	0	220	2.0
(*Loma Linda* Big Franks Low Fat) .	80	12.0	3.0	2.5	0	240	2.0
frozen/refrigerated:							
(*Morningstar Farms Veggie Dogs*), 2 oz.	80	11.0	6.0	.5	0	580	1.0
(*Quorn* Dogs), 1.5 oz.	70	5.0	3.0	4.0	5	250	2.0
(*Worthington Leanies*), 1.4 oz.	100	8.0	2.0	7.0	0	430	1.0
(*Yves* The Good Dog), 1.8 oz.	100	11.0	2.0	5.0	0	550	0

Food and Measure	cal.	prot. (gms)	carbo. (gms)	fat (gms)	chol. (mgs)	sod. (mgs)	fiber (gms)
(*Yves* Tofu Dogs), 1.3 oz.	45	9.0	2.0	.5	0	240	0
(*Yves* Veggie Dogs), 1.6 oz.	60	11.0	1.0	0	0	400	1.0
(*Yves* Veggie Dogs Jumbo), 2.7 oz. . .	100	16.0	7.0	1.5	0	480	2.0
hot and spicy (*Yves* Chili Dogs), 1.8 oz.	70	13.0	3.0	1.0	0	400	2.0
wrapped (*Moringstar Farms* Corn Dogs), 2.5 oz.	150	7.0	22.0	4.0	0	500	3.0
wrapped (*Loma Linda* Corn Dogs), 2.5 oz.	150	7.0	22.0	4.0	0	500	3.0
wrapped, mini (*Morningstar Farms* Corn Dogs), 4 pcs., 2.7 oz.	170	11.0	21.0	4.5	0	580	1.0
Frankfurter, wrapped:							
(*Hebrew National* Franks in a Blanket), 5 pcs., 2.9 oz.	290	9.0	8.0	24.0	40	690	1.0
corn dogs (*Oscar Mayer*), 3.2-oz. pc.	260	7.0	25.0	15.0	35	720	1.0
Franks and beans, see "Beans and franks"							
French toast (see also "Breakfast pocket/ sandwich"), frozen:							
(*Aunt Jemima* Home-style), 2 pcs.	240	7.0	39.0	6.0	70	340	2.0
(*Pepperidge Farm* Homestyle), 1 pc. . . .	160	5.0	23.0	5.0	35	200	1.0
cinnamon:							
(*Aunt Jemima*), 3 pcs.	220	8.0	34.0	6.0	75	300	2.0
swirl (*Pepperidge Farm*), 1 pc.	170	5.0	24.0	6.0	35	190	2.0
sticks (*Aunt Jemima*), 5 pcs.	330	6.0	50.0	12.0	0	400	2.0
sticks, 6 pcs. w/syrup:							
(*Pillsbury* Original) .	350	4.0	68.0	6.0	10	640	1.0
cinnamon (*Pillsbury*)	350	4.0	69.0	6.0	5	580	1.0
sticks, toaster, 2 pcs.:							
(*Eggo* French Toaster Sticks Original) .	220	5.0	36.0	6.0	20	530	1.0

Food and Measure	cal.	prot. (gms)	carbo. (gms)	fat (gms)	chol. (mgs)	sod. (mgs)	fiber (gms)
French toast, sticks, toaster *(cont.)*							
cinnamon (*Eggo French Toaster Sticks*)	220	4.0	37.0	6.0	20	510	1.0
Frog's legs, raw, 2 oz.	41	9.2	0	.2	28	32	0
Frosting, ready-to-spread, 2 tbsp.:							
butter cream:							
(*Betty Crocker* Rich & Creamy)	150	0	20.0	8.0	0	80	0
(*Betty Crocker* Whipped)	110	0	14.0	6.0	0	25	0
(*Duncan Hines*) . . .	140	0	22.0	5.0	0	60	0
caramel (*Betty Crocker* Rich & Creamy) . . .	150	0	20.0	8.0	0	90	0
cherry:							
(*Betty Crocker* Rich & Creamy)	150	0	20.0	8.0	0	80	0
chocolate:							
(*Betty Crocker* Pour & Frost)	140	0	18.0	8.0	0	90	1.0
(*Betty Crocker* Rich & Creamy)	150	0	18.0	8.0	0	95	0
(*Betty Crocker* Whipped)	100	<1.0	13.0	5.0	0	55	1.0
(*Duncan Hines* Classic)	140	0	22.0	5.0	0	95	0
almond or milk (*Betty Crocker* Rich & Creamy)	150	0	18.0	8.0	0	95	0
dark (*Betty Crocker* Rich & Creamy) .	150	1.0	17.0	9.0	0	105	0
dark, fudge (*Duncan Hines*)	130	0	20.0	5.0	0	95	0
milk (*Betty Crocker* Pour & Frost) . . .	150	0	18.0	8.0	0	90	0
milk (*Betty Crocker* Whipped)	100	0	14.0	5.0	0	50	0
milk (*Duncan Hines*)	140	0	22.0	5.0	0	95	0
chocolate chip:							
triple fudge (*Betty Crocker* Rich & Creamy)	140	1.0	22.0	5.0	0	85	1.0

Food and Measure	cal.	prot. (gms)	carbo. (gms)	fat (gms)	chol. (mgs)	sod. (mgs)	fiber (gms)
vanilla (*Betty Crocker* Rich & Creamy) .	140	0	23.0	5.0	0	65	0
coconut:							
(*Duncan Hines* Supreme)	150	0	24.0	6.0	0	65	0
pecan (*Betty Crocker* Rich & Creamy) .	140	1.0	17.0	8.0	0	50	0
cream cheese:							
(*Betty Crocker* Rich & Creamy)	150	0	20.0	8.0	0	80	0
(*Betty Crocker* Whipped)	110	0	14.0	6.0	0	45	0
strawberry (*Betty Crocker* Rich & Creamy)	150	0	20.0	8.0	0	80	0
lemon:							
(*Betty Crocker* Rich & Creamy)	150	0	20.0	8.0	0	80	0
(*Betty Crocker* Whipped)	110	0	14.0	6.0	0	25	0
(*Duncan Hines* Supreme)	140	0	24.0	5.0	0	65	0
rainbow chip (*Betty Crocker* Rich & Creamy)	140	0	20.0	5.0	0	65	0
sour cream:							
chocolate (*Betty Crocker* Rich & Creamy)	150	0	18.0	8.0	0	95	0
white (*Betty Crocker* Rich & Creamy) .	150	0	20.0	8.0	0	80	0
strawberry (*Betty Crocker* Whipped) .	110	0	14.0	6.0	0	25	0
vanilla:							
(*Betty Crocker* Pour & Frost)	150	0	20.0	8.0	0	85	0
(*Betty Crocker* Rich & Creamy)	150	0	20.0	8.0	0	80	0
(*Betty Crocker* Whipped)	110	0	14.0	6.0	0	25	0
(*Duncan Hines* Classic)	140	0	24.0	5.0	0	65	0
w/rainbow sprinkles (*Betty Crocker* Toppers)	160	0	21.0	8.0	0	80	0

Food and Measure	cal.	prot. (gms)	carbo. (gms)	fat (gms)	chol. (mgs)	sod. (mgs)	fiber (gms)
Frosting *(cont.)*							
vanilla, French:							
(*Betty Crocker* Rich & Creamy)	140	0	23.0	5.0	0	70	0
(*Betty Crocker* Whipped)	110	0	14.0	6.0	0	25	0
(*Duncan Hines*) ...	140	0	24.0	5.0	0	65	0
white, fluffy (*Betty Crocker* Whipped) .	110	0	14.0	6.0	0	25	0
Frosting mix:							
fudge (*"Jiffy"*), ¼ cup	150	<1.0	28.0	4.0	0	150	<1.0
white:							
(*"Jiffy"*), ¼ cup ...	150	0	27.0	4.5	0	150	0
fluffy (*Betty Crocker* Homestyle), 3 tbsp.	100	<1.0	24.0	0	0	55	0
Frozen desserts, see "Ice cream" and specific listings							
Fructose:							
(*Estee*), 1 tsp.	15	0	4.0	0	0	0	0
(*Featherweight*), 1 tsp.	15	0	4.0	0	0	0	0
(*Tree of Life*), 1 tbsp. .	68	0	1.0	4.0	0	2	0
Fruit, see specific listings							
Fruit, mixed, can or jar (see also "Fruit cocktail"), ½ cup, except as noted:							
(*Dole FruitBowls*), 4 oz.	90	<1.0	22.0	0	0	10	1.0
in juice:							
(*Del Monte*), 4-oz. cup	50	0	13.0	0	0	10	<1.0
(*Del Monte Fruit Naturals Fruit Cup*), 4.5 oz.	50	0	13.0	0	0	10	<1.0
(*Del Monte Orchard Select*)	80	<1.0	19.0	0	0	10	<1.0
chunky (*Del Monte*)	60	0	15.0	0	0	10	1.0
chunky (*S&W* Natural Style)	80	<1.0	19.0	0	0	20	3.0
tropical (*Del Monte*), 4-oz. cup	70	<1.0	18.0	0	0	5	<1.0
tropical (*Del Monte Fruit Naturals*) ..	70	<1.0	18.0	0	0	5	<1.0

Food and Measure	cal.	prot. (gms)	carbo. (gms)	fat (gms)	chol. (mgs)	sod. (mgs)	fiber (gms)
in extra light syrup:							
(*Del Monte Fruit Cup Lite*), 4.5 oz.	50	0	13.0	0	0	10	<1.0
Ambrosia (*Del Monte Sunfresh*)	70	0	16.0	0	0	5	2.0
chunky (*Del Monte*)	60	0	15.0	0	0	10	1.0
citrus (*Del Monte Sunfresh*)	80	0	20.0	0	0	20	0
in gelatin, cherry (*Del Monte*), 4.5-oz. cup	90	0	23.0	0	0	40	0
in light syrup:							
(*Del Monte*), 4-oz. cup	70	<1.0	18.0	0	0	5	<1.0
cherry (*Del Monte*)	90	<1.0	22.0	0	0	10	<1.0
cherry (*Del Monte*), 4-oz. cup	70	<1.0	18.0	0	0	10	<1.0
cherry (*Del Monte Very Cherry*) . . .	90	1.0	22.0	0	0	10	<1.0
citrus (*Del Monte*) .	80	0	20.0	0	0	20	0
tropical (*Del Monte Sunfresh*)	80	0	20.0	0	0	10	0
tropical (*Dole*)	80	<1.0	20.0	0	0	10	1.0
tropical, w/passion fruit juice (*Del Monte Sunfresh*)	80	0	21.0	0	0	10	1.0
in heavy syrup:							
(*Del Monte Fruit Cup*), 4.5 oz. . . .	80	0	20.0	0	0	10	<1.0
chunky (*Del Monte*)	100	0	24.0	0	0	10	1.0
tropical (*Dole Fruit-Bowls*), 4 oz.	60	<1.0	16.0	0	0	10	2.0
Fruit, mixed, candied, 1 oz.	91	.1	23.4	0	0	28	.5
Fruit, mixed, dried, ¼ cup, 1.4 oz.:							
(*Express*)	100	1.0	24.0	0	0	15	3.0
(*SunRidge Farms Tropical Mix*)	130	0	30.0	.5	0	20	1.0
(*Sunsweet* Morsels) . .	120	1.0	28.0	0	0	55	2.0
(*Sunsweet* Tropical Mix)	140	0	32.0	1.0	0	50	2.0
(*Sunsweet* Orchard Mix)	100	1.0	25.0	0	0	60	3.0
Fruit, mixed, frozen (*McKenzie's*), ⅓ of 16-oz. pkg.	60	1.0	13.0	0	0	20	2.0

Food and Measure	cal.	prot. (gms)	carbo. (gms)	fat (gms)	chol. (mgs)	sod. (mgs)	fiber (gms)
Fruit bar, frozen (see also "Ice bar," "Iced confection bar," and "Sorbet bar"), 1 pc., except as noted:							
all varieties:							
(*Breyer's* Bars No Sugar)	25	0	5.0	0	0	5	0
(*Breyer's* Swirl) ...	50	0	13.0	0	0	5	0
(*Minute Maid* Juice Bars)	60	0	15.0	0	0	15	0
(*Popsicle* All Natural)	50	0	12.0	0	0	5	0
(*Popsicle* Mini Bars)	70	<1.0	19.0	0	<5	15	0
(*Popsicle* Fantastic Fruity)	50	0	13.0	0	0	5	0
(*Popsicle Scribblers* Juice Pops), 2 pcs.	60	0	16.0	0	0	0	0
(*Welch's* No Sugar Variety Pack) ...	25	0	6.0	0	0	0	0
except orange (*Tropicana* Real Fruit Variety Pack)	50	0	12.0	0	0	5	0
except orange (*Tropicana* Real Fruit Variety Pack No Sugar)	25	0	6.0	0	0	5	0
except tropical (*Welch's* Variety Pack)	45	0	11.0	0	0	0	0
banana, creamy:							
(*FrozFruit* Cream) ..	150	1.0	20.0	8.0	30	20	<1.0
(*Fruit-a-Freeze*) ...	100	1.0	18.0	3.5	15	40	<1.0
(*Fruit-a-Freeze* Single)	140	1.0	24.0	4.5	20	55	<1.0
chocolate dipped (*FrozFruit*)	210	1.0	22.0	14.0	20	15	1.0
chocolate dipped (*Fruit-a-Freeze*) .	170	2.0	21.0	10.0	10	40	1.0
berry, wild (*Whole Fruit*)	80	0	20.0	0	0	0	0
cantaloupe:							
(*FrozFruit*)	60	0	15.0	0	0	5	0
(*Fruit-a-Freeze*) ...	50	0	14.0	0	0	5	0
cappuccino (*Fruit-a-Freeze*)	120	2.0	19.0	5.0	20	55	0
cherry (*FrozFruit*)	70	1.0	16.0	0	0	55	<1.0

Food and Measure	cal.	prot. (gms)	carbo. (gms)	fat (gms)	chol. (mgs)	sod. (mgs)	fiber (gms)
coconut, creamy:							
(*FrozFruit* Cream) ..	200	2.0	18.0	14.0	35	25	2.0
(*Fruit-a-Freeze*) ...	150	2.0	19.0	8.0	15	50	<1.0
(*Fruit-a-Freeze* Single)	190	3.0	26.0	11.0	20	70	<1.0
(*Tropicana* Chunks of Fruit)	110	2.0	16.0	4.5	15	25	0
(*Whole Fruit*)	120	3.0	21.0	3.0	0	40	0
chocolate dipped (*FrozFruit*)	240	2.0	24.0	17.0	20	35	8.0
chocolate dipped (*Fruit-a-Freeze*) .	210	2.0	22.0	13.0	15	45	1.0
grape:							
(*Welch's*)	80	0	19.0	0	0	0	0
(*Whole Fruit*)	80	0	20.0	0	0	0	0
lemon:							
(*Dr. Praeger's* Sensible Treats) .	90	0	24.0	0	0	7	0
(*FrozFruit*)	80	0	19.0	0	0	75	0
(*Fruit-a-Freeze* Single)	80	0	21.0	0	0	25	0
lemonade:							
(*Tropicana* Cooler) .	70	0	18.0	0	0	5	0
(*Whole Fruit*)	80	0	20.0	0	0	0	0
soft (*Minute Maid* Tubes)	100	0	25.0	0	0	20	0
lime:							
(*FrozFruit*)	90	0	22.0	0	0	85	0
(*Fruit-a-Freeze*) ...	60	0	15.0	0	0	0	0
(*Fruit-a-Freeze* Single)	80	0	21.0	0	0	25	0
(*Whole Fruit*)	80	0	20.0	0	0	0	0
key, creamy (*Fruit-a-Freeze*)	140	2.0	20.0	6.0	15	60	0
mango:							
(*FrozFruit*)	110	0	26.0	0	0	5	<1.0
(*Fruit-a-Freeze* Single)	100	0	26.0	0	0	20	0
mango pineapple (*Fruit-a-Freeze*)	60	0	15.0	0	0	15	0
orange:							
(*Tropicana* Real Fruit)	60	0	16.0	0	0	0	0
(*Tropicana* Real Fruit Variety Pack) ...	50	0	13.0	0	0	5	0
(*Tropicana* Real Fruit Variety Pack No Sugar)	25	0	7.0	0	0	5	0

Food and Measure	cal.	prot. (gms)	carbo. (gms)	fat (gms)	chol. (mgs)	sod. (mgs)	fiber (gms)
Fruit bar, orange *(cont.)*							
w/light ice cream (*Whole Fruit* Orange & Cream)	80	1.0	16.0	1.5	5	30	0
peach:							
(*Dr. Praeger's* Sensible Treats) .	100	0	25.0	0	0	7	<1.0
(*FrozFruit Smoothie. Yum* Give Peach a Chance)	80	0	21.0	0	0	15	0
(*Whole Fruit*)	90	0	23.0	0	0	0	0
pina colada (*FrozFruit* Cream)	180	2.0	22.0	10.0	30	20	1.0
pineapple:							
(*FrozFruit*)	80	0	20.0	0	0	0	0
(*Fruit-a-Freeze* Single)	80	0	21.0	0	0	20	0
strawberry:							
(*Breyer's*), 1.75 fl. oz.	45	0	12.0	0	0	5	0
(*Breyer's*), 3.75 fl. oz.	120	0	30.0	0	0	10	<1.0
(*Dr. Praeger's* Sensible Treats)	60	0	16.0	0	0	5	<1.0
(*FrozFruit*)	90	0	23.0	0	0	5	<1.0
(*Fruit-a-Freeze*)	60	0	15.0	0	0	20	0
(*Fruit-a-Freeze* Single)	80	0	20.0	0	0	25	0
(*Tropicana* Chunks of Fruit)	50	0	14.0	0	0	0	<1.0
(*Whole Fruit*)	80	0	21.0	0	0	0	0
strawberry, chocolate coated (*Dr. Praeger's* Sensible Treats) . . .	170	<1.0	31.0	5.0	0	9	<1.0
strawberry, creamy:							
(*FrozFruit* Cream) . .	150	1.0	22.0	7.0	25	20	<1.0
(*Fruit-a-Freeze*) . . .	110	1.0	18.0	3.5	15	40	0
chocolate dipped (*Fruit-a-Freeze*) .	170	2.0	21.0	9.0	10	40	<1.0
chocolate dipped (*FrozFruit*)	200	2.0	18.0	17.0	20	15	1.0
strawberry banana (*FrozFruit Smoothie. Yum Yumtonic*) . . .	130	1.0	34.0	0	0	15	1.0
tangerine (*Whole Fruit*)	80	0	20.0	0	0	0	0
tropical:							
(*Breyer's*)	80	0	20.0	0	0	10	0
(*FrozFruit*)	90	0	21.0	0	0	55	<1.0

Food and Measure	cal.	prot. (gms)	carbo. (gms)	fat (gms)	chol. (mgs)	sod. (mgs)	fiber (gms)
(*Welch's Tropical Coolers* Variety Pack)	45	0	11.0	0	0	0	0
(*Whole Fruit*)	100	0	26.0	0	0	0	0
watermelon:							
(*FrozFruit*)	70	0	17.0	0	0	0	0
(*Fruit-a-Freeze*)	50	0	14.0	0	0	15	0
Fruit cocktail, can or jar, ½ cup:							
(*Del Monte Carb Clever*)	40	0	11.0	0	0	10	<1.0
in juice:							
(*Del Monte Fruit Naturals*)	60	0	15.0	0	0	10	1.0
(*S&W* Natural Style)	80	0	20.0	0	0	20	2.0
w/liquid	55	.6	14.1	0	0	5	1.2
in extra light syrup (*Del Monte* Lite)	60	0	15.0	0	0	10	1.0
in light syrup:							
(*S&W*)	70	0	18.0	0	0	15	1.0
w/liquid	72	.5	18.8	.1	0	7	1.4
in heavy syrup:							
(*Del Monte*)	100	0	24.0	0	0	10	1.0
(*S&W*)	90	0	23.0	0	0	15	1.0
w/liquid	91	.5	23.4	.1	0	7	1.2
Fruit dip, 2 tbsp.:							
caramel:							
(*Litehouse* Lowfat)	110	1.0	28.0	0	0	150	0
(*Litehouse* Original)	110	1.0	25.0	1.5	0	125	0
(*Litehouse* Premium Dip Sleeve)	120	1.0	20.0	4.5	0	115	0
chocolate (*Litehouse*)	120	1.0	24.0	3.0	0	120	0
toffee (*Litehouse*)	120	1.0	27.0	1.5	0	150	0
chocolate:							
(*Litehouse*)	70	0	19.0	0	0	25	0
milk (*Baker's* Dipping Real)	80	1.0	9.0	5.0	0	10	0
semisweet, dark (*Baker's* Dipping Real)	70	1.0	9.0	4.5	0	5	1.0
strawberry creme (*Litehouse*)	90	1.0	9.0	6.0	5	50	0
vanilla creme, plain or cinnamon (*Litehouse*)	90	1.0	9.0	6.0	5	50	0

Food and Measure	cal.	prot. (gms)	carbo. (gms)	fat (gms)	chol. (mgs)	sod. (mgs)	fiber (gms)
Fruit drink blend (see also "Citrus drink" and specific listings), 8 fl. oz., except as noted:							
(*Capri Sun* Splash Cooler), 6.75 fl. oz.	100	0	27.0	0	0	15	0
(*R.W. Knudsen* Razzleberry)	130	<1.0	33.0	0	0	35	0
(*R.W. Knudsen* Razzleberry Box)	120	1.0	28.0	0	0	20	0
(*Simply Nutritious* Mega Antioxidant) .	120	0	29.0	0	0	20	0
(*Simply Nutritious* Mega C)	140	<1.0	31.0	0	0	15	0
(*Simply Nutritious* Mega Green)	120	1.0	30.0	0	0	35	0
(*Simply Nutritious* Morning Blend) . . .	120	1.0	31.0	0	0	15	0
(*Simply Nutritious* Vita Juice)	120	2.0	29.0	0	0	35	0
(*V8 Splash Medley*) . .	110	0	28.0	0	0	40	0
lemon ginger echinacea (*Simply Nutritious*)	110	0	29.0	0	0	15	0
punch:							
(*Hood*)	130	0	32.0	0	0	7	0
(*Langers* Cocktail) .	120	0	30.0	0	0	15	0
(*Lincoln*)	140	0	34.0	0	0	45	0
(*Minute Maid* Carton/ Jug)	120	0	31.0	0	0	15	0
(*Minute Maid* Plastic)	100	0	28.0	0	0	80	0
(*Minute Maid Coolers*), 6.75-fl.-oz. pouch	100	0	26.0	0	0	15	0
(*Nantucket Nectars*)	130	0	32.0	0	0	5	0
(*Ocean Spray*)	130	0	32.0	0	0	35	0
(*Snapple*)	110	0	29.0	0	0	10	0
canned	117	0	29.5	0	0	55	.3
frozen* (*Minute Maid*)	110	0	30.0	0	0	0	0
frozen*	114	0	28.9	0	0	10	.4
herbal (*AriZona* Rx Power)	100	0	26.0	0	0	25	0
tropical:							
(*Ocean Spray Cravin' Less Sugar*)	80	0	20.0	0	0	60	0

Food and Measure	cal.	prot. (gms)	carbo. (gms)	fat (gms)	chol. (mgs)	sod. (mgs)	fiber (gms)
(*Santa Cruz Organic* Box)	120	0	31.0	0	0	0	0
(*Snapple-a-Day*), 11.5 fl. oz.	210	7.0	43.0	0	0	110	5.0
(*Sobe* Lizard Lightning)	130	0	33.0	0	0	20	0
(*V8 Splash*)	110	0	27.0	0	0	40	0
colada (*V8 Splash* Smoothies)	130	3.0	30.0	0	0	50	1.0
tropical punch:							
(*Capri Sun*), 6.75 fl. oz.	90	0	25.0	0	0	15	0
(*Minute Maid*)	110	0	30.0	0	0	15	0
(*Minute Maid Coolers*), 6.75-fl.-oz. pouch	100	0	26.0	0	0	15	0
(*R.W. Knudsen* Box)	120	1.0	29.0	0	0	20	0
frozen* (*Minute Maid*)	100	0	28.0	0	0	0	0
Fruit glaze, see specific fruit listings							
Fruit juice blend (see also specific listings), 8 fl. oz., except as noted:							
(*Bolthouse Farms* Green Goddess)	140	2.0	33.0	0	0	25	1.0
(*Ceres* Medley)	130	0	31.0	0	0	10	2.0
(*Langers* Autumn/ Spring/Winter Blend)	120	0	30.0	0	0	10	0
(*Langers* Summer Blend)	125	0	31.0	0	0	10	0
(*Minute Maid* Medley), 11.5-fl.-oz. can	170	0	42.0	0	0	30	0
(*Minute Maid* Medley), 12-fl.-oz. bottle ...	170	0	43.0	0	0	31	0
punch:							
(*Juicy Juice*)	120	0	29.0	0	0	20	0
(*Minute Maid*), 6.75-fl.-oz. box .	100	0	24.0	0	0	15	0
tropical (*Santa Cruz Organic*)	140	1.0	33.0	0	0	10	0
Fruit pectin, 1/8 tsp.:							
(*Sure-Jell/Slim Set*) ..	0	0	0	0	0	0	0
(*Sure-Jell* for Lower Sugar Recipes) ...	0	0	0	0	0	5	0

Food and Measure	cal.	prot. (gms)	carbo. (gms)	fat (gms)	chol. (mgs)	sod. (mgs)	fiber (gms)
Fruit protector (*Sure-Jell Ever Fresh*), ⅛ tsp.	5	0	<1.0	0	0	0	0
Fruit sauce, Asian, four (*Heaven and Earth*), 1 tbsp.	100	10.0	5.0	16.0	0	90	0
Fruit snack (see also specific listings), all fruits:							
(*Animal Planet*), . 8-oz. pouch	70	1.0	17.0	0	0	35	0
(*Fruit by the Foot*), ¾-oz. roll	80	0	17.0	1.5	0	50	0
(*Fruit Gushers*), . 8-oz. pouch	90	0	20.0	1.0	0	55	0
(*Fruit Rippers*), . 6-oz. pouch	60	2.0	11.0	0	0	15	0
(*Fruit Roll-Ups*), .5-oz. roll	50	0	12.0	1.0	0	55	0
except apricot, blackberry, mango, and tropical (*Stretch Island* Fruit Leather), .5-oz. bar	45	0	12.0	0	0	0	1.0
except strawberry (*Stretch Island* Fruit Leather Organic), .5-oz. bar	45	0	12.0	0	0	5	1.0
all shapes/characters (*Betty Crocker* Fruit Snacks), .8-oz. pouch	.80	0	21.0	0	0	50	0
apricot, mango, or tropical (*Stretch Island* Fruit Leather), .5-oz. bar	45	0	11.0	0	0	0	1.0
blackberry, berry (*Stretch Island* Fruit Leather), .5-oz. bar	45	0	12.0	0	0	0	2.0
strawberry (*Stretch Island* Fruit Leather Organic), .5-oz. bar	45	0	11.0	0	0	0	1.0
Fruit spread (see also "Jam and preserves" and specific listings),							

Food and Measure	cal.	prot. (gms)	carbo. (gms)	fat (gms)	chol. (mgs)	sod. (mgs)	fiber (gms)
all fruits, 1 tbsp.:							
(*Cascadian Farm*) ..	40	0	10.0	0	0	0	0
(*Harvest Moon*) ...	30	0	8.0	0	0	0	0
(*Smucker's Simply 100% Fruit*)	40	0	10.0	0	0	0	0
except apricot (*Tree of Life*)	35	0	9.0	0	0	0	0
apricot (*Tree of Life*) .	35	0	9.0	0	0	0	<1.0
Fruit-nut mix, see "Trail mix"							
Fudge, see "Candy"							
Fudge topping, see "Chocolate topping"							
Fuki, see "Butterbur"							
Furikake, see "Sesame seed condiment"							
Fuzzy navel, drink mixer, frozen (*Bacardi*), 2 fl. oz. .	110	0	29.0	0	0	0	0

G

Food and Measure	cal.	prot. (gms)	carbo. (gms)	fat (gms)	chol. (mgs)	sod. (mgs)	fiber (gms)
Gai choy, see "Cabbage, mustard"							
Gai lan, see "Kale, Chinese"							
Galanga, raw (*Frieda's*), ⅔ cup, 3 oz.	60	1.0	13.0	.5	0	10	2.0
Garbanzo bean:							
dry, ¼ cup:							
(*Arrowhead Mills*) .	160	9.0	27.0	2.5	0	10	8.0
(*Shiloh Farms*)	170	10.0	29.0	2.0	0	10	6.0
boiled, ½ cup	134	7.3	22.5	2.1	0	6	2.9
presoaked (*Frieda's*), ⅓ cup	150	7.0	23.0	3.0	0	230	22.0
Garbanzo bean, canned, ½ cup:							
(*Allens/East Texas Fair* Chick Peas)	120	5.0	19.0	2.5	0	330	8.0
(*Bush's*)	130	6.0	22.0	2.0	0	500	9.0
(*Eden* Organic)	120	7.0	19.0	1.5	0	10	5.0
(*Old El Paso*)	100	6.0	16.0	1.5	0	340	4.0
(*Progresso* Chick Peas)	120	5.0	20.0	2.5	0	280	5.0
(*S&W*)	80	7.0	19.0	1.0	0	460	5.0
(*S&W* 50% Less Salt)	80	7.0	19.0	1.0	0	220	5.0
(*Westbrae Natural* Organic)	110	6.0	18.0	2.0	0	140	5.0
(*Zapata*)	120	6.0	20.0	2.0	0	290	8.0
Garlic, fresh:							
(*Frieda's* Elephant), chopped, 1 tbsp. ...	5	0	1.0	0	0	0	0
trimmed, 1 oz.	42	1.8	9.4	.1	0	5	.6
1 clove, .1 oz.	4	.2	1.0	<.1	0	1	.1
granulated/minced, 1 tsp.	13	.7	2.9	0	0	1	0

Food and Measure	cal.	prot. (gms)	carbo. (gms)	fat (gms)	chol. (mgs)	sod. (mgs)	fiber (gms)
Garlic, in jars:							
crushed, 1 tsp.:							
(*Christopher Ranch*)	10	0	1.0	0	0	0	0
(*McCormick* California Style) .	15	0	0	.5	0	0	0
marinated (*Frieda's*), 1 oz.	30	1.0	7.0	0	0	140	0
minced (*McCormick* California Style), 1 tsp.	15	0	1.0	.5	0	0	0
Garlic bread, see "Bread, frozen"							
Garlic bread sprinkle (*McCormick*), ¼ tsp.	5	0	0	0	0	30	0
Garlic and herb sauce mix (*Golden Dipt Bag 'n Season*), 1 tbsp. . .	25	0	3.0	0	0	370	0
Garlic juice (*McCormick*), ¼ tsp. . . .	0	0	0	0	0	0	0
Garlic oil (*Watkins* Liquid Spice), 1 tsp. .	40	0	0	4.5	0	0	0
Garlic paste (*Italia In Tavola*), 1 tbsp. . . .	60	0	3.0	6.0	0	520	0
Garlic pepper:							
(*Lawry's*), ¼ tsp.	0	0	0	0	0	70	0
(*McCormick* California Style), ¼ tsp.	0	0	0	0	0	105	0
(*McCormick* Grinder), ¼ tsp.	0	0	0	0	0	75	0
1 tsp.	8	.3	1.8	0	0	360	.3
Garlic powder:							
1 tsp.	10	.5	2.3	0	0	1	0
w/parsley (*Lawry's*), ¼ tsp.	0	0	<1.0	0	0	0	0
Garlic relish, Indian, medium (*Patak's*), 1 tbsp.	40	1.0	3.0	3.0	0	55	0
Garlic salt, ¼ tsp.:							
(*Lawry's*)	0	0	0	0	0	240	0
(*McCormick*)	0	0	0	0	0	450	0
(*McCormick* California Style)	0	0	0	0	0	220	0
(*McCormick Season-All*)	0	0	0	0	0	260	0
and parsley (*McCormick*)	0	0	0	0	0	225	0

Food and Measure	cal.	prot. (gms)	carbo. (gms)	fat (gms)	chol. (mgs)	sod. (mgs)	fiber (gms)
Garlic seasoning:							
herb (*McCormick 1 Step*), ¾ tsp.	10	0	1.0	0	0	115	0
roasted, and bell pepper (*McCormick 1 Step*), 1 tsp.	10	0	2.0	0	0	460	0
Garlic spread:							
(*Lawry's*), 1 tbsp.	100	0	2.0	10.0	0	190	0
(*Lawry's* Concentrate), 2 tsp.	50	0	1.0	6.0	0	80	0
(*McCormick*), ½ tbsp.	45	0	1.0	4.0	0	140	0
and herb (*McCormick*), ½ tbsp.	45	0	1.0	4.5	0	125	0
Garlic sprouts, fresh (*Jonathan's*), 1 cup	70	5.0	14.0	.5	0	10	3.0
Garlic-herb dip mix (*Fantastic* Soup/Dip), 2¼ tsp.	20	0	5.0	0	0	540	0
Gefilte fish, in jars, w/out gel:							
(*Manischewitz*), 2.3-oz. pc.	70	6.0	1.0	5.0	30	320	<1.0
(*Manischewitz* Fishlets), 7 pcs., 2 oz.	50	5.0	2.0	2.5	20	270	<1.0
(*Rokeach*), 2-oz. pc. .	60	6.0	2.0	3.0	35	290	1.0
sweet, 2-oz. pc.	47	5.1	4.1	1.0	17	293	0
whitefish/pike: (*Manischewitz*), 2.3-oz. pc.	50	7.0	3.0	1.5	15	350	<1.0
(*Rokeach* Old Vienna), 2-oz. pc.	50	5.0	4.0	2.0	30	240	1.0
Gefilte fish, frozen, cooked (*A&B Famous*), 2 oz.	80	6.2	9.0	2.5	40	170	1.0
Gefilte fish, frozen, uncooked:							
(*BenZ's*), 3 oz.	140	10.0	19.0	2.0	0	160	0
(*Dr. Praeger's*), 1.8 oz.	85	6.0	6.0	4.0	20	185	0
(*Ungar's*), 1.8 oz.	83	6.0	4.5	4.5	41	263	0
(*Ungar's* Lite), 2.4 oz.	80	7.0	5.0	3.0	20	190	2.0
gluten free (*A&B Famous*), 2 oz.	80	6.0	7.0	3.5	50	220	1.0
low cholesterol (*A&B Famous*), 2 oz.	90	6.0	8.0	3.5	10	220	1.0

Food and Measure	cal.	prot. (gms)	carbo. (gms)	fat (gms)	chol. (mgs)	sod. (mgs)	fiber (gms)
salmon:							
(*A&B Famous*), 2 oz.	140	12.0	4.0	8.0	20	260	1.0
(*Ungar's*), 1.8 oz. . .	88	6.0	6.0	4.5	33	324	0
sugar free:							
(*A&B Famous*), 2 oz.	80	0	4.0	5.5	50	220	1.0
(*A&B Famous*							
Gourmet), 2 oz. .	80	6.0	2.0	5.0	25	350	<1.0
(*Ungar's*), 1.8 oz. . .	70	6.0	3.0	3.5	15	180	0
sweet, 2 oz.:							
(*A&B Famous*)	80	6.0	7.0	3.5	50	220	<1.0
and savory (*A&B*							
Famous Hungarian							
Style)	80	6.0	9.0	2.5	40	170	1.0
Gelatin, unflavored							
(*Knox*), ¼ pkt.	5	2.0	0	0	0	0	0
Gelatin dessert, ready-to-eat, 3.5 oz.:							
all fruit flavors:							
(*Hunt's Snack Packs*							
Juicy Gels)	100	0	24.0	0	0	40	0
(*Jell-O*)	70	1.0	17.0	0	0	40	0
(*Jell-O* Sugar Free) .	10	1.0	0	0	0	45	0
cherry and blue raspberry (*Jell-O X-Treme*)	70	0	17.0	0	0	40	0
w/fruit, see specific fruit listings							
watermelon and green apple (*Jell-O X-Treme*)	100	0	24.0	0	0	45	0
Gelatin dessert mix, ½ cup*:							
all fruit flavors:							
(*Jell-O*) . . . . : .	80	2.0	19.0	0	0	-¹	0
(*Jell-O* Sugar Free) .	10	1.0	0	0	0	-²	0
Gelatin sticks, all flavors (*Jell-O X-Treme*), 1 pc. . . .	60	0	16.0	0	0	35	0
Gemelli pasta dish, mix, w/roasted garlic, Parmesan sauce (*Annie's*), 1 cup* . .	360	12.0	50.0	13.0	35	700	1.0

1. Sodium values vary between 75 and 120 mgs. according to flavor.
2. Sodium values vary between 45 and 80 mgs. according to flavor.

Food and Measure	cal.	prot. (gms)	carbo. (gms)	fat (gms)	chol. (mgs)	sod. (mgs)	fiber (gms)
Ginger, trimmed root:							
1 oz.	20	.5	4.3	.2	0	4	.6
sliced, ¼ cup	17	.4	3.6	.2	0	3	.5
Ginger, candied or crystallized:							
(*Frieda's*), 9 pcs., 1.1 oz.	100	0	26.0	0	0	10	0
(*Tree of Life*), 7 pcs., 1.4 oz.	150	0	37.0	0	0	25	1.0
Ginger, ground, 1 tsp.	6	.2	1.3	.1	0	1	.2
Ginger, pickled:							
Japanese, 1 oz.	10	.1	2.1	<.1	0	105	0
w/shiso leaves (*Eden*), 1 tbsp., .5 oz.	15	0	3.0	0	0	340	1.0
Ginger, Thai, see "Galanga"							
Ginger-garlic oil (*Watkins* Liquid Spice), 1 tsp.	40	0	0	4.5	0	0	0
Ginkgo nut, shelled:							
raw, 1 oz.	52	1.2	10.7	.5	0	2	<1.0
canned, drained, 1 oz.	32	.6	6.3	.5	0	87	2.6
dried, 1 oz.	99	2.9	20.6	.8	0	4	n.a.
Glacé, cake, see "Fruit, mixed, candied"							
Glaze, see "Ham glaze" and specific fruit listings							
Glaze sauce, see "Grilling sauce" and "Marinade"							
Gluten, see "Wheat gluten"							
Gnocchi, potato:							
pkg.:							
(*Bellino*), 1 cup . . .	210	5.0	46.0	1.0	0	440	3.0
w/spinach (*Bellino*), ¾ cup	180	4.0	41.0	0	0	460	2.0
refrigerated, 1½ cups:							
(*Rienzi*)	280	5.0	30.0	.5	0	590	2.0
w/cheese (*Rienzi*) .	320	5.0	30.0	1.0	0	590	0
Goat, meat only, roasted, 4 oz.	162	30.7	0	3.4	85	98	0
Gobo root, see "Burdock root"							

Food and Measure	cal.	prot. (gms)	carbo. (gms)	fat (gms)	chol. (mgs)	sod. (mgs)	fiber (gms)
Godfather's Pizza:							
original, medium, ⅛ pie:							
all meat combo ...	373	19.0	35.0	16.0	39	905	2.0
bacon cheeseburger	328	16.0	35.0	13.0	35	795	2.0
cheese	260	12.0	34.0	7.0	15	455	1.0
combo	352	17.0	36.0	14.0	31	847	3.0
combo, super	387	19.0	37.0	17.0	41	938	3.0
Hawaiian	281	13.0	37.0	8.0	19	549	2.0
Hawaiian, super ...	277	13.0	36.0	8.0	19	549	2.0
hot stuff	360	17.0	35.0	16.0	39	773	2.0
humble pie	379	16.0	34.0	18.0	37	752	2.0
pepperoni	294	13.0	34.0	10.0	22	579	1.0
taco	362	18.0	36.0	16.0	42	810	2.0
taco, super	392	19.0	36.0	18.0	47	846	3.0
veggie	275	12.0	36.0	8.0	15	524	2.0
original, large, 1/10 pie:							
all meat combo ...	383	19.0	38.0	16.0	38	911	2.0
bacon cheeseburger	355	18.0	37.0	15.0	40	870	2.0
cheese	293	14.0	36.0	9.0	19	451	1.0
combo	366	18.0	37.0	15.0	40	870	2.0
combo, super	432	22.0	39.0	19.0	47	1037	3.0
Hawaiian	316	15.0	39.0	9.0	23	616	2.0
Hawaiian, super ...	311	15.0	38.0	9.0	23	615	2.0
hot stuff	401	19.0	37.0	18.0	40	854	2.0
humble pie	420	18.0	38.0	20.0	43	832	2.0
pepperoni	330	15.0	36.0	12.0	26	648	1.0
taco	418	22.0	38.0	19.0	53	913	2.0
taco, super	450	22.0	39.0	22.0	60	952	3.0
veggie	310	14.0	45.0	8.0	17	543	3.0
golden, medium, ⅛ pie:							
all meat combo ...	285	14.0	27.0	13.0	27	654	1.0
bacon cheeseburger	267	13.0	26.0	12.0	27	620	1.0
cheese	221	10.0	26.0	8.0	13	371	1.0
combo	288	13.0	27.0	13.0	25	653	2.0
combo, super	322	16.0	28.0	15.0	34	744	2.0
Hawaiian	238	11.0	28.0	8.0	16	464	1.0
Hawaiian, super ...	235	11.0	27.0	8.0	16	464	1.0
hot stuff	294	13.0	27.0	14.0	27	603	1.0
humble pie	306	13.0	27.0	15.0	29	589	1.0
pepperoni	255	11.0	26.0	11.0	19	495	1.0
taco	300	15.0	27.0	14.0	35	619	2.0
taco, super	328	15.0	28.0	17.0	39	645	2.0
veggie	232	10.0	27.0	8.0	13	416	2.0

Food and Measure	cal.	prot. (gms)	carbo. (gms)	fat (gms)	chol. (mgs)	sod. (mgs)	fiber (gms)
Godfather's Pizza *(cont.)*							
golden, large, 1/10 pie:							
all meat combo ...	325	16.0	29.0	15.0	31	751	2.0
bacon cheeseburger	307	15.0	29.0	14.0	32	709	1.0
cheese	252	11.0	28.0	9.0	15	425	1.0
combo	328	15.0	30.0	15.0	29	710	2.0
combo, super	371	18.0	31.0	18.0	40	859	2.0
Hawaiian	268	12.0	30.0	10.0	19	525	1.0
Hawaiian, super ...	267	12.0	30.0	10.0	19	525	1.0
hot stuff	337	15.0	29.0	17.0	32	696	1.0
humble pie	352	15.0	29.0	18.0	34	679	1.0
pepperoni	289	12.0	28.0	13.0	22	588	1.0
taco	346	17.0	30.0	17.0	41	723	2.0
taco, super	377	17.0	30.0	20.0	46	753	2.0
veggie	264	11.0	30.0	11.0	15	480	2.0
thin, medium, 1/8 pie:							
all meat combo ...	282	13.0	20.0	15.0	31	607	1.0
bacon cheeseburger	246	11.0	19.0	13.0	28	521	1.0
cheese	200	8.0	19.0	9.0	14	271	>1.0
combo	266	12.0	21.0	14.0	26	553	2.0
combo, super	301	14.0	21.0	16.0	35	644	2.0
Hawaiian	217	10.0	21.0	9.0	17	365	1.0
Hawaiian, super ...	213	10.0	20.0	9.0	17	364	1.0
hot stuff	272	12.0	20.0	15.0	28	503	0
humble pie	285	12.0	20.0	16.0	30	490	1.0
pepperoni	234	10.0	19.0	12.0	20	395	>1.0
taco	278	13.0	20.0	15.0	35	520	1.0
taco, super	306	14.0	21.0	18.0	40	546	2.0
veggie	209	9.0	20.0	9.0	14	317	1.0
thin, large, 1/10 pie:							
all meat combo ...	311	15.0	20.0	17.0	37	697	1.0
bacon cheeseburger	293	14.0	20.0	17.0	38	655	1.0
cheese	215	9.0	19.0	10.0	16	308	>1.0
combo	293	14.0	21.0	16.0	30	639	2.0
combo, super	334	16.0	22.0	19.0	41	741	2.0
Hawaiian	234	11.0	22.0	10.0	20	408	1.0
Hawaiian, super ...	230	11.0	21.0	10.0	20	407	1.0
hot stuff	300	13.0	20.0	17.0	33	579	1.0
humble pie	315	13.0	20.0	19.0	35	562	1.0
pepperoni	252	11.0	19.0	13.0	23	440	>1.0
taco	309	15.0	21.0	18.0	42	605	1.0
taco, super	339	16.0	21.0	21.0	47	635	2.0
veggie	227	10.0	21.0	10.0	16	264	1.0

Food and Measure	cal.	prot. (gms)	carbo. (gms)	fat (gms)	chol. (mgs)	sod. (mgs)	fiber (gms)
extras:							
bread stick, 1 pc. . . .	80	2.0	14.0	2.0	0	71	1.0
cheese sticks	132	5.0	18.0	4.0	6	197	1.0
potato wedges, 4 oz.	192	3.0	24.0	9.0	0	342	4.0
apple dessert:							
alum pan, 1/6	139	3.0	28.0	2.0	0	142	1.0
small, 1/6	202	4.0	37.0	5.0	0	200	1.0
medium, 1/8	206	4.0	39.0	4.0	0	204	1.0
large, 1/10	229	5.0	42.0	5.0	0	225	1.0
cherry dessert:							
alum pan, 1/6	142	3.0	29.0	2.0	0	135	1.0
small, 1/6	206	4.0	38.0	5.0	0	190	1.0
medium, 1/8	210	4.0	40.0	4.0	0	193	1.0
large, 1/10	233	5.0	44.0	5.0	0	213	1.0
chocolate chip cookie,							
alum pan, 1/6	195	2.0	30.0	8.0	21	157	0
cinnamon streusel:							
alum pan, 1/6	161	3.0	30.0	3.0	0	150	1.0
small, 1/6 . . . . :	226	4.0	39.0	6.0	0	205	1.0
medium, 1/8	228	5.0	40.0	6.0	0	208	1.0
large, 1/10	258	5.0	45.0	7.0	0	231	1.0
M&M's **streusel:**							
alum pan, 1/6	173	4.0	31.0	4.0	0	152	1.0
small, 1/6	249	5.0	42.0	7.0	1	208	1.0
medium, 1/8	263	5.0	45.0	7.0	1	212	1.0
large, 1/10	300	5.0	51.0	8.0	1	236	1.0
Golden nugget squash (*Frieda's*), 3/4 cup,							
3 oz.	30	1.0	7.0	0	0	0	1.0
Goose, roasted:							
meat w/skin, 4 oz. . . .	346	28.5	0	24.9	103	79	0
meat only, 4 oz.	270	32.9	0	14.4	109	86	0
Goose fat, 1 tbsp. . . .	115	0	0	12.8	13	0	0
Goose liver, see "Liver" and "Pâté"							
Gooseberries, fresh,							
1/2 cup	34	.7	7.6	.4	0	1	3.2
Gordita entree kit (*Old El Paso* Dinner Kit), 1/4 pkg.:							
w/ranch sauce:							
as packaged	300	4.0	34.0	16.0	0	1010	1.0
w/meat and cheese*	390	20.0	34.0	19.0	45	1070	1.0

Food and Measure	cal.	prot. (gms)	carbo. (gms)	fat (gms)	chol. (mgs)	sod. (mgs)	fiber (gms)
Gordita entree kit *(cont.)*							
w/red sauce:							
as packaged	210	4.0	36.0	5.0	0	950	1.0
w/meat and cheese*	310	21.0	36.0	9.0	45	1010	1.0
Gourd, boiled, ½ cup:							
dishcloth, 1" slices ...	50	.6	12.8	.3	0	18	<1.0
white-flower, 1" cubes	11	.4	2.7	<.1	0	1	<1.0
Gourd, dried, see "Kanpyo"							
Grain salad, see "Tabouli," "Wheat salad," and specific listings							
Grains, mixed, dish, mix (see also specific listings), 1 cup*:							
brown rice/wheat:							
barley, chicken herb:							
(*Near East*), 2 oz.	240	8.0	51.0	2.0	0	780	6.0
(*Near East*), 1 cup*	270	8.0	51.0	6.0	0	780	6.0
bulgur, roasted garlic:							
(*Near East*), 2 oz.	190	6.0	41.0	2.0	0	570	5.0
(*Near East*), 1 cup*	220	6.0	41.0	5.0	0	570	5.0
pecan and garlic:							
(*Near East*), 2 oz. ..	210	6.0	37.0	5.0	0	540	4.0
(*Near East*), 1 cup*	240	6.0	37.0	9.0	0	540	4.0
white rice/pearled wheat, creamy Parmesan:							
(*Near East*), 2 oz. ..	240	8.0	48.0	3.0	5	790	3.0
(*Near East*), 1 cup*	280	8.0	48.0	8.0	20	840	3.0
Granadilla, see "Passion fruit"							
Granola, see "Cereal"							
Granola/cereal bar, 1 bar, except as noted:							
(*Cascadian Farm* Harvest Berry Granola)	130	2.0	27.0	2.0	0	130	1.0
(*Froot Loops*)	100	2.0	16.0	3.0	0	75	<1.0
(*Frosted Flakes*)	110	2.0	19.0	3.0	0	90	<1.0
all varieties:							
(*Health Valley* Fat Free Granola) ...	140	2.0	35.0	0	0	10	3.0

Food and Measure	cal.	prot. (gms)	carbo. (gms)	fat (gms)	chol. (mgs)	sod. (mgs)	fiber (gms)
(*Health Valley* Fat Free Bakes)	70	2.0	19.0	0	0	30	3.0
(*Health Valley* Cobbler Cereal) .	130	2.0	27.0	2.0	0	50	1.0
(*Health Valley* Low Fat Cobbler Cereal)	130	2.0	27.0	2.0	0	50	1.0
(*Health Valley* Low Fat Tarts/Creme Sandwich)	130	2.0	28.0	2.0	0	80	1.0
(*Nature Valley* Chewy Granola)	140	2.0	26.0	3.5	0	130	1.0
(*Nutri-Grain* Cereal)	140	2.0	27.0	3.0	0	110	1.0
(*Nutri-Grain* Minis), 1 pouch	160	2.0	32.0	3.0	0	115	<1.0
except peanut butter chocolate chip and dipped varieties (*PowerBar Harvest*)	240	7.0	45.0	4.0	0	80	4.0
almond, roasted (*Nature Valley* Crunchy Granola), 2 bars ...	190	4.0	28.0	7.0	0	180	2.0
apple:							
cobbler (*Nutri-Grain Twists*)	140	1.0	27.0	3.0	0	105	1.0
crisp (*Nature Valley* Crunchy Granola), 2 bars	180	4.0	29.0	6.0	0	160	2.0
Dutch (*Health Valley* Moist & Chewy Granola)	100	2.0	22.0	1.0	0	15	2.0
apple berry (*Uncle Sam* Cereal)	180	9.0	28.0	3.0	0	125	3.0
apple cinnamon:							
(*Nature Valley* Chewy Trail Mix)	140	2.0	25.0	4.0	0	120	1.0
(*PowerBar*)	230	10.0	45.0	2.5	0	90	3.0
banana:							
(*Nutri-Grain* Muffin)	160	3.0	30.0	4.0	0	110	1.0
(*PowerBar*)	230	9.0	45.0	2.0	0	90	3.0
banana nut:							
(*Nature Valley* Crunchy Granola), 2 bars	190	4.0	28.0	7.0	0	160	2.0

Food and Measure	cal.	prot. (gms)	carbo. (gms)	fat (gms)	chol. (mgs)	sod. (mgs)	fiber (gms)
Granola/cereal bar, banana *(cont.)*							
(*PowerBar Harvest* Dipped)	250	7.0	45.0	5.0	0	125	4.0
chocolate (*Save the Forest* Trail Mix) .	110	2.0	19.0	4.0	0	0	1.0
berry:							
mixed (*Nature Valley* Chewy Trail Mix)	140	2.0	26.0	3.5	0	90	1.0
wild (*Health Valley* Moist & Chewy Granola)	100	2.0	22.0	1.0	0	5	2.0
wild (*PowerBar*) ...	230	9.0	45.0	2.5	0	90	3.0
blueberry:							
(*Honey Maid* Soft Baked)	150	2.0	27.0	4.5	0	130	1.0
(*Nutri-Grain* Muffin)	170	2.0	31.0	4.0	0	100	<1.0
and yogurt (*Barbara's Puffins* Cereal & Milk)	120	5.0	24.0	1.5	0	90	3.0
brown sugar cinnamon (*All-Bran* Cereal) ..	130	2.0	27.0	3.0	0	170	5.0
cappuccino and cream (*Nutri-Grain Twists*)	140	1.0	28.0	3.0	0	90	1.0
caramel nut crunch (*Nutri-Grain* Chewy Granola Bites), 1 pouch	130	2.0	18.0	6.0	0	60	1.0
carob chip (*Barbara's Nature's Choice* Granola)	80	2.0	15.0	2.0	0	0	<1.0
carrot cake (*PowerBar Harvest* Dipped) ...	260	7.0	45.0	5.0	0	100	3.0
chocolate:							
(*PowerBar*)	230	10.0	45.0	2.0	0	95	3.0
almond toffee (*Go-Lean* Cereal)	290	13.0	45.0	6.0	0	250	6.0
caramel (*GoLean Crunchy!* Cereal Karma)	140	8.0	26.0	3.0	20	180	5.0
cookie, double (*PowerBar Pria*) .	110	5.0	16.0	3.0	0	90	0
crème (*Hershey's SnackBarz*)	130	<1.0	17.0	6.0	0	80	0

Food and Measure	cal.	prot. (gms)	carbo. (gms)	fat (gms)	chol. (mgs)	sod. (mgs)	fiber (gms)
double (*PowerBar Harvest* Dipped) .	260	7.0	45.0	5.0	0	100	3.0
espresso (*Café Creations*)	130	2.0	27.0	3.0	0	60	2.0
fudge brownie (*PowerBar Protein Plus*)	270	24.0	36.0	5.0	5	140	2.0
honey graham (*PowerBar Pria*) .	110	5.0	16.0	3.0	0	80	0
peanut (*GoLean* Crunchy! Cereal Bliss)	170	9.0	30.0	4.0	0	220	5.0
peanut butter (*PowerBar*)	240	10.0	45.0	3.0	0	95	3.0
peanut butter (*PowerBar Protein Plus*)	290	24.0	38.0	5.0	5	220	1.0
peanut crunch (*PowerBar Pria*) .	110	5.0	16.0	3.5	0	80	0
raspberry (*Café Creations*)	130	1.0	27.0	3.0	0	50	2.0
cinnamon (*Café Creations* Danish)	130	2.0	27.0	2.5	0	80	2.0
chocolate chip/chunk:							
(*Nutri-Grain* Chewy Granola)	110	1.0	18.0	3.5	0	55	<1.0
(*Nutri-Grain* Chewy Granola Bites), 1 pouch	120	1.0	20.0	4.5	0	65	1.0
cinnamon:							
(*Nature Valley* Crunchy Granola), 2 bars	180	4.0	29.0	6.0	0	160	2.0
raisin (*Barbara's Nature's Choice* Granola)	80	2.0	14.0	2.0	0	0	<1.0
(*Nutri-Grain* Muffin)	170	2.0	32.0	4.0	0	100	1.0
raisin (*Save the Forest* Cereal) . . .	120	3.0	19.0	4.0	0	20	2.0
roll (*PowerBar Harvest* Dipped)	250	7.0	45.0	5.0	0	125	3.0
cocoa (*Rice Krispies*) .	100	1.0	17.0	2.5	0	70	<1.0
cookies and cream:							
(*GoLean* Cereal) . . .	290	13.0	50.0	6.0	0	200	6.0

Food and Measure	cal.	prot. (gms)	carbo. (gms)	fat (gms)	chol. (mgs)	sod. (mgs)	fiber (gms)
Granola/cereal bar, cookies and cream *(cont.)*							
(*PowerBar*)	240	9.0	45.0	3.5	0	120	2.0
(*PowerBar Protein Plus*)	290	24.0	38.0	5.0	5	160	1.0
cranberry crunch (*Save the Forest* Trail Mix)	130	4.0	14.0	7.0	0	0	2.0
crème caramel crisp (*PowerBar Pria*) ...	110	5.0	17.0	3.0	0	80	0
French toast (*Barbara's Puffins* Cereal & Milk)	130	5.0	25.0	1.5	0	100	3.0
fruit and nut:							
(*Cascadian Farm* Granola)	140	2.0	24.0	4.0	0	110	1.0
(*Nature Valley* Chewy Trail Mix)	140	3.0	25.0	4.0	0	95	2.0
honey oat:							
(*All-Bran* Cereal) ..	130	2.0	27.0	3.0	0	170	5.0
raisin (*Nutri-Grain* Chewy Granola) .	110	2.0	18.0	3.0	0	60	1.0
honey vanilla yogurt (*GoLean* Cereal) ...	290	13.0	49.0	5.0	0	160	6.0
lemon lime (*GoLean* Crunchy! Cereal) ..	160	9.0	32.0	3.0	0	150	5.0
malt nut (*PowerBar*) .	230	10.0	45.0	2.5	0	90	3.0
malted chocolate crisp (*GoLean* Cereal) ...	290	13.0	49.0	6.0	0	200	6.0
maple brown sugar (*Nature Valley* Crunchy Granola), 2 bars	180	4.0	29.0	6.0	0	160	2.0
marshmallow crème (*Hershey's Snack-Barz* S'Mores)	110	1.0	18.0	4.0	0	90	0
mint chocolate cookie (*PowerBar Pria*) ...	110	5.0	16.0	3.0	0	90	1.0
mocha java (*GoLean* Cereal)	290	13.0	50.0	6.0	0	190	6.0
multigrain:							
(*Cascadian Farm* Granola)	130	2.0	27.0	2.0	0	150	1.0
all fruit varieties (*Barbara's Nature's Choice* Cereal) ..	120	1.0	25.0	1.5	0	65	2.0

Food and Measure	cal.	prot. (gms)	carbo. (gms)	fat (gms)	chol. (mgs)	sod. (mgs)	fiber (gms)
nut, triple (*Skippy* Trail Mix)	170	4.0	19.0	9.0	0	80	2.0
nutty S'mores (*Skippy* Trail Mix)	150	3.0	23.0	6.0	0	105	1.0
oatmeal (*Honey Maid*)	150	2.0	24.0	6.0	0	160	1.0
oatmeal raisin:							
(*GoLean* Cereal) . . .	280	13.0	49.0	5.0	0	140	6.0
(*Honey Maid* Soft Baked)	150	2.0	27.0	3.0	0	135	1.0
(*PowerBar*)	230	10.0	45.0	2.5	0	110	3.0
(*Uncle Sam* Cereal)	180	9.0	28.0	3.0	0	135	3.0
iced (*PowerBar Harvest* Dipped) .	250	7.0	45.0	5.0	0	100	3.0
oats and honey:							
(*Barbara's Nature's Choice* Granola) .	80	2.0	14.0	2.0	0	0	<1.0
(*Nature Valley* Crunchy Granola), 2 bars	180	4.0	29.0	6.0	0	160	2.0
peanut butter:							
(*Barbara's Nature's Choice* Granola) .	80	2.0	13.0	3.0	0	0	<1.0
(*Hershey's Snack-Barz*)	130	2.0	16.0	6.0	0	115	<1.0
(*Nature Valley* Crunchy Granola), 2 bars .	180	5.0	30.0	7.0	0	190	2.0
(*PowerBar*)	240	10.0	45.0	3.5	0	120	3.0
(*Skippy* Snack Bar Granola)	180	4.0	18.0	11.0	0	95	1.0
all varieties (*Health Valley* Peanut Butter Bars)	130	2.0	26.0	2.5	0	140	1.0
chocolate (*GoLean* Cereal)	290	13.0	48.0	6.0	0	280	6.0
chocolate chip (*Barbara's Puffins* Cereal & Milk) . .	140	6.0	22.0	3.5	0	190	3.0
chocolate chip (*PowerBar Harvest*)	240	7.0	45.0	4.5	0	80	4.0
and fudge (*Skippy* Snack Bar Granola)	190	4.0	18.0	12.0	0	95	1.0
and strawberry (*Skippy* Snack Bar Granola)	170	4.0	14.0	12.0	0	170	1.0

Food and Measure	cal.	prot. (gms)	carbo. (gms)	fat (gms)	chol. (mgs)	sod. (mgs)	fiber (gms)
Granola/cereal bar *(cont.)*							
peanut crunch (*Health Valley* Moist & Chewy Granola) ...	110	3.0	19.0	3.0	0	80	2.0
raspberry:							
(*Save the Forest* Cereal)	120	3.0	19.0	4.0	0	25	2.0
creme stripe (*Power-Bar*)	230	9.0	45.0	2.0	0	100	2.0
spice cake, frosted (*Go-Lean* Cereal)	290	13.0	49.0	5.0	0	200	6.0
strawberry:							
cheesecake (*Nutri-Grain Twists*) ...	140	2.0	26.0	3.0	0	100	<1.0
shortcake (*PowerBar Pria*)	110	5.0	17.0	3.0	0	70	0
toffee chocolate chip (*PowerBar Harvest* Dipped)	250	7.0	45.0	5.0	0	100	4.0
vanilla crisp:							
(*PowerBar*)	230	9.0	45.0	2.5	0	90	3.0
French (*PowerBar Pria*)	110	5.0	16.0	3.0	0	80	0
yogurt:							
strawberry (*Barbara's Puffins* Cereal & Milk)	130	5.0	24.0	2.0	0	90	3.0
strawberry or vanilla (*Nutri-Grain*) ...	140	2.0	27.0	3.0	0	110	1.0
strawberry vanilla (*GoLean* Cereal) .	290	13.0	50.0	5.0	0	200	6.0
vanilla (*PowerBar Protein Plus*) ...	290	24.0	37.0	5.0	5	150	1.0
Grape, fresh:							
(*Chiquita*), 1½ cups ..	90	1.0	24.0	1.0	0	0	1.0
(*Del Monte*), 1½ cups	90	1.0	24.0	1.0	0	0	1.0
(*Dole* Green), 1½ cups	90	1.0	24.0	1.0	0	0	1.0
(*Frieda's* Champagne), ½ cup, 3 oz.......	50	1.0	15.0	0	0	0	1.0
American type (slipskin):							
10 medium	15	.2	4.1	.1	0	tr.	.3
peeled and seeded, ½ cup	29	.3	7.9	.2	0	1	.6

Food and Measure	cal.	prot. (gms)	carbo. (gms)	fat (gms)	chol. (mgs)	sod. (mgs)	fiber (gms)
European type (adherent skin):							
seeded, 1 lb.	287	2.7	72.0	2.3	0	7	2.7
seedless, 10 medium	36	.3	8.9	.3	0	1	.3
seedless or seeded, ½ cup	57	.5	14.2	.5	0	2	.5
Grape, canned, seedless, in heavy syrup w/liquid, ½ cup . . .	94	.6	25.1	.1	0	6	.5
Grape drink, 8 fl. oz.:							
(*Nantucket Nectars* Organic Concord) . .	130	0	31.0	0	0	35	0
(*Newman's Own* Gorilla Grape)	140	0	34.0	0	0	40	0
(*Ocean Spray Cravin' Less Sugar*)	90	0	22.0	0	0	60	0
(*R.W. Knudsen* Box) .	150	1.0	38.0	0	0	30	0
(*Santa Cruz Organic* Box)	100	0	24.0	0	0	10	0
(*Sobe Grape Grog*) . . .	120	0	30.0	0	0	15	0
canned	113	0	28.8	0	0	15	0
cocktail, frozen* (*Minute Maid*)	120	0	33.0	0	0	5	0
grapeade:							
(*AriZona*)	120	0	31.0	0	0	20	0
(*Nantucket Nectars*)	130	0	33.0	0	0	5	0
(*Snapple*)	120	0	29.0	0	0	10	0
punch (*Minute Maid*) .	120	0	32.0	0	0	15	0
Grape drink mix (*Lincoln*), 8 fl. oz.*	130	0	32.0	0	0	45	0
Grape juice, 8 fl. oz., except as noted:							
(*Juicy Juice*)	130	0	34.0	0	0	20	0
(*L&A* Plus)	160	0	40.0	0	0	15	0
(*Langers* Cocktail/Plus)	160	0	40.0	0	0	15	0
(*Nantucket Nectars*) . .	160	0	39.0	0	0	20	0
(*R.W. Knudsen*)	150	0	37.0	0	0	30	0
(*R.W. Knudsen* Concord)	160	<1.0	40.0	0	0	15	0
(*R.W. Knudsen* Organic)	160	<1.0	39.0	0	0	15	0
(*Santa Cruz Organic* Concord)	160	<1.0	40.0	0	0	15	0
(*Walnut Acres* Concord)	120	0	31.0	0	0	0	0
blend:							
(*Minute Maid*), 6.75-fl.-oz. box .	100	0	26.0	0	0	15	0

Food and Measure	cal.	prot. (gms)	carbo. (gms)	fat (gms)	chol. (mgs)	sod. (mgs)	fiber (gms)
Grape juice, blend *(cont.)*							
(*Minute Maid*),							
11.5-fl.-oz. can ..	180	0	45.0	0	0	30	0
(*Minute Maid*),							
12-fl.-oz. bottle .	180	0	47.0	0	0	31	0
canned or bottled	154	1.4	37.9	.2	0	8	.3
frozen*:							
(*Cascadian Farm*							
Concord)	130	0	32.0	0	0	5	0
sweetened	128	.5	31.9	.2	0	5	.3
white grape:							
(*Ceres* Hanport) ...	130	0	30.0	0	0	10	0
(*Juicy Juice*)	150	0	38.0	0	0	25	0
(*Langers* Plus)	160	0	40.0	0	0	15	0
(*Santa Cruz Organic*)	160	<1.0	39.0	0	0	10	0
Grape juice concen-							
trate, Concord (*Tree*							
of Life), 9 tsp.	160	<1.0	40.0	0	0	15	0
Grape leaves, fresh:							
1 cup	13	.8	2.4	.3	0	1	1.5
1 leaf	3	.2	.5	<.1	0	<1	.3
Grape leaves, in jar:							
(*Fanci Food*), 2 leaves	5	0	0	0	0	100	0
(*Krinos*), 1 leaf	5	0	0	0	0	200	1.0
Grape leaves, stuffed,							
6 pcs., 4.9 oz.:							
(*Cedar's*)	180	4.0	22.0	8.0	0	870	8.0
(*Peloponnese*)	200	2.0	27.0	9.0	0	1000	3.0
Grapefruit, fresh:							
(*Chiquita*), ½ medium	60	1.0	16.0	0	0	0	6.0
(*Dole*), ½ medium ...	60	1.0	16.0	0	0	0	6.0
(*Sunkist*), ½ medium,							
5.4 oz.	60	1.0	16.0	0	0	0	6.0
all areas/varieties:							
½ large, 4.7 oz.	53	1.1	13.4	.2	0	0	1.8
sections, 1 cup ...	74	1.5	18.6	.2	0	0	2.5
all areas, pink/red:							
½ medium, 3¾" ...	37	.7	9.5	.1	0	0	n.a.
sections, 1 cup ...	69	1.3	17.7	.2	0	0	n.a.
all areas, white:							
½ medium, 3¾" ...	39	.8	9.9	.1	0	0	1.3
sections, 1 cup ...	76	1.3	17.7	.2	0	0	2.5
California/Arizona:							
pink/red, ½ medium,							
3¾"	46	.6	11.9	.1	0	1	1.4

Food and Measure	cal.	prot. (gms)	carbo. (gms)	fat (gms)	chol. (mgs)	sod. (mgs)	fiber (gms)
pink/red, sections w/juice, 1 cup ..	85	1.2	22.3	.2	0	2	2.6
white, ½ medium, 3¾"	43	1.0	10.7	.1	0	0	1.3
white, sections, w/juice, 1 cup ..	85	2.0	20.9	.2	0	0	2.6
Florida:							
pink/red, ½ medium, 3¾"	37	.7	9.2	.1	0	0	1.4
pink/red, sections w/juice, 1 cup ..	69	1.3	17.3	.2	0	0	2.5
white, ½ medium, 3¾"	38	.7	9.7	.1	0	0	.2
white, sections w/juice, 1 cup ..	74	1.5	18.8	.2	0	0	.4
Grapefruit, can or jar, ½ cup, except as noted:							
in juice:							
(*Fanci Food*), ⅔ cup	50	0	14.0	0	0	25	0
white (*Del Monte Sunfresh*)	45	1.0	9.0	0	0	15	2.0
with liquid	46	.9	11.4	.1	0	9	.5
in extra light syrup, red (*Del Monte Fruit Naturals*)	60	0	16.0	0	0	15	<1.0
red (*Del Monte Sunfresh*)	60	1.0	14.0	0	0	15	<1.0
in light syrup:							
red (*Del Monte Sunfresh*)	80	1.0	19.0	0	0	10	2.0
w/liquid	76	.7	19.6	.1	0	3	.5
Grapefruit, Chinese, see "Pummelo"							
Grapefruit drink, ruby red, 8 fl. oz.:							
(*Hood Carb Countdown*)	25	0	5.0	0	0	130	0
(*Langers*)	130	0	33.0	0	0	10	0
(*Langers* Diet)	40	0	10.0	0	0	10	0
(*Langers* Low Carb) ..	30	0	8.0	0	0	10	0
(*Minute Maid*)	130	0	34.0	0	0	20	0
(*Ocean Spray*)	120	0	30.0	0	0	35	0
(*Ocean Spray* Cocktail)	120	0	30.0	0	0	65	0

Food and Measure	cal.	prot. (gms)	carbo. (gms)	fat (gms)	chol. (mgs)	sod. (mgs)	fiber (gms)
Grapefruit drink *(cont.)*							
(Ocean Spray Light Ruby)	40	0	10.0	0	0	65	0
Grapefruit drink blend, ruby red, 8 fl. oz.:							
lemonade *(Ocean Spray Ruby•Lemonade)* ..	120	0	31.0	0	0	35	0
mango *(Ocean Spray Ruby•Mango)*	120	0	30.0	0	0	65	0
strawberry *(Ocean Spray Ruby• Strawberry)*	130	0	31.0	0	0	65	0
tangerine *(Ocean Spray Ruby•Tangerine)* ..	120	0	31.0	0	0	65	0
tropical *(Langers)* ...	135	0	34.0	0	0	10	0
Grapefruit juice, 8 fl. oz.:							
(Nantucket Nectars) ..	100	0	23.0	0	0	0	0
(Ocean Spray Premium)	100	0	24.0	0	0	35	0
(S&W)	100	0	25.0	0	0	10	0
pink:							
(Ocean Spray Premium)	110	0	28.0	0	0	35	0
(Organic Valley) ...	90	1.0	21.0	0	0	0	0
(Tree Ripe)	100	1.0	24.0	0	0	0	0
ruby red:							
(Ocean Spray Premium)	130	0	32.0	0	0	35	0
(R.W. Knudsen Rio Red)*	140	1.0	35.0	0	0	0	0
canned, unsweetened	94	1.3	22.1	.3	0	3	.3
fresh, pink or white ·..	96	1.2	22.7	.3	0	3	.3
frozen*:							
(Minute Maid w/Calcium)	100	0	25.0	0	0	0	0
unsweetened	101	1.4	24.0	.3	0	3	.3
Gravlax, see "Salmon, marinated"							
Gravy, see specific listings							
Gravy, country, in jars, ¼ cup:							
cream *(Campbell's)* ..	50	1.0	3.0	3.5	5	190	0
sausage *(Campbell's)* .	70	2.0	3.0	6.0	10	270	0

Food and Measure	cal.	prot. (gms)	carbo. (gms)	fat (gms)	chol. (mgs)	sod. (mgs)	fiber (gms)
Gravy mix (see also specific listings), ¼ cup*:							
country style:							
(*McCormick*)	50	0	4.0	3.5	0	260	0
(*McCormick* Lowfat)	40	0	5.0	2.0	0	280	0
sausage flavor							
(*McCormick*) . . .	45	0	4.0	3.0	0	300	0
golden (*Road's End Organics*)	25	<1.0	5.0	0	0	230	0
homestyle (*McCormick*)	25	0	4.0	1.0	0	280	0
savory (*Road's End Organics*)	25	<1.0	5.0	0	0	210	0
Gravy seasoning, see "Browning sauce"							
Great northern bean:							
dry (*Shiloh Farms*), ¼ cup	160	10.0	29.0	.5	0	5	18.0
boiled, ½ cup	104	7.3	18.6	.4	0	2	6.2
Great northern bean, canned, ½ cup:							
(*Allens*)	100	6.0	19.0	.5	0	310	7.0
(*Bush's*)	110	7.0	18.0	.5	0	400	7.0
(*Eden* Organic)	110	5.0	20.0	1.0	0	65	8.0
(*Westbrae Natural* Organic)	100	7.0	19.0	0	0	140	6.0
w/sausage (*Trappey's*)	100	6.0	18.0	1.0	0	460	7.0
seasoned (*Glory*)	90	6.0	15.0	.5	0	850	3.0
Green bean (see also "Snap bean"), fresh:							
raw:							
cut (*Glory*), 2 cups	25	2.0	5.0	0	0	0	3.0
½ cup	17	1.0	3.9	.1	0	3	1.9
boiled, drained, ½ cup	22	1.2	4.9	.2	0	2	2.0
Green bean, can or jar, ½ cup:							
all styles (*Del Monte*) .	20	1.0	4.0	0	0	390	2.0
whole:							
(*Allens*)	30	1.0	6.0	0	0	460	3.0
(*Freshlike* Selects) .	35	2.0	7.0	0	0	380	3.0
whole or cut (*S&W*) .	20	1.0	4.0	0	0	390	2.0
cut:							
(*Allens* No Salt) . . .	15	0	3.0	0	0	10	2.0
(*Allens/Sunshine*) .	30	0	6.0	0	0	320	3.0

Food and Measure	cal.	prot. (gms)	carbo. (gms)	fat (gms)	chol. (mgs)	sod. (mgs)	fiber (gms)
Green bean, can or jar, cut *(cont.)*							
(*Freshlike*)	35	2.0	7.0	0	0	380	3.0
(*Freshlike* No Salt) .	25	2.0	4.0	0	0	0	2.0
(*Freshlike* Selects) .	30	2.0	5.0	0	0	370	2.0
(*Green Giant* Low Sodium)	20	<1.0	4.0	0	0	200	1.0
(*Green Giant/Green Giant* Kitchen Sliced)	20	<1.0	4.0	0	0	400	1.0
(*Veg-All*)	20	<1.0	4.0	0	0	400	2.0
(*Westbrae Natural Organic*)	20	1.0	4.0	0	0	370	1.0
dilled (*S&W*)	20	0	5.0	0	0	125	1.0
w/liquid	18	1.0	4.2	.1	0	311	1.8
cut or French (*Del Monte* No Salt)	20	1.0	4.0	0	0	10	2.0
French style:							
(*Allens/Sunshine*) .	25	1.0	4.0	0	0	300	2.0
(*Freshlike*)	20	1.0	3.0	0	0	380	3.0
(*Freshlike* No Salt) .	20	1.0	4.0	0	0	0	2.0
(*Green Giant*)	20	<1.0	4.0	0	0	390	1.0
(*Veg-All*)	20	<1.0	4.0	0	0	400	1.0
(*Westbrae Natural Organic*)	20	1.0	4.0	0	0	370	1.0
seasoned (*Del Monte*)	20	1.0	4.0	0	0	360	2.0
Italian cut:							
(*Allens* Shellouts) . .	50	3.0	9.0	0	0	320	3.0
(*Allens/Sunshine*) .	35	1.0	7.0	0	0	320	3.0
(*Del Monte*)	30	1.0	6.0	0	0	390	3.0
seasoned (*Allens/ Sunshine*)	45	2.0	8.0	0	0	370	3.0
seasoned:							
(*Glory* Pole Beans) .	45	2.0	9.0	0	0	430	2.0
(*Glory* String Beans)	30	1.0	6.0	.5	0	410	2.0
Green bean, freeze-dried, 1 serving:							
(*Mountain House*) . . .	30	1.0	6.0	0	0	0	2.0
almondine (*AlpineAire*)	100	4.0	13.0	3.0	0	560	5.0
Green bean, frozen:							
whole:							
(*Birds Eye*), 1 cup .	35	1.0	5.0	0	0	0	2.0
(*Cascadian Farm* Petite), 1 cup . . .	25	1.0	5.0	0	0	90	2.0

Food and Measure	cal.	prot. (gms)	carbo. (gms)	fat (gms)	chol. (mgs)	sod. (mgs)	fiber (gms)
(*C&W* Haricots Verts/ Petite), ¾ cup ..	25	1.0	4.0	0	0	10	2.0
(*Green Giant Select*), 1 cup	20	1.0	4.0	0	0	10	2.0
cut:							
(*Birds Eye*), ⅔ cup	30	1.0	5.0	0	0	0	2.0
(*Cascadian Farm*), ¾ cup	30	2.0	6.0	0	0	0	2.0
(*Green Giant*), ½ cup cooked	20	1.0	4.0	0	0	10	2.0
(*McKenzie's* Pole Beans), ½ cup ..	25	1.0	4.0	0	0	10	2.0
(*Dr. Praeger's*), ⅔ cup	30	1.0	5.0	0	0	0	2.0
(*Tree of Life*), ⅔ cup	25	1.0	4.0	0	0	10	2.0
French (*C&W*), ⅔ cup	25	1.0	4.0	0	0	10	2.0
Italian cut:							
(*Birds Eye*), ¾ cup .	35	1.0	5.0	0	0	0	2.0
(*C&W*), ¾ cup	25	1.0	4.0	0	0	10	2.0
boiled, drained, ½ cup	19	1.0	4.4	.1	0	6	2.0
in garlic butter (*Green Giant*), ½ cup cooked	45	2.0	6.0	1.5	<5	450	2.0
Green bean, pickled, in jars, hot (*Tillen Farms*), ¼ cup	15	1.0	3.0	0	0	250	0
Green bean combinations, canned, ½ cup:							
casserole:							
(*Allens*)	40	2.0	6.0	1.0	0	270	1.0
(*Del Monte Savory Sides*)	70	2.0	11.0	2.5	5	540	2.0
(*Glory*)	45	2.0	9.0	.5	0	480	2.0
and potatoes:							
(*Allens/Sunshine*) .	50	2.0	10.0	0	0	160	2.0
(*Glory* String Beans)	50	2.0	10.0	.5	0	580	2.0
w/ham flavor (*Del Monte*)	30	1.0	6.0	0	0	330	<1.0
Green bean combinations, frozen:							
w/almonds:							
(*Cascadian Farm* Bag), ¾ cup	70	3.0	10.0	3.0	0	115	4.0
(*Cascadian Farm* Box), ⅔ cup	70	3.0	8.0	3.0	0	180	2.0

Food and Measure	cal.	prot. (gms)	carbo. (gms)	fat (gms)	chol. (mgs)	sod. (mgs)	fiber (gms)
Green bean combinations, frozen, w/almonds *(cont.)*							
(*C&W*), 1 cup	80	3.0	9.0	3.5	0	470	3.0
(*Green Giant*), ½ cup cooked	50	2.0	4.0	3.0	0	100	2.0
toasted (*Birds Eye Medley*), 1 cup ..	100	3.0	10.0	5.0	5	360	5.0
toasted, lightly (*Birds Eye*), ¾ cup	80	3.0	8.0	4.0	0	410	3.0
baby, mixed, w/carrots (*Birds Eye*), 1 cup .	35	1.0	6.0	0	0	20	2.0
casserole (*Green Giant*), ⅔ cup	110	2.0	7.0	8.0	0	470	2.0
and spaetzle, in sauce (*Birds Eye Bavarian*), 1 cup	150	5.0	16.0	7.0	30	390	3.0
stir-fry (*Birds Eye Crisp*), 1 cup cooked	100	4.0	19.0	0	0	30	2.0
Green peas, see "Peas, green"							
Greens, see specific listings							
Greens, mixed, salad, see "Salad blend"							
Greens, mixed, canned, ½ cup:							
(*Allens No Salt*)	30	1.0	8.0	.5	0	10	4.0
all varieties (*Bush's*) ..	25	2.0	3.0	0	0	300	2.0
seasoned:							
(*Allens/Sunshine*) .	45	4.0	6.0	.5	0	830	1.0
(*Glory*)	50	4.0	7.0	.5	0	470	3.0
Grenadine syrup:							
(*Angostura*), 1 tsp....	15	0	4.0	0	0	390	0
(*Giroux*), 2 tbsp.	100	0	26.0	0	0	30	0
(*Trader Vic's*), 2 tbsp.	90	0	23.0	0	0	15	0
Grilling sauce (see also "Barbecue sauce," "Marinade," and specific listings), 2 tbsp., except as noted:							
garlic, roasted, and herb (*McCormick Grill Mates*)	35	0	7.0	0	0	440	0

Food and Measure	cal.	prot. (gms)	carbo. (gms)	fat (gms)	chol. (mgs)	sod. (mgs)	fiber (gms)
hickory barbecue (*McCormick Grill Mates*)	80	0	17.0	.5	0	500	0
honey mustard (*McCormick Grill Mates*)	70	0	15.0	.5	0	600	0
Hunan (*House of Tsang* Hibachi Smokehut), 1 tbsp.	40	0	8.0	.5	0	410	0
Italian grill (*World Harbors*)	25	0	4.0	1.0	0	300	0
lemon butter dill:							
(*Golden Dipt*)	120	0	4.0	10.0	0	210	0
(*Golden Dipt* Fat Free)	35	0	7.0	0	0	210	0
mesquite (*McCormick Grill Mates*)	60	0	12.0	.5	0	750	0
peanut, Thai (*House of Tsang* Hibachi), 1 tbsp.	50	1.0	4.0	3.0	0	280	0
pepper, cracked (*San-J*)	25	1.0	5.0	0	0	560	<1.0
sesame, sweet ginger (*House of Tsang* Hibachi), 1 tbsp. ..	40	0	8.0	1.0	0	410	0
steak:							
kobe (*House of Tsang* Hibachi), 1 tbsp.	50	0	2.0	4.0	0	560	0
Montreal (*McCormick Grill Mates*)	35	0	7.0	0	0	730	0
sweet and hot chili (*San-J*)	30	<1.0	6.0	.5	0	370	<1.0
teriyaki:							
(*House of Tsang* Hibachi), 1 tbsp.	40	0	10.0	0	0	520	0
(*McCormick Grill Mates*)	60	0	12.0	1.0	0	610	0
Grilling seasoning (*Watkins*), ¼ tsp. ...	0	0	0	0	0	210	0
Grits, see "Corn grits"							
Grog mixer, see "Navy grog drink mixer"							
Ground cherry, ½ cup	37	1.3	7.8	.5	0	n.a.	2.0
Grouper, meat only:							
raw, 4 oz.	104	22.0	0	1.2	42	60	0

Food and Measure	cal.	prot. (gms)	carbo. (gms)	fat (gms)	chol. (mgs)	sod. (mgs)	fiber (gms)
Grouper *(cont.)*							
baked, broiled, or							
microwaved, 4 oz. .	134	28.2	0	1.5	53	60	0
Guacamole, frozen or							
refrigerated, 2 tbsp.,							
except as noted:							
(*Calavo* Fiesta)	60	<1.0	2.0	5.0	0	140	2.0
(*Calvao* Homestyle) . .	50	<1.0	3.0	4.0	0	90	2.0
(*Calavo* Original)	50	<1.0	3.0	4.5	0	140	0
(*Kraft*)	50	1.0	3.0	4.5	0	240	0
(*Tofutti Sour Supreme*)	50	1.0	1.0	5.0	0	120	0
Mexican or Western							
(*Calavo*)	50	<1.0	3.0	4.5	0	170	0
mild (*Calavo*)	50	<1.0	4.0	4.0	0	120	2.0
w/salsa (*San Pedro's*							
Holy Guacamole!),							
1 oz.	30	1.0	3.0	2.0	0	110	0
spicy:							
(*Calavo*)	50	<1.0	3.0	4.0	0	160	2.0
(*Goya*)	57	1.0	3.0	5.0	0	147	2.0
Guacamole seasoning							
(*Lawry's*), ½ tsp. . . .	0	0	1.0	0	0	130	0
Guava (see also							
"Feijoas"):							
(*Frieda's*), 3-oz. pc. . .	45	1.0	10.0	.5	0	0	5.0
1 medium, 4 oz.	45	.7	10.7	.5	0	2	4.9
½ cup	42	.7	9.8	.5	0	2	4.5
strawberry, ½ cup . . .	85	.7	21.2	.7	0	45	7.8
Guava, in jars, whole							
in syrup, (*Herdez*),							
4 pcs., 4.5 oz.	190	0	32.0	0	0	10	5.0
Guava drink blend,							
8 fl. oz.:							
(*Nantucket Nectars*) . .	130	0	33.0	0	0	5	0
passion fruit (*V8 Splash*)	110	0	27.0	0	0	40	0
strawberry (*R.W.*							
Knudsen)	110	<1.0	27.0	0	0	25	0
Guava juice (*Ceres*),							
8 fl. oz.	120	0	29.0	0	0	5	0
Guava nectar (*Goya*),							
12 fl. oz.	240	1.0	59.0	0	0	25	2.0
Guava sauce, ½ cup .	43	.4	11.3	.2	0	4	4.3
Guavadilla, see							
"Passionfruit"							

Food and Measure	cal.	prot. (gms)	carbo. (gms)	fat (gms)	chol. (mgs)	sod. (mgs)	fiber (gms)
Guinea hen, raw:							
meat w/skin, 4 oz. . . .	179	26.5	0	7.3	84	86	0
meat only, 4 oz.	125	23.4	0	2.8	71	78	0
Gyros mix, dry							
(*Casbah*), .65 oz. . .	64	2.0	12.0	0	0	470	0

H

Food and Measure	cal.	prot. (gms)	carbo. (gms)	fat (gms)	chol. (mgs)	sod. (mgs)	fiber (gms)
Habas, see "Broad bean, mature"							
Haddock, meat only:							
raw, 4 oz.	99	21.5	0	.8	65	78	0
baked, broiled, or microwaved, 4 oz. . .	127	27.5	0	1.1	84	99	0
smoked, 4 oz.	132	28.6	0	1.1	87	865	0
Haddock entree, frozen:							
fillet:							
battered (*Van de Kamp's*), 2 pcs., 3.7 oz.	220	10.0	20.0	11.0	25	590	0
breaded (*Mrs. Paul's*), 4 oz. pc.	220	14.0	17.0	10.0	40	320	0
w/shrimp, crab, and vegetables (*Oven Poppers*), 5-oz. pc.	210	19.0	12.0	9.0	85	310	1.0
Hake, see "Whiting"							
Halibut, meat only:							
Atlantic/Pacific, 4 oz.:							
raw	124	23.6	0	2.6	37	61	0
baked, broiled, or microwaved	159	30.3	0	3.3	46	78	0
Greenland, 4 oz.							
raw	211	16.3	0	15.7	52	91	0
baked, broiled, or microwaved	271	20.9	0	20.1	67	117	0
Halvah, chocolate, vanilla, or marble (*Joyva*), 2 oz.	390	6.0	18.0	25.0	0	120	2.0
Ham, fresh, meat only, 4 oz., except as noted:							
whole leg, roasted:							
lean w/fat	310	30.4	0	20.0	107	68	0

Food and Measure	cal.	prot. (gms)	carbo. (gms)	fat (gms)	chol. (mgs)	sod. (mgs)	fiber (gms)
lean w/fat, diced, 1 cup	369	36.2	0	23.8	127	81	0
lean only	239	33.4	0	10.7	107	73	0
lean only, diced, 1 cup	285	39.7	0	12.7	127	86	0
rump half, roasted:							
lean w/fat	286	32.7	0	16.2	109	70	0
lean only	235	35.1	0	9.2	109	74	0
shank half, roasted:							
lean w/fat	328	28.7	0	22.7	104	67	0
lean only	244	32.0	0	11.9	104	73	0
Ham, cured:							
whole leg, lean w/fat:							
unheated, 4 oz. ...	279	21.0	.1	21.0	64	1456	0
unheated, chopped or diced, 1 cup ..	344	25.9	.1	25.9	78	1798	0
roasted, 4 oz.	276	24.5	0	19.0	70	1346	0
roasted, chopped or diced, 1 cup	341	30.2	0	23.5	86	1661	0
whole leg, lean only:							
unheated, 4 oz. ...	167	25.3	.1	6.5	59	1719	0
unheated, chopped or diced, 1 cup ..	206	31.3	0	8.0	73	2122	0
roasted, 4 oz.	178	28.4	0	6.2	62	1505	0
roasted, chopped or diced, 1 cup	219	35.1	0	7.7	77	1858	0
boneless (11% fat):							
unheated, 4 oz. ...	206	19.9	3.5	12.0	65	1493	0
roasted, 4 oz.	202	25.7	0	10.2	67	1701	0
roasted, chopped or diced, 1 cup	249	31.7	0	12.6	83	2100	0
boneless, extra lean (5% fat):							
unheated, 4 oz. ...	149	21.9	1.1	5.6	53	1620	0
roasted, 4 oz.	164	23.7	1.7	6.3	60	1364	0
roasted, chopped or diced, 1 cup	203	29.3	2.1	7.7	74	1684	0
Ham, deviled, see "Ham spread"							
Ham, refrigerated or canned, 3 oz., except as noted:							
(*Black Label* Refrigerator Can)	100	14.0	1.0	4.5	40	1020	0

Food and Measure	cal.	prot. (gms)	carbo. (gms)	fat (gms)	chol. (mgs)	sod. (mgs)	fiber (gms)
Ham, refrigerated or canned *(cont.)*							
(Bilinski Champagne Ham)	150	11.0	1.0	12.0	45	390	0
(Cure 81)	100	15.0	0	4.5	45	890	0
(Curemaster)	80	14.0	0	2.5	40	950	0
(Spiral Cure 81)	130	16.0	1.0	7.0	45	1060	0
chunk *(Hormel)*, 2 oz.	50	9.0	0	6.0	30	620	0
extra lean (4% fat):							
unheated, 4 oz. ...	136	21.0	0	5.2	43	1423	0
unheated, 1 cup ...	202	25.2	0	10.4	53	1786	0
roasted, 4 oz.	154	24.0	.6	5.5	34	1287	0
roasted , 1 cup	234	29.3	.7	11.8	57	1495	0
smoked *(Organic Valley)*	110	16.0	1.0	4.0	55	1460	0
steak, cooked:							
(Hatfield Traditional)	100	14.0	3.0	4.0	40	970	0
honey *(Hatfield)* ...	100	13.0	5.0	3.0	25	870	0
maple *(Hatfield)* ...	90	12.0	6.0	2.5	20	740	0
"Ham," vegetarian,							
slices *(Yves)*, 2.2 oz.	80	14.0	6.0	0	0	480	1.0
Ham and cheese loaf:							
(Hansel 'n Gretel), 2 oz.	130	7.0	3.0	14.0	30	840	0
(Oscar Mayer), 1 oz. .	60	4.0	1.0	4.5	20	350	0
Ham and cheese pocket/sandwich, frozen, 4.5-oz. pc., except as noted:							
(Hot Pockets)	310	14.0	33.0	13.0	30	770	3.0
(Lean Pockets Ultra) .	200	25.0	19.0	6.0	20	570	7.0
cheddar:							
(Croissant Pockets)	340	12.0	36.0	16.0	25	760	3.0
(Lean Pockets)	280	14.0	40.0	7.0	25	700	3.0
(Smart Ones Smartwich)	270	14.0	38.0	6.0	30	600	1.0
sub *(Michelina's Hot Subs)*, 2.1-oz. pc. .	280	16.0	32.0	10.0	35	1020	1.0
Ham entree, frozen, sausage Jambalaya:							
(Glory Savory Singles), 11-oz. pkg.	400	17.0	42.0	18.0	50	1320	2.0
(Glory Savory Singles Family Size), 1 cup	370	16.0	38.0	16.0	45	1210	2.0
Ham entree mix, and au gratin potatoes *(Betty Crocker Complete Meals)*, 1/5 pkg.	300	9.0	37.0	13.0	25	1110	2.0

Food and Measure	cal.	prot. (gms)	carbo. (gms)	fat (gms)	chol. (mgs)	sod. (mgs)	fiber (gms)
Ham glaze:							
(*Boar's Head* Sugar & Spice), 2 tbsp.	120	0	30.0	0	0	95	0
(*Crosse & Blackwell*), 1 tbsp.	30	0	8.0	0	0	25	0
(*Reese's*), 1 tbsp.	20	0	5.0	0	0	55	0
Ham lunch meat (see also "Prosciutto"), 2 oz., except as noted:							
(*Boar's Head* Deluxe) .	60	9.0	2.0	1.0	25	590	0
(*Boar's Head* Deluxe 42% Lower Sodium)	60	10.0	2.0	1.0	25	460	0
(*Deli Delight*)	60	9.0	2.0	1.5	20	330	0
(*Dietz & Watson* Gourmet Lite)	50	10.0	1.0	1.0	25	420	0
(*Dietz & Watson* Tiffany)	60	10.0	1.0	1.5	25	480	0
(*Hansel 'n Gretel* Deluxe)	65	9.0	1.0	2.0	25	560	0
(*Hatfield Deli Choice* Ham Off the Bone) .	60	9.0	2.0	2.0	25	490	0
(*Healthy Deli* Zero Carb Deluxe)	60	9.0	0	1.5	20	480	0
(*Healthy Deli* Zero Carb Less Sodium Fat Free)	45	10.0	0	0	5	480	0
(*Williams* Old Fashion)	70	10.0	1.0	3.0	30	590	0
baked:							
(*Healthy Choice* Hearty Slices), 1 oz.	30	5.0	1.0	1.0	15	240	0
(*Healthy Choice* Tub), 2 slices, 2 oz. . . .	60	10.0	1.0	1.5	25	460	0
(*Healthy Choice* Deli Thin), 6 slices, 2 oz.	60	9.0	1.0	1.5	25	470	0
(*Sara Lee* Homestyle)	60	10.0	2.0	2.0	25	600	0
(*Williams* Home) . .	70	9.0	2.0	1.5	25	650	0
brown sugar:							
(*Oscar Mayer* Deli Style Shaved), 1.8 oz.	60	9.0	3.0	1.5	25	740	0
(*Oscar Mayer* Deli Style Thin Sliced)	70	10.0	4.0	1.5	25	830	0
(*Sara Lee*)	70	10.0	5.0	1.5	20	600	0

Food and Measure	cal.	prot. (gms)	carbo. (gms)	fat (gms)	chol. (mgs)	sod. (mgs)	fiber (gms)
Ham lunch meat, brown sugar *(cont.)*							
(*Sara Lee* Sliced),							
2 slices, 1.6 oz. . .	60	8.0	4.0	1.5	10	480	0
(*Tyson* Bag),							
.9-oz. slice	35	5.0	1.0	1.0	15	280	0
Black Forest:							
(*Boar's Head*)	60	10.0	2.0	1.0	30	580	0
(*Dietz & Watson*) . .	60	10.0	2.0	1.5	25	420	0
(*Healthy Deli*)	60	10.0	1.0	1.5	20	480	0
(*Hormel*)	60	10.0	.0	2.0	25	700	0
(*Sara Lee*)	60	10.0	1.0	1.0	20	520	0
(*Tyson*), 1-oz. slice	30	5.0	0	1.0	10	300	0
boiled (*Oscar Mayer*							
96% Fat Free), 2.2 oz.	60	10.0	1.0	2.0	30	820	0
capicola/cappy:							
(*Black Bear*							
Capocollo), 1 oz.	80	8.0	<1.0	5.0	17	540	0
(*Boar's Head* Cappy)	60	10.0	3.0	1.5	15	530	0
(*Hansel 'n Gretel*) .	60	9.0	2.0	1.5	20	280	0
(*Healthy Deli*)	60	9.0	2.0	1.5	20	480	0
Italian (*Boar's Head*							
Capocollo), 1 oz.	80	7.0	0	5.0	15	590	0
chopped:							
(*Hormel Black Label*)	140	7.0	3.0	11.0	30	690	0
(*Oscar Mayer*), 1 oz.	50	4.0	1.0	3.0	15	340	0
cinnamon apple							
(*Healthy Deli*)	70	9.0	4.0	1.5	20	480	0
cooked:							
(*Alpine Lace* 97%							
Fat Free)	60	9.0	2.0	1.5	25	600	0
(*Hatfield Deli Choice*							
Imported)	70	10.0	1.0	1.5	30	410	0
(*Hatfield Deli Choice*							
Premium)	60	10.0	2.0	2.0	25	730	0
(*Healthy Choice*) . .	60	9.0	1.0	1.5	25	460	0
(*Healthy Choice*							
Hearty Slices),							
1 oz.	30	5.0	1.0	1.0	15	240	0
(*Healthy Choice Deli*							
Thin), 4 slices,							
1.8 oz.	60	9.0	2.0	1.5	25	450	0
(*Hormel*)	60	9.0	0	3.0	30	690	0
(*Oscar Mayer* 96%							
Fat Free), 2.2 oz.	60	10.0	1.0	2.0	30	760	0

Food and Measure	cal.	prot. (gms)	carbo. (gms)	fat (gms)	chol. (mgs)	sod. (mgs)	fiber (gms)
(*Sara Lee* Old Fashioned)	50	10.0	1.0	1.0	25	780	0
(*Tyson* Bag), 2 slices, 1.6 oz.	45	9.0	0	1.5	20	740	0
(*Tyson* Box), 5 slices, 1.8 oz.	60	10.0	0	1.5	25	760	0
fresh, seasoned (*Boar's Head*)	80	14.0	0	3.0	35	310	0
glazed:							
(*Hansel 'n Gretel*) .	60	10.0	2.0	1.5	20	620	0
(*Healthy Deli* Deluxe)	60	10.0	2.0	1.5	20	480	0
honey/honey cured:							
(*Alpine Lace* 97% Fat Free)	60	9.0	2.0	1.5	25	600	0
(*Healthy Choice*) . .	60	9.0	2.0	1.5	25	480	0
(*Healthy Choice* Hearty Slices), 1 oz.	35	5.0	1.0	1.0	15	240	0
(*Healthy Choice* Tub), 5 slices, 1.9 oz. .	60	9.0	2.0	1.5	25	450	0
(*Healthy Choice* Deli Thin), 4 slices, 1.8 oz.	60	9.0	2.0	1.5	25	450	0
(*Healthy Deli*)	60	9.0	2.0	1.5	20	480	0
(*Hormel*)	70	3.0	3.0	3.0	30	600	0
(*Louis Rich Carving Board* 97% Fat Free), 2.1 oz. . . .	70	11.0	2.0	1.5	30	760	0
(*Oscar Mayer*), 2.2 oz.	70	11.0	2.0	2.0	30	770	0
(*Sara Lee*)	60	10.0	2.0	1.5	25	520	0
(*Sara Lee* Sliced), 2 slices, 1.6 oz. .	45	8.0	1.0	1.0	20	420	0
(*Sara Lee* Bavarian)	70	9.0	2.0	3.5	40	560	0
(*Tyson* Bag), 2 slices, 1.6 oz.	50	9.0	1.0	1.5	25	740	0
(*Tyson* Box), 5 slices, 1.8 oz.	50	9.0	1.0	1.5	30	760	0
chopped (*Oscar Mayer* 96% Fat Free), 1 oz.	60	4.0	4.0	3.5	15	320	0
cured (*Tyson*), .9-oz. slice	35	5.0	2.0	1.0	15	250	0

Ham lunch meat (cont.)

Food and Measure	cal.	prot. (gms)	carbo. (gms)	fat (gms)	chol. (mgs)	sod. (mgs)	fiber (gms)
honey maple:							
(*Healthy Choice Hearty Slices*), 1 oz.	30	5.0	1.0	1.0	15	170	0
(*Healthy Choice Deli Thin*), 4 slices, 1.8 oz.	60	9.0	1.0	1.5	25	450	0
honey mustard							
(*Healthy Choice Deli Thin*), 4 slices, 1.8 oz.	60	9.0	3.0	1.5	25	450	0
jalapeño (*Healthy Deli*)	60	8.0	3.0	1.5	15	480	0
loaf (*Deli Delight*) ...	150	9.0	3.0	11.0	30	400	0
maple:							
(*Healthy Choice*) ..	60	10.0	3.0	1.5	25	480	0
(*Healthy Deli Vermont*)	60	9.0	3.0	1.5	20	460	0
(*Williams* Buffet) ..	70	10.0	1.0	3.0	30	590	0
glazed (*Boar's Head Honey Coat*)	60	10.0	3.0	1.0	20	570	0
honey (*Sara Lee*) ..	70	9.0	4.0	1.5	20	520	0
peppered:							
(*Boar's Head Gourmet*)	60	10.0	2.0	1.0	20	610	0
(*Dietz & Watson*) ..	50	9.0	0	1.5	25	590	0
(*Hatfield Deli Choice*)	70	10.0	2.0	2.5	30	650	0
(*Healthy Deli*)	60	9.0	2.0	1.5	20	470	0
(*Sara Lee*)	60	10.0	2.0	1.0	20	530	0
spiced, see "Lunch meat"							
pesto Parmesan oven roasted (*Boar's Head*)	90	14.0	0	4.0	30	320	0
rosemary sun-dried tomato (*Boar's Head*)	70	10.0	2.0	2.5	10	590	0
smoked:							
(*Boar's Head Sweet Slice*)	100	15.0	1.0	3.5	30	780	0
(*Healthy Choice*) ..	60	9.0	2.0	1.5	30	430	0
(*Sara Lee Smokehouse*) ...	60	10.0	1.0	1.5	20	620	0
(*Oscar Mayer* Deli Style Thin Sliced)	50	10.0	0	1.5	25	720	

Food and Measure	cal.	prot. (gms)	carbo. (gms)	fat (gms)	chol. (mgs)	sod. (mgs)	fiber (gms)
(*Oscar Mayer* 96% Fat Free Wallet Pack), 2.2 oz. . . .	60	11.0	0	1.5	30	790	0
double (*Healthy Deli*)	60	10.0	1.0	1.5	20	470	0
double (*Hormel*) . .	70	10.0	0	3.0	30	590	0
maple glaze (*Dietz & Watson*)	60	9.0	2.0	1.5	30	450	0
tavern:							
(*Boar's Head*)	60	10.0	2.0	1.0	30	580	0
(*Dietz & Watson* Gourmet Lite) . . .	60	10.0	1.0	1.5	30	460	0
(*Hatfield Deli Choice*), 3 oz.	110	16.0	3.0	3.0	45	900	0
(*Healthy Deli*)	60	10.0	1.0	1.5	20	470	0
honey (*Sara Lee*) . .	60	9.0	2.0	1.0	20	500	0
Virginia:							
(*Boar's Head*)	60	9.0	2.0	1.0	25	590	0
(*Deli Delight*)	70	9.0	3.0	1.5	20	330	0
(*Dietz & Watson* Gourmet Lite) . . .	60	10.0	2.0	1.5	25	420	0
(*Hansel 'n Gretel*) .	65	10.0	2.0	2.0	25	600	0
(*Hatfield Deli Choice*)	70	9.0	4.0	1.5	25	500	0
(*Healthy Choice*) . .	60	9.0	2.0	1.5	25	480	0
(*Healthy Choice* Hearty Slices), 1 oz.	30	5.0	1.0	1.0	15	240	0
(*Healthy Deli* Zero Carb)	50	9.0	0	1.5	20	480	0
(*Sara Lee* Sliced), 2 slices, 1.6 oz. .	50	8.0	2.0	1.5	20	480	0
(*Tyson*), .9-oz. slice	30	5.0	0	1.0	10	300	0
oven baked (*Healthy Deli*)	70	10.0	3.0	1.5	20	480	0
smoked (*Healthy Choice*), 2 slices, 2 oz.	60	9.0	2.0	1.5	25	470	0
smoked (*Healthy Choice Deli Thin*), 4 slices, 1.8 oz. .	60	9.0	2.0	1.5	25	450	0
smoked (*Healthy Deli*)	60	9.0	2.0	1.5	20	480	0
Ham patties, 2-oz. patty:							
(*Hormel*)	180	7.0	1.0	16.0	40	620	0
and cheese (*Hormel*) .	180	7.0	0	17.0	40	520	0

Food and Measure	cal.	prot. (gms)	carbo. (gms)	fat (gms)	chol. (mgs)	sod. (mgs)	fiber (gms)
Ham spread, deviled:							
(*Hormel Cure 81*),							
4 tbsp.	150	9.0	2.0	12.0	40	430	0
(*Underwood*), ¼ cup .	150	9.0	0	12.0	35	460	0
Hamburger, see "Beef pocket/sandwich"							
"Hamburger," vege-tarian, see "Burger, vegetarian"							
Hamburger entree mix, 1 cup*, except as noted:							
cheddar melt (*Hamburger Helper*)	290	19.0	28.0	12.0	50	820	1.0
cheese, three (*Hamburger Helper*)	350	23.0	30.0	16.0	60	800	1.0
cheeseburger:							
bacon (*Hamburger Helper*)	380	24.0	33.0	17.0	60	960	1.0
macaroni (*Annie's Organic Skillet Meal*)	350	28.0	27.0	13.0	50	670	1.0
macaroni (*Ham-burger Helper*) . .	350	21.0	34.0	15.0	50	890	1.0
chili macaroni (*Hamburger Helper*)	290	20.0	28.0	11.0	55	750	1.0
enchilada, cheesy (*Hamburger Helper*)	360	21.0	38.0	15.0	60	740	<1.0
fettuccine Alfredo (*Hamburger Helper*)	300	20.0	24.0	14.0	55	870	1.0
hash browns, cheesy (*Hamburger Helper*)	400	21.0	38.0	20.0	55	540	2.0
Italian, zesty (*Ham-burger Helper*)	300	20.0	30.0	11.0	55	770	1.0
lasagna:							
(*Betty Crocker Complete Meals Pasta Bake*), 1/5 pkg.	240	9.0	35.0	8.0	10	1060	2.0
(*Hamburger Helper Oven Favorites*), 1/6 pkg.*	290	18.0	29.0	11.0	50	1000	1.0

Food and Measure	cal.	prot. (gms)	carbo. (gms)	fat (gms)	chol. (mgs)	sod. (mgs)	fiber (gms)
cheesy (*Annie's Organic Skillet Meal*)	280	23.0	26.0	9.0	35	670	1.0
four cheese (*Hamburger Helper*) ..	320	22.0	27.0	15.0	60	710	1.0
meat loaf, mashed potato (*Hamburger Helper Oven Favorites*), 1/6 pkg.*	360	19.0	30.0	19.0	85	880	2.0
Parmesan, Italian (*Hamburger Helper*)	300	21.0	29.0	12.0	55	810	1.0
pasta (*Hamburger Helper*)	280	20.0	25.0	11.0	55	810	1.0
penne, tomato basil (*Hamburger Helper*)	300	21.0	30.0	11.0	55	780	1.0
Philly cheesesteak (*Hamburger Helper*)	330	21.0	24.0	17.0	55	890	1.0
pizza, double cheese (*Hamburger Helper*)	320	21.0	33.0	12.0	55	950	1.0
potato:							
baked, cheesy (*Hamburger Helper*) ..	310	20.0	27.0	14.0	60	960	1.0
garlic (*Hamburger Helper*)	290	20.0	27.0	12.0	55	870	1.0
quesadilla, double cheese (*Hamburger Helper*)	370	22.0	37.0	15.0	60	960	<1.0
ravioli and cheese (*Hamburger Helper*)	320	21.0	32.0	12.0	55	940	1.0
rice Oriental (*Hamburger Helper*)	300	19.0	31.0	11.0	55	960	0
Romanoff (*Hamburger Helper*)	300	22.0	26.0	12.0	55	910	1.0
Salisbury (*Hamburger Helper*)	280	20.0	24.0	12.0	55	790	1.0
shells, cheesy (*Hamburger Helper*)	340	23.0	29.0	16.0	60	810	1.0
spaghetti (*Hamburger Helper*)	280	20.0	26.0	11.0	55	870	1.0
Stroganoff:							
(*Annie's* Organic Skillet Meal)	320	25.0	24.0	13.0	45	620	1.0
(*Hamburger Helper*)	320	23.0	26.0	14.0	60	900	1.0

Food and Measure	cal.	prot. (gms)	carbo. (gms)	fat (gms)	chol. (mgs)	sod. (mgs)	fiber (gms)
Hamburger entree mix, Stroganoff *(cont.)*							
creamy, w/pasta (*Campbell's Supper Bakes*), 1/6 pkg. mix	190	6.0	31.0	4.0	10	650	1.0
potatoes (*Hamburger Helper*)	290	20.0	23.0	14.0	60	830	1.0
taco:							
(*Hamburger Helper*)	280	18..0	28.0	11.0	50	890	1.0
crunchy (*Hamburger Helper*)	330	19.0	32.0	14.0	55	960	1.0
soft, bake (*Hamburger Helper Oven Favorites*), 1/6 pkg.*	420	25.0	32.0	21.0	75	980	0
Hard sauce (*Crosse & Blackwell*), 2 tbsp. ..	180	0	24.0	9.0	25	20	0
Hardee's, 1 serving:							
breakfast:							
big country platter, no syrup/butter:							
bacon	980	28.0	90.0	56.0	435	2080	3.0
chicken	1140	44.0	104.0	61.0	480	2580	4.0
ham, breakfast ..	970	34.0	90.0	52.0	455	2450	3.0
ham, country ...	970	33.0	90.0	53.0	460	2600	3.0
sausage	1060	30.0	91.0	64.0	455	2140	4.0
steak, country ..	1150	36.0	98.0	68.0	455	2260	4.0
biscuit:							
bacon	340	8.0	35.0	28.0	10	1110	0
bacon/egg/cheese	560	16.0	37.0	38.0	225	1360	0
chicken fillet	600	24.0	50.0	34.0	55	1680	1.0
ham, country ...	440	14.0	36.0	26.0	35	1710	0
ham/egg/cheese .	560	23.0	37.0	35.0	245	1800	0
omelet, loaded ..	640	21.0	37.0	44.0	245	1510	0
sausage	530	11.0	36.0	38.0	30	1240	0
sausage, smoked	620	15.0	37.0	46.0	40	1680	0
sausage/egg	610	17.0	36.0	44.0	235	1290	0
steak, country ..	620	16.0	44.0	41.0	35	1360	0
biscuit, *Made From Scratch*	370	5.0	35.0	23.0	0	890	0
Biscuit 'n Gravy ...	530	8.0	47.0	34.0	10	1550	0
Biscuit 'n Gravy bowl, loaded	770	20.0	49.0	54.0	245	1950	0

Food and Measure	cal.	prot. (gms)	carbo. (gms)	fat (gms)	chol. (mgs)	sod. (mgs)	fiber (gms)
breakfast bowl, low							
carb	620	36.0	6.0	50.0	325	1380	2.0
burrito, loaded	781	40.2	38.4	51.1	495	1625	n.a.
croissant, sunrise:							
bacon	450	19.0	28.0	29.0	240	900	0
ham	430	23.0	28.0	26.0	250	1050	0
sausage	550	22.0	29.0	38.0	265	1030	0
Frisco sandwich ...	410	27.0	39.0	17.0	245	870	2.0
pancakes, 3 pcs. ...	300	8.0	55.0	5.0	25	830	2.0
tortilla scrambler ..	230	9.0	18.0	13.0	30	520	0
breakfast sides:							
biscuit gravy	160	3.0	12.0	11.0	10	660	0
butter blend pkt. ..	25	0	0	3.0	0	45	0
Cinnamon 'n Raisin							
biscuit	280	3.0	40.0	12.0	0	650	0
Cinnamon 'n Raisin							
biscuit, apple ...	250	2.0	42.0	8.0	0	350	0
croissant	210	4.0	26.0	10.0	5	200	0
grits	110	2.0	16.0	5.0	0	480	0
Hash Rounds:							
large	460	5.0	45.0	29.0	0	650	2.0
medium	350	4.0	34.0	22.0	0	490	1.0
small	260	3.0	25.0	16.0	0	360	1.0
pancake syrup	90	0	21.0	0	0	0	0
burgers:							
⅓ lb. cheeseburger	680	29.0	52.0	39.0	90	1450	2.0
⅓ lb. *Thickburger* .	850	30.0	54.0	57.0	105	1470	3.0
bacon cheese ...	910	33.0	50.0	63.0	115	1490	3.0
chili cheese	870	41.0	55.0	54.0	135	1840	4.0
low carb	420	30.0	5.0	32.0	115	1010	2.0
mushroom Swiss	720	35.0	48.0	42.0	100	1570	2.0
Western bacon ..	876	33.9	69.6	50.3	105	1900	3.0
½ lb. six dollar							
burger	1060	40.0	60.0	72.0	150	1860	3.0
½ lb. grilled sour-							
dough *Thickburger*	1040	45.0	49.0	73.0	155	1420	3.0
⅔ lb. *Thickburger*:							
double	1230	52.0	53.0	90.0	195	2090	3.0
double bacon							
cheese	1300	55.0	51.0	96.0	205	2110	3.0
monster	1418	63.6	48.7	107.2	230	2651	n.a.
slammer	240	13.0	19.0	12.0	35	300	0
slammer w/cheese .	280	15.0	20.0	16.0	45	500	0

Food and Measure	cal.	prot. (gms)	carbo. (gms)	fat (gms)	chol. (mgs)	sod. (mgs)	fiber (gms)
Hardee's *(cont.)*							
sandwiches:							
beef, roast	330	19.0	29.0	16.0	40	860	2.0
Big Roast Beef	470	29.0	38.0	23.0	60	1290	2.0
chicken, big fillet ..	770	39.0	73.0	36.0	95	2000	4.0
chicken, charbroiled	590	36.0	53.0	26.0	80	1180	4.0
barbecued	310	26.0	45.0	3.5	60	730	2.0
low carb club ...	420	41.0	11.0	24.0	95	1230	2.0
chicken, spicy	470	14.0	46.0	26.0	40	1220	2.0
hot dog	420	16.0	22.0	30.0	55	1200	1.0
Hot Ham 'n Cheese	287	20.0	30.0	13.0	37	1110	2.0
Hot Ham 'n Cheese,							
big	435	36.0	40.0	20.0	74	2009	2.0
chicken:							
fried, breast	370	29.0	29.0	15.0	75	1190	0
fried, leg	170	13.0	15.0	7.0	45	570	0
fried, thigh	330	19.0	30.0	15.0	60	1000	0
fried, wing	200	10.0	23.0	8.0	30	740	0
strips, 3 pcs.	380	22.0	27.0	21.0	55	1360	1.0
strips, 5 pcs.	630	37.0	45.0	34.0	90	2260	2.0
sides:							
chili cheese fries ..	700	22.0	67.0	39.0	50	780	7.0
coleslaw, small	170	1.0	20.0	10.0	10	140	2.0
Crispy Curls:							
large	480	6.0	60.0	23.0	0	1190	5.0
medium	410	5.0	52.0	20.0	0	1020	4.0
small	340	4.0	43.0	17.0	0	840	4.0
fries, large	610	10.0	78.0	28.0	0	370	6.0
fries, medium	520	8.0	67.0	24.0	0	320	5.0
fries, small	390	6.0	51.0	19.0	0	240	4.0
gravy, chicken	20	0	3.0	1.0	0	220	0
potatoes, mashed,							
small	90	1.0	17.0	2.0	0	410	0
sauce/condiments:							
dipping, 1 oz.:							
barbecue	45	1.0	10.0	0	0	250	0
honey mustard ..	110	0	6.0	9.0	10	220	0
ranch	160	0	2.0	16.0	15	240	0
sweet and sour .	45	0	11.0	0	0	85	0
horseradish pkt. ...	25	0	1.0	2.0	5	35	0
hot sauce pkt.	0	0	0	0	0	210	0
ketchup pkt.	10	0	2.0	0	0	105	0
mayo pkt.	90	0	1.0	9.0	5	70	0

Food and Measure	cal.	prot. (gms)	carbo. (gms)	fat (gms)	chol. (mgs)	sod. (mgs)	fiber (gms)
shakes, 16 fl. oz.:							
chocolate:							
hand-dipped	510	11.0	61.0	27.0	105	230	0
soft-serve	710	27.0	137.0	7.0	20	550	0
strawberry:							
hand-dipped	480	11.0	58.0	27.0	105	230	0
soft-serve	720	22.0	128.0	14.0	40	430	0
vanilla:							
hand-dipped	480	14.0	52.0	27.0	120	240	0
soft-serve	650	27.0	98.0	17.0	50	550	0
desserts:							
apple turnover	290	2.0	36.0	15.0	5	350	1.0
chocolate chip cookie	290	4.0	44.0	11.0	20	270	0
twist cone	180	4.0	34.0	2.0	10	120	0
Hash, see "Beef hash"							
Hazelnut, shelled:							
chopped (*Planters*),							
2-oz. pkg.	350	7.0	9.0	2.5	0	0	5.0
raw, ¼ cup:							
(*Shiloh Farms*)	190	5.0	5.0	16.0	0	0	4.0
(*Tree of Life*)	210	4.0	5.0	21.0	0	0	3.0
dried:							
1 oz.	179	3.7	4.4	17.8	0	1	1.7
chopped, 1 cup ...	727	15.0	17.6	72.0	0	3	7.0
dry-roasted, salted, 1 oz.	188	2.8	5.1	18.8	0	221	<2.0
oil-roasted, salted, 1 oz.	187	4.1	5.4	18.1	0	223	1.8
Hazelnut spread:							
(*Nutella*), 2 tbsp.	160	2.0	19.0	9.0	0	30	0
butter (*Kettle Roaster*							
Fresh Unsalted), 1 oz.	188	4.0	5.0	19.0	0	1	0
Hazelnut syrup (*Ferrara*),							
2 oz.	130	0	32.0	0	0	12	0
Head cheese, 2 oz.:							
(*Hansel 'n Gretel*) ...	90	9.0	2.0	5.0	35	960	0
pork	88	7.7	0	6.1	39	465	0
Heart, braised or							
simmered, 4 oz.:							
beef	199	32.6	.5	6.4	219	71	0
chicken, broiler-fryer .	210	30.0	.1	9.0	274	54	0
lamb	210	28.3	2.2	9.0	282	71	0
pork	168	26.8	.5	5.7	251	40	0
turkey	201	30.3	2.3	6.9	256	62	0
veal	211	33.0	.1	7.7	200	66	0

Food and Measure	cal.	prot. (gms)	carbo. (gms)	fat (gms)	chol. (mgs)	sod. (mgs)	fiber (gms)
Herbs, see specific listings							
Herbs, mixed, seasoning (*Lawry's* Pinch of Herbs), ¼ tsp.	0	0	0	0	0	125	0
Herring, fresh:							
Atlantic, meat only:							
raw, 4 oz.	180	20.4	0	10.3	68	102	0
baked, broiled, or microwaved, 4 oz.	230	26.1	0	13.1	87	130	0
kippered, 4 oz.	246	27.9	0	14.0	93	1041	0
pickled, 4 oz.	297	16.1	10.9	20.4	15	987	0
lake, see "Cisco"							
Pacific, meat only:							
raw, 4 oz.	224	18.6	0	15.8	87	84	0
baked, broiled, or microwaved, 4 oz.	284	23.8	0	20.2	112	108	0
Herring, canned (see also "Sardine"):							
in hot sauce, 1 can:							
(*Beach Cliff/Brunswick* Fish Steaks Louisiana), 3.75 oz.	160	19.0	2.0	7.0	75	480	0
(*Brunswick* Seafood Snacks Louisiana), 3.25 oz.	140	16.0	2.0	8.0	70	450	0
kippered:							
(*Beach Cliff* 4 oz.), 3.3 oz.	220	19.0	0	16.0	135	490	0
(*Brunswick* Seafood Snacks 3.5 oz.), 3.2 oz.	160	18.0	0	9.0	55	490	0
(*Crown Prince* Kipper Snacks Low Sodium), ¼ cup .	110	11.0	0	8.0	35	40	0
mustard sauce (*Crown Prince* Kipper Snacks), ¼ cup	100	9.0	0	8.0	40	290	0
lemon/cracked pepper (*Brunswick* Seafood Snacks 3.5 oz.), 3.2 oz.	160	19.0	0	10.0	55	270	0

Food and Measure	cal.	prot. (gms)	carbo. (gms)	fat (gms)	chol. (mgs)	sod. (mgs)	fiber (gms)
mustard sauce (*Beach Cliff/Brunswick* Fish Steaks), 3.75-oz. can	160	21.0	2.0	9.0	80	420	0
smoked, golden (*Brunswick* Seafood Snacks), 3.25-oz. can	170	19.0	0	11.0	55	270	0
in soybean oil, drained: (*Beach Cliff/ Brunswick* Fish Steaks 3.75 oz.), 3.4 oz.	200	20.0	1.0	13.0	80	310	0
w/hot green chili (*Beach Cliff* Fish Steaks 3.75 oz.), 3.4 oz.	160	17.0	1.0	10.0	65	390	0
w/jalapeño (*Beach Cliff* Fish Steaks 3.75 oz.), 3.4 oz.	220	20.0	1.0	14.0	80	240	0
w/hot tabasco pepper (*Brunswick* Fish Steaks 3.75 oz.), 3.4 oz.	220	20.0	1.0	14.0	80	240	0
teriyaki sauce (*Brunswick* Seafood Snacks), 3.5-oz. can	160	6.0	5.0	8.0	70	800	0
tomato basil sauce (*Brunswick* Seafood Snacks), 3.5-oz. can	140	16.0	2.0	8.0	70	420	0
in water, drained (*Brunswick* Fish Steaks 3.75 oz.), 3.3 oz.	150	19.0	0	8.0	115	240	0
Herring, kippered, see "Herring" and "Herring, canned"							
Herring, pickled, in jars:							
in cream sauce (*Acme*), 5 pcs., 2 oz.	90	5.0	7.0	5.0	13	450	1.0
in wine sauce:							
(*Acme*), 5 pcs., 2 oz.	85	8.0	7.0	3.0	18	550	1.0
(*Nathan's*), ¼ cup .	90	5.0	7.0	4.0	25	420	0
tidbits (*Skansen*), 5 pcs., 2 oz.	85	8.0	7.0	3.0	18	550	<1.0

Food and Measure	cal.	prot. (gms)	carbo. (gms)	fat (gms)	chol. (mgs)	sod. (mgs)	fiber (gms)
Herring oil, see "Oil"							
Hibiscus cooler (*Santa Cruz Organic*), 8 fl. oz.	100	<1.0	24.0	0	0	40	0
Hickory nut, dried, shelled, 1 oz.	187	3.6	5.2	18.3	0	tr.	1.8
Hiziki, see "Seaweed"							
Hoisin sauce:							
(*House of Tsang*), 1 tsp.	15	0	4.0	0	0	120	0
(*Ka-Me*), 2 tbsp.	70	1.0	15.0	0	0	370	0
(*Kikkoman*), 2 tbsp. . . .	80	1.0	17.0	1.5	0	460	0
1 tbsp.	35	.5	7.1	.5	0	258	.4
Hollandaise sauce, in jars, 2 tbsp.:							
(*Melba*)	90	1.0	1.0	9.0	80	410	0
(*Reese*)	110	0	1.0	11.0	30	60	0
Hollandaise sauce mix:							
(*McCormick*), 1 tsp. .	15	0	1.0	0	15	110	0
(*Produce Partners*), 2 tsp.	20	0	2.0	.5	0	160	0
Hominy, dry, white (*Goya*), ¼ cup	180	4.0	39.0	0	0	0	0
Hominy, canned:							
golden, ½ cup:							
(*Allens/Allens Pepi-Hominy*)	120	2.0	27.0	.5	0	340	4.0
(*Bush's*)	60	1.0	13.0	0	0	550	3.0
white, ½ cup:							
(*Allens*)	100	2.0	22.0	.5	0	340	4.0
(*Bush's*)	70	1.0	14.0	1.0	0	530	4.0
Hominy grits, see "Corn grits"							
Hommus, see "Hummus"							
Honey, 1 tbsp.:							
(*Aunt Sue's/Grandma's/ Sue Bee*)	60	0	17.0	0	0	0	0
(*Miel H*)	70	0	17.0	0	0	0	0
raw, all varieties (*Tree of Life*)	60	0	17.0	0	0	0	0
Honey bun, see "Bun, sweet"							
Honey butter, see "Butter, flavored"							

Food and Measure	cal.	prot. (gms)	carbo. (gms)	fat (gms)	chol. (mgs)	sod. (mgs)	fiber (gms)
Honey mustard, see "Mustard blend" and "Pretzel dip"							
Honey pepper sauce (*Neera's* Barbados), 2 tsp.	23	0	5.0	1.0	0	101	0
Honey roll sausage, beef, 1 oz.	52	5.3	.6	3.0	14	375	0
Honeycomb (*Frieda's*), ½ cup, 3 oz.	260	0	70.0	0	0	0	0
Honeydew melon:							
(*Chiquita*), 1/10 melon	50	1.0	13.0	0	0	35	1.0
(*Del Monte*), 1/10 melon, 4.7 oz.	50	1.0	13.0	0	0	35	1.0
(*Dole*), 1/10 melon . .	50	1.0	13.0	0	0	35	1.0
1/10 melon, 7" x 2" . .	46	.6	11.8	.1	0	13	.8
cubed, 1 cup	60	.8	15.6	.2	0	17	1.0
Horned melon (*Frieda's*), 3.5-oz. melon	25	1.0	3.0	0	0	0	1.0
Horseradish, fresh:							
leafy tips, ½ cup:							
raw, chopped	6	.9	.8	.1	0	1	.2
boiled, drained, chopped	13	1.1	2.3	.2	0	2	.4
pods, ½ cup:							
raw, sliced	19	1.1	4.3	.1	0	21	1.6
boiled, drained, sliced	21	1.2	4.8	.1	0	25	2.5
Horseradish, prepared, 1 tsp.:							
(*Boar's Head*)	0	0	0	0	0	30	0
extra hot (*Silver Spring*)	0	0	0	0	0	10	0
Horseradish mustard, see "Mustard blend"							
Horseradish sauce, 1 tsp.:							
(*Boar's Head* Pub Style)	15	0	1.0	1.5	5	15	0
(*Heinz*)	25	0	1.0	2.0	0	35	0
(*Kraft*)	20	0	1.0	1.5	5	35	0
(*Sara Lee*)	20	0	0	2.0	0	45	0
Hot dog, see "Frankfurter"							
Hot dog sauce, see "Chili sauce"							

Food and Measure	cal.	prot. (gms)	carbo. (gms)	fat (gms)	chol. (mgs)	sod. (mgs)	fiber (gms)
Hot fudge sauce, see "Chocolate topping"							
Hot sauce, 1 tsp., except as noted:							
(*Búfalo* Especial)	0	0	0	0	0	140	0
(*Búfalo* Picante Clasica)	0	0	0	0	0	210	0
(*Cajun Bayou* Gator Swamp Sauce), 1 tbsp.	0	0	1.0	0	0	75	0
(*D.L. Jardine's* Texas Kicker XX)	25	1.0	<1.0	0	0	10	<1.0
(*Da'Bomb* The Final Answer), 2 tsp. . . .	10	0	2.0	0	0	0	0
(*Frank's* Red Hot Xtra Hot)	0	0	0	0	0	210	0
(*Glory*)	0	0	0	0	0	130	0
(*Fiesta* Quest for Fire)	5	0	1.0	0	0	40	0
(*Tabasco*)	0	0	0	0	0	30	0
(*Taco Bell*)	0	0	0	0	0	50	0
(*TryMe* Tennessee Sunshine)	0	0	0	0	0	160	0
(*TryMe* Yucatan Sunshine)	0	0	0	0	0	125	0
(*TryMe* Tiger Sauce Original)	10	0	2.0	0	0	140	0
(*World Harbors*), 2 tbsp.	30	0	7.0	0	0	390	0
(*Zapata*)	0	0	0	0	0	125	0
cayenne (*D.L. Jardine's* Texas Champagne) .	0	0	0	0	0	240	0
cayenne (*Cajun Bayou*)	0	0	1.0	0	0	199	0
chipotle:							
(*Búfalo*)	0	0	0	0	0	150	0
(*Tabasco*)	0	0	<1.0	0	0	115	0
garlic (*Tabasco*)	0	0	0	0	0	140	0
garlic pepper (*Cajun Bayou*), 1 tbsp. . . .	5	0	1.0	0	0	75	0
habanero:							
(*D.L. Jardine's* Blazin' Saddle XXX)	25	1.0	<1.0	0	0	10	<1.0
(*Tabasco*)	5	0	1.0	0	0	140	0
jalapeño:							
(*Búfalo*)	0	0	0	0	0	115	0
(*Cajun Bayou*)	0	0	1.0	0	0	100	0

Food and Measure	cal.	prot. (gms)	carbo. (gms)	fat (gms)	chol. (mgs)	sod. (mgs)	fiber (gms)
(*D.L. Jardine's* Texapeppa)	0	0	0	0	0	240	0
(*Tabasco*)	0	0	0	0	0	140	0
Hubbard squash:							
raw:							
(*Frieda's* Blue/Orange), ¾ cup, 3 oz.	35	2.0	7.0	0	0	5	2.0
1 cup	46	2.3	10.1	.6	0	8	2.7
baked, cubed, ½ cup .	51	2.5	11.0	.6	0	8	2.9
boiled, drained, mashed, ½ cup	35	1.8	7.6	.4	0	6	3.4
Hummus, 2 tbsp., except as noted:							
(*Athenos* Greek)	50	2.0	5.0	3.0	0	160	<1.0
(*Athenos* Original) . . .	50	1.0	5.0	3.0	0	160	1.0
(*Guiltless Gourmet* Original)	35	1.0	4.0	1.5	0	115	1.0
all varieties (*Cedar's*) .	50	3.0	5.0	2.0	0	120	3.0
artichoke garlic (*Athenos*)	45	2.0	4.0	2.5	0	160	<1.0
cucumber dill (*Athenos*)	50	1.0	5.0	3.0	0	160	1.0
eggplant, roasted (*Athenos*)	45	1.0	5.0	2.0	0	160	1.0
garlic, roasted:							
(*Athenos*)	50	1.0	6.0	3.0	0	160	<.10
(*Guiltless Gourmet*)	35	1.0	4.0	1.5	0	115	1.0
olive, black (*Athenos*)	50	1.0	5.0	3.0	0	180	1.0
pesto, spicy three pepper, or scallion (*Athenos*)	50	1.0	5.0	3.0	0	160	1.0
Hummus, mix, dry:							
(*Fantastic* Original), 2 tbsp.	80	3.0	11.0	3.0	0	280	1.0
spinach Parmesan (*Fantastic*), 2 tbsp. .	80	3.0	11.0	3.0	0	280	1.0
Hunter sauce mix (*McCormick*), 1 tsp.	25	0	4.0	0	0	270	0
Hush puppies, frozen:							
(*Delta Pride*), 3 pcs. . . .	140	2.0	21.0	5.0	0	470	n.a.
(*McKenzie's*), 2 oz.	190	2.0	23.0	10.0	0	470	2.0
jalapeño (*Delta Pride*), 3 pcs.	130	2.0	20.0	5.0	0	470	n.a.
Hush puppy mix (*Golden Dipt* Fry Easy), ¼ cup	130	2.0	25.0	.5	0	530	0

Food and Measure	cal.	prot. (gms)	carbo. (gms)	fat (gms)	chol. (mgs)	sod. (mgs)	fiber (gms)
Hyacinth bean, immature, boiled, drained, ½ cup ...	22	1.3	4.1	.1	0	1	n.a.
Hyacinth bean, dried, boiled, ½ cup	114	7.9	20.1	.6	0	7	n.a.

I

Food and Measure	cal.	prot. (gms)	carbo. (gms)	fat (gms)	chol. (mgs)	sod. (mgs)	fiber (gms)
Ice:							
all flavors (*Luigi's* Swirls), 6 fl. oz. . . .	150	0	39.0	0	0	10	0
cherry:							
(*Luigi's* Italian), 6 fl. oz.	130	0	32.0	0	0	15	<1.0
(*Popsicle Zone*), 12 fl. oz.	240	0	62.0	0	0	10	0
slush (*Popsicle Screwball*), 3.75 fl. oz.	110	0	27.0	0	0	15	0
chocolate fudge (*Luigi's* Italian), 6 fl. oz. . . .	160	0	40.0	0	0	25	<1.0
grape (*Luigi's* Italian), 6 fl. oz.	120	0	31.0	0	0	15	<1.0
lemon:							
(*Chill* Soft Serve), 6 fl. oz.	150	0	38.0	0	0	35	0
(*Luigi's* Italian), 6 fl. oz.	120	0	30.0	0	0	10	<1.0
(*Popsicle Zone*), 12 fl. oz.	230	0	60.0	0	0	10	0
lemonade, soft:							
(*Breyer's*), 12 fl. oz.	290	0	74.0	0	0	25	0
(*Minute Maid*), 4-oz. tube	110	0	25.0	0	0	20	0
(*Minute Maid*), 12 fl. oz.	300	0	77.0	0	0	55	0
strawberry (*Minute Maid*), 4-oz. tube	100	0	26.0	0	0	15	0
strawberry (*Minute Maid*), 12 fl. oz. .	300	0	78.0	0	0	45	0
orange:							
(*Chill* Soft Serve), 6 fl. oz.	160	0	41.0	0	0	35	0

Food and Measure	cal.	prot. (gms)	carbo. (gms)	fat (gms)	chol. (mgs)	sod. (mgs)	fiber (gms)
Ice, orange *(cont.)*							
(Chill Orange Overload), ¾ of 6-fl.-oz. cup	100	0	24.0	0	0	20	0
rainbow *(Popsicle Snow Cone)*, 7 fl. oz.	30	0	7.0	0	0	5	0
raspberry *(Chill Blue Raspberry Blast)*, ¾ of 6-oz. cup	100	0	26.0	0	0	20	0
strawberry:							
(Chill Soft Serve), 6 fl. oz.	140	0	36.0	0	0	30	0
(Chill Very Strawberry), ¾ of 6-oz. cup	90	0	23.0	0	0	20	0
(Luigi's Italian), 6 fl. oz.	120	0	31.0	0	0	10	<1.0
Ice bar (see also "Iced confection bar" and "Fruit bar"), 1 pc.:							
(Eskimo Pie Great American Chilly Pops 12 Pack)	40	0	10.0	0	0	0	0
(Eskimo Pie Great American Jr. Single)	40	0	10.0	0	0	0	0
(Eskimo Pie Great American Single) ..	100	0	26.0	0	0	0	0
(Popsicle Big Stick Big Reds)	70	0	17.0	0	0	0	0
(Popsicle Firecracker), 1.6 fl. oz.	40	0	10.0	0	0	0	0
(Popsicle Firecracker), 4.5 fl. oz.	80	0	20.0	0	0	0	0
(Popsicle Firecracker Jr.), 1.6 fl. oz.	40	0	10.0	0	0	0	0
(Popsicle Great White), 1.75 fl. oz.	45	0	11.0	0	0	0	0
(Popsicle Great White), 3 fl. oz.	70	0	18.0	0	0	0	0
(Popsicle Hyper Stripe)	80	0	19.0	0	0	10	0
all flavors:							
(Darigold Super Pops)	90	0	23.0	0	0	15	0
(Hendrie's Stix) ...	40	0	9.0	0	0	5	0
(Hoodsie Pops) ...	60	0	16.0	0	0	0	0

Food and Measure	cal.	prot. (gms)	carbo. (gms)	fat (gms)	chol. (mgs)	sod. (mgs)	fiber (gms)
(*Lifesavers* Pops) . .	40	0	10.0	0	0	0	0
(*Lifesavers* Sugar Free Pops)	10	0	2.0	0	0	0	0
(*Popsicle* Ice Pops)	45	0	11.0	0	0	0	0
(*Popsicle* Sugar Free)	15	0	4.0	0	0	0	0
(*Popsicle* Sugar Free), 2 bars	25	0	9.0	0	0	0	2.0
(*Popsicle* Swirl Bar)	60	0	13.0	0	0	0	0
(*Popsicle* Lick-a-Color), 2 fl. oz. .	50	0	13.0	0	0	0	0
(*Popsicle* Lick-a-Color), 3.5 fl. oz.	90	0	22.0	0	0	0	0
(*Popsicle* Rainbow), 1.75 fl. oz.	45	0	11.0	0	0	0	0
(*Popsicle* Rainbow), 3.5 fl. oz.	90	0	22.0	0	0	0	0
(*Popsicle* Super Twin)	70	0	16.0	0	0	5	0
(*Popsicle* Tingle Twister)	50	0	13.0	0	0	0	0
(*Popsicle* Towering Tornado)	90	0	21.0	0	0	0	0
cherry:							
(*Eskimo Pie* Red Rocket Single) . .	40	0	10.0	0	0	0	0
(*Popsicle* Red Zone)	80	0	19.0	0	0	15	0
(*Popsicle* Torpedo) .	35	0	8.0	0	0	0	0
cherry pineapple swirl (*Popsicle* Big Stick)	50	0	12.0	0	0	5	0
citrus:							
(*Hendrie's* Stix) . . .	40	0	10.0	0	0	5	0
berry (*Hendrie's* No Sugar)	15	0	2.0	0	0	5	0
tropical (*Popsicle* Sugar Free)	15	0	4.0	0	0	0	0
Ice cream, ½ cup:							
(*Ben & Jerry's Chubby Hubby*)	330	7.0	31.0	20.0	55	150	1.0
(*Ben & Jerry's Dublin Mudslide*)	270	4.0	28.0	16.0	65	80	≾1.0
(*Ben & Jerry's Everything But The . . .*) .	310	5.0	30.0	19.0	50	85	1.0
(*Ben & Jerry's Fossil Fuel*)	280	4.0	30.0	17.0	60	75	1.0

Food and Measure	cal.	prot. (gms)	carbo. (gms)	fat (gms)	chol. (mgs)	sod. (mgs)	fiber (gms)
Ice cream *(cont.)*							
(*Ben & Jerry's* Fudge Central)	300	4.0	31.0	18.0	55	60	1.0
(*Ben & Jerry's* the Gobfather)	270	4.0	32.0	14.0	30	50	2.0
(*Ben & Jerry's* In a Crunch)	350	6.0	30.0	23.0	55	150	1.0
(*Ben & Jerry's* Half Baked)	280	5.0	34.0	14.0	50	90	<1.0
(*Ben & Jerry's* Karamel Sutra)	280	4.0	32.0	15.0	50	75	1.0
(*Ben & Jerry's* Marsha Marsha Marshmallow)	270	4.0	32.0	14.0	30	50	2.0
(*Creamy Commotions* Moose Tracks)	190	3.0	21.0	12.0	25	60	1.0
(*Dreyer's/Edy's* Grand Turtle Sundae)	160	3.0	18.0	9.0	25	50	0
(*Dreyer's/Edy's* Grand Light *French Silk*) .	130	3.0	19.0	4.5	15	50	0
(*Healthy Choice* Double Karma)	140	2.0	28.0	2.0	10	90	<1.0
(*Healthy Choice* Happy Together)	150	2.0	29.0	2.0	10	70	<1.0
(*Hood* Heavenly Hash)	140	2.0	21.0	6.0	15	40	0
(*Hood* Heavenly Hash Light)	130	2.0	22.0	5.0	15	60	0
(*Turkey Hill* Turtle) . . .	170	2.0	21.0	9.0	25	85	1.0
almond:							
(*Darigold* Avalanche)	170	3.0	17.0	10.0	25	50	1.0
toasted (*Dreyer's* Grand)	150	3.0	15.0	9.0	25	30	0
almond hazelnut swirl (*Häagen-Dazs*)	320	5.0	26.0	22.0	100	100	<1.0
almond praline:							
(*Dreyer's* Grand) . .	170	3.0	21.0	8.0	25	85	0
(*Hood* Delight Light)	140	3.0	23.0	4.5	15	75	0
apple pie (*Dreamery* Deep Dish)	280	3.0	34.0	15.0	75	95	0
Baily's Irish Cream (*Häagen-Dazs*)	270	5.0	23.0	17.0	115	70	0
banana:							
(*Breyer's* Fresa) . . .	140	2.0	20.0	5.0	15	35	0
split (*Dreamery*) . .	240	3.0	31.0	11.0	60	45	1.0
split (*Häagen-Dazs*)	280	4.0	31.0	16.0	90	70	0

Food and Measure	cal.	prot. (gms)	carbo. (gms)	fat (gms)	chol. (mgs)	sod. (mgs)	fiber (gms)
split (*Turkey Hill*) ..	150	2.0	19.0	8.0	25	55	1.0
foster (*Häagen-Dazs*)	260	4.0	28.0	15.0	100	90	0
banana fudge chunk:							
(*Breyer's*)	160	3.0	21.0	8.0	20	40	<1.0
walnut (*Ben & Jerry's*							
Chunky Monkey)	300	5.0	30.0	18.0	55	45	1.0
berry:							
(*Dreamery* Blue							
Ribbon Pie)	260	4.0	31.0	15.0	75	105	<1.0
(*Turkey Hill* Berried							
Treasure)	160	2.0	22.0	6.0	20	130	0
brownie sundae:							
(*Hood* Light)	140	2.0	23.0	4.0	15	60	0
double (*Hood* Fat							
Free)	120	2.0	27.0	0	0	60	0
butter almond:							
(*Breyer's*)	160	4.0	14.0	10.0	20	85	<1.0
(*Turkey Hill* Philadel-							
phia Style)	170	4.0	15.0	10.0	30	120	0
butter brickle (*Turkey*							
Hill)	150	2.0	18.0	8.0	30	70	0
butter crunch, toffee:							
(*Hood* Light)	140	2.0	23.0	4.5	15	95	0
(*Peak Pleasures*) ..	160	2.0	21.0	8.0	30	100	0
butter pecan:							
(*Ben & Jerry's*) ...	280	4.0	20.0	21.0	65	105	0
(*Breyer's*)	170	3.0	14.0	11.0	20	115	0
(*Breyer's* Light) ...	120	3.0	15.0	7.0	10	115	4.0
(*Creamy Commotions*							
Janas Sticky Bun)	150	2.0	21.0	8.0	25	100	0
(*Dreamery* Triple) ..	300	4.0	30.0	18.0	70	160	1.0
(*Dreyer's/Edy's* Grand)	170	3.0	16.0	10.0	25	70	0
(*Dreyer's/Edy's* Grand							
Light)	120	3.0	16.0	5.0	20	80	0
(*Dreyer's/Edy's*							
Homemade Old							
Fashioned)	150	3.0	15.0	9.0	30	120	0
(*Dreyer's/Edys* No							
Sugar)	110	3.0	15.0	4.5	10	70	0
(*Dreyer's/Edy's* Carb							
Benefit)	170	2.0	13.0	12.0	30	55	6.0
(*Endulge*)	170	2.0	12.0	15.0	40	40	4.0
(*Green's* Light)	140	3.0	16.0	7.0	10	100	0
(*Green's* No Sugar)	120	4.0	4.0	7.0	15	105	0

Food and Measure	cal.	prot. (gms)	carbo. (gms)	fat (gms)	chol. (mgs)	sod. (mgs)	fiber (gms)
Ice cream, butter pecan *(cont.)*							
(*Green's* Southern) .	170	3.0	16.0	11.0	30	85	<1.0
(*Häagen-Dazs*)	310	5.0	21.0	23.0	110	110	<1.0
(*Healthy Choice*) . .	120	3.0	20.0	2.0	10	70	1.0
(*Healthy Choice* No Sugar)	110	2.0	18.0	2.5	10	65	3.0
(*Hood* Light)	140	2.0	19.0	6.0	10	90	0
(*Turkey Hill*)	160	2.0	15.0	11.0	30	95	0
(*Turkey Hill CarbIQ*)	130	2.0	11.0	11.0	25	90	4.0
butterscotch (*Hood* Blast)	160	2.0	20.0	7.0	25	60	0
w/candy:							
(*Breyer's Almond Joy*)	170	3.0	19.0	9.0	15	75	1.0
(*Breyer's Snickers*) .	160	3.0	20.0	8.0	20	50	0
(*Breyer's Snickers Cruncher*)	160	3.0	20.0	8.0	20	40	0
cappuccino, see "coffee," below							
caramel:							
(*Darigold Killer*) . . .	140	2.0	21.0	6.0	25	65	0
(*Green's Snapper*) .	160	2.0	19.0	8.0	25	70	0
(*Healthy Choice* Crazy for Caramel)	120	2.0	23.0	2.0	10	70	<1.0
(*Peak Pleasures* Caramel Cup Goldmine)	170	2.0	22.0	8.0	25	60	0
w/chocolate (*Dreyer's/ Edy's* Grand Ultimate Caramel Cup)	170	2.0	22.0	8.0	20.0	55	0
caramel cone (*Häagen-Dazs*)	320	4.0	32.0	19.0	100	190	0
caramel fudge:							
(*Breyer's*)	160	3.0	20.0	7.0	20	80	0
brownie (*Healthy Choice*)	120	3.0	21.0	2.0	10	70	1.0
caramel praline crunch (*Breyer's*)	170	3.0	22.0	7.0	20	110	0
caramel toffee bar (*Dreamery* Heaven)	290	4.0	32.0	16.0	75	90	0
cashew praline (*Dreamery*)	280	4.0	30.0	16.0	75	75	0
cherry:							
(*Green's* Whitehouse)	140	2.0	18.0	7.0	30	55	0
black (*Darigold*) . . .	140	2.0	18.0	7.0	25	50	0

Food and Measure	cal.	prot. (gms)	carbo. (gms)	fat (gms)	chol. (mgs)	sod. (mgs)	fiber (gms)
black (*Turkey Hill*) .	140	2.0	18.0	7.0	25	40	0
cherry chocolate chip:							
(*Ben & Jerry's Cherry Garcia*)	250	4.0	26.0	14.0	60	50	<1.0
(*Breyer's*)	150	3.0	18.0	7.0	20	40	0
(*Dreamery* ba da Bing)	280	3.0	33.0	15.0	65	50	1.0
(*Edy's* Grand)	160	2.0	19.0	8.0	25	40	0
(*Healthy Choice* Mambo)	120	3.0	21.0	2.0	5	70	<1.0
cherry fudge:							
ripple (*Turkey Hill* Fat Free No Sugar) . .	80	3.0	22.0	0	0	70	4.0
truffle (*Häagen-Dazs* Light)	230	5.0	37.0	7.0	50	40	0
cherry vanilla:							
(*Breyer's*)	140	3.0	17.0	8.0	20	45	0
(*Häagen-Dazs*)	240	4.0	23.0	15.0	100	60	0
(*Stonyfield* Organic)	250	2.0	24.0	16.0	60	35	0
sweet (*Turkey Hill* Philadelphia Style)	140	3.0	18.0	7.0	25	45	0
chocolate:							
(*Ben & Jerry's*) . . .	260	4.0	25.0	16.0	50	50	2.0
(*Ben & Jerry's* Therapy)	270	4.0	30.0	15.0	35	70	2.0
(*Breyer's*)	150	3.0	17.0	8.0	20	35	<1.0
(*Breyer's* Extra Creamy)	140	3.0	18.0	7.0	20	35	<1.0
(*Breyer's* 98% Fat Free)	90	3.0	20.0	1.5	5	50	4.0
(*Darigold* Totally) . .	140	2.0	17.0	7.0	25	65	1.0
(*Dreyer's/Edy's* Grand)	150	3.0	16.0	8.0	25	35	0
(*Dreyer's/Edy's* Grand Light)	110	3.0	16.0	3.5	20	45	0
(*Dreyer's/Edy's* Homemade)	150	3.0	19.0	7.0	30	55	0
(*Dreyer's/Edys* No Sugar)	90	3.0	13.0	3.0	10	45	0
(*Dreyer's/Edy's* Carb Benefit)	150	2.0	13.0	10.0	30	35	7.0
(*Endulge*)	140	2.0	13.0	12.0	45	20	5.0
(*Green's*)	140	2.0	17.0	8.0	30	45	<1.0
(*Häagen-Dazs*)	270	5.0	22.0	18.0	115	60	1.0
(*Hood*)	140	2.0	17.0	7.0	25	45	0

Food and Measure	cal.	prot. (gms)	carbo. (gms)	fat (gms)	chol. (mgs)	sod. (mgs)	fiber (gms)
Ice cream, chocolate *(cont.)*							
(*Hood* Fat Free Passion)	100	2.0	23.0	0	0	50	0
(*Stonyfield* Organic)	270	3.0	22.0	18.0	65	30	1.0
(*Turkey Hill* Philadelphia Style)	150	3.0	18.0	8.0	30	40	0
(*Turkey Hill CarbIQ*)	110	2.0	11.0	8.0	30	40	4.0
Belgian dark (*Godiva*)	280	5.0	26.0	17.0	65	40	2.0
brownie (*Healthy Choice* Brownie Bliss)	130	2.0	25.0	2.0	10	60	1.0
w/cake (*Dreyer's/ Edy's* Grand *Blue Ribbon Chocolate Cake*)	180	3.0	20.0	10.0	25	60	0
w/chocolate hearts (*Godiva*)	330	5.0	32.0	20.0	60	45	2.0
Dutch (*Häagen-Dazs* Light)	190	4.0	33.0	5.0	55	95	<1.0
Dutch (*Turkey Hill*)	150	2.0	18.0	8.0	30	40	1.0
Dutch (*Turkey Hill* Fat Free No Sugar)	70	3.0	20.0	0	0	75	6.0
French (*Breyer's* Light)	140	4.0	20.0	5.0	30	50	<1.0
milk (*Godiva* Classic)	290	5.0	28.0	18.0	65	50	1.0
pecan, brownie, caramel (*Healthy Choice* Turtle Fudge Cake)	130	2.0	23.0	2.0	10	70	<1.0
triple (*Dreyer's/Edy's* Grand *Triple Chocolate Thunder*) . .	160	2.0	18.0	9.0	25	35	0
triple (*Dreyer's/Edy's* No Sugar)	100	3.0	16.0	3.0	10	55	0
truffle (*Dreamery* Explosion)	280	5.0	31.0	15.0	55	85	1.0
chocolate brownie:							
(*Peak Pleasures*) . .	170	2.0	23.0	8.0	25	50	0
w/candy (*M&M's*) .	180	3.0	22.0	9.0	25	55	0
chocolate brownie, fudge:							
(*Ben & Jerry's*) . . .	260	5.0	32.0	13.0	35	80	2.0
(*Ben & Jerry's* Organic) . . . . :	270	4.0	30.0	13.0	35	55	2.0

Food and Measure	cal.	prot. (gms)	carbo. (gms)	fat (gms)	chol. (mgs)	sod. (mgs)	fiber (gms)
(*Breyer's* 98% Fat Free No Sugar) . .	90	3.0	20.0	1.5	5	85	4.0
(*Dreamery* Brownie Turtle Sundae) . .	310	5.0	33.0	17.0	55	70	2.0
(*Endulge*)	150	2.0	15.0	12.0	45	45	5.0
(*Healthy Choice* No Sugar)	120	3.0	21.0	2.0	5	60	1.0
double (*Dreyer's/Edys* No Sugar)	110	3.0	17.0	3.5	10	55	0
chocolate cake, German (*Turkey Hill*)	160	2.0	22.0	7.0	25	105	1.0
chocolate caramel: (*Breyer's* No Sugar)	100	3.0	18.0	4.0	10	60	3.0
fudge (*Darigold* Gooey Cluster) . .	150	2.0	21.0	7.0	20	75	0
swirl (*Dreyer's/Edy's* Grand)	170	2.0	19.0	9.0	25	45	0
chocolate cheesecake (*Godiva*)	310	4.0	36.0	17.0	60	190	1.0
chocolate chip: (*Breyer's*)	160	3.0	17.0	9.0	20	40	0
(*Dreyer's/Edy's* Grand)	170	3.0	18.0	9.0	25	45	0
(*Dreyer's/Edy's* Grand Light)	120	3.0	17.0	4.5	20	50	0
(*Dreyer's/Edy's* Carb Benefit*)	160	2.0	14.0	11.0	30	30	6.0
(*Hood* Chippedy Chocolaty)	150	2.0	18.0	9.0	25	45	0
(*Hood* Low Fat No Sugar)	100	3.0	30.0	2.5	5	65	0
(*Peak Pleasures*) . .	150	2.0	20.0	9.0	25	40	0
chocolate (*Häagen-Dazs*)	300	5.0	26.0	20.0	105	55	2.0
chocolate chip cookie dough: (*Ben & Jerry's*) . . .	270	4.0	32.0	15.0	65	85	0
(*Breyer's*)	170	3.0	20.0	9.0	25	55	0
(*Dreamery* Grandma's)	290	4.0	32.0	17.0	75	80	0
(*Dreyer's/Edy's* Grand)	180	3.0	21.0	9.0	25	65	0
(*Dreyer's/Edy's* Grand Light)	130	3.0	19.0	4.5	20	65	0
(*Dreyer's/Edys* No Sugar)	110	3.0	16.0	4.0	15	65	0
(*Green's*)	180	3.0	21.0	9.0	30	60	0

Food and Measure	cal.	prot. (gms)	carbo. (gms)	fat (gms)	chol. (mgs)	sod. (mgs)	fiber (gms)
Ice cream, chocolate chip cookie dough *(cont.)*							
(*Häagen-Dazs*)	310	4.0	29.0	20.0	95	125	0
(*Hood* Delight)	160	2.0	20.0	8.0	25	60	0
(*Turkey Hill*)	160	2.0	20.0	9.0	30	80	0
chocolate (*Hood* Light)	140	3.0	21.0	5.0	15	70	0
swirl (*Dreyer's/Edy's* Grand *Nestlé* Toll House)	170	2.0	21.0	9.0	25	60	0
chocolate chunk:							
chocolate (*Healthy Choice*)	120	3.0	21.0	2.0	5	60	1.0
milk (*Dreyer's/Edy's* Homemade)	160	3.0	18.0	8.0	25	55	0
chocolate fudge:							
(*Breyer's Fudgsicle*)	140	3.0	17.0	7.0	20	55	1.0
(*Dreyer's/Edy's* Fat/ Sugar Free)	100	4.0	22.0	0	0	60	0
chunks w/nuts (*Ben & Jerry's New York Super Fudge Chunk*)	310	5.0	29.0	20.0	40	55	2.0
mousse (*Edy's* Grand)	160	2.0	19.0	9.0	25	45	0
sundae (*Edy's* Grand)	170	3.0	20.0	9.0	20	50	0
chocolate malt:							
chips (*Creamy Commotions* Choco Malt Chip)	170	2.0	22.0	9.0	25	80	0
nuts (*Dreamery* Nuts About Malt)	290	5.0	29.0	17.0	70	65	1.0
chocolate marshmallow:							
(*Turkey Hill*)	160	2.0	23.0	7.0	25	100	1.0
caramel fudge (*Ben & Jerry's Phish Food*)	280	4.0	37.0	13.0	30	85	1.0
swirl (*Green's*)	150	2.0	21.0	7.0	25	105	<1.0
chocolate mocha silk (*Healthy Choice*) ..	120	2.0	24.0	1.5	5	50	1.0
chocolate peanut butter:							
(*Dreyer's/Edy's* Grand)	200	4.0	17.0	13.0	25	75	0
(*Häagen-Dazs*)	360	8.0	27.0	24.0	100	100	2.0
(*Peak Pleasures*) ..	170	2.0	21.0	9.0	25	55	0
swirl (*Endulge*) ...	170	3.0	14.0	14.0	40	70	5.0

Food and Measure	cal.	prot. (gms)	carbo. (gms)	fat (gms)	chol. (mgs)	sod. (mgs)	fiber (gms)
chocolate pretzel:							
(*Creamy Commotions Snyder's*)	180	2.0	22.0	9.0	25	80	0
(*Turkey Hill*)	170	2.0	21.0	9.0	25	85	1.0
chocolate rainbow							
(*Breyer's*)	140	3.0	16.0	7.0	20	35	0
chocolate raspberry:							
(*Stonyfield* Organic)	250	3.0	25.0	15.0	55	30	1.0
truffle (*Godiva*)	290	4.0	32.0	16.0	55	60	2.0
truffle, white (*Häagen-Dazs*)	310	5.0	32.0	18.0	105	65	1.0
white (*Godiva*)	260	5.0	32.0	12.0	55	65	0
coconut crème pie							
(*Turkey Hill*)	170	2.0	21.0	9.0	20	120	1.0
coffee:							
(*Ben & Jerry's*)	240	4.0	21.0	15.0	75	60	0
(*Breyer's*)	140	3.0	15.0	8.0	20	40	0
(*Dreyer's/Edy's* Grand)	140	2.0	15.0	8.0	25	40	0
(*Häagen-Dazs*)	270	5.0	21.0	18.0	120	70	0
(*Häagen-Dazs* Light)	210	5.0	32.0	7.0	65	85	0
(*Hood Caribbean Coffee Royale* Light)	110	2.0	18.0	3.5	15	50	0
(*Starbucks* Classic)	230	5.0	26.0	12.0	65	50	0
(*Stonyfield* Organic Decaf)	250	3.0	21.0	18.0	65	40	0
(*Turkey Hill* Philadelphia Style)	150	3.0	16.0	8.0	30	50	0
almond fudge (*Healthy Choice* Jumpin' Java)	130	2.0	25.0	2.0	5	75	<1.0
almond fudge (*Healthy Choice* No Sugar)	110	3.0	20.0	2.0	5	55	1.0
almond fudge (*Starbucks*)	250	5.0	29.0	13.0	60	65	1.0
caramel, espresso chips (*Creamy Commotions* Alpine Espresso)	160	2.0	20.0	8.0	50	90	0
caramel cappuccino swirl (*Starbucks*)	240	4.0	30.0	12.0	65	100	0
cappuccino chocolate chunk (*Healthy Choice*)	120	3.0	20.0	2.0	10	70	<1.0

Food and Measure	cal.	prot. (gms)	carbo. (gms)	fat (gms)	chol. (mgs)	sod. (mgs)	fiber (gms)
Ice cream, coffee *(cont.)*							
chocolate chip (*Peak Pleasures* Java Chip Trails)	160	2.0	19.0	9.0	25	40	0
chocolate chip (*Starbucks* Java Chip)	250	4.0	29.0	13.0	60	55	0
Colombian (*Turkey Hill*)	140	2.0	16.0	8.0	30	45	0
creamy (*Hood*) . . .	140	2.0	16.0	7.0	25	45	0
espresso chip (*Edy's* Grand)	150	2.0	17.0	8.0	25	50	0
fudge swirl (*Dreamery* Mudslide)	260	4.0	28.0	15.0	75	45	1.0
latte (*Starbucks* Low Fat)	170	5.0	30.0	3.0	10	60	0
latte, white chocolate (*Starbucks*)	280	5.0	31.0	15.0	60	60	0
toffee (*Ben & Jerry's Heath* Crunch) . .	290	4.0	29.0	18.0	65	115	0
cookie dough, see "chocolate chip cookie dough," above							
w/cookies:							
(*Breyer's Oreo*)	160	3.0	20.0	8.0	20	80	0
(*Breyer's Twix*)	160	2.0	21.0	7.0	15	45	0
cookies and cream:							
(*Ben & Jerry's* Sweet Cream Organic) .	250	4.0	24.0	15.0	60	95	0
(*Breyer's*)	160	3.0	18.0	8.0	20	45	<1.0
(*Darigold*)	140	2.0	18.0	7.0	25	65	0
(*Dreyer's/Edy's* Grand)	160	3.0	19.0	8.0	25	50	0
(*Dreyer's/Edy's* Grand Light)	120	3.0	18.0	4.0	15	60	0
(*Green's*)	150	2.0	18.0	8.0	30	50	0
(*Häagen-Dazs*)	270	5.0	23.0	17.0	105	95	0
(*Healthy Choice*) . .	120	3.0	21.0	2.0	5	90	<1.0
(*Hood*)	160	2.0	19.0	8.0	25	65	0
(*Hood* Light)	130	2.0	21.0	4.0	15	70	0
(*Turkey Hill*)	160	2.0	19.0	8.0	25	60	0
chocolate covered (*Godiva*)	300	4.0	32.0	18.0	85	55	<1.0
cookie sandwich (*Peak Pleasures*)	170	2.0	21.0	9.0	25	75	0

Food and Measure	cal.	prot. (gms)	carbo. (gms)	fat (gms)	chol. (mgs)	sod. (mgs)	fiber (gms)
crème brûlée (*Häagen-Dazs*)	280	4.0	23.0	19.0	120	75	0
crème caramel (*Stonyfield* Organic)	250	3.0	26.0	15.0	55	75	0
dulce de leche							
(*Breyer's*)	150	3.0	20.0	7.0	20	105	0
(*Häagen-Dazs*)	290	5.0	28.0	17.0	100	95	0
(*Häagen-Dazs* Light)	220	5.0	33.0	7.0	60	110	0
eggnog:							
(*Hood* Holiday)	150	2.0	16.0	8.0	45	50	0
(*Turkey Hill*)	150	2.0	17.0	8.0	45	45	0
espresso, see "coffee," above							
fudge:							
(*Peak Pleasures* River Rapids) ...	150	2.0	20.0	7.0	25	45	0
double (*Dreyer's/ Edy's* Grand) ...	170	2.0	19.0	9.0	30	45	0
hot, sundae (*Dreamery*)	310	5.0	29.0	20.0	75	80	<1.0
ripple (*Turkey Hill*) .	150	2.0	20.0	7.0	25	55	0
twister (*Hood*)	140	2.0	20.0	7.0	25	45	0
latte, see "coffee," above							
lemon pie (*Turkey Hill* Southern)	160	2.0	22.0	7.0	25	105	0
macadamia brittle (*Häagen-Dazs*)	300	4.0	25.0	20.0	110	110	0
maple walnut (*Hood*) .	150	2.0	17.0	8.0	25	55	0
mango (*Häagen-Dazs*)	250	4.0	28.0	14.0	85	50	<1.0
mint:							
w/candy (*Breyer's M&M's*)	170	2.0	19.0	9.0	15	50	0
w/candy (*M&M's*) .	190	3.0	20.0	11.0	25	55	0
w/cookies (*Breyer's Oreo*)	170	2.0	23.0	7.0	15	75	0
w/cookies (*Peak Pleasures* Cookie Caverns)	170	2.0	21.0	9.0	25	70	0
mint chocolate chip:							
(*Breyer's*)	160	3.0	17.0	9.0	20	40	0
(*Breyer's* Light) ...	130	3.0	19.0	4.5	10	45	0
(*Darigold* Cool) ...	140	2.0	17.0	7.0	25	55	0
(*Dreyer's/Edy's* Grand)	170	3.0	18.0	9.0	25	45	0

Food and Measure	cal.	prot. (gms)	carbo. (gms)	fat (gms)	chol. (mgs)	sod. (mgs)	fiber (gms)
Ice cream, mint chocolate chip *(cont.)*							
(*Dreyer's/Edy's* Grand Light)	120	3.0	17.0	4.5	20	50	0
(*Dreyer's/Edys* No Sugar)	90	3.0	13.0	3.0	10	50	0
(*Dreyer's/Edy's Carb Benefit*)	160	2.0	14.0	11.0	30	30	6.0
(*Endulge*)	160	2.0	14.0	12.0	45	20	4.0
(*Green's*)	150	2.0	17.0	8.0	30	55	0
(*Häagen-Dazs*)	300	5.0	26.0	19.0	105	85	<1.0
(*Häagen-Dazs* Light)	230	6.0	34.0	8.0	55	65	0
(*Healthy Choice*)	120	3.0	20.0	2.0	10	70	<1.0
(*Healthy Choice* No Sugar)	110	3.0	18.0	2.0	10	50	1.0
(*Hood* Grasshopper Pie)	160	2.0	22.0	7.0	20	65	0
(*Turkey Hill* Premium)	160	2.0	17.0	10.0	25	45	1.0
(*Turkey Hill* Philadelphia Style)	170	3.0	18.0	9.0	30	45	0
(*Turkey Hill CarbIQ*)	120	2.0	14.0	9.0	25	40	4.0
fudge swirl (*Dreyer's/ Edy's* Grand *Andes Cool Mint*)	170	2.0	19.0	9.0	25	40	0
mint chocolate cookie (*Ben & Jerry's*)	260	4.0	26.0	16.0	65	100	0
mocha almond fudge:							
(*Breyer's*)	170	4.0	18.0	9.0	15	45	2.0
(*Darigold*)	140	2.0	18.0	7.0	25	55	1.0
(*Dreyer's* Grand)	160	3.0	17.0	9.0	25	45	0
(*Dreyer's* Grand Light)	120	3.0	16.0	4.5	20	45	0
(*Häagen-Dazs*)	340	5.0	28.0	23.0	100	85	<1.0
mud pie:							
(*Darigold*)	140	2.0	21.0	6.0	20	65	1.0
(*Hood* Medley Light)	140	3.0	20.0	5.0	15	60	0
(*Starbucks*)	240	4.0	32.0	11.0	55	85	1.0
Neapolitan:							
(*Darigold*)	130	2.0	16.0	7.0	25	55	0
(*Dreyer's/Edy's* Grand)	140	2.0	16.0	7.0	25	35	0
(*Dreyer's/Edy's* Grand Light)	100	3.0	15.0	3.0	20	40	0
(*Dreyer's/Edys* No Sugar)	90	3.0	13.0	3.0	10	50	0
(*Green's* Metropolitan)	140	2.0	17.0	7.0	30	50	0

Food and Measure	cal.	prot. (gms)	carbo. (gms)	fat (gms)	chol. (mgs)	sod. (mgs)	fiber (gms)
(*Turkey Hill*)	140	2.0	17.0	8.0	30	40	0
(*Turkey Hill* Philadelphia Style)	140	3.0	17.0	8.0	30	45	0
oatmeal cookie chunk (*Ben & Jerry's*)	270	4.0	31.0	15.0	55	120	<1.0
peach:							
(*Breyer's*)	120	2.0	17.0	5.0	15	30	0
(*Dreyer's/Edy's* Homemade Grovestand)	120	2.0	17.0	5.0	20	45	0
(*Green's* Just Peachy!)	140	2.0	17.0	7.0	30	55	0
and cream (*Häagen-Dazs*)	240	3.0	29.0	12.0	75	55	0
and cream (*Turkey Hill*)	130	2.0	17.0	6.0	25	35	0
peanut brittle (*Turkey Hill* Light No Sugar)	120	5.0	19.0	6.0	0	105	5.0
peanut butter:							
(*Breyer's Twix*)	170	3.0	18.0	10.0	15	75	<1.0
(*Turkey Hill* Mania)	180	2.0	20.0	11.0	25	85	0
(*Turkey Hill CarbIQ* Paradise)	150	3.0	13.0	12.0	25	110	4.0
chunk, chocolate (*Dreamery*)	310	7.0	29.0	18.0	50	110	2.0
fudge (*Breyer's*)	170	4.0	17.0	10.0	20	80	<1.0
ripple (*Turkey Hill*)	180	3.0	16.0	11.0	25	90	1.0
twirl (*Greens*)	180	3.0	16.0	11.0	25	85	<1.0
peanut butter cup:							
(*Ben & Jerry's*)	360	7.0	27.0	26.0	60	125	1.0
(*Breyer's Reese's Peanut Butter Cups*)	180	3.0	22.0	9.0	15	75	0
(*Dreyer's/Edy's* Grand)	180	3.0	19.0	10.0	20	75	0
(*Healthy Choice*)	120	3.0	21.0	2.0	5	70	<1.0
chocolate (*Turkey Hill*)	180	3.0	18.0	11.0	25	85	1.0
fudge (*Dreyer's/Edy's* Grand Fudge Tracks)	180	3.0	18.0	11.0	25	60	0
fudge (*Dreyer's/Edy's* Grand Light Fudge Tracks)	120	3.0	18.0	4.0	15	50	0
peppermint stick:							
(*Hood*)	140	2.0	22.0	5.0	20	45	0
(*Turkey Hill*)	150	2.0	19.0	8.0	30	55	0

Food and Measure	cal.	prot. (gms)	carbo. (gms)	fat (gms)	chol. (mgs)	sod. (mgs)	fiber (gms)
Ice cream (cont.)							
pineapple coconut							
(*Häagen-Dazs*)	230	4.0	25.0	13.0	90	55	0
pineapple upside down							
cake (*Turkey Hill*) ..	150	2.0	21.0	7.0	20	85	0
pistachio:							
(*Ben & Jerry's*) ...	260	5.0	21.0	17.0	65	55	<1.0
(*Häagen-Dazs*)	290	5.0	22.0	20.0	110	80	<1.0
praline and caramel							
(*Healthy Choice*) ..	120	2.0	23.0	2.0	10	80	<1.0
raspberry:							
black (*Dreamery*							
Avalanche*)	270	4.0	27.0	16.0	80	50	1.0
black (*Green's* Blast)	150	2.0	20.0	8.0	25	55	0
black (*Turkey Hill*) .	140	2.0	18.0	7.0	30	35	0
black, ripple (*Peak							
Pleasures*)	150	2.0	20.0	7.0	25	50	0
raspberry brownie							
(*Dreamery* à la Mode)	270	3.0	27.0	14.0	75	60	1.0
raspberry cheesecake							
(*Turkey Hill CarbIQ*)	120	2.0	16.0	7.0	25	95	4.0
raspberry vanilla swirl							
(*Dreyer's/Edy's* Fat/							
Sugar Free)	90	3.0	19.0	0	0	50	0
rocky road:							
(*Breyer's*)	170	3.0	20.0	8.0	20	60	<1.0
(*Darigold*)	160	3.0	19.0	8.0	25	65	<1.0
(*Dreyer's/Edy's* Grand)	170	3.0	17.0	10.0	25	30	0
(*Dreyer's/Edy's* Grand							
Light)	120	3.0	17.0	4.0	20	40	0
(*Green's*)	160	3.0	19.0	9.0	25	40	1.0
(*Häagen-Dazs*)	300	5.0	29.0	18.0	90	75	1.0
(*Healthy Choice*) ..	130	3.0	25.0	2.0	5	60	<1.0
(*Turkey Hill*)	180	3.0	22.0	8.0	25	120	1.0
rum raisin:							
(*Häagen-Dazs*)	270	4.0	22.0	17.0	110	60	0
(*Turkey Hill*)	165	2.0	19.0	7.0	25	55	0
S'mores:							
(*Dreamery*)	280	5.0	39.0	13.0	45	120	1.0
(*Häagen-Dazs* Light)	240	4.0	42.0	6.0	45	105	<1.0
spumoni:							
(*Dreyer's/Edy's*							
Grand)	150	3.0	16.0	8.0	25	40	0
(*Hood*)	140	2.0	17.0	7.0	25	45	0

Food and Measure	cal.	prot. (gms)	carbo. (gms)	fat (gms)	chol. (mgs)	sod. (mgs)	fiber (gms)
strawberry:							
(*Ben & Jerry's*) ...	230	4.0	26.0	13.0	65	50	0
(*Ben & Jerry's* Organic)	210	3.0	21.0	12.0	55	40	0
(*Breyer's*)	120	2.0	15.0	6.0	15	30	0
(*Darigold* Summer)	120	2.0	16.0	6.0	25	45	0
(*Dreamery Strawberry Fields*)	220	3.0	26.0	12.0	65	35	1.0
(*Dreyer's/Edy's* Grand Light)	100	2.0	17.0	2.5	15	40	0
(*Dreyer's/Edy's* Grand Real)	130	2.0	16.0	6.0	20	30	0
(*Dreyer's/Edys* No Sugar)	90	3.0	13.0	3.0	10	50	0
(*Green's*)	140	2.0	17.0	7.0	30	50	0
(*Häagen-Dazs*)	250	4.0	23.0	16.0	95	65	<1.0
(*Hood*)	130	2.0	17.0	7.0	25	40	0
and cream (*Dreyer's/Edy's* Homemade)	130	2.0	17.0	6.0	25	50	0
and cream (*Turkey Hill*)	130	2.0	16.0	6.0	25	35	1.0
strawberry cheesecake:							
(*Dreamery* New York)	260	4.0	27.0	15.0	80	70	0
(*Häagen-Dazs*)	270	4.0	28.0	16.0	100	130	0
(*Creamy Commotions Janas*)	170	2.0	22.0	8.0	30	100	0
graham swirl (*Ben & Jerry's* Primary Berry Graham) ..	270	3.0	29.0	15.0	60	110	1.0
strawberry shortcake (*Breyer's*)	160	2.0	23.0	6.0	15	40	0
tin roof sundae:							
(*Darigold*)	150	2.0	19.0	7.0	25	70	0
(*Healthy Choice*) ..	120	3.0	21.0	2.0	10	60	1.0
(*Turkey Hill*)	160	2.0	19.0	8.0	25	65	0
tiramisu (*Dreamery*) .	260	4.0	31.0	13.0	75	150	0
toffee bar:							
(*Breyer's Heath*) ...	180	2.0	22.0	9.0	20	120	0
(*Dreyer's/Edy's* Grand Crunch)	170	2.0	19.0	9.0	25	65	0
vanilla:							
(*Ben & Jerry's*) ...	240	4.0	21.0	16.0	75	60	0
(*Ben & Jerry's* Organic)	220	3.0	18.0	14.0	65	50	0

Food and Measure	cal.	prot. (gms)	carbo. (gms)	fat (gms)	chol. (mgs)	sod. (mgs)	fiber (gms)
Ice cream, vanilla *(cont.)*							
(*Breyer's*)	140	3.0	15.0	8.0	20	40	0
(*Breyer's* Calcium Rich)	130	3.0	14.0	7.0	20	40	0
(*Breyer's* Extra Creamy)	150	3.0	17.0	8.0	20	45	0
(*Breyer's* Homemade)	140	3.0	16.0	7.0	35	50	0
(*Breyer's* Lactose Free)	130	2.0	14.0	7.0	20	35	0
(*Breyer's* Light) ...	130	3.0	18.0	4.5	30	60	0
(*Breyer's* Light All Natural)	110	3.0	17.0	3.0	10	50	0
(*Breyer's* 98% Fat Free)	90	2.0	20.0	1.5	5	50	4.0
(*Breyer's* No Sugar)	100	3.0	15.0	4.5	15	45	3.0
(*Darigold* Very) ...	130	2.0	16.0	7.0	25	50	0
(*Dreamery*)	260	5.0	25.0	15.0	70	55	0
(*Dreamery* Fortunate)	300	4.0	33.0	17.0	70	60	1.0
(*Dreyer's/Edy's* Fat/ Sugar Free)	90	3.0	20.0	0	0	50	0
(*Dreyer's* Grand) ..	150	2.0	14.0	10.0	35	35	0
(*Dreyer's/Edy's* Grand Light)	100	3.0	15.0	3.5	20	45	0
(*Dreyer's/Edy's* Homemade)	140	3.0	15.0	7.0	30	60	0
(*Dreyer's/Edy's* No Sugar)	100	3.0	14.0	3.0	10	50	0
(*Edy's* Grand)	140	2.0	15.0	8.0	25	30	0
(*Endulge*)	140	2.0	13.0	12.0	45	20	4.0
(*Green's*)	150	2.0	17.0	8.0	35	60	0
(*Green's* Light)	110	3.0	17.0	3.5	10	70	0
(*Green's* No Sugar)	90	3.0	3.0	4.0	15	60	0
(*Häagen-Dazs*)	270	5.0	21.0	18.0	120	70	0
(*Healthy Choice*) ..	110	3.0	19.0	2.0	10	60	<1.0
(*Healthy Choice* No Sugar)	100	3.0	17.0	2.0	10	55	1.0
(*Hood* Fat Free Very)	100	2.0	23.0	0	0	50	0
(*Hood* Low Fat No Sugar Dream) ..	90	3.0	19.0	1.5	5	65	0
(*Peak Pleasures* Snowdrift)	150	2.0	17.0	8.0	30	45	0
(*Stonyfield* Organic)	250	3.0	20.0	18.0	65	40	0
(*Turkey Hill* Original)	140	2.0	16.0	8.0	30	45	0

Food and Measure	cal.	prot. (gms)	carbo. (gms)	fat (gms)	chol. (mgs)	sod. (mgs)	fiber (gms)
bean (*Dreyer's/Edy's Grand*)	140	2.0	15.0	8.0	25	35	0
bean (*Dreyer's/Edy's Carb Benefit*) ...	140	2.0	13.0	9.0	30	30	6.0
bean (*Green's Philly*)	150	2.0	17.0	8.0	35	70	0
bean (*Häagen-Dazs Light*)	200	5.0	29.0	7.0	65	55	0
bean (*Heathy Choice In the Beginning*)	110	2.0	21.0	2.0	5	50	<1.0
bean (*Hood*)	140	2.0	16.0	7.0	30	45	0
bean (*Turkey Hill*) .	140	2.0	16.0	8.0	30	45	0
bean (*Turkey Hill* Fat Free No Sugar) ..	70	3.0	19.0	0	0	75	5.0
bean (*Turkey Hill* Philadelphia Style)	150	3.0	16.0	8.0	30	50	0
bean (*Turkey Hill CarbIQ*)	110	2.0	11.0	8.0	30	40	4.0
creamy (*Hood* Light)	110	2.0	18.0	3.5	15	50	0
French (*Breyer's*) ..	150	3.0	15.0	8.0	50	45	0
French (*Breyer's Light*)	120	3.0	18.0	4.0	35	50	0
French (*Breyer's* No Sugar)	100	3.0	14.0	4.5	25	60	3.0
French (*Darigold*) .	140	2.0	17.0	7.0	45	50	0
French (*Dreyer's/Edy's Grand*)	160	2.0	17.0	9.0	50	40	0
French (*Dreyer's/Edy's Grand Light*)	100	3.0	15.0	3.5	30	45	0
French (*Green's*) ..	150	3.0	18.0	8.0	60	60	0
French (*Peak Pleasures Summit*)	160	2.0	18.0	8.0	60	60	0
French (*Turkey Hill*)	140	2.0	16.0	8.0	55	45	0
golden (*Hood*)	140	2.0	16.0	7.0	30	65	0
vanilla, w/candy (*M&M's*)	180	3.0	22.0	9.0	25	50	0
vanilla, w/chocolate caramel hearts (*Godiva*)	310	5.0	32.0	18.0	80	55	1.0
vanilla, w/chocolate dip cone (*Dreamery Coney Island Waffle Cone*)	310	4.0	32.0	18.0	70	55	1.0
vanilla, w/chocolate wafers (*Edy's* Grand Ice Cream Sandwich)	150	3.0	19.0	7.0	25	75	0

Food and Measure	cal.	prot. (gms)	carbo. (gms)	fat (gms)	chol. (mgs)	sod. (mgs)	fiber (gms)
Ice cream *(cont.)*							
vanilla, w/raspberry:							
brownie swirl (*Ben & Jerry's Dave Matthews Band Magic Brownie*) .	250	4.0	29.0	13.0	60	75	0
swirl (*Hood* Light) .	120	2.0	22.0	3.0	10	55	0
vanilla caramel:							
fudge (*Ben & Jerry's*)	280	4.0	31.0	15.0	67	10	0
pecan (*Godiva*)	290	4.0	33.0	16.0	75	125	0
vanilla and chocolate:							
(*Breyer's* Light) . . .	110	3.0	18.0	3.0	10	45	0
(*Breyer's* No Sugar)	90	3.0	15.0	4.0	10	45	3.0
(*Breyer's* Take Two)	140	3.0	16.0	8.0	20	40	0
(*Dreyer's/Edy's* Grand)	150	3.0	16.0	8.0	25	30	0
(*Green's*)	140	2.0	17.0	8.0	30	50	0
(*Hood Patchwork*) .	140	2.0	17.0	7.0	25	45	0
(*Peak Pleasures* Twin Peaks)	140	2.0	16.0	8.0	30	45	0
(*Turkey Hill*)	150	2.0	17.0	8.0	30	40	0
swirl (*Dreyer's/Edy's* Fat/Sugar Free) .	100	4.0	20.0	0	0	50	0
vanilla chocolate chip (*Häagen-Dazs*)	310	5.0	26.0	20.0	105	75	<1.0
vanilla chocolate and strawberry:							
(*Breyer's*)	140	3.0	16.0	7.0	20	35	0
(*Hood Classic Trio*)	140	2.0	17.0	7.0	25	45	0
(*Hood Classic Trio* Light)	110	2.0	18.0	3.5	15	45	0
(*Hood Classic Trio* Fat Free)	100	2.0	23.0	0	0	50	0
(*Hood Classic Trio* Low Fat No Sugar)	90	3.0	19.0	1.5	5	65	0
(*Peak Pleasures* Triple Peaks) . . .	140	2.0	17.0	8.0	30	40	0
vanilla custard (*Dreyer's/Edy's* Homemade)	150	3.0	17.0	8.0	55	70	0
vanilla fudge:							
(*Breyer's* Checks) . .	170	3.0	19.0	9.0	25	50	0
(*Dreyer's/Edy's* Grand French Vanilla Fudge Pie)	160	2.0	20.0	8.0	45	55	0

Food and Measure	cal.	prot. (gms)	carbo. (gms)	fat (gms)	chol. (mgs)	sod. (mgs)	fiber (gms)
(*Häagen-Dazs*)	290	5.0	26.0	18.0	100	95	0
brownie (*Breyer's*) .	160	3.0	19.0	9.0	25	80	<1.0
brownie (*Stonyfield Organic*)	260	3.0	28.0	15.0	65	60	0
w/candy (*Breyer's M&M's*)	170	3.0	20.0	10.0	15	50	0
swirl (*Endulge*) ...	140	2.0	14.0	10.0	40	30	4.0
swirl (*Green's*)	150	2.0	21.0	6.0	25	50	0
twirl (*Breyer's*)	140	3.0	18.0	7.0	20	45	<1.0
twirl (*Breyer's* No Sugar)	110	3.0	19.0	4.0	10	50	3.0
vanilla peanut butter fudge (*Green's* Pocono Paws)	18-	3.0	21.0	11.0	25	75	0
vanilla Swiss almond:							
(*Endulge*)	160	2.0	14.0	13.0	40	20	5.0
(*Häagen-Dazs*)	300	5.0	24.0	20.0	105	75	<1.0
vanilla toffee (*Ben & Jerry's* Heath)	290	4.0	29.0	18.0	65	120	0
"Ice cream," nondairy, ½ cup:							
(*Purely Decadent Soy Delicious* Turtle Tracks)	200	1.0	31.0	8.0	0	35	5.0
almond pecan (*It's Soy Delicious*)	160	2.0	24.0	6.0	0	75	1.0
banana, w/chocolate (*Purely Decadent Soy Delicious* Swinging Anna) ...	230	2.0	31.0	13.0	0	15	5.0
"butter" pecan:							
(*Organic Soy Delicious*)	170	2.0	22.0	8.0	0	85	1.0
(*Tofutti* Better Pecan)	210	1.0	22.0	13.0	0	200	0
cappuccino (*Rice-Dream*) 150	0	23.0	6.0	0	100	1.0	
carob:							
(*RiceDream*)	150	1.0	24.0	6.0	0	100	2.0
almond (*RiceDream*)	170	1.0	24.0	8.0	0	95	2.0
peppermint (*It's Soy Delicious*)	130	2.0	24.0	3.0	0	30	1.0
chai (*It's Soy Delicious* Tiger)	110	2.0	24.0	1.5	0	160	2.0

Food and Measure	cal.	prot. (gms)	carbo. (gms)	fat (gms)	chol. (mgs)	sod. (mgs)	fiber (gms)
"Ice cream," nondairy *(cont.)*							
cheesecake, blueberry, chocolate, or strawberry (*Tofutti* Cheesecake Supreme)	200	2.0	20.0	12.0	0	200	0
cherry (*Purely Decadent Soy Delicious* Nirvana)	190	1.0	32.0	9.0	0	15	5.0
chocolate:							
(*It's Soy Delicious* Awesome)	130	2.0	24.0	3.0	0	25	1.0
(*Organic Soy Delicious* Velvet) . . .	130	2.0	23.0	4.0	0	35	2.0
(*Purely Decadent Soy Delicious* Obsession)	210	2.0	36.0	9.0	0	15	5.0
(*Sweet Nothings*) . .	100	1.0	27.0	0	0	135	3.0
(*Tofutti* No Sugar) .	115	1.0	12.0	5.0	0	90	0
(*Tofutti* Super Soy Supreme New York, New York) .	170	4.0	22.0	9.0	0	180	0
(*Tofutti* Supreme) . .	180	3.0	18.0	11.0	0	180	0
Swiss (*Dr. Praeger's* Sensible Treats) .	125	3.0	21.0	3.0	0	65	3.0
chocolate almond (*It's Soy Delicious*)	160	2.0	24.0	6.0	0	65	2.0
chocolate brownie almond (*Purely Decadent Soy Delicious*)	210	3.0	34.0	10.0	0	75	6.0
chocolate coffee (*It's Soy Delicious* Mexican)	110	2.0	22.0	2.0	0	80	1.0
chocolate cookie crunch (*Tofutti*)	190	3.0	26.0	11.0	0	100	0
chocolate fudge (*Tofutti* Low Fat) . .	145	2.0	25.0	4.0	0	98	0
chocolate peanut butter:							
(*It's Soy Delicious*) .	150	3.0	25.0	5.0	0	50	1.0
(*Organic Soy Delicious*)	150	2.0	23.0	5.0	0	65	1.0
cocoa marble fudge (*RiceDream*)	150	1.0	25.0	6.0	0	100	2.0
coffee marshmallow swirl (*Tofutti* Low Fat)	120	1.0	24.0	3.0	0	77	0

Food and Measure	cal.	prot. (gms)	carbo. (gms)	fat (gms)	chol. (mgs)	sod. (mgs)	fiber (gms)
cookie:							
(*Purely Decadent Soy Delicious* Avalanche)	190	1.0	32.0	9.0	0	15	5.0
(*RiceDream* Cookies 'n Dream)	170	1.0	26.0	7.0	0	100	1.0
and "cream" (*Organic Soy Delicious*) ..	160	2.0	25.0	5.0	0	70	4.0
dulce de leche (*Organic Soy Delicious*)	150	2.0	25.0	4.0	0	12	4.0
espresso (*It's Soy Delicious*)	130	2.0	25.0	3.0	0	30	1.0
green tea (*It's Soy Delicious*)	110	2.0	24.0	1.5	0	130	2.0
mango raspberry:							
(*It's Soy Delicious*) .	110	1.0	25.0	1.5	0	105	2.0
(*Sweet Nothings*) ..	110	0	29.0	0	0	120	2.0
mint, chunky, w/chocolate (*Purely Decadent Soy Delicious Madness*)	200	2.0	35.0	8.0	0	30	6.0
mint chocolate chip:							
(*Tofutti*)	210	3.0	21.0	13.0	0	130	0
or carob chip (*RiceDream*)	170	1.0	26.0	8.0	0	95	1.0
mint fudge:							
(*Sweet Nothings*) ..	110	0	30.0	0	0	170	3.0
marble (*Organic Soy Delicious*)	140	2.0	25.0	3.0	0	35	1.0
mocha fudge:							
(*Dr. Praeger's Sensible Treats*) .	110	2.0	21.0	2.5	0	45	1.0
(*Organic Soy Delicious*)	150	2.0	27.0	3.5	0	60	1.0
(*Sweet Nothings*) ..	110	0	30.0	0	0	180	3.0
almond (*Purely Decadent Soy Delicious*)	200	3.0	32.0	9.0	0	45	6.0
Neapolitan:							
(*Organic Soy Delicious*)	130	2.0	23.0	4.0	0	40	1.0
(*RiceDream*)	150	1.0	24.0	6.0	0	100	2.0
orange vanilla swirl (*RiceDream*)	150	0	24.0	6.0	0	90	1.0

Food and Measure	cal.	prot. (gms)	carbo. (gms)	fat (gms)	chol. (mgs)	sod. (mgs)	fiber (gms)
"Ice cream," nondairy *(cont.)*							
peanut butter (*Purely Decadent Soy Delicious* Zig Zag) . .	230	3.0	32.0	13.0	0	50	5.0
pistachio almond (*It's Soy Delicious*)	130	3.0	23.0	4.5	0	200	3.0
praline:							
(*RiceDream* Supreme Pralines 'n Dream)	180	1.0	24.0	9.0	0	95	1.0
pecan (*Purely Decadent Soy Delicious*) . . .210		2.0	33.0	10.0	0	50	5.0
raspberry:							
(*It's Soy Delicious*) .	130	1.0	25.0	3.0	0	25	1.0
à la mode (*Purely Decadent Soy Delicious*)	200	2.0	34.0	7.0	0	70	5.0
rocky road (*Purely Decadent Soy Delicious*)	190	2.0	31.0	8.0	0	85	5.0
strawberry:							
(*Dr. Praeger's Sensible Treats*) .	120	2.0	20.0	1.0	0	60	<1.0
(*Organic Soy Delicious*)	130	2.0	23.0	4.0	0	55	1.0
(*RiceDream*)	140	0	24.0	5.0	0	85	1.0
(*Sweet Nothings* Cool)	120	0	30.0	0	0	130	2.0
(*Tofutti* No Sugar) .	110	1.0	12.0	5.0	0	100	0
vanilla:							
(*Dr. Praeger's Sensible Treats*) .	120	2.0	25.0	1.0	0	90	2.0
(*It's Soy Delicious*) .	130	2.0	25.0	3.0	0	30	1.0
(*Organic Soy Delicious* Old Fashioned)	120	2.0	24.0	4.0	0	55	5.0
(*Purely Decadent Soy Delicious* Purely)	170	1.0	29.0	8.0	0	20	6.0
(*RiceDream*)	150	0	23.0	6.0	0	100	1.0
(*SoyDream*)	140	1.0	17.0	7.0	0	70	1.0
(*Sweet Nothings*) . .	100	0	28.0	0	0	150	3.0
(*Tofutti*)	190	2.0	20.0	11.0	0	210	0

Food and Measure	cal.	prot. (gms)	carbo. (gms)	fat (gms)	chol. (mgs)	sod. (mgs)	fiber (gms)
(*Tofutti* Super Soy Supreme Bella) .	160	4.0	20.0	8.0	0	190	0
creamy (*Organic Soy Delicious*)	130	2.0	23.0	4.0	0	55	1.0
vanilla almond:							
bark (*Tofutti*)	210	3.0	21.0	9.0	0	130	0
Swiss (*Purely Decadent Soy Delicious*)	200	2.0	31.0	9.0	0	90	6.0
Swiss (*RiceDream*)	180	1.0	25.0	8.0	0	95	1.0
vanilla fudge:							
(*It's Soy Delicious*) .	120	2.0	25.0	1.5	0	130	2.0
(*Sweet Nothings*) . . .	110	0	30.0	0	0	140	3.0
(*Tofutti*)	190	2.0	25.0	9.0	0	130	0
(*Tofutti* Low Fat) . .	140	2.0	24.0	4.0	0	90	0
vanilla orange (*Organic Soy Delicious* Twisted)	120	2.0	24.0	2.0	0	35	4.0
wildberry (*Tofutti* Supreme) . . . . . . , . :	190	2.0	24.0	9.0	0	190	0
Ice cream bar (see also "Iced confection bar"), 1 pc., except as noted:							
(*Ben & Jerry's Half Baked*)	340	5.0	46.0	16.0	40	125	2.0
(*Scribblers* Ice Cream Pops), 2 pcs.	130	3.0	17.0	5.0	15	45	0
almond, toasted:							
(*Eskimo Pie*)	220	2.0	27.0	12.0	15	35	0
(*Eskimo Pie* King Size)	230	3.0	21.0	16.0	25	80	0
(*Eskimo Pie* Premium Single)	220	2.0	27.0	12.0	15	35	0
(*Good Humor*), 3 fl. oz.	180	2.0	22.0	10.0	5	35	<1.0
(*Good Humor*), 4 fl. oz.	230	2.0	30.0	12.0	10	45	<1.0
butter pecan (*Endulge* Single)	180	3.0	11.0	16.0	30	35	3.0
candy center, w/chocolate, crisps: (*Eskimo Pie* Crunch Bar)	230	3.0	21.0	16.0	25	80	0

Food and Measure	cal.	prot. (gms)	carbo. (gms)	fat (gms)	chol. (mgs)	sod. (mgs)	fiber (gms)
Ice cream bar, candy center, w/chocolate, crisps *(cont.)*							
(*Good Humor* Crunch Bar)	310	3.0	24.0	23.0	15	85	<1.0
caramel fudge swirl (*Endulge* Caramel Turtle Sundae)	180	2.0	12.0	16.0	30	35	4.0
caramel and peanuts, w/chocolate:							
(*Klondike Planters*)	300	4.0	28.0	20.0	15	150	1.0
(*Klondike Planters* Single)	290	4.0	25.0	19.0	15	150	<1.0
caramel crunch (*Klondike*)	270	3.0	26.0	17.0	25	80	0
cherry, w/chocolate (*Ben & Jerry's* Cherry Garcia) ..	280	4.0	29.0	18.0	35	55	2.0
chocolate, w/chocolate:							
(*Dove* Original 4-Pack)	260	4.0	27.0	17.0	25	30	3.0
(*Dove* Original Single)	320	4.0	32.0	21.0	30	40	3.0
(*Klondike*)	280	3.0	23.0	19.0	20	55	<1.0
dark (*Häagen-Dazs*)	300	4.0	24.0	21.0	70	40	<1.0
chocolate éclair:							
(*Eskimo Pie*)	220	2.0	26.0	12.0	15	45	<1.0
(*Eskimo Pie* King Size)	240	3.0	31.0	13.0	15	125	1.0
(*Eskimo Pie* Premium King Size Single)	220	2.0	26.0	12.0	15	45	<1.0
(*Good Humor*), 3 fl. oz.	160	2.0	20.0	8.0	5	60	<1.0
(*Good Humor*), 4 fl. oz.	220	2.0	30.0	11.0	10	85	<1.0
(*Hood*)	150	1.0	14.0	10.0	5	45	0
(*No Pudge*)	110	3.0	23.0	1.5	<5	95	4.0
(*Popsicle Col. Crunch*)	160	2.0	20.0	8.0	5	70	<1.0
chocolate fudge swirl:							
(*Endulge*)	180	2.0	12.0	16.0	30	25	4.0
(*Endulge* Single) ..	180	3.0	12.0	16.0	30	25	4.0
coffee, w/chocolate (*Klondike* Cappuccino Bar)	280	3.0	24.0	19.0	20	70	0
coffee almond crunch (*Häagen-Dazs*)	310	4.0	23.0	22.0	75	65	<1.0

Food and Measure	cal.	prot. (gms)	carbo. (gms)	fat (gms)	chol. (mgs)	sod. (mgs)	fiber (gms)
cookies and cream:							
(*Eskimo Pie* No Sugar)	130	3.0	15.0	8.0	5	70	3.0
(*Good Humor*)	190	2.0	21.0	12.0	10	120	<1.0
(*No Pudge*)	110	6.0	21.0	2.5	<5	95	6.0
cookie coated (*Good Humor Oreo*) ...	250	3.0	28.0	15.0	15	160	<1.0
dulce de leche (*Häagen-Dazs*)	300	4.0	28.0	19.0	60	70	0
fudge, w/chocolate (*Darigold* Fudge & Cream)	170	2.0	17.0	11.0	15	60	0
mint, w/chocolate:							
(*Eskimo Pie* Peppermint Pattie)	250	3.0	24.0	16.0	25	55	1.0
(*Eskimo Pie* Thin Mint)	250	3.0	23.0	17.0	25	50	1.0
(*Klondike* York Peppermint Pattie)	280	3.0	24.0	19.0	20	55	<1.0
Neapolitan, w/chocolate (*Klondike*)	280	3.0	24.0	19.0	20	65	<1.0
peanut butter:							
(*Darigold* Cup)	200	3.0	13.0	15.0	15	50	0
(*Good Humor Reese's*)	310	4.0	27.0	21.0	20	90	<1.0
w/chocolate (*Butterfinger*) ...	210	2.0	17.0	15.0	15	50	0
swirl (*Endulge*) ...	180	3.0	12.0	16.0	30	40	4.0
strawberry shortcake:							
(*Eskimo Pie*)	220	3.0	26.0	12.0	15	70	0
(*Eskimo Pie* King Size)	250	2.0	30.0	13.0	15	105	<1.0
(*Eskimo Pie* Premium Single)	220	2.0	26.0	12.0	15	70	0
(*Eskimo Pie* Reduced Fat)	110	2.0	15.0	7.0	5	15	3.0
(*Good Humor*), 3 fl. oz.	170	1.0	21.0	9.0	5	60	0
(*Good Humor*), 4 fl. oz.	230	2.0	30.0	12.0	10	90	<1.0
(*No Pudge*)	110	3.0	23.0	1.5	<5	85	4.0
(*Popsicle Col. Crunch*)	170	1.0	21.0	9.0	5	60	0
toffee w/chocolate (*Klondike Heath*) ..	300	3.0	26.0	20.0	20	100	0

Food and Measure	cal.	prot. (gms)	carbo. (gms)	fat (gms)	chol. (mgs)	sod. (mgs)	fiber (gms)
Ice cream bar *(cont.)*							
vanilla w/chocolate:							
(*Darigold*)	180	2.0	14.0	13.0	20	40	0
(*Good Humor*), 2.75 fl. oz.	180	2.0	19.0	11.0	10	30	<1.0
(*Good Humor*), 4 fl. oz.	260	3.0	23.0	17.0	15	55	<1.0
(*Hood*)	160	1.0	11.0	12.0	15	45	0
(*Klondike* Original) .	280	3.0	24.0	19.0	20	75	0
(*Klondike* Slim-a Bear No Sugar Reduced Fat) ...	170	4.0	21.0	9.0	5	65	4.0
(*Popsicle*)	160	2.0	15.0	11.0	15	35	1.0
(*Popsicle Sprinklers*), 2.1 fl. oz.	130	1.0	18.0	6.0	10	25	0
(*Popsicle Sprinklers*), 3 fl. oz.	180	1.0	26.0	8.0	10	35	0
almond (*Klondike Hershey*)	250	4.0	20.0	18.0	20	80	<1.0
chocolate stripe (*Good Humor Number 1 Bar*) ..	200	2.0	21.0	11.0	10	50	<1.0
crisps (*Eskimo Pie* No Sugar)	120	3.0	13.0	8.0	10	40	0
crisps (*Klondike Krunch*), 4 fl. oz.	260	3.0	24.0	17.0	15	75	0
crisps (*Klondike Krunch*), 5 fl. oz.	280	3.0	25.0	19.0	20	90	0
dark (*Eskimo Pie*) .	160	2.0	15.0	10.0	15	35	0
dark (*Dove* Original 4-Pack)	260	3.0	26.0	17.0	30	35	2.0
dark (*Dove* Original Single)	320	4.0	32.0	21.0	35	45	2.0
dark (*Endulge*)	180	3.0	11.0	16.0	30	35	3.0
dark (*Eskimo Pie* Giant King Size Single)	410	5.0	35.0	29.0	35	80	2.0
dark (*Eskimo Pie* King Size)	220	3.0	21.0	14.0	25	50	<1.0
dark (*Eskimo Pie* No Sugar)	120	3.0	13.0	8.0	10	40	0
dark (*Good Humor*)	190	2.0	15.0	13.0	10	35	<1.0
dark (*Häagen-Dazs*)	300	4.0	23.0	21.0	70	45	<1.0
dark (*Klondike*) ...	280	3.0	24.0	19.0	20	55	<1.0

Food and Measure	cal.	prot. (gms)	carbo. (gms)	fat (gms)	chol. (mgs)	sod. (mgs)	fiber (gms)
dark, miniatures (*Dove* Original), 5 pcs.	320	4.0	32.0	20.0	45	40	2.0
milk (*Dove* 4-Pack)	260	3.0	25.0	17.0	30	60	1.0
milk (*Dove* Single)	330	4.0	31.0	21.0	40	60	1.0
milk (*Endulge*)	180	3.0	12.0	16.0	30	25	4.0
milk (*Endulge* Single)	180	2.0	12.0	16.0	30	20	5.0
milk (*Eskimo Pie*)	160	2.0	14.0	11.0	20	35	0
milk (*Eskimo Pie* King Size/Premium)	220	3.0	21.0	15.0	25	50	0
milk (*Eskimo Pie* King Size Single)	250	3.0	23.0	17.0	30	55	0
milk (*Good Humor*)	180	2.0	15.0	13.0	15	45	0
milk (*Häagen-Dazs*)	290	4.0	22.0	21.0	75	55	0
milk, w/almonds (*Dove* 4-Pack)	270	5.0	23.0	18.0	30	110	1.0
milk, w/almonds (*Dove* Single)	340	6.0	28.0	23.0	35	135	1.0
milk, caramel toffee crunch (*Dove* 4-Pack)	270	3.0	29.0	16.0	30	90	1.0
milk, caramel toffee crunch (*Dove* Single)	330	4.0	35.0	20.0	35	110	1.0
milk, w/crunchy cookies (*Dove* 4-Pack)	280	3.0	27.0	18.0	25	75	1.0
milk, miniatures (*Dove* Original), 5 pcs.	320	4.0	30.0	20.0	30	55	1.0
mini (*Klondike* Snack Size), 2 pcs.	170	2.0	15.0	11.0	15	45	0
mini (*Klondike* Movie Bites), 4.48-fl.-oz. pkg.	310	4.0	26.0	22.0	25	70	0
mini (*Popsicle*), 2 pcs.	200	2.0	18.0	13.0	15	40	0
vanilla cookie (*Popsicle WWE*)	180	2.0	23.0	9.0	10	95	<1.0
vanilla almond (*Ben & Jerry's*)	340	5.0	30.0	23.0	65	135	2.0
vanilla w/chocolate ice cream (*Endulge* Fudge & Cream)	70	2.0	7.0	6.0	20	10	2.0

Food and Measure	cal.	prot. (gms)	carbo. (gms)	fat (gms)	chol. (mgs)	sod. (mgs)	fiber (gms)
Ice cream bar *(cont.)*							
vanilla fudge swirl							
(*Endulge*)	180	2.0	12.0	16.0	30	25	4.0
"Ice cream" bar,							
nondairy, 1 bar:							
chocolate:							
(*RiceDream*)	270	2.0	32.0	15.0	0	95	2.0
w/nuts (*RiceDream*							
Nutty Bar)	270	4.0	23.0	18.0	0	55	2.0
chocolate fudge:							
(*Tofutti* Coffee Break)	30	1.0	6.0	0	0	86	0
(*Tofutti* Totally Fudge)	95	1.0	19.0	1.5	0	53	0
(*Tofutti* Treats)	30	1.0	6.0	0	0	86	0
chocolate center:							
peanut butter, dark							
chocolate (*Tofutti*							
Monkey Bars) . . .	220	3.0	22.0	13.0	0	105	0
vanilla, dark choco-							
late (*Tofutti* Hooray							
Hooray No Sugar)	150	2.0	10.0	9.0	0	90	0
vanilla:							
(*RiceDream*)	270	1.0	33.0	14.0	0	95	1.0
w/dark chocolate							
(*Tofutti* Marry Me)	160	2.0	22.0	8.0	0	105	0
w/fruit ice coating							
(*Tofutti* Kid Sticks)	110	1.0	15.0	4.0	0	80	0
w/nuts (*RiceDream*							
Nutty Bar)	260	4.0	23.0	18.0	0	55	2.0
vanilla, chocolate, or							
strawberry, w/dark							
chocolate (*Tofutti*							
Delights)	120	2.0	7.0	7.0	0	80	0
Ice cream cone, filled,							
1 pc.:							
(*Choco Taco*)	290	4.0	35.0	16.0	10	115	1.0
chocolate, w/chocolate							
(*Klondike* Slim-a-							
Bear 96% Fat Free)	180	3.0	36.0	3.0	0	125	3.0
chocolate, w/nuts:							
(*Drumstick* Sundae)	360	5.0	33.0	23.0	25	100	<1.0
(*Klondike*)	280	5.0	29.0	16.0	15	75	1.0
cookies and cream:							
(*Eskimo Pie*)	140	4.0	28.0	4.5	5	130	5.0
(*No Pudge*)	140	4.0	29.0	3.0	<5	130	3.0

Food and Measure	cal.	prot. (gms)	carbo. (gms)	fat (gms)	chol. (mgs)	sod. (mgs)	fiber (gms)
mint, w/nuts (*Drumstick* Sundae)	330	4.0	38.0	18.0	25	135	<1.0
vanilla, w/chocolate: (Klondike Slim-a-Bear 96% Fat Free)	170	3.0	35.0	3.0	0	125	3.0
and brownie (*No Pudge* Fudgy Brownie Cones) .	140	4.0	32.0	2.5	<5	115	4.0
and candy (*M&M's*)	230	3.0	32.0	11.0	20	95	1.0
vanilla, w/chocolate, nuts:							
(*Drumstick* Sundae)	340	5.0	33.0	21.0	20	90	<1.0
(*Endulge*)	230	5.0	19.0	18.0	35	30	7.0
(*Eskimo Pie* Giant Sundae)	250	4.0	30.0	13.0	15	100	1.0
(*Eskimo Pie* No Sugar)	200	5.0	24.0	12.0	15	100	<1.0
(*Good Humor* Sundae), 4 fl. oz.	270	4.0	31.0	15.0	15	90	1.0
(*Good Humor* Sundae), 4.3 fl. oz.	270	4.0	29.0	15.0	15	95	<1.0
(*Good Humor* Giant King Cone)	400	7.0	44.0	22.0	35	130	1.0
(*Good Humor* King Cone)	250	4.0	30.0	13.0	15	100	<1.0
(*Hood Nutty Royale*)	220	4.0	26.0	12.0	20	80	<1.0
(*Klondike*)	280	5.0	29.0	16.0	15	85	<1.0
(*Klondike Big Bear* Sundae)	300	5.0	31.0	17.0	15	90	<1.0
(*No Pudge* Sundae)	110	7.0	22.0	3.5	<5	55	5.0
w/caramel (*Drumstick* Sundae) . . .	360	5.0	36.0	22.0	25	100	<1.0
w/caramel (*Klondike*)	300	5.0	34.0	16.0	15	110	<1.0
w/caramel (*Klondike Big Bear* Sundae)	320	5.0	35.0	18.0	15	115	<1.0
w/fudge (*Klondike*)	300	5.0	34.0	16.0	15	80	<1.0
w/fudge (*Klondike Big Bear* Sundae)	320	5.0	36.0	17.0	15	85	<1.0
vanilla fudge (*Turkey Hill* Sundae)	320	6.0	33.0	18.0	20	120	2.0
Ice cream cone/cup, unfilled, 1 pc.:							
bowl (*Keebler*)	50	<1.0	10.0	1.0	0	25	0

Food and Measure	cal.	prot. (gms)	carbo. (gms)	fat (gms)	chol. (mgs)	sod. (mgs)	fiber (gms)
Ice cream cone/cup *(cont.)*							
cone:							
chocolate (*Oreo*) ..	60	1.0	12.0	.5	0	75	0
sugar (*Comet*)	60	1.0	12.0	0	0	5	0
sugar (*Keebler*) ...	50	1.0	10.0	.5	0	55	0
waffle (*Keebler*) ...	50	<1.0	10.0	1.0	0	25	0
cup:							
(*Comet*)	20	0	4.0	0	0	10	0
(*Keebler*)	15	0	4.0	0	0	20	0
fudge dipped							
(*Keebler Fudge*							
Shoppe)	35	0	6.0	1.5	0	20	0
rainbow (*Comet*) ..	20	0	4.0	0	1	10	0
Ice cream cup, filled,							
1 cup:							
sundae:							
(*Hoodsie*), 3 fl. oz. .	120	1.0	19.0	5.0	15	40	0
(*Klondike*), 6 fl. oz.	280	6.0	26.0	17.0	35	75	<1.0
vanilla (*Hoodsie*),							
3 fl. oz.	100	2.0	12.0	5.0	20	35	0
vanilla, w/chocolate							
strawberry swirl							
(*Good Humor*							
Swirland), 6 fl. oz. .	160	4.0	31.0	2.5	10	110	0
vanilla, w/root beer							
(*Barq's Floatz*),							
4 fl. oz.	120	<1.0	22.0	3.0	10	25	0
Ice cream dessert:							
brownie:							
à la mode (*Smart*							
Ones), 3.1 oz. ..	190	5.0	33.0	4.0	30	190	2.0
parfait, double fudge							
(*Smart Ones*),							
3.8 oz.	260	5.0	43.0	3.0	10	200	1.0
chocolate chip cookie							
dough sundae							
(*Smart Ones*), 2.6 oz.	190	3.0	35.0	4.5	5	120	1.0
Ice cream pie, see							
"Ice cream sandwich"							
Ice cream sandwich,							
w/chocolate wafers,							
except as noted, 1 pc:							
chocolate (*Endulge*) ..	150	6.0	16.0	10.0	25	80	5.0

Food and Measure	cal.	prot. (gms)	carbo. (gms)	fat (gms)	chol. (mgs)	sod. (mgs)	fiber (gms)
chocolate chip:							
malt (*Turkey Hill*) ..	210	3.0	32.0	8.0	20	190	1.0
mint (*Turkey Hill* No Sugar)	160	4.0	31.0	4.5	5	140	5.0
vanilla:							
(*Chipwich*)	250	4.0	37.0	11.0	15	115	0
(*Chipwich* King) .	310	4.0	45.0	13.0	20	140	<1.0
(*Chipwich* No Sugar)	190	4.0	36.0	8.0	<5	60	3.0
vanilla fudge (*Chipwich*)	200	4.0	36.0	5.0	5	130	2.0
cookies and cream:							
(*Eskimo Pie*)	230	3.0	34.0	9.0	10	310	1.0
w/sugar cookies (*Chilly Bears*) ...	180	2.0	24.0	9.0	25	115	<1.0
mint (*Klondike* Slim-a-Bear 98% Fat Free)	130	4.0	28.0	1.5	5	120	3.0
mint chocolate chip (*Hood*)	100	2.0	15.0	4.0	10	85	0
Neapolitan:							
(*Darigold*)	190	3.0	28.0	7.0	20	170	0
(*Good Humor* Giant)	250	4.0	37.0	10.0	20	210	<1.0
(*Klondike Big Bear*), 4.23 fl. oz.	190	3.0	28.0	7.0	15	170	<1.0
(*Klondike Big Bear*), 7 fl. oz.	300	5.0	42.0	12.0	25	230	1.0
peanut butter ripple (*Turkey Hill*)	220	4.0	28.0	10.0	20	200	1.0
vanilla:							
(*Darigold*)	190	3.0	28.0	8.0	20	170	0
(*Endulge*)	150	5.0	15.0	10.0	25	80	4.0
(*Eskimo Pie* Giant King Size)	250	4.0	36.0	10.0	20	210	0
(*Eskimo Pie* No Sugar)	160	4.0	27.0	4.0	10	135	<1.0
(*Eskimo Pie* Slender Pie Clamshell No Sugar)	120	4.0	28.0	1.5	<5	130	4.0
(*Good Humor*), 3 fl. oz.	160	2.0	25.0	6.0	10	140	<1.0
(*Good Humor*), 3.5 fl. oz.	160	3.0	25.0	6.0	10	160	0
(*Good Humor* Giant), 6 fl. oz.	250	4.0	36.0	10.0	20	210	0

Food and Measure	cal.	prot. (gms)	carbo. (gms)	fat (gms)	chol. (mgs)	sod. (mgs)	fiber (gms)
Ice cream sandwich, vanilla *(cont.)*							
(*Healthy Choice*) . .	130	2.0	24.0	3.0	5	150	<1.0
(*Hood*)	180	3.0	27.0	7.0	20	170	1.0
(*Hood* Light)	160	3.0	29.0	3.5	10	160	1.0
(*Hood* Lowfat)	90	2.0	15.0	1.5	5	75	0
(*Klondike* Slim-a-Bear 98% Fat Free)	130	4.0	28.0	1.5	5	120	3.0
(*Klondike* Slim-a-Bear No Sugar) .	120	4.0	25.0	3.0	5	230	2.0
(*Klondike Big Bear*), 4.23 fl. oz.	190	3.0	28.0	7.0	15	170	0
(*Klondike Big Bear*), 7 fl. oz.	300	5.0	42.0	12.0	25	240	<1.0
(*Popsicle* Mini)	100	2.0	15.0	3.5	5	95	0
(*Turkey Hill*)	190	3.0	26.0	8.0	25	180	0
(*Turkey Hill* Double Decker)	200	3.0	29.0	8.0	20	170	1.0
brownie, w/candy (*M&M's*)	220	3.0	28.0	10.0	25	135	0
brownie batter swirl (*No Pudge*)	140	4.0	30.0	2.0	<5	160	3.0
brownie chunk (*No Pudge*)	140	4.0	30.0	2.0	<5	150	4.0
chocolate chip cookie (*Good Humor*) . .	290	3.0	41.0	13.0	20	210	1.0
chocolate chip cookie, giant (*Klondike Hershey*)	470	7.0	66.0	20.0	30	65	2.0
chocolate chip cookie (*Klondike Big Bear*)	270	3.0	38.0	12.0	15	210	1.0
gingerbread cookie (*Eskimo Pie* Gingerbread Men)	160	2.0	26.0	6.0	15	180	<1.0
peanut butter candy (*Klondike Reese's Pieces*)	260	4.0	37.0	12.0	10	180	1.0
vanilla cookie, w/candy (*M&M's*)	220	3.0	29.0	11.0	25	170	1.0
vanilla, w/cookie pieces (*Klondike Oreo* Cookie)	230	3.0	34.0	9.0	10	310	2.0
vanilla caramel swirl, vanilla cookie (*Healthy Choice*) . .	140	2.0	27.0	3.0	5	120	<1.0

Food and Measure	cal.	prot. (gms)	carbo. (gms)	fat (gms)	chol. (mgs)	sod. (mgs)	fiber (gms)
vanilla fudge:							
(*Eskimo Pie* Slender Pie Clamshell No Sugar)	120	4.0	28.0	1.5	<5	130	4.0
swirl (*Healthy Choice*)	140	2.0	27.0	3.0	5	150	<1.0
vanilla fudge chip, w/fudge swirl cookie (*Ben & Jerry's* 'Wich)	350	4.0	45.0	18.0	55	220	1.0
vanilla strawberry chocolate (*Eskimo Pie* Giant King Size)	250	4.0	37.0	10.0	20	210	1.0
"Ice cream" sandwich, nondairy, w/wafers, 1 pc.:							
blueberry swirl, mini (*Tofutti Cuties*)	140	2.0	20.0	6.0	0	130	0
chocolate:							
(*RiceDream* Pie) . . .	320	3.0	39.0	18.0	0	80	2.0
(*SoyDelicious* Li'l Buddies)	150	3.0	28.0	4.5	0	25	3.0
mini (*Tofutti Cuties*)	130	2.0	16.0	5.0	0	110	0
swirl, mini (*Tofutti Cuties* Wave) . . .	140	2.0	20.0	6.0	0	130	0
chocolate chip, w/chocolate chip wafers (*Tofutti* Too Too's)	230	3.0	30.0	11.0	0	155	0
coffee, mini (*Tofutti Cuties* Coffee Break)	130	2.0	16.0	5.0	0	110	0
cookies and cream, mini (*Tofutti Cuties*)	120	2.0	17.0	6.0	0	135	0
mint:							
(*RiceDream* Pie) . . .	320	3.0	39.0	18.0	0	80	2.0
chocolate chip, mini (*Tofutti Cuties*) . .	120	2.0	19.0	5.0	0	110	0
mocha (*RiceDream* Pie)	320	3.0	40.0	17.0	0	80	1.0
peanut butter, mini (*Tofutti Cuties*)	165	3.0	20.0	8.0	0	135	0
strawberry swirl, mini (*Tofutti Cuties* Wave)	140	2.0	20.0	6.0	0	130	0
vanilla:							
(*RiceDream* Pie) . . .	320	3.0	40.0	17.0	0	80	1.0
(*Soy Delicious* Li'l Buddies)	160	3.0	28.0	4.5	0	30	3.0

Food and Measure	cal.	prot. (gms)	carbo. (gms)	fat (gms)	chol. (mgs)	sod. (mgs)	fiber (gms)
"Ice cream" sandwich, nondairy, vanilla *(cont.)*							
mini (*Tofutti Cuties*)	120	2.0	17.0	5.0	0	121	0
mini (*Tofutti Cuties No Sugar*)	100	1.0	11.0	5.0	0	86	0
w/vanilla wafer, mini (*Tofutti Cuties*) ..	120	2.0	16.0	5.0	0	110	0
wildberry, mini (*Tofutti Cuties*)	120	2.0	17.0	5.0	0	121	0
Ice cream and sherbet or sorbet, see "Sherbet" and "Sorbet"							
Iced confection bar, dairy (see also "Ice bar" and "Fruit bar"), 1 pc.:							
all varieties:							
(*CarbSmart Creamsicle*)	20	1.0	5.0	1.0	0	0	1.0
(*Hawaiian Punch Arctic Surfer Pops*)	50	0	12.0	0	0	5	0
(*Popsicle Rainbow Floats*)	60	1.0	11.0	1.5	5	15	0
(*Popsicle Sherbet Cyclone*)	50	1.0	11.0	.5	0	10	0
coffee:							
(*Frappuccino*)	110	4.0	20.0	1.5	5	45	9.0
fudge (*Frappuccino Java Fudge*)	130	4.0	25.0	2.0	5	50	4.0
fudge (*Hood* Java Smoothie)	90	1.0	17.0	2.5	10	30	0
fudge:							
(*Darigold* Super Fudge)	180	5.0	30.0	5.0	20	135	1.0
(*Eskimo Pie* No Sugar)	60	2.0	11.0	1.0	10	60	0
(*Fudgsicle*), 1.75 fl. oz.	60	2.0	11.0	1.0	5	45	<1.0
(*Fudgsicle*), 2.5 fl. oz.	100	2.0	18.0	2.0	0	65	1.0
(*Fudgsicle*), 2.7 fl. oz.	90	3.0	17.0	1.5	5	65	<1.0
(*Fudgsicle* Fat Free)	60	3.0	14.0	0	0	50	<1.0
(*Fudgsicle* Mini), 2 bars	80	3.0	16.0	1.5	0	60	<1.0
(*Fudgsicle* No Sugar 12 Pack), 2 bars	70	1.0	12.0	1.5	0	95	0

Food and Measure	cal.	prot. (gms)	carbo. (gms)	fat (gms)	chol. (mgs)	sod. (mgs)	fiber (gms)
(*Fudgsicle* No Sugar 20 Pack), 2 bars	80	3.0	18.0	1.5	0	95	4.0
(*Fudgsicle* Sugar Free), 2 bars ...	70	4.0	9.0	0	0	0	2.0
(*Healthy Choice*) ..	80	3.0	13.0	1.0	5	60	0
(*Hendrie's* Fat Free Stix)	60	1.0	15.0	0	0	50	1.0
(*Klondike* Slim-a-Bear)	90	3.0	22.0	1.5	5	90	4.0
(*Simply Slender*), 1.75 fl. oz.	50	2.0	9.0	1.5	5	40	0
(*Simply Slender*), 2.5 fl. oz.	85	2.0	21.0	.5	0	70	1.0
chocolate (*Endulge*)	130	2.0	12.0	11.0	40	20	5.0
double (*Superscile* Firecracker)	150	5.0	29.0	2.0	10	95	<1.0
mocha (*Frappuccino*) .	120	4.0	22.0	2.0	10	50	3.0
orange sherbet (*Popsicle Pop-Ups*)	80	<1.0	19.0	1.0	<5	15	0
orange sherbet/vanilla ice cream:							
(*Creamsicle*), 1.75 fl. oz.	70	1.0	13.0	2.0	5	20	0
(*Creamsicle*), 2.5 fl. oz.	100	1.0	18.0	2.5	5	30	0
(*Creamsicle*), 2.7 fl. oz.	110	1.0	20.0	3.0	10	30	0
(*Creamsicle* No Sugar)	25	1.0	5.0	0	0	10	1.0
(*Creamsicle* Sugar Free), 2 bars ...	40	1.0	10.0	2.0	0	0	6.0
(*Hood* Orange Cream)	90	1.0	18.0	1.5	5	30	0
(*Minute Maid* Swirl Bars), 3-oz. tube	90	0	16.0	3.0	10	25	0
rainbow (*Popsicle Pop-Ups*)	90	<1.0	19.0	1.0	<5	15	0
Icing, cake, see "Frosting"							
Irish cream syrup (*Ferrara*), 2 oz.	130	0	32.0	0	0	12	0

J

Food and Measure	cal.	prot. (gms)	carbo. (gms)	fat (gms)	chol. (mgs)	sod. (mgs)	fiber (gms)
Jack in the Box, 1 serving:							
breakfast:							
biscuit, sausage . . .	600	13.0	41.0	36.0	35	1200	2.0
w/egg, cheese . .	970	26.0	50.0	68.0	280	1905	2.0
burrito	580	34.0	32.0	38.0	440	1410	22.0
w/salsa	580	35.0	34.0	38.0	440	1530	22.0
meaty	480	25.0	29.0	29.0	345	1190	2.0
meaty, w/salsa . .	490	25.0	30.0	29.0	345	1310	2.0
Breakfast Jack	305	13.0	34.0	14.0	205	715	0
croissant, sausage .	605	18.0	42.0	40.5	240	725	1.0
croissant, supreme	475	16.0	41.0	27.0	220	815	1.0
hash browns	150	1.0	13.0	10.0	0	230	2.0
sausage sandwich,							
extreme	690	25.0	37.0	50.0	280	1265	0
sourdough sandwich	445	16.0	37.0	26.0	215	875	2.0
ultimate sandwich .	605	26.0	58.0	30.5	425	1630	2.0
burgers:							
cheeseburger:							
bacon bacon . . .	780	33.0	50.0	49.5	90	1545	2.0
junior bacon	525	21.0	32.0	36.0	70	880	0
ultimate	945	39.0	52.0	64.5	120	1525	2.0
ultimate, bacon .	1025	46.0	53.0	70.5	135	1985	2.0
hamburger	310	17.0	30.0	14.0	45	590	0
w/cheese	355	19.0	31.0	17.5	55	770	0
deluxe	370	17.0	32.0	21.0	50	545	0
deluxe w/cheese .	460	21.0	34.0	28.0	75	915	0
Jumbo Jack	600	20.0	52.0	34.5	45	935	2.0
w/cheese	695	24.0	55.0	41.5	70	1305	2.0
Sourdough Jack . . .	715	26.0	36.0	51.0	75	1165	2.0
chicken/fish:							
chicken breast strips	630	35.0	39.0	38.0	90	1470	3.0
chicken ciabatta:							
bruschetta	660	41.0	69.0	26.0	85	1880	4.0
classic	510	36.0	69.0	13.0	65	1700	4.0

Food and Measure	cal.	prot. (gms)	carbo. (gms)	fat (gms)	chol. (mgs)	sod. (mgs)	fiber (gms)
chicken fajita pita ..	315	22.0	33.0	9.0	65	1080	0
chicken sandwich ..	390	15.0	39.0	21.0	35	730	1.0
w/bacon	440	19.0	39.0	24.0	40	970	2.0
w/cheese	430	17.0	40.0	24.0	45	880	1.0
Cordon Blue	555	40.0	33.0	28.0	100	1335	2.0
fish & chips	840	16.0	69.0	56.0	55	1600	4.0
Jack's Spicy Chicken	615	24.0	62.0	30.5	50	1090	3.0
w/cheese	695	29.0	63.0	36.5	70	1400	3.0
sourdough grilled chicken club	505	29.0	35.0	27.0	75	1220	2.0
Southwest pita	260	20.0	35.0	4.5	40	880	4.0
sandwiches:							
Pannido:							
deli trio	645	30.0	53.0	34.0	95	2530	2.0
ham & turkey ...	610	36.0	54.0	29.0	110	1785	2.0
zesty turkey	740	40.0	51.0	43.5	135	1880	2.0
ultimate club	630	36.0	52.0	29.0	105	1985	2.0
tacos/snacks:							
bacon cheddar potato wedges ..	620	18.0	45.0	41.0	55	1300	5.0
egg roll, 1 pc......	175	5.0	26.0	6.0	5	470	2.0
egg roll, 3 pcs.....	445	14.0	55.0	19.0	15	1080	6.0
jalapeños, stuffed:							
3 pcs.	230	7.0	22.0	13.0	20	690	2.0
7 pcs.	530	15.0	51.0	30.0	45	1600	4.0
taco	160	5.0	15.0	8.0	15	270	2.0
taco, monster	240	8.0	20.0	14.0	20	390	3.0
fries:							
natural:							
large	530	8.0	69.0	25.0	0	870	5.0
medium	360	5.0	47.0	17.0	0	590	4.0
small	270	4.0	35.0	12.0	0	440	3.0
seasoned curly:							
large	550	8.0	60.0	31.0	0	1200	6.0
medium	400	6.0	45.0	23.0	0	890	5.0
small	270	4.0	30.0	15.0	0	590	3.0
onion rings	500	6.0	51.0	30.0	0	420	3.0
salad:							
chicken, Asian	595	20.0	58.0	32.5	25	1315	8.0
chicken, Southwest	735	29.0	56.0	44.5	95	2135	7.0
chicken Caesar	220	26.0	10.0	8.0	55	1030	3.0
chicken club	825	34.0	34.0	61.5	95	2065	5.0
side salad	155	5.0	16.0	7.5	10	290	0

Food and Measure	cal.	prot. (gms)	carbo. (gms)	fat (gms)	chol. (mgs)	sod. (mgs)	fiber (gms)
Jack in the Box *(cont.)*							
sauces/dressing:							
dipping sauce:							
barbecue	45	0	11.0	0	0	330	0
buttermilk house	130	0	3.0	13.0	10	210	0
Franks Red Hot							
Buffalo	10	0	2.0	0	0	840	0
tartar	210	0	2.0	22.0	20	370	0
sweet and sour .	45	0	11.0	0	0	160	0
dressing:							
balsamic, low fat	40	0	6.0	2.0	0	600	0
creamy Caesar ..	310	3.0	6.0	30.0	35	800	0
ranch	390	1.0	4.0	41.0	30	590	0
ranch, light	190	1.0	3.0	18.0	25	700	0
herb mayo, reduced							
fat	15	0	1.0	1.0	0	110	0
mayo onion sauce .	60	0	1.0	7.0	5	60	0
soy sauce	5	1.0	1.0	0	0	480	0
taco sauce	90	0	0	0	0	80	0
shakes, ice cream:							
caramel, creamy:							
large	1330	22.0	173.0	59.0	235	570	1.0
medium	860	15.0	109.0	40.0	155	360	0
small	670	11.0	87.0	30.0	115	290	0
chocolate:							
large	1310	23.0	178.0	57.0	225	540	2.0
medium	850	15.0	111.0	38.0	150	340	1.0
small	660	11.0	89.0	29.0	110	270	1.0
Oreo cookie:							
large	1350	22.0	161.0	66.0	225	700	2.0
medium	870	15.0	103.0	43.0	150	420	1.0
small	670	11.0	81.0	33.0	110	350	1.0
strawberry:							
large	1270	21.0	167.0	56.0	225	440	0
medium	830	14.0	106.0	38.0	150	300	0
small	640	10.0	84.0	28.0	110	220	0
strawberry banana:							
large	1410	21.0	199.0	56.0	225	1260	0
medium	900	14.0	122.0	38.0	150	850	0
small	700	10.0	100.0	28.0	110	630	0
vanilla:							
large	1140	22.0	129.0	58.0	230	440	0
medium	750	14.0	85.0	38.0	150	290	0
small	570	11.0	65.0	29.0	115	220	0

Food and Measure	cal.	prot. (gms)	carbo. (gms)	fat (gms)	chol. (mgs)	sod. (mgs)	fiber (gms)
desserts:							
cheesecake	310	7.0	34.0	16.0	55	220	0
double fudge cake .	310	3.0	49.0	11.0	25	270	4.0
Jackfruit, fresh,							
trimmed, 1 oz.	27	.4	6.8	.1	0	1	.5
Jackfruit, canned, in							
syrup, ½ cup	82	.3	21.3	.1	0	10	.8
Jackson wonder bean,							
canned (*Westbrae*							
Natural Organic Heir-							
loom Beans), ½ cup	100	5.0	19.0	0	0	135	5.0
Jalapeño, see "Pepper,							
jalapeño"							
Jalapeño sauce, see							
"Hot sauce" and							
specific listings							
Jam and preserves (see							
also "Fruit spreads"),							
1 tbsp.:							
all fruits:							
(*Smucker's*)	50	0	13.0	0	0	0	0
(*Smucker's* Low							
Sugar)	25	0	6.0	0	0	0	0
except boysenberry							
(*Smucker's* Sugar							
Free)	10	0	5.0	0	0	0	0
boysenberry (*Smucker's*							
Sugar Free)	10	0	5.0	0	0	5	0
grapefruit marmalade,							
pink (*Bellisimo*) . . .	50	0	12.0	0	0	0	0
orange marmalade:							
(*Cascadian Farm*) . .	40	0	11.0	0	0	0	0
(*Dundee*)	50	0	14.0	0	0	0	0
Java plum:							
3 medium, .4 oz.	5	.1	1.4	<.1	0	1	<1.0
seeded, ½ cup	41	.5	10.5	.2	0	9	<1.0
Jelly, fruit, 1 tbsp.:							
all fruits (*Smucker's*) .	50	0	13.0	0	0	0	0
apple mint (*Great*							
Expectations)	50	0	13.0	0	0	5	0
guava (*Goya*)	58	0	14.0	0	0	0	0
Jelly, hot pepper							
(*Reese*), 1 tbsp. . . .	50	0	13.0	0	0	35	0

Food and Measure	cal.	prot. (gms)	carbo. (gms)	fat (gms)	chol. (mgs)	sod. (mgs)	fiber (gms)
Jerk sauce, see "Barbecue sauce" and "Marinade"							
Jerk seasoning:							
(*McCormick* Caribbean), ¼ tsp.	0	0	0	0	0	70	0
dry rub (*Neera's* Jamaican), 1 tsp. . .	5	0	2.0	0	0	185	0
spice paste (*Neera's* Jamaican), 2 tsp. . .	15	1.0	4.0	0	0	290	1.0
Jerusalem artichoke:							
(*Frieda's Sunchoke*), ½ cup, 3 oz.	70	2.0	14.0	0	0	0	1.0
sliced, ½ cup	57	1.5	13.1	<.1	0	3	1.2
Jew's ear, see "Pepeao"							
Jicama, see "Yam bean"							
Jujube:							
raw, seeded, 1 oz. . . .	22	.3	5.7	.1	0	1	n.a.
dried, 1 oz.	81	1.0	20.1	.3	0	3	n.a.
Jute, potherb, ½ cup:							
raw	5	.7	.8	<.1	0	1	n.a.
boiled, drained	16	1.6	3.1	.1	0	5	.9

K

Food and Measure	cal.	prot. (gms)	carbo. (gms)	fat (gms)	chol. (mgs)	sod. (mgs)	fiber (gms)
Kabocha squash (*Frieda's*), ¾ cup, 3 oz.	30	1.0	7.0	0	0	0	1.0
Kahn choy, see "Celery, Chinese"							
Kale, fresh:							
(*Glory*), 2.8 oz.	40	3.0	8.0	.5	0	35	2.0
raw, chopped, ½ cup .	17	1.1	3.4	.2	0	15	.7
boiled, drained, chopped, ½ cup . . .	18	1.2	3.7	.3	0	5	3.6
Kale, canned, ½ cup:							
(*Allens* No Salt)	30	2.0	3.0	.5	0	20	2.0
(*Bush's*)	30	2.0	4.0	0	0	330	2.0
seasoned:							
(*Allens/Sunshine*) .	35	3.0	5.0	.5	0	830	1.0
(*Glory*)	50	4.0	6.0	.5	0	440	3.0
Kale, frozen, boiled, drained, chopped, ½ cup	20	1.9	3.4	.3	0	10	1.3
Kale, Chinese, fresh:							
(*Frieda's* Chinese Broccoli), 1 cup, 3 oz.	15	2.0	3.0	0	0	15	0
cooked, 1 cup	19	1.0	3.3	.6	0	6	2.2
Kale, Scotch, ½ cup:							
raw, chopped	14	1.0	2.8	.2	0	24	.6
boiled, drained, chopped	18	1.2	3.7	.3	0	29	.8
Kamranga, see "Carambola"							
Kamut, grain (*Shiloh Farms*), ¼ cup	170	6.0	35.0	1.0	0	0	9.0
Kamut flakes, see "Cereal"							

Food and Measure	cal.	prot. (gms)	carbo. (gms)	fat (gms)	chol. (mgs)	sod. (mgs)	fiber (gms)
Kamut flour (*Arrowhead Mills*), ⅓ cup .	130	5.0	25.0	1.0	0	0	4.0
Kanpo, dried:							
.2-oz. strip	16	.5	4.1	<.1	0	1	n.a.
½ cup	70	2.3	15.6	.1	0	4	n.a.
Kasha, see "Buckwheat groats"							
Kefir, 8 fl. oz.:							
plain:							
(*Lifeway* Nonfat) . .	80	11.0	8.0	0	5	125	0
(*Lifeway* Original) . .	150	8.0	12.0	8.0	30	125	0
(*Lifeway* Organic/							
Lifeway Lowfat) .	110	14.0	8.0	2.5	10	125	0
(*Lifeway Slim6*) . . .	110	14.0	3.0	2.0	10	125	2.0
flavored, all varieties:							
(*Lifeway* Nonfat) . .	150	10.0	28.0	0	5	120	0
(*Lifeway* Organic/							
Lifeway Lowfat) .	160	14.0	21.0	2.0	10	125	0
(*Lifeway Slim6*) . . .	110	14.0	8.0	2.0	10	125	2.0
soy blend, see "Soy beverage"							
Ketchup, 1 tbsp.:							
(*Annie's Naturals* Organic)	15	0	3.0	0	0	150	0
(*Del Monte*)	15	0	4.0	0	0	190	0
(*Heinz*)	15	0	4.0	0	0	190	0
(*Hunt's*)	15	0	4.0	0	0	180	0
(*Hunt's* No Salt)	20	0	4.0	0	0	0	0
(*Muir Glen*)	15	0	4.0	0	0	240	0
(*Red Gold*)	20	0	5.0	0	0	180	0
(*Red Pack*)	15	0	4.0	0	0	190	0
(*S&W*)	20	0	4.0	0	0	150	0
(*Tree of Life*)	10	0	3.0	0	0	25	0
fruit sweetened:							
(*Westbrae Natural*)	10	0	3.0	0	0	90	0
(*Westbrae Natural* No Salt)	10	0	3.0	0	0	5	0
(*Westbrae Natural* Squeeze)	20	0	4.0	0	0	210	0
garlic, zesty (*Heinz*) . .	20	0	5.0	0	0	200	0
hot and spicy (*Heinz Kick'rs*)	20	0	4.0	0	0	200	0
jalapeño, smoked, spicy (*Fiesta*)	15	0	3.0	0	0	210	0

Food and Measure	cal.	prot. (gms)	carbo. (gms)	fat (gms)	chol. (mgs)	sod. (mgs)	fiber (gms)
unsweetened (*Westbrae Natural* UnKetchup)	5	0	1.0	0	0	60	0
KFC, 1 serving:							
chicken:							
Extra Crispy:							
breast	460	34.0	19.0	28.0	135	1230	0
drumstick	160	12.0	5.0	10.0	70	420	0
thigh	370	21.0	12.0	26.0	120	710	0
whole wing	190	10.0	10.0	12.0	55	390	0
hot and spicy:							
breast	460	33.0	20.0	27.0	130	1450	0
drumstick	150	13.0	4.0	9.0	65	380	0
thigh	400	22.0	14.0	28.0	125	1240	0
whole wing	180	11.0	9.0	11.0	60	420	0
Original Recipe:							
breast	380	40.0	11.0	19.0	145	1150	0
drumstick	140	14.0	4.0	8.0	75	440	0
thigh	360	22.0	12.0	25.0	165	1060	0
whole wing	150	110	5.0	9.0	60	370	0
chicken, popcorn:							
family	1210	77.0	73.0	68.0	200	3870	1.0
individual	380	24.0	23.0	21.0	60	1200	0
large	560	36.0	34.0	31.0	90	1790	1.0
chicken pot pie	770	33.0	70.0	40.0	115	1680	5.0
chicken strips, 3 pcs. .	400	29.0	17.0	24.0	75	1250	0
chicken wings, 6 pcs.:							
honey barbecue sauced	540	25.0	12.0	33.0	150	1130	1.0
Hot Wings	450	24.0	8.0	29.0	145	1120	1.0
meal, w/green beans, rice:							
strips, oven roasted	420	38.0	50.0	7.0	90	2410	6.0
Tender Roast fillet .	360	33.0	41.0	7.0	85	2010	4.0
sides, individual:							
baked beans	230	8.0	46.0	1.0	0	720	7.0
biscuit, 2 oz.	190	2.0	23.0	10.0	2	580	0
coleslaw	190	1.0	22.0	11.0	5	300	3.0
corn on cob, 3" . . .	70	2.0	13.0	1.5	0	5	3.0
corn on cob, 5.5" . .	150	5.0	26.0	3.0	0	10	7.0
green beans	50	2.0	7.0	1.5	5	570	2.0
macaroni and cheese	400	15.0	30.0	18.0	15	1920	4.0
potato salad	180	2.0	22.0	9.0	5	470	1.0
potato wedges	240	4.0	30.0	12.0	0	830	3.0

Food and Measure	cal.	prot. (gms)	carbo. (gms)	fat (gms)	chol. (mgs)	sod. (mgs)	fiber (gms)
KFC, sides *(cont.)*							
potatoes, mashed	110	2.0	16.0	4.0	0	260	1.0
w/gravy	120	2.0	18.0	4.5	0	380	1.0
rice, seasoned	150	4.0	32.0	1.0	0	640	2.0
sandwiches:							
crunch, double	530	6.0	42.0	28.0	55	1240	3.0
crunch, triple	650	8.0	49.0	34.0	75	1640	3.0
honey barbecue	300	22.0	41.0	6.0	55	920	1.0
KFC snacker	320	14.0	31.0	16.0	25	700	2.0
honey barbecue	220	15.0	32.0	3.5	35	490	2.0
Tender Roast	390	31.0	24.0	19.0	70	810	1.0
no sauce	260	31.0	23.0	5.0	65	690	1.0
Twister, crispy	670	27.0	55.0	38.0	60	1650	3.0
Twister, oven roast	510	29.0	50.0	22.0	70	1400	4.0
salad, no dressing or croutons:							
BLT, crispy	350	27.0	21.0	17.0	60	1170	4.0
BLT, roasted	210	28.0	8.0	7.0	70	900	4.0
Caesar, crispy	370	29.0	20.0	19.0	65	1110	3.0
Caesar, roasted	220	29.0	6.0	9.0	75	850	3.0
salad croutons, 1 pkt.	70	1.0	9.0	3.0	0	160	0
salad dressing, 1 pkt.:							
Caesar, Parmesan	260	2.0	4.0	26.0	15	530	0
Italian, light	40	<1.0	8.0	0	0	350	0
ranch	180	1.0	3.0	18.0	20	5	0
ranch, fat free	40	<1.0	8.0	0	0	370	0
dessert:							
apple pie, mini, 3	400	3.0	46.0	22.0	0	250	2.0
applesauce	100	0	24.0	0	0	0	1.0
cake, double chocolate chip	400	4.0	31.0	29.0	45	230	2.0
Lil' Bucket:							
chocolate cream	270	2.0	37.0	13.0	0	180	2.0
fudge brownie	270	2.0	44.0	9.0	30	170	1.0
lemon creme	400	4.0	65.0	14.0	5	210	2.0
strawberry short-cake	200	2.0	34.0	6.0	20	110	0
pie, 1 slice:							
apple	290	2.0	44.0	11.0	0	230	2.0
lemon meringue	240	1.0	40.0	9.0	0	230	1.0
pecan	480	5.0	68.0	21.0	40	360	2.0
sweet potato	340	5.0	44.0	16.0	5	210	1.0
Kidney beans:							
dry, dark *(Shiloh Farms),* ¼ cup	160	11.0	29.0	.5	0	0	10.0

Food and Measure	cal.	prot. (gms)	carbo. (gms)	fat (gms)	chol. (mgs)	sod. (mgs)	fiber (gms)
boiled, ½ cup	112	7.6	20.1	.4	0	2	6.5
Kidney beans, canned, ½ cup:							
red:							
(*Eden* Organic)	100	8.0	18.0	0	0	15	10.0
(*Progresso*)	110	7.0	20.0	.5	0	280	8.0
(*S&W*)	100	7.0	23.0	.5	0	460	6.0
(*S&W* 50% Less Salt)	120	7.0	21.0	.5	0	220	6.0
(*Westbrae Natural* Organic)	100	6.0	18.0	0	0	140	5.0
red, dark:							
(*Allens*)	130	8.0	22.0	.5	0	310	8.0
(*Bush's*)	130	8.0	21.0	1.0	0	260	7.0
(*Progresso*)	110	8.0	20.0	0	0	340	6.0
(*Trappey's*)	120	1.0	28.0	0	0	470	5.0
red, light:							
(*Allens/Trappey's*) .	120	6.0	22.0	.5	0	340	8.0
(*Bush's*)	110	7.0	20.0	0	0	260	7.0
w/bacon (*Trappey's*)	130	7.0	23.0	1.0	0	350	7.0
w/chili (*Trappey's*) .	110	6.0	20.0	1.0	0	510	7.0
w/jalapeno (*Trappey's*)	110	6.0	19.0	1.0	0	420	6.0
white (cannellini):							
(*Bush's*)	110	7.0	18.0	.5	0	300	6.0
(*Eden* Organic)	100	6.0	17.0	1.0	0	40	5.0
(*Goya*)	80	6.0	18.0	0	0	390	7.0
(*Progresso*)	100	5.0	16.0	.5	0	270	5.0
Kidney beans, sprouted, raw, ½ cup	27	3.9	3.8	.5	0	6	<1.0
Kidneys, braised:							
beef, 4 oz.	163	28.9	1.1	3.9	439	152	0
lamb, 4 oz.	155	26.8	1.1	4.1	641	171	0
pork, 4 oz.	171	28.8	0	5.3	544	91	0
pork, chopped, 1 cup .	211	35.6	0	6.6	673	111	0
veal, 4 oz.	185	29.8	0	6.4	897	125	0
Kielbasa, 2 oz.:							
(*Boar's Head*)	120	9.0	0	10.0	50	440	0
(*Healthy Choice* Polska)	80	7.0	6.0	2.5	25	480	0
turkey (*Louis Rich* Polska)	90	8.0	2.0	5.0	35	500	0
Kimchee (*Frieda's*), ¼ cup, 2 oz.	15	1.0	2.0	0	0	340	1.0
Kippers, see "Herring"							
Kiwi, fresh:							
(*Chiquita*), 2 medium, 5.2 oz.	100	2.0	24.0	1.0	0	0	4.0

Food and Measure	cal.	prot. (gms)	carbo. (gms)	fat (gms)	chol. (mgs)	sod. (mgs)	fiber (gms)
Kiwi *(cont.)*							
(*Del Monte*), 2 medium, 5.2 oz.	100	2.0	24.0	1.0	0	0	4.0
(*Dole*), 2 medium, 5.2 oz.	100	2.0	24.0	1.0	0	0	4.0
(*Frieda's/Frieda's* Baby/ Gold), 5 oz.	90	1.0	21.0 ·	.5	0	5	5.0
1 large, 3.7 oz.	55	.9	13.5	.4	0	4	3.1
1 medium, 3.1 oz. . . .	46	.8	11.3	.3	0	4	2.6
Kiwi drink blend, 8 fl. oz.:							
berry (*Nantucket Nectars*)	120	0	30.0	0	0	5	0
raspberry or strawberry (*Langers* Juice Cocktail)	120	0	29.0	0	0	0	0
strawberry:							
(*AriZona*)	120	0	29.0	0	0	20	0
(*Ocean Spray*)	120	0	31.0	0	0	35	0
(*Ocean Spray Cravin'* Less Sugar)	70	0	19.0	0	0	70	0
(*R.W. Knudsen*) . . .	120	<1.0	30.0	0	0	25	0
(*Snapple*)	110	0	28.0	0	0	10	0
(*Snapple* Diet)	20	0	5.0	0	0	10	0
Kiwi-strawberry juice (*Juicy Juice*), 8 fl. oz.	120	0	29.0	0	0	20	0
Knockwurst, 1 link:							
(*Karl Ehmer*), 4 oz. . .	250	15.0	1.0	20.0	65	850	0
(*Schaller & Weber* Knackwurst), 2 oz. .	140	8.0	2.0	11.0	30	380	0
beef:							
(*Boar's Head*), 4 oz.	310	15.0	1.0	27.0	70	950	0
(*Hebrew National*), 3 oz.	260	2.0	1.0	24.0	55	670	0
Kohlrabi:							
raw:							
(*Frieda's*), ⅔ cup, sliced, ½ cup . . .	19	1.2	4.3	.1	0	14	2.5
boiled, drained, sliced, ½ cup	24	1.5	5.5	.1	0	17	.9
Krispy Kreme:							
doughnuts, 1 pc.:							
blueberry, glazed . .	330	3.0	43.0	17.0	20	290	<1.0
blueberry filled, powdered	290	3.0	33.0	16.0	5	140	<1.0

Food and Measure	cal.	prot. (gms)	carbo. (gms)	fat (gms)	chol. (mgs)	sod. (mgs)	fiber (gms)
cake, powdered ...	280	3.0	37.0	14.0	20	320	<1.0
cake, traditional ...	230	3.0	25.0	13.0	20	320	<1.0
caramel kreme crunch	350	4.0	43.0	19.0	5	170	<1.0
cheesecake, New York	320	4.0	35.0	19.0	10	190	<1.0
chocolate, glazed:							
cake	300	3.0	41.0	15.0	5	310	2.0
cruller	290	2.0	37.0	15.0	15	240	<1.0
chocolate, iced:							
cake	270	3.0	37.0	14.0	20	320	<1.0
custard filled ...	300	3.0	35.0	17.0	5	140	<1.0
glazed	250	3.0	33.0	12.0	5	100	<1.0
kreme filled	350	3.0	38.0	20.0	5	140	<1.0
w/sprinkles	260	3.0	38.0	12.0	5	100	<1.0
chocolate brownie deluxe	290	4.0	33.0	17.0	15	350	2.0
cinnamon, glazed ..	210	2.0	24.0	12.0	5	100	<1.0
cinnamon apple filled	290	3.0	32.0	16.0	5	150	<1.0
cinnamon bun	260	3.0	28.0	16.0	5	125	<1.0
cinnamon twist ...	230	3.0	33.0	9.0	5	85	1.0
cruller, glazed	240	2.0	26.0	14.0	15	240	<1.0
dulce de leche	290	3.0	30.0	18.0	5	160	<1.0
key lime pie	320	3.0	40.0	17.0	5	150	<1.0
kreme filled, glazed	340	3.0	38.0	20.0	5	140	<1.0
lemon filled, glazed	290	3.0	35.0	16.0	5	135	<1.0
maple iced glazed .	240	2.0	32.0	12.0	5	100	<1.0
pumpkin spice cake	340	3.0	42.0	18.0	20	310	<1.0
raspberry filled, glazed	300	3.0	39.0	16.0	5	125	<1.0
sour cream, glazed	340	3.0	42.0	18.0	20	310	<1.0
strawberry filled, powdered	290	3.0	33.0	16.0	5	135	<1.0
sugar	200	2.0	21.0	12.0	5	95	0
frozen blends, w/out whipped cream:							
chocolate, double:							
12 oz.	440	7.0	69.0	16.0	25	210	0
16 oz.	610	9.0	93.0	22.0	35	280	0
20 oz.	740	11.0	116.0	26.0	35	340	0
chocolate, double, w/coffee:							
12 oz.	440	6.0	69.0	16.0	25	210	0
16 oz.	600	8.0	93.0	22.0	35	280	0
20 oz.	730	10.0	116.0	26.0	35	340	0

Food and Measure	cal.	prot. (gms)	carbo. (gms)	fat (gms)	chol. (mgs)	sod. (mgs)	fiber (gms)
Krispy Kreme, frozen blends *(cont.)*							
latte:							
12 oz.	440	8.0	69.0	16.0	25	210	0
16 oz.	610	10.0	92.0	22.0	35	280	0
20 oz.	740	13.0	114.0	28.0	35	340	0
original:							
12 oz.	440	6.0	70.0	15.0	25	200	0
16 oz.	600	8.0	95.0	21.0	35	270	0
20 oz.	730	10.0	117.0	24.0	35	330	0
original, w/coffee:							
12 oz.	440	6.0	70.0	15.0	25	210	0
16 oz.	600	8.0	95.0	21.0	35	280	0
20 oz.	730	10.0	117.0	24.0	35	340	0
raspberry:							
12 oz.	430	5.0	74.0	13.0	25	160	0
16 oz.	590	6.0	99.0	19.0	35	230	0
20 oz.	710	8.0	123.0	22.0	35	270	0
Kumquat:							
(*Frieda's*), 5 oz.	90	1.0	23.0	0	0	10	9.0
1 medium, .7 oz.	12	.2	3.1	<.1	0	1	1.3
seeded, 1 oz.	18	.3	4.7	<.1	0	2	1.9
Kuri squash, see "Red kuri squash"							
Kuzu root (*Eden Organic*), .3 oz. . . .	30	0	8.0	0	0	0	0

L

Food and Measure	cal.	prot. (gms)	carbo. (gms)	fat (gms)	chol. (mgs)	sod. (mgs)	fiber (gms)
Lamb, choice grade, trimmed to ¼" fat, meat only, 4 oz., except as noted:							
cubed, leg/shoulder:							
braised or stewed .	253	38.2	0	10.0	122	79	0
broiled	211	31.8	0	8.3	102	86	0
foreshank, braised:							
lean w/fat	276	32.2	0	15.3	120	82	0
lean only	212	35.2	0	6.8	118	84	0
ground:							
raw	320	18.8	0	26.5	83	67	0
broiled	321	28.1	0	22.3	110	92	0
broiled, 1 cup	328	28.7	0	23.1	113	94	0
leg, whole, roasted:							
lean w/fat	293	29.0	0	18.7	105	75	0
lean w/fat, 1 slice, 3" diam. x ¼" . . .	73	7.2	0	4.7	26	19	0
lean only	217	32.1	0	8.8	101	77	0
lean only, 3" slice . .	54	8.0	0	2.2	25	19	0
leg, shank, roasted:							
lean w/fat	255	29.9	0	14.1	102	74	0
lean w/fat, 1 slice, 3" diam. x ¼" . . .	64	7.5	0	3.5	26	18	0
lean only	204	31.9	0	7.6	99	75	0
lean only, 3" slice . .	51	8.0	0	1.9	25	19	0
leg, sirloin, roasted:							
lean w/fat	331	27.9	0	23.4	110	77	0
lean w/fat, 1 slice, 3" diam. x ¼" . . .	83	7.0	0	5.9	27	19	0
lean only	231	32.1	0	10.4	104	81	0
lean only, 3" slice . .	58	8.0	0	2.6	26	20	0
loin chop, broiled:							
lean w/fat, 2¼ oz. (4.2 oz. raw w/bone)	201	16.1	0	14.7	64	49	0

Food and Measure	cal.	prot. (gms)	carbo. (gms)	fat (gms)	chol. (mgs)	sod. (mgs)	fiber (gms)
Lamb, loin chop, broiled *(cont.)*							
lean w/fat	358	28.5	0	26.2	113	87	0
lean only, 1.6 oz. (4.2 oz. raw w/bone and							
fat)	100	13.9	0	4.5	44	39	0
lean only	245	34.0	0	11.0	108	95	0
loin, roasted:							
lean w/fat	350	25.6	0	26.8	108	73	0
lean only	229	30.2	0	11.1	99	75	0
rib:							
broiled, lean w/fat .	409	25.1	0	33.6	112	86	0
broiled, lean only ..	266	31.5	0	14.7	103	96	0
roasted, lean w/fat .	407	24.0	0	33.8	110	83	0
roasted, lean only .	263	29.7	0	15.1	100	92	0
shoulder, whole:							
braised, lean w/fat .	390	32.5	0	27.8	132	85	0
braised, lean only ..	321	37.2	0	10.0	133	90	0
roasted, lean w/fat .	313	25.5	0	22.6	104	75	0
roasted, lean only .	231	28.3	0	12.2	99	77	0
Lamb, New Zealand, meat only, 4 oz.:							
foreshank:							
braised, lean w/fat .	293	30.6	0	18.0	116	53	0
braised, lean only ..	211	34.9	0	6.8	115	56	0
leg, whole:							
roasted, lean w/fat .	279	28.1	0	17.6	115	49	0
roasted, lean only .	205	31.4	0	7.9	113	51	0
loin chop:							
broiled, lean w/fat .	357	26.6	0	27.1	127	56	0
broiled, lean only ..	226	33.2	0	9.3	129	62	0
rib:							
roasted, lean w/fat .	386	21.5	0	32.6	113	49	0
roasted, lean only .	222	27.7	0	11.5	107	54	0
shoulder:							
braised, lean w/fat .	405	32.0	0	29.8	139	58	0
braised, lean only ..	323	38.6	0	17.6	144	64	0
Lamb's quarters, boiled, drained, chopped, ½ cup ...	29	2.9	4.5	.6	0	26	1.9
Lard, 1 tbsp.:							
(*Goya* Achiotina)	120	0	0	13.0	0	10	0
pork	115	0	0	12.8	12	<1	0

Food and Measure	cal.	prot. (gms)	carbo. (gms)	fat (gms)	chol. (mgs)	sod. (mgs)	fiber (gms)
Lasagna entree, freeze-dried, 1 serving:							
meat sauce:							
(*Mountain House Can*), 1 cup	250	13.0	29.0	9.0	20	470	2.0
(*Mountain House Double*), ½ pouch	310	16.0	36.0	12.0	30	580	2.0
(*Mountain House Four*), 1 cup	240	13.0	29.0	9.0	20	470	2.0
(*Mountain House Single*)	380	20.0	45.0	15.0	35	730	3.0
vegetable (*Mountain House*), ½ pouch ..	210	9.0	35.0	5.0	5	430	3.0
Lasagna entree, frozen, 1 pkg., except as noted:							
Alfredo (*Michelina's Authentico*), 9 oz...	340	13.0	38.0	16.0	45	730	2.0
bake:							
(*Healthy Choice*), 9 oz.	270	14.0	36.0	7.0	20	600	5.0
(*Stouffer's*), 11.5 oz.	450	24.0	47.0	18.0	50	1070	4.0
Bolognese (*Smart Ones*), 9 oz.	240	13.0	43.0	2.5	10	560	4.0
cheese:							
(*Amy's*), 10.3 oz. ..	390	17.0	35.0	20.0	45	680	4.0
(*Ian's* Natural Low Carb), ½ of 12-oz. pkg.	250	20.0	9.0	15.0	30	410	3.0
five (*Lean Cuisine Everyday Favorites Classic*), 11.5 oz.	330	18.0	48.0	7.0	25	690	4.0
five (*Michelina's Lean Gourmet*), 8.5 oz.	220	10.0	38.0	5.0	10	760	5.0
five (*Stouffer's*), 10.75 oz.	370	21.0	39.0	14.0	35	960	4.0
five (*Stouffer's* Family Style Recipes), 1/11 of 96-oz. pkg.	290	15.0	32.0	11.0	30	780	3.0
four (*Michelina's Authentico*), 8 oz.	280	13.0	43.0	7.0	25	550	3.0
four (*Uncle Ben's* Pasta Bowl), 12 oz.	330	24.0	41.0	7.0	30	830	7.0

Food and Measure	cal.	prot. (gms)	carbo. (gms)	fat (gms)	chol. (mgs)	sod. (mgs)	fiber (gms)
Lasagna entree, frozen, cheese *(cont.)*							
four, layered (*Michelina's* Authentico), 8 oz.	260	13.0	30.0	11.0	30	690	1.0
w/chicken (*Lean Cuisine* Café Classics), 10 oz.	290	18.0	36.0	8.0	30	570	4.0
w/meatless ground round (*Cedarlane*), 10 oz.	380	25.0	45.0	12.0	35	570	3.0
chicken:							
(*Stouffer's* Family Style Recipes), 1/5 of 39-oz. pkg.	330	14.0	29.0	17.0	25	840	2.0
(*Stouffer's* Family Style Recipes), 1/11 of 96-oz. pkg.	320	16.0	34.0	13.0	30	840	3.0
Florentine (*Lean Cuisine* Everyday Favorites), 10 oz.	270	19.0	35.0	6.0	25	710	3.0
Florentine:							
(*Smart Ones*), 10.5 oz.	290	15.0	36.0	8.0	30	650	5.0
bake (*Lean Cuisine* Café Classics), 10 oz.	270	19.0	35.0	6.0	25	690	3.0
meat sauce:							
(*Lean Cuisine* Everyday Favorites), 10.5 oz.	310	19.0	43.0	7.0	30	650	4.0
(*Smart Ones* Traditional), 10.5 oz.	300	22.0	38.0	7.0	40	790	3.0
(*Stouffer's*), 10.5 oz.	360	28.0	37.0	11.0	35	800	3.0
(*Stouffer's*), 1/3 of 21-oz. pkg.	250	17.0	27.0	8.0	30	720	2.0
(*Stouffer's* Family Style Recipes), 1/5 of 40-oz. pkg.	270	16.0	28.0	10.0	30	730	2.0
(*Stouffer's* Family Style Recipes), 1/7 of 57-oz. pkg.	320	20.0	31.0	13.0	40	840	2.0
(*Stouffer's* Family Style Recipes), 1/12 of 96-oz. pkg.	320	22.0	27.0	14.0	45	700	2.0

Food and Measure	cal.	prot. (gms)	carbo. (gms)	fat (gms)	chol. (mgs)	sod. (mgs)	fiber (gms)
four cheese (*Michelina's* Authentico), 9 oz.	280	15.0	40.0	7.0	35	800	3.0
layered (*Michelina's Lean Gourmet*), 8 oz.	250	14.0	34.0	7.0	25	890	5.0
meatless (*Boca*), 10.5 oz.	270	20.0	41.0	5.0	2	880	5.0
mozzarella (*Michelina's* Zap'ems), 8 oz. . . .	260	10.0	39.0	8.0	15	650	3.0
primavera (*Michelina's* Zap'ems), 8 oz. . . .	260	9.0	35.0	10.0	25	710	3.0
seafood (*Contessa* Minute Meal Bowl), 10 oz.	430	26.0	35.0	21.0	65	720	3.0
tomato sauce, sausage (*Stouffer's*), 10⅞ oz.	410	18.0	41.0	19.0	50	520	4.0
vegetable:							
(*Amy's*), 9.5 oz. . . .	300	14.0	35.0	12.0	20	680	5.0
(*Amy's* Family Size), 1/7 of 45-oz. pkg.	200	11.0	25.0	8.0	10	480	4.0
(*Cedarlane Carb Buster*), 9.5 oz. .	504	22.0	19.0	40.0	98	834	9.0
(*Stouffer's*), 10.5 oz.	420	19.0	43.0	19.0	25	810	5.0
(*Stouffer's* Family Style Recipes), 1/12 of 96-oz. pkg.	370	16.0	36.0	18.0	30	790	3.0
(*Yves* Veggie), 10.5 oz.	300	17.0	51.0	3.0	0	650	4.0
garden (*Amy's*), 10.25 oz.	290	13.0	41.0	9.0	20	720	5.0
garden (*Cedarlane* Low Fat), ½ of 10-oz. pkg.	180	10.0	26.0	3.0	10	390	2.0
tofu (*Amy's*), 9.5 oz.	300	13.0	41.0	10.0	0	630	6.0
Lasagna entree mix, see "Hamburger entree mix"							
Lecithin granules:							
(*Shiloh Farms*), 2 tbsp.	70	0	1.0	5.0	0	0	0
(*Tree of Life*), 1 tbsp. .	55	0	1.0	4.0	0	2	0
Leek, w/lower leaf portion, fresh:							
raw:							
(*Frieda's*), 1 cup, 3 oz.	50	1.0	12.0	0	0	15	2.0

Food and Measure	cal.	prot. (gms)	carbo. (gms)	fat (gms)	chol. (mgs)	sod. (mgs)	fiber (gms)
Leek, raw *(cont.)*							
9.9-oz. leek	76	1.9	17.6	.4	0	25	2.2
chopped, ½ cup . . .	32	.8	7.4	.2	0	10	.9
boiled, drained:							
4.4-oz. leek	38	.2	9.5	.3	0	12	1.2
chopped, ½ cup . . .	16	.4	4.0	.1	0	5	.5
Leek, freeze-dried,							
1 tbsp.	1	<.1	.2	tr.	0	<1	<1.0
Lemon, fresh:							
(*Dole*), 2-oz. fruit	15	0	5.0	0	0	5	1.0
(*Del Monte*), 2-oz. fruit	15	0	5.0	0	0	5	1.0
(*Sunkist*), 2-oz. fruit .	15	0	5.0	0	0	0	<1.0
2⅛" lemon, 3.8 oz. . . .	22	1.3	11.6	.3	0	3	n.a.
1 wedge, ¼ medium .	5	.3	2.9	.1	0	1	n.a.
peeled, 2⅛" lemon . . .	17	.6	5.4	.2	0	1	1.6
Lemon butter dill sauce, see "Grilling sauce"							
Lemon curd, 1 tbsp.:							
(*Crosse & Blackwell*) .	50	0	13.0	0	0	0	0
(*Dickenson's*)	70	0	14.0	1.0	15	15	0
(*Grant's*)	40	0	10.0	0	0	15	0
(*Laird's Larder*)	60	0	15.0	1.0	0	25	0
Lemon dill sauce mix (*Golden Dipt Bag 'n Season*), 1 tbsp.	35	0	6.0	0	0	190	0
Lemon drink (see also "Lemonade") (*Santa Cruz Organic* Box), 8 fl. oz.	110	0	28.0	0	0	0	0
Lemon drink blend:							
ginger echinacea (*Santa Cruz Organic*), 8 fl. oz.	110	<1.0	25.0	0	0	70	0
Lemon garlic herb sauce (*Litehouse*), 2 tbsp.	45	0	8.0	1.5	0	290	0
Lemon herb seasoning (*McCormick 1 Step*), 1 tsp.	10	0	1.0	0	0	550	0
Lemon juice:							
fresh:							
½ cup	31	.5	10.5	0	0	1	.5
1 tbsp.	4	.1	1.3	0	0	<1	.1
bottled (*Santa Cruz Organic*), 1 tsp. . . .	0	0	0	0	0	0	0

Food and Measure	cal.	prot. (gms)	carbo. (gms)	fat (gms)	chol. (mgs)	sod. (mgs)	fiber (gms)
Lemon peel, fresh,							
1 tbsp.	-[1]	.1	1.0	<.1	0	0	.6
Lemon pepper, ¼ tsp.,							
except as noted:							
(*Lawry's*)	0	0	0	0	0	80	0
(*McCormick* California							
Style)	0	0	0	0	0	30	0
1 tsp.	7	.2	1.5	0	0	425	.3
and lime seasoning rub							
(*Ducks Unlimited*) .	0	0	0	0	0	120	0
salt (*McCormick*)	0	0	0	0	0	130	0
Lemonade, 8 fl. oz.,							
except as noted:							
(*AriZona*)	110	0	27.0	0	0	25	0
(*Hood*)	110	0	28.0	0	0	5	0
(*Minute Maid*),							
12-fl.-oz. cont.	150	0	42.0	0	0	115	0
(*Minute Maid*),							
6.75-fl.-oz. box . . .	90	0	25.0	0	0	15	0
(*Minute Maid* Carton/							
Jug)	110	0	31.0	0	0	15	0
(*Minute Maid* Plastic/							
Can)	100	0	28.0	0	0	80	0
(*Nantucket Nectars*							
Squeezed)	130	0	32.0	0	0	5	0
(*Newman's Own* Virgin)	110	0	27.0	0	0	40	0
(*R.W. Knudsen* Juice							
Box)	110	1.0	28.0	0	0	15	0
(*Santa Cruz Organic*) .	100	0	24.0	0	0	45	0
(*Snapple*)	110	0	28.0	0	0	50	0
(*Snapple* Super Sour)	130	0	33.0	0	0	50	0
(*Sobe MacLizard's*							
Special Recipe) . . .	120	0	30.0	0	0	15	0
(*Tropicana*)	100	0	27.0	0	0	60	0
(*Turkey Hill*)	120	0	29.0	0	0	10	0
(*Walnut Acres*)	110	0	29.0	0	0	5	0
pink:							
(*Hi-C Blast*)	120	0	32.0	0	0	140	0
(*Hood*)	110	0	28.0	0	0	5	0
(*Minute Maid*),							
12-fl.-oz. cont. . .	150	0	42.0	0	0	115	0
(*Minute Maid* Carton/							
Jug)	110	0	30.0	0	0	15	0

1. *Cannot be calculated; no digestibility value for fresh peel.*

Food and Measure	cal.	prot. (gms)	carbo. (gms)	fat (gms)	chol. (mgs)	sod. (mgs)	fiber (gms)
Lemonade, pink *(cont.)*							
(*Minute Maid* Plastic/							
Can)	100	0	28.0	0	0	80	0
(*Minute Maid Cooler*),							
6.75-fl.-oz. box . .	90	0	25.0	0	0	15	0
(*Nantucket Nectars*							
Squeezed)	120	0	29.0	0	0	10	0
(*Newman's Own*) . .	110	0	27.0	0	0	40	0
(*Snapple*)	110	0	28.0	0	0	50	0
(*Walnut Acres*)	110	0	29.0	0	0	5	0
frozen*:							
(*Cascadian Farm*) . .	110	0	28.0	0	0	9	0
(*Minute Maid*)	110	0	29.0	0	0	0	0
pink	99	.3	25.9	0	0	7	0
white	99	.3	26.0	0	0	7	.3
sparkling (*Santa Cruz*							
Organic), 12 fl. oz. .	100	0	26.0	0	0	0	0
tea, see "Tea, iced"							
Lemonade fruit blend,							
8 fl. oz.:							
cranberry:							
(*Nantucket Nectars*							
Squeezed)	120	0	30.0	0	0	5	0
white (*Langers*) . . .	120	0	30.0	0	0	15	0
limeade (*Nantucket*							
Nectars)	120	0	29.0	0	0	30	0
mango (*Bolthouse*							
Farms)	120	<1.0	30.0	0	0	0	<1.0
peach:							
(*Nantucket Nectars*							
Squeezed)	140	0	35.0	0	0	0	0
(*V8 Splash*)	110	0	27.0	0	0	45	0
raspberry:							
(*Langers*)	120	0	29.0	0	0	0	0
(*Minute Maid* Carton)	120	0	32.0	0	0	15	0
(*Minute Maid* Plastic)	110	0	28.0	0	0	75	0
(*Santa Cruz Organic*)	90	0	23.0	0	0	5	0
(*Turkey Hill*)	120	0	29.0	0	0	10	0
(*V8 Splash*)	110	0	27.0	0	0	45	0
frozen* (*Minute*							
Maid)	110	0	29.0	0	0	0	0
strawberry (*Santa Cruz*							
Organic)	100	0	24.0	0	0	0	0

Food and Measure	cal.	prot. (gms)	carbo. (gms)	fat (gms)	chol. (mgs)	sod. (mgs)	fiber (gms)
strawberry kiwi (*Turkey Hill*)	120	0	29.0	0	0	10	0
watermelon (*Nantucket Nectars*)	110	0	30.0	0	0	0	0
Lemonade, mix*, 8 fl. oz.:							
(*Country Time*)	60	0	16.0	0	0	25	0
(*Country Time* Sugar Free)	5	0	0	0	0	0	0
raspberry:							
(*Country Time*) ...	80	0	19.0	0	0	0	0
strawberry (*Country Time*)	80	0	20.0	0	0	0	0
Lemongrass, fresh:							
1 tbsp.	5	.1	1.2	<.1	0	<1	n.a.
1 cup	66	.5	16.9	.3	0	4	n.a.
Lemongrass sauce, see "Marinade"							
Lentil:							
dry, ¼ cup:							
black Beluga (*Shiloh Farms*)	200	12.0	34.0	3.0	0	9	9.0
French (*Shiloh Farms*)	160	10.0	30.0	0	0	0	3.0
green (*Arrowhead Mills*)	150	10.0	27.0	1.0	0	5	7.0
green (*Shiloh Farms*)	150	11.0	27.0	0	0	15	7.0
green	162	13.5	27.4	.5	0	5	14.6
pink	166	11.9	28.4	1.0	0	3	5.2
red (*Arrowhead Mills*)	170	13.0	28.0	1.0	0	5	7.0
red, split (*Shiloh Farms*)	150	11.0	27.0	0	0	15	7.0
cooked, ½ cup	115	8.9	19.9	.4	0	2	7.8
Lentil, canned, ½ cup:							
(*Goya*)	80	6.0	16.0	0	0	310	4.0
(*Westbrae Natural* Organic)	100	8.0	17.0	0	0	150	9.0
black Beluga (*Westbrae Natural* Organic Heirloom)	100	6.0	16.0	0	0	120	4.0
w/onion, bay leaf (*Eden* Organic)	90	8.0	13.0	0	0	210	4.0
Lentil, sprouted, raw, ½ cup	40	3.4	8.4	.2	0	4	n.a.

Food and Measure	cal.	prot. (gms)	carbo. (gms)	fat (gms)	chol. (mgs)	sod. (mgs)	fiber (gms)
Lentil dish, mix:							
(*Neera's* Dal and							
Seasoning), 1 cup*	140	11.0	23.0	1.0	0	4	12.0
(*Neera's* Urad and							
Channa Dal), 1 cup*	104	8.0	18.0	1.0	0	4	9.0
pilaf, w/rice:							
(*Near East*), 2 oz. . . .	180	11.0	36.0	.5	0	630	8.0
(*Near East*), 1 cup*	200	11.0	36.0	3.5	10	660	8.0
Lentil entree, frozen,							
garlic stew (*Ethnic*							
Gourmet Dal Bahaar),							
12 oz.	300	11.0	53.0	6.0	0	640	4.0
Lentil entree, pkg.:							
(*Tasty Bite* Bengal),							
½ of 10-oz. pkg. . .	158	6.0	16.0	8.0	0	439	8.0
(*Tasty Bite* Jodhpur),							
½ of 10-oz. pkg. . .	106	6.0	12.0	4.0	0	664	7.0
(*Tasty Bite* Madras),							
½ of 10-oz. pkg. . .	127	6.0	14.0	5.0	3	455	5.0
w/rice, 9.25-oz. pkg.:							
chili (*Tamarind Tree*							
Dal Makhani) . . .	330	14.0	55.0	6.0	5	670	14.0
vegetables (*Tamarind*							
Tree Channa Dal							
Masala)	340	13.0	62.0	5.0	0	700	10.0
Lettuce (see also							
"Salad blend"							
and "Salad kit"):							
bibb or Boston:							
1 head, 5" diam. . . .	21	2.1	3.8	.4	0	8	1.6
2 inner leaves	2	.2	.4	<.1	0	1	.5
butterhead (*Frieda's*							
Limestone), ⅔ cup,							
3 oz.	10	1.0	2.0	0	0	10	1.0
iceberg:							
(*Dole*), 1/6 medium	15	1.0	3.0	0	0	10	1.0
1 head, 6" diam. . . .	70	5.4	11.3	1.0	0	48	7.5
1 leaf, .7 oz.	3	.2	.4	<.1	0	2	.3
shredded (*Dole*), 3 oz.	15	1.0	3.0	0	0	10	1.0
shredded (*Fresh*							
Express Shreds!),							
1½ cups, 3 oz. . .	15	1.0	3.0	0	0	10	1.0
shredded, 1 cup . . .	7	.6	1.2	.1	0	3	.8

Food and Measure	cal.	prot. (gms)	carbo. (gms)	fat (gms)	chol. (mgs)	sod. (mgs)	fiber (gms)
leaf/loose-leaf, shredded:							
(*Dole*), 1½ cups, 3 oz.	15	1.0	4.0	0	0	30	2.0
½ cup	5	.4	1.0	.1	0	3	.5
romaine or cos:							
(*Dole*), 6 leaves, 3 oz.	20	1.0	3.0	.5	0	0	1.0
(*Ready Pac* Bella), 1½ cups, 3 oz. . . .	15	1.0	2.0	0	0	5	1.0
(*Ready Pac* Caesar), 2½ cups, 2.9 oz.	20	1.0	3.0	.5	0	0	1.0
(*Ready Pac* Caesar Organic), 2¾ cups, 3 oz.	15	<1.0	2.0	0	0	10	<1.0
hearts (*Fresh Express*), 3 oz.	15	1.0	2.0	0	0	5	1.0
1 inner leaf	1	.2	.2	0	0	1	.2
shredded, ½ cup . .	4	.5	.7	.1	0	2	.5
romaine hearts, 3 oz.:							
(*Andy Boy*), 6 leaves	20	1.0	3.0	0	0	0	1.0
(*Dole*)	15	1.0	3.0	0	0	10	1.0
(*Dole* Organic)	15	1.0	3.0	0	0	5	1.0
Lima beans:							
immature, ½ cup:							
raw, trimmed	88	5.3	15.7	.7	0	6	3.8
boiled, drained	104	5.8	20.1	.3	0	14	4.5
mature, dry:							
baby, ¼ cup:							
(*Goya*)	70	8.0	23.0	0	0	15	15.0
(*Shiloh Farms*)	70	8.0	23.0	0	0	15	15.0
baby, boiled, ½ cup	115	7.3	21.2	.3	0	2	7.0
large (*Shiloh Farms*), ¼ cup	70	7.0	22.0	0	0	20	12.0
boiled, ½ cup	108	7.3	19.6	.4	0	2	6.6
Lima beans, canned (see also "Butter beans"), ½ cup:							
baby:							
(*Eden* Organic)	100	6.0	17.0	1.0	0	35	4.0
seasoned (*Glory*) . .	140	8.0	24.0	1.0	0	620	7.0
green:							
(*Allens/East Texas Fair*)	120	7.0	23.0	0	0	370	8.0

Food and Measure	cal.	prot. (gms)	carbo. (gms)	fat (gms)	chol. (mgs)	sod. (mgs)	fiber (gms)
Lima beans, canned, green *(cont.)*							
(*Del Monte*)	80	4.0	15.0	0	0	390	4.0
w/bacon (*Trappey's*)	120	6.0	22.0	1.0	0	330	6.0
green, baby:							
(*Freshlike/Freshlike*							
Selects)	140	9.0	26.0	.5	0	270	7.0
(*Veg-All*)	90	4.0	15.0	1.0	0	330	3.0
green and white (*Allens*)	110	6.0	20.0	1.0	0	280	9.0
white, w/bacon							
(*Trappey's*)	130	8.0	21.0	1.5	0	350	6.0
Lima beans, frozen,							
½ cup, except as							
noted:							
baby:							
(*Birds Eye*)	110	6.0	20.0	0	0	240	5.0
(*C&W/C&W* Petite)	90	6.0	15.0	.5	0	80	5.0
(*Green Giant*)	80	5.0	16.0	0	0	140	3.0
(*McKenzie's*)	110	6.0	22.0	.5	0	140	5.0
baby, in butter sauce							
(*Green Giant*), ⅔ cup	110	5.0	20.0	1.5	<5	390	4.0
Fordhook:							
(*Birds Eye*)	100	6.0	18.0	0	0	5	4.0
Lime, fresh:							
(*Del Monte*), 2.4-oz.							
lime	20	0	7.0	0	0	0	2.0
(*Frieda's* Key Lime),							
3-oz. lime	25	1.0	9.0	0	0	0	2.0
2"-diam. lime	20	.5	7.1	.1	0	1	1.9
peeled, seeded, 1 oz. . .	9	.2	3.0	.1	0	1	.8
Lime curd, 1 tbsp.:							
(*Crosse & Blackwell*) .	50	0	13.0	0	0	0	0
(*Dickenson's*)	70	0	14.0	1.0	15	15	0
Lime drink, see							
"Limeade"							
Lime juice:							
fresh:							
½ cup	33	.5	11.1	.1	0	1	.5
1 tbsp.	4	.1	1.4	<.1	0	tr.	.1
bottled:							
(*Angostura*), 1 tsp. . .	5	0	1.0	0	0	0	0
(*Santa Cruz Organic*),							
1 tsp.	0	0	0	0	0	0	0
sweetened (*Rose's*),							
1 tsp.	10	0	2.0	0	0	0	0

Food and Measure	cal.	prot. (gms)	carbo. (gms)	fat (gms)	chol. (mgs)	sod. (mgs)	fiber (gms)
unsweetened:							
(*Rose's*), 2 tbsp.	10	0	2.0	0	0	0	0
2 tbsp.	6	<.1	2.0	<.1	0	5	.1
Lime relish, Indian, 1 tbsp.:							
hot (*Patak's*)	30	<1.0	.5	3.0	0	520	<1.0
mild (*Patak's*)	30	0	0	3.0	0	530	0
Limeade, 8 fl. oz., except as noted:							
(*Nantucket Nectars Squeezed*)	110	0	28.0	0	0	80	0
(*Santa Cruz Organic*) .	100	0	26.0	0	0	35	0
(*Walnut Acres*)	110	0	27.0	0	0	5	0
cherry (*Minute Maid*) .	120	0	34.0	0	0	15	0
sparkling (*Santa Cruz Organic*), 12 fl. oz. . .	100	0	26.0	0	0	0	0
Ling, meat only:							
raw, 4 oz.	99	21.5	0	.7	45	153	0
baked, broiled, micro-waved, 4 oz.	126	27.6	0	.9	58	196	0
Ling cod, meat only:							
raw, 4 oz.	96	20.0	0	1.2	59	67	0
baked, broiled, or micro-waved, 4 oz.	124	25.7	0	1.5	76	86	0
Linguica sausage (*Caspar's*), 2 oz. . . .	120	10.0	1.0	9.0	30	360	0
Linguine:							
dry, see "Pasta"							
refrigerated:							
(*Buitoni*), 1¼ cups	240	10.0	45.0	2.5	55	20	2.0
(*Monterey Carb Smart* Egg Recipe), 3.5 oz.	200	12.0	27.0	5.0	140	70	5.0
Linguine entree, frozen, w/clams (*Michelina's* Authentico), 8.5- oz. pkg.	290	11.0	50.0	3.5	10	560	2.0
Liquor[1], 1 fl. oz.:							
80 proof	64	0	0	0	0	tr.	0
90 proof	73	0	0	0	0	tr.	0
100 proof	82	0	0	0	0	tr.	0

1. Includes all pure distilled liquors: bourbon, brandy, gin, rum, Scotch, tequila, vodka, etc.

Food and Measure	cal.	prot. (gms)	carbo. (gms)	fat (gms)	chol. (mgs)	sod. (mgs)	fiber (gms)
Litchi, see "Lychee"							
Little Caesars:							
⅛ of 12" pizza:							
cheese only	180	10.0	23.0	6.1	15	290	1.0
pepperoni	210	11.0	23.0	7.6	20	400	1.0
add toppings:							
bacon	36	1.7	.1	3.1	6	110	0
beef	19	.9	.4	1.4	2	51	.2
extra cheese	22	1.8	.2	1.5	5	48	0
green pepper ...	2	.1	.4	0	0	0	.1
ham	6	.9	.5	.2	2	66	0
hot peppers	0	0	0	0	0	93	0
mushrooms	2	.2	.5	0	0	39	.2
olives, black	12	.2	.2	1.6	0	46	.2
onions	2	.1	.1	0	0	0	.1
pepperoni	25	1.1	.1	1.5	4	105	0
pineapple	7	0	1.7	0	0	0	.1
sausage, Italian .	19	.8	.1	1.7	5	61	0
tomato	2	.1	.4	0	0	1	.1
1/10 of 14" pizza:							
cheese only	200	10.0	25.0	6.5	15	320	1.0
meatsa	280	15.0	26.0	12.9	30	630	2.0
pepperoni	230	12.0	25.0	8.0	20	430	1.0
supreme	270	13.0	31.0	10.4	25	510	3.0
veggie	240	12.0	32.0	7.6	15	710	3.0
add toppings:							
bacon	41	2.0	.1	3.6	7	125	.1
beef	20	1.0	.4	1.5	2	55	.2
extra cheese	26	2.2	.2	1.8	6	48	0
green pepper ...	2	.1	.4	0	0	0	.1
ham	5	.9	.1	.2	2	66	0
hot peppers	0	0	0	0	0	93	0
mushrooms	2	.2	.4	0	0	40	.2
olives, black	12	.3	.2	1.6	0	47	.2
onions	3	.1	.6	0	0	0	.1
pepperoni	26	1.1	.1	1.5	4	110	0
pineapple	7	.1	1.7	0	0	0	0
sausage, Italian .	22	.9	.2	1.9	5	68	.1
tomato	2	.1	.5	0	0	1	.1
deep dish, ⅛ pie:							
large, cheese	320	15.0	37.0	12.2	20	460	2.0
large, pepperoni ...	350	17.0	38.0	14.2	25	610	2.0
medium, cheese ...	230	11.0	27.0	9.2	15	340	1.0
medium, pepperoni	260	12.0	27.0	10.8	20	450	1.0

Food and Measure	cal.	prot. (gms)	carbo. (gms)	fat (gms)	chol. (mgs)	sod. (mgs)	fiber (gms)
slice, 1/6 of 14" pie:							
cheese	330	17.0	42.0	10.9	25	530	2.0
pepperoni	390	20.0	42.0	13.0	35	750	2.0
deli sandwiches:							
ham and cheese ...	640	32.0	66.0	28.8	50	1540	3.0
Italian	800	35.0	66.0	44.5	90	1950	3.0
veggie	600	24.0	67.0	27.5	30	980	3.0
other items, 1 pc.,							
except as noted:							
Baby Pan!Pan!	360	17.0	34.0	16.0	30	630	2.0
cheese bread, Italian	130	7.0	13.0	6.2	10	310	0
chicken wing	70	5.0	0	4.9	25	210	0
Crazy Bread	90	3.0	15.0	2.5	<1	140	0
Crazy Bread, cinna-							
mon, 2 pcs.	100	3.0	19.0	1.9	<1	95	0
Crazy Sauce, 4 oz. .	45	0	9.0	0	0	380	3.0
salad:							
antipasto	140	9.0	6.0	7.5	20	560	2.0
Caesar	90	4.0	12.0	2.9	0	190	3.0
Greek	120	6.0	11.0	6.5	25	590	3.0
tossed	100	2.0	15.0	3.1	0	190	3.0
salad dressing:							
Caesar	230	1.0	1.0	25.0	55	360	0
Greek	270	0	0	29.0	0	200	0
Italian	220	0	2.0	23.0	0	370	0
Italian, fat free	25	0	5.0	0	0	390	0
ranch	230	1.0	2.0	24.0	10	380	0
Liver:							
beef, panfried, 4 oz. ...	246	30.3	8.9	9.1	547	120	0
calves (veal), 4 oz.:							
braised	218	32.2	4.3	7.1	579	88	0
panfried	219	31.0	5.1	7.4	550	96	0
chicken, simmered:							
4 oz.	189	27.7	1.0	7.4	638	86	0
chopped, 1 cup ...	219	34.1	1.2	7.6	883	71	0
chicken, panfried, 4 oz.	195	29.2	1.3	7.3	640	104	0
duck, raw, 1 oz.	39	5.3	1.0	1.3	146	n.a.	0
goose, raw, 1 oz.	38	4.6	1.8	1.2	146	40	0
lamb, 4 oz.:							
braised	249	34.7	2.9	10.0	568	64	0
panfried	270	29.0	4.3	14.3	559	141	0
pork, braised, 4 oz. ..	187	29.5	4.3	5.0	403	56	0
turkey, simmered:							
4 oz.	192	27.2	3.9	6.7	710	73	0
chopped, 1 cup ...	237	33.6	4.8	8.3	876	89	0

Food and Measure	cal.	prot. (gms)	carbo. (gms)	fat (gms)	chol. (mgs)	sod. (mgs)	fiber (gms)
Liver cheese:							
(*Oscar Mayer*), 1.3 oz.	120	6.0	1.0	10.0	80	420	0
pork, 2 oz.	170	8.5	1.8	14.3	97	686	0
Liver pâté, see "Pâté"							
Liver sausage, see "Braunschweiger" and "Liverwurst"							
Liver steak, beef, organic (*Organic Valley*), 2 oz.	80	11.0	3.0	2.0	200	40	0
Liverwurst (see also "Braunschweiger" and "Pâté"), 2 oz.:							
(*Boar's Head* Strassburger)	170	8.0	1.0	15.0	85	560	0
(*Dietz & Watson*)	180	9.0	0	15.0	55	500	0
(*Hansel & Gretel*)	170	9.0	4.0	13.0	95	730	0
(*Hatfield Deli Choice*) .	170	8.0	3.0	14.0	130	520	0
onion (*Boar's Head*) . .	160	8.0	1.0	13.0	75	580	0
smoked (*Boar's Head*)	170	8.0	1.0	15.0	45	620	0
Liverwurst spread, ¼ cup, 2 oz.	168	6.8	3.2	14.0	65	385	1.4
Lo bok, see "Radish, Oriental"							
Lobster, northern, meat only:							
raw, 4 oz.	102	21.3	.6	1.0	108	n.a.	0
boiled or steamed:							
4 oz.	111	23.2	1.5	.7	82	431	0
1 cup, 5.1 oz.	142	29.7	1.9	.9	104	551	0
"Lobster," imitation, chunk or salad style (*Louis Kemp Lobster Delights*), ½ cup, 3 oz.	80	8.0	12.0	0	10	420	0
Lobster, spiny, see "Spiny lobster"							
Lobster sauce, canned (*Progresso*), ½ cup	100	3.0	6.0	7.0	5	430	2.0
Loganberries, fresh, 1 cup	89	1.4	21.5	.9	0	1	n.a.
Loganberries, frozen, ½ cup	40	1.1	9.6	.2	0	1	3.6

Food and Measure	cal.	prot. (gms)	carbo. (gms)	fat (gms)	chol. (mgs)	sod. (mgs)	fiber (gms)
Long bean, see "Yard-long bean"							
Long John Silver's:							
fish/seafood:							
cod, baked, 1 pc. . . .	120	22.0	1.0	4.5	90	240	0
clams, breaded, 3 oz.	240	8.0	22.0	13.0	10	1110	1.0
fish, battered, 1 pc.	260	12.0	17.0	16.0	35	790	<1.0
shrimp:							
battered, 1 pc. . . .	45	2.0	3.0	3.0	15	160	0
crunchy, basket,							
21 pcs.	380	12.0	34.0	22.0	110	850	2.0
giant, 1 pc.	80	2.0	5.0	5.0	20	250	0
Chicken Plank, 1 pc. .	140	8.0	9.0	8.0	20	480	<1.0
dipping sauce, 1 oz.:							
cocktail	25	0	6.0	0	0	250	0
tartar	100	0	4.0	9.0	15	250	0
sandwich:							
chicken	360	13.0	41.0	15.0	25	810	3.0
fish	440	17.0	48.0	20.0	35	1120	3.0
Ultimate Fish	500	20.0	48.0	25.0	50	1310	3.0
salad, no dressing:							
chicken club	510	28.0	35.0	30.0	65	1550	5.0
shrimp and seafood	260	18.0	22.0	12.0	85	820	4.0
salad dressing, 1 pkt.:							
French, fat free	50	0	12.0	0	0	240	<1.0
Italian, light	20	0	3.0	1.0	0	780	0
ranch, garden	230	1.0	2.0	24.0	10	400	0
Thousand Island . .	220	0	7.0	21.0	25	350	0
sides/starters:							
clam chowder, bowl	220	9.0	23.0	10.0	25	810	0
coleslaw, 4 oz.	200	1.0	15.0	15.0	20	340	3.0
cheesesticks, 3 pcs.	140	4.0	12.0	8.0	10	320	1.0
corn cobbette, 1 pc.	90	3.0	14.0	3.0	0	0	3.0
Crumblies, 1 oz. . . .	170	1.0	14.0	12.0	0	420	1.0
fries, large	390	4.0	56.0	17.0	0	580	5.0
fries, regular	230	3.0	34.0	10.0	0	350	3.0
hush puppies, 1 pc.	60	1.0	9.0	2.5	0	200	1.0
lobster stuffed crab							
cake, 1 pc.	170	6.0	16.0	10	30	390	1.0
rice, 4 oz.	180	3.0	34.0	3.5	0	540	3.0
dessert pie:							
chocolate cream . . .	310	5.0	24.0	22.0	15	170	1.0
pecan	370	4.0	55.0	15.0	40	190	2.0
pineapple cream . . .	290	4.0	39.0	13.0	15	210	1.0

Food and Measure	cal.	prot. (gms)	carbo. (gms)	fat (gms)	chol. (mgs)	sod. (mgs)	fiber (gms)
Longan, fresh:							
1 medium	2	<.1	.5	0	0	0	tr.
seeded, 1 oz.	17	.4	4.3	<.1	0	<1	.3
Longan, dried, 1 oz. .	81	1.4	21.0	.1	0	14	<1.0
Loquat:							
(*Frieda's*), 5 oz.	70	1.0	17.0	0	0	0	2.0
1 large, .7 oz.	9	<.1	2.4	0	0	tr.	.3
cubed, 1 cup	70	.6	18.1	.3	0	1	2.5
peeled, seeded, 1 oz. .	13	.1	3.4	.1	0	<1	.5
Lotus root:							
raw:							
(*Frieda's*), 1 cup,							
3 oz.	50	2.0	15.0	0	0	35	4.0
10 slices	60	2.1	14.0	.1	0	32	4.0
trimmed, 1 oz.	16	.7	4.9	<.1	0	11	1.4
boiled, drained, ½ cup	40	1.0	9.6	<.1	0	27	1.9
Lotus root, sun-dried							
(*Eden*), .4 oz.	35	1.0	8.0	0	0	25	2.0
Lotus seeds:							
raw, 1 oz.	25	1.2	4.9	.2	0	<1	n.a.
dried, 1 oz.	94	4.4	18.3	.6	0	1	n.a.
fried, 1 cup	106	4.9	20.6	.6	0	1	n.a.
Lox, see "Salmon, smoked"							
Lunch meat, loaf (see also specific listings), 2 oz., except as noted:							
(*Hatfield Deli Choice* Original)	130	7.0	4.0	9.0	20	400	0
barbecue (*Deli Delight*)	150	7.0	6.0	11.0	25	400	0
deluxe (*Deli Delight*) .	160	7.0	7.0	11.0	25	390	0
Dutch brand:							
(*Boar's Head*)	150	7.0	2.0	12.0	25	610	0
(*Deli Delight*)	160	8.0	4.0	12.0	30	400	0
pepper (*Hatfield Deli Choice*)	120	7.0	3.0	9.0	25	560	0
Italian (*Deli Delight*) . .	150	7.0	5.0	11.0	30	400	0
jalapeño (*Hansel 'n Gretel*)	150	5.0	6.0	12.0	30	910	0
macaroni and cheese (*Hansel 'n Gretel*) .	160	7.0	8.0	12.0	30	890	0
olive:							
(*Boar's Head*)	130	6.0	<1.0	12.0	20	630	0

Food and Measure	cal.	prot. (gms)	carbo. (gms)	fat (gms)	chol. (mgs)	sod. (mgs)	fiber (gms)
(*Hansel 'n Gretel*) .	180	6.0	7.0	14.0	35	850	0
(*Hatfield Deli*							
Choice)	120	6.0	6.0	8.0	15	430	0
(*Oscar Mayer*), 1 oz.	70	3.0	2.0	6.0	20	360	0
(*Tyson* Bag), .9-oz.							
slice	70	9.0	3.0	5.0	10	330	0
pepper (*Deli Delight*) .	110	8.0	5.0	6.0	25	400	0
pickle:							
(*Deli Delight*)	110	7.0	7.0	6.0	25	400	0
(*Tyson* Bag), .9-oz.							
slice	70	3.0	5.0	5.0	10	210	0
pickle and pepper							
(*Boar's Head*)	150	6.0	2.0	13.0	30	500	0
pickle and pimento:							
(*Hatfield Deli*							
Choice)	120	7.0	2.0	9.0	25	570	0
(*Oscar Mayer*), 1 oz.	80	3.0	2.0	6.0	20	360	0
spiced:							
(*Hansel 'n Gretel*) .	180	7.0	6.0	15.0	40	840	0
(*Oscar Mayer*							
Luncheon), 1 oz.	60	4.0	2.0	4.5	20	340	0
spiced ham:							
(*Boar's Head*)	120	7.0	1.0	10.0	30	570	0
(*Hormel*)	140	8.0	1.0	11.0	35	690	0
Lunch meat, canned,							
2 oz.:							
(*Spam* Classic)	180	7.0	1.0	16.0	40	790	0
(*Spam* Less Salt)	180	7.0	1.0	16.0	40	580	0
(*Spam* Lite)	110	9.0	1.0	8.0	40	580	0
barbecue (*Spam*)	160	7.0	4.0	13.0	40	650	0
w/cheese (*Spam*)	170	8.0	2.0	15.0	35	710	0
garlic (*Spam*)	160	8.0	1.0	14.0	40	600	0
hot and spicy (*Spam*)	180	7.0	2.0	16.0	40	600	0
smoked (*Spam*)	170	8.0	2.0	15.0	40	610	0
turkey (*Spam*)	80	8.0	2.0	4.0	30	450	0
Lunch "meat,"							
vegetarian, frozen							
(*Worthington Wham*),							
3 slices, 2 oz.	110	10.0	3.0	7.0	0	400	0
Lupin, boiled, ½ cup .	98	12.9	8.2	2.4	0	3	2.3
Lychee, fresh:							
(*Frieda's*), 6-8 pcs.,							
3.5 oz.	60	1.0	14.0	0	0	0	1.0
1 fruit, .3 oz.	6	.1	1.6	0	0	0	.1

Food and Measure	cal.	prot. (gms)	carbo. (gms)	fat (gms)	chol. (mgs)	sod. (mgs)	fiber (gms)
Lychee *(cont.)*							
shelled:							
1 cup	125	1.6	31.4	.8	0	2	2.5
1 oz.	19	.2	4.7	.1	0	<1	.4
Lychee, dried, 10 fruits,							
.7 oz.	69	1.0	17.7	.3	0	0	1.2
Lychee juice *(Ceres),*							
8 fl. oz.	120	0	30.0	0	0	10	0

M

Food and Measure	cal.	prot. (gms)	carbo. (gms)	fat (gms)	chol. (mgs)	sod. (mgs)	fiber (gms)
Macadamia nut:							
(*Planters*), 1 oz.	200	2.0	4.0	21.0	0	55	3.0
raw, whole or halves:							
(*Tree of Life*), ¼ cup	230	3.0	5.0	24.0	0	0	2.0
1 oz.	204	2.2	3.9	21.5	0	1	2.4
¼ cup	241	2.7	4.6	25.4	0	2	2.9
chopped (*Planters*),							
2-oz. pkg.	400	5.0	8.0	42.0	0	0	5.0
dried, shelled:							
1 oz.	199	2.4	3.9	20.9	0	1	2.6
¼ cup	235	2.8	4.6	24.7	0	2	3.1
dry-roasted:							
(*Mauna Loa*), 1 oz. . .	200	2.0	4.0	21.0	0	60	2.0
(*Mauna Loa* Unsalted),							
1 oz.	200	2.0	4.0	21.0	0	0	2.0
1 oz.	204	2.2	3.8	21.8	0	1	2.3
whole or halves,							
¼ cup	241	2.6	4.5	25.5	0	1	2.7
oil-roasted, 1 oz.	204	2.1	3.7	21.7	0	2	n.a.
Macadamia nut,							
flavored (see also							
"Candy"), 1 oz.:							
coated (*Beer Nuts*) . . .	120	1.0	24.0	2.0	0	20	1.0
coffee glazed (*Mauna*							
Loa Kona)	190	2.0	10.0	15.0	<5	55	1.0
honey roasted (*Mauna*							
Loa)	210	2.0	6.0	21.0	0	35	2.0
onion garlic (*Mauna*							
Loa)	210	2.0	4.0	21.0	0	135	2.0
Macaroni (see also							
"Pasta"):							
uncooked:							
2 oz.	210	7.3	42.4	.9	0	4	1.4
elbow, 1 cup	389	13.4	78.4	1.7	0	8	2.5

Food and Measure	cal.	prot. (gms)	carbo. (gms)	fat (gms)	chol. (mgs)	sod. (mgs)	fiber (gms)
Macaroni, uncooked *(cont.)*							
enriched, 2 oz.	213	11.3	38.3	1.3	0	5	1.4
whole wheat, 2 oz. .	198	.3	42.8	.8	0	5	4.7
cooked, 1 cup:							
enriched, elbows ..	197	6.7	39.7	.9	0	1	1.8
enriched, spirals ..	189	6.4	38.0	.9	0	1	1.7
small shells, 1 cup .	162	5.5	32.6	.8	0	1	1.8
vegetable, enriched,							
spirals	172	6.1	35.7	.2	0	8	5.8
whole-wheat, elbows	174	7.5	37.2	.8	0	4	3.9
Macaroni entree, can or pkg., 1 cup, except as noted:							
and beef:							
(*Kid's Kitchen* Beefy Macaroni)	170	8.0	24.0	5.0	20	800	2.0
(*Kid's Kitchen* Cheezy)	260	14.0	34.0	3.0	25	840	1.0
and cheese:							
(*Bowl Appétit!*), 1 cont.	370	11.0	56.0	12.0	10	930	1.0
(*Kid's Kitchen* Cheezy)	270	12.0	32.0	11.0	35	710	1.0
(*Hormel*), 7.5-oz. can	270	12.0	32.0	11.0	35	710	1.0
w/ham (*Hormel Cure 81* Bowl), 10 oz. .	330	18.0	32.0	14.0	30	1070	1.0
and franks (*Kid's Kitchen* Cheezy) ...	300	12.0	26.0	16.0	45	930	1.0
Macaroni entree, freeze-dried, and cheese:							
(*Mountain House* Can), 1 cup	340	15.0	33.0	16.0	40	970	<1.0
(*Mountain House* Double), ½ pouch .	450	20.0	45.0	21.0	50	1310	1.0
w/beef (*Mountain House* Double), 1 cup	260	13.0	32.0	9.0	35	820	3.0
w/veggies (*AlpineAire Forever Young*), 1 serving	370	17.0	55.0	10.0	n.a.	1420	2.0
Macaroni entree, frozen, 1 pkg., except as noted:							
and beef:							
(*Lean Cuisine Everyday Favorites*), 9.5 oz.	270	16.0	39.0	5.0	20	600	3.0

Food and Measure	cal.	prot. (gms)	carbo. (gms)	fat (gms)	chol. (mgs)	sod. (mgs)	fiber (gms)
(*Michelina's* Zap'ems), 8 oz.	240	12.0	36.0	7.0	20	680	2.0
(*Stouffer's*), 11.5 oz.	360	21.0	39.0	13.0	40	1070	4.0
and cheese:							
(*Amy's*), 9 oz.	410	16.0	47.0	16.0	40	590	3.0
(*Amy's* Large Size), 8 oz.	360	14.0	41.0	14.0	45	590	3.0
(*Glory* Savory Singles), 11 oz. .	480	21.0	47.0	23.0	90	1300	1.0
(*Glory* Savory Singles Family Size), 1 cup	390	17.0	38.0	18.0	70	1050	<1.0
(*Healthy Choice*), 9 oz.	270	13.0	40.0	6.0	25	600	3.0
(*Lean Cuisine Everyday Favorites*), 10 oz.	300	16.0	43.0	7.0	20	650	1.0
(*Linda McCartney*), 10 oz.	420	14.0	32.0	21.0	65	980	3.0
(*Michelina's* Authentico), 8 oz.	240	11.0	41.0	4.0	10	540	2.0
(*Michelina's* Zap'ems), 8 oz.	320	14.0	41.0	11.0	25	620	2.0
(*Michelina's* Lean Gourmet*), 10 oz.	300	14.0	51.0	5.0	15	670	3.0
(*Smart Ones*), 10 oz.	240	10.0	45.0	2.5	10	800	3.0
(*Stouffer's*), ½ of 12-oz. pkg.	320	14.0	32.0	15.0	25	950	2.0
(*Stouffer's* Family Style Recipes), 1/5 of 40-oz. pkg.	150	16.0	37.0	18.0	30	970	2.0
(*Stouffer's* Family Style Recipes), 1/9 of 76-oz. pkg.	380	16.0	38.0	18.0	30	990	2.0
(*Stouffer's Maxaroni*), 9 oz.	320	13.0	36.0	14.0	30	700	2.0
w/broccoli (*Stouffer's*), 10.5 oz.	350	15.0	39.0	15.0	20	940	4.0
cheddar, sharp (*Michelina's* Authentico), 10 oz. .	400	18.0	50.0	15.0	30	820	3.0
w/dessert (*Ian's* Natural Kids Meal), 9 oz.	835	18.0	118.0	13.0	30	625	3.0
w/ham (*Michelina's* Authentico), 8 oz.	310	18.0	34.0	13.0	40	870	2.0

Food and Measure	cal.	prot. (gms)	carbo. (gms)	fat (gms)	chol. (mgs)	sod. (mgs)	fiber (gms)
Macaroni entree, frozen, and cheese *(cont.)*							
w/rice pasta (*Amy's* Rice Mac & Cheese), 9 oz. . .	410	16.0	47.0	16.0	50	590	3.0
and cheese, three:							
(*Moosewood*), 10 oz.	420	16.0	44.0	19.0	45	980	1.0
(*Smart Ones*), 9 oz.	290	12.0	45.0	7.0	10	630	2.0
and chili, see "Chili entree"							
and meat sauce (*Organic Classics*), 10 oz.	340	16.0	49.0	9.0	20	580	3.0
vegetarian, soy cheese:							
(*Amy's*), 9 oz.	370	16.0	42.0	15.0	0	500	4.0
(*Yves* The Good Bowl), 10.5 oz. . .	350	13.0	52.0	9.0	5	880	3.0
Macaroni entree mix:							
Alfredo:							
cheesy (*Kraft*), ⅓ of 7.25-oz. pkg. . . .	260	11.0	44.0	2.5	10	610	2.0
nondairy (*Road's End Organics Mac & Chreese*), ½ cup mix	290	9.0	50.0	1.0	0	260	6.0
and cheddar:							
(*Kraft* Deluxe), ¼ of 14-oz. pkg.	320	13.0	44.0	10.0	15	910	2.0
(*Kraft* Deluxe 2% Milk), ¼ of 14-oz. pkg.	290	13.0	49.0	4.5	15	870	1.0
sharp (*Kraft* Deluxe), ¼ of 14-oz. pkg.	320	12.0	45.0	10.0	15	880	1.0
white (*Kraft*), 2 oz. .	260	11.0	48.0	2.5	10	570	2.0
and cheese:							
(*Annie's* Mac & Cheese Single Serve), ¾ cup* .	230	9.0	40.0	4.5	10	570	<1.0
(*DeBoles* Homestyle), ⅓ pkg.	300	10.0	53.0	6.0	10	320	5.0
(*Kraft* The Cheesiest), 2 oz.	260	11.0	47.0	2.5	10	560	1.0
(*Kraft* Deluxe Family Size), 3.5 oz. . . .	320	13.0	44.0	10.0	35	870	2.0
(*Kraft* Thick 'n Creamy), 2 oz. . .	260	11.0	48.0	2.5	10	560	2.0

Food and Measure	cal.	prot. (gms)	carbo. (gms)	fat (gms)	chol. (mgs)	sod. (mgs)	fiber (gms)
3 cheese (*Kraft*), 2 oz.	260	11.0	48.0	2.5	10	600	2.0
4 cheese (*Annie's* Creamy Deluxe), 1 cup*	320	14.0	45.0	11.0	30	750	2.0
4 cheese (*Kraft* Deluxe), ¼ of 14-oz. pkg.	320	12.0	44.0	10.0	15	920	1.0
rice pasta (*DeBoles*), ¼ pkg.	100	3.0	19.0	1.5	5	100	0
whole wheat pasta (*DeBoles* Organic), ⅓ pkg.	280	11.0	47.0	5.0	10	290	8.0
whole wheat pasta (*Hodgson Mill*), 2 oz.	250	11.0	45.0	.5	<5	570	6.0
and "cheese," nondairy, whole wheat (*Road's End Organics Mac & Chreese*), ½ cup ..	220	9.0	42.0	1.5	0	270	5.0
shells and cheese, see "Shells, pasta, mix"							
Macaroni and cheese, see "Macaroni dish" and "Macaroni entree"							
Macaroni salad, refrigerated:							
(*Blue Ridge Farm*), 4 oz.	240	3.0	25.0	14.0	10	1020	1.0
(*Hellmann's* Classic), 4.9 oz.	500	4.0	59.0	25.0	15	720	3.0
(*Reser's*), ¾ cup	320	5.0	28.0	22.0	15	780	2.0
Mace, ground, 1 tsp. ..	8	.1	.9	.6	0	1	.1
Mackerel, meat only: Atlantic, 4 oz.:							
raw	230	21.1	0	15.8	80	102	0
baked, broiled, or microwaved	297	27.0	0	20.2	85	94	0
king, 4 oz.:							
raw	119	23.0	0	2.3	61	179	0
baked, broiled, or microwaved	152	29.5	0	2.9	77	230	0
Pacific/jack, 4 oz.:							
raw	179	22.8	0	9.0	53	98	0
baked, broiled, or microwaved	228	29.2	0	11.5	68	125	0

Food and Measure	cal.	prot. (gms)	carbo. (gms)	fat (gms)	chol. (mgs)	sod. (mgs)	fiber (gms)
Mackerel *(cont.)*							
Spanish, 4 oz.:							
raw	158	21.9	0	7.2	86	67	0
baked, broiled, or							
microwaved	179	26.8	0	7.2	83	75	0
Mackerel, canned,							
jack, drained:							
(*Brunswick*), 2 oz. . . .	100	13.0	0	5.0	50	80	0
(*Bumble Bee*), 2 oz. . .	90	13.0	0	4.0	55	280	0
Mackerel, salted, 2 oz.	171	10.4	0	14.1	53	2492	0
Mackerel, smoked,							
fillets (*Anchor Bay*							
Seafood), 2 oz. . . .	75	10.0	0	4.0	10	560	0
Mahimahi, see							
"Dolphin fish"							
Mai Tai drink mixer							
(*Trader Vic's*), 4 fl. oz.	130	0	32.0	0	0	20	0
Malanga, fresh:							
(*Frieda's*), ⅔ cup, 3 oz.	90	1.0	23.0	0	0	10	2.0
sliced, ½ cup	66	1.0	16.0	.3	0	14	1.0
Malt cooler (*Bartles &*							
Jaymes), 12 fl. oz.:							
berry, exotic	210	0	33.0	0	0	5	0
blackberry, luscious . .	228	0	39.0	0	0	4	0
blue Hawaiian	179	0	28.0	0	0	7	0
cherry, black	200	0	32.0	0	0	5	0
classic original	190	0	29.0	0	0	0	0
fuzzy navel	230	0	39.0	0	0	5	0
kiwi strawberry	214	0	39.0	0	0	4	0
lemonade, hard	230	0	39.0	0	0	0	0
Margarita	260	0	46.0	0	0	40	0
melon splash	229	0	38.0	0	0	0	0
orange sunset	240	0	38.0	0	0	0	0
peach, juicy	210	0	33.0	0	0	5	0
piña colada	270	0	48.0	0	0	5	0
raspberry daiquiri . . .	216	0	36.0	0	0	4	0
strawberry:							
cosmopolitan	219	0	37.0	0	0	2	0
daiquiri	220	0	36.0	0	0	5	0
tropical burst	230	0	37.0	0	0	5	0
Malt syrup, see							
"Barley malt syrup"							
Malted milk powder,							
3 tbsp.:							
natural (*Carnation*) . . .	90	3.0	15.0	2.0	5	85	<1.0

Food and Measure	cal.	prot. (gms)	carbo. (gms)	fat (gms)	chol. (mgs)	sod. (mgs)	fiber (gms)
chocolate (*Carnation*) .	90	1.0	18.0	1.0	0	40	<1.0
Mammy apple:							
½ of 25-oz. fruit	216	2.1	52.9	2.1	0	63	12.7
peeled, seeded, 1 oz. .	14	.1	3.5	.1	0	4	.9
Mandarin orange, see "Tangerine"							
Mango, fresh:							
(*Dole*), ½ medium . . .	70	0	17.0	.5	0	0	1.0
(*Del Monte*), ½ medium, 4.9 oz.	70	0	17.0	0	0	0	1.0
10.6-oz. fruit, 7.3 oz. trimmed	135	1.1	35.2	.6	0	4	3.7
sliced, 1 cup	107	8.4	28.1	.5	0	2	3.0
Mango, in jars:							
in light syrup (*Del Monte Sunfresh*), ½ cup	70	0	19.0	0	0	15	<1.0
in syrup, sliced (*Herdez*), 2 pcs. . . .	170	0	30.0	0	0	10	5.0
Mango, dried:							
(*Sunsweet*), ⅓ cup, 1.4 oz.	140	0	34.0	0	0	20	1.0
slices, unsweetened: (*SunRidge Farms Organic*), 3 pcs., 1.4 oz.	45	1.0	11.0	0	0	0	<1.0
(*Tree of Life*), 1.4 oz.	30	0	7.0	0	0	0	1.0
spears (*SunRidge Farms*), 4 pcs., 1.4 oz. . .	130	0	34.0	0	0	20	1.0
Mango, frozen, chunks:							
(*Contessa*), 1 cup . . .	90	1.0	21.0	0	0	25	2.0
(*C&W*), 1 cup	90	<1.0	21.0	0	0	0	2.0
Mango drink, 8 fl. oz., except as noted:							
(*AriZona* Mucho Mango)	100	0	27.0	0	0	20	0
(*Langers* Mongo)	120	0	30.0	0	0	0	0
(*Snapple* Mango Madness)	110	0	29.0	0	0	10	0
nectar (*Goya*), 12 fl. oz.	230	0	56.0	0	0	15	2.0
nectar (*Walnut Acres*)	120	0	29.0	0	0	10	0
Mango drink blend, 8 fl. oz.:							
melon (*Sobe* Nirvana)	120	0	31.0	0	0	15	0

Food and Measure	cal.	prot. (gms)	carbo. (gms)	fat (gms)	chol. (mgs)	sod. (mgs)	fiber (gms)
Mango drink blend *(cont.)*							
orange (*Langers*)	130	0	33.0	0	0	0	0
peach:							
(*R.W. Knudsen*) ...	120	<1.0	30.0	0	0	50	0
(*V8 Splash*)	110	0	27.0	0	0	40	0
Mango juice, 8 fl. oz.:							
(*After the Fall* Montage)	150	1.0	37.0	0	0	15	0
(*Ceres*)	120	0	30.0	0	0	10	1.0
Mango nectar, see "Mango drink"							
Mango relish (see also "Chutney"), Indian, 1 tbsp.:							
hot (*Patak's*)	40	<1.0	1.5	4.0	0	640	<1.0
mild (*Patak's*)	40	0	1.0	4.0	0	660	0
Mangosteen, canned in syrup, ½ cup	70	.4	6.7	5.7	0	7	1.8
Manhattan drink mixer (*Holland House*), 4 fl. oz.	150	0	29.0	0	0	25	0
Manicotti entree, frozen, cheese, 1 pkg.:							
(*Michelina's Lean Gourmet*), 8.5 oz.	290	12.0	48.0	5.0	25	780	3.0
three cheese:							
(*Healthy Choice*), 11 oz.	290	14.0	46.0	5.0	35	600	3.0
(*Stouffer's*), 9 oz. ..	360	18.0	41.0	14.0	70	920	2.0
Manioc, see "Yuca"							
Maple syrup, pure, ¼ cup:							
(*Cary's/MacDonald's/ Maple Orchard's*)	210	0	52.0	0	0	15	0
(*Great Expectations*) .	200	0	53.0	0	0	5	0
(*Tree of Life*)	200	0	53.0	0	0	10	0
Margarine, 1 tbsp., except as noted:							
(*Blue Bonnet*)	80	0	0	9.0	0	110	0
(*Blue Bonnet Light*) ..	50	0	0	5.0	0	80	0
(*Country Morning Blend*)	100	0	0	11.0	0	90	0
(*I Can't Believe It's Not Butter!*)	90	0	0	10.0	0	95	0
(*I Can't Believe It's Not Butter! Light*)	50	0	0	6.0	0	85	0

Food and Measure	cal.	prot. (gms)	carbo. (gms)	fat (gms)	chol. (mgs)	sod. (mgs)	fiber (gms)
(*Parkay* Light)	50	0	0	5.0	0	75	0
(*Parkay* Original)	90	0	0	10.0	0	105	0
(*Shedd's Country Crock*)	60	0	0	7.0	0	110	0
soft or stick (*Land O Lakes*)	100	0	0	11.0	0	105	0
spread/soft tub:							
(*Blue Bonnet*)	60	0	0	7.0	0	125	0
(*Blue Bonnet* Light)	40	0	0	4.5	0	90	0
(*Country Morning Blend*)	100	0	0	11.0	0	80	0
(*I Can't Believe It's Not Butter!*)	80	0	0	9.0	0	90	0
(*I Can't Believe It's Not Butter! Calcium*)	50	0	0	5.0	0	90	0
(*I Can't Believe It's Not Butter! Fat Free*)	5	0	0	0	0	90	0
(*I Can't Believe It's Not Butter! Light*)	50	0	0	5.0	0	85	0
(*Parkay*)	60	0	0	7.0	0	100	0
(*Parkay* Light)	50	0	0	5.0	0	130	0
(*Shedd's Country Crock*)	60	0	0	7.0	0	110	0
(*Shedd's Country Crock* Churn Style)	80	0	0	8.0	0	95	0
(*Shedd's Country Crock* Light)	50	0	0	5.0	0	85	0
(*Shedd's Country Crock* Plus Yogurt)	40	0	0	4.0	0	110	0
spread, flavored:							
cinnamon (*Shedd's Country Crock*) .	60	0	3.0	6.0	0	45	0
strawberry (*Shedd's Country Crock*) .	50	0	2.0	5.0	0	35	0
squeeze:							
(*I Can't Believe It's Not Butter!*)	60	0	0	7.0	0	85	0
whipped (*Shedd's Country Crock*) .	60	0	0	7.0	0	85	0
Margarita drink mixer (see also "Daiquiri/ Margarita drink mixer"):							
(*Angostura*), 4 fl. oz. .	100	0	25.0	0	0	20	0

Food and Measure	cal.	prot. (gms)	carbo. (gms)	fat (gms)	chol. (mgs)	sod. (mgs)	fiber (gms)
Margarita drink mixer *(cont.)*							
(*Bacardi*), 3.2 fl. oz. . . .	130	0	35.0	0	0	75	0
(*D.L. Jardine's* Texarita), 3.5 fl. oz.	100	0	30.0	0	0	90	0
frozen (*Bacardi*), 2 fl. oz.	90	0	25.0	0	0	0	0
strawberry (*Trader Vic's*), 4 fl. oz.	160	0	40.0	0	0	20	0
Marinade (see also "Grilling sauce" and specific listings), 1 tbsp., except as noted:							
(*A.1.* Chicago)	20	0	2.0	1.0	0	280	0
(*A.1.* New York Steakhouse)	20	0	5.0	0	0	230	0
(*Annie's Naturals* Organic Paradise), 2 tbsp.	50	<1.0	5.0	3.5	0	470	0
(*Badias* Mojo)	10	0	2.5	0	0	270	0
(*Neera's* Kashmiri), 1 tsp.	18	0	5.0	1.0	0	69	0
(*TryMe Dragon Sauce*), 1 tsp.	5	1.0	1.0	0	0	260	0
Cajun:							
(*A.1.* New Orleans) .	25	0	5.0	0	0	180	0
(*Golden Dipt*)	60	0	2.0	4.5	0	230	0
(*Litehouse*), 2 tbsp.	35	0	7.0	.5	0	410	0
cherry soy (*World Harbors* Cheriyaki), 2 tbsp.	50	0	14.0	0	0	390	0
chimichurri (*World Harbors*), 2 tbsp. . . .	40	0	9.0	0	0	180	0
chipotle (*Lawry's* Baja)	15	0	4.0	0	0	390	0
citrus (*Lawry's* Citrus Grill)	15	0	3.0	0	0	220	0
fajita:							
(*D.L. Jardine's*) . . .	5	0	1.0	0	0	190	0
(*Litehouse*), 2 tbsp.	15	0	3.0	0	0	540	0
(*S&W* Southwest) .	10	0	2.0	0	0	230	<1.0
(*World Harbors*), 2 tbsp.	45	0	10.0	0	0	230	0
medium (*Zapata*) . .	5	0	<1.0	0	0	125	0
garlic herb (*Golden Dipt*)	60	0	1.0	6.0	0	140	0

Food and Measure	cal.	prot. (gms)	carbo. (gms)	fat (gms)	chol. (mgs)	sod. (mgs)	fiber (gms)
garlic and lime (*Lawry's*)	10	0	2.0	0	0	330	0
ginger:							
spicy (*Annie's Naturals* Organic), 2 tbsp.	35	1.0	3.0	2.0	0	450	0
Thai (*Lawry's*)	10	0	2.0	0	0	400	0
Hawaiian (*Lawry's*) ..	25	0	5.0	0	0	250	0
herb and garlic (*Lawry's*)	10	0	2.0	0	0	420	0
honey mustard:							
(*Golden Dipt*)	25	0	4.0	0	0	60	0
Dijon (*Lawry's*) ...	20	0	4.0	0	0	440	0
Dijon (*Litehouse*), 2 tbsp.	80	1.0	6.0	7.0	0	280	0
honey soy (*Golden Dipt*)	30	0	7.0	0	0	390	0
jerk:							
(*Lawry's* Caribbean)	25	0	5.0	0	0	430	0
(*Litehouse* Jamaican), 2 tbsp.	60	0	1.0	4.5	0	410	<1.0
(*World Harbors*), 2 tbsp.	70	0	18.0	0	0	200	0
lemongrass:							
(*Thai Kitchen* Splash)	10	2.0	<1.0	0	0	690	0
herb (*Annie Chun's*)	25	0	4.0	1.5	0	105	0
lemon herb (*Golden Dipt*)	80	0	0	8.0	0	125	0
lemon pepper:							
(*Golden Dipt*)	25	0	1.0	2.0	0	130	0
(*Lawry's*)	10	0	2.0	0	0	390	0
and garlic (*World Harbors*), 2 tbsp.	35	0	8.0	0	0	140	0
mango (*World Harbors* Island), 2 tbsp.	60	0	14.0	0	0	190	0
mesquite:							
(*Golden Dipt*)	10	0	1.0	.5	0	250	0
(*Lawry's*)	5	0	1.0	0	0	350	0
(*S&W*)	10	0	3.0	0	0	400	0
grill (*Litehouse*), 2 tbsp.	15	0	4.0	0	0	460	0
mojo (*World Harbors*), 2 tbsp.	25	0	5.0	1.0	0	300	0
pepper, red (*Lawry's* Louisiana)	10	0	2.0	0	0	390	0

Food and Measure	cal.	prot. (gms)	carbo. (gms)	fat (gms)	chol. (mgs)	sod. (mgs)	fiber (gms)
Marinade *(cont.)*							
sesame ginger :							
(*Lawry's*)	30	0	7.0	0	0	580	0
(*World Harbors* Mandarin)	70	0	16.0	0	0	500	0
sesame, toasted (*Kikkoman Quick & Easy Marinade*) ...	40	1.0	7.0	.5	0	560	0
smokey (*Annie's Naturals* Organic Campfire), 2 tbsp.	60	0	1.0	6.0	0	160	0
tequila lime (*Lawry's*)	15	0	4.0	0	0	490	0
teriyaki:							
(*A.1.* Steakhouse) .	25	0	5.0	1.0	0	490	0
(*Angostura*)	20	0	4.0	0	0	350	0
(*Angostura* All Natural)	10	1.0	1.0	0	0	280	0
(*Annie's Naturals* Organic)	30	0	6.0	.5	0	340	0
(*Kikkoman*)	15	1.0	2.0	0	0	610	0
(*Kikkoman* Lite) ...	15	<1.0	3.0	0	0	320	0
(*Kikkoman Quick & Easy Marinade* Gourmet)	30	1.0	7.0	0	0	450	0
(*Lawry's*)	20	0	5.0	0	0	560	0
(*Litehouse* Marinade & Sauce), 2 tbsp.	35	1.0	6.0	.5	0	470	0
(*S&W*)	25	<1.0	5.0	0	0	480	0
(*S&W* Lite)	25	1.0	5.0	0	0	220	0
(*World Harbors*), 2 tbsp.	70	0	14.0	0	0	270	0
ginger (*Golden Dipt*)	60	0	5.0	3.0	0	560	0
hickory (*Ducks Unlimited*)	15	0	3.0	0	0	720	0
honey (*Ducks Unlimited*)	30	0	6.0	0	0	620	0
honey mustard (*Kikkoman Quick & Easy Marinade*)	35	1.0	7.0	0	0	450	0
hot (*World Harbors*), 2 tbsp.	70	0	17.0	0	0	300	0
roasted garlic (*Kikkoman*)	25	1.0	5.0	0	0	730	0

Food and Measure	cal.	prot. (gms)	carbo. (gms)	fat (gms)	chol. (mgs)	sod. (mgs)	fiber (gms)
roasted garlic herb (*Kikkoman Quick & Easy Marinade*)	20	1.0	4.0	0	0	610	0
white wine (*Golden Dipt*)	10	0	1.0	0	0	125	0
Marinade seasoning mix, ¾ tsp.:							
(*Adolph's Marinade in Minutes*)	5	0	1.0	0	0	380	0
beef, tenderizing (*Lawry's*)	0	0	<1.0	0	0	560	0
Marionberry, see "Blackberry, dried"							
Marjoram, dried, 1 tsp.	2	.1	.4	<.1	0	<1	.1
Marmalade, see "Jam and preserves"							
Marrow squash, raw, trimmed, 1 oz.	4	.2	1.0	<.1	0	n.a.	<1.0
Marshmallow topping, 2 tbsp.:							
(*Marshmallow Fluff*) .	60	0	15.0	0	0	10	0
(*Smucker's*)	120	0	29.0	0	0	0	0
raspberry or strawberry (*Marshmallow Fluff*)	60	0	15.0	0	0	10	0
Masa, see "Cornmeal"							
Matai, see "Water chestnut"							
Matzo, see "Cracker"							
Matzo ball, in jars:							
(*Manischewitz*), 1 cup	220	7.0	27.0	9.0	80	880	3.0
(*Mrs. Adler's*), 1 cup, 3 pcs. w/liquid	190	5.0	24.0	8.0	0	710	1.0
Matzo ball mix, dry (*Manischewitz*), 1½ tbsp.	45	1.0	9.0	0	0	660	<1.0
Matzo meal, see "Cracker crumbs/ meal"							
Mayonnaise, 1 tbsp.:							
(*Blue Plate*)	100	0	0	11.0	10	80	0
(*Cains*)	100	0	0	11.0	5	75	0
(*Cains Fat Free*)	10	0	3.0	0	0	140	0
(*Cains Light*)	50	0	2.0	4.5	5	125	0
(*Cains Reduced Fat*) ..	30	0	3.0	2.0	0	130	0
(*Hain*)	100	0	0	11.0	5	100	0

Food and Measure	cal.	prot. (gms)	carbo. (gms)	fat (gms)	chol. (mgs)	sod. (mgs)	fiber (gms)
Mayonnaise *(cont.)*							
(*Hain* Lite)	45	0	2.0	4.0	5	130	0
(*Hellmann's/Best Foods* Real)	100	0	0	11.0	5	90	0
(*Hellmann's/Best Foods* Light)	50	0	1.0	5.0	5	120	0
(*Henri's*)	100	0	0	11.0	5	85	0
(*Hollywood* Canola) ..	100	0	0	11.0	5	100	0
(*Kraft* Light)	40	0	2.0	3.5	5	90	0
(*Kraft* Real)	100	0	0	11.0	5	75	0
(*Smart Balance* Light)	50	0	2.0	5.0	5	125	0
(*Smart Beat* Fat Free) .	10	0	3.0	0	0	135	0
(*Vegenaise*)	90	0	1.0	9.0	0	80	0
bacon and tomato (*Hellmann's*)	50	0	1.0	5.0	5	210	0
chipotle:							
chili (*French's GourMayo*)	50	0	1.0	5.0	10	95	0
smokey (*French's GourMayo*)	50	0	1.0	5.0	10	115	0
dressing:							
(*Kraft* Fat Free)	10	0	2.0	0	0	120	0
(*Miracle Whip*)	40	0	2.0	3.5	5	125	0
(*Miracle Whip* Fat Free)	15	0	3.0	0	0	125	0
(*Miracle Whip* Light)	25	0	3.0	1.5	5	140	0
hot and spicy (*Miracle Whip*) ..	45	0	2.0	4.0	5	140	0
fresh, refrigerated:							
(*Delouis Fils*)	110	0	0	12.0	30	70	0
garlic, fresh, refrigerated (*Delouis Fils* Aioli)	102	0	0	11.2	27	97	0
hot and spicy (*Kraft*) .	100	0	0	11.0	5	85	0
sun-dried tomato (*French's GourMayo*)	45	0	2.0	4.0	10	100	0
spicy, smoked jalapeno (*Fiesta*)	60	3.0	12.0	.5	0	390	0
wasabi horseradish (*French's GourMayo*)	50	0	2.0	5.0	10	115	0
Mayonnaise dressing, see "Mayonnaise"							
McDonald's, 1 serving:							
breakfast:							
Big Breakfast	730	27.0	53.0	46.0	465	1460	3.0

Food and Measure	cal.	prot. (gms)	carbo. (gms)	fat (gms)	chol. (mgs)	sod. (mgs)	fiber (gms)
biscuit, plain	240	4.0	31.0	11.0	0	680	1.0
bacon/egg/cheese	440	19.0	36.0	24.0	245	1250	1.0
sausage	410	10.0	34.0	26.0	30	990	1.0
sausage/egg	500	18.0	36.0	32.0	250	1080	1.0
burrito, sausage ...	300	13.0	26.0	16.0	175	760	1.0
cinnamon roll	420	8.0	57.0	18.0	60	400	2.0
cinnamon roll deluxe	590	9.0	86.0	24.0	55	660	4.0
deluxe breakfast ...	1220	33.0	136.0	60.0	480	1900	4.0
eggs, scrambled, 2	180	15.0	5.0	11.0	435	180	0
hash browns	140	1.0	15.0	8.0	0	290	2.0
hotcakes w/sausage	770	15.0	104.0	33.0	50	930	2.0
hotcakes, w/syrup, 2 pats margarine	600	9.0	102.0	17.0	20	620	2.0
jam or preserves ..	35	0	9.0	0	0	0	0
McGriddles:							
bacon/egg/cheese	450	16.0	46.0	21.0	245	1260	1.0
sausage	420	15.0	44.0	22.0	30	990	1.0
sausage/egg/ cheese	560	16.0	48.0	32.0	260	1290	1.0
McMuffin:							
egg	290	17.0	30.0	11.0	235	850	2.0
sausage	370	14.0	31.0	21.0	45	790	2.0
sausage/egg	450	20.0	39.0	26.0	260	930	2.0
muffin, English	150	5.0	27.0	2.0	0	260	2.0
sausage patty	170	7.0	2.0	15.0	30	310	0
sandwiches:							
Big Mac	560	25.0	46.0	30.0	80	1010	3.0
Big N' Tasty	520	24.0	41.0	29.0	80	730	3.0
w/cheese	570	27.0	43.0	33.0	90	960	3.0
cheeseburger	310	15.0	35.0	12.0	40	740	1.0
double	460	25.0	37.0	23.0	80	1140	1.0
chicken, crispy	500	24.0	50.0	23.0	50	1090	3.0
Chicken McGrill ...	400	27.0	38.0	16.0	70	1010	3.0
Filet-O-Fish	400	14.0	42.0	18.0	40	640	1.0
hamburger	260	13.0	33.0	9.0	30	530	1.0
McChicken	420	15.0	41.0	22.0	45	760	1.0
hot and spicy ...	440	14.0	42.0	24.0	45	920	1.0
Quarter Pounder ..	420	24.0	40.0	18.0	70	730	3.0
w/cheese	510	29.0	43.0	25.0	95	1150	3.0
w/cheese, double	730	47.0	46.0	40.0	160	1330	3.0
Chicken McNuggets:							
4 pcs.	170	10.0	10.0	10.0	25	450	0
6 pcs.	250	15.0	15.0	15.0	35	670	0

Food and Measure	cal.	prot. (gms)	carbo. (gms)	fat (gms)	chol. (mgs)	sod. (mgs)	fiber (gms)
McDonald's, Chicken McNuggets (cont.)							
10 pcs.	420	25.0	26.0	24.0	60	1120	0
20 pcs.	840	50.0	51.0	49.0	125	2240	0
McNuggets sauce:							
barbecue	45	0	11.0	0	0	260	0
honey	50	0	12.0	0	0	0	0
hot mustard	50	1.0	9.0	2.0	0	260	1.0
sweet 'n sour . . .	50	0	11.0	0	0	160	0
Chicken Selects, breast:							
3 pcs.	380	23.0	28.0	20.0	55	930	0
5 pcs.	630	39.0	46.0	33.0	90	1550	0
10 pcs.	1270	77.0	92.0	66.0	180	3100	0
Selects sauce:							
barbecue, chipotle	70	0	16.0	0	0	260	0
Buffalo, spicy . . .	60	0	1.0	6.0	0	910	<.10
honey mustard . .	70	1.0	13.0	2.0	0	160	1.0
ranch, creamy . .	200	0	3.0	21.0	10	300	0
fries:							
large	520	6.0	70.0	25.0	0	330	7.0
medium	350	4.0	47.0	16.0	0	220	5.0
small	230	2.0	30.0	11.0	0	140	3.0
ketchup, pkt.	10	0	3.0	0	0	100	0
salad, no dressing:							
bacon ranch, plain .	130	9.0	9.0	7.0	25	290	3.0
w/crispy chicken	350	27.0	23.0	17.0	65	1030	3.0
w/grilled chicken	250	31.0	12.0	9.0	85	950	3.0
Caesar, plain	90	7.0	8.0	4.0	10	180	3.0
w/crispy chicken	310	25.0	23.0	14.0	50	910	3.0
w/grilled chicken	210	28.0	11.0	6.0	70	830	3.0
Cobb, plain	150	11.0	8.0	9.0	85	410	3.0
w/crispy chicken	370	29.0	23.0	18.0	125	1150	3.0
w/grilled chicken	270	33.0	11.0	11.0	145	1060	3.0
side salad	15	1.0	3.0	0	0	10	1.0
butter garlic croutons	60	2.0	10.0	1.0	0	160	<1.0
salad dressing (*Newman's Own*), 2 fl. oz.:							
balsamic vinaigrette	40	0	4.0	3.0	0	730	0
Caesar, creamy	190	2.0	4.0	18.0	20	500	0
Cobb	120	1.0	9.0	9.0	10	440	0
ranch	170	1.0	9.0	15.0	20	530	0
dessert/shakes:							
apple dippers	35	0	8.0	0	0	0	0
w/caramel dip . .	100	0	22.0	1.0	5	35	0
apple pie	250	3.0	39.0	11.0	0	150	2.0

Food and Measure	cal.	prot. (gms)	carbo. (gms)	fat (gms)	chol. (mgs)	sod. (mgs)	fiber (gms)
caramel dip	70	0	14.0	1.0	5	35	0
cone, vanilla, reduced fat	150	4.0	24.0	3.5	15	60	0
cookies:							
chocolate chip ..	160	2.0	22.0	7.0	10	95	<1.0
McDonaldland ..	250	4.0	42.0	8.0	0	270	<1.0
McDonaldland chocolate chip	270	3.0	39.0	11.0	35	170	1.0
oatmeal raisin ..	140	2.0	22.0	5.0	10	125	1.0
sugar	150	2.0	22.0	6.0	5	115	0
fruit 'n yogurt parfait	160	4.0	31.0	2.0	5	85	<1.0
w/out granola ...	130	4.0	25.0	2.0	5	55	0
McFlurry, 12 fl. oz.:							
M&M's	620	14.0	96.0	20.0	55	190	<1.0
Oreo	560	14.0	88.0	16.0	50	250	0
sundaes:							
hot caramel	340	7.0	62.0	7.0	30	140	0
hot fudge	330	8.0	55.0	9.0	25	170	<1.0
strawberry	280	6.0	51.0	6.0	25	85	0
sundae peanuts .	45	2.0	2.0	3.5	0	0	1.0
Triple Thick shake:							
chocolate, 12 oz.	440	10.0	76.0	10.0	40	190	<1.0
chocolate, 16 oz.	580	13.0	102.0	14.0	50	250	<1.0
chocolate, 21 oz.	770	18.0	134.0	18.0	70	330	1.0
chocolate, 32 oz.	1160	27.0	203.0	27.0	100	510	2.0
strawberry, 12 oz.	420	10.0	73.0	10.0	40	130	0
strawberry, 16 oz.	560	13.0	97.0	13.0	50	170	0
strawberry, 21 oz.	740	17.0	128.0	18.0	70	230	0
strawberry, 32 oz.	1110	25.0	194.0	26.0	100	350	0
vanilla, 12 oz. ...	420	9.0	72.0	10.0	40	140	0
vanilla, 16 oz. ...	550	13.0	96.0	13.0	50	190	0
vanilla, 21 oz. ...	740	17.0	128.0	18.0	70	250	0
vanilla, 32 oz. ...	1110	25.0	193.0	26.0	100	370	0
Meat, potted, see "Meat spread"							
Meat loaf, refrigerated, 5 oz.:							
(Hormel)	120	20.0	13.0	13.0	55	790	2.0
seasoned (Tyson)	320	14.0	16.0	23.0	60	940	0
Meat loaf dinner, frozen, 1 pkg.:							
(Healthy Choice Dinners), 12 oz. ...	300	18.0	36.0	9.0	40	600	6.0

Food and Measure	cal.	prot. (gms)	carbo. (gms)	fat (gms)	chol. (mgs)	sod. (mgs)	fiber (gms)
Meat loaf dinner *(cont.)*							
(*Stouffer's* Homestyle),							
17 oz.	560	29.0	46.0	29.0	95	1350	6.0
(*Swanson Hungry-Man*),							
16.5 oz.	850	34.0	87.0	43.0	105	2500	6.0
"Meat" loaf dinner,							
vegetarian, frozen							
(*Amy's* Veggie Loaf							
Meal), 10-oz. pkg. .	280	8.0	47.0	7.0	0	690	7.0
Meat loaf entree,							
frozen, 1 pkg.,							
except as noted:							
(*Michelina's Lean*							
Gourmet), 8 oz. . . .	210	13.0	22.0	8.0	50	1170	2.0
(*Stouffer's* Homestyle),							
9⅞ oz.	350	24.0	23.0	18.0	60	860	2.0
and gravy:							
(*Stouffer's* Family							
Style Recipes),							
1/6 of 33-oz. pkg.	210	15.0	10.0	12.0	50	560	1.0
w/mashed potato							
(*Michelina's* Au-							
thentico), 8 oz. . . .	270	11.0	20.0	16.0	55	1380	2.0
w/vegetable medley							
(*Organic Classics*),							
9.5 oz.	290	23.0	19.0	14.0	40	690	4.0
w/mashed potato:							
(*Boston Market*),							
12 oz.	530	21.0	38.0	33.0	105	1360	3.0
(*Smart Ones Bistro*							
Selections), 9.5 oz.	260	24.0	22.0	8.0	35	760	5.0
w/potato and green							
beans (*Swanson*							
Angus), 11 oz.	380	15.0	30.0	22.0	45	1210	4.0
and whipped potato							
(*Lean Cuisine* Café							
Classics), 9⅜ oz. . .	280	20.0	29.0	9.0	45	580	3.0
"Meat" loaf entree,							
vegetarian, frozen:							
(*Amy's* Veggie Loaf							
Family Size), ¼ of							
23-oz. pkg.	220	7.0	32.0	7.0	0	650	6.0
(*Hain Vegetarian Clas-*							
sics Homestyle),							
10-oz. pkg.	300	32.0	39.0	6.0	0	400	16.0

Food and Measure	cal.	prot. (gms)	carbo. (gms)	fat (gms)	chol. (mgs)	sod. (mgs)	fiber (gms)
Meat loaf seasoning mix, dry:							
(*Adolph's Meal Makers*), 1 tbsp.	25	<1.0	5.0	0	0	380	0
(*Lawry's*). 1 tbsp.	30	<1.0	7.0	0	0	470	<1.0
(*McCormick*), 1 tsp. .	15	0	2.0	0	0	350	0
(*McCormick Bag 'n Season*), 2 tsp.	15	1.0	2.0	0	0	390	0
(*Mrs. Cubbison's*), 1 tbsp.	30	0	4.0	.5	0	430	0
Meat marinade mix (*McCormick*), 1 tsp.	15	0	2.0	0	0	240	0
Meat spread (see also specific listings):							
(*Oscar Mayer* Sandwich Spread), 2 oz.	130	4.0	9.0	9.0	25	460	0
(*Spam* Spread), 4 tbsp.	140	8.0	1.0	12.0	40	570	0
w/crackers (*Spam* Spread), 1 kit	300	14.0	14.0	22.0	60	1040	1.0
potted meat:							
(*Goya*), ¼ cup	80	8.0	0	5.0	55	550	0
(*Hormel*), 4 tbsp. . . .	100	7.0	0	8.0	50	610	0
Meat tenderizer:							
(*Adolph's* Original), ¼ tsp.	0	0	0	0	0	380	0
(*McCormick*), ¼ tsp. .	0	0	0	0	0	400	0
(*Tone's*), 1 tsp.	7	0	1.2	.2	0	1760	tr.
(*Watkins* Meat Magic), 1 tsp.	5	0	1.0	0	0	180	0
seasoned, ¼ tsp.:							
(*Adolph's*)	0	0	0	0	0	450	0
(*McCormick*)	0	0	0	0	0	300	0
Meatball, frozen:							
(*Ian's* Natural Italian), 3 pcs., 3 oz.	145	16.0	10.0	4.0	70	250	1.0
(*Mama Lucia*), 4 pcs., 3.2 oz.	280	11.0	8.0	23.0	50	640	0
(*On the Go Bistro* Gourmet), 2 pcs., 3 oz. .	300	16.0	6.0	23.0	60	530	0
(*Organic Classics*), 3 pcs., 3 oz.	180	17.0	5.0	11.0	50	430	1.0
(*Prima Familia*), 4 pcs., 3.2 oz.	250	17.0	6.0	18.0	60	620	<1.0

Food and Measure	cal.	prot. (gms)	carbo. (gms)	fat (gms)	chol. (mgs)	sod. (mgs)	fiber (gms)
"Meatball," vegetarian, frozen (*Quorn*), 4 pcs., 2.4 oz.	110	14.0	7.0	3.0	5	430	1.0
Meatball entree, canned, stew (*Dinty Moore*), 1 cup	250	13.0	19.0	15.0	40	1050	1.0
Meatball entree, frozen, 1 pkg.:							
and mashed potato (*Michelina's* Authentico), 8.5 oz. . .	270	11.0	26.0	14.0	35	1150	3.0
penne and, see "Penne entree"							
spaghetti and, see "Spaghetti entree"							
Swedish:							
(*Lean Cuisine Everyday Favorites*), 9⅛ oz.	290	22.0	33.0	8.0	50	640	2.0
(*Michelina's Lean Gourmet*), 9 oz. . .	290	17.0	40.0	7.0	30	850	3.0
(*Smart Ones*), 9 oz.	280	19.0	34.0	7.0	30	740	3.0
(*Stouffer's*), 11.5 oz.	570	28.0	39.0	33.0	110	1150	2.0
w/gravy, pasta (*Michelina's* Authentico), 10 oz. . .	390	19.0	41.0	17.0	50	950	3.0
Meatball pocket, frozen 4.5-oz. pc.:							
cheese, three (*Smart Ones Smartwich*) . .	270	10.0	39.0	7.0	15	520	2.0
and mozzarella:							
(*Croissant Pockets*)	330	14.0	45.0	15.0	15	810	3.0
(*Hot Pockets*)	330	12.0	39.0	14.0	30	770	2.0
(*Lean Pockets*)	290	13.0	44.0	7.0	20	700	3.0
(*Lean Pockets* Ultra)	200	24.0	19.0	6.0	25	570	7.0
Meatball seasoning and sauce mix, Swedish (*McCormick*), 2 tsp. seasoning and 1 tsp. sauce mix . .	45	0	4.0	1.0	0	790	0
Melba sauce (*Roland*), 2 tbsp.	100	0	25.0	0	0	10	0
Melogold (*Frieda's*), ½ fruit, 5.9 oz.	50	0	13.0	0	0	0	2.0

Food and Measure	cal.	prot. (gms)	carbo. (gms)	fat (gms)	chol. (mgs)	sod. (mgs)	fiber (gms)
Melon, see specific melon listings							
Melon balls, frozen, cantaloupe/honeydew, ½ cup	28	.7	6.9	.2	0	27	.6
Melon drink, see "Watermelon drink"							
Mesclun, see "Salad blend"							
Mexican beans, see "Pinto beans" and specific listings							
Mexican seasoning mix (*Chi-Chi's* Fiesta Restaurante), 1 tsp.	10	0	2.0	0	0	290	0
Mexican squash (*Frieda's*), ½ cup, 3 oz.	35	1.0	9.0	0	0	0	2.0
Mexican entree, frozen casserole (*Amy's* Bowls), 9.5-oz. pkg.	480	10.0	70.0	18.0	20	780	7.0
Mexican sauce (see also specific listings), cooking:							
cilantro lime (*Pace Mexican Creations*), 1 cup	160	7.0	17.0	7.0	10	890	7.0
onion and garlic, roasted (*Pace Mexican Creations*), 1 cup	230	12.0	15.0	13.0	25	880	1.0
roasted ranchero (*Pace Mexican Creations*), ¼ cup	35	1.0	6.0	1.0	0	500	1.0
verde (*Pace Mexican Creations*), 1 cup ..	120	9.0	14.0	3.0	15	890	3.0
Mexican snack rolls, frozen (*Health is Wealth Munchees*), 6 pcs., 3 oz.	190	5.0	32.0	5.0	0	560	3.0
Milk, 8 fl. oz.:							
buttermilk:							
(*Darigold* Lowfat) ..	110	9.0	13.0	2.5	15	270	0

Food and Measure	cal.	prot. (gms)	carbo. (gms)	fat (gms)	chol. (mgs)	sod. (mgs)	fiber (gms)
Milk, buttermilk *(cont.)*							
(Hood)	90	9.0	13.0	0	<5	220	0
(Organic Valley							
Lowfat)*	100	8.0	12.0	2.5	15	250	0
cultured	99	8.1	11.7	2.2	9	257	0
whole:							
(Cool Moos)	160	8.0	12.0	8.0	35	120	0
(Darigold)	150	8.0	12.0	8.0	35	125	0
(Hood)	150	8.0	12.0	8.0	35	125	0
(Organic Valley) ...	150	8.0	12.0	8.0	35	125	0
3.3% fat	150	8.0	11.4	8.2	33	120	0
reduced fat (2%):							
(Cool Moos)	130	8.0	12.0	5.0	20	120	0
(Darigold)	130	8.0	13.0	5.0	20	125	0
(Darigold White) ..	140	10.0	14.0	5.0	25	140	0
(Hood)	130	8.0	13.0	5.0	20	125	0
(Organic Valley) ...	130	8.0	12.0	5.0	20	120	0
2% fat	121	8.1	11.7	4.7	18	122	0
2%, protein fortified	137	9.7	13.5	4.9	19	145	0
low fat (1%):							
(Cool Moos)	100	8.0	12.0	2.5	10	125	0
(Darigold)	110	9.0	13.0	2.5	10	130	0
(Darigold Acidophilus/							
Calcium Extra)* ..	110	9.0	13.0	2.5	15	130	0
(Hood)	110	8.0	13.0	2.5	15	125	0
(Organic Valley) ...	110	8.0	13.0	2.5	15	125	0
(Organic Valley							
Lactose Free)* ...	100	8.0	12.0	2.5	10	125	0
(Simply Smart) ...	120	10.0	13.0	2.5	15	130	0
1% fat	102	8.0	11.7	2.6	10	123	0
1%, protein fortified	119	9.7	13.6	2.9	10	143	0
skim/fat free:							
(Darigold)	90	9.0	13.0	0	5	130	0
(Darigold Acidophilus/							
Trim Deluxe)* ...	100	10.0	14.0	0	5	140	0
(Hood)	80	8.0	13.0	0	<5	125	0
(Organic Valley) ...	90	8.0	13.0	0	5	125	0
(Simply Smart) ...	90	10.0	13.0	0	<5	130	0
8 fl. oz.	86	8.4	11.9	.4	4	126	0
Milk, canned, 2 tbs.:							
condensed, sweetened:							
(Carnation)	130	3.0	22.0	3.0	10	45	0
(Eagle Brand)	130	3.0	23.0	3.0	10	40	0
(Eagle Brand Fat Free)*	110	3.0	24.0	0	<5	40	0

Food and Measure	cal.	prot. (gms)	carbo. (gms)	fat (gms)	chol. (mgs)	sod. (mgs)	fiber (gms)
(*Eagle Brand* Lowfat)	130	3.0	23.0	1.5	5	40	0
(*Magnolia*)	130	3.0	23.0	3.0	10	40	0
evaporated:							
(*Carnation*)	40	2.0	3.0	2.0	10	30	0
(*Carnation* Fat Free)	25	2.0	4.0	0	0	40	0
(*Carnation* Lowfat) .	25	2.0	3.0	.5	5	35	0
(*Pet*)	40	2.0	3.0	2.0	10	30	0
skim (*Pet*)	25	2.0	4.0	0	0	40	0
Milk, chocolate, see "Milk, flavored"							
Milk, dry:							
buttermilk:							
sweet cream, 1 cup	464	41.2	58.8	6.9	83	620	0
sweet cream, 1 tbsp.	25	2.2	3.2	.4	4	34	0
buttermilk blend (*Organic Valley*), 3 tbsp.	110	10.0	16.0	1.0	25	45	0
whole, 1 oz.	141	7.5	10.9	7.6	27	105	0
whole, 1 cup	635	33.7	49.2	34.2	124	475	0
nonfat:							
(*Organic Valley*), 3 tbsp.	90	9.0	13.0	0	<5	130	0
regular, 1 cup	435	43.4	62.4	.9	24	642	0
instant, 3.2-oz. pkt.	244	23.9	35.5	.5	12	373	0
Milk, flavored, 8 fl. oz.:							
banana, reduced fat (*Nesquik*)	200	7.0	30.0	5.0	20	120	0
chocolate:							
(*Hershey's* Creamy MilkShake)	270	10.0	43.0	8.0	20	140	1.0
whole (*Darigold* Extra)	240	8.0	33.0	9.0	40	270	<1.0
whole (*Hood*)	230	9.0	31.0	8.0	35	250	<1.0
reduced fat (*Darigold* Smooth)	210	9.0	33.0	5.0	25	250	<1.0
reduced fat (*Hershey's*)	200	8.0	31.0	5.0	20	135	1.0
reduced fat (*Nesquik*)	200	8.0	32.0	5.0	15	150	<1.0
reduced fat (*Nesquik* Milkshake)	170	8.0	26.0	5.0	15	180	<1.0
reduced fat (*Organic Valley*)	170	8.0	23.0	5.0	20	250	<1.0
reduced fat (*Organic Valley* Ultra)	240	12.0	33.0	7.0	30	320	2.0
low fat (*Cool Moos*)	180	8.0	32.0	2.5	10	210	0

Food and Measure	cal.	prot. (gms)	carbo. (gms)	fat (gms)	chol. (mgs)	sod. (mgs)	fiber (gms)
Milk, flavored, chocolate *(cont.)*							
low fat (*Hershey's* No Sugar)	120	11.0	15.0	2.5	5	170	1.0
low fat (*Hood*)	170	9.0	28.0	3.0	15	170	<1.0
nonfat (*Nesquik*) ..	160	8.0	32.0	0	0	150	<1.0
chocolate, double, re-duced fat (*Nesquik*)	200	8.0	30.0	5.0	15	170	<1.0
chocolate mint (*Hershey's York* Milk-Shake)	300	10.0	52.0	7.0	20	220	<1.0
coffee, low fat (*Hood*)	170	8.0	28.0	2.5	15	125	0
cookies and cream (*Hershey's* Shake) .	280	10.0	45.0	7.0	20	180	0
mocha, reduced fat (*Nesquik*)	200	8.0	32.0	5.0	15	240	0
strawberry:							
(*Hershey's* Shake) .	280	9.0	44.0	7.0	20	220	0
reduced fat (*Darigold*)	210	9.0	33.0	5.0	25	140	0
reduced fat (*Hershey's*)	200	8.0	30.0	5.0	15	130	0
reduced fat (*Nesquik*)	200	8.0	33.0	5.0	15	120	0
reduced fat (*Nesquik* Milkshake)	170	8.0	25.0	5.0	20	140	<1.0
low fat (*Cool Moos*)	160	8.0	27.0	2.5	10	125	0
low fat (*Organic Valley*)	180	10.0	30.0	3.0	10	150	3.0
vanilla:							
(*Darigold*)	210	9.0	33.0	5.0	25	140	0
(*Hershey's* Shake) .	320	9.0	55.0	7.0	20	240	0
reduced fat (*Hood*)	190	8.0	28.0	5.0	20	130	0
reduced fat (*Nesquik* Very)	200	8.0	30.0	5.0	15	120	0
low fat (*Cool Moos*)	160	8.0	26.0	2.5	10	125	0
low fat (*Organic Valley*)	170	10.0	28.0	3.0	10	150	2.0
Milk, goat, 8 fl. oz.:							
(*Meyenberg*)	140	8.0	11.0	7.0	25	115	0
fresh	168	8.7	10.9	10.1	28	122	0
"Milk," nondairy, see "Rice beverage" and "Soy beverage"							
Milk, human, 8 fl. oz.	172	2.9	16.9	10.8	34	42	0
Milk, sheep, 8 fl. oz. .	265	14.7	13.1	17.2	66	108	0

Food and Measure	cal.	prot. (gms)	carbo. (gms)	fat (gms)	chol. (mgs)	sod. (mgs)	fiber (gms)
Milkfish, meat only:							
raw, 4 oz.	168	23.3	0	7.6	59	82	0
baked, broiled, or							
microwaved, 4 oz. .	215	29.8	0	9.8	76	104	0
Millet:							
dry:							
(*Shiloh Farms*),							
¼ cup	150	5.0	34.0	1.5	0	0	3.0
1 oz.	107	3.1	20.7	1.2	0	1	2.4
cooked, 4 oz.	135	4.0	26.8	1.1	0	2	1.5
Millet flour (*Arrow-*							
head Mills), ⅓ cup .	130	4.0	26.0	1.5	0	0	3.0
Mincemeat, see "Pie							
filling"							
Mint, fresh:							
peppermint, 2 tbsp. . .	2	.1	.5	0	0	.1	<.1
spearmint, 2 tbsp. . . .	5	.4	.9	.1	0	3	.7
Mint, dried, spearmint,							
1 tbsp.	5	.3	.8	.1	0	6	.5
Mint sauce (*Crosse &*							
Blackwell), 1 tsp. . . .	5	0	1.0	0	0	0	0
Mirin rice wine, see							
"Wine, cooking"							
Miso, soy paste:							
(*Eden* Organic Hacho),							
1 tbsp.	35	3.0	2.0	1.5	0	600	1.0
(*Eden* Organic Shiro),							
1 tbsp.	35	2.0	5.0	1.0	0	410	1.0
(*Westbrae Natural* Bag),							
1 tsp.	10	<1.0	0	.5	0	280	0
1 oz.	58	3.3	7.9	1.7	0	1034	1.5
½ cup	284	16.3	38.6	8.4	0	5032	7.6
w/barley (*Westbrae*							
Natural Bag), 1 tsp.	10	0	2.0	0	0	310	0
w/brown rice:							
(*Eden* Organic Gen-							
mai), 1 tbsp. . . .	25	2.0	3.0	1.0	0	810	1.0
(*Westbrae Natural*							
Bag), 1 tsp.	10	<1.0	<1.0	0	0	250	0
(*Westbrae Natural*							
Organic Mellow),							
1 tsp.	10	<1.0	2.0	0	0	220	<1.0
red or white (*Westbrae*							
Natural Organic							
Mellow), 1 tsp.	10	<1.0	2.0	0	0	180	<1.0

Food and Measure	cal.	prot. (gms)	carbo. (gms)	fat (gms)	chol. (mgs)	sod. (mgs)	fiber (gms)
Miso *(cont.)*							
w/soybean and barley							
(*Eden* Organic Mugi),							
1 tbsp.	25	2.0	3.0	1.0	0	760	1.0
Miso condiment, see							
"Tekka"							
Mocha drink (*Yoo-hoo*							
Dyna-Mocha), 8 fl. oz.	150	2.0	34.0	.5	0	100	1.0
Mochi, see "Rice snack"							
Molasses, 1 tbsp.:							
(*Brer Rabbit* Full							
Flavored)	60	0	15.0	0	0	10	0
(*Grandma's*)	50	0	12.0	0	0	0	0
blackstrap:							
(*Brer Rabbit*)	60	1.0	13.0	0	0	65	0
(*New Morning*)	60	<1.0	13.0	0	0	20	0
(*Tree of Life*)	45	0	11.0	0	0	15	0
mild:							
(*Brer Rabbit*)	60	0	15.0	0	0	10	0
(*Grandma's*)	50	0	14.0	0	0	0	0
robust (*Grandma's*) . .	50	0	12.0	0	0	0	0
Mole sauce:							
(*Doña Maria*), 2 tbsp. .	230	3.0	12.0	15.0	0	460	2.0
(*Doña Maria* Verde),							
2 tbsp.	240	5.0	6.0	18.0	0	660	2.0
green (*La Costeña*),							
1 tbsp	90	3.0	8.0	5.0	0	750	<1.0
hot (*La Costeña*), 1 tbsp.	120	1.0	13.0	8.0	0	130	1.0
Monkfish, meat only:							
raw, 4 oz.	86	16.4	0	1.7	29	21	0
baked, broiled, or micro-							
waved, 4 oz.	110	21.0	0	2.2	36	26	0
Monosodium glutamate							
(MSG):							
(*McCormick*), ¼ tsp. .	0	0	0	0	0	125	0
(*Tone's*), 1 tsp.	0	0	0	0	0	638	0
Moose, meat only,							
roasted, 4 oz.	152	33.2	0	1.1	88	78	0
Mortadella, 2 oz.:							
(*Boar's Head*)	160	9.0	0	14.0	30	560	0
beef and pork	174	9.2	1.7	14.2	31	698	0
w/pistachios (*Boar's							
Head*)	170	10.0	2.0	14.0	30	560	0
Mothbean, boiled, 4 oz.	133	8.9	23.8	.6	0	11	n.a.

Food and Measure	cal.	prot. (gms)	carbo. (gms)	fat (gms)	chol. (mgs)	sod. (mgs)	fiber (gms)
MSG, see "Monosodium glutamate"							
Muffin, 1 pc., 2 oz., except as noted:							
banana walnut, mini (*Hostess*), 2-oz. pkg.	230	2.0	24.0	14.0	30	125	<1.0
blueberry:							
gluten free (*Foods by George*), 2.8 oz. .	220	3.0	34.0	8.0	25	390	<1.0
mini (*Hostess*), 3 pcs., 1.2 oz.	160	2.0	19.0	8.0	30	120	0
chocolate chip, mini (*Hostess*), 2-oz. pkg.	250	3.0	28.0	14.0	35	150	0
corn:							
(*Foods by George*), 2.8 oz.	240	4.0	36.0	9.0	30	420	1.0
2 oz.	174	3.6	29.0	4.8	15	297	1.9
English:							
(*Bays* Original)	140	5.0	27.0	1.5	0	530	1.0
(*Pepperidge Farm*) .	130	5.0	25.0	1.0	0	170	1.0
(*Thomas'* Original) .	120	4.0	25.0	1.0	0	200	1.0
cinnamon raisin (*Thomas'*), 2.2 oz.	150	4.0	31.0	1.0	0	180	2.0
honey wheat (*Thomas'*)	130	5.0	27.0	1.0	0	190	2.0
multigrain (*Thomas'*)	130	5.0	25.0	1.5	0	160	1.0
multigrain (*Thomas' Light*)	100	7.0	22.0	1.0	<5	210	8.0
plain, wheat or raisin (*Country Kitchen Reduced Calorie*)	100	5.0	22.0	1.0	0	150	5.0
sourdough (*Bays*) .	130	5.0	26.0	1.0	0	470	2.0
sourdough (*Thomas'*)	120	4.0	25.0	1.0	0	190	1.0
whole wheat (*Pepperidge Farm*) . .	130	6.0	26.0	.5	0	210	3.0
whole wheat (*Thomas'*), 2.2 oz.	120	6.0	22.0	1.0	0	200	3.0
English, gluten free, 3.6 oz.:							
(*Foods by George*) .	210	4.0	39.0	3.5	0	270	1.0
cinnamon currant (*Foods by George*)	220	4.0	42.0	3.5	0	220	2.0
rye (*Foods by George No-Rye*)	210	4.0	40.0	4.0	0	270	2.0
oat bran	154	4.0	27.5	4.2	0	224	2.6

Food and Measure	cal.	prot. (gms)	carbo. (gms)	fat (gms)	chol. (mgs)	sod. (mgs)	fiber (gms)
Muffin, frozen, chocolate chip (*Smart Ones*), 2.5-oz. pc. .	190	3.0	39.0	2.0	0	350	4.0
Muffin, toaster, see "Toaster pastry and muffin"							
Muffin mix (see also "Bread mix, sweet"), 1 pc.*, except as noted:							
apple cinnamon:							
(*Betty Crocker*) . . .	130	2.0	21.0	4.0	15	210	0
(*"Jiffy"*), ¼ cup . . .	170	2.0	28.0	5.0	0	300	1.0
apple streusel (*Betty Crocker*)	210	2.0	33.0	8.0	20	220	0
banana nut:							
(*Betty Crocker*) . . .	130	2.0	21.0	5.0	0	190	0
(*"Jiffy"*), ¼ cup . . .	160	2.0	25.0	5.0	0	300	2.0
berry, triple (*Betty Crocker*)	120	2.0	23.0	3.0	15	220	0
blueberry:							
(*Betty Crocker*) . . .	180	2.0	30.0	6.0	20	210	0
(*Betty Crocker Twice the Blueberries*) .	140	2.0	25.0	4.0	20	180	1.0
(*Duncan Hines Bakery Style*) . . .	150	2.0	25.0	4.5	20	250	1.0
(*"Jiffy"*), ¼ cup . . .	160	2.0	28.0	5.0	0	270	1.0
wild (*Betty Crocker*)	170	2.0	28.0	5.0	20	210	<1.0
wild, whole wheat (*Hodgson Mill*), ¼ cup	145	5.0	32.0	1.0	0	206	4.0
bran, ¼ cup:							
(*Hodgson Mill*) . . .	130	4.0	27.0	.5	0	150	3.0
w/dates (*"Jiffy"*) . .	150	2.0	26.0	4.0	0	240	3.0
chocolate, double (*Betty Crocker*) .	200	3.0	30.0	8.0	20	220	0
chocolate chip:							
(*Betty Crocker*) . . .	130	2.0	21.0	5.0	15	210	0
(*Duncan Hines*) . . .	190	3.0	31.0	6.0	20	300	1.0
corn, ¼ cup:							
(*Glory*)	150	2.0	25.0	4.0	0	340	<1.0
(*Hodgson Mill*)	130	4.0	28.0	.5	0	240	3.0
(*"Jiffy"*)	160	2.0	28.0	4.0	0	320	1.0
cranberry orange (*Betty Crocker*)	150	2.0	25.0	5.0	20	180	0

Food and Measure	cal.	prot. (gms)	carbo. (gms)	fat (gms)	chol. (mgs)	sod. (mgs)	fiber (gms)
lemon poppy seed:							
(*Betty Crocker*) . . .	130	2.0	22.0	3.5	0	190	0
(*Betty Crocker Sunkist*)	190	2.0	29.0	7.0	20	230	0
raspberry ("*Jiffy*"), ¼ cup	170	2.0	26.0	6.0	0	310	<1.0
whole wheat (*Hodgson Mill*), ¼ cup	130	4.0	27.0	.5	0	206	3.0
Muffin sandwich, see "Breakfast sandwich"							
Mulberries, fresh:							
10 berries, ½ oz.	7	.2	1.5	.1	0	2	.3
½ cup	31	1.0	6.9	.3	0	7	1.2
Mullet, striped, meat only:							
raw , 4 oz.	133	22.0	0	4.3	56	74	0
baked, broiled, or microwaved, 4 oz. .	170	28.1	0	5.5	71	81	0
Multigrain chips, see "Snack chips"							
Mung bean:							
dry (*Shiloh Farms*), ¼ cup	160	11.0	28.0	.5	0	0	9.0
boiled, ½ cup	106	7.1	19.3	.4	0	2	7.7
Mung bean sprouts:							
raw:							
(*Jonathan's*), 1 cup	30	3.0	4.0	.5	0	5	.5
1 cup	31	3.2	6.2	.2	0	6	1.9
1 oz.	9	.9	1.7	.1	0	2	.5
boiled, drained, ½ cup	13	1.3	2.6	.1	0	6	.5
Mung bean sprouts, canned, drained, 1 cup	15	1.8	2.7	<.1	0	175	1.0
Mungo bean, boiled, ½ cup	95	6.8	16.5	.5	0	7	5.8
Mushroom (see also specific listings), common, ½ cup:							
raw, pcs. or slices . . .	9	1.0	1.5	.2	0	1	.4
boiled, drained, pcs. .	21	1.7	4.0	.4	0	2	1.7
Mushroom, breaded, frozen (*Empire* Kosher), 7 pcs., 2.85 oz.	90	4.0	16.0	1.0	0	390	1.0

Food and Measure	cal.	prot. (gms)	carbo. (gms)	fat (gms)	chol. (mgs)	sod. (mgs)	fiber (gms)
Mushroom, can or jar (see also "Mushroom, straw"), ½ cup, except as noted:							
whole or sliced:							
(*Green Giant*)	30	3.0	4.0	0	0	440	2.0
drained	19	1.5	3.9	.5	0	332	1.9
w/liquid	20	2.0	3.0	0	0	400	<1.0
in butter (*BinB*), 3-oz. can	40	2.0	4.0	1.5	<5	460	1.0
sliced, w/garlic:							
(*Green Giant*)	25	2.0	4.0	0	0	530	1.0
in butter (*BinB*), 3-oz. can	40	2.0	5.0	1.5	<5	410	1.0
sliced, random (*Fanci Food*)	20	2.0	3.0	0	0	400	<1.0
stems and pieces:							
(*Green Giant*)	30	3.0	4.0	0	0	440	2.0
Mushroom, chanterelle, dried (*Frieda's*), 2 pcs., .14 oz.	15	1.0	2.0	0	0	0	1.0
Mushroom, cloud ear, dried:							
.2-oz. pc.	13	.4	3.3	<.1	0	2	3.2
½ cup	39	1.3	10.2	.1	0	5	9.8
Mushroom, crimini, brown, or Italian, raw, .5-oz. pc.	3	.4	.6	0	0	1	<.1
Mushroom, enoki, fresh:							
(*Frieda's*), ¼ pkg., .9 oz.	10	1.0	2.0	0	0	0	1.0
trimmed, 1 oz.	10	.2	2.0	.1	0	1	.7
1 large, 4⅛" long	2	.1	.4	<.1	0	<1	<1.0
Mushroom, maitake, dried (*Eden*), .4 oz., about 10 pcs.	35	2.0	7.0	0	0	0	4.0
Mushroom, morel, dried (*Frieda's*), 3 pcs. .14 oz.	15	1.0	2.0	0	0	0	0
Mushroom, oyster: fresh:							
1 large, 5.2 oz.	55	6.1	9.2	.8	0	46	3.6
1 small, .5 oz.	6	.6	.9	.1	0	5	.4
dried (*Frieda's*), 3 pcs.	15	1.0	2.0	0	0	0	0

Food and Measure	cal.	prot. (gms)	carbo. (gms)	fat (gms)	chol. (mgs)	sod. (mgs)	fiber (gms)
Mushroom, pickled, cocktail (*Fanci Food*), 1 oz.	10	1.0	0	0	0	360	0
Mushroom, porcini, dried:							
(*Epicurean Specialty*), ⅓ oz.	12	1.0	2.0	0	0	6	0
(*Frieda's*), 5 pcs.	15	1.0	2.0	0	0	0	1.0
Mushroom, portobello:							
fresh, 1 oz.	7	.7	1.4	<.1	0	2	.4
dried (*Frieda's*), 7 pcs., .14 oz.	0	1.0	1.0	0	0	0	0
Mushroom, shiitake:							
fresh, raw (*Frieda's*), 3.5 oz.	290	9.0	75.0	1.0	0	15	11.0
fresh, cooked, 4 medium or ½ cup pcs.	40	1.1	10.4	.2	0	3	1.5
dried:							
(*Frieda's*), ¼ cup, .14 oz.	10	0	3.0	0	0	0	0
4 medium, .5 oz. . .	44	1.4	11.3	.2	0	2	1.7
whole or sliced (*Eden*), 6 pcs., .4 oz. . . .	35	2.0	7.0	0	0	0	5.0
Mushroom, straw:							
canned:							
drained, ½ cup . . .	29	3.5	4.2	.6	0	350	2.3
sliced, stir-fry (*Port Arthur*), ½ cup .	20	2.0	3.0	0	0	380	2.0
dried (*Frieda's* Padi Straw), 6 pcs.	15	1.0	2.0	0	0	0	0
Mushroom, wood ear, dried (*Frieda's*), 3 pcs., .14 oz.	15	0	2.0	0	0	0	0
Mushroom batter mix (*Don's Chuck Wagon*), ¼ cup	95	3.0	21.0	0	0	706	1.0
Mushroom gravy, in jars, ¼ cup:							
(*Campbell's*)	20	0	3.0	1.0	<5	280	0
(*Pacific Foods*)	20	1.0	4.0	.5	0	270	1.0
creamy (*Campbell's*) .	20	0	4.0	.5	<5	350	0
rich (*Heinz* Home Style)	20	<1.0	3.0	.5	0	320	0
Mushroom gravy mix, ¼ cup*:							
(*McCormick*)	20	0	2.0	.5	0	260	0

Food and Measure	cal.	prot. (gms)	carbo. (gms)	fat (gms)	chol. (mgs)	sod. (mgs)	fiber (gms)
Mushroom gravy mix *(cont.)*							
shiitake (*Road's End Organics*)	25	<1.0	5.0	0	0	200	<1.0
Mushroom sauce, shiitake (*Annie Chun's*), 1 tbsp.	15	1.0	3.0	0	0	190	0
Muskrat, meat only, roasted, 4 oz.	265	34.1	0	13.3	88	78	0
Mussels, blue, meat only:							
raw, 4 oz.	98	13.5	4.2	2.5	32	324	0
raw, 1 cup	129	17.9	3.4	5.5	42	429	0
boiled or steamed, 4 oz.	195	27.0	8.4	5.1	64	418	0
Mussels, canned, in red sauce (*Reese*), 4-oz. can drained ..	120	11.0	4.0	5.0	20	560	0
Mussels, smoked:							
(*SeaBear*), 2 oz.	60	6.0	0	3.0	60	400	0
(*Ducktrap River*), ¼ cup	140	9.0	3.0	10.0	60	560	0
(*Roland*), ⅓ cup	90	9.0	3.0	5.0	50	250	0
Mustard, prepared, 1 tsp., except as noted:							
Asian style (*Westbrae Natural*)	5	0	0	0	0	110	0
brown:							
(*Eden* Organic)	0	0	1.0	0	0	65	0
(*Eden* Organic Squeeze)	0	0	1.0	0	0	80	0
spicy (*Grey Poupon*) .	5	0	0	0	0	50	0
spicy (*Gulden's*)	5	0	0	0	0	50	0
Chinese, hot (*Port Arthur*)	0	0	0	0	0	75	0
Creole (*Luzianne*), 1 tbsp.	10	1.0	2.0	0	0	320	0
deli style:							
(*Boar's Head*)	0	0	0	0	0	40	0
(*French's*)	0	0	0	0	0	80	0
(*Grey Poupon*)	5	0	0	0	0	50	0
(*Hebrew National*) .	0	0	0	0	0	65	0
Dijon:							
(*Annie's Naturals* Organic)	0	0	0	0	0	120	0

Food and Measure	cal.	prot. (gms)	carbo. (gms)	fat (gms)	chol. (mgs)	sod. (mgs)	fiber (gms)
(*Grey Poupon/Grey Poupon* Country)	5	0	1.0	0	0	120	0
(*Maille* Original) ...	5	0	0	.5	0	105	0
(*Sara Lee* French Country)	5	0	0	0	0	105	0
(*Tree of Life*)	0	0	0	0	0	65	0
(*Westbrae Natural*)	0	0	0	0	0	65	0
extra hot (*Maille*) ..	10	0	1.0	.5	0	115	0
green pepper, strong (*Delouis Fils*)	5	<1.0	<1.0	0	0	120	0
stone ground:							
(*Sara Lee* Bavarian)	5	0	0	0	0	55	0
(*Westbrae Natural*)	0	0	0	0	0	65	0
(*Westbrae Natural* No Salt)	0	0	0	0	0	0	0
w/herbs (*Tree of Life*)	3	<1.0	<1.0	0	0	50	0
or yellow (*Tree of Life* Organic)	0	0	0	0	0	55	0
yellow:							
(*Annie's Naturals* Organic)	0	0	0	0	0	55	0
(*Eden* Organic)	0	0	0	0	0	80	0
(*French's*)	0	0	0	0	0	55	0
(*Westbrae Natural* Organic)	0	0	0	0	0	75	0
Mustard blend (see also "Pretzel dip"), 1 tsp.:							
honey:							
(*Annie's Naturals* Organic)	10	0	2.0	0	0	40	0
(*Boar's Head*)	10	0	2.0	0	0	25	0
(*French's*)	5	0	1.0	0	0	30	0
(*Sara Lee* Country)	10	0	2.0	0	0	25	0
(*Westbrae Natural* Organic)	5	0	1.0	0	0	50	0
cranberry (*Sara Lee*)	10	0	2.0	0	0	25	0
horseradish:							
(*Annie's Naturals* Organic)	5	0	1.0	0	0	90	0
(*Watkins*)	5	0	1.0	0	0	75	0
onion, sweet (*French's*)	10	0	2.0	0	0	70	0
pepper, garden, trio (*Sara Lee*)	10	0	1.0	0	0	40	0

Food and Measure	cal.	prot. (gms)	carbo. (gms)	fat (gms)	chol. (mgs)	sod. (mgs)	fiber (gms)
Mustard blend *(cont.)*							
raspberry (*Annie's Naturals* Organic) ..	5	0	1.0	0	0	35	0
Mustard cabbage, see "Cabbage, mustard"							
Mustard greens, fresh:							
raw (*Glory*), 2 cups ...	20	2.0	4.0	0	0	20	3.0
raw, chopped:							
(*Del Monte*), 2 cups	25	1.0	5.0	0	0	30	1.0
1 oz. or ½ cup	7	.8	1.4	.1	0	7	.6
boiled, drained,							
½ cup	11	1.6	1.5	.2	0	11	1.4
Mustard greens, canned, ½ cup:							
(*Allens* No Salt)	30	1.0	5.0	.5	0	10	3.0
(*Bush's*)	25	2.0	3.0	0	0	400	2.0
seasoned:							
(*Allens/Sunshine*) .	45	4.0	6.0	.5	0	830	1.0
(*Glory*)	50	3.0	7.0	.5	0	460	3.0
Mustard greens, frozen, chopped boiled,							
drained, 1 cup	30	3.4	4.7	.4	0	38	4.2
Mustard powder, 1 tsp.	9	.5	.3	.6	0	<1	<1.0
Mustard seeds, 1 tsp.	15	.8	1.2	1.0	0	<1	<1.0
Mustard spinach:							
raw, chopped, 1 cup .	33	3.3	5.9	.5	0	32	4.2
boiled, drained,							
chopped, 1 cup ...	29	3.1	5.0	.4	0	25	3.6
Mustard tallow, 1 tbsp.	115	0	0	12.8	13	0	0

N

Food and Measure	cal.	prot. (gms)	carbo. (gms)	fat (gms)	chol. (mgs)	sod. (mgs)	fiber (gms)
Nacho snack, frozen (*Amy's*), 5-6 pcs. . . .	210	9.0	26.0	8.0	20	460	<1.0
Nacho snack kit, w/beans, sauce, chips, salsa (*Taco Bell Ultimate Nachos*), ¼ of 18.5-oz. pkg. . .	280	7.0	29.0	15.0	10	920	4.0
Name yam (*Frieda's*), ¾ cup, 3 oz.	100	1.0	24.0	0	0	10	3.0
Nathans Famous, 1 serving:							
burgers:							
bacon cheeseburger	707	32.2	43.3	43.6	128	1340	1.7
¼ lb. burger	537	24.5	42.3	30.1	90	813	1.7
¼ lb. burger w/cheese	850	29.6	45.4	61.5	136	1239	1.7
super burger	864	30.2	42.2	61.7	136	1245	2.6
fish sandwich	469	14.3	41.7	20.2	34	750	13.3
cheese steak:							
original	741	44.5	50.3	42.8	124	1239	4.0
supreme	786	45.4	60.8	43.0	124	1525	4.8
cheese steak, chicken	565	38.4	62.5	19.0	81	1786	4.8
chili, *Nathan's*, 9 oz. . .	290	17.0	32.0	10.0	n.a.	n.a.	.9
hot dog	309	10.6	22.7	20.1	35	684	1.3
hot dog nuggets, 6 . .	351	5.0	20.0	27.6	20	400	0
fries:							
large	759	8.1	64.8	52.2	0	278	8.1
regular	547	5.8	46.4	37.7	0	200	5.8
super	1188	12.6	101.0	81.9	0	433	12.6
onion rings:							
large	745	4.2	47.7	58.6	0	768	2.1
small	559	3.1	35.8	44.0	0	576	1.6
sauce, cheese, 2 oz. . .	82	1.8	6.4	5.5	n.a.	n.a.	.9
sauerkraut, ½ cup . . .	25	1.0	5.0	0	0	n.a.	3.0

Food and Measure	cal.	prot. (gms)	carbo. (gms)	fat (gms)	chol. (mgs)	sod. (mgs)	fiber (gms)
Natto, ½ cup	187	15.6	12.6	9.7	0	6	4.8
Navy beans:							
dry (*Shiloh Farms*),							
¼ cup	170	12.0	32.0	.5	0	5	13.0
boiled, ½ cup	129	7.9	24.0	.5	0	1	3.3
Navy beans, canned,							
½ cup:							
(*Allens*)	110	6.0	19.0	1.0	0	380	6.0
(*Bush's*)	110	5.0	19.0	.5	0	450	6.0
(*Eden* Organic)	110	7.0	20.0	.5	0	15	7.0
w/bacon:							
(*Trappey's*)	110	5.0	18.0	1.5	0	420	6.0
jalapeño (*Trappey's*)	110	5.0	17.0	1.5	0	420	6.0
sweet (*Glory*)	140	7.0	27.0	0	0	470	7.0
Navy beans, sprouted,							
½ cup	35	3.2	6.8	.4	0	14	n.a.
Nectarine:							
(*Chiquita*), 1 medium,							
4.9 oz.	70	1.0	16.0	.5	0	0	2.0
(*Del Monte*), 1 medium,							
4.9 oz.	70	1.0	16.0	0	0	0	2.0
(*Dole*), 1 medium,							
4.9 oz.	70	1.0	16.0	.5	0	0	2.0
1 medium, 2½" diam.	67	1.3	16.0	.6	0	<1	2.2
sliced, ½ cup	34	.7	8.1	.3	0	<1	1.1
Noni juice (*Tree of Life*),							
2 tbsp.	15	0	4.0	0	0	10	0
Noodle, Asian, 2 oz.							
dry, except as noted:							
cellophane (*Port Arthur*							
Bean Thread*), 1 cup							
dry	190	0	50.0	0	0	0	1.0
cellophane or long rice	200	.1	48.8	<.1	0	6	<1.0
chow mein:							
(*Annie Chun's*)	200	8.0	39.0	1.0	0	350	3.0
fresh (*Frieda's*), 4 oz.	332	9.0	70.0	6.0	0	160	1.0
chow mein, dried,							
½ cup	119	1.9	13.0	6.9	0	99	.9
crispy (*Frieda's*), ½ cup,							
1 oz.	160	1.0	17.0	6.0	0	160	1.0
kuzu (*Eden*)	200	0	48.0	0	0	0	2.0
rice:							
(*Annie Chun's* Hunan/							
Original/Thai Basil)	210	2.0	50.0	0	0	75	0

Food and Measure	cal.	prot. (gms)	carbo. (gms)	fat (gms)	chol. (mgs)	sod. (mgs)	fiber (gms)
(*A Taste of Thai* Original/Thin/Wide)	200	3.0	46.0	0	0	20	2.0
(*Thai Kitchen* Stirfry/ Thin/Wide)	196	3.0	46.0	0	0	0	2.0
sticks (*Port Arthur*), 1 cup dry	195	4.0	48.0	0	0	30	1.0
soba:							
(*Annie Chun's*)	200	8.0	39.0	1.0	0	390	3.0
buckwheat (*Eden*) .	200	6.0	43.0	1.0	0	5	3.0
buckwheat, 40% (*Eden*)	190	8.0	37.0	1.0	0	490	3.0
lotus root (*Eden*) . .	190	9.0	37.0	1.0	0	470	4.0
mugwort (*Eden*) . . .	190	8.0	37.0	.5	0	550	2.0
spelt (*Eden* Organic)	200	9.0	37.0	1.5	0	50	2.0
whole grain, 70% (*Eden* Organic) . .	200	8.0	38.0	1.5	0	70	2.0
wild yam (*Eden* Jinenjo)	190	9.0	37.0	.5	0	510	2.0
soba, cooked, 1 cup . .	113	5.8	24.4	.1	0	40	n.a.
somen:							
uncooked	203	6.5	42.2	.5	0	1049	2.4
whole grain 80% (*Eden* Organic) . .	200	8.0	38.0	1.5	0	80	3.0
somen, cooked, 1 cup	230	7.0	48.5	.3	0	284	n.a.
thin cut, fresh (*Azumaya*), 1 cup . .	210	8.0	43.0	.5	0	400	2.0
udon:							
(*Eden*)	190	8.0	37.0	1.5	0	660	3.0
brown rice (*Eden*) .	190	8.0	38.0	1.0	0	510	2.0
brown rice (*Eden* Organic)	200	8.0	38.0	2.0	0	80	3.0
kamut (*Eden* Organic)	200	10.0	37.0	1.5	0	55	3.0
whole grain, 80% (*Eden* Organic) . .	200	8.0	38.0	1.5	0	80	3.0
udon, cooked, 4 oz. . . .	115	2.8	23.0	.6	0	51	n.a.
wide cut (*Azumaya*), 1 cup	210	8.0	43.0	.5	0	410	2.0
Noodle, egg:							
dry, 2 oz.:							
enriched	216	7.9	40.3	2.4	54	12	1.5
whole wheat (*Hodgson Mill*) .	190	10.0	34.0	2.0	30	20	4.0
whole wheat, spinach (*Hodgson Mill*) .	190	10.0	32.0	1.0	30	45	5.0

Food and Measure	cal.	prot. (gms)	carbo. (gms)	fat (gms)	chol. (mgs)	sod. (mgs)	fiber (gms)
Noodle, egg *(cont.)*							
cooked:							
1 cup	212	7.6	39.7	2.4	53	11	1.8
spinach, 1 cup	211	8.1	38.8	2.5	52	20	3.7
Noodle, Chinese,							
Japanese, or Thai,							
see "Noodle, Asian"							
Noodle entree, frozen,							
1 pkg.:							
Asian, stir-fry *(Amy's)*,							
10 oz.	240	7.0	41.0	4.5	0	680	4.0
and chicken, see							
"Chicken entree,							
frozen"							
w/chicken, peas, carrots							
(Michelina's Au-							
thentico), 8 oz.	260	13.0	34.0	10.0	70	760	2.0
lo mein, vegetable,							
w/tofu *(Ethnic Gour-*							
met), 11 oz.	410	19.0	60.0	11.0	35	870	6.0
pad Thai, w/tofu *(Ethnic*							
Gourmet), 11 oz. ..	460	13.0	84.0	8.0	0	890	4.0
Romanoff, w/meatballs							
(Michelina's Au-							
thentico), 10 oz.	300	15.0	42.0	7.0	65	1550	2.0
Stroganoff *(Michelina's*							
Authentico), 8 oz. ..	320	14.0	35.0	14.0	75	760	2.0
Noodle entree, pkg.:							
and chicken *(Kid's*							
Kitchen), 1 cup ...	140	8.0	18.0	4.0	25	950	1.0
ginger shiitake *(Fan-*							
tastic Fast Naturals),							
1 pkg.	340	8.0	58.0	10.0	0	690	4.0
pad Thai:							
(Fantastic Fast Natu-							
rals), 1 pkg.	400	18.0	59.0	11.0	0	680	5.0
sauce *(Tasty Bite)*,							
⅓ pkg.	260	5.0	49.0	5.0	0	420	2.0
peanut sauce *(Tasty Bite)*,							
⅓ pkg.	270	5.0	42.0	9.0	0	160	1.0
stir-fry sauce *(Tasty Bite)*,							
⅓ pkg.	200	4.0	40.0	3.5	0	660	2.0
Thai lemongrass *(Fan-*							
tastic Fast Naturals),							
1 pkg.	340	8.0	48.0	10.0	0	690	5.0

Food and Measure	cal.	prot. (gms)	carbo. (gms)	fat (gms)	chol. (mgs)	sod. (mgs)	fiber (gms)
vegetables and, see "Vegetable entree, pkg." and "Vegetarian entree, pkg."							
Noodle entree mix:							
chow mein, w/sauce:							
black bean (*Annie Chun's*), ⅓ pkg. .	230	8.0	42.0	2.5	0	690	2.0
garlic scallion (*Annie Chun's*), ⅓ pkg. .	240	8.0	39.0	5.0	0	940	2.0
peanut sesame (*Annie Chun's*), ⅓ pkg.	270	9.0	42.0	7.0	0	600	2.0
curry stir-fry (*Thai Kitchen* Noodles & Sauce), 1 cup*	290	5.0	59.0	4.0	0	1325	0
garlic:							
roasted (*Thai Kitchen* Noodle Cart), 1 pkg.	230	4.0	47.0	3.0	0	840	0
savory stir-fry (*Thai Kitchen* Noodles & Sauce), 1 cup* . .	220	3.0	46.0	3.0	0	443	<1.0
lemongrass and chili stir-fry (*Thai Kitchen* Noodles & Sauce), 1 cup*	285	4.0	60.0	3.0	0	530	0
pad Thai, w/sauce:							
(*Annie Chun's*), ⅓ pkg.	210	3.0	48.0	1.0	0	570	0
(*A Taste of Thai* for Two), ½ pkg. . . .	345	5.0	89.0	.5	0	395	3.5
(*Thai Kitchen* Noodle Cart), 1 pkg.	235	3.0	49.0	3.0	0	450	<1.0
w/chili stir fry (*Thai Kitchen* Noodles & Sauce), 1 cup*	310	3.0	73.0	1.0	0	1149	<1.0
stir-fry (*Thai Kitchen* Noodles & Sauce), 1 cup*	400	5.0	93.0	1.0	0	621	<1.0
peanut, Thai:							
(*Thai Kitchen* Noodle Cart), 1 pkg.	265	4.0	47.0	7.0	0	200	0

Food and Measure	cal.	prot. (gms)	carbo. (gms)	fat (gms)	chol. (mgs)	sod. (mgs)	fiber (gms)
Noodle entree mix, peanut, Thai *(cont.)*							
stir-fry (*Thai Kitchen* Noodles & Sauce), 1 cup*	310	7.0	55.0	7.0	0	629	0
sesame, toasted, stir-fry (*Thai Kitchen* Noodles & Sauce), 1 cup*	280	5.0	54.0	5.0	0	1016	.5
soba, w/soy ginger sauce (*Annie Chun's*), ⅓ pkg.	210	8.0	41.0	2.0	0	920	3.0
Nopales/Nopalitos, see "Cactus pads"							
Nori, see "Seaweed"							
Nut topping, see specific nut listings							
Nutmeg, ground, 1 tsp.	12	.1	1.1	.8	0	tr.	.1
Nuts, see specific listings							
Nuts, mixed, 1 oz., except as noted:							
(*Fisher* Less Than 50% Peanuts	180	6.0	5.0	16.0	0	110	2.0
(*Frito Lay* Deluxe), ¼ cup, 1 oz.	170	4.0	6.0	16.0	0	115	2.0
(*Planters*)	170	6.0	6.0	15.0	0	115	2.0
(*Planters* Deluxe)	170	5.0	6.0	16.0	0	110	2.0
(*Planters* Lightly Salted)	170	6.0	6.0	15.0	0	55	2.0
(*Planters* Unsalted)	170	6.0	6.0	15.0	0	0	2.0
(*Tree of Life* Just Nuts Trail Mix), 1.1 oz.	180	2.0	5.0	17.0	0	0	2.0
cashews:							
almonds, macadamias (*Planters*), ¾ oz.	170	5.0	6.0	15.0	0	50	2.0
almonds, pecans (*Planters*)	170	4.0	7.0	15.0	0	95	2.0
jumbo, and mixed nuts (*Planters*)	170	5.0	8.0	14.0	0	120	1.0
glazed (*Beer Nuts*)	180	7.0	4.0	15.0	0	60	2.0
honey roasted:							
(*Kettle*)	160	6.0	8.0	13.0	0	120	2.0
(*Planters*)	160	5.0	9.0	13.0	0	120	2.0
macadamia mix:							
(*Mauna Loa* Mixed Nuts)	190	5.0	8.0	15.0	0	60	2.0

Food and Measure	cal.	prot. (gms)	carbo. (gms)	fat (gms)	chol. (mgs)	sod. (mgs)	fiber (gms)
cashew mix (*Mauna Loa*)	180	4.0	8.0	15.0	0	65	1.0
cashew, almonds (*Planters*)	180	4.0	6.0	17.0	0	100	2.0
peanuts:							
almonds, pecans, hazelnuts, pistachios (*Planters*) .	170	6.0	5.0	16.0	0	55	3.0
and cashews, honey (*Planters*)	160	5.0	10.0	12.0	0	120	2.0

O

Food and Measure	cal.	prot. (gms)	carbo. (gms)	fat (gms)	chol. (mgs)	sod. (mgs)	fiber (gms)
Oat (see also "Cereal"):							
(*Shiloh Farms* Steel Cut),							
¼ cup	170	6.0	29.0	3.0	0	0	5.0
whole grain, 1 oz. . . .	110	4.8	18.8	2.0	0	1	3.0
rolled or oatmeal:							
dry (*Shiloh Farms*							
Rolled), ⅓ cup . .	130	6.0	23.0	2.5	0	0	4.0
dry, 1 oz.	109	4.5	19.0	1.8	0	1	2.9
cooked, 1 cup	145	6.1	25.3	2.3	0	2	4.0
Oat bran, dry:							
(*Shiloh Farms* 1 lb.),							
⅓ cup	150	8.0	23.0	2.5	0	0	7.0
(*Tree of Life*), ½ cup .	120	3.0	31.0	3.5	0	0	7.0
(*Tree of Life* Organic),							
½ cup	120	8.0	31.0	3.5	0	0	7.0
1 oz.	70	4.9	18.8	2.0	0	1	4.5
Oat flour:							
(*Arrowhead Mills*),							
⅓ cup	120	4.0	21.0	3.0	0	0	3.0
(*Shiloh Farms*), ⅓ cup	120	5.0	20.0	2.0	0	0	4.0
bran (*Hodgson Mill*),							
¼ cup	110	3.0	23.0	2.0	0	4	3.0
bran (*Hodgson Mill*							
Organic), ¼ cup . . .	110	3.0	24.0	2.0	0	0	3.0
bran blend (*Hodgson*							
Mill), <¼ cup	110	3.0	24.0	1.0	0	0	3.0
Oat groats, ¼ cup:							
(*Arrowhead Mills*) . . .	160	7.0	28.0	3.0	0	0	4.0
(*Shiloh Farms*)	160	6.0	29.0	3.0	0	0	4.0
Oco (*Frieda's*), ½ cup,							
3 oz.	70	2.0	15.0	0	0	5	1.0
Ocean perch, Atlantic,							
meat only:							
raw, 4 oz.	107	21.1	0	1.9	48	85	0

Food and Measure	cal.	prot. (gms)	carbo. (gms)	fat (gms)	chol. (mgs)	sod. (mgs)	fiber (gms)
baked, broiled, or microwaved, 4 oz. . .	137	27.1	0	2.4	61	109	0
Octopus, meat only:							
raw, 4 oz.	93	16.9	2.5	1.2	54	261	0
boiled or steamed, 4 oz.	186	33.8	5.0	2.4	109	522	0
Octopus, canned:							
in olive oil (*Goya*), ¼ cup	110	12.0	3.0	6.0	30	360	0
spiced, in red sauce (*Reese*), 2 oz.	120	7.0	4.0	8.0	0	430	0
Oheloberry, ½ cup . .	20	.3	4.8	.2	0	1	n.a.
Oil, 1 tbsp., except as noted:							
(*Arrowhead Mills Essential Balance*) .	130	0	0	14.0	0	0	0
(*House of Tsang Mongolian Fire*), 1 tsp. .	45	0	0	5.0	0	0	0
all varieties:							
(*Eden*)	120	0	0	14.0	0	0	0
(*Hain*)	120	0	0	14.0	0	0	0
almond, canola, cocoa butter, corn, cottonseed, hazelnut, oat, palm, or poppy seed	120	0	0	13.6	0	0	0
avocado or mustard . .	124	0	0	14.0	0	0	0
butter oil	112	<.1	0	12.7	33	0	0
coconut	117	0	0	13.6	0	0	0
cod liver	123	0	0	13.6	78	0	0
flax seed (*Arrowhead Mills*)	130	0	0	14.0	0	0	0
herring	123	0	0	13.6	104	0	0
menhaden	123	0	0	16.3	85	0	0
olive, peanut, safflower, sesame, soybean, sunflower, vegetable, or walnut	120	0	0	14.0	0	0	0
salmon	123	0	0	13.6	66	0	0
sardine	123	0	0	13.6	97	0	0
sesame, regular or hot chili (*House of Tsang*), 1 tsp.	45	0	0	5.0	0	0	0
wok (*House of Tsang*)	130	0	0	14.0	0	0	0
Okra, fresh:							
raw:							
red (*Frieda's*), 3.5 oz.	33	2.0	8.0	.2	0	8	3.0

Food and Measure	cal.	prot. (gms)	carbo. (gms)	fat (gms)	chol. (mgs)	sod. (mgs)	fiber (gms)
Okra, raw *(cont.)*							
sliced, ½ cup	19	1.0	3.8	.1	0	4	1.3
boiled, drained, 8 pods,							
3" x ⅝"	27	1.6	6.1	.1	0	5	2.1
boiled drained, sliced,							
½ cup	25	1.5	5.8	.1	0	4	2.0
Okra, canned, ½ cup:							
(*Allens/Trappey's*) . . .	30	1.0	6.0	0	0	400	3.0
(*Glory*)	25	2.0	6.0	0	0	n.a.	2.0
Creole gumbo							
(*Trappey's*)	35	2.0	6.0	0	0	290	3.0
and tomatoes:							
(*Allens/Trappey's*) .	30	1.0	5.0	0	0	380	3.0
and corn (*Allens*) . .	30	1.0	6.0	0	0	280	4.0
and corn (*Trappey's*)	30	<1.0	6.0	0	0	280	4.0
Okra, frozen, ½ cup:							
whole or cut							
(*McKenzies*)	25	1.0	5.0	0	0	35	3.0
boiled, drained, sliced	34	1.9	7.5	.3	0	3	2.6
breaded (*McKenzie's*							
Gold King)	90	3.0	n.a.	.5	0	350	n.a.
w/tomatoes, onions							
(*McKenzie's*)	20	1.0	4.0	0	0	30	2.0
Old-fashioned drink							
mixer (*Holland*							
House), 4 fl. oz. . . .	180	0	39.0	0	0	30	0
Olive, pickled:							
(*D.L. Jardine's* Martini),							
.5-oz. pc.	15	0	0	1.5	0	510	0
black, see "ripe," below							
Calamata (*Krinos*),							
3 pcs., .5 oz.	45	0	2.0	4.0	0	230	0
Greek, black:							
10 medium	65	.4	1.7	6.9	0	631	0
10 extra large	89	.6	2.3	9.5	0	868	0
pitted, 1 oz.	96	.6	2.5	10.2	0	932	0
green, w/pits:							
10 small	33	.4	.4	3.6	0	686	.7
10 large	45	.5	.5	4.9	0	926	1.0
10 giant	76	.9	.9	8.3	0	1572	1.7
green, cracked (*Krinos*),							
2 pcs., .5 oz.	20	0	2.0	1.0	0	220	0
green, pitted:							
(*Lindsay*), 5 medium,							
.5 oz.	25	0	1.0	2.5	0	115	0

Food and Measure	cal.	prot. (gms)	carbo. (gms)	fat (gms)	chol. (mgs)	sod. (mgs)	fiber (gms)
1 oz.	33	.4	.4	3.6	0	680	.7
w/pimento, sliced (*Lindsay*), 2 tbsp.	25	0	<1.0	2.5	0	330	0
ripe, pitted: (*Lindsay*), 4 large, .5 oz.	25	0	1.0	2.5	0	115	0
sliced (*Lindsay*), 2 tbsp.	25	0	1.0	2.5	0	125	0
salad, w/pimento (*Pompeian*), 1 tbsp., .5 oz.	25	0	1.0	2.5	0	240	0
stuffed, green: w/almonds (*Reese*), 4 pcs., .5 oz. . . .	35	0	<1.0	3.5	0	310	0
w/anchovies (*Goya*), 4 pcs., .5 oz. . . .	25	0	<1.0	2.5	<1	240	0
w/anchovies (*Reese*), 4 pcs., .5 oz.	20	0	<1.0	2.0	0	220	0
w/jalapeños (*D.L. Jardine's* Texas Caviar), 2 pcs., .5 oz.	15	0	0	1.5	0	510	0
w/sun-dried tomato (*Byzantine*), 5 pcs.	17	.5	1.5	1.3	0	281	.7
stuffed, w/pimento: (*Pompeian*), 6 pcs., .5 oz.	25	0	1.0	2.5	0	350	0
Manzanilla (*Lindsay*), 5 pcs., .5 oz. . . .	25	0	<1.0	2.5	0	330	0
queen (*Goya*), 1 pc.	20	0	1.0	1.5	0	160	0
queen (*Lindsay*), 2 pcs., .5 oz. . . .	15	0	<1.0	1.5	0	310	0
Olive loaf, see "Lunch meat"							
Olive oil, see "Oil"							
Olive paste, black (*Roland*), 1 tbsp. . . .	60	0	3.0	6.0	0	220	1.0
Olive sauce, green (*Italia In Tavola*), 2 tbsp.	90	0	0	10.0	0	970	0
Olive spread, 2 tbsp., except as noted: (*Lindsay Olivada* Taste of Greece)	60	0	2.0	6.0	0	250	0

Food and Measure	cal.	prot. (gms)	carbo. (gms)	fat (gms)	chol. (mgs)	sod. (mgs)	fiber (gms)
Olive spread *(cont.)*							
(*Lindsay Olivada* Taste of Sicily)	60	0	3.0	5.0	0	240	0
(*Lindsay Olivada* Taste of Tuscany)	45	0	3.0	4.0	0	230	0
tapanade (*Cantare*), 1 tbsp.	30	0	1.0	2.5	0	160	0
Omelette, see "Egg breakfast"							
Onion, fresh/stored:							
raw:							
(*Del Monte*), 1 medium, 5.2 oz.	60	1.0	16.0	0	0	5	3.0
(*Frieda's* Boiler/ Cipolline), 3 pcs., 3 oz.	30	1.0	7.0	0	0	0	2.0
(*Frieda's* Hawaiian Maui), ⅓ cup, 1.1 oz.	10	0	3.0	0	0	0	1.0
(*Frieda's* Pearl), ⅔ cup, 3 oz. . . .	30	1.0	7.0	0	0	0	2.0
1 oz.	11	.3	2.4	<.1	0	1	.5
chopped, ½ cup . . .	30	.9	6.9	0.1	0	2	1.4
chopped, 1 tbsp. . .	4	.1	.9	<.1	0	tr.	.2
boiled, drained:							
chopped, ½ cup . . .	46	1.4	10.7	.2	0	3	1.5
chopped, 1 tbsp. . .	7	.2	1.5	<.1	0	<1	.2
Onion, can or jar:							
cocktail (*Crosse & Blackwell*), 1 tbsp. .	0	0	1.0	0	0	250	0
pickled, sour (*London Pub*), ¼ cup, 1.1 oz.	0	2.0	2.0	0	0	130	0
Onion, dried:							
flakes, 1 tbsp.	16	.5	4.2	<.1	0	1	.5
minced (*Lawry's*), ¼ tsp.	0	0	<1.0	0	0	0	0
minced, 1 tsp.	7	.2	1.9	0	0	<1	.2
Onion, french fried, canned (*French's* Original), 2 tbsp. . .	45	0	3.0	3.5	0	60	0
Onion, frozen:							
whole:							
(*C&W* Petite), ⅔ cup	30	0	7.0	0	0	10	1.0
boiled, drained, ½ cup	30	.7	7.0	0	0	8	1.5

Food and Measure	cal.	prot. (gms)	carbo. (gms)	fat (gms)	chol. (mgs)	sod. (mgs)	fiber (gms)
pearl, white (*Birds Eye*), ⅔ cup	30	0	6.0	0	0	10	1.0
chopped:							
boiled, drained, 1 tbsp.	4	.1	1.0	<.1	0	2	.2
w/peppers (*Mc-Kenzie's* Seasoning Mix), 1 oz.	10	1.0	2.0	0	0	10	0
rings, see "Onion rings"							
Onion, green, raw, trimmed, w/top:							
(*Dole*), ¼ cup	10	0	2.0	0	0	5	1.0
chopped, ½ cup	16	.9	3.7	.1	0	8	1.3
chopped, 1 tbsp.	2	.1	.4	<.1	0	1	.2
Onion, pickled, see "Onion, can or jar"							
Onion, Welsh, 1 oz. .	10	.5	1.8	.1	0	5	<1.0
Onion dip, 2 tbsp., except as noted:							
(*Litehouse*)	110	1.0	2.0	11.0	10	180	0
French:							
(*Cabot*)	50	1.0	1.0	5.0	15	190	0
(*Kraft*)	60	1.0	3.0	4.5	0	210	0
(*Ruffles*), 4 tbsp. ...	200	7.0	9.0	15.0	0	100	2.0
green (*Kraft*)	60	1.0	3.0	4.5	0	170	0
Onion dip mix, dry:							
(*Fantastic* Soup/Dip), 2½ tsp.	25	1.0	6.0	0	0	480	1.0
French (*McCormick*), ¾ tsp.	5	0	0	0	0	140	0
mushroom (*Fantastic* Soup/Dip), 1½ tbsp.	25	0	6.0	0	0	480	<1.0
spring (*McCormick*), ½ tsp.	5	0	1.0	0	0	130	0
Onion flavor chips, see "Corn chips/crisps"							
Onion gravy mix (*Mc-Cormick*), ¼ cup* .	20	0	3.0	.5	0	340	0
Onion nuggets, frozen, w/cheese, breaded (*Kineret*), 3½ pcs., 2.8 oz.	150	5.0	20.0	5.0	10	490	6.0
Onion oil (*Watkins* Liquid Spice), 1 tsp.	40	0	0	4.5	0	0	0

Food and Measure	cal.	prot. (gms)	carbo. (gms)	fat (gms)	chol. (mgs)	sod. (mgs)	fiber (gms)
Onion powder:							
(*Tone's*), ¼ tsp.	5	.0	1.0	0	0	0	0
1 tsp.	7	.2	1.7	0	0	1	.1
Onion ring batter mix, ¼ cup dry:							
(*Don's Chuck Wagon*)	100	3.0	21.0	0	0	690	1.0
(*Golden Dipt* Fry Easy)	100	1.0	20.0	0	0	660	0
(*Hodgson Mill*)	100	3.0	21.0	0	0	690	1.0
(*Produce Partners Zebbie's*)	110	2.0	18.0	.5	0	610	0
Onion rings, frozen, breaded:							
(*Kineret*), 6 pcs., 3.2 oz.	180	3.0	26.0	8.0	0	250	2.0
(*McKenzie's*), 3.25 oz.	220	3.0	28.0	10.0	0	210	6.0
(*Ore-Ida Onion Ringers*), 5 pcs., 2.9 oz.	190	2.0	21.0	11.0	0	190	2.0
and strings (*Ian's* Natural), 6-8 pcs., 2.5 oz.	152	2.0	16.0	7.0	0	180	1.0
heated, 10 rings	289	3.8	27.1	19.0	0	17	2.9
Onion salt (*McCormick* California Style), ¼ tsp.	0	0	0	0	0	170	0
Onion sauce (*Boar's Head* Sweet Vidalia), 1 tbsp.	10	0	2.0	0	0	15	0
Onion snack chips, see "Snack chips"							
Onion sprouts (*Jonathan's*), 1 cup	30	1.0	5.0	0	0	5	2.0
Opo squash (*Frieda's*), ⅔ cup, 3 oz.	10	1.0	3.0	0	0	0	0
Opossum, meat only, roasted, 4 oz.	251	34.3	0	11.6	146	66	0
Orange, fresh:							
(*Dole*), 5.4-oz. fruit . .	70	1.0	21.0	0	0	0	7.0
(*Frieda's* Blood Moro/ Cara Cara), 5 oz. . .	70	1.0	16.0	0	0	0	3.0
(*Frieda's* Seville), 3 oz.	40	1.0	10.0	0	0	0	2.0
(*Sunkist*), 5.4-oz. fruit	80	1.0	21.0	0	0	0	7.0
all varieties:							
3-1/16" fruit, 6.5 oz.	87	1.7	21.6	.2	0	0	4.4
sections, 1 cup . . .	85	1.7	21.2	.2	0	0	4.3
California navel:							
2⅞" fruit, 5 oz.	65	1.4	16.3	.1	0	1	3.4
sections, 1 cup . . .	76	1.7	19.2	.2	0	2	4.0

Food and Measure	cal.	prot. (gms)	carbo. (gms)	fat (gms)	chol. (mgs)	sod. (mgs)	fiber (gms)
California Valencia:							
2⅝" fruit, 4.25 oz. . .	59	1.3	14.4	.4	0	0	3.0
sections, 1 cup . . .	88	1.9	21.4	.5	0	0	4.5
Florida:							
2-11/16" fruit, 5 oz.	65	1.0	16.3	.3	0	1	3.4
sections, 1 cup . . .	85	1.3	21.4	.4	0	1	4.4
Orange, mandarin, see "Tangerine"							
Orange drink, 8 fl. oz.:							
(*Hi-C Blast*)	120	0	31.0	0	0	75	0
(*Hood Carb Countdown*)	25	0	5.0	0	0	130	0
(*Minute Maid* Light) . .	50	0	13.0	0	0	15	0
(*Santa Cruz Organic* Box)	100	0	25.0	0	0	70	0
orange flavor:							
(*Bright & Early*) . . .	110	0	30.0	0	0	20	0
frozen* (*Bright & Early*)	110	0	29.0	0	0	10	0
orangeade:							
(*AriZona*)	120	0	27.0	0	0	25	0
(*Snapple*)	120	0	29.0	0	0	10	0
(*Tropicana*)	100	0	28.0	0	0	60	0
(*Turkey Hill*)	120	0	30.0	0	0	10	0
Orange drink blend, 8 fl. oz., except as noted:							
apricot (*Lincoln* Breakfast Cocktail)	120	0	29.0	0	0	45	0
carrot (*Sobe Elixer 3C*)	90	0	24.0	0	0	15	0
crème (*V8 Splash* Smoothies)	130	3.0	29.0	0	0	50	1.0
grapefruit (*Langers* Ruby)	130	0	33.0	0	0	10	0
mango:							
(*Nantucket Nectars*)	130	0	32.0	0	0	5	0
(*Newman's Own* Tango)	150	0	37.0	0	0	5	0
(*R.W. Knudsen*) . . .	120	<1.0	30.0	0	0	50	0
(*Santa Cruz Organic*)	130	1.0	31.0	0	0	15	0
pineapple:							
(*Hood Carb Countdown*)	25	0	5.0	0	0	140	0
(*Lincoln*)	130	0	32.0	0	0	70	0
(*V8 Splash*)	110	0	28.0	0	0	40	0

Food and Measure	cal.	prot. (gms)	carbo. (gms)	fat (gms)	chol. (mgs)	sod. (mgs)	fiber (gms)
Orange drink blend *(cont.)*							
strawberry (*Minute Maid Coolers*),							
6.75-fl. oz. pouch ..	100	0	26.0	0	0	15	0
Orange juice, 8 fl. oz., except as noted:							
(*Bolthouse Farms*) ...	110	3.0	24.0	0	0	95	>1.0
(*Hood*)	120	0	30.0	0	0	20	0
(*Langers* Plus)	120	0	29.0	0	0	15	0
(*Minute Maid*)	110	2.0	27.0	0	0	15	0
(*Minute Maid*), 11.5-fl.-oz. can	170	2.0	38.0	0	0	25	0
(*Minute Maid* Calcium/ Country Style/Home Squeezed/Pulp Free/ Extra Vitamins) ...	110	2.0	27.0	0	0	15	0
(*Minute Maid* Heartwise/ Low Acid)	110	2.0	27.0	0	0	20	0
(*Nantucket Nectars* Premium)	120	0	27.0	0	0	0	0
(*Ocean Spray*)	120	0	31.0	0	0	35	0
(*Organic Valley*)	120	2.0	26.0	0	0	0	0
(*Organic Valley* Calcium)	110	2.0	26.0	0	0	0	0
(*R.W. Knudsen*)	100	2.0	23.0	0	0	35	0
(*S&W*)	120	0	30.0	0	0	10	0
canned	105	1.5	24.5	.4	0	5	.5
chilled	110	2.0	25.1	.7	0	3	.5
fresh	112	1.7	25.8	.5	0	2	.5
frozen*:							
(*Cascadian Farm*) ..	120	1.0	29.0	0	0	5	0
(*Minute Maid*)	110	0	27.0	0	0	0	0
(*Minute Maid* Calcium/ Vitamins)	120	0	27.0	0	0	0	0
Orange juice blend, 8 fl. oz., except as noted:							
carrot (*After the Fall* 24 Karrot)	120	1.0	28.0	0	0	55	0
carrot (*Walnut Acres*)	110	0	27.0	0	0	30	0
passion fruit (*Minute Maid*)	130	1.0	31.0	0	0	20	0
tangerine (*Minute Maid*)	110	2.0	27.0	0	0	15	0
tropical:							
(*Minute Maid*), 6.75-fl.-oz. box .	110	0	27.0	0	0	15	0

Food and Measure	cal.	prot. (gms)	carbo. (gms)	fat (gms)	chol. (mgs)	sod. (mgs)	fiber (gms)
(Minute Maid), 11.5-fl.-oz. can ..	180	0	46.0	0	0	30	0
frozen*:							
passion fruit (Minute Maid)	130	0	31.0	0	0	5	0
tangerine (Minute Maid)	110	0	27.0	0	0	0	0
Orange peel, fresh, 1 tbsp.	-[1]	.1	1.5	<.1	0	0	.2
Oregano, dried, 1 tsp.	3	.1	.5	0	0	0	.1
Oriental 5-spice (Tone's), 1 tsp.	9	.3	1.9	.3	0	2	.5
Ostrich, ground, pan-broiled, 4 oz.	187	22.9	0	10.0	81	82	0
Oyster, meat only, 4 oz., except as noted:							
Eastern, wild:							
raw, 1 lb.	310	32.0	17.7	11.1	238	957	0
raw, 6 medium, 3 oz.	57	5.9	3.3	2.1	44	177	0
baked, broiled, or microwaved	82	9.4	5.4	2.2	56	277	0
steamed or poached	155	16.0	8.9	5.6	119	478	0
Eastern, farmed:							
raw	67	5.9	6.3	1.8	29	202	0
baked, broiled, or microwaved	90	7.9	8.3	2.4	43	185	0
Pacific:							
raw	92	10.7	5.6	2.6	57	120	0
raw, steamed or poached, 1 medium	41	4.7	2.5	1.2	25	53	0
boiled or steamed .	185	21.4	11.2	5.2	113	240	0
Oyster, canned:							
whole (Bumble Bee), 2 oz.	70	7.0	3.0	3.0	45	140	
Eastern, wild:							
w/liquid, 4 oz.	78	8.0	4.4	2.8	62	127	0
w/liquid, 1 cup	170	17.5	9.7	6.1	136	277	0
Oyster, smoked, canned, in olive oil, 3-oz. can:							
(Crown Prince)	290	12.0	11.0	22.0	45	220	<1.0

1. Cannot be calculated; no digestibility value for peel.

Food and Measure	cal.	prot. (gms)	carbo. (gms)	fat (gms)	chol. (mgs)	sod. (mgs)	fiber (gms)
Oyster, smoked *(cont.)*							
drained *(Brunswick)*,							
2.3 oz.	140	11.0	7.0	8.0	23	230	1.0
Oyster dish, frozen,							
breaded *(Hillman)*,							
7 pcs., 3 oz.	220	7.0	20.0	12.0	15	390	<1.0
Oyster plant, see							
"Salsify"							
Oyster sauce, Asian:							
(Ka•Me), 1 tbsp.	10	0	3.0	0	0	260	0
1 tbsp.	9	.2	2.0	0	0	492	0
Oyster and shrimp							
sauce *(TryMe*							
Caribbean Clipper),							
1 tsp.	10	0	2.0	0	0	140	0
Oyster stew, see "Soup,							
condensed"							

P

Food and Measure	cal.	prot. (gms)	carbo. (gms)	fat (gms)	chol. (mgs)	sod. (mgs)	fiber (gms)
Pad Thai entree, see "Noodle entree"							
Pad Thai sauce, see "Thai sauce"							
Paella, see "Rice entree, frozen"							
Palak paneer, see "Spinach entree"							
Palm, hearts of, can or jar:							
marinated (*Fanci Food*), ½ cup	60	4.0	8.0	1.0	0	770	4.0
nuggets (*Fanci Food* for Salad), ½ cup	40	3.0	4.0	1.0	0	550	2.0
sliced or whole (*Island Blaze*), ⅓ cup	25	3.0	4.0	0	0	220	2.0
spears (*Fanci Food* Jar), ½ cup	40	3.0	5.0	1.0	0	560	3.0
sticks (*Fanci Food* Can), 2 pcs.	20	2.0	3.0	0	0	450	<1.0
1.2-oz. pc.	9	.8	1.5	.2	0	141	.8
1 cup	41	3.7	6.8	.9	0	622	3.5
Pancake, freeze-dried, blueberry (*AlpineAire*), ½ pkg.	340	13.0	52.0	9.0	n.a.	1280	7.0
Pancake, frozen, 3 pcs., except as noted:							
(*Aunt Jemima* Homestyle)	200	6.0	37.0	3.5	15	460	1.0
(*Aunt Jemima* Low Fat)	190	6.0	35.0	2.5	30	380	2.0
(*Aunt Jemima* Mini), 5 pcs.	240	6.0	46.0	4.0	25	640	2.0
(*Ian's* Natural), 1 pc. .	100	3.0	19.0	2.0	<5	150	1.0
(*Pillsbury* Original) ...	240	5.0	46.0	4.0	10	640	1.0

Food and Measure	cal.	prot. (gms)	carbo. (gms)	fat (gms)	chol. (mgs)	sod. (mgs)	fiber (gms)
Pancake, frozen *(cont.)*							
blueberry:							
(*Ian's* Natural), 1 pc.	100	3.0	19.0	2.0	<5	150	1.0
(*Pillsbury*)	240	5.0	45.0	4.0	10	590	1.0
mini (*Pillsbury*),							
14 pcs. w/syrup .	430	4.0	89.0	7.0	5	500	1.0
buttermilk:							
(*Aunt Jemima*)	200	6.0	37.0	3.5	15	410	0
(*Eggo*)	320	7.0	51.0	10.0	15	640	1.0
(*Pillsbury*)	260	5.0	51.0	4.5	10	630	1.0
mini (*Pillsbury*),							
14 pcs. w/syrup .	410	4.0	84.0	7.0	10	540	1.0
Pancake mix, 3 cakes*,							
except as noted:							
(*Betty Crocker* Original							
Complete)	200	6.0	39.0	3.0	10	540	1.0
(*Betty Crocker* Pouch),							
3.3 cakes*	250	9.0	39.0	7.0	70	660	1.0
(*Shake 'n Pour* Original)	210	5.0	39.0	4.0	0	710	<1.0
blueberry (*Shake 'n*							
Pour)	210	6.0	40.0	3.5	0	640	1.0
buckwheat, 1/3 cup:							
(*Don's Chuck Wagon*)	160	5.0	33.0	1.0	0	457	1.0
(*Hodgson Mill*) . . .	190	5.0	40.0	1.0	0	380	3.0
buttermilk:							
(*Betty Crocker*							
Complete)	200	5.0	39.0	2.5	10	540	1.0
(*Betty Crocker*							
Complete Pouch),							
3.3 cakes*	210	6.0	39.0	4.0	25	780	1.0
(*"Jiffy"* Complete),							
1/4 cup	160	4.0	32.0	2.5	0	530	<1.0
and honey (*Maple							
Grove Farms*),							
1/3 cup	130	4.0	28.0	.5	0	550	3.0
multigrain, w/flax							
seed, soy (*Hodg-							
son Mill*), 1/3 cup	150	10.0	31.0	2.0	0	321	5.0
whole wheat (*Hodg-							
son Mill*), 1/3 cup	120	4.0	28.0	1.0	0	321	4.0
Pancake syrup, 4 tbsp.							
or 1/4 cup:							
(*Aunt Jemima*)	210	0	52.0	0	0	120	0
(*Aunt Jemima* Lite) . .	100	0	26.0	0	0	190	0

Food and Measure	cal.	prot. (gms)	carbo. (gms)	fat (gms)	chol. (mgs)	sod. (mgs)	fiber (gms)
(*Eggo*)	240	0	60.0	0	0	35	0
(*Eggo* Butter Flavor) . .	160	0	41.0	0	0	90	0
(*Eggo* Lite)	110	0	27.0	0	0	180	0
(*Hungry Jack*)	210	0	51.0	0	0	80	0
(*Karo*)	240	0	63.0	0	0	85	0
(*Log Cabin*)	210	0	53.0	0	0	100	0
(*Log Cabin* Lite)	100	0	25.0	0	0	130	0
(*Mrs. Butterworth's*) .	220	0	55.0	0	0	130	0
(*Mrs. Butterworth's* Lite)	100	0	24.0	0	0	130	0
(*Smucker's* No Sugar)	30	0	8.0	0	0	60	0
(*Vermont Maid*)	210	0	53.0	0	0	25	0
(*Vermont Maid* Butter Lite)	100	0	26.0	0	0	100	0
Pancetta, see "Bacon, Italian"							
Pancreas, braised:							
beef, 4 oz.	307	30.7	0	19.5	297	68	0
lamb, 4 oz.	265	25.9	0	17.1	454	59	0
pork, 4 oz.	248	32.3	0	12.2	357	48	0
veal (calves), 4 oz. . . .	290	33.0	0	16.6	n.a.	77	0
Paneer entree, see "Cheese entree" and "Spinach entree"							
Panera Bread:							
bread, artisan, 2 oz.:							
cheese, three	120	5.0	21.0	1.5	5	270	<1.0
cheese demi loaf . .	140	7.0	21.0	3.5	10	310	<1.0
country	120	5.0	25.0	0	0	290	1.0
focaccia, cheese . . .	150	5.0	19.0	6.0	5	300	1.0
French	110	4.0	23.0	0	0	310	<1.0
kalamata olive	140	5.0	26.0	2.0	0	270	1.0
multigrain	120	4.0	24.0	.5	0	230	1.0
raisin pecan	140	4.0	25.0	0	0	280	1.0
rye, stone-milled . .	110	4.0	22.0	0	0	320	2.0
sesame semolina . .	120	4.0	24.0	0	0	300	1.0
three seed	130	5.0	23.0	2.0	0	250	1.0
bread/rolls, 2 oz., except as noted:							
asiago, demi, loaf . .	140	7.0	21.0	3.5	10	310	<1.0
breadstick, lower carb, 1.2 oz.	120	9.0	13.0	2.5	0	230	7.0
ciabatta, 6 oz.	430	14.0	70.0	10.0	0	990	3.0
cinnamon raisin . . .	160	4.0	31.0	3.0	0	300	1.0

Food and Measure	cal.	prot. (gms)	carbo. (gms)	fat (gms)	chol. (mgs)	sod. (mgs)	fiber (gms)
Panera Bread, bread/rolls (cont.)							
croissant, 3 oz. ...	260	5.0	26.0	15.0	40	190	1.0
focaccio:							
asiago cheese ..	150	5.0	19.0	6.0	5	300	1.0
basil pesto	150	4.0	19.0	6.0	5	300	1.0
rosemary onion .	140	4.0	19.0	4.5	5	280	1.0
French:							
baguette, loaf ...	130	5.0	24.0	.5	0	270	1.0
roll, 2.25 oz.	140	6.0	28.0	1.0	0	310	1.0
golden original, lower carb, 1.1-oz. slice	80	7.0	10.0	1.0	0	170	4.0
honey wheat	140	5.0	25.0	2.5	0	310	1.0
Italian herb, lower carb, 1.1-oz. slice	80	7.0	10.0	1.0	0	160	4.0
nine grain	150	5.0	26.0	2.5	0	270	2.0
rosemary walnut, lower carb, 1.1-oz. slice	80	7.0	9.0	2.5	0	160	5.0
rye	140	5.0	25.0	2.5	0	290	1.0
sourdough:							
baguette, loaf, round	120	5.0	25.0	0	0	270	1.0
roll, 2.5 oz.	160	6.0	32.0	0	0	340	1.0
soup bowl, 8 oz.	500	20.0	102.0	1.5	0	1090	4.0
sunflower	160	6.0	24.0	1.0	0	320	1.0
tomato basil	130	5.0	27.0	0	0	350	1.0
bagel, 1 pc.:							
plain	280	11.0	57.0	1.0	0	450	2.0
plain, lower carb ..	200	18.0	25.0	2.0	0	460	12.0
apple, Dutch, raisin	340	10.0	70.0	2.5	0	410	3.0
asiago	330	15.0	58.0	5.0	15	480	2.0
asiago, lower carb .	240	19.0	20.0	9.0	20	500	9.0
blueberry	320	12.0	67.0	1.5	0	490	3.0
chocolate hazelnut .	400	12.0	72.0	4.5	0	490	3.0
chocolate raspberry	370	11.0	67.0	7.0	0	460	2.0
cinnamon crunch ..	420	10.0	78.0	7.0	0	430	3.0
everything	290	11.0	58.0	1.5	0	540	2.0
French toast	340	10.0	65.0	4.5	0	610	2.0
nine grain	290	11.0	58.0	1.0	0	390	3.0
pumpkin spice	360	11.0	76.0	1.5	0	670	3.0
sesame	310	12.0	60.0	2.5	0	460	3.0
spinach Parmesan .	340	15.0	83.0	3.5	5	590	3.0
cream cheese, 2 oz.:							
plain	190	3.0	2.0	18.0	55	210	0

Food and Measure	cal.	prot. (gms)	carbo. (gms)	fat (gms)	chol. (mgs)	sod. (mgs)	fiber (gms)
reduced calorie:							
plain	130	5.0	2.0	12.0	35	230	<1.0
hazelnut	150	5.0	6.0	11.0	35	210	<1.0
honey walnut . . .	150	4.0	9.0	11.0	30	200	<1.0
mocha	160	5.0	10.0	11.0	30	180	<1.0
raspberry	120	4.0	3.0	10.0	30	200	0
sun-dried tomato	140	5.0	4.0	11.0	35	220	<1.0
veggie	130	5.0	4.0	11.0	35	230	1.0
soup, 8 oz.:							
asparagus chicken							
Florentine	230	10.0	12.0	16.0	50	870	3.0
black bean:							
chicken chorizo .	220	14.0	33.0	4.5	10	800	15.0
low fat	160	9.0	31.0	1.0	0	820	11.0
broccoli cheddar . .	230	8.0	13.0	16.0	45	1000	1.0
chicken, cream of,							
and wild rice . . .	200	5.0	19.0	12.0	35	970	<1.0
chicken noodle, low							
fat	100	5.0	15.0	2.0	15	1080	1.0
clam chowder,							
Boston	210	6.0	19.0	11.0	40	990	<1.0
mushroom bisque .	210	5.0	17.0	14.0	45	820	1.0
onion, French	220	9.0	23.0	10.0	20	1810	2.0
potato, baked	260	6.0	23.0	16.0	35	750	1.0
tomato basil, low fat	110	3.0	17.0	3.0	0	910	3.0
vegetable, garden,							
low fat	90	4.0	17.0	.5	0	860	2.0
sandwiches:							
asiago roast beef . .	730	50.0	54.0	35.0	115	1620	2.0
Bacon Turkey Bravo	770	47.0	84.0	28.0	45	2850	5.0
carnitas panini,							
Coronado	810	47.0	77.0	35.0	95	2210	3.0
chicken, Tuscan . . .	720	41.0	77.0	27.0	80	1790	6.0
chicken salad:							
nine grain	640	35.0	56.0	29.0	90	1340	4.0
sesame semolina	730	39.0	80.0	26.0	90	1750	6.0
Frontago Chicken							
Panini	860	49.0	71.0	42.0	110	2260	5.0
ham and Swiss:							
artisan rye	930	52.0	106.0	31.0	110	3000	6.0
rye	650	42.0	47.0	34.0	110	2350	4.0
Italian combo	1050	60.0	80.0	54.0	165	3570	5.0
peanut butter/jelly:							
artisan French . .	570	18.0	90.0	15.0	0	1030	5.0
French	450	15.0	63.0	15.0	0	580	3.0

Food and Measure	cal.	prot. (gms)	carbo. (gms)	fat (gms)	chol. (mgs)	sod. (mgs)	fiber (gms)
Panera Bread, sandwiches *(cont.)*							
Pepperblue Steak . .	780	40.0	78.0	38.0	75	2070	4.0
pesto Roma club . .	650	49.0	27.0	38.0	85	2440	11.0
portobello mozzarella							
panini	670	27.0	69.0	33.0	45	1020	7.0
Smokehouse Turkey Panini:							
artisan three cheese	670	47.0	68.0	23.0	50	2320	4.0
asiago focaccia .	840	50.0	73.0	38.0	60	2740	5.0
tuna salad:							
artisan multigrain	830	32.0	78.0	41.0	65	1790	5.0
honey wheat	720	26.0	50.0	43.0	65	1570	4.0
turkey, Sierra	950	40.0	71.0	55.0	40	2360	4.0
turkey artichoke panini	810	41.0	76.0	38.0	25	1470	6.0
turkey breast, smoked:							
artisan country . .	590	34.0	73.0	16.0	10	2320	5.0
sourdough	440	29.0	44.0	15.0	10	1950	3.0
veggie, garden	570	15.0	74.0	23.0	15	1490	5.0
salad, w/dressing:							
Bistro Steak Salad .	630	16.0	10.0	58.0	55	940	4.0
Caesar	390	13.0	22.0	26.0	110	750	3.0
Caesar, grilled chicken	500	36.0	19.0	33.0	125	1530	3.0
classic café	390	3.0	14.0	37.0	0	350	4.0
chicken, Asian sesame	330	32.0	34.0	17.0	65	1170	5.0
Fandango Salad . . .	400	7.0	21.0	28.0	25	480	6.0
Greek	520	9.0	17.0	48.0	20	1560	5.0
tomato mozzarella .	790	30.0	50.0	55.0	85	790	6.0
pastries/sweets:							
apple croissant	260	4.0	34.0	11.0	30	230	1.0
apple Danish	510	9.0	50.0	30.0	85	350	2.0
apple raisin strudel	390	4.0	40.0	22.0	0	330	1.0
banana nut muffin:							
3 oz.	260	5.0	34.0	12.0	15	250	3.0
5.75 oz.	470	9.0	67.0	20.0	30	500	5.0
bear claw	380	7.0	37.0	21.0	70	310	1.0
blueberry muffin . .	450	8.0	73.0	15.0	35	570	4.0
brownie:							
caramel pecan . .	470	5.0	60.0	24.0	80	150	2.0

Food and Measure	cal.	prot. (gms)	carbo. (gms)	fat (gms)	chol. (mgs)	sod. (mgs)	fiber (gms)
chocolate raspberry	370	2.0	47.0	18.0	75	130	2.0
very chocolate ..	460	5.0	62.0	22.0	80	150	2.0
butter Danish, gooey	770	11.0	88.0	43.0	100	480	2.0
carrot walnut mini Bundt cake	430	6.0	51.0	21.0	75	340	2.0
cheese croissant ..	300	6.0	34.0	16.0	45	220	1.0
cheese Danish	590	10.0	55.0	35.0	110	430	1.0
cherry Danish	520	8.0	60.0	36.0	85	340	1.0
cherry strudel	400	5.0	38.0	24.0	0	290	1.0
chocolate chip muffin:							
2.5 oz.	240	4.0	36.0	10.0	15	240	2.0
5.75 oz.	540	8.0	83.0	22.0	30	550	5.0
chocolate cookie:							
chipper	420	5.0	51.0	22.0	60	320	2.0
duet, w/walnuts .	410	3.0	30.0	25.0	60	320	3.0
nutty chipper ...	440	6.0	46.0	26.0	55	300	3.0
chocolate croissant	440	7.0	56.0	23.0	35	180	4.0
chocolate Danish, German	770	10.0	83.0	46.0	85	570	4.0
chocolate hazelnut macaroon	270	3.0	30.0	15.0	0	90	3.0
cinnamon chip scone	560	10.0	70.0	27.0	150	440	2.0
cinnamon roll	500	12.0	64.0	26.0	90	480	3.0
cobblestone	560	8.0	100.0	9.0	0	620	4.0
coffeecake, cherry-cheese	190	3.0	21.0	10.0	30	130	1.0
lemon poppy mini Bundt cake	460	6.0	62.0	20.0	90	430	1.0
nutty oatmeal raisin cookie	350	5.0	51.0	14.0	45	260	3.0
orange scone	530	10.0	67.0	25.0	140	370	3.0
peach Danish, Georgia	580	9.0	67.0	30.0	85	390	2.0
pecan roll	520	6.0	60.0	31.0	40	260	2.0
pineapple upside-down mini Bundt cake	450	5.0	64.0	20.0	70	490	2.0
pumpkin muffin:							
3 oz.	270	3.0	43.0	6.0	30	270	1.0
5.75 oz.	510	6.0	80.0	12.0	60	530	1.0
raspberry cheese croissant	280	5.0	37.0	13.0	35	190	1.0
shortbread cookie .	340	3.0	36.0	21.0	60	160	1.0

Food and Measure	cal.	prot. (gms)	carbo. (gms)	fat (gms)	chol. (mgs)	sod. (mgs)	fiber (gms)
Panera Bread, pastries/sweets *(cont.)*							
triple-berry muffin, low fat	300	6.0	63.0	3.0	30	320	3.0
beverages:							
caffee latte	120	7.0	12.0	4.5	20	120	0
caffee mocha	360	11.0	47.0	16.0	55	190	2.0
cappuccino	120	7.0	12.0	6.5	20	120	0
caramel latte	400	9.0	54.0	16.0	55	450	0
chai tea latte	210	7.0	37.0	4.5	15	115	0
hot chocolate	350	11.0	45.0	15.0	50	190	2.0
house latte	320	8.0	43.0	13.0	50	135	0
I.C., 16 oz.:							
cappuccino chip .	590	5.0	64.0	35.0	70	125	0
caramel	550	6.0	77.0	24.0	80	400	0
mocha	520	7.0	70.0	24.0	75	140	2.0
spice	470	4.0	66.0	22.0	70	80	0
iced chai tea latte ..	170	6.0	29.0	3.5	15	95	0
Panko, flakes (*Shirakiku*), ⅓ cup .	80	2.0	15.0	.5	0	75	0
Papa John's, ⅛ pizza, except as noted:							
original crust, 12":							
barbecued chicken:							
and bacon	240	11.0	32.0	8.0	20	690	1.0
Hawaiian	240	11.0	33.0	8.0	20	690	1.0
cheese	210	9.0	27.0	8.0	15	520	1.0
chicken Alfredo ...	210	11.0	26.0	8.0	20	510	1.0
chicken club	230	11.0	28.0	8.0	20	590	1.0
garden fresh	200	8.0	28.0	7.0	10	500	2.0
Italian, spicy	260	11.0	27.0	8.0	20	690	3.0
meatball, spicy	240	11.0	28.0	10.0	25	640	1.0
the meats	240	11.0	27.0	11.0	20	650	2.0
the meats, w/beef .	250	11.0	27.0	11.0	25	670	2.0
pepperoni	220	9.0	27.0	9.0	15	580	1.0
sausage	240	9.0	27.0	11.0	15	590	2.0
spinach Alfredo ...	210	8.0	26.0	8.0	15	450	1.0
spinach Alfredo chicken tomato .	220	11.0	28.0	8.0	20	490	2.0
the works	230	10.0	28.0	8.0	15	620	2.0
original crust, 14":							
barbecued chicken:							
and bacon	340	15.0	44.0	11.0	30	960	2.0
Hawaiian	340	16.0	46.0	11.0	30	960	2.0
cheese	310	13.0	39.0	12.0	20	770	2.0

Food and Measure	cal.	prot. (gms)	carbo. (gms)	fat (gms)	chol. (mgs)	sod. (mgs)	fiber (gms)
chicken Alfredo ...	300	15.0	36.0	11.0	30	700	2.0
chicken club	320	16.0	40.0	12.0	30	840	2.0
garden fresh	280	11.0	40.0	9.0	15	680	2.0
Italian, spicy	370	15.0	39.0	11.0	30	970	4.0
meatball, spicy	330	15.0	40.0	13.0	35	880	2.0
the meats	350	15.0	38.0	16.0	30	940	2.0
the meats, w/beef .	370	17.0	38.0	17.0	35	980	3.0
pepperoni	320	13.0	38.0	13.0	20	820	2.0
sausage	330	13.0	38.0	15.0	20	820	3.0
spinach Alfredo ...	290	11.0	36.0	11.0	20	630	2.0
spinach Alfredo							
chicken tomato .	300	13.0	37.0	11.0	25	680	2.0
the works	330	14.0	40.0	11.0	25	900	3.0
thin crust, 14":							
barbecued chicken:							
and bacon	280	13.0	29.0	14.0	30	740	<1.0
Hawaiian	290	13.0	31.0	14.0	30	740	1.0
cheese	260	11.0	24.0	14.0	20	550	1.0
chicken Alfredo ...	250	12.0	21.0	13.0	30	480	1.0
chicken club	270	13.0	25.0	14.0	30	620	1.0
garden fresh	230	9.0	25.0	12.0	15	480	2.0
Italian, spicy	320	12.0	24.0	14.0	30	750	3.0
meatball, spicy	280	12.0	25.0	16.0	35	660	1.0
the meats	300	13.0	23.0	18.0	30	720	2.0
the meats, w/beef .	320	14.0	23.0	20.0	35	760	2.0
pepperoni	270	10.0	23.0	15.0	20	600	1.0
sausage	280	10.0	23.0	18.0	20	600	2.0
spinach Alfredo ...	240	9.0	21.0	14.0	20	410	1.0
spinach Alfredo							
chicken tomato .	250	12.0	24.0	14.0	25	460	1.0
the works	280	12.0	25.0	14.0	25	680	2.0
sides:							
breadstick, 1	140	4.0	26.0	2.0	0	260	1.0
cheese sticks, 2 ...	360	15.0	42.0	16.0	25	830	2.0
chicken strips, 2 ..	160	10.0	10.0	8.0	25	350	0
dipping sauce, 1 oz.:							
barbecue	40	0	11.0	0	0	240	0
blue cheese	170	1.0	1.0	18.0	20	240	0
Buffalo	15	0	2.0	.5	0	890	0
cheese	70	1.0	1.0	6.0	0	150	0
garlic	150	0	0	17.0	0	310	0
honey mustard ..	150	0	5.0	15.0	10	120	0
pizza	20	0	3.0	0	0	140	0
ranch	110	1.0	1.0	11.0	10	250	0

Food and Measure	cal.	prot. (gms)	carbo. (gms)	fat (gms)	chol. (mgs)	sod. (mgs)	fiber (gms)
Papa John's, sides *(cont.)*							
Papa's wings, 2 pcs.:							
Buffalo, spicy . . .	160	14.0	1.0	11.0	90	n.a.	<1.0
chipotle, mild . . .	160	14.0	5.0	10.0	85	n.a.	0
Papa's Cinnaple, 2 .	200	3.0	29.0	8.0	0	320	<1.0
Papaya, fresh:							
(*Del Monte*), ½ medium,							
4.9 oz.	70	0	19.0	0	0	10	2.0
(*Dole*), ½ medium,							
4.9 oz.	70	0	19.0	0	0	10	2.0
(*Frieda's* Golden Sunrise/							
Mexican), 1 cup, 5 oz.	50	0	14.0	0	0	0	3.0
1-lb., 3½" x 5⅛"	117	1.9	29.8	.4	0	8	5.5
cubed, 1 cup	55	.9	13.7	.2	0	4	2.5
mashed, 1 cup	90	1.4	22.6	.3	0	7	4.1
Papaya, dried (*Sun-Ridge Farms* Organic),							
1.4-oz. pc.	100	2.0	26.0	0	0	10	5.0
Papaya, frozen, (*Goya*),							
⅓ pkg.	50	1.0	11.0	0	0	12	2.0
Papaya, in jars, in extra light syrup (*Del Monte Sunfresh*),							
½ cup	70	1.0	17.0	0	0	5	1.0
Papaya drink (*Lincoln*),							
8 fl. oz.	130	0	32.0	0	0	75	0
Papaya juice, 8 fl. oz.:							
(*Ceres*)	120	0	30.0	0	0	5	0
(*R.W. Knudsen* Nectar)	140	<1.0	35.0	0	0	35	0
creamed (*R.W. Knudsen*)	40	<1.0	10.0	0	0	10	0
Papaya juice blend, 8 fl. oz.:							
(*L&A* Delight)	130	1.0	32.0	0	0	10	0
pineapple (*L&A* Delight)	130	0	31.0	0	0	10	0
Papaya nectar:							
(*Goya*), 12 fl. oz.	220	0	56.0	0	0	25	1.0
canned, 8 fl. oz.	143	.4	36.3	.4	0	12	1.5
Paprika, 1 tsp.	6	.3	1.2	.3	0	1	.6
Parsley, fresh:							
10 sprigs	4	.3	.6	.1	0	6	.3
chopped, ½ cup	11	.9	1.9	.2	0	17	1.0
Parsley, dried:							
1 tsp.	1	.1	.2	.1	0	1	.2
freeze-dried, 1 tbsp. . . .	1	.1	.2	<.1	0	2	.2

Food and Measure	cal.	prot. (gms)	carbo. (gms)	fat (gms)	chol. (mgs)	sod. (mgs)	fiber (gms)
Parsley root:							
(*Frieda's*), ⅔ cup, 3 oz.	10	2.0	2.0	.5	0	70	1.0
1 oz.	3	.8	.7	.2	0	28	.4
Parsnip:							
raw, sliced:							
(*Frieda's*), 1 cup . . .	100	2.0	24.0	0	0	10	7.0
½ cup	50	.8	12.1	.2	0	7	3.3
boiled, drained:							
1 medium, 9"	130	2.1	31.3	.5	0	17	6.4
sliced, ½ cup	63	1.0	15.2	.2	0	8	3.1
Passion fruit, fresh:							
(*Frieda's*), 5 oz.	140	3.0	33.0	1.0	0	40	15.0
purple:							
1 medium	18	.4	4.2	.1	0	5	1.9
trimmed, ½ cup . . .	115	.3	27.5	.8	0	33	12.2
Passion fruit, frozen							
(*Goya*), ⅓ pkg.	70	2.0	15.0	0	0	35	2.0
Passion fruit juice,							
8 fl. oz.:							
(*Ceres*)	120	0	31.0	0	0	10	0
fresh:							
purple	126	1.0	33.6	.1	0	15	.5
yellow	148	1.7	35.7	.4	0	15	.5
Passion fruit juice							
blend, apple and							
carrot (*Bolthouse*							
Farms), 8 fl. oz. . . .	120	2.0	29.0	0	0	95	2.0
Passion fruit nectar							
(*Goya*), 12 fl. oz. . .	230	0	57.0	0	0	5	0
Passion fruit syrup							
(*Trader Vic's*), 2 tbsp.	80	0	21.0	0	0	15	0
Pasta (see also							
"Macaroni" and							
"Noodles"), dry,							
2 oz., except as noted:							
plain	211	7.3	42.6	.9	0	4	1.4
all styles:							
(*Delverde*)	200	7.0	41.0	.5	0	0	1.0
(*Venecia*)	210	7.0	41.0	1.0	0	0	2.0
unflavored (*DeBoles*)	210	7.0	41.0	1.0	0	0	1.0
unflavored (*DeBoles*							
Organic)	210	7.0	43.0	1.0	0	5	1.0
veggie (*Hodgson*							
Mills)	200	8.0	41.0	1.0	0	15	1.0

Food and Measure	cal.	prot. (gms)	carbo. (gms)	fat (gms)	chol. (mgs)	sod. (mgs)	fiber (gms)
Pasta *(cont.)*							
alphabets, vegetable							
(*Eden* Organic)	200	8.0	40.0	1.0	0	15	2.0
angel hair:							
garlic and parsley							
(*DeBoles*)	210	7.0	41.0	1.0	0	5	2.0
garlic and parsley							
(*DeBoles* Organic)	210	7.0	42.0	1.0	0	15	2.0
tomato and basil							
(*DeBoles*)	210	7.0	41.0	1.0	0	0	2.0
tomato and basil							
(*DeBoles* Organic)	210	7.0	43.0	1.0	0	5	2.0
tomato and pesto							
(*DeBoles* Organic)	210	7.0	42.0	1.0	0	10	1.0
artichoke ribbons (*Eden*							
Organic)	210	9.0	40.0	1.5	0	10	2.0
elbows, whole wheat							
(*Hodgson Mill*) ...	190	9.0	40.0	1.0	0	10	6.0
extra fine (*Eden* Organic)	210	9.0	40.0	1.5	0	0	3.0
corn:							
angel hair (*Westbrae*							
Natural)	210	4.0	46.0	1.5	0	15	0
elbow or spaghetti							
(*DeBoles*)	200	4.0	43.0	2.0	0	15	5.0
gemelli twists:							
pesto (*Eden* Organic)	210	8.0	41.0	1.0	0	0	4.0
quinoa/kamut (*Eden*							
Organic)	210	8.0	2.0	2.0	0	0	5.0
lasagna, 2 pcs.:							
spinach (*Westbrae*							
Natural Organic) .	180	9.0	35.0	2.0	0	20	8.0
whole wheat (*West-*							
brae Natural							
Organic)	180	8.0	34.0	1.5	0	5	7.0
mung bean (*Eden*							
Harusame)	190	0	47.0	0	0	5	0
penne:							
(*Annie's* Organic) ..	200	7.0	41.0	1.0	0	0	2.0
whole wheat (*Annie's*							
Organic)	195	7.0	41.0	1.0	0	5	5.0
ribbons:							
parsley garlic, pesto,							
saffron, or vege-							
table (*Eden*							
Organic)	210	9.0	40.0	1.5	0	0	3.0

Food and Measure	cal.	prot. (gms)	carbo. (gms)	fat (gms)	chol. (mgs)	sod. (mgs)	fiber (gms)
spelt (*Eden* Organic)	210	7.0	41.0	2.0	0	10	5.0
spinach (*Eden* Organic)	210	8.0	41.0	1.0	0	30	4.0
yolkless, whole wheat (*Hodgson Mill*)	190	10.0	34.0	1.0	0	15	5.0
rice:							
(*Eden* Bifun)	200	5.0	44.0	.5	0	5	0
all styles, except lasagna (*DeBoles*)	210	4.0	46.0	.5	0	15	<1.0
lasagna (*DeBoles*), ¼ pkg., 2.5 oz. ...	260	5.0	56.0	.5	0	15	1.0
rotini, spaghetti, or penne (*Lundberg* Organic)	210	4.0	44.0	2.0	0	5	3.0
rigatoni:							
(*Eden* Organic Endless Tubes)	210	8.0	41.0	1.0	0	0	4.0
rotini (*Annie's* Organic)	200	7.0	41.0	1.0	0	0	2.0
shells, vegetable:							
(*Eden* Organic)	200	8.0	40.0	1.0	0	0	3.0
small (*Eden* Organic)	210	9.0	40.0	2.0	0	20	4.0
spaghetti:							
(*Annie's* Organic) ..	195	7.0	41.0	1.0	0	0	2.0
garlic parsley (*Eden* Organic)	210	8.0	41.0	1.0	0	0	4.0
kamut (*Eden* Organic)	190	10.0	38.0	1.5	0	0	6.0
semolina (*Eden* Organic)	200	8.0	40.0	1.0	0	0	2.0
spinach (*Westbrae Natural* Organic) .	180	9.0	38.0	2.0	0	20	8.0
spinach, whole wheat (*Hodgson Mill*) .	190	9.0	35.0	1.0	0	25	5.0
whole grain, 60% (*Eden* Organic) ..	210	8.0	41.0	1.0	0	0	4.0
whole grain, 100% (*Eden* Organic) ..	210	10.0	40.0	1.5	0	0	6.0
whole wheat (*Annie's* Organic)	195	7.0	41.0	1.0	0	5	5.0
whole wheat (*Westbrae Natural* Organic)	200	9.0	39.0	1.5	0	10	9.0
spelt:							
white (*Vita Spelt*) ..	210	9.0	42.0	.5	0	0	2.0

Food and Measure	cal.	prot. (gms)	carbo. (gms)	fat (gms)	chol. (mgs)	sod. (mgs)	fiber (gms)
Pasta, spelt *(cont.)*							
whole grain (*Vita Spelt*)	190	8.0	40.0	1.5	0	0	5.0
spinach, fettuccine or spaghetti (*DeBoles Organic*)	210	7.0	43.0	1.0	0	20	0
spirals:							
flax rice (*Eden Organic*)	200	9.0	40.0	~2.0	0	10	4.0
kamut (*Eden* Organic)	190	10.0	33.0	1.5	0	0	6.0
kamut vegetable (*Eden* Organic) ..	210	8.0	40.0	2.0	0	45	6.0
mixed grain (*Eden* Organic)	210	8.0	41.0	2.0	0	15	7.0
rye (*Eden* Organic) .	200	6.0	44.0	0	0	10	8.0
spinach (*Eden* Organic)	210	8.0	41.0	1.0	0	30	4.0
vegetable (*Eden* Organic)	200	8.0	40.0	1.0	0	0	3.0
whole wheat, all styles:							
(*DeBoles* Organic) .	210	7.0	42.0	1.5	0	10	5.0
except elbows, spinach spaghetti and yolkless ribbons (*Hodgson Mills*)	190	9.0	34.0	1.0	0	10	6.0
w/flax seed (*Hodgson Mills Organic*) ..	200	9.0	40.0	2.0	0	10	6.0
ziti rigati:							
garlic parsley (*Eden Organic*)	210	8.0	41.0	1.0	0	0	5.0
spelt (*Eden* Organic)	210	7.0	41.0	2.0	0	10	5.0
Pasta, cooked (see also "Macaroni"):							
corn, 1 cup	176	3.7	39.1	1.0	0	1	3.4
spaghetti, 1 cup:							
plain	197	6.7	39.7	.9	0	1	2.4
protein fortified ...	230	11.3	44.3	.3	0	7	2.4
spinach	182	6.4	36.6	.9	0	20	n.a.
whole wheat	174	7.5	37.2	.6	0	4	6.3
Pasta, refrigerated (see also specific listings) plain:							
uncooked:							
w/egg, 2 oz.	163	6.4	31.0	1.3	41	15	2.0

Food and Measure	cal.	prot. (gms)	carbo. (gms)	fat (gms)	chol. (mgs)	sod. (mgs)	fiber (gms)
spinach (*Azumaya*), 1 cup	210	8.0	42.0	.5	0	370	2.0
spinach, w/egg, 2 oz.	164	6.4	31.6	1.2	41	15	n.a.
cooked, 4 oz.:							
w/egg	149	5.8	28.3	1.2	37	7	n.a.
spinach, w/egg	147	5.7	28.4	1.1	37	7	n.a.
Pasta dish, frozen (see also "Pasta entree, frozen" and specific pasta listings), w/vegetables:							
broccoli Alfredo (*Green Giant Pasta Accents*), 1 cup cooked	210	10.0	34.0	4.0	<5	770	3.0
cheddar:							
creamy (*Green Giant Pasta Accents*), 1 cup cooked ...	250	9.0	640	8.0	15	640	3.0
white (*Green Giant Pasta Accents*), 1 cup cooked ...	290	10.0	37.0	11.0	15	710	3.0
cheese, three (*Green Giant Pasta Accents*), 1 cup cooked	350	13.0	42.0	14.0	20	920	4.0
cheese sauce, creamy (*Birds Eye*), 1 cup .	170	7.0	27.0	4.0	0	380	1.0
garlic (*Green Giant Pasta Accents*), 1 cup cooked	260	7.0	36.0	10.0	15	640	3.0
herb, garden (*Green Giant Pasta Accents*), 1 cup cooked	230	9.0	32.0	7.0	15	750	7.0
Pasta dish, mix (see also "Pasta salad mix" and specific pasta listings), 1 cup*:							
butter and herb (*Annie's Organic*)	290	11.0	43.0	9.0	25	770	2.0
w/cheese:							
(*Annie's Bunny*) ...	370	11.0	49.0	15.0	40	650	1.0
Parmesan (*Annie's Peace Pasta*) ...	270	12.0	48.0	4.0	10	610	1.0
garlic, roasted, and herb (*Annie's Organic*)	270	10.0	39.0	9.0	25	670	2.0

Food and Measure	cal.	prot. (gms)	carbo. (gms)	fat (gms)	chol. (mgs)	sod. (mgs)	fiber (gms)
Pasta dish, mix *(cont.)*							
Parmesan (*Annie's* Organic)	300	11.0	45.0	9.0	25	820	2.0
Pasta entree, can or cont. (see also "Pasta entree, pkg." and specific listings):							
garden salsa (*Hormel* Pasta Cup), 1 cont.	120	5.0	23.0	.5	0	650	2.0
Italian style (*Hormel* Pasta Cup), 1 cont.	220	7.0	26.0	10.0	10	1540	1.0
lemon pepper:							
(*Hormel* Bowl), 10 oz.	310	12.0	33.0	13.0	45	1630	2.0
(*Hormel* Pasta Cup), 1 cont.	240	9.0	25.0	10.0	35	1220	2.0
Mediterranean (*Hormel* Pasta Cup), 1 cont.	200	7.0	24.0	8.0	10	710	2.0
tomato cheese sauce, 1 cup:							
(*Annie's* Organic All Stars/BernieO's) .	150	4.0	31.0	1.0	0	680	<1.0
(*Annie's* Artrhur Organic Loops) .	150	5.0	32.0	1.0	0	670	1.0
w/soy "meatballs" (*Annie's* Organic P'Sghetti Loops)	190	9.0	29.0	4.0	0	650	2.0
Pasta entree, freeze-dried, 1 serving:							
primavera:							
(*Mountain House* Can/Four), 1 cup	230	9.0	32.0	7.0	25	860	2.0
(*Mountain House* Double), ½ pouch	300	11.0	42.0	9.0	35	1140	3.0
(*Mountain House* Single)	380	14.0	52.0	12.0	40	1420	3.0
Roma (*AlpineAire*) . . .	390	19.0	54.0	11.0	n.a.	730	3.0
Pasta entree, frozen (see also "Pasta dish, frozen" and specific listings), 1 pkg.:							
Alfredo:							
w/chicken and broccoli (*Lean Cuisine Everyday Favorites*), 10 oz.	270	17.0	38.0	6.0	40	690	3.0

Food and Measure	cal.	prot. (gms)	carbo. (gms)	fat (gms)	chol. (mgs)	sod. (mgs)	fiber (gms)
w/vegetables (*Green Giant*), 9 oz.	300	14.0	38.0	8.0	10	980	3.0
broccoli, Parmesan (*Moosewood*), 10 oz.	360	14.0	48.0	13.0	30	580	3.0
cheese, three (*Green Giant*), 9 oz.	270	10.0	40.0	8.0	25	1230	3.0
w/chicken, wine/ mushroom sauce (*Michelina's Lean Gourmet*), 8.5 oz. .	290	12.0	46.0	6.0	10	550	3.0
and beans (*Moosewood* Pasta e Fagioli), 10 oz.	260	10.0	47.0	3.5	0	340	6.0
peanut, spicy, w/vegetarian chicken (*Linda McCartney*), 10 oz.	340	15.0	44.0	5.0	0	810	4.0
portobello mushroom (*Uncle Ben's* Pasta Bowl Savory), 12 oz.	280	15.0	43.0	4.5	15	1050	3.0
primavera:							
(*Amy's*), 9 oz.	300	15.0	37.0	11.0	45	670	3.0
(*Green Giant*), 9 oz.	300	14.0	39.0	10.0	10	930	3.0
(*Michelina's* Zap'ems), 8 oz.	220	9.0	36.0	4.0	10	520	2.0
w/vegetables:							
cheese sauce (*Amy's* Bowls Country Cheddar), 9.5 oz.	400	15.0	41.0	19.0	20	690	4.0
garlic, roasted (*Green Giant*), 9 oz.	250	9.0	41.0	6.0	15	960	3.0
wheels and cheese (*Michelina's* Zap'ems), 8 oz.	350	15.0	48.0	12.0	25	650	3.0
Pasta entree, pkg., (see also specific listings), 1 cont.:							
Alfredo (*Bowl Appétit!*)	360	13.0	52.0	12.0	15	840	1.0
chicken flavored (*Bowl Appétit!* Homestyle)	260	10.0	42.0	6.0	10	830	2.0
pesto primavera, vegetarian (*Fantastic Carb 'Tastic*), 8 oz. .	270	23.0	22.0	13.0	10	750	14.0

Food and Measure	cal.	prot. (gms)	carbo. (gms)	fat (gms)	chol. (mgs)	sod. (mgs)	fiber (gms)
Pasta flour, see "Semolina flour"							
Pasta salad, refrigerated, Italian (*Reser's*), ½ cup	160	4.0	18.0	9.0	0	670	3.0
Pasta salad mix, approx. 1 cup*, except as noted: (*Suddenly Salad* Classic)	240	6.0	37.0	7.0	0	880	2.0
Caesar (*Suddenly Salad*)	350	6.0	34.0	10.0	0	650	1.0
Parmesan: creamy (*Suddenly Salad*)	360	7.0	30.0	24.0	20	520	1.0
roasted garlic (*Suddenly Salad*), ¾ cup*	330	7.0	34.0	23.0	15	520	1.0
ranch and bacon (*Suddenly Salad*), ¾ cup*	340	7.0	31.0	20.0	15	520	1.0
Pasta salad sauce mix, dry: Meditarranean (*McCormick*), 1 tbsp.	25	1.0	4.0	0	0	460	0
vinaigrette (*McCormick*), 1 tsp.	15	0	2.0	0	0	590	0
Pasta sauce (see also "Tomato sauce" and specific sauce listings), tomato, ½ cup, except as noted: (*Amy's* Pomodoro Zucca)	30	1.0	6.0	.5	0	590	1.0
(*Del Monte* Traditional)	60	2.0	15.0	.5	0	590	3.0
(*Eden* Organic)	80	3.0	12.0	2.5	0	320	3.0
(*Eden* Organic No Salt)	80	3.0	12.0	2.5	0	10	3.0
(*Healthy Choice* Traditional)	60	3.0	13.0	0	0	370	3.0
(*Hunt's* Light)	45	2.0	9.0	0	0	430	3.0
(*Hunt's* No Sugar)	45	2.0	9.0	1.0	0	580	3.0
(*Hunt's* Traditional)	50	2.0	10.0	.5	0	580	3.0
(*Prego* Chunky Garden)	90	2.0	17.0	1.5	0	470	3.0
(*Prego* Traditional)	120	2.0	19.0	3.5	0	580	3.0

Food and Measure	cal.	prot. (gms)	carbo. (gms)	fat (gms)	chol. (mgs)	sod. (mgs)	fiber (gms)
(*Prego* Traditional Plastic)	130	2.0	20.0	4.5	0	590	3.0
(*Ragú* Old World Traditional)	70	2.0	8.0	3.0	0	770	2.0
(*Red Pack* Spaghetti) .	80	2.0	11.0	3.0	0	610	2.0
(*Tree of Life* Classic Tomato Fat Free) ..	40	2.0	9.0	0	0	180	<1.0
(*Tree of Life* Pasta Sauce)	50	2.0	9.0	2.0	0	380	<1.0
arrabiata:							
(*Mama Capri*)	80	3.0	6.0	5.0	0	650	2.0
(*Pasta Cosi*)	70	1.0	6.0	4.5	0	310	1.0
basil, tomato:							
(*Amy's*)	110	2.0	11.0	6.0	0	580	3.0
(*Classico* di Napoli)	60	2.0	11.0	1.0	0	310	2.0
(*Del Monte*)	70	2.0	16.0	1.0	0	600	3.0
(*Muir Glen*)	50	2.0	12.0	1.0	0	370	0
(*Newman's Own* Bombolina)	100	1.0	13.0	4.0	0	590	<1.0
(*Walnut Acres*)	50	2.0	9.0	1.0	0	330	1.0
(*Walnut Acres* Low Sodium)	40	2.0	9.0	0	0	20	<1.0
basil and garlic:							
(*Mama Capri* Basilico)	90	1.0	5.0	7.0	0	450	2.0
(*Prego*)	90	2.0	17.0	2.0	0	420	3.0
beef, w/onion, garlic (*Classico* Bolognese)	130	5.0	14.0	5.0	15	660	3.0
w/cheese:							
five (*Newman's Own*)	90	2.0	10.0	3.0	<5	510	<1.0
four (*Classico* di Parma)	90	3.0	10.0	5.0	<5	570	1.0
four (*Del Monte*) ..	70	2.0	15.0	1.5	0	680	3.0
four (*Hunt's*)	50	3.0	10.0	1.0	0	600	3.0
three (*Prego*)	90	2.0	17.0	2.0	5	430	3.0
w/cheese and garlic (*Hunt's*)	50	3.0	9.0	1.0	0	600	2.0
chicken, roasted, w/Parmesan, garlic (*Classico* di Romagna)	90	5.0	13.0	2.0	10	470	2.0
garlic:							
(*Prego* Supreme) ..	120	2.0	17.0	4.5	0	470	3.0

Food and Measure	cal.	prot. (gms)	carbo. (gms)	fat (gms)	chol. (mgs)	sod. (mgs)	fiber (gms)
Pasta sauce, garlic *(cont.)*							
(*Walnut Acres* Garlic-Garlic)	50	2.0	10.0	1.0	0	280	1.0
garlic, roasted:							
(*Amy's*)	130	2.0	13.0	8.0	0	470	3.0
(*Classico* di Sorrento)	60	2.0	11.0	1.0	0	220	2.0
(*Muir Glen*)	50	2.0	10.0	.5	0	320	0
(*Pasta Cosi*)	90	2.0	9.0	5.0	0	140	2.0
(*Walnut Acres*)	60	2.0	11.0	1.0	0	280	1.0
and herb (*Prego*) . .	110	2.0	17.0	4.0	0	530	2.0
and onion (*Hunt's*) .	50	2.0	10.0	1.0	0	540	3.0
Parmesan (*Prego*) .	110	3.0	20.0	2.0	5	550	3.0
and peppers							
(*Newman's Own*)	70	2.0	11.0	2.5	0	460	4.0
tomato and							
(*Newman's Own*)	70	2.0	11.0	2.5	0	580	<1.0
garlic and:							
basil (*Prego* Pasta							
Bake), ⅛ jar	80	1.0	11.0	3.5	0	530	2.0
herb (*Del Monte*							
Chunky)	60	2.0	11.0	1.5	0	490	<1.0
herb (*Healthy Choice*)	60	2.0	13.0	0	0	320	3.0
herb (*Hunt's*)	40	2.0	8.0	.5	0	610	3.0
mushroom (*Amy's*)	120	3.0	10.0	7.0	5	680	3.0
onion (*Del Monte*) .	80	2.0	16.0	1.0	0	490	2.0
onion (*Muir Glen*) .	55	2.0	12.0	.5	0	320	0
onion (*Ragú* Chunky)	110	2.0	21.0	3.0	0	510	2.0
green pepper/mushroom							
(*Del Monte*)	80	2.0	16.0	1.0	0	490	3.0
herb:							
(*Muir Glen*)	50	2.0	12.0	.5	0	320	0
Italian (*Del Monte*							
Chunky)	60	2.0	12.0	1.0	0	520	<1.0
Italian (*Muir Glen*) .	55	2.0	12.0	.5	0	320	0
7 (*Ragú Robusto*) .	80	2.0	12.0	3.5	0	550	2.0
hot and spicy							
(*Newman's Own* Fra							
Diavolo)	70	0	10.0	3.0	0	510	0
marinara:							
(*Amy's* Family)	50	1.0	8.0	1.0	0	590	3.0
(*Amy's* Low Sodium)	40	1.0	7.0	1.0	0	100	1.0
(*Mama Capri*)	120	2.0	5.0	10.0	0	440	2.0
(*Newman's Own*) . .	60	2.0	12.0	2.0	0	590	<1.0

Food and Measure	cal.	prot. (gms)	carbo. (gms)	fat (gms)	chol. (mgs)	sod. (mgs)	fiber (gms)
(*Pasta Cosi*)	70	1.0	6.0	4.5	0	310	1.0
(*Prego*)	100	2.0	11.0	5.0	0	550	4.0
(*Red Pack*)	60	3.0	8.0	3.5	<5	480	6.0
basil, sweet (*Classico di Campania*) . . .	70	2.0	13.0	1.0	0	280	1.0
Cabernet (*Muir Glen*)	50	2.0	11.0	.5	0	330	0
Cabernet, w/herbs (*Classico di Piedmont*)	60	1.0	10.0	2.0	0	400	2.0
w/cheese (*Prego*) . .	100	3.0	11.0	5.0	<5	550	4.0
cheese, three (*Prego Pasta Bake*), ⅛ jar	100	3.0	11.0	4.5	5	650	2.0
w/herbs or zinfadel (*Walnut Acres*) . .	50	2.0	9.0	1.0	0	330	1.0
mushroom (*Newman's Own*)	60	2.0	12.0	2.0	0	590	<1.0
w/mushroom (*Prego*)	100	2.0	11.0	5.0	0	550	4.0
meat:							
(*Del Monte*)	60	3.0	14.0	1.0	2	720	3.0
(*Hunt's*)	60	3.0	11.0	1.0	0	610	3.0
(*Prego*)	130	2.0	19.0	5.0	5	570	3.0
(*Prego* Pasta Bakes Hearty), ⅛ jar . .	50	4.0	12.0	6.0	10	790	2.0
(*Ragú* Old World) . .	70	2.0	7.0	3.0	0	750	2.0
(*Ragú* Rich & Meaty)	110	6.0	10.0	5.0	15	540	2.0
w/fresh mushrooms (*Prego Hearty Meat* Classic) . . .	130	6.0	14.0	6.0	10	660	2.0
three (*Prego Hearty Meat* Supreme) .	170	7.0	12.0	10.0	15	600	3.0
w/meatballs:							
mini (*Prego*)	150	4.0	20.0	6.0	10	650	3.0
Parmesan (*Prego Hearty Meat*) . . .	160	7.0	16.0	8.0	10	690	2.0
mushroom:							
(*Del Monte*)	60	2.0	14.0	.5	0	630	2.0
(*Hunt's*)	50	2.0	10.0	1.0	0	600	3.0
(*Prego* Chunky Garden Supreme)	120	2.0	20.0	4.0	0	470	4.0
(*Prego* Zesty)	110	2.0	18.0	3.5	0	530	3.0
(*Ragú* Old World) . .	70	2.0	8.0	3.0	0	760	2.0
fresh (*Prego*)	110	2.0	18.0	3.5	0	550	3.0
fresh (*Prego* Plastic)	130	2.0	21.0	4.5	0	590	3.0
marinara (*Muir Glen*)	45	2.0	10.0	0	0	320	0

Food and Measure	cal.	prot. (gms)	carbo. (gms)	fat (gms)	chol. (mgs)	sod. (mgs)	fiber (gms)
Pasta sauce, mushroom *(cont.)*							
portobello *(Muir Glen)*	50	2.0	11.0	0	0	330	0
tomato and *(Walnut Acres)*	50	2.0	9.0	1.0	0	330	1.0
triple *(Classico di Toscana)*	80	3.0	12.0	2.0	0	390	3.0
wild *(Amy's)*	60	2.0	7.0	2.5	0	580	2.0
mushroom and:							
garlic *(Healthy Choice* Super Chunky)	45	2.0	10.0	0	0	340	3.0
garlic *(Prego)*	110	2.0	20.0	2.0	0	510	2.0
green pepper *(Prego Chunky Garden)* .	110	2.0	17.0	4.0	0	470	4.0
olive, ripe *(Classico di Sicillia)*	60	2.0	11.0	1.0	0	390	2.0
Parmesan *(Prego)* .	130	3.0	22.0	3.5	5	480	3.0
onion:							
diced, and garlic *(Prego)*	120	2.0	18.0	4.5	0	480	3.0
and garlic *(Prego Chunky Garden)* .	110	2.0	18.0	3.5	0	490	4.0
and garlic *(Tree of Life* Fat Free) ...	40	2.0	8.0	0	0	260	<1.0
roasted, balsamic *(Muir Glen)*	50	2.0	12.0	.5	0	320	0
pepper, red:							
roasted, and garlic *(Prego)*	120	2.0	19.0	4.0	0	530	3.0
spicy *(Classico di Roma Arrabbiata)*	60	2.0	7.0	1.5	0	300	2.0
tomatoes and spices *(Newman's Own)*	60	2.0	12.0	2.0	0	590	<1.0
pepper, sweet:							
(Tree of Life Fat Free)	35	2.0	8.0	0	0	310	<1.0
and onion *(Walnut Acres)*	50	2.0	9.0	1.0	0	280	1.0
puttanesca:							
(Amy's)	40	1.0	5.0	2.0	0	680	1.0
(Pasta Cosi)	70	1.0	6.0	5.0	0	390	1.0
ricotta Parmesan *(Prego)*	120	3.0	20.0	3.5	5	500	3.0
sausage, Italian:							
(Hunt's)	60	2.0	10.0	1.5	0	590	3.0

Food and Measure	cal.	prot. (gms)	carbo. (gms)	fat (gms)	chol. (mgs)	sod. (mgs)	fiber (gms)
(*Prego* Pasta Bakes), ⅛ jar	90	3.0	12.0	3.5	5	760	3.0
(*Prego Hearty Meat*)	150	6.0	16.0	7.0	15	600	2.0
and garlic (*Prego*) .	120	3.0	16.0	5.0	10	500	3.0
w/pepper, onion (*Classico* d'Abruzzi)	90	5.0	13.0	2.0	5	470	2.0
spinach and cheese (*Classico* di Firenze)	80	3.0	6.0	5.0	<5	560	2.0
steak, hearty, w/Burgundy (*Classico*)	120	5.0	13.0	5.0	15	660	3.0
tomato:							
fire-roasted, and garlic (*Classico* di Siena)	50	2.0	10.0	.5	0	320	2.0
spicy, and pesto (*Classico* di Genoa)	90	3.0	11.0	4.0	0	470	2.0
sun-dried (*Classico* di Capri)	80	2.0	11.0	3.0	0	390	2.0
sun-dried (*Muir Glen*)	55	2.0	10.0	1.0	0	370	0
vegetable:							
chunky (*Hunt's*) ...	50	2.0	11.0	1.0	0	560	3.0
garden (*Muir Glen*)	50	2.0	10.0	1.0	0	320	0
garden, primavera (*Classico* di Lazio)	60	2.0	11.0	1.0	0	610	2.0
primavera (*Healthy Choice* Super Chunky)	60	2.0	13.0	0	0	390	3.0
vodka:							
(*Bove's*)	100	1.0	7.0	6.0	10	390	1.0
(*Mama Capri*)	140	3.0	5.0	10.0	0	440	2.0
(*Newman's Own*) ..	110	5.0	11.0	5.0	5	440	0
(*Pasta Cosi*)	110	2.0	8.0	7.0	5	140	2.0
Pasta sauce, refrige-rated (see also specific sauce list-ings), tomato, ½ cup:							
marinara:							
(*Buitoni*)	80	2.0	11.0	3.0	0	580	2.0
(*DiGiorno*)	70	2.0	15.0	0	0	220	2.0
garlic, roasted (*Buitoni*)	60	2.0	9.0	1.5	5	580	1.0

Food and Measure	cal.	prot. (gms)	carbo. (gms)	fat (gms)	chol. (mgs)	sod. (mgs)	fiber (gms)
Pasta sauce, refrigerated, marinara *(cont.)*							
portobello mushroom (*Buitoni*)	80	2.0	11.0	3.0	0	520	2.0
tomato herb Parmesan (*Buitoni*)	120	0	9.0	8.0	10	790	2.0
Pasta sauce mix, 1 tbsp. dry, except as noted:							
(*Lawry's* Spaghetti Extra Rich & Thick)	30	<1.0	7.0	0	0	620	<1.0
(*Lawry's* Spaghetti Original), 1½ tbsp. .	25	0	6.0	0	0	600	0
(*McCormick* Pasta Rosa)	40	1.0	4.0	2.0	5	540	0
herb and garlic (*McCormick*)	20	1.0	2.0	0	0	500	0
primavera (*McCormick*)	30	0	4.0	1.0	0	490	0
spaghetti sauce: (*McCormick* Thick & Zesty)	25	0	6.0	0	0	620	0
Italian style (*McCormick*) ...	25	0	5.0	0	0	490	0
mild (*McCormick*) .	25	1.0	5.0	.5	0	410	0
tomato basil (*McCormick*)	25	0	5.0	0	0	210	0
Pastrami, beef, 2 oz., except as noted:							
(*Black Bear* Brisket) ..	80	10.0	2.0	4.0	30	610	0
(*Boar's Head* Brisket) .	90	12.0	2.0	4.0	30	670	0
(*Boar's Head* Red) ...	80	12.0	1.0	3.0	35	610	0
(*Boar's Head* Round) .	70	12.0	1.0	2.5	30	580	0
(*Boar's Head* Top Round Cap-off)	70	13.0	1.0	2.5	30	600	0
(*Dietz & Watson* Brisket)	90	10.0	0	4.0	30	610	0
(*Healthy Choice*)	60	10.0	2.0	1.5	30	410	0
(*Healthy Choice Deli Thin*), 4 slices, 1.8 oz.	60	10.0	2.0	1.5	25	450	0
(*Healthy Deli*)	80	11.0	3.0	3.0	30	480	0
(*Hebrew National*) ...	90	13.0	1.0	4.0	35	500	0
(*Hormel*)	70	10.0	0	3.0	30	650	0
(*Sara Lee*)	70	11.0	1.0	2.5	30	390	0
(*Sara Lee* Pre-sliced), 2 slices, 1.6 oz.	60	9.0	0	2.5	25	380	0
(*Tyson* Bag), 2 slices, 2.25 oz.	70	13.0	0	2.0	20	530	0

Food and Measure	cal.	prot. (gms)	carbo. (gms)	fat (gms)	chol. (mgs)	sod. (mgs)	fiber (gms)
Pastry, puff (see also "Fillo dough" and "Pie crust"):							
frozen (*Kineret* Ready to Bake), 2-oz. sq. . .	250	3.0	20.0	18.0	0	140	<1.0
patty shell (*Pepperidge Farm*), 1 pc.	190	4.0	16.0	13.0	0	230	<1.0
sheet (*Pepperidge Farm*), 1/6 sheet	170	3.0	14.0	11.0	0	200	<1.0
Pastry filling (see also "Pie filling"), canned, 2 tbsp.:							
almond (*Solo*)	120	1.0	23.0	2.5	0	45	2.0
apple, Dutch (*Solo*) . .	80	0	20.0	0	0	45	1.0
apricot (*Solo*)	80	0	17.0	0	0	20	1.0
blueberry (*Solo*)	80	0	17.0	0	0	25	1.0
cherry (*Solo*)	80	0	20.0	0	0	25	1.0
date (*Solo*)	100	0	22.0	0	0	40	3.0
nut, fancy (*Solo*)	140	1.0	25.0	5.0	0	55	5.0
pecan (*Solo*)	130	1.0	24.0	4.0	0	50	1.0
pineapple (*Solo*)	80	0	19.0	0	0	20	1.0
poppy seed (*Solo*) . . .	140	2.0	30.0	4.0	0	30	3.0
prune plum (*Solo*) . . .	70	0	18.0	0	0	25	1.0
raspberry (*Solo*)	80	0	19.0	0	0	25	1.0
strawberry (*Solo*)	70	0	18.0	0	0	20	1.0
Pâté, can or jar:							
2 oz.	179	8.0	.6	15.7	143	390	0
1 tbsp.	41	1.9	.2	3.6	33	91	0
chicken liver:							
2 oz.	113	7.5	3.7	7.3	219	216	0
1 tbsp.	26	1.8	.9	1.7	51	51	0
goose liver:							
smoked, 2 oz.	259	6.4	2.6	24.6	84	390	0
smoked, 1 tbsp. . . .	60	1.5	.6	5.7	20	91	0
truffle flavor, 2 oz. . . .	183	6.3	3.5	16.0	59	452	0
Pâté, refrigerated (see also "Salmon pâté"), 2 oz.:							
duck mousse, w/truffles:							
(*Chef Georges*)	192	5.0	5.0	17.0	56	375	0
and port wine (*Marcel & Henri*)	240	6.0	<1.0	24.0	95	340	0
w/goose fat and liver (*Shaller & Weber*) .	190	8.0	1.0	17.0	80	230	0

Food and Measure	cal.	prot. (gms)	carbo. (gms)	fat (gms)	chol. (mgs)	sod. (mgs)	fiber (gms)
Pâté, refrigerated *(cont.)*							
pork, w/champagne							
(*Marcel & Henri* Pâté							
de Campagne)	210	7.0	1.0	19.0	80	370	<1.0
Pea pods, see "Peas,							
edible-podded"							
Peach, fresh:							
(*Chiquita*), 1 medium,							
3.5 oz.	40	1.0	10.0	0	0	0	2.0
(*Del Monte*), 1 medium,							
3.5 oz.	40	1.0	10.0	0	0	0	2.0
(*Dole*), 1 medium,							
3.5 oz.	40	1.0	10.0	0	0	0	2.0
(*Frieda's Donut/Frieda's*							
Late Season), 5 oz.	60	1.0	16.0	0	0	0	3.0
2½" peach, 4 per lb. .	37	.6	9.7	.1	0	0	1.7
sliced, 1 cup	73	1.2	18.9	.2	0	0	3.4
Peach, can or jar,							
halves or slices,							
½ cup, except as							
noted:							
(*Del Monte Carb Clever*)	30	1.0	7.0	0	0	10	1.0
diced (*Dole Fruit-Bowls*),							
4 oz.	80	<1.0	16.0	0	0	15	1.0
in juice:							
(*Del Monte/Del Monte*							
Fruit Naturals) . .	60	0	15.0	0	0	10	1.0
(*S&W* Natural Style)	80	1.0	19.0	0	0	20	1.0
chunks (*Del Monte*							
Fruit Naturals) . .	70	<1.0	17.0	0	0	10	<1.0
diced (*Del Monte*							
Fruit Naturals							
Fruit Cup), 4.5 oz.	50	0	13.0	0	0	10	<1.0
w/liquid	55	.8	14.5	<.1	0	5	1.6
in extra light syrup:							
(*Del Monte* Lite Cling)	60	0	15.0	0	0	10	1.0
(*Del Monte* Lite							
Freestone)	60	0	14.0	0	0	10	1.0
diced (*Del Monte*							
Fruit Cup Lite),							
4.5 oz.	50	0	13.0	0	0	10	<1.0
in gelatin:							
peach gel (*Del Monte*),							
4.5-oz. cup	90	0	22.0	0	0	40	0

Food and Measure	cal.	prot. (gms)	carbo. (gms)	fat (gms)	chol. (mgs)	sod. (mgs)	fiber (gms)
raspberry gel (*Del Monte*), 4.5-oz. cup	90	0	23.0	0	0	40	0
strawberry-banana (*Del Monte* Lite), 4.5-oz. cup	60	0	14.0	0	0	40	0
in light syrup:							
(*Del Monte Orchard Select*)	80	<1.0	20.0	0	0	10	<1.0
(*S&W*)	70	0	17.0	0	0	10	1.0
w/liquid	68	.6	18.3	<.1	0	5	1.6
raspberry flavor (*Del Monte*)	80	<1.0	20.0	0	0	10	<1.0
spiced (*Del Monte Harvest Spice*) . .	80	<1.0	21.0	0	0	10	<1.0
strawberry-banana flavor (*Del Monte*)	70	<1.0	17.0	0	0	10	<1.0
in light syrup, chunks:							
(*S&W* Sun)	80	<1.0	20.0	0	0	20	1.0
(*S&W* Tropical) . . .	80	<1.0	19.0	0	0	15	<1.0
cinnamon (*Del Monte*)	80	0	20.0	0	0	10	1.0
cinnamon, brown sugar (*S&W Sweet Memory*) .	80	<1.0	19.0	0	0	15	<1.0
hybrid (*S&W* Snow)	80	<1.0	20.0	0	0	15	1.0
raspberry flavor (*Del Monte*)	80	<1.0	20.0	0	0	10	<1.0
in heavy syrup:							
(*Del Monte*)	100	0	24.0	0	0	10	1.0
(*S&W*)	100	0	24.0	0	0	10	1.0
w/liquid	97	.6	26.1	.1	0	8	1.7
diced (*Del Monte*) .	80	0	20.0	0	0	10	<1.0
diced (*Del Monte Fruit Cup*), 4.5 oz.	80	0	20.0	0	0	10	<1.0
spiced, whole (*Del Monte*)	100	0	24.0	0	0	10	<1.0
Peach, dried:							
(*Sun•Maid*), ¼ cup . .	100	2.0	25.0	0	0	0	3.0
(*Sunsweet*), 3 pcs., 1.4 oz.	110	2.0	25.0	0	0	0	3.0
sulfured:							
halves, ½ cup	191	2.9	49.1	.6	0	6	6.6
10 halves, 4.6 oz. . .	311	4.7	79.7	1.0	0	9	10.7

Food and Measure	cal.	prot. (gms)	carbo. (gms)	fat (gms)	chol. (mgs)	sod. (mgs)	fiber (gms)
Peach, freeze-dried, diced (*AlpineAire*), .4 oz.	40	1.0	9.0	0	0	0	0
Peach, frozen, sliced:							
(*Cascadian Farm*), 1 cup	60	1.0	14.0	0	0	0	1.0
(*C&W*), ⅔ cup	50	1.0	13.0	0	0	0	2.0
sweetened, ½ cup . . .	118	.8	30.0	.2	0	8	1.8
Peach drink, 8 fl. oz., except as noted:							
(*Snapple* Summer Peach)	120	0	30.0	0	0	10	0
(*Snapple-a-Day*), 11.5 fl. oz.	210	7.0	43.0	0	0	110	5.0
(*Walnut Acres*)	120	0	32.0	0	0	15	0
nectar:							
(*Goya*), 6 fl. oz. . . .	110	<1.0	27.0	0	0	30	1.0
(*Goya*), 12 fl. oz. . .	220	1.0	54.0	0	0	25	2.0
(*R.W. Knudsen*) . . .	120	<1.0	30.0	0	0	25	0
(*Santa Cruz Organic*)	120	1.0	29.0	0	0	10	0
canned	135	.7	34.7	<.1	0	17	1.5
Peach dumpling, frozen (*Pepperidge Farm*), 3-oz. pc.	320	3.0	50.0	11.0	0	150	4.0
Peach glaze (*Litehouse*), 3 tbsp.	70	0	18.0	0	0	25	0
Peach juice, 8 fl. oz.:							
(*After the Fall* Georgia)	130	1.0	31.0	0	0	15	0
(*Ceres*).	120	0	30.0	0	0	5	0
Peach nectar, see "Peach drink"							
Peach-mango drink (*V8 Splash* Smoothies), 8 fl. oz	120	3.0	27.0	0	0	60	0
Peach-orange juice, (*Nantucket Nectars*), 8 fl. oz.	130	0	31.0	0	0	25	0
Peanut, shelled, 1 oz., except as noted:							
(*Beer Nuts* Kettle Cooked)	185	8.0	6.0	15.0	0	60	2.0
(*Beer Nuts* Original) . .	170	7.0	7.0	14.0	0	80	2.0
(*Frito Lay* Salted)	160	7.0	6.0	14.0	0	170	2.0
(*Planters* Cocktail) . . .	170	7.0	6.0	14.0	0	115	2.0

Food and Measure	cal.	prot. (gms)	carbo. (gms)	fat (gms)	chol. (mgs)	sod. (mgs)	fiber (gms)
(*Planters* Cocktail Lightly Salted)	170	7.0	5.0	15.0	0	55	2.0
(*Planters* Cocktail Unsalted)	170	7.0	6.0	14.0	0	0	2.0
(*Shiloh Farms* Raw Redskin), ¼ cup ..	190	9.0	7.0	16.0	0	0	3.0
barbecue (*Beer Nuts* Crunch Nuts)	130	4.0	18.0	4.5	0	110	2.0
boiled, salted	90	3.8	6.0	6.2	0	213	2.5
Cajun (*Beer Nuts* Crunch Nuts)	140	4.0	15.0	6.0	0	140	1.0
dry-roasted:							
(*Fisher*)	170	7.0	6.0	14.0	0	190	2.0
(*Planters*)	160	7.0	6.0	13.0	0	190	2.0
(*Planters*), 1.75-oz. pkg. ...	290	8.0	9.0	26.0	0	230	4.0
(*Planters* Lightly Salted)	170	8.0	5.0	14.0	0	95	2.0
(*Planters* Unsalted)	160	8.0	6.0	14.0	0	0	2.0
½ cup	428	17.3	15.7	36.3	0	4	5.8
honey (*Planters*) ..	150	7.0	8.0	12.0	0	95	2.0
glazed (*Beer Nuts* Old Fashioned)	140	8.0	6.0	14.0	0	60	2.0
honey mustard (*Beer Nuts* Crunch Nuts) .	140	4.0	19.0	5.0	0	55	1.0
honey roasted:							
(*Fisher*)	170	7.0	7.0	13.0	0	70	2.0
(*Kettle*)	160	6.0	8.0	12.0	0	120	2.0
(*Planters*)	160	6.0	8.0	13.0	0	95	2.0
hot and spicy:							
(*D.L. Jardine's* Texacali), ¼ cup .	160	8.0	5.0	14.0	0	220	<2.0
(*Frito-Lay*), 1.1 oz. .	190	7.0	6.0	16.0	0	250	2.0
oil-roasted:							
(*Fisher*)	170	7.0	6.0	15.0	0	130	2.0
½ cup	419	19.0	13.6	35.5	0	4	6.6
sesame (*Beer Nuts* Crunch Nuts)	130	4.0	15.0	6.0	0	90	2.0
Spanish:							
(*Kettle* Jumbo Salted)	160	8.0	5.0	14.0	0	125	2.0
(*Planters* Redskin) .	180	8.0	5.0	14.0	0	100	2.0
raw (*Kettle*)	160	7.0	4.0	14.0	0	5	3.0
raw (*Planters*)	150	7.0	6.0	13.0	0	5	3.0

Food and Measure	cal.	prot. (gms)	carbo. (gms)	fat (gms)	chol. (mgs)	sod. (mgs)	fiber (gms)
Peanut *(cont.)*							
sweet and crunchy:							
(*Planters*)	140	4.0	16.0	7.0	0	20	2.0
honey roasted							
(*Planters*)	170	7.0	6.0	14.0	0	115	2.0
Peanut butter (see also "Peanut Spread"), 2 tbsp., except as noted:							
(*Kettle Roaster Fresh Unsalted*), 1 oz. ...	166	8.0	5.0	14.0	0	2	0
(*Simply Jif*)	190	8.0	6.0	16.0	0	65	2.0
chunky or creamy:							
(*Arrowhead Mills*) .	190	8.0	6.0	16.5	0	0	2.0
(*Smucker's*)	210	8.0	6.0	16.0	0	120	2.0
(*Tree of Life*)	190	8.0	7.0	16.0	0	45	1.0
(*Tree of Life* No Salt)	190	8.0	7.0	16.0	0	0	1.0
blended (*Tree of Life*) .	190	7.0	7.0	15.0	0	55	2.0
chunky/crunchy:							
(*Jif* Reduced Fat) ..	190	8.0	15.0	12.0	0	220	2.0
(*Reese's*)	200	8.0	7.0	15.0	0	110	2.0
(*Skippy Super Chunk*)	190	7.0	7.0	17.0	0	140	2.0
(*Skippy Super Chunk Reduced Fat*) ...	190	7.0	14.0	12.0	0	170	2.0
extra (*Jif*)	190	8.0	7.0	16.0	0	130	2.0
creamy:							
(*Jif*)	190	8.0	7.0	16.0	0	150	2.0
(*Jif* Reduced Fat) ..	190	8.0	15.0	12.0	0	250	2.0
(*Reese's*)	200	7.0	8.0	15.0	0	140	2.0
(*Skippy*)	190	7.0	7.0	17.0	0	150	2.0
(*Skippy* Natural) ...	190	8.0	6.0	16.0	0	150	2.0
(*Skippy* Reduced Fat)	190	7.0	15.0	12.0	0	190	2.0
(*Skippy Carb Options*)	190	7.0	5.0	17.0	0	150	2.0
(*Smucker's* No Salt)	210	7.0	6.0	16.0	0	0	2.0
(*Smucker's* Reduced Fat)	200	9.0	12.0	12.0	0	120	2.0
honey:							
(*Smucker's*)	200	7.0	9.0	16.0	0	30	2.0
creamy (*Jif*)	190	6.0	11.0	15.0	0	120	2.0
roasted, chunky or creamy (*Skippy*)	190	7.0	7.0	17.0	0	125	2.0
Peanut butter baking chips, 1 tbsp., .5 oz.:							
(*Hershey's Bake Shoppe Reese's*) ..	80	2.0	8.0	4.0	0	40	<1.0

Food and Measure	cal.	prot. (gms)	carbo. (gms)	fat (gms)	chol. (mgs)	sod. (mgs)	fiber (gms)
and milk (*Hershey's Bake Shoppe Reese's*)	80	2.0	8.0	4.5	0	25	0
Peanut butter sprinkles (*Reese's*), 2 tbsp. ...	90	1.0	12.0	4.0	0	45	<1.0
Peanut butter topping (*Reese's* Shell), 2 tbsp.	220	<1.0	17.0	17.0	0	70	1.0
Peanut butter-jelly: grape or strawberry (*Smucker's Goober*), 3 tbsp.	240	7.0	24.0	13.0	0	140	2.0
Peanut butter-jelly sandwich, frozen, grape or strawberry (*Smucker's Uncrustables*), 2-oz. pc. ...	210	7.0	25.0	9.0	0	260	2.0
Peanut coating mix (*Thai Kitchen* Peanut Bake), dry, .75 oz. .	95	2.5	13.9	4.9	9	458	0
Peanut flour, 1 cup:							
defatted	196	31.3	20.8	.3	0	9	9.5
low fat	257	20.3	18.8	13.1	0	0	9.5
Peanut sauce, 2 tbsp., except as noted:							
(*Annie Chun's*)	120	4.0	10.0	7.0	0	230	1.0
(*Heaven and Earth*), 1 tbsp.	100	<10.0	5.0	16.0	0	90	0
(*San-J* Thai)	70	3.0	7.0	3.0	0	710	1.0
satay:							
(*A Taste of Thai*) ..	80	1.0	9.0	4.5	0	180	1.0
(*Thai Kitchen*)	85	2.0	7.0	5.0	0	100	<1.0
spicy (*Thai Kitchen*)	90	2.0	8.0	6.0	0	140	0
Peanut sauce mix:							
(*Thai Kitchen*), ¼ cup*	70	2.0	7.0	3.0	0	284	0
plain or spicy Thai bake (*A Taste of Thai*), ¼ pkg	45	1.0	7.0	1.5	0	190	1.0
Peanut spread, 2 tbsp.:							
(*Peanut Wonder*)	100	4.0	13.0	2.5	0	190	0
(*Peanut Wonder* Low Sodium)	100	4.0	13.0	2.5	0	95	0
Pear, fresh, w/peel: (*Chiquita*), 1 medium, 5.9 oz.	100	1.0	25.0	1.0	0	0	4.0

Food and Measure	cal.	prot. (gms)	carbo. (gms)	fat (gms)	chol. (mgs)	sod. (mgs)	fiber (gms)
Pear *(cont.)*							
(*Del Monte*), 1 medium, 5.9 oz.	100	1.0	25.0	1.0	0	0	4.0
(*Dole*), 1 medium, 5.9 oz.	100	1.0	25.0	1.0	0	0	4.0
1 large, 2 per lb.	123	.8	31.6	.8	0	0	5.0
Bartlett, 1 medium, 2½ per lb.	98	.7	25.1	.7	0	1	4.0
sliced, ½ cup	49	.3	12.5	.3	0	1	2.0
Pear, Asian:							
(*Frieda's*), 5 oz.	60	1.0	15.0	0	0	0	5.0
1 medium, 2¼" x 2½" diam.	51	.6	13.0	.3	0	0	4.4
Pear, can or jar, halves or slices, ½ cup, except as noted:							
(*Del Monte Carb Clever*)	40	0	10.0	0	0	10	1.0
in juice:							
(*Del Monte/Del Monte Fruit Naturals*)	60	0	15.0	0	0	10	1.0
(*S&W* Natural Style)	80	0	21.0	0	0	10	2.0
w/liquid	62	.4	16.0	.1	0	5	2.0
in extra light syrup:							
(*Del Monte Lite*) . . .	60	0	15.0	0	0	10	1.0
diced (*Del Monte Lite*), 4-oz. can . .	50	0	13.0	0	0	10	<1.0
diced (*Del Monte Fruit Cup Lite*), 4.5 oz.	50	0	13.0	0	0	10	<1.0
in light syrup:							
(*Del Monte Orchard Select*)	80	<1.0	20.0	0	0	10	2.0
(*S&W*)	80	0	19.0	0	0	10	2.0
w/liquid	72	.2	19.0	<.1	0	6	2.0
chunks (*S&W* Sun)	80	<1.0	20.0	0	0	10	<1.0
cinnamon (*Del Monte*)	80	0	21.0	0	0	10	1.0
ginger (*Del Monte*)	90	0	22.0	0	0	10	1.0
in heavy syrup:							
(*Del Monte*)	100	0	24.0	0	0	10	1.0
(*S&W*)	100	0	24.0	0	0	10	1.0
w/liquid	98	.3	25.5	.2	0	7	2.1
diced (*Del Monte*), 4-oz. can	80	0	20.0	0	0	10	<1.0

Food and Measure	cal.	prot. (gms)	carbo. (gms)	fat (gms)	chol. (mgs)	sod. (mgs)	fiber (gms)
diced (*Del Monte Fruit Cup*), 4.5 oz.	80	0	20.0	0	0	10	<1.0
Pear, dried:							
2 oz.	149	1.1	39.5	.4	0	4	4.3
sulfured:							
halves, ½ cup	236	1.7	62.7	.6	0	5	6.8
stewed, ½ cup	162	1.2	43.1	.4	0	4	8.2
Pear juice, 8 fl. oz.:							
(*Ceres*)	120	0	30.0	0	0	10	0
(*R.W. Knudsen* Organic)	120	<1.0	30.0	0	0	25	0
sparkling (*R.W. Knudsen*)	120	0	29.0	0	0	5	0
Pear nectar:							
(*Goya*), 12 fl. oz.	240	1.0	59.0	0	0	20	2.0
(*Santa Cruz Organic*), 8 fl. oz.	120	0	30.0	0	0	30	0
canned, 8 fl. oz.	150	.3	39.4	<.1	0	10	1.5
Peas, see specific listings							
Peas, black-eyed, see "Black-eyed peas"							
Peas, cream, canned, (*East Texas Fair*), ½ cup	100	6.0	17.0	1.0	0	460	5.0
Peas, crowder, canned, ½ cup:							
(*Allens/East Texas Fair*)	110	6.0	19.0	1.0	0	460	8.0
(*Bush's*)	110	7.0	18.0	1.0	0	500	5.0
Peas, edible-podded, fresh:							
raw:							
(*Frieda's* Snow), 1 cup, 3 oz.	35	2.0	6.0	0	0	0	2.0
in pods (*Frieda's* Sugar Snap), ⅔ cup, 3 oz. . . .	35	2.0	6.0	0	0	0	2.0
raw, w/sauce, ½ cup:							
(*Frieda's* Snow) . . .	40	2.0	8.0	0	0	180	2.0
(*Frieda's* Sugar Snap)	35	2.0	8.0	0	0	180	2.0
boiled, drained, ½ cup	34	2.6	5.6	.2	0	3	2.2
Peas, edible podded, frozen:							
snow peas (*C&W* Baby Pea Pods), ⅔ cup .	40	3.0	7.0	0	0	45	3.0

Food and Measure	cal.	prot. (gms)	carbo. (gms)	fat (gms)	chol. (mgs)	sod. (mgs)	fiber (gms)
Peas, edible podded, frozen *(cont.)*							
sugar snap:							
(*Birds Eye*), ⅔ cup	40	2.0	7.0	0	0	0	2.0
(*Cascadian Farm* Bag), ¾ cup	35	2.0	6.0	0	0	140	2.0
(*Cascadian Farm* Box), ¾ cup	35	2.0	6.0	0	0	160	2.0
(*C&W Sugar Snap*), ⅔ cup	35	2.0	6.0	0	0	5	2.0
(*Green Giant*), ½ cup	50	3.0	10.0	0	0	95	3.0
(*Green Giant Select*), ¾ cup	35	2.0	7.0	0	0	0	3.0
boiled, drained, ½ cup	42	2.8	7.2	.3	0	4	2.5
Peas, edible podded, combinations, frozen, sugar snap, 1 cup:							
baby carrots, cauli-flower, broccoli (*C&W*)	30	2.0	5.0	0	0	30	2.0
stir-fry, w/carrots, onion, mushrooms (*Birds Eye*)	40	1.0	7.0	0	0	30	2.0
Peas, field, canned, (see also "Peas, crowder" and "Peas, purple hull"), ½ cup:							
w/bacon (*Trappey's*) ..	90	6.0	15.0	1.0	0	380	5.0
w/jalapeno (*East Texas Fair* Pepper Peas) ..	120	6.0	22.0	1.0	0	580	6.0
w/pork (*East Texas Fair* Peas & Pork)	110	6.0	19.0	1.5	0	540	5.0
seasoned (*Glory*)	80	5.0	14.0	0	0	830	4.0
w/snaps:							
(*Allens East Texas Fair/Sunshine*) ..	120	6.0	21.0	1.0	0	300	6.0
(*Bush's*)	110	7.0	17.0	.5	0	550	5.0
and bacon (*Trappey's*)	110	6.0	19.0	1.0	0	380	4.0
seasoned (*Glory*) ..	70	5.0	12.0	0	0	830	5.0
Peas, field, frozen (*McKenzie's*), ½ cup	110	7.0	21.0	.5	0	10	4.0
Peas, green, fresh:							
raw:							
in pod, 1 lb.	140	9.3	24.9	.7	0	8	8.8
shelled, ½ cup	59	3.9	10.4	.3	0	3	3.7

Food and Measure	cal.	prot. (gms)	carbo. (gms)	fat (gms)	chol. (mgs)	sod. (mgs)	fiber (gms)
boiled, drained, ½ cup	67	4.3	12.5	.2	0	2	4.4
Peas, green, can or jar, ½ cup:							
(*Del Monte*)	60	3.0	13.0	0	0	390	4.0
(*Del Monte* No Salt) . .	60	3.0	11.0	0	0	10	4.0
(*Del Monte* Very Young Small)	60	3.0	10.0	0	0	360	4.0
(*Freshlike* Selects Petite)	90	5.0	16.0	.5	0	410	5.0
(*Freshlike* Tender Garden)	110	6.0	19.0	.5	0	370	6.0
(*Freshlike* Tender Garden No Salt) . . .	110	6.0	19.0	.5	0	10	6.0
(*Green Giant*)	60	4.0	11.0	0	0	390	3.0
(*Green Giant* 50% Less Sodium)	60	4.0	11.0	0	0	195	3.0
(*LeSueur*)	60	4.0	12.0	0	0	380	3.0
(*S&W* Petit Pois)	60	3.0	10.0	0	0	360	4.0
(*S&W* Young)	60	3.0	13.0	0	0	390	4.0
(*Veg-All* Tender)	60	4.0	10.0	.5	0	370	3.0
(*Westbrae* Natural Organic)	60	4.0	10.0	0	0	360	3.0
drained	59	3.8	10.7	.3	0	214	3.5
in onion sauce (*Glory* Creamed Peas)	80	4.0	13.0	1.0	5	530	3.0
seasoned, w/liquid . . .	57	3.5	10.5	.3	0	288	2.8
Peas, green, combinations, can or jar:							
and carrots, ½ cup:							
(*Del Monte*)	60	2.0	11.0	0	0	360	2.0
(*Freshlike*)	60	4.0	11.0	0	0	350	3.0
(*S&W*)	60	2.0	11.0	0	0	360	2.0
(*Veg-All*)	60	2.0	12.0	0	0	330	4.0
w/liquid	48	2.8	10.8	.3	0	332	2.6
and onions, ½ cup:							
(*Freshlike* Selects) .	60	3.0	11.0	0	0	440	3.0
(*Green Giant*)	60	4.0	11.0	0	0	440	3.0
(*S&W*)	40	3.0	11.0	0	0	530	3.0
w/liquid	31	2.0	5.1	.2	0	265	1.4
Peas, green, combinations, frozen, ⅔ cup, except as noted:							
and carrots:							
(*Cascadian Farm*) . .	50	3.0	10.0	0	0	75	3.0

Food and Measure	cal.	prot. (gms)	carbo. (gms)	fat (gms)	chol. (mgs)	sod. (mgs)	fiber (gms)
Peas, green, combinations, frozen, and carrots *(cont.)*							
(*C&W Early Harvest* Petite/Baby)	60	4.0	12.0	0	0	95	3.0
boiled, drained, ½ cup	38	2.7	8.1	.3	0	54	2.5
and pearl onions:							
(*Cascadian Farm*), ¾ cup	60	4.0	11.0	0	0	160	3.0
(*C&W* Petite)	70	4.0	11.0	0	0	90	4.0
(*Green Giant*), ½ cup	50	3.0	10.0	0	0	160	3.0
baby (*Birds Eye*) ..	60	4.0	12.0	0	0	0	3.0
baby, and vegetables (*Birds Eye*), ¾ cup	40	2.0	7.0	0	0	20	2.0
in sauce (*Birds Eye*)	90	5.0	17.0	0	0	510	4.0
boiled, drained, ½ cup	41	2.3	7.8	.2	0	33	2.0
Peas, green, dried:							
rehydrated (*Frieda's*), ⅓ cup, 3 oz.	130	9.0	22.0	0	0	290	9.0
wasabi (*Anne's House of Nuts*), ⅓ cup ...	124	5.0	17.0	4.0	0	100	2.0
Peas, green, freeze-dried:							
(*AlpineAire*), ¾ oz.	80	5.0	14.0	0	0	115	5.0
(*Mountain House* Can), ½ cup	80	6.0	14.0	.5	0	75	5.0
Peas, green, frozen, ⅔ cup, except as noted:							
(*Birds Eye* Baby)	70	4.0	12.0	0	0	0	4.0
(*Birds Eye* Garden) ...	70	5.0	12.0	0	0	0	4.0
(*Cascadian Farm* Garden/Sweet)	70	4.0	12.0	0	0	95	4.0
(*Cascadian Farm* Petite)	50	4.0	11.0	0	0	140	4.0
(*C&W* Petite)	70	5.0	12.0	.5	0	105	4.0
(*C&W Early Harvest/ Organic/No Salt* Petite)	70	5.0	12.0	.5	0	10	4.0
(*Green Giant* Baby Sweet)	70	4.0	12.0	.5	0	190	4.0
(*Green Giant* Sweet) ..	70	5.0	12.0	.5	0	135	4.0
(*Green Giant Select* Early June)	60	4.0	11.0	.5	0	150	4.0
(*Tree of Life*)	70	5.0	12.0	0	0	100	4.0

Food and Measure	cal.	prot. (gms)	carbo. (gms)	fat (gms)	chol. (mgs)	sod. (mgs)	fiber (gms)
boiled, drained, ½ cup	62	4.1	11.4	.2	0	70	4.4
Peas, pigeon, see "Pigeon peas"							
Peas, purple hull, canned, ½ cup:							
(*Allens/East Texas Fair*)	120	7.0	21.0	1.0	0	350	6.0
(*Bush's*)	110	7.0	18.0	1.0	0	500	5.0
Peas, purple hull, frozen (*McKenzie's*), ½ cup	110	7.0	21.0	.5	0	1	4.0
Peas, split, see "Split peas"							
Peas, sprouted:							
raw, ½ cup	77	5.3	17.0	.4	0	12	n.a.
boiled, drained, 4 oz.	134	8.0	24.8	.6	0	3	3.7
Peas, sugar snap or snow, see "Peas, edible-podded"							
Peas, sweet, see "Peas, green"							
Peas, wasabi, see "Peas, green, dried"							
Peas, white acre, canned (*East Texas Fair*), ½ cup	100	6.0	17.0	1.0	0	460	5.0
Peas and carrots or onions, see "Peas, green, combinations"							
Pecan, shelled:							
(*Fisher*), 1 oz.	200	3.0	4.0	20.0	0	0	2.0
1 oz.	190	2.2	5.2	19.2	0	<1	2.2
halves:							
(*Shiloh Farms*), ⅓ cup, 1.2 oz.	220	3.0	6.0	22.0	0	0	3.0
1 cup	721	8.4	19.7	73.1	0	1	8.2
halves or pieces:							
(*Planters*), 1 oz.	190	3.0	4.0	20.0	0	0	3.0
(*Planters*), 2-oz. pkg.	390	5.0	9.0	40.0	0	5	7.0
chips (*Planters*), 2-oz. pkg.	390	5.0	9.0	40.0	0	5	7.0
chopped, 1 cup	794	9.2	21.7	80.5	0	1	9.0
dry-roasted:							
unsalted, 1 oz.	201	2.7	3.8	21.1	0	<1	2.7
unsalted, 1 cup	781	10.5	14.9	81.7	0	11	10.5

Food and Measure	cal.	prot. (gms)	carbo. (gms)	fat (gms)	chol. (mgs)	sod. (mgs)	fiber (gms)
Pecan *(cont.)*							
oil-roasted:							
unsalted, 1 oz.	203	2.7	3.7	21.3	0	<1	2.7
unsalted, 1 cup . . .	787	10.5	14.3	82.8	0	11	10.5
Pecan flour, 1 oz. . . .	93	9.1	14.4	.4	0	tr.	n.a.
Pecan topping, in syrup (*Smucker's* Spoonable), 1 tbsp.	170	1.0	20.0	10.0	0	0	0
Pectin, see "Fruit pectin"							
Penne, dry, see "Pasta"							
Penne entree, frozen, 1 pkg.:							
(*Jeff Nathan Creations* Siciliano), 12 oz. . .	340	16.0	41.0	12.0	30	840	5.0
w/chicken, see "Chicken entree, frozen"							
puttanesca, spicy (*Moosewood*), 10 oz.	300	8.0	45.0	10.0	0	380	2.0
w/sauce and meatballs (*Organic Classics*), 10 oz.	360	19.0	45.0	12.0	35	690	4.0
w/tomato (*Lean Cuisine Everyday Favorites*), 10 oz.	270	9.0	51.0	3.0	0	390	5.0
vegetarian (*Yves* Veggie), 10.5 oz.	220	12.0	36.0	1.5	0	730	4.0
Penne entree, pkg.:							
Alfredo:							
(*Annie's*), 1 cup* . .	360	13.0	49.0	13.0	35	610	1.0
(*Fantastic Carb 'Tastic*), 8-oz. pkg.	280	25.0	25.0	15.0	25	870	21.0
"meat" sauce, vegetarian (*Fantastic Carb 'Tastic*), 8-oz. pkg. .	240	20.0	22.0	14.0	0	790	14.0
tomato Parmesan (*Bowl Appétit!*), 1 cont.	350	12.0	59.0	8.0	5	870	2.0
Pepeao, raw, sliced, 1 cup	25	.5	6.7	0	0	9	n.a.
Pepeao, dried, 1 cup	72	1.2	19.5	.1	0	17	n.a.
Peppadew (*Frieda's*), ⅓ cup, 1.1 oz.	40	0	10.0	0	0	80	3.0
Pepper, seasoning:							
black, 1 tsp.:							
ground	6	.3	1.7	.1	0	1	.7

Food and Measure	cal.	prot. (gms)	carbo. (gms)	fat (gms)	chol. (mgs)	sod. (mgs)	fiber (gms)
whole	8	.3	1.9	0	0	1	.8
chili, 1 tsp.	9	.3	1.2	.3	0	<1	.7
red or cayenne, 1 tsp.	6	.2	1.0	.3	0	1	.7
seasoned (*Lawry's*), ¼ tsp.	0	0	1.0	0	0	0	0
Szechuan blend (*McCormick*), ¼ tsp. . . .	0	0	0	0	0	15	0
white, 1 tsp.	7	.3	1.7	.1	0	0	.2
Pepper, ancho, dried, .6-oz. pepper	48	2.0	8.7	1.4	0	7	3..7
Pepper, banana, fresh, 1.2-oz. pc.	9	.6	1.8	.2	0	4	1.1
Pepper, banana, in jars, wax (*Fanci Food*), 2 pcs., 1 oz.	10	0	2.0	0	0	290	0
Pepper, bell, see "Pepper, sweet"							
Pepper, cherry, in jars:							
(*Fanci Food*), 2-3 pcs.	15	1.0	0	.5	0	290	0
(*Vlasic*), 2 pcs., 1 oz. .	10	0	2.0	0	0	480	0
Pepper, cherry, stuffed, w/proscuitto and provolone, marinated (*Boar's Head*), 2 oz.	60	2.0	1.0	5.0	10	490	0
Pepper, chili, fresh, green and red:							
1 medium, 1.6 oz. . . .	18	.9	4.3	.1	0	3	.7
chopped, ½ cup	30	1.5	7.1	.2	0	5	1.1
Pepper, chili, can or jar (see also specific listings):							
whole, green, 1 pc.:							
(*Chi-Chi's*), 1.2 oz. . .	10	0	2.0	0	0	100	0
(*La Victoria*), 1.2 oz.	5	0	1.0	0	0	190	<1.0
(*Las Palmas*), 1.2 oz.	10	0	2.0	0	0	230	1.0
(*Old El Paso*), 1.2 oz.	10	0	2.0	0	0	230	1.0
mild (*Zapata*)	5	0	1.0	0	0	85	0
large, 2.6 oz.	15	.7	3.7	<.1	0	856	1.0
whole, green, ½ cup .	15	.5	3.2	.1	0	276	1.2
chopped:							
(*Old El Paso*), 2 tbsp.	5	0	1.0	0	0	110	1.0
w/liquid, ½ cup . . .	17	.6	4.2	.1	0	n.a.	1.3
diced, green, 2 tbsp.:							
(*Chi-Chi's*)	10	0	2.0	0	0	60	0

Food and Measure	cal.	prot. (gms)	carbo. (gms)	fat (gms)	chol. (mgs)	sod. (mgs)	fiber (gms)
Pepper, chili, can or jar, diced, green *(cont.)*							
(*La Victoria*)	0	0	<1.0	0	0	70	0
(*Las Palmas*)	5	0	1.0	0	0	110	1.0
mild (*Zapata*)	5	0	1.0	0	0	75	0
strips, green (*Las Palmas*), 1.3-oz. pc.	10	0	2.0	0	0	240	1.0
Pepper, chili, dried:							
(*Frieda's* Ancho/Guajillo Chiles), .5 oz.	50	2.0	8.0	0	0	5	2.0
(*Frieda's* California Chiles), 2 tbsp.	15	0	2.0	0	0	15	0
(*Frieda's* Japones Chiles), .5 oz.	50	4.0	7.0	0	0	5	2.0
sun-dried, hot, 2 pcs.	3	.1	.8	.1	0	1	.3
Pepper, Greek, golden (*Fanci Food*), 3 pcs.	10	0	2.0	0	0	490	0
Pepper, green or red, sweet, see "Pepper, sweet"							
Pepper, güerito, in jars (*Embasa*), 7 pcs., 1.1 oz.	10	0	1.0	.5	0	550	2.0
Pepper, Hungarian, fresh, .94-oz. pc. . .	8	.2	1.8	.1	0	<1	n.a.
Pepper, jalapeño, fresh, .5-oz. pc.	4	.2	.8	.1	0	<1	.4
Pepper, jalapeño, can or jar:							
whole:							
(*Chi-Chi's*), 2 pcs., 1.1 oz.	10	0	2.0	0	0	190	0
(*Herdez*), 3 pcs., 1.25 oz.	15	0	1.0	0	0	670	1.0
(*Las Palmas*), 2 pcs., 1.3 oz.	15	<1.0	2.0	0	0	190	0
(*Old El Paso*), 2 pcs., .9 oz.	5	0	1.0	0	0	380	0
(*Zapata* Very Hot), 1½ pcs.	5	0	1.0	0	0	420	0
chopped, w/liquid, ¼ cup	7	.2	1.2	.2	0	434	.8
diced:							
(*La Victoria*), 2 tbsp.	0	0	<1.0	0	0	150	0
(*Zapata*), 4 tbsp. . .	5	0	1.0	0	0	250	0

Food and Measure	cal.	prot. (gms)	carbo. (gms)	fat (gms)	chol. (mgs)	sod. (mgs)	fiber (gms)
marinated (*La Victoria*), 1½ tbsp.	10	0	2.0	0	0	280	<1.0
sliced:							
(*Herdez*), ¼ cup ..	10	0	1.0	0	0	630	0
(*La Victoria* Nacho), 14 pcs., 1.1 oz. ..	5	0	<1.0	0	0	350	0
(*Las Palmas*), 3 tbsp.	10	<1.0	2.0	0	0	210	0
(*Zapata* Nacho), 4 tbsp.	5	0	<1.0	0	0	530	0
w/liquid, ¼ cup ...	9	.3	1.6	.3	0	568	.9
wheels (*Chi-Chi's*), ¼ cup	10	0	2.0	0	0	190	0
Pepper, pablanos, in jars (*Herdez*), ½ pc., 1.2 oz.	10	0	1.0	0	0	160	0
Pepper, pasilla, dried, 2 pcs., .5 oz.	48	1.7	7.2	2.2	0	12	3.8
Pepper, poblano, see "Pepper, chili, can or jar"							
Pepper, roasted, see "Pepper, sweet, can or jar"							
Pepper, Serrano, fresh:							
whole, .2-oz. pc.	2	.1	.4	<.1	0	2	.2
chopped, ½ cup	17	.9	3.5	.5	0	5	1.9
Pepper, Serrano, in jars (*Herdez*), 4 pcs, 1.25 oz.	15	0	1.0	0	0	570	0
Pepper, stuffed, entree, frozen, w/beef, tomato sauce:							
(*Stouffer's*), 10-oz. pkg.	230	11.0	25.0	9.0	25	920	2.0
(*Stouffer's*), ½ of 15.5-oz. pkg.	180	8.0	21.0	7.0	20	670	2.0
(*Stouffer's* Family Style Recipes), ¼ of 32-oz. pkg.	180	8.0	20.0	7.0	20	1050	2.0
Pepper, sweet, fresh:							
green and red:							
raw (*Chiquita*), 5.2-oz. pc.	30	1.0	7.0	0	0	0	2.0
raw (*Dole*), 5.2-oz. pc.	30	1.0	7.0	0	0	0	2.0

Food and Measure	cal.	prot. (gms)	carbo. (gms)	fat (gms)	chol. (mgs)	sod. (mgs)	fiber (gms)
Pepper, sweet, green and red *(cont.)*							
raw, 1 medium, 3¾" x 3" or ½ cup chopped	20	.7	4.8	.1	0	1	1.3
raw, sliced, 1 cup	25	.8	5.9	.2	0	2	1.7
boiled, drained, 1 medium	20	.7	4.9	.1	0	1	.9
boiled, drained, chopped, 1 tbsp.	3	.1	.8	<.1	0	<1	.1
boiled, drained, strips, ½ cup	19	.6	4.6	.1	0	1	.8
yellow, raw:							
1 large, 5" x 3"	50	1.9	11.8	.4	0	4	1.7
10 strips, 1.8 oz.	14	.5	3.3	.1	0	1	.5
Pepper, sweet, can or jar (see also "Pimento"), red:							
drained, ½ cup	13	.6	2.7	.2	0	958	.8
fire-roasted:							
(*Pompeian*), ½ cup	30	1.0	5.0	.0	0	310	1.0
w/garlic, oil (*Paesana*), 2 tbsp.	20	0	2.0	1.0	0	125	0
roasted (*Frieda's*), 1-oz. pc.	35	1.0	5.0	0	0	280	0
Pepper, sweet, freeze-dried, red or green, ¼ cup	5	.3	1.1	<.1	0	3	.3
Pepper, sweet, frozen:							
sliced, stir-fry, w/onion (*Birds Eye*), 1 cup	25	1.0	5.0	0	0	10	1.0
strips (*C&W*), ¾ cup	20	1.0	4.0	0	0	10	2.0
chopped, 1 oz.	6	.3	1.2	.1	0	1	.5
Pepper, tempero, see "Pepperoncini"							
Pepper relish, 1 tbsp.:							
hot (*Cains*)	20	0	5.0	0	0	60	0
jalapeño (*Old El Paso*)	5	0	1.0	0	0	110	0
sweet (*Cains*)	20	0	5.0	0	0	45	0
Pepper rings, marinated (*Vlasic*), 3 pcs., 1 oz.	5	0	1.0	0	0	480	0
Pepper sauce, see "Hot sauce," and specific listings							

Food and Measure	cal.	prot. (gms)	carbo. (gms)	fat (gms)	chol. (mgs)	sod. (mgs)	fiber (gms)
Pepper spread, red, w/eggplant and garlic (*Marco Polo*), 2 tbsp.	10	0	2.0	0	0	10	<1.0
Pepper steak, see "Beef entree, frozen"							
Peppercorns, green (*Fanci Food*), 2 tbsp.	15	0	3.0	0	0	430	1.0
Pepperoncini:							
(*Krinos*), ¼ cup	5	0	2.0	0	0	950	0
(*Trappey's* Tempero), 1 oz.	5	0	1.0	0	0	470	0
(*Zorba*), 5 pcs., 1.1 oz.	15	1.0	2.0	0	0	450	0
Pepperoni, 1 oz., except as noted:							
(*Hansel & Gretel*), 2 oz.	240	12.0	2.0	20.0	50	860	0
(*Hormel* Chunk or Sliced)	140	5.0	0	13.0	35	490	0
(*Hormel* Twin)	140	5.0	0	13.0	35	500	0
(*Hormel* Pillow Pack) .	140	5.0	0	13.0	35	490	0
(*Rosa Grande*)	140	5.0	0	13.0	35	490	0
sandwich style:							
(*Boar's Head*)	130	5.0	1.0	12.0	25	460	0
(*Fiorucci*)	120	6.0	1.0	11.0	25	480	0
(*Sara Lee* Sliced) . .	140	6.0	0	13.0	30	530	0
(*Tyson* Sliced)	130	6.0	0	12.0	25	470	0
turkey, see "Turkey pepperoni"							
"Pepperoni," vege-tarian, pizza slices (*Yves*), 1.7 oz.	70	14.0	4.0	0	0	390	3.0
Pepperoni pocket, see "Pizza, stuffed/ pocket"							
Perch, meat only:							
raw, 4 oz.	103	22.0	0	1.1	102	70	0
baked, broiled, or microwaved, 4 oz. .	133	28.2	0	1.3	130	90	0
ocean, see "Ocean perch"							
Persimmon, fresh:							
(*Frieda's* Fuyu/Hachiya/ Sharon), 5 oz.	100	1.0	26.0	0	0	0	5.0
Japanese, 1 medium .	118	1.0	31.2	.3	0	3	6.0

Food and Measure	cal.	prot. (gms)	carbo. (gms)	fat (gms)	chol. (mgs)	sod. (mgs)	fiber (gms)
Persimmon *(cont.)*							
native, 1 medium, 1.1 oz.	32	.2	8.4	.1	0	<1	n.a.
Persimmon, dried:							
(*Frieda's* Fuyu), ⅓ cup, 1.4 oz.	140	1.0	35.0	0	0	10	3.0
Japanese, 1 oz.	78	.4	20.8	.2	0	1	4.1
Pesto paste (*Amore*), 2 tbsp.	110	<1.0	3.0	10.0	0	630	0
Pesto sauce, in jars, ¼ cup, except as noted:							
basil:							
(*Bellino*)	130	2.0	3.0	13.0	5	270	1.0
(*Classico* di Genova)	230	3.0	6.0	21.0	0	720	1.0
(*Sacla*)	210	3.0	2.0	21.0	0	560	3.0
tomato, sun-dried:							
(*Classico* di Capri) .	90	3.0	8.0	5.0	0	630	1.0
and garlic (*Sacla*) . .	80	1.0	5.0	6.0	0	380	1.0
Pesto sauce, refrigerated, ¼ cup:							
basil:							
(*Buitoni*)	300	7.0	9.0	26.0	20	560	2.0
(*Buitoni* Family Size)	330	10.0	11.0	27.0	20	560	6.0
(*Buitoni* Reduced Fat)	230	7.0	9.0	18.0	15	560	2.0
(*DiGiorno*)	320	7.0	2.0	31.0	15	530	1.0
tomato, sun-dried							
(*Buitoni*)	210	4.0	9.0	18.0	5	400	2.0
Pesto sauce mix (*Mc-Cormick*), 2 tsp.	10	1.0	1.0	0	0	480	0
Pheasant:							
raw, meat w/skin, 4 oz.	205	25.7	0	10.5	81	45	0
raw, meat only:							
4 oz.	151	26.7	0	4.1	75	42	0
½ breast, 6.4 oz. . .	243	44.4	0	5.9	106	60	0
1 leg, 3.8 oz.	143	23.8	0	4.6	112	48	0
cooked, meat w/skin, 4 oz.	280	36.7	0	13.7	101	49	0
Phyllo, see "Fillo dough"							
Picante sauce (see also "Salsa"), 2 tbsp.:							
(*Pace*)	10	0	2.0	0	0	230	<1.0
(*Taco Bell* Smooth & Zesty Mild)	15	0	3.0	0	0	190	1.0

Food and Measure	cal.	prot. (gms)	carbo. (gms)	fat (gms)	chol. (mgs)	sod. (mgs)	fiber (gms)
mild or medium:							
(*Chi-Chi's*)	10	0	2.0	0	0	170	0
(*Old El Paso*)	10	0	2.0	0	0	230	0
Piccalilli, see "Tomato relish"							
Pickle, cucumber, 1 oz., except as noted:							
bread and butter:							
(*Cascadian Farm*) . .	25	0	6.0	0	0	180	0
(*Claussen* Chips) . .	30	0	4.0	0	0	180	0
(*D.L. Jardine's* Texas)	50	0	14.0	0	0	210	0
(*Mrs. Fannings*), 3 pcs., 1 oz.	25	0	6.0	0	0	190	0
(*Vlasic* Chips)	25	0	6.0	0	0	170	0
cornichon:							
(*Italica*), 7 pcs., 1.1 oz.	0	0	0	0	0	330	0
(*Maille*)	4	0	.3	.1	0	200	.5
(*Trois Petits Cochons*), 1 oz., about 6 pcs.	0	0	0	0	0	300	0
dill:							
baby or kosher (*Cascadian Farm*)	5	0	1.0	0	0	300	1.0
chips, hamburger (*Del Monte*)	5	0	0	0	0	300	0
chips, hamburger (*Vlasic*)	5	0	3.0	0	0	390	0
whole or halves (*Del Monte*)	5	0	1.0	0	0	370	<1.0
dill, kosher:							
(*Cascadian Farm* Reduced Sodium)	5	1.0	0	0	0	135	0
baby (*Vlasic/Vlasic Snack'mms*)	5	0	1.0	0	0	280	0
burger slices (*Claussen*), .8 oz.	5	0	1.0	0	0	300	0
halves (*Claussen*) . .	5	0	1.0	0	0	330	0
mini (*Claussen*), .8 oz.	5	0	1.0	0	0	290	0
sandwich slices (*Claussen*), 1.2 oz.	5	0	1.0	0	0	420	0
spears (*Claussen*) .	5	0	1.0	0	0	330	0
tiny (*Del Monte*) . . .	5	0	1.0	0	0	250	<1.0
whole (*Hebrew National*), 1 large	23	1.0	4.0	0	0	1570	0

Food and Measure	cal.	prot. (gms)	carbo. (gms)	fat (gms)	chol. (mgs)	sod. (mgs)	fiber (gms)
Pickle, dill, kosher *(cont.)*							
whole or spears (*Vlasic*)	5	0	1.0	0	0	210	0
garlic, slices (*Claussen Hearty Deli Style*), 1.2 oz.	5	0	1.0	0	0	320	0
sour, half (*Claussen New York Deli Style Wholes*)	5	0	1.0	0	0	260	0
sweet:							
all styles (*Del Monte*)	40	0	10.0	0	0	210	<1.0
gherkins (*Claussen*), .9 oz.	30	0	7.0	0	0	210	0
gherkins (*Vlasic*), 3 pcs., 1 oz.	35	0	9.0	0	0	170	0
Pickle relish (see also specific listings), cucumber, 1 tbsp.:							
(*Crosse & Blackwell Branston*)	25	0	6.0	0	0	125	0
dill (*Vlasic*)	5	0	1.0	0	0	240	0
hamburger (*Del Monte*)	20	0	6.0	0	0	220	<1.0
hot dog:							
(*Del Monte*)	15	0	4.0	0	0	140	<1.0
(*Heinz*)	15	0	4.0	0	0	150	0
India (*Heinz*)	20	0	5.0	0	0	100	0
sweet:							
(*Cascadian Farm*) . .	20	0	5.0	0	0	75	0
(*Claussen*)	15	0	3.0	0	0	85	0
(*Del Monte*)	20	0	5.0	0	0	125	0
(*Heinz*)	20	0	5.0	0	0	95	0
(*Vlasic*)	15	0	4.0	0	0	140	0
Pickle relish cubes, sweet (*Vlasic*), 1 oz.	20	0	5.0	0	0	220	0
Pickling spice (*Tone's*), 1 tsp.	10	.3	1.2	.6	0	1	.3
Pie, fresh, apple (*Entenmann's*), 1/6 pie	380	3.0	57.0	16.0	0	410	2.0
Pie, frozen (see also "Cobbler"), 1/8 pie, except as noted:							
apple:							
(*Amy's*), 1/2 of 8-oz. pie	240	2.0	37.0	8.0	25	135	2.0

Food and Measure	cal.	prot. (gms)	carbo. (gms)	fat (gms)	chol. (mgs)	sod. (mgs)	fiber (gms)
(*Mrs. Smith's*)	340	3.0	46.0	17.0	0	380	2.0
(*Sara Lee Oven Fresh*)	340	3.0	46.0	16.0	0	310	1.0
cinnamon French, deep dish (*Sara Lee Signature Selection*), 1/10 pie	360	7.0	48.0	15.0	15	260	2.0
crumb (*Mrs. Smith's*)	360	3.0	52.0	16.0	0	360	2.0
deep dish (*Mrs. Smith's*), 1/12 pie	330	2.0	45.0	16.0	0	340	2.0
deep dish (*Sara Lee Signature Selection Orchard*), 1/10 pie	400	3.0	43.0	24.0	15	440	3.0
Dutch (*Sara Lee Oven Fresh*)	350	3.0	53.0	15.0	0	320	2.0
berry (*Marie Callender's Razzleberry*), 1/10 pie	360	2.0	43.0	21.0	0	180	5.0
blueberry (*Sara Lee Oven Fresh*)	360	3.0	53.0	15.0	0	260	2.0
caramel apple nut, deep dish (*Sara Lee Signature Selection*), 1/9 pie	370	9.0	45.0	18.0	15	170	2.0
cherry:							
(*Mrs. Smith's*)	330	3.0	45.0	16.0	0	370	2.0
(*Sara Lee Oven Fresh*)	320	4.0	44.0	14.0	0	260	0
deep dish (*Sara Lee Signature Selection Gourmet*), 1/10 pie	340	3.0	46.0	16.0	20	360	2.0
chocolate cream (*Sara Lee French Silk*), 1/5 pie	340	4.0	34.0	21.0	10	230	2.0
coconut cream (*Sara Lee*), 1/5 pie	330	3.0	37.0	19.0	5	190	2.0
dulce de leche caramel swirl (*Sara Lee Signature Selection*) ..	400	7.0	37.0	15.0	5	100	2.0
fruit, mixed, deep dish (*Sara Lee Signature Selection Fruits of the Forest*), 1/9 pie	340	5.0	41.0	17.0	15	190	0
lemon meringue:							
(*Mrs. Smith's*)	290	2.0	47.0	11.0	40	190	<1.0
(*Sara Lee*), 1/6 pie .	220	1.0	41.0	5.0	0	160	1.0

Food and Measure	cal.	prot. (gms)	carbo. (gms)	fat (gms)	chol. (mgs)	sod. (mgs)	fiber (gms)
Pie, frozen *(cont.)*							
lime, key:							
(*Smart Ones*),							
2.8-oz. pc.	200	4.0	34.0	6.0	10	80	0
(*Sara Lee Signature*							
Selection)	400	7.0	41.0	25.0	5	95	2.0
mince (*Sara Lee Oven*							
Fresh)	370	3.0	55.0	15.0	0	400	2.0
Mississippi mud (*Smart*							
Ones), 2.4-oz. pc. .	160	4.0	26.0	5.0	5	120	1.0
peach:							
(*Mrs. Smith's*)	320	3.0	40.0	17.0	0	450	2.0
(*Sara Lee Oven Fresh*)	330	3.0	50.0	13.0	0	250	2.0
deep dish (*Sara Lee*							
Signature Selection							
Golden), 1/10 pie	340	3.0	46.0	16.0	20	360	2.0
peanut butter (*Smart*							
Ones), 2.6-oz. pc. .	210	6.0	27.0	6.0	<5	240	1.0
pecan:							
(*Mrs. Smith's*),							
1/5 pie	560	6.0	75.0	27.0	65	450	<2.0
(*Sara Lee Signature*							
Selection Southern)	520	5.0	70.0	24.0	45	480	3.0
pumpkin:							
(*Sara Lee Oven Fresh*)	260	4.0	37.0	11.0	30	460	2.0
(*Sara Lee Signature*							
Selection Tradi-							
tional), 1/10 pie .	250	7.0	34.0	9.0	40	290	2.0
custard (*Mrs. Smith's*)	270	5.0	35.0	13.0	40	330	2.0
raspberry (*Sara Lee*							
Oven Fresh)	360	4.0	50.0	16.0	0	250	3.0
strawberry and cream							
(*Sara Lee Signature*							
Selection)	400	8.0	33.0	27.0	5	60	2.0
sweet potato:							
(*Mrs. Smith's*)	340	4.0	44.0	17.0	40	240	2.0
(*Sara Lee Oven Fresh*							
Southern)	280	4.0	45.0	10.0	35	420	2.0
Pie, mix, 1/6 pkg.,							
except as noted:							
chocolate silk (*Jell-O*							
No Bake)	180	2.0	34.0	6.0	0	390	2.0
cookie:							
(*Jell-O Chips Ahoy!*							
No Bake)	260	2.0	46.0	9.0	0	360	1.0

Food and Measure	cal.	prot. (gms)	carbo. (gms)	fat (gms)	chol. (mgs)	sod. (mgs)	fiber (gms)
(*Jell-O Oreo* No Bake)	270	2.0	48.0	9.0	0	460	2.0
peanut butter cup (*Jell-O* No Bake), ⅛ pkg.	290	3.0	38.0	15.0	0	310	2.0
pumpkin pie style (*Jell-O* No Bake), ⅛ pkg.	130	1.0	29.0	1.5	0	350	1.0
Pie, snack, fruit:							
apple:							
(*Drake's*), 2 pies, 4 oz.	400	3.0	60.0	16.0	0	240	3.0
(*Little Debbie*), 4-oz. pie	430	3.0	62.0	19.0	0	530	1.0
cherry:							
(*Drake's*), 2 pies, 4 oz.	420	3.0	60.0	18.0	0	260	3.0
(*Little Debbie*), 4-oz. pie	430	3.0	64.0	18.0	0	520	1.0
lemon (*Drakes*), 4.5-oz. pie	500	3.0	66.0	24.0	20	430	0
Pie crust (see also "Pastry shell"), ⅛ crust, except as noted:							
(*Nilla*), 1/6 crust	140	1.0	18.0	7.0	5	65	1.0
(*Oreo*), 1/6 crust	140	2.0	18.0	7.0	0	170	1.0
(*Pet•Ritz*)	80	1.0	9.0	4.5	0	75	0
(*Pet•Ritz* Extra Large)	110	1.0	13.0	6.0	5	110	0
(*Pillsbury*)	120	<1.0	13.0	7.0	5	110	0
chocolate (*Ready Crust*)	100	1.0	14.0	4.5	0	110	<1.0
deep dish (*Pet•Ritz*) . .	90	1.0	11.0	5.0	0	85	0
graham:							
(*Honey Maid*), 1/6 crust	140	1.0	18.0	7.0	0	125	1.0
(*Ready Crust* 9") . .	110	1.0	14.0	5.0	0	115	<1.0
(*Ready Crust* 10"), 1/10 crust	140	1.0	18.0	6.0	0	140	<1.0
(*Ready Crust* Reduced Fat) . . .	90	1.0	15.0	3.5	0	100	0
tart (*Ready Crust*), .8-oz. pc.	120	1.0	15.0	6.0	0	150	<1.0
shortbread (*Ready Crust*)	100	1.0	14.0	5.0	0	110	0

Food and Measure	cal.	prot. (gms)	carbo. (gms)	fat (gms)	chol. (mgs)	sod. (mgs)	fiber (gms)
Pie crust mix:							
(*Betty Crocker*), ⅛ of							
9" crust*	110	1.0	9.0	8.0	0	135	0
("*Jiffy*"), ¼ cup mix . .	180	2.0	19.0	10.0	<5	250	<1.0
Pie filling (see also							
"Pastry filling"),							
⅓ cup, except as							
noted:							
apple:							
(*Lucky Leaf/Lucky*							
Leaf Premium) . .	90	0	22.0	0	0	40	2.0
(*Lucky Leaf* Lite) . .	30	0	7.0	0	0	10	0
apricot (*Lucky Leaf*) . .	90	0	22.0	0	0	55	0
blueberry:							
(*Lucky Leaf*)	90	0	22.0	0	0	50	1.0
(*Lucky Leaf* Premium)	100	0	24.0	0	0	45	1.0
cherry:							
(*Lucky Leaf*)	100	0	24.0	0	0	40	0
(*Lucky Leaf* Lite) . .	35	0	8.0	0	0	15	0
(*Lucky Leaf* Premium)	100	0	24.0	0	0	40	1.0
coconut crème (*Lucky*							
Leaf)	110	1.0	25.0	2.0	0	140	3.0
lemon:							
(*Lucky Leaf*)	120	0	29.0	1.0	15	220	0
crème (*Lucky Leaf*)	130	0	31.0	1.0	0	220	0
mince/mincemeat:							
(*Crosse & Blackwell*),							
¼ cup	180	<1.0	43.0	0	0	220	0
(*None Such* Original)	190	0	45.0	.5	0	230	0
w/brandy and rum							
(*Crosse & Black-*							
well), ¼ cup . . .	180	<1.0	43.0	0	0	230	0
w/brandy and rum							
(*None Such*)	200	0	47.0	1.0	0	250	0
condensed (*None*							
Such), 4 tsp. . . .	150	0	36.0	.5	0	230	1.0
peach (*Lucky Leaf*) . .	80	0	21.0	0	0	30	0
pineapple (*Lucky Leaf*)	100	–0	23.0	0	0	35	1.0
pumpkin (*Libby's* Mix)	90	1.0	20.0	.5	0	120	3.0
raisin (*Lucky Leaf*) . . .	90	0	22.0	0	0	75	1.0
raspberry (*Lucky Leaf*							
Premium)	80	0	19.0	0	0	35	2.0
strawberry (*Lucky Leaf*)	80	0	20.0	0	0	50	1.0

Food and Measure	cal.	prot. (gms)	carbo. (gms)	fat (gms)	chol. (mgs)	sod. (mgs)	fiber (gms)
Pie filling mix, see "Pudding and pie filling mix"							
Pierogi, frozen, 3 pcs., 4.25 oz., except as noted:							
potato and cheddar:							
bacon, mini (*Mrs. T.'s*), 7 pcs., 3 oz.	140	5.0	25.0	3.0	5	450	1.0
broccoli (*Mrs. T.'s*)	200	6.0	33.0	4.0	5	560	2.0
jalapeno (*Mrs. T.'s*)	180	6.0	34.0	2.5	10	540	1.0
mini (*Mrs. T.'s*), 7 pcs., 3 oz.	130	4.0	25.0	1.5	5	360	1.0
potato and cheese:							
(*Empire* Kosher), ½ pkg., 5.3 oz. . .	247	7.0	44.0	4.0	60	233	.7
American (*Mrs. T.'s*)	180	6.0	32.0	3.5	10	450	1.0
four (*Mrs. T.'s*)	230	6.0	36.0	7.0	10	570	1.0
four, mini (*Mrs. T.'s*), 7 pcs., 3 oz.	160	4.0	27.0	4.5	5	390	1.0
potato and onion:							
(*Empire* Kosher), ½ pkg., 5.3 oz. . .	243	5.0	47.0	4.0	48	260	.7
(*Mrs. T.'s*)	170	5.0	33.0	2.0	5	420	1.0
potato, sour cream, and chive (*Mrs. T.'s*) . . .	200	6.0	34.0	5.0	15	520	1.0
sauerkraut (*Mrs. T.'s*) .	150	5.0	30.0	1.5	5	770	3.0
Pig's feet:							
simmered, 4 oz.	220	21.8	0	14.1	113	34	0
pickled:							
(*Hormel*), 2 oz. . . .	80	7.0	0	6.0	45	590	0
cured, 1 oz.	58	3.8	<.1	4.6	26	262	0
jalapeño (*Hormel*), 2 oz.	80	7.0	0	6.0	45	580	0
Pigeon peas, fresh:							
raw, ½ cup	105	5.5	18.4	1.3	0	4	3.2
boiled, drained, ½ cup	86	4.6	15.0	1.1	0	3	2.5
Pigeon peas, canned, green (*Goya*), 8 oz.	110	10.0	26.0	0	0	560	8.0
Pigeon peas, dried, boiled, ½ cup	102	5.7	19.5	.3	0	5	3.9
Pignolia nuts, see "Pine nuts"							

Food and Measure	cal.	prot. (gms)	carbo. (gms)	fat (gms)	chol. (mgs)	sod. (mgs)	fiber (gms)
Pike, meat only:							
northern, 4 oz.:							
raw	100	21.8	0	.8	44	44	0
baked, broiled, or							
microwaved	128	28.0	0	1.0	57	56	0
walleye, 4 oz.:							
raw	105	21.7	0	1.4	98	58	0
baked, broiled, or							
microwaved	135	27.8	0	1.8	125	74	0
Pili nuts, shelled:							
dried, 1 oz.	204	3.1	1.1	22.6	0	4	<1.0
dried, 1 cup	863	13.0	4.8	95.5	0	4	3.4
Pimento, in jars, (*Goya*							
Fancy), ¼ pc., .5 oz.	0	0	1.0	0	0	40	0
Piña colada drink, see							
"Pineapple drink							
blend"							
Piña colada drink							
mixer:							
(*Bacardi*), 3.2 fl. oz. ..	140	0	39.0	0	0	65	0
(*Daily's*), 3 fl. oz.	170	0	44.0	0	0	40	0
(*Holland House*),							
4 fl. oz.	170	0	44.0	0	0	40	0.
frozen (*Bacardi*), 2 fl. oz.	170	0	35.0	4.0	0	20	0
Pine nuts, dried:							
(*Frieda's*), ¼ cup, 1.1 oz.	150	7.0	4.0	15.0	0	0	1.0
(*Planters*), 2-oz. pkg. ..	320	13.0	8.0	28.0	0	0	3.0
pignolia:							
(*Shiloh Farms*),							
¼ cup, 1.3 oz. ..	190	4.0	9.0	15.0	0	0	4.0
1 oz.	160	6.8	4.0	14.2	0	1	1.3
1 tbsp.	49	2.1	1.2	4.4	0	<1	.4
pinyon:							
1 oz.	178	3.3	5.5	17.3	0	20	3.0
10 kernels	6	.1	.2	.6	0	1	.1
Pineapple, fresh:							
(*Del Monte*), 2 slices,							
4 oz.	65	0	17.0	0	0	10	1.0
(*Dole* Fresh Cut),							
2 slices,							
3" diam. x ¾"	60	1.0	16.0	.5	0	10	1.0
(*Dole* Whole), 2 slices,							
3" diam x ¾"	60	1.0	16.0	0	0	10	1.0

Food and Measure	cal.	prot. (gms)	carbo. (gms)	fat (gms)	chol. (mgs)	sod. (mgs)	fiber (gms)
(*Frieda's* South African Baby), 1 cup, 5 oz. . .	70	1.0	17.0	.5	0	0	2.0
whole, 1 lb.	231	1.8	58.5	2.0	0	5	5.7
diced, ½ cup	38	.3	9.6	.3	0	<1	.9
Pineapple, can or jar, ½ cup, except as noted:							
(*Dole FruitBowls*), 4 oz.	60	<1.0	16.0	0	0	10	1.0
in juice:							
all styles, except sliced (*Del Monte*)	70	0	17.0	0	0	10	1.0
chunks (*Del Monte Fruit Naturals*) . .	70	<1.0	18.0	0	0	5	<1.0
chunks or tidbits (*Dole*)	60	<1.0	15.0	0	0	10	1.0
crushed (*Dole*)	70	<1.0	17.0	0	0	10	1.0
sliced (*Del Monte*), 2 pcs.	60	0	16.0	0	0	10	1.0
sliced (*Dole*), 2 pcs.	60	<1.0	15.0	0	0	10	1.0
sliced (*S&W*), 2 pcs.	60	0	16.0	0	0	10	1.0
tidbits (*Del Monte* Plastic), 4 oz. . . .	70	<1.0	18.0	0	0	5	<1.0
tidbits (*Del Monte* Pull-Top), 4 oz. .	50	0	15.0	0	0	10	<1.0
tidbits (*Del Monte* Fruit Cup), 4.5 oz.	50	0	15.0	0	0	10	<1.0
wedges (*Dole*)	60	0	15.0	0	0	10	1.0
in light syrup:							
(*Del Monte Sunfresh*)	70	0	18.0	0	0	10	<1.0
crushed or chunks .	66	.5	17.0	.2	0	1	1.0
in heavy syrup:							
chunks or crushed (*Del Monte*)	90	0	24.0	0	0	10	1.0
chunks or tidbits (*Dole*)	90	<1.0	24.0	0	0	10	1.0
chunks, tidbits or crushed	100	.5	25.8	.1	0	2	.9
sliced (*Del Monte*), 2 pcs.	90	0	23.0	0	0	10	1.0
sliced (*Dole*), 2 pcs.	90	<1.0	24.0	0	0	10	1.0
Pineapple, dried:							
(*Shiloh Farms*), 6-7 rings, 1.4 oz. . .	130	1.0	32.0	0	0	5	1.0

Food and Measure	cal.	prot. (gms)	carbo. (gms)	fat (gms)	chol. (mgs)	sod. (mgs)	fiber (gms)
Pineapple, dried *(cont.)*							
(*SunRidge Farms*),							
1.5 rings, 1.4 oz. ..	130	1.0	30.0	1.0	0	5	2.0
(*Sunsweet*), ⅓ cup,							
1.4 oz.	130	0	34.0	0	0	20	1.0
Pineapple, freeze-dried,							
chunks (*AlpineAire*), .							
4 oz.	45	0	10.0	0	0	0	1.0
Pineapple, frozen,							
chunks, sweetened,							
½ cup	104	.5	27.1	.1	0	2	1.3
Pineapple drink blend,							
8 fl. oz.:							
coconut:							
(*AriZona* Pina Colada)	140	0	34.0	1.0	0	30	0
(*R.W. Knudsen*) ...	130	1.0	31.0	1.0	0	50	0
orange (*Hood Carb*							
Countdown)	25	0	5.0	0	0	140	0
orange guava:							
(*Langers*)	130	0	30.0	0	0	0	0
(*Nantucket Nectars*)	120	0	31.0	0	0	5	0
Pineapple guava, see							
"Feijoas"							
Pineapple juice,							
8 fl. oz.:							
(*Ceres*)	120	0	29.0	0	0	5	2.0
(*Del Monte*)	110	1.0	29.0	0	0	15	2.0
(*Del Monte* From							
Concentrate)	130	1.0	32.0	0	0	10	1.0
(*Dole*)	120	<1.0	29.0	0	0	10	0
(*R.W. Knudsen* Nectar)	140	<1.0	34.0	0	0	20	0
(*S&W*)	110	1.0	29.0	0	0	15	2.0
(*Walnut Acres*)	130	0	32.0	0	0	5	0
canned	140	.8	34.5	.2	0	3	.5
frozen*	130	1.0	31.9	<.1	0	3	.5
Pineapple juice blend,							
8 fl. oz.:							
coconut:							
(*L&A*)	140	0	28.0	3.0	0	55	0
(*Langers*)	140	0	28.0	3.0	0	55	0
orange banana (*Nan-*							
tucket Nectars)	140	<1.0	35.0	0	0	15	0
Pineapple topping							
(*Smucker's*), 2 tbsp.	100	0	26.0	0	0	0	0

Food and Measure	cal.	prot. (gms)	carbo. (gms)	fat (gms)	chol. (mgs)	sod. (mgs)	fiber (gms)
Pink bean, dried, boiled, ½ cup	125	7.6	23.5	.4	0	2	4.5
Pinquito bean, canned, (*S&W* California), ½ cup	80	6.0	20.0	.5	0	480	6.0
Pinto bean:							
dry, ¼ cup:							
(*Arrowhead Mills*) .	150	9.0	27.0	0	0	0	10.0
(*Shiloh Farms*)	160	10.0	31.0	.5	0	0	12.0
boiled, ½ cup	117	7.0	21.8	.4	0	1	7.3
Pinto bean, canned (see also "Chili Beans" and "Refried beans"), ½ cup:							
(*Allens*)	110	5.0	20.0	1.0	0	290	7.0
(*Bush's*)	110	6.0	19.0	0	0	390	6.0
(*Eden* Organic)	100	6.0	18.0	0	0	15	6.0
(*Progresso*)	110	7.0	16.0	1.0	0	250	7.0
(*S&W*)	100	6.0	22.0	0	0	220	7.0
(*Westbrae Natural* Organic)	100	6.0	19.0	0	0	140	7.0
w/bacon:							
(*Trappey's*)	120	6.0	20.0	1.0	0	270	7.0
and jalapeño (*Trappey's Jala- pinto*)	120	6.0	22.0	1.0	0	540	8.0
seasoned (*Bush's*) .	120	6.0	17.0	2.5	5	530	6.0
in chili sauce, red (*Old El Paso* Mexe Beans)	110	7.0	19.0	0	0	630	7.0
w/pork (*Bush's*)	120	6.0	17.0	2.5	5	530	6.0
seasoned (*Glory*)	90	5.0	15.0	.5	0	850	5.0
spicy (*Eden* Organic) .	125	6.0	24.0	0	0	195	7.0
w/tomato, corn, chili (*Del Monte Savory Sides* Rio Grande) .	70	2.0	14.0	0	0	470	2.0
Pinto bean, frozen, boiled, drained, ⅓ of 10-oz. pkg. ..	152	8.8	29.0	.5	0	78	8.1
Pipian sauce (*Doña Maria*), 2 tbsp.	250	4.0	5.0	20.0	0	580	3.0
Pistachio nut, shelled, except as noted:							
(*Shiloh Farms*), ¼ cup	190	6.0	9.0	15.0	0	5	1.0
(*Sunkist*), ½ cup in shell, ¼ cup shelled	180	6.0	9.0	14.0	0	220	3.0

Food and Measure	cal.	prot. (gms)	carbo. (gms)	fat (gms)	chol. (mgs)	sod. (mgs)	fiber (gms)
Pistachio nut *(cont.)*							
dried, 1 oz.	164	5.8	7.1	13.7	0	2	3.1
dry-roasted:							
(*Planters*), 1 oz. . . .	170	4.0	7.0	15.0	0	190	3.0
unsalted, 1 oz.	162	6.1	7.8	13.0	0	2	2.9
unsalted, ¼ cup . . .	183	6.8	8.9	14.7	0	3	3.3
Pita, see "Bread"							
Pitanga:							
1 medium, .3 oz.	2	.1	.5	<.1	0	<1	<1.0
½ cup	29	.7	6.5	.3	0	3	<1.0
Pizza, frozen, 1 pie or pkg., except as noted:							
artichoke and roasted garlic (*Linda Mc-Cartney*), ½ pie . . .	400	13.0	33.0	20.0	35	560	4.0
bacon burger (*Totino's Crisp Crust Party Pizza*), ½ pie	390	14.0	35.0	21.0	15	810	2.0
Canadian bacon:							
(*Jenos Crisp 'N Tasty*)	440	16.0	51.0	19.0	15	1120	2.0
(*Totino's Crisp Crust Party Pizza*), ½ pie	330	13.0	35.0	15.0	10	860	1.0
cheese:							
(*Amy's*), ⅓ pie	300	12.0	38.0	12.0	15	590	2.0
(*Elio's*), ⅓ pie	340	15.0	47.0	11.0	20	780	2.0
(*Elio's* Rectangle 24 oz.), 1/9 pie . .	170	7.0	25.0	4.0	10	270	2.0
(*Ian's* Natural), 1/6 pie	100	4.0	14.0	3.0	10	200	1.0
(*Linda McCartney*), ½ pie	340	14.0	35.0	11.0	30	610	4.0
(*Michelina's* Zap'ems)	420	15.0	44.0	21.0	30	820	2.0
(*Totino's* Family Size), ⅓ pie	370	17.0	39.0	16.0	20	740	2.0
(*Totino's Crisp Crust Party Pizza*), ½ pie	320	15.0	34.0	14.0	20	620	2.0
extra (*Tombstone* Original)	580	21.0	74.0	22.0	50	1800	4.0
rice crust (*Amy's*), ⅓ pie	300	11.0	31.0	14.0	15	590	2.0
cheese, five, tomato:							
(*California Pizza Kitchen* 12.58 oz.), ⅓ pie	320	6.0	29.0	15.0	35	720	1.0

Food and Measure	cal.	prot. (gms)	carbo. (gms)	fat (gms)	chol. (mgs)	sod. (mgs)	fiber (gms)
(*California Pizza Kitchen* 27.2 oz.), 1/6 pie	350	18.0	35.0	15.0	35	770	2.0
cheese, four:							
(*Di Giorno* Thin Crispy Crust), 1/5 pie	300	15.0	34.0	11.0	25	660	3.0
(*Di Giorno* Rising Crust), 1/6 pie ..	310	15.0	40.0	11.0	20	830	3.0
(*Di Giorno* Rising Crust Microwave), ½ pie	370	15.0	44.0	15.0	15	720	3.0
(*Health is Wealth*) .	360	23.0	54.0	17.0	45	820	6.0
(*Ian's* Natural Low Carb), 1/3 pie	275	18.0	8.0	18.0	40	450	3.0
(*Lean Cuisine* Café Classics)	380	18.0	60.0	7.0	15	690	3.0
(*Smart Ones*)	330	16.0	49.0	8.0	15	720	3.0
cheese, three:							
(*Heaven's Bistro*), 1/3 pie	240	13.0	42.0	2.0	5	630	4.0
cornmeal crust (*Amy's*), 1/3 pie ..	370	10.0	41.0	19.0	10	580	2.0
"cheese," vegetarian:							
(*Amy's* Soy Cheeze), 1/3 pie	290	12.0	37.0	11.0	0	590	2.0
(*Tofutti* Pizza Pizzaz), 1/3 pkg.	175	7.0	24.0	5.0	0	320	0
cheese/pesto, whole wheat crust (*Amy's*), 1/3 pie	360	13.0	37.0	18.0	15	680	2.0
chicken:							
barbecue (*California Pizza Kitchen* 12.96 oz.), 1/3 pie	280	17.0	33.0	9.0	30	700	1.0
barbecue (*California Pizza Kitchen* 28 oz.), 1/6 pie ..	310	17.0	38.0	9.0	30	780	2.0
barbecue (*Heaven's Bistro*), 1/3 pie ...	270	16.0	48.0	2.0	15	790	4.0
Jamaican jerk (*California Pizza Kitchen*), 1/3 pie .	270	15.0	33.0	3.5	25	730	2.0

Food and Measure	cal.	prot. (gms)	carbo. (gms)	fat (gms)	chol. (mgs)	sod. (mgs)	fiber (gms)
Pizza, chicken *(cont.)*							
sausage (*Heaven's Bistro*), ⅓ pie ...	250	14.0	42.0	3.0	10	630	4.0
Thai (*California Pizza Kitchen* 12.98 oz.), ⅓ pie	290	16.0	33.0	10.0	20	740	3.0
Thai (*California Pizza Kitchen* 27.9 oz.), 1/6 pie	310	16.0	38.0	11.0	20	790	2.0
tomato and spinach, grilled (*Di Giorno* Thin Crispy Crust), 1/5 pie	260	16.0	33.0	8.0	25	550	2.0
deluxe:							
(*Lean Cuisine* Café Classics)	370	17.0	55.0	9.0	25	590	3.0
(*Smart Ones*)	360	22.0	47.0	10.0	30	700	4.0
ham and shrimp, Hawaiian (*Contessa*), ⅓ pie	320	13.0	45.0	10.0	25	890	2.0
hamburger:							
(*Jenos Crisp 'N Tasty*)	500	18.0	51.0	25.0	25	1040	2.0
(*Totino's Crisp Crust Party Pizza*), ½ pie	380	14.0	35.0	20.0	15	790	2.0
Margherita (*Lean Cuisine* Café Classics) .	320	14.0	48.0	9.0	5	540	4.0
meat, four (*Di Giorno* Thin Crispy Crust), 1/5 pie	320	13.0	37.0	13.0	35	830	2.0
meat, three:							
(*Di Giorno Rising Crust* Microwave), ½ pie	420	17.0	44.0	19.0	25	900	3.0
(*Lean Cuisine* Café Classics)	350	21.0	48.0	9.0	25	670	4.0
(*Jenos Crisp 'N Tasty*)	490	17.0	49.0	25.0	25	1150	2.0
(*Totino's Crisp Crust Party Pizza*), ½ pie	360	13.0	34.0	19.0	15	860	2.0
cheese stuffed (*Di Giorno*), 1/6 pie .	390	21.0	37.0	19.0	45	1100	3.0
Mexican style (*Health is Wealth*)	330	14.0	50.0	9.0	20	560	3.0
mushroom and olive (*Amy's*), ⅓ pie	250	10.0	33.0	9.0	10	560	2.0

Food and Measure	cal.	prot. (gms)	carbo. (gms)	fat (gms)	chol. (mgs)	sod. (mgs)	fiber (gms)
mushroom and spinach (*Linda McCartney*), ½ pie	320	12.0	34.0	10.0	20	480	4.0
pepperoni:							
(*Di Giorno* Deep Dish), 1/6 pie	390	17.0	33.0	22.0	45	1010	2.0
(*Di Giorno* Thin Crispy Crust), 1/5 pie	310	15.0	34.0	12.0	35	790	2.0
(*Di Giorno Rising Crust*), 1/6 pie ..	360	17.0	40.0	16.0	35	1010	2.0
(*Di Giorno Rising Crust* Microwave), ½ pie	390	16.0	43.0	18.0	20	840	3.0
(*Elio's* Rectangle 24 oz.), 1/9 pie ..	180	7.0	24.0	6.0	10	340	1.0
(*Heaven's Bistro*), ⅓ pie	250	15.0	42.0	2.0	10	730	4.0
(*Jenos Crisp 'N Tasty*)	510	16.0	50.0	27.0	25	1130	2.0
(*Lean Cuisine* Café Classics)	380	20.0	55.0	9.0	25	680	3.0
(*Michelina's* Zap'ems)	440	14.0	44.0	24.0	30	960	2.0
(*Smart Ones*)	350	17.0	49.0	9.0	20	760	3.0
(*Tombstone* Brick-oven), ¼ pie	310	14.0	29.0	16.0	35	740	2.0
(*Totino's* Family Size), ⅓ pie	420	14.0	38.0	23.0	20	940	2.0
(*Totino's Crisp Crust Party Pizza*), ½ pie	380	13.0	34.0	21.0	20	910	2.0
cheese (*Tombstone* Deep Dish), ½ pie	500	16.0	51.0	25.0	35	1030	3.0
sliced (*Totino's Crisp Crust Party Pizza*), ½ pie	380	13.0	35.0	21.0	20	860	1.0
"pepperoni," meatless:							
(*Boca*), ⅓ pie	260	13.0	36.0	7.0	10	660	2.0
and "sausage" (*Boca*), ⅓ pie	260	13.0	36.0	8.0	10	740	2.0
pepperoni/cheese (*Di Giorno Rising Crust* Half & Half), 1/6 pie	390	19.0	40.0	18.0	40	1090	3.0
pesto (*Amy's*), ⅓ pie .	310	12.0	39.0	12.0	10	480	2.0
sausage:							
(*Jenos Crisp 'N Tasty*)	480	16.0	51.0	24.0	20	1050	2.0

Food and Measure	cal.	prot. (gms)	carbo. (gms)	fat (gms)	chol. (mgs)	sod. (mgs)	fiber (gms)
Pizza, sausage *(cont.)*							
(*Totino's* Family Size), ¼ pie	300	11.0	29.0	16.0	10	680	1.0
(*Totino's Crisp Crust Party Pizza*), ½ pie	380	13.0	36.0	19.0	15	780	2.0
spicy (*Smart Ones*)	350	20.0	48.0	9.0	20	690	4.0
sausage/mushroom (*Totino's Crisp Crust Party Pizza*), ½ pie .	360	13.0	34.0	19.0	15	780	2.0
sausage/pepperoni:							
(*Jenos Crisp 'N Tasty*)	500	17.0	50.0	26.0	20	1100	2.0
(*Tombstone* Brick-oven), ¼ pie	320	15.0	30.0	16.0	40	740	3.0
(*Totino's* Family Size), ¼ pie	310	11.0	29.0	17.0	15	700	1.0
(*Totino's Crisp Crust Party Pizza*), ½ pie	380	13.0	35.0	21.0	15	850	2.0
zesty Italiano (*Totino's Crisp Crust Party Pizza*), ½ pie . . .	390	13.0	36.0	21.0	15	850	2.0
shrimp and, ⅓ pie:							
basil pesto (*Contessa*)	300	12.0	37.0	11.0	20	700	2.0
roasted red pesto (*Contessa*)	300	11.0	38.0	12.0	15	690	2.0
roasted vegetables (*Contessa*)	280	10.0	38.0	9.0	15	650	2.0
spinach:							
(*Amy's*), ⅓ pie	300	12.0	38.0	12.0	15	590	2.0
and 4 cheese (*Ian's* Natural Low Carb), ⅓ pie	210	15.0	8.0	13.0	25	375	4.0
and mushroom (*Lean Cuisine* Café Classics)	310	17.0	46.0	7.0	15	430	4.0
supreme:							
(*Di Giorno* Deep Dish), ⅛ pie	310	14.0	25.0	17.0	35	760	2.0
(*Di Giorno Rising Crust* 14.3 oz.), ⅓ pie	320	15.0	35.0	14.0	30	900	3.0
(*Di Giorno Rising Crust* 32.7 oz.), 1/6 pie	370	17.0	41.0	15.0	30	1000	3.0

Food and Measure	cal.	prot. (gms)	carbo. (gms)	fat (gms)	chol. (mgs)	sod. (mgs)	fiber (gms)
(*Di Giorno Rising Crust* Microwave), ½ pie	410	17.0	44.0	18.0	25	860	3.0
(*Jenos Crisp 'N Tasty*)	500	17.0	50.0	26.0	20	1090	2.0
(*Tombstone* Brick-oven), ¼ pie	320	14.0	30.0	16.0	35	720	3.0
†(*Totino's Crisp Crust Party Pizza*), ½ pie	380	13.0	35.0	21.0	15	840	2.0
vegetable/veggie:							
(*Heaven's Bistro*), ⅓ pie	230	13.0	42.0	1.0	0	590	4.0
(*Smart Ones* Ultimate)	340	19.0	50.0	7.0	15	610	4.0
combo (*Amy's*), ⅓ pie	290	10.0	36.0	11.0	10	580	1.0
roasted (*Amy's*), ⅓ pie	260	6.0	42.0	8.0	0	490	2.0
roasted (*Lean Cuisine* Café Classics)	330	15.0	57.0	4.5	10	560	3.0
Thai, spicy (*Linda McCartney*), ½ pie	320	13.0	36.0	9.0	20	540	4.0
Pizza, bagel, frozen:							
(*Health is Wealth*), 4 pcs., 3.1 oz.	150	8.0	28.0	0	0	490	3.0
(*Dr. Praeger's*), 2-oz. pc.	110	3.0	20.0	2.0	5	280	2.0
cheese, three (*Bagel Bites*), 4 pcs., 3 oz.	200	8.0	28.0	6.0	15	540	2.0
Pizza, French bread, frozen, 1 pc.:							
cheese:							
(*Healthy Choice*) ..	360	20.0	57.0	5.0	10	600	5.0
(*Lean Cuisine*)	320	16.0	47.0	7.0	20	520	3.0
(*Stouffer's*)	380	15.0	43.0	16.0	30	660	3.0
extra (*Stouffer's*) ..	400	16.0	44.0	18.0	35	770	3.0
five (*Stouffer's*)	410	15.0	47.0	18.0	35	880	3.0
deluxe:							
(*Lean Cuisine*)	310	16.0	44.0	9.0	20	700	3.0
(*Stouffer's*)	430	15.0	45.0	21.0	30	880	3.0
meat, three (*Stouffer's*)	480	16.0	47.0	25.0	40	1130	4.0
pepperoni:							
(*Healthy Choice*) ..	360	21.0	56.0	5.0	30	600	6.0
(*Lean Cuisine*)	300	16.0	44.0	7.0	15	560	2.0
(*Stouffer's*)	430	16.0	44.0	21.0	30	930	3.0
pepperoni and mushroom (*Stouffer's*) ..	410	12.0	47.0	19.0	25	990	4.0
sausage (*Stouffer's*) ..	420	16.0	45.0	20.0	35	820	3.0

Food and Measure	cal.	prot. (gms)	carbo. (gms)	fat (gms)	chol. (mgs)	sod. (mgs)	fiber (gms)
Pizza, French bread *(cont.)*							
sausage and pepperoni							
(*Stouffer's*)	460	15.0	47.0	24.0	35	1040	4.0
supreme (*Healthy*							
Choice) :	330	21.0	51.0	5.0	20	600	6.0
vegetable:							
(*Healthy Choice*) ..	320	18.0	50.0	5.0	10	600	4.0
grilled (*Stouffer's*) .	340	10.0	49.0	12.0	15	760	3.0
white (*Stouffer's*)	470	22.0	44.0	23.0	40	900	4.0
Pizza, stuffed/pocket,							
frozen, 1 pc., 4.5 oz.,							
except as noted:							
cheese:							
(*Amy's*)	300	14.0	42.0	9.0	15	450	4.0
(*Amy's* Toaster Pops),							
1.9 oz.	150	5.0	23.0	4.5	5	220	<1.0
(*Jack's Pizza Bursts*							
Super), 3 oz. ...	250	9.0	25.0	13.0	20	440	1.0
five (*Croissant*							
Pockets)	390	14.0	37.0	20.0	20	880	3.0
"cheese," soy (*Amy's*							
Cheeze)	260	9.0	39.0	8.0	0	520	6.0
pepperoni:							
(*Croissant Pockets*)	390	12.0	39.0	20.0	20	810	3.0
(*Hot Pockets*)	360	11.0	41.0	17.0	25	730	3.0
(*Jack's Pizza Bursts*),							
3 oz.	260	8.0	25.0	15.0	15	550	1.0
(*Lean Pockets*)	280	14.0	42.0	7.0	25	720	4.0
(*Smart Ones*							
Smartwich)	270	12.0	39.0	7.0	20	580	2.0
sausage/pepperoni:							
(*Jack's Pizza Bursts*),							
3 oz.	250	8.0	25.0	13.0	10	470	1.0
(*Lean Pockets*)	280	13.0	41.0	7.0	45	630	3.0
supreme:							
(*Jack's Pizza Bursts*),							
3 oz.	260	8.0	25.0	14.0	15	490	1.0
(*Lean Pockets* Ultra)	200	24.0	19.0	6.0	25	540	7.0
vegetarian (*Amy's*) ...	250	11.0	39.0	6.0	10	360	4.0
Pizza crust, frozen,							
dough (*Rhodes*),							
1/6 pkg.	180	5.0	32.0	3.0	0	250	1.0
Pizza crust mix:							
(*Betty Crocker*),							
¼ crust*	160	4.0	33.0	2.0	0	340	1.0

Food and Measure	cal.	prot. (gms)	carbo. (gms)	fat (gms)	chol. (mgs)	sod. (mgs)	fiber (gms)
("Jiffy"), ⅓ cup mix . .	160	4.0	31.0	2.5	0	280	2.0
Pizza entree, frozen, w/dessert (*Ian's* Natural Kids Meal), 9 oz.	340	9.0	60.0	7.0	25	290	4.0
Pizza Hut, 1 slice, except as noted:							
Dippin' Sticks, 2 pcs.:							
cheese only	270	11.0	29.0	12.0	25	520	2.0
chicken supreme . .	260	12.0	30.0	10.0	25	540	2.0
ham, quartered . . .	250	11.0	28.0	10.0	20	580	2.0
Meat Lover's	370	16.0	29.0	21.0	45	890	2.0
pepperoni	280	11.0	28.0	13.0	25	570	2.0
Pepperoni Lover's .	330	14.0	29.0	17.0	40	720	2.0
Pepperoni Trio	310	14.0	30.0	15.0	30	630	1.0
supreme	300	12.0	30.0	15.0	30	660	2.0
super supreme	320	14.0	30.0	16.0	35	770	2.0
Veggie Lover's	250	9.0	30.0	10.0	15	490	2.0
dipping sauce:							
garlic, 1½ oz. . . .	100	0	3.0	10.0	0	250	0
marinara, 3 oz. . . .	45	2.0	9.0	0	0	380	2.0
ranch, 1½ oz. . . .	210	<1.0	4.0	22.0	10	340	0
Fit 'N Delicious, 12"							
chicken/onion/pepper	170	10.0	23.0	4.5	15	460	2.0
chicken/mushroom	170	10.0	22.0	5.0	15	690	2.0
ham/mushroom . . .	160	8.0	22.0	4.5	15	470	2.0
ham/pineapple	160	8.0	24.0	4.0	15	470	2.0
pepper/onion	150	6.0	24.0	4.0	10	360	2.0
tomato/mushroom .	150	6.0	22.0	4.0	10	590	2.0
Fit 'N Delicious, 14"							
chicken/onion/pepper	160	9.0	22.0	4.0	15	420	2.0
chicken/mushroom	160	9.0	20.0	4.5	15	630	2.0
ham/mushroom . . .	150	8.0	21.0	4.0	15	440	2.0
ham/pineapple	150	7.0	22.0	4.0	15	440	1.0
pepper/onion	140	6.0	22.0	3.5	10	330	2.0
tomato/mushroom .	140	6.0	21.0	4.0	10	540	2.0
extra large, 16":							
cheese only	420	20.0	51.0	15.0	45	1080	3.0
chicken supreme . .	400	22.0	52.0	12.0	40	1070	3.0
ham, quartered . . .	380	19.0	50.0	12.0	40	1110	3.0
Meat Lover's	500	24.0	51.0	22.0	60	1400	3.0
pepperoni	430	19.0	50.0	17.0	45	1130	3.0
Pepperoni Lover's .	520	25.0	51.0	24.0	65	1370	3.0
Sausage Lover's . . .	510	23.0	51.0	23.0	55	1330	3.0
supreme	460	22.0	52.0	19.0	45	1250	4.0

Food and Measure	cal.	prot. (gms)	carbo. (gms)	fat (gms)	chol. (mgs)	sod. (mgs)	fiber (gms)
***Pizza Hut*, extra large** *(cont.)*							
super supreme	490	23.0	53.0	21.0	55	1430	4.0
Veggie Lover's	390	17.0	53.0	12.0	30	1030	4.0
hand-tossed, 12":							
cheese only	240	12.0	30.0	8.0	25	520	2.0
chicken supreme ..	230	14.0	30.0	6.0	25	550	2.0
ham, quartered ...	220	12.0	29.0	6.0	20	550	2.0
Meat Lover's	300	15.0	29.0	13.0	35	760	2.0
pepperoni	250	12.0	29.0	9.0	25	570	2.0
Pepperoni Lover's .	300	15.0	30.0	13.0	40	710	2.0
Pepperoni Trio	280	14.0	30.0	11.0	30	640	2.0
Sausage Lover's ...	280	13.0	30.0	12.0	30	650	2.0
supreme	270	13.0	30.0	11.0	25	660	2.0
super supreme	300	15.0	31.0	13.0	35	780	2.0
Veggie Lover's	220	10.0	31.0	6.0	15	490	2.0
hand-tossed, 14":							
cheese only	220	11.0	27.0	8.0	25	480	1.0
chicken supreme ..	210	13.0	28.0	6.0	20	500	2.0
ham, quartered ...	200	11.0	27.0	6.0	20	520	1.0
Meat Lover's	280	14.0	27.0	12.0	35	710	2.0
pepperoni	230	11.0	27.0	9.0	25	540	2.0
Pepperoni Lover's .	280	14.0	27.0	13.0	35	680	2.0
Pepperoni Trio	270	14.0	28.0	11.0	30	610	2.0
Sausage Lover's ...	260	12.0	27.0	11.0	30	600	2.0
supreme	250	13.0	28.0	10.0	25	620	2.0
super supreme	270	14.0	28.0	12.0	30	720	2.0
Veggie Lover's	200	9.0	28.0	6.0	15	460	2.0
pan pizza, 12":							
cheese only	280	11.0	29.0	13.0	25	500	1.0
chicken supreme ..	280	13.0	30.0	12.0	25	530	2.0
ham, quartered ...	260	11.0	29.0	11.0	20	540	1.0
Meat Lover's	340	15.0	29.0	19.0	35	750	2.0
pepperoni	290	11.0	29.0	15.0	25	560	2.0
Pepperoni Lover's .	340	15.0	29.0	19.0	40	700	2.0
Pepperoni Trio	320	14.0	29.0	17.0	30	620	1.0
Sausage Lover's ...	330	13.0	29.0	17.0	30	640	2.0
supreme	320	13.0	30.0	16.0	25	650	2.0
super supreme	340	14.0	30.0	18.0	35	760	2.0
Veggie Lover's	260	10.0	30.0	12.0	15	470	4.0
pan pizza, 14":							
cheese only	270	11.0	27.0	13.0	25	470	1.0
chicken supreme ..	260	12.0	27.0	11.0	20	490	2.0
ham, quartered ...	250	11.0	26.0	11.0	20	510	1.0
Meat Lover's	320	14.0	27.0	18.0	35	690	2.0

Food and Measure	cal.	prot. (gms)	carbo. (gms)	fat (gms)	chol. (mgs)	sod. (mgs)	fiber (gms)
pepperoni	280	11.0	26.0	14.0	25	530	1.0
Pepperoni Lover's .	330	14.0	27.0	18.0	35	670	2.0
Pepperoni Trio	300	13.0	27.0	16.0	30	590	1.0
Sausage Lover's . . .	300	12.0	27.0	17.0	30	590	2.0
supreme	300	12.0	27.0	16.0	25	600	2.0
super supreme	320	13.0	28.0	17.0	30	700	2.0
Veggie Lover's	250	9.0	28.0	11.0	15	440	4.0
Personal Pan Pizza, ¼ of 6" pie:							
cheese only	160	7.0	18.0	7.0	15	310	<1.0
chicken supreme . .	160	8.0	19.0	6.0	15	320	<1.0
ham, quartered . . .	150	7.0	18.0	6.0	15	330	<1.0
Meat Lover's	200	9.0	18.0	10.0	20	470	1.0
pepperoni	170	7.0	18.0	8.0	15	340	<1.0
Pepperoni Lover's .	200	9.0	18.0	10.0	25	440	1.0
Sausage Lover's . . .	190	8.0	18.0	10.0	20	400	1.0
supreme	190	8.0	19.0	9.0	20	420	1.0
super supreme	200	9.0	19.0	10.0	20	480	1.0
Veggie Lover's	150	6.0	19.0	6.0	10	280	1.0
stuffed crust, 14":							
cheese only	360	18.0	43.0	13.0	40	920	2.0
chicken supreme . .	380	20.0	44.0	13.0	40	1020	3.0
ham, quartered . . .	340	18.0	42.0	11.0	40	960	2.0
Meat Lover's	450	21.0	43.0	21.0	55	1250	3.0
pepperoni	370	18.0	42.0	15.0	45	970	3.0
Pepperoni Lover's .	420	19.0	43.0	19.0	55	1120	3.0
Pepperoni Trio	450	23.0	45.0	19.0	55	1190	3.0
Sausage Lover's . . .	430	19.0	43.0	19.0	50	1130	3.0
supreme	400	20.0	44.0	16.0	45	1070	3.0
super supreme	440	21.0	45.0	20.0	50	1270	3.0
Veggie Lover's	360	16.0	45.0	14.0	35	980	3.0
stuffed crust, 3Cheese:							
cheese only	350	17.0	43.0	13.0	35	940	3.0
chicken supreme . .	370	19.0	44.0	13.0	35	1040	3.0
ham, quartered . . .	330	17.0	42.0	11.0	35	970	3.0
Meat Lover's	440	21.0	43.0	20.0	50	1270	3.0
pepperoni	360	17.0	42.0	14.0	35	990	3.0
Pepperoni Lover's .	420	20.0	43.0	18.0	50	1130	3.0
supreme	390	19.0	43.0	16.0	40	1080	4.0
super supreme	430	20.0	45.0	19.0	45	1280	4.0
Veggie Lover's	360	16.0	45.0	13.0	30	1000	3.0
The Full House XL Pizza:							
cheese	280	12.0	30.0	12.0	25	760	3.0
chicken supreme . .	270	13.0	31.0	10.0	25	770	3.0

Food and Measure	cal.	prot. (gms)	carbo. (gms)	fat (gms)	chol. (mgs)	sod. (mgs)	fiber (gms)
Pizza Hut, The Full House XL Pizza *(cont.)*							
ham, quartered ...	260	12.0	30.0	10.0	25	790	3.0
Meat Lover's	380	17.0	30.0	21.0	45	1120	3.0
pepperoni	290	12.0	30.0	13.0	25	810	3.0
Pepperoni Lover's .	310	13.0	30.0	15.0	30	880	3.0
Pepperoni Trio	320	14.0	30.0	15.0	35	870	3.0
supreme	310	13.0	31.0	15.0	30	890	3.0
super supreme	330	15.0	32.0	16.0	35	1000	3.0
Veggie Lover's	260	10.0	32.0	11.0	20	740	3.0
Thin 'N Crispy, 12":							
cheese	200	10.0	21.0	8.0	25	490	1.0
chicken supreme ..	200	12.0	22.0	7.0	25	520	1.0
ham, quartered ...	180	9.0	21.0	6.0	20	530	1.0
Meat Lover's	270	13.0	21.0	14.0	35	740	2.0
pepperoni	210	10.0	21.0	10.0	25	550	1.0
Pepperoni Lover's .	260	13.0	21.0	14.0	40	690	2.0
Pepperoni Trio	240	12.0	21.0	12.0	30	610	1.0
Sausage Lover's ...	240	11.0	21.0	13.0	30	630	2.0
supreme	240	11.0	22.0	11.0	25	640	2.0
super supreme	260	13.0	23.0	13.0	35	760	2.0
Veggie Lover's	180	8.0	23.0	7.0	15	480	2.0
Thin 'N Crispy, 14":							
cheese	190	9.0	20.0	8.0	25	460	1.0
chicken supreme ..	180	11.0	21.0	6.0	20	480	1.0
ham, quartered ...	170	9.0	19.0	6.0	20	500	1.0
Meat Lover's	250	12.0	20.0	13.0	35	700	2.0
pepperoni	200	9.0	19.0	9.0	25	520	1.0
Pepperoni Lover's .	250	12.0	20.0	14.0	35	660	1.0
Pepperoni Trio	220	11.0	19.0	11.0	30	570	1.0
Sausage Lover's ...	230	10.0	20.0	12.0	30	580	1.0
supreme	220	11.0	21.0	11.0	25	600	2.0
super supreme	240	12.0	21.0	12.0	30	710	2.0
Veggie Lover's	170	8.0	21.0	7.0	15	450	2.0
appetizers:							
bread stick, 1 pc.:							
regular	150	4.0	20.0	6.0	0	220	<1.0
cheese	200	7.0	21.0	10.0	15	340	<1.0
dipping sauce ...	50	1.0	11.0	0	0	370	2.0
wings, hot 2 pcs. ..	110	11.0	1.0	6.0	70	450	0
wings, mild, 2 pcs.	110	11.0	<1.0	7.0	70	320	0
wings dipping sauce:							
blue cheese	230	2.0	2.0	24.0	25	550	0
ranch	210	<1.0	4.0	22.0	10	340	0

Food and Measure	cal.	prot. (gms)	carbo. (gms)	fat (gms)	chol. (mgs)	sod. (mgs)	fiber (gms)
desserts:							
apple pizza, 1 slice .	260	4.0	53.0	3.5	0	250	1.0
cherry pizza, 1 slice .	240	4.0	47.0	3.5	0	250	1.0
cinnamon sticks, 2 .	170	4.0	27.0	5.0	0	170	<1.0
icing dipping	190	0	46.0	0	0	0	0
Pizza kit, taco, cheesy (*Old El Paso* Dinner Kit):							
as packaged, ⅛ pkg. .	130	2.0	16.0	6.0	0	450	1.0
prepared, ⅛ pizza* ..	350	19.0	17.0	23.0	70	660	1.0
Pizza pocket, see "Pizza, stuffed/ pocket"							
Pizza rolls, see "Pizza snack"							
Pizza sauce, ¼ cup, except as noted:							
(*Contadina* Original/ Squeeze)	30	1.0	6.0	0	0	340	1.0
(*Eden* Organic Pizza/ Pasta), ½ cup	80	3.0	12.0	2.5	0	320	3.0
(*Hunt's* Family Favorites)	25	1.0	5.0	0	0	270	1.0
(*Muir Glen*)	40	1.0	6.0	1.0	0	230	2.0
w/basil (*Red Pack*) ..	30	1.0	6.0	0	0	180	1.0
w/cheese, four (*Contadina*)	30	<1.0	6.0	.5	0	390	<1.0
pepperoni flavor (*Contadina*)	35	1.0	5.0	1.0	0	390	<1.0
Pizza snack, frozen:							
(*Cedarlane* Mini Bistro), 3 pcs., 4 oz.	280	10.0	27.0	15.0	25	660	2.0
(*Health is Wealth*), 2 pcs., 3 oz.	190	5.0	32.0	5.0	0	560	3.0
(*Health is Wealth* Supreme), 10 pcs., 5 oz.	290	13.0	46.0	7.0	0	760	7.0
(*Ian's Pizzetta*), 7 pcs., 4.75 oz.	340	15.0	38.0	15.0	25	690	4.0
(*Michelina's* Zap'ems), 5-oz. pkg.	470	16.0	41.0	27.0	65	850	2.0
cheese:							
(*Amy's*), 5-6 pcs. ...	190	9.0	22.0	7.0	10	390	2.0
double (*Pizza Mini's*), 5 pcs., 3 oz.	240	5.0	30.0	11.0	10	410	2.0

Food and Measure	cal.	prot. (gms)	carbo. (gms)	fat (gms)	chol. (mgs)	sod. (mgs)	fiber (gms)
Pizza snack *(cont.)*							
pepperoni (*Pizza Mini's*),							
5 pcs., 3 oz.	240	6.0	29.0	12.0	15	510	2.0
"pepperoni," meatless							
(*Health is Wealth*),							
10 pcs., 5 oz.	310	14.0	46.0	9.0	0	870	6.0
rolls, 6 pcs., 3 oz.:							
cheese (*Totino's* Pizza							
Rolls)	200	9.0	26.0	7.0	10	420	1.0
cheesy taco (*Totino's*							
Pizza Rolls)	210	7.0	23.0	10.0	20	450	1.0
hamburger (*Totino's*							
Pizza Rolls)	210	8.0	24.0	9.0	10	490	1.0
meat, three (*Totino's*							
Pizza Rolls)	220	8.0	24.0	10.0	15	450	1.0
pepperoni (*Totino's*							
Pizza Rolls)	230	8.0	24.0	11.0	10	530	1.0
pepperoni sausage,							
spicy (*Totino's*							
Pizza Rolls)	230	8.0	24.0	11.0	10	540	1.0
pepperoni supreme							
(*Totino's* Pizza							
Rolls)	220	8.0	24.0	10.0	10	450	1.0
sausage (*Totino's*							
Pizza Rolls)	230	8.0	24.0	11.0	10	370	1.0
sausage/pepperoni							
(*Totino's* Pizza							
Rolls)	230	8.0	23.0	12.0	15	470	1.0
supreme (*Totino's*							
Pizza Rolls)	220	7.0	25.0	10.0	10	350	1.0
sausage and pepperoni							
(*Pizza Mini's*), 5 pcs.,							
3 oz.	230	6.0	29.0	10.0	10	440	2.0
spinach (*Amy's*),							
5-6 pcs.	190	8.0	26.0	6.0	15	420	<1.0
Plantain, fresh:							
raw:							
(*Del Monte*),							
½ medium, 3.9 oz.	180	0	22.0	0	0	0	5.0
(*Frieda's*), 3 oz.	100	1.0	27.0	0	0	0	2.0
1 medium, 6.3 oz.	218	2.3	57.1	.6	0	7	4.1
sliced, ½ cup	91	1.0	23.6	.3	0	3	1.7
cooked, sliced, ½ cup	89	.6	24.0	.1	0	4	1.8

Food and Measure	cal.	prot. (gms)	carbo. (gms)	fat (gms)	chol. (mgs)	sod. (mgs)	fiber (gms)
Plantain, frozen:							
baked, ripe (*Goya* Plátanos Maduros Horneados), 3 oz., 3 pcs.	237	1.0	56.0	1.0	0	68	3.0
fried:							
(*Goya* Tostones), 3 oz., 3 pcs.	170	1.0	37.0	2.0	0	480	9.0
ripe (*Goya* Platanos Maduros), 2 oz., 2 pcs.	110	0	22.0	2.0	0	319	2.0
Plum, fresh:							
(*Del Monte*), 2 medium, 4.7 oz.	80	1.0	19.0	1.0	0	0	2.0
(*Chiquita*), 2 medium, 4.7 oz.	80	1.0	19.0	1.0	0	0	2.0
Japanese or hybrid, 2⅛" fruit	36	.5	8.6	.4	0	tr.	<1.0
sliced, ½ cup	46	.7	10.7	.5	0	1	1.2
Plum, can or jar, purple:							
in juice:							
½ cup	73	.7	19.1	<.1	0	2	1.3
3 plums and 2 tbsp. liquid	55	.5	14.4	<.1	0	1	1.0
in light syrup:							
½ cup	79	.5	20.5	.1	0	25	1.3
3 plums and 2¾ tbsp. liquid	83	.5	21.7	.1	0	26	1.3
in heavy syrup, ½ cup	115	.5	30.0	.1	0	25	1.3
in extra heavy syrup, whole (*S&W*)	130	0	33.0	0	0	15	2.0
Plum, dried (prune):							
(*Dole*), ¼ cup, 1.4 oz.	110	1.0	26.0	0	0	5	2.0
w/pits, 1.4 oz.:							
extra large (*Sunsweet*), 3 pcs.	100	1.0	26.0	0	0	5	3.0
large (*Sunsweet*), 5 pcs.	100	1.0	26.0	0	0	5	3.0
medium (*Sunsweet*), 6 pcs.	100	1.0	26.0	0	0	5	3.0
pitted:							
(*Shiloh Farms*), 1.4 oz., 5 pcs.	124	1.0	29.0	0	0	6	3.0

Food and Measure	cal.	prot. (gms)	carbo. (gms)	fat (gms)	chol. (mgs)	sod. (mgs)	fiber (gms)
Plum, dried, pitted *(cont.)*							
(*Sunsweet*), ⅓ cup,							
1.4 oz.	90	1.0	24.0	0	0	5	3.0
10 pcs.	201	2.2	52.7	.4	0	3	6.0
bite size (*Sunsweet*),							
7 pcs., 1.4 oz. ...	100	1.0	26.0	0	0	5	3.0
cherry, lemon, or							
orange essence							
(*Sunsweet*), 5 pcs.,							
1.4 oz.	100	1.0	26.0	0	0	5	3.0
stewed, w/pits, un-							
sweetened, ½ cup .	113	1.2	29.8	.2	0	2	7.0
Plum, dried, canned,							
in heavy syrup:							
pitted, 4 oz.	119	1.0	31.5	.2	0	3	4.3
½ cup	123	1.0	32.5	.2	0	3	4.4
5 pcs., 2 tbsp. liquid .	90	.8	23.9	.2	0	2	3.3
Plum, pickled, see							
"Umeboshi plum"							
Plum butter (*Lost Acres*),							
1 tbsp.	45	0	11.0	0	0	0	0
Plum drink, red							
(*Nantucket Nectars*),							
8 fl. oz.	120	0	31.0	0	0	30	0
Plum pudding (*Crosse*							
& Blackwell), ⅓ pkg.	460	6.0	87.0	10.0	0	240	5.0
Plum sauce, 2 tbsp.,							
except as noted:							
(*Ka•Me*)	70	0	16.0	0	0	360	0
(*Kikkoman*)	80	0	18.0	.5	0	280	0
(*Ty Ling* Duck)	80	0	20.0	0	0	150	0
dipping (*Trader Vic's*) .	70	0	16.0	0	0	220	0
light, sweet (*Thai*							
Kitchen), 1 tbsp. ..	10	2.0	<1.0	0	0	690	0
Poi, ½ cup	134	.5	32.7	.2	0	14	.5
Pocket sandwich, see							
specific listings							
Pokeberry shoots:							
raw, ½ cup	18	2.1	3.0	.3	0	18	1.4
boiled, drained, ½ cup	16	1.9	2.5	.3	0	15	1.2
Pole beans, see "Green							
beans"							
Polenta (see also "Corn							
meal"), ¼ cup:							
(*Shiloh Farms*)	110	3.0	22.0	1.5	0	10	1.0

Food and Measure	cal.	prot. (gms)	carbo. (gms)	fat (gms)	chol. (mgs)	sod. (mgs)	fiber (gms)
instant (*Bellino*)	140	3.0	32.0	0	0	0	4.0
Polenta, refrigerated, prepared:							
(*Frieda's* Organic Traditional), 2 slices, ½", 3.5 oz.	70	2.0	15.0	0	0	310	1.0
(*San Gennaro* Traditional), 2½" slice, 3.5 oz.	70	2.0	15.0	0	0	310	1.0
basil and garlic (*San Gennaro*), 2½" slice, 3.5 oz.	71	2.0	15.0	0	0	310	1.0
sun-dried tomato and garlic (*San Gennaro*), 2½" slice, 3.5 oz. . . .	74	2.0	16.0	0	0	310	1.0
Polish sausage, see "Sausage"							
Pollock, meat only:							
Atlantic, 4 oz.:							
raw	104	22.1	0	1.1	80	98	0
baked, broiled, or microwaved	134	28.3	0	1.4	103	125	0
walleye, 4 oz.:							
raw	91	19.5	0	.9	81	112	0
baked, broiled, or microwaved	128	26.7	0	1.3	109	132	0
Pomegranate:							
(*Frieda's*), 5 oz.	100	1.0	24.0	0	0	0	1.0
w/peel, 9.7-oz. fruit . .	104	1.5	26.4	.5	0	5	.9
Pomegranate drink blend, 8 fl. oz.:							
cranberry (*Sobe Elixer 3C*)	100	0	26.0	0	0	27	0
pear (*Nantucket Nectars*)	110	0	28.0	0	0	30	0
Pomegranate juice, 8 fl. oz.:							
(*Pom*)	140	1.0	35.0	0	0	30	0
(*R.W. Knudsen*)	150	<1.0	37.0	0	0	10	0
(*R.W. Knudsen* Just Pomegranate)	150	<1.0	38.0	0	0	20	0
Pomegranate juice blend, 8 fl. oz.:							
blueberry (*Pom*)	140	1.0	34.0	0	0	45	0
cherry (*Pom*)	140	1.0	33.0	0	0	35	0

Food and Measure	cal.	prot. (gms)	carbo. (gms)	fat (gms)	chol. (mgs)	sod. (mgs)	fiber (gms)
Pomegranate juice blend *(cont.)*							
mango (*Pom*)	140	1.0	34.0	0	0	70	0
tangerine (*Pom*)	150	0	37.0	0	0	75	0
Pomegranate juice concentrate (*Tree of Life*), 8 tsp.	110	2.0	41.0	0	0	5	0
Pomegranate syrup, see "Grenadine syrup"							
Pompano, Florida, meat only:							
raw, 4 oz.	186	21.0	0	10.7	57	74	0
baked, broiled, or microwaved, 4 oz. .	239	26.4	0	13.8	73	86	0
Ponzu sauce (*Eden*), 1 tbsp.	5	0	1.0	0	0	340	0
Popcorn, unpopped, 2 tbsp., except as noted:							
(*America's Best*)	90	3.0	23.0	2.0	0	210	9.0
(*Arrowhead Mills*), ¼ cup	170	5.0	33.0	2.0	0	0	7.0
(*B. K. Heuermann's* Kettle Korn)	140	2.0	17.0	8.0	0	190	3.0
(*B. K. Heuermann's Exclusive*)	120	2.0	16.0	8.0	0	115	4.0
(*Healthy Choice* Natural Flavor), 3 tbsp.	120	4.0	26.0	2.5	0	330	5.0
(*Jolly Time* Mallow Magic)	180	2.0	15.0	13.0	0	200	3.0
(*Jolly Time* Crispy & White)	150	3.0	16.0	10.0	0	410	6.0
(*Jolly Time* Crispy & White Light)	120	3.0	20.0	5.0	0	320	7.0
(*Jolly Time* Healthy Pop Kettle Corn Regular or Minis)	90	3.0	23.0	2.0	0	280	8.0
(*Jolly Time* KettleMania)	170	2.0	15.0	13.0	0	270	3.0
(*Newman's Own* Natural), 1.1 oz., 3½ cups*	170	2.0	16.0	11.0	0	180	3.0
(*Orville Redenbacher's*), 3 tbsp.	120	4.0	29.0	1.5	0	0	6.0
(*Orville Redenbacher's* Corn on the Cob) . .	170	2.0	15.0	13.0	0	290	4.0

Food and Measure	cal.	prot. (gms)	carbo. (gms)	fat (gms)	chol. (mgs)	sod. (mgs)	fiber (gms)
(*Orville Redenbacher's Natural*)	170	2.0	17.0	11.0	0	500	4.0
(*Orville Redenbacher's Natural Light*)	110	3.0	19.0	5.0	0	360	4.0
(*Orville Redenbacher's Smart Pop! Kettle Korn*), 3 tbsp.	120	4.0	27.0	3.0	0	350	6.0
(*Pop•Secret Homestyle*), 3 tbsp.	170	3.0	17.0	12.0	0	430	3.0
(*Pop•Secret Kettle Corn*), 3 tbsp.	190	2.0	15.0	13.0	0	160	3.0
(*Simple Snacks Organic Lightly Salted 94% Fat Free*), 1 oz., 4 cups*	100	3.0	21.0	2.0	0	350	5.0
butter flavor:							
(*B. K. Heuermann's Exclusive*)	140	2.0	16.0	8.0	0	115	4.0
(*B. K. Heuermann's Exclusive Intense Butter Taste*) ...	160	2.0	16.0	9.0	0	270	4.0
(*B. K. Heuermann's Exclusive Low Fat*)	120	2.0	16.0	2.0	0	115	4.0
(*Healthy Choice*), 3 tbsp.	120	4.0	25.0	3.0	0	330	5.0
(*Jolly Time Blast O Butter Light*)	130	3.0	21.0	6.0	0	340	6.0
(*Jolly Time Blast O Butter Minis*), 3 tbsp.	190	3.0	21.0	15.0	0	410	10.0
(*Jolly Time Blast O Butter Ultimate Theater Style Butter*)	150	3.0	19.0	11.0	0	340	9.0
(*Jolly Time Butter-Licious*)	150	2.0	16.0	10.0	0	390	5.0
(*Jolly Time Butter-Licious Light*) ...	130	4.0	22.0	5.0	0	230	4.0
(*Jolly Time Healthy Pop Regular or Minis*)	90	3.0	23.0	2.0	0	210	9.0
(*Jolly Time White & Buttery*)	150	4.0	16.0	9.0	0	350	4.0

Food and Measure	cal.	prot. (gms)	carbo. (gms)	fat (gms)	chol. (mgs)	sod. (mgs)	fiber (gms)
Popcorn, butter flavor *(cont.)*							
(*Newman's Own*), 1.1 oz., 3½ cups*	170	2.0	16.0	11.0	0	180	3.0
(*Newman's Own Butter Boom*), 1.1 oz., 3½ cups*	170	2.0	15.0	11.0	0	630	3.0
(*Newman's Own Light*), 1.1 oz., 3½ cups*	110	2.0	20.0	3.0	0	90	3.0
(*Newman's Own 99% Fat Free*), 1.1 oz., 3½ cups*	110	2.0	22.0	1.5	0	250	2.0
(*Orville Redenbacher's*)	160	2.0	17.0	12.0	0	390	4.0
(*Orville Redenbacher's Kettle Korn*)	180	2.0	16.0	12.0	<5	230	3.0
(*Orville Redenbacher's Light*)	110	3.0	19.0	5.0	0	330	4.0
(*Orville Redenbacher's Movie Theater Light*)	120	3.0	19.0	4.5	0	320	5.0
(*Orville Redenbacher's Movie Theater Pour Over*)	170	2.0	14.0	14.0	0	330	3.0
(*Orville Redenbacher's Old Fashioned*)	160	2.0	17.0	11.0	0	330	4.0
(*Orville Redenbacher's Pour Over*)	170	2.0	14.0	14.0	0	320	3.0
(*Orville Redenbacher's Smart Pop!*), 3 tbsp.	110	4.0	26.0	2.0	0	360	6.0
(*Orville Redenbacher's Smart Pop! Movie Theater*), 3 tbsp.	120	4.0	28.0	2.0	0	420	7.0
(*Orville Redenbacher's Sweet & Buttery*)	180	2.0	16.0	14.0	<5	270	3.0
(*Orville Redenbacher's Ultimate!*)	160	2.0	16.0	11.0	0	440	4.0
(*Pop•Secret*), 3 tbsp.	180	3.0	17.0	12.0	0	330	3.0
(*Pop•Secret Jumbo Pop*), 3 tbsp.	170	2.0	18.0	11.0	0	280	3.0
(*Pop•Secret Jumbo Pop Movie Theater*), 3 tbsp.	170	2.0	18.0	11.0	0	320	3.0

Food and Measure	cal.	prot. (gms)	carbo. (gms)	fat (gms)	chol. (mgs)	sod. (mgs)	fiber (gms)
(*Pop•Secret* Light), 3 tbsp.	140	3.0	23.0	6.0	0	390	4.0
(*Pop•Secret* Movie Theater), 3 tbsp.	180	2.0	17.0	13.0	0	300	3.0
(*Pop•Secret* 94% Fat Free), 3 tbsp.	120	4.0	26.0	2.0	0	380	4.0
(*Simple Snacks* Organic), 1 oz., 4 cups*	160	3.0	19.0	8.0	0	320	3.0
extra (*Orville Redenbacher's* Movie Theater)	170	2.0	16.0	12.0	0	360	4.0
extra (*Pop•Secret*), 3 tbsp.	180	2.0	17.0	13.0	0	360	3.0
caramel:							
(*Orville Redenbacher's*)	180	1.0	23.0	10.0	0	45	2.0
apple (*Jolly Time Healthy Pop*)	110	4.0	23.0	2.0	0	380	6.0
cheddar:							
(*Orville Redenbacher's* Pour Over)	150	2.0	12.0	12.0	0	280	3.0
white (*Newman's Own*), 1.1 oz., 3½ cups*	190	5.0	18.0	10.0	5	550	3.0
cheese (*Jolly Time The Big Cheez*)	140	2.0	17.0	9.0	0	340	6.0
cinnamon butter (*Orville Redenbacher's Cinnabon*)	180	2.0	15.0	14.0	0	90	2.0
honey butter (*Orville Redenbacher's*)	180	2.0	16.0	12.0	0	170	3.0
honey or toffee butter (*Pop•Secret*), 3 tbsp.	190	2.0	15.0	13.0	0	160	3.0
yellow:							
(*Shiloh Farms*), ¼ cup	110	4.0	27.0	1.0	0	0	6.0
or white (*Jolly Time*)	100	4.0	24.0	1.0	0	0	6.0
white (*Orville Redenbacher's*), 3 tbsp.	120	4.0	29.0	1.5	0	0	6.0
Popcorn, popped:							
(*Chester's*), 3 cups	170	2.0	16.0	12.0	0	330	3.0
(*Hain PureSnax* Kettle Corn), 1½ cups	120	2.0	24.0	2.0	0	240	3.0

Food and Measure	cal.	prot. (gms)	carbo. (gms)	fat (gms)	chol. (mgs)	sod. (mgs)	fiber (gms)
Popcorn, popped *(cont.)*							
(*Shiloh Farms* Organic No Salt), 3½ cups .	130	2.0	19.0	5.0	0	0	3.0
(*Shiloh Farms* Organic Lite), 3½ cups	130	2.0	19.0	5.0	0	210	3.0
butter flavor:							
(*Orville Redenbacher's*), 2¾ cups	160	3.0	10.0	10.0	0	190	3.0
(*Snyder's*), ⅝ oz. ..	110	1.0	6.0	10.0	0	150	n.a.
(*Wise*), .5 oz.	80	1.0	7.0	5.0	0	190	1.0
caramel (*Jays* Fat Free), ¾ cup	110	<1.0	26.0	0	0	80	1.0
caramel nut, ½ cup:							
(*Cracker Jack*)	120	2.0	23.0	2.0	0	70	1.0
(*Orville Redenbacher's* Clusters)	130	2.0	22.0	4.5	<5	140	1.0
cheddar, white:							
(*Cape Cod*), 3 cups	170	4.0	13.0	12.0	8	270	2.0
(*Orville Redenbacher's*), 2¾ cups	150	3.0	16.0	9.0	<5	330	2.0
(*Shiloh Farms*), 3 cups	140	3.0	18.0	6.0	0	190	3.0
(*Smartfood*), 3 cups	140	4.0	19.0	6.0	<5	280	3.0
(*Wise*), .5 oz.	80	1.0	6.0	6.0	<5	200	1.0
cheddar, zesty (*Orville Redenbacher's*), 2¾ cups	170	3.0	15.0	12.0	<5	330	2.0
cheese:							
(*Chester's*), 3 cups .	200	3.0	17.0	13.0	<5	340	2.0
(*O-Ke-Doke*), 1 oz. ..	160	2.0	13.0	11.0	10	270	2.0
hot (*Wise*), .5 oz. ..	80	1.0	7.0	5.0	0	140	1.0
chocolate, milk (*Orville Redenbacher's* Drizzlers), ⅔ cup ..	150	1.0	23.0	6.0	<5	125	2.0
fudge, white (*Orville Redenbacher's* Drizzlers), ⅔ cups .	150	2.0	24.0	6.0	<5	140	<1.0
toffee, butter:							
(*Cracker Jack*), ¾ cup	140	2.0	22.0	4.0	0	100	1.0
(*Orville Redenbacher's* Clusters), ½ cup	130	3.0	20.0	5.0	<5	190	1.0
white (*Orville Redenbacher's* Tender), 2 tbsp.	180	3.0	14.0	13.0	0	340	2.0

Food and Measure	cal.	prot. (gms)	carbo. (gms)	fat (gms)	chol. (mgs)	sod. (mgs)	fiber (gms)
Popcorn cake:							
butter:							
(*Orville Redenbacher's*), 2 pcs., .6 oz. . . .	60	2.0	14.0	1.0	0	65	2.0
mini (*Orville Redenbacher's*), 6 pcs., .5 oz.	60	2.0	12.0	1.0	0	70	1.0
caramel:							
(*Orville Redenbacher's*), .4-oz. pc.	40	<1.0	10.0	0	0	15	<1.0
mini (*Orville Redenbacher's*), 6 pcs., .5 oz.	60	1.0	13.0	0	0	35	1.0
cheddar, white (*Orville Redenbacher's*), 2 pcs., .6 oz.	60	2.0	13.0	1.0	0	65	2.0
chocolate (*Orville Redenbacher's*), .4-oz. pc.	45	<1.0	10.0	0	0	20	<1.0
chocolate peanut crunch, mini (*Orville Redenbacher's*), 6 pcs., .5 oz.	60	2.0	12.0	.5	0	25	2.0
peanut caramel crunch, mini (*Orville Redenbacher's*), 6 pcs., .5 oz.	60	1.0	12.0	.5	0	30	1.0
and rice (*Lundberg Organic*), .7-oz. pc.	70	1.0	16.0	0	0	55	0
sour cream/onion, mini (*Orville Redenbacher's*), 6 pcs., .5 oz.	60	2.0	12.0	1.0	0	105	2.0
Popcorn seasoning:							
butter flavor, ½ tsp.:							
(*Fanci Food*)	0	0	0	0	0	630	0
(*Fanci Food Pop'n Topper*)	5	0	2.0	1.0	0	160	0
buttery (*Jolly Time*), ¼ tsp.	0	4.0	0	0	0	610	0
cheddar flavor (*Fanci Food*), ½ tsp.	5	0	<1.0	0	0	125	0
Poppy seeds:							
(*Shiloh Farms*), 1 tsp.	20	1.0	1.0	2.0	0	0	1.0
1 tsp.	15	.5	.7	1.3	0	1	.8

Food and Measure	cal.	prot. (gms)	carbo. (gms)	fat (gms)	chol. (mgs)	sod. (mgs)	fiber (gms)
Porgy, see "Scup"							
Pork (see also "Pork, refrigerated"), meat only, 4 oz.:							
back ribs, roasted, lean w/fat	420	27.5	0	33.5	134	115	0
ground, cooked	337	29.1	0	23.6	107	83	0
leg, see "Ham"							
loin, whole:							
braised, lean w/fat .	271	30.9	0	15.4	90	54	0
braised, lean only . .	231	32.4	0	10.3	90	57	0
broiled, lean w/fat .	274	30.9	0	15.8	90	70	0
broiled, lean only . .	238	32.4	0	11.1	90	73	0
roasted, lean w/fat .	281	30.7	0	16.6	93	67	0
roasted, lean only .	237	32.5	0	10.9	92	66	0
loin, blade:							
braised, lean w/fat .	366	24.8	0	28.8	96	62	0
braised, lean only . .	255	28.4	0	14.8	94	70	0
broiled, lean w/fat .	363	25.5	0	28.2	98	79	0
broiled, lean only . .	265	28.8	0	15.8	95	91	0
roasted, lean w/fat .	366	26.9	0	27.9	106	34	0
roasted, lean only .	280	30.2	0	16.8	106	33	0
loin, center:							
braised, lean w/fat .	280	31.7	0	16.0	98	67	0
braised, lean only . .	229	33.8	0	9.4	96	70	0
broiled, lean w/fat .	272	32.6	0	14.8	93	66	0
broiled, lean only . .	229	34.2	0	9.2	93	68	0
pan-fried, lean w/fat	314	33.9	0	18.8	104	91	0
pan-fried, lean only	263	36.5	0	11.9	104	97	
roasted, lean w/fat .	265	29.8	0	15.3	91	71	0
roasted, lean only .	226	31.2	0	10.2	90	75	0
loin, center rib:							
braised, lean w/fat .	284	30.2	0	17.1	83	45	0
braised, lean only . .	234	32.1	0	10.7	81	47	0
broiled, lean w/fat .	298	32.6	0	17.6	93	70	0
broiled, lean only . .	248	34.9	0	11.0	92	74	0
roasted, lean w/fat .	289	31.1	0	17.3	83	52	0
roasted, lean only .	253	32.6	0	12.6	81	53	0
loin, top, bone-in:							
braised, lean w/fat .	264	31.5	0	14.4	85	48	0
braised, lean only . .	229	33.0	0	9.7	83	48	0
broiled, lean w/fat .	260	34.0	0	12.7	92	71	0
broiled, lean only . .	230	35.3	0	8.8	91	74	0
roasted, lean w/fat .	256	31.9	0	13.0	89	50	0
roasted, lean only .	220	34.3	0	8.2	89	51	0

Food and Measure	cal.	prot. (gms)	carbo. (gms)	fat (gms)	chol. (mgs)	sod. (mgs)	fiber (gms)
loin, top, boneless:							
pan-fried, lean w/fat	291	32.9	0	16.8	89	62	0
pan-fried, lean only	255	34.6	0	11.9	87	65	0
ribs, country-style:							
braised, lean w/fat .	336	27.1	0	24.4	99	67	0
braised, lean only . .	265	29.5	0	15.4	98	71	0
roasted, lean w/fat .	372	26.5	0	28.7	104	59	0
roasted, lean only .	280	30.2	0	16.8	106	33	0
shoulder, whole:							
roasted, lean w/fat .	331	26.4	0	24.3	102	77	0
roasted, lean only .	261	28.7	0	15.4	102	85	0
shoulder, arm (picnic):							
braised, lean w/fat .	374	31.7	0	26.3	124	100	0
braised, lean only . .	281	36.6	0	13.8	129	116	0
roasted, lean w/fat .	360	26.6	0	27.2	107	79	0
roasted, lean only .	259	30.3	0	14.3	108	91	0
shoulder, Boston blade:							
braised, lean w/fat .	362	32.5	0	24.7	128	79	0
braised, lean only . .	310	35.3	0	17.6	132	85	0
broiled, lean w/fat .	294	29.0	0	18.8	108	78	0
broiled, lean only . .	257	30.3	0	14.2	107	84	0
roasted, lean w/fat .	305	26.2	0	21.4	98	76	0
roasted, lean only .	263	27.5	0	16.2	96	100	0
sirloin, bone-in:							
braised, lean w/fat .	278	28.8	0	17.1	93	58	0
braised, lean only . .	223	30.6	0	10.2	92	60	0
broiled, lean w/fat .	294	30.2	0	18.2	98	77	0
broiled, lean only . .	242	32.3	0	11.5	96	82	0
roasted, lean w/fat .	296	30.9	0	28.2	99	68	0
roasted, lean only .	245	32.7	0	11.7	98	71	0
sirloin, boneless:							
braised, lean w/fat .	214	30.1	0	9.5	92	52	0
braised, lean only . .	198	30.6	0	7.5	92	52	0
broiled, lean w/fat .	236	34.6	0	9.8	103	64	0
broiled, lean only . .	219	35.3	0	7.6	104	64	0
roasted, lean w/fat .	235	32.3	0	10.7	98	64	0
roasted, lean only .	225	32.7	0	9.4	98	64	0
spareribs, lean w/fat,							
braised	450	33.0	0	34.4	137	106	0
tenderloin:							
broiled, lean w/fat .	228	33.9	0	9.2	107	73	0
roasted, lean w/fat .	196	31.5	0	6.9	90	62	0
roasted, lean only .	186	31.9	0	5.5	90	64	0

Food and Measure	cal.	prot. (gms)	carbo. (gms)	fat (gms)	chol. (mgs)	sod. (mgs)	fiber (gms)
Pork, cured:							
arm (picnic), roasted:							
lean w/fat, 4 oz. . . .	318	23.2	0	24.2	66	1216	0
lean w/fat, chopped							
or diced, 1 cup . .	392	28.6	0	29.9	81	1501	0
lean only, 4 oz.	193	28.3	0	8.0	54	1396	0
lean only, chopped							
or diced, 1 cup . .	238	34.9	0	9.9	67	1723	0
blade roll, lean w/fat,							
roasted, 4 oz.	325	19.6	.4	26.6	76	1103	0
leg, see "Ham"							
Pork, freeze-dried,							
cooked, diced (*Mountain House*), ¾ cup	190	27.0	1.0	21.0	100	490	0
Pork, frozen or refrigerated, raw, 4 oz., except as noted:							
butts (*Always Tender*)	250	18.0	0	20.0	65	330	0
chop (see also "loin," below):							
(*Tyson*)	200	20.0	0	13.0	45	290	0
center cut (*Organic Valley*), 6-oz. chop	390	54.0	0	18.0	155	140	0
chop, boneless, center cut, marinated:							
(*Hatfield Simply Tender*), 4.25-oz. chop	160	23.0	0	6.0	65	380	0
(*Hatfield Simply Tender* Family Pack), 4.25-oz. chop . . .	150	24.0	0	6.0	709	340	0
thin (*Hatfield Simply Tender*), 2 chops, 4.4 oz.	160	24.0	0	7.0	65	380	0
chop, breaded, 1 chop:							
(*Tyson*), 6.25 oz. . .	180	20.0	10.0	7.0	55	220	0
lemon pepper (*Tyson*), 6.25 oz.	190	19.0	5.0	11.0	60	280	2.0
crown roast (*Always Tender*)	190	21.0	0	12.0	60	330	0
fresh, roast:							
(*Always Tender*) . . .	170	20.0	0	10.0	60	330	0
(*Tyson*)	130	21.0	0	4.5	65	300	0
ground, reduced fat (*Tyson*)	260	18.0	0	20.0	65	320	0

Food and Measure	cal.	prot. (gms)	carbo. (gms)	fat (gms)	chol. (mgs)	sod. (mgs)	fiber (gms)
loin, bone-in:							
(*Always Tender*) ...	190	18.0	0	12.0	54	277	0
center cut (*Tyson*) .	190	20.0	0	13.0	45	330	0
loin, boneless:							
(*Hatfield Simply Tender*)	140	22.0	0	5.0	65	310	0
center cut (*Always Tender*)	160	21.0	0	9.0	60	330	0
center cut chop (*Tyson*)	180	20.0	0	12.0	45	330	0
center cut chop, butterfly or thick (*Tyson*)	190	20.0	0	13.0	45	330	0
half loin (*Tyson*) ...	190	20.0	0	12.0	45	270	0
roast (*Tyson*)	190	20.0	0	12.0	45	290	0
roast, rib eye (*Tyson*)	200	20.0	0	13.0	45	290	0
loin fillet, marinated:							
honey mustard (*Always Tender*) .	140	20.0	4.0	5.0	45	510	0
mojo (*Always Tender*)	140	20.0	3.0	5.0	45	520	0
picnic (*Always Tender*)	230	19.0	0	18.0	70	330	0
rib ends, boneless (*Always Tender*) ...	160	21.0	0	9.0	60	330	0
ribs:							
(*Tyson*)	200	20.0	0	13.0	45	290	0
baby back (*Always Tender*)	240	18.0	0	18.0	80	330	0
country style (*Tyson*)	180	20.0	0	12.0	45	330	0
loin back ribs (*Tyson*)	250	17.0	0	20.0	70	360	0
spareribs (*Always Tender*)	280	17.0	0	18.0	80	330	0
spareribs (*Hatfield Simply Tender*) .	160	21.0	0	8.0	60	350	0
spareribs (*Tyson*) ..	290	16.0	0	24.0	80	330	0
roast, marinated (*Hatfield Simply Tender Chef's Prime*)	160	21.0	0	8.0	60	350	0
shoulder roast:							
(*Always Tender*) ...	180	19.0	0	11.0	60	480	0
onion garlic (*Always Tender*)	180	19.0	2.0	11.0	60	550	0
shoulder steak (*Tyson*)	260	17.0	0	21.0	70	320	0
sirloin roast:							
(*Always Tender*) ...	130	22.0	0	4.5	60	330	0
(*Tyson*)	140	21.0	0	6.0	65	300	0

Food and Measure	cal.	prot. (gms)	carbo. (gms)	fat (gms)	chol. (mgs)	sod. (mgs)	fiber (gms)
Pork, frozen or refrigerated, raw *(cont.)*							
stewing (*Tyson*)	130	21.0	0	4.5	65	300	0
tenderloin:							
(*Always Tender*) ...	120	22.0	0	3.0	60	330	0
(*Hatfield Simply*							
Tender)	120	21.0	0	3.0	65	340	0
(*Tyson*)	120	21.0	0	3.5	65	300	0
tenderloin, marinated:							
garlic (*Always Tender*)	130	19.0	1.0	5.0	45	690	0
mesquite (*Always*							
Tender)	130	19.0	2.0	5.0	45	780	0
peppercorn (*Always*							
Tender)	120	18.0	2.0	4.0	50	630	0
teriyaki (*Always*							
Tender)	140	20.0	5.0	4.0	50	500	0
Pork, frozen or refrigerated, cooked:							
w/barbecue sauce:							
pulled (*Hormel*), 2 oz.	90	8.0	10.0	2.5	25	510	0
pulled, w/sauce							
(*Smithfield*), 2 oz.	90	9.0	7.0	4.0	20	220	0
shredded, honey							
sauce w/ (*Lloyd's*),							
¼ cup	90	6.0	13.0	2.0	15	430	0
shredded, original							
sauce w/ (*Lloyd's*),							
¼ cup	90	6.0	11.0	2.0	15	380	0
sliced (*Hormel*), 5 oz.	200	23.0	23.0	4.5	50	1460	0
carnitas, Southwestern							
(*Hormel*), 2 oz. ...	60	7.0	2.0	2.0	25	380	0
patties, breaded (*Tyson*),							
3.2-oz. patty	260	11.0	17.0	16.0	25	600	2.0
ribs, barbecue sauce:							
baby back (*Lloyd's*),							
2 ribs w/honey							
hickory sauce,							
4.1 oz.	290	18.0	16.0	17.0	70	690	0
baby back (*Lloyd's*),							
2 ribs w/original							
sauce, 5 oz.	340	21.0	18.0	20.0	85	950	0
spareribs (*Boar's*							
Head), 3 ribs							
w/sauce, 5 oz. ..	400	22.0	9.0	31.0	70	430	0

Food and Measure	cal.	prot. (gms)	carbo. (gms)	fat (gms)	chol. (mgs)	sod. (mgs)	fiber (gms)
spareribs (*Lloyd's*), 2 ribs w/original sauce, 4.25 oz. . .	320	19.0	13.0	21.0	80	790	0
roast, 5 oz.:							
(*Hormel*)	180	29.0	0	7.0	85	570	0
in gravy (*Tyson*) . . .	140	22.0	3.0	4.5	55	840	0
chops, w/gravy (*Hormel*), 5 oz. . . .	160	22.0	3.0	5.0	55	750	0
strips, teriyaki (*Tyson*), 3 oz.	120	19.0	0	5.0	50	490	0
sweet and sour (*Simply Simmered*), 5 oz. . . .	150	14.0	21.0	1.5	5	840	5.0
Pork, pickled (see also "Pig's feet"), 2 oz.:							
hocks (*Hormel*)	110	9.0	0	8.0	45	530	0
tidbits (*Hormel*)	100	8.0	0	8.0	45	530	0
Pork back fat, 1 oz. . .	230	2.6	0	25.3	16	3	0
Pork belly, raw, 1 oz.	147	2.7	0	15.0	20	9	0
Pork coating mix, seasoned, ⅛ pkg., except as noted:							
(*Oven Fry* Extra Crispy)	60	2.0	11.0	1.5	0	340	0
(*Shake 'n Bake*), 1/16 of 6-oz. pkg. .	45	1.0	8.0	.5	0	230	0
chops (*McCormick Bag 'n Season*), 2 tsp. . .	15	0	4.0	0	0	590	0
herb roasted tenderloin (*McCormick Bag 'n Season*)	5	0	0	0	0	180	0
Pork entree, freeze-dried, sweet/sour, w/rice, 1 serving:							
(*Mountain House* Can), 1 cup	290	11.0	43.0	8.0	25	810	2.0
(*Mountain House*), ½ pouch	380	14.0	56.0	11.0	35	1060	3.0
Pork entree, frozen (see also "Pork, frozen or refrigerated, cooked"), 1 pkg.:							
apple glazed medallions (*Healthy Choice*), 10.8 oz.	310	16.0	46.0	6.0	35	450	4.0

Food and Measure	cal.	prot. (gms)	carbo. (gms)	fat (gms)	chol. (mgs)	sod. (mgs)	fiber (gms)
Pork entree, frozen *(cont.)*							
boneless, w/potato and corn (*Swanson*), 10.5 oz.	410	16.0	67.0	15.0	50	1250	4.0
w/cherry sauce (*Lean Cuisine Spa Cuisine*), 8.25 oz.	260	15.0	38.0	5.0	35	540	4.0
cutlet, boneless, breaded (*Stouffer's Homestyle*), 10 oz. .	370	15.0	33.0	20	40	1150	4.0
roast/roasted:							
(*Stouffer's Homestyle*), 9.5 oz.	350	20.0	43.0	11.0	50	960	4.0
honey (*Lean Cuisine Café Classics*), 9.5 oz.	230	18.0	18.0	9.0	50	580	5.0
sweet and sour (*Contessa* Minute Meal Bowl), 10.5 oz.	320	13.0	58.0	3.5	25	440	2.0
Pork entree mix:							
chops:							
breaded, mashed potato (*Pork Helper Oven Favorites*), 1/6 pkg.*	340	18.0	28.0	18.0	45	830	1.0
w/herb stuffing (*Campbell's Supper Bakes*), 1/6 pkg. mix	160	5.0	31.0	1.0	<5	770	2.0
and stuffing (*Pork Helper*), 1 cup* .	320	25.0	23.0	14.0	60	610	1.0
fried rice (*Pork Helper*), 1 cup*	340	27.0	24.0	15.0	145	680	<1.0
Pork fat, roasted, 1 oz.	167	2.2	0	17.5	24	177	0
Pork gravy, in jars, golden (*Campbell's*), 1/4 cup	40	1.0	3.0	3.0	10	320	0
Pork gravy mix (*McCormick*), 1/4 cup* .	20	0	4.0	0	0	370	0
Pork hocks, pickled (*Hormel*), 2 oz. . . .	100	8.0	0	8.0	45	690	0
Pork lunch meat (see also "Ham lunch meat"), roast, 2 oz.:							
(*Hatfield Deli Choice*) .	100	17.0	1.0	3.0	45	350	0

Food and Measure	cal.	prot. (gms)	carbo. (gms)	fat (gms)	chol. (mgs)	sod. (mgs)	fiber (gms)
barbecue flavor (*Dietz & Watson*)	60	9.0	3.0	1.0	30	290	0
black pepper crust, loin (*Hatfield Deli Choice*)	70	10.0	1.0	2.5	30	270	0
garlic, roasted, and onion, loin (*Hatfield Del Choice*)	70	10.0	1.0	2.5	30	340	0
Italian style:							
(*Dietz & Watson*) ..	50	9.0	1.0	1.0	30	290	0
loin (*Hatfield Deli Choice*)	70	10.0	1.0	2.5	30	390	0
oven roasted (*Sara Lee*)	70	9.0	1.0	3.0	40	440	0
sirloin (*Dietz & Watson*)	70	12.0	0	2.0	30	320	0
Pork rind snack, .5 oz., except as noted:							
(*Baken-ets* Cracklins) .	90	7.0	<1.0	6.0	15	550	<1.0
(*Baken-ets* Fried Skins)	80	7.0	0	5.0	20	310	0
(*Wise Original*), .6 oz.	90	9.0	1.0	6.0	25	330	0
barbecue:							
(*Baken-ets* Sweet & Tangy)	80	7.0	1.0	5.0	20	400	1.0
(*Wise* Hot & Spicy), .6 oz.	90	9.0	1.0	5.0	20	480	0
(*Wise* Sweet & Mild), .6 oz.	90	9.0	1.0	8.0	20	300	0
hot:							
(*Baken-ets* Hot 'n Spicy Cracklins) .	80	7.0	<1.0	5.0	20	330	<1.0
(*Baken-ets* Hot 'n Spicy Skins)	80	7.0	<1.0	5.0	20	470	<1.0
Pork seasoning mix, see "Pork coating mix"							
Pork tidbits, pickled (*Hormel*), 2 oz. ...	100	8.0	0	8.0	45	690	0
Portugese sausage, see "Linguica sausage"							
Pot pie, see specific entree listings							
Pot roast, see "Beef dinner, frozen" and "Beef entree, frozen"							

Food and Measure	cal.	prot. (gms)	carbo. (gms)	fat (gms)	chol. (mgs)	sod. (mgs)	fiber (gms)
Pot stickers, see "Dumplings" and "Chicken entree, frozen"							
Potato:							
raw:							
(*Del Monte*), 1 medium, 5.2 oz.	100	4.0	26.0	0	0	0	3.0
(*Frieda's* Baby/ Fingerling/Red/ Purple/Yukon Gold/ Yellow Finnish), ½ cup, 3 oz.	70	2.0	15.0	0	0	5	1.0
(*Frieda's* Fingerling Bag), 4 pcs., 5.2 oz.	100	4.0	25.0	0	0	0	3.0
unpeeled:							
1 large, 6.5 oz. . . .	145	3.8	33.1	.2	0	11	2.9
1 long, 7.1 oz. . . .	160	4.2	36.3	.2	0	12	3.2
peeled, 2½" potato .	88	2.3	20.1	.1	0	7	1.8
peeled, diced, ½ cup	59	1.6	13.5	.1	0	5	1.2
baked:							
in skin, 4¾" x 2⅓" .	220	4.7	51.0	.2	0	16	4.8
w/out skin, 2⅓" . . .	145	3.1	33.6	.2	0	8	2.3
w/out skin, ½ cup .	57	1.2	13.2	.1	0	3	.9
skin only, 1 oz.	56	1.2	13.1	0	0	6	2.2
boiled in skin, peeled:							
2½" potato, 4.8 oz.	118	2.5	27.4	.1	0	6	2.4
½ cup	68	1.5	15.7	.1	0	3	1.4
boiled w/out skin:							
2½" potato	116	2.3	27.0	.1	0	7	2.4
½ cup	67	1.3	15.6	.1	0	4	1.4
microwaved in skin:							
w/skin, 4¾" x 2⅓" potato	212	4.9	48.7	.2	0	16	4.7
peeled, ½ cup	78	1.6	18.2	.1	0	5	1.2
skin only, 2 oz.	75	2.5	16.8	.1	0	9	3.2
mashed, w/whole milk:							
½ cup	81	2.0	18.4	.6	2	318	2.1
w/butter, ½ cup . . .	111	2.0	17.5	4.4	13	309	2.1
w/margarine, ½ cup	111	2.0	17.5	4.4	2	309	2.1
Potato, can or jar:							
w/liquid, 1 cup	132	3.6	29.7	.3	0	651	4.2
drained, 1 cup	108	2.5	24.5	.4	0	394	4.1

Food and Measure	cal.	prot. (gms)	carbo. (gms)	fat (gms)	chol. (mgs)	sod. (mgs)	fiber (gms)
whole:							
(*Butterfield* New),							
3½ pcs.	90	2.0	20.0	0	0	330	2.0
(*Del Monte* New),							
2 pcs.	60	1.0	13.0	0	0	360	2.0
(*Sunshine*), 3 pcs. .	90	2.0	20.0	0	0	330	2.0
(*S&W* Small), 2 pcs.	60	1.0	13.0	0	0	360	2.0
1.2-oz. potato	21	.5	4.8	.1	0	77	.8
diced:							
(*Butterfield* New),							
⅔ cup	100	2.0	22.0	0	0	350	3.0
(*Del Monte* New),							
½ cup	45	1.0	11.0	0	0	280	<1.0
sliced:							
(*Butterfield* New),							
½ cup	100	2.0	22.0	0	0	390	4.0
(*Del Monte* New),							
⅔ cup	60	1.0	13.0	0	0	360	2.0
Potato, dried, see							
"Potato dish, freeze-							
dried" and "Potato							
dish, mix"							
Potato, frozen (see also							
"Potato dish, frozen"),							
3 oz., except as							
noted:							
whole, baby (*Birds Eye*),							
7 pcs., 4 oz.	80	2.0	17.0	0	0	25	1.0
fried/fries:							
(*Cascadian Farm*							
Oven French Fries)	100	2.0	14.0	4.0	0	20	0
(*Ian's* Natural							
Harvest Fries),							
2.5 oz.	78	1.0	13.0	2.5	0	5	1.0
(*Ian's* Natural Quick							
Fries)	150	2.0	23.0	6.0	0	100	2.0
(*Ian's Alphatots*							
Natural), 3.5 oz. .	155	2.0	23.0	7.0	0	160	.5
(*McCain Smiles*)	170	2.0	24.0	6.5	0	390	2.0
(*Ore-Ida Golden Fries*)	120	2.0	17.0	3.0	0	340	2.0
(*Tree of Life*)	110	2.0	19.0	3.0	0	75	1.0
cheddar cheese (*Ian's*							
Natural)	180	4.0	29.0	6.0	5	500	2.0
crinkle cut (*Kineret*)	120	2.0	20.0	4.0	0	25	2.0

Food and Measure	cal.	prot. (gms)	carbo. (gms)	fat (gms)	chol. (mgs)	sod. (mgs)	fiber (gms)
Potato, frozen, fried/fries *(cont.)*							
crinkle cut (*McCain*)	130	2.0	21.0	4.0	0	320	2.0
crinkle cut (*McCain Premium Golden Crisp*)	150	2.0	23.0	5.0	0	380	2.0
crinkle cut (*Ore-Ida Golden Crinkles*)	130	2.0	17.0	4.0	0	340	2.0
crinkle cut, seasoned (*McCain Premium Golden Crisp*) . . .	150	2.0	20.0	7.0	0	410	2.0
cross cut, w/skin (*McCain Premium Golden Crisp*) . . .	170	2.0	21.0	9.0	0	490	2.0
shoestring (*Cascadian Farm*)	140	2.0	21.0	5.0	0	380	2.0
shoestring (*McCain*)	140	2.0	21.0	5.5	0	290	2.0
shoestring (*McCain 5-Minute Fries!*) .	200	2.0	32.0	7.5	0	340	3.0
shoestring (*McCain Premium Golden Crisp*)	150	2.0	20.0	7.0	0	400	2.0
shoestring (*Ore-Ida*)	150	2.0	19.0	6.0	0	370	2.0
spirals, seasoned (*McCain Premium Golden Crisp*) . . .	150	2.0	18.0	7.5	0	390	2.0
steak (*McCain*)	120	2.0	21.0	3.0	0	330	2.0
steak (*McCain Premium Golden Crisp*)	130	2.0	23.0	3.0	0	380	1.0
steak (*Ore-Ida*)	120	2.0	17.0	3.0	0	340	2.0
straight cut (*McCain*)	120	2.0	20.0	4.0	0	360	2.0
straight cut (*McCain Premium Golden Crisp*)	150	2.0	23.0	5.0	0	380	2.0
waffle (*Ore-Ida*) . . .	160	2.0	22.0	6.0	0	300	2.0
wedges, w/skin (*McCain Premium Golden Crisp*) . . .	130	2.0	17.0	6.0	0	390	2.0
hash browns:							
(*Cascadian Farm*) . .	70	1.0	17.0	0	0	0	2.0
(*Ore-Ida Golden Patties*), 2.4-oz. patty	140	1.0	15.0	8.0	0	170	2.0

Food and Measure	cal.	prot. (gms)	carbo. (gms)	fat (gms)	chol. (mgs)	sod. (mgs)	fiber (gms)
w/onions and peppers (*Cascadian Farm* Country Style)	35	1.0	9.0	0	0	10	2.0
mashed:							
(*Ore-Ida*), ⅔ cup ..	100	2.0	18.0	3.0	<5	180	2.0
creamy (*Reser's* Deluxe), ½ cup .	160	3.0	18.0	8.0	15	500	2.0
garlic (*Reser's*), ½ cup	150	3.0	19.0	6.0	15	430	2.0
garlic or plain (*Diner's* Choice), ⅔ cup .	170	3.0	19.0	10.0	20	520	1.0
onion, caramelized (*Reser's*), ½ cup	160	3.0	21.0	8.0	10	440	2.0
puffs:							
(*Cascadian Farm* Spud Puppies) ..	130	2.0	14.0	8.0	0	480	0
(*McCain Tasti Tater*)	160	2.0	20.0	7.5	0	410	3.0
(*Ore-Ida Tater Tots*)	150	2.0	20.0	7.0	0	420	2.0
roasting, seasoned:							
(*McCain Roasters* All-American) ...	120	2.0	21.0	3.0	0	370	2.0
(*McCain Roasters* South of the Border)	140	2.0	25.0	3.0	0	360	2.0
and vegetable blend (*Birds Eye*), ¾ cup .	40	1.0	8.0	0	0	20	1.0
Potato, mix, see "Potato dish, mix"							
Potato, sweet, see "Sweet potato"							
Potato chips/crisps (see also "Potato soy crisps" and "Sweet potato chips"), 1 oz., except as noted:							
(*Barbara's* Unsalted) .	150	2.0	15.0	10.0	0	20	1.0
(*Barbara's/Barbara's* Ripple)	150	2.0	15.0	10.0	0	180	1.0
(*Cape Cod* Classic) ...	150	2.0	17.0	8.0	0	110	1.0
(*Cape Cod* 40% Reduced Fat)	130	2.0	18.0	6.0	0	110	1.0
(*Cape Cod* No Salt) ..	150	2.0	14.0	10.0	0	0	<1.0

Food and Measure	cal.	prot. (gms)	carbo. (gms)	fat (gms)	chol. (mgs)	sod. (mgs)	fiber (gms)
Potato chips/crisps *(cont.)*							
(*Cape Cod* Robust Russet)	150	2.0	16.0	8.0	0	150	1.0
(*Cape Cod* Whole Earth Classic)	150	2.0	17.0	8.0	0	110	1.0
(*Cape Cod* Whole Earth 40% Reduced Fat) .	130	2.0	18.0	6.0	0	110	1.0
(*Garden of Eatin'*) . . .	150	2.0	16.0	9.0	0	140	1.0
(*Herr's/Herr's* Ripples)	140	2.0	16.0	8.0	0	180	1.0
(*Jays*)	150	2.0	14.0	10.0	0	190	1.0
(*Kettle Chips* Lightly Salted)	150	2.0	15.0	9.0	0	110	1.0
(*Kettle Chips* Lightly Salted Low Fat) . . .	110	3.0	22.0	1.5	0	160	2.0
(*Kettle Chips* Unsalted)	150	2.0	15.0	9.0	0	0	1.0
(*Krunchers!* Original) .	140	2.0	16.0	8.0	0	160	1.0
(*Lay's* Chicago Steakhouse)	150	2.0	15.0	9.0	0	230	1.0
(*Lay's* Classic)	150	2.0	15.0	10.0	0	180	1.0
(*Lay's* Deli Style)	150	1.0	16.0	10.0	0	180	1.0
(*Lay's* Original Baked!)	110	2.0	23.0	1.5	0	150	2.0
(*Lay's* Original Light) .	75	2.0	18.0	0	0	200	1.0
(*Lay's* Original Wavy) .	150	2.0	15.0	10.0	0	180	1.0
(*Lay's Stax* Original) . .	160	1.0	16.0	10.0	0	180	1.0
(*Miss Vickie's* Original), 1 pkg.	200	2.0	22.0	13.0	0	170	1.0
(*Munchos*)	160	1.0	16.0	10.0	0	230	1.0
(*Pringles* Original) . . .	160	1.0	15.0	11.0	0	170	1.0
(*Pringles* Reduced Fat)	140	2.0	19.0	7.0	0	135	1.0
(*Ruffles* Original)	160	2.0	14.0	10.0	0	160	1.0
(*Ruffles* Original Baked!)	120	2.0	21.0	3.0	0	200	2.0
(*Ruffles* Original Light)	70	2.0	17.0	0	0	190	1.0
(*Snyder's*)	140	2.0	19.0	6.0	0	90	n.a.
(*Snyder's* Coney Island)	150	2.0	20.0	7.0	0	240	n.a.
(*Snyder's* Ripple)	140	2.0	18.0	6.0	0	100	n.a.
(*Snyder's* Unsalted) . .	140	2.0	19.0	6.0	0	0	n.a.
(*Terra* Potpourri)	140	2.0	17.0	7.0	0	110	4.0
(*Terra* Yukon Gold) . . .	130	2.0	19.0	5.0	0	80	0
(*Terra* Blues)	140	3.0	17.0	6.0	0	110	1.0
(*Terra* Red Bliss)	140	1.0	18.0	7.0	0	110	2.0
(*Wise* Original)	150	2.0	14.0	10.0	0	190	1.0
(*Wise* Choice Crisps) .	110	2.0	19.0	3.0	0	250	1.0
(*Wise* New York Deli)	130	2.0	13.0	8.0	0	150	<1.0
aioli (*Terra Frites*)	150	2.0	18.0	8.0	0	160	3.0

Food and Measure	cal.	prot. (gms)	carbo. (gms)	fat (gms)	chol. (mgs)	sod. (mgs)	fiber (gms)
au gratin (*Lay's* Wavy)	150	2.0	14.0	10.0	<5	200	1.0
barbecue:							
(*Cape Cod* Beachside)	150	2.0	17.0	8.0	0	160	1.0
(*Kettle Chips* Classic)	150	2.0	16.0	8.0	0	190	1.0
(*Kettle Chips Chipotle Chili Barbecue Organic*)	150	2.0	16.0	8.0	0	160	2.0
(*Lay's* Country Natural)	150	2.0	15.0	9.0	0	150	1.0
(*Lay's* KC Masterpiece)	150	2.0	15.0	10.0	0	200	1.0
(*Lay's K.C. Masterpiece* Baked!) ...	120	2.0	22.0	3.0	0	210	2.0
(*Lay's K.C. Masterpiece* Light)	75	2.0	17.0	0	0	250	1.0
(*Ruffles KC Masterpiece*)	150	2.0	16.0	10.0	0	190	1.0
(*Snyder's*)	150	2.0	21.0	6.0	0	230	n.a.
(*Snyder's* Rib)	140	2.0	17.0	7.0	0	290	n.a.
(*Terra* Yukon Gold) .	130	3.0	19.0	5.0	0	90	2.0
(*Wise*)	160	2.0	15.0	10.0	0	210	1.0
hickory (*Kettle Chips* Low Fat)	110	3.0	22.0	1.5	0	170	2.0
hickory (*Lay's* Wavy)	150	2.0	16.0	9.0	0	210	1.0
mesquite (*Lay's* Kettle Cooked) ..	140	2.0	16.0	8.0	0	210	<1.0
mesquite, w/soy (*Wise Choice* Crisps)	110	7.0	14.0	3.0	0	370	3.0
mesquite, sweet (*Pringles*)	150	2.0	15.0	10.0	0	200	1.0
Cajun (*Pringles*)	160	1.0	14.0	11.0	0	200	1.0
cheddar, white (*Pringles*)	160	2.0	15.0	10.0	0	180	0
cheddar w/herbs (*Kettle Chips* New York)	150	2.0	15.0	8.0	0	190	1.0
cheddar and bacon (*T.G.I. Friday's*)	150	<1.0	17.0	9.0	0	170	1.0
cheddar and sour cream:							
(*Ruffles*)	160	2.0	14.0	10.0	0	230	1.0
(*Ruffles* Baked!) ...	120	2.0	22.0	3.0	0	220	2.0
(*Ruffles* Light)	75	3.0	16.0	0	0	230	1.0
(*Wise* Ridgies)	150	2.0	15.0	9.0	0	190	1.0

Food and Measure	cal.	prot. (gms)	carbo. (gms)	fat (gms)	chol. (mgs)	sod. (mgs)	fiber (gms)
Potato chips/crisps *(cont.)*							
cheese flavor:							
(*Pringles* Cheezums)	150	2.0	15.0	10.0	0	180	0
(*Wise Cheez Doodles*)	150	2.0	14.0	10.0	0	200	1.0
chili cheese (*Pringles*)	160	1.0	15.0	11.0	0	230	1.0
chipotle (*Wise*)	150	2.0	14.0	10.0	0	200	1.0
cottage cut (*Wise*) . . .	140	2.0	12.0	9.0	0	170	<1.0
dill:							
(*Snyder's* Kosher) .	140	2.0	20.0	6.0	0	360	n.a.
pickle (*Lay's*)	160	2.0	13.0	10.0	0	360	1.0
and sour cream							
(*Kettle Chips*							
Krinkle Cut)	140	2.0	15.0	8.0	0	170	1.0
garlic, roasted:							
and chive (*Wise*							
Choice Crisps) . .	110	2.0	20.0	3.0	0	200	1.0
Parmesan (*Yukon*							
Red Bliss)	140	2.0	16.0	7.0	0	115	2.0
guacamole (*Lay's Cool*							
Guacamole)	160	2.0	15.0	11.0	0	250	1.0
herb:							
fine (*Terra Red Bliss*)	140	2.0	18.0	7.0	0	70	3.0
garden (*Cape Cod*)	130	2.0	19.0	6.0	0	160	1.0
Italian, w/soy (*Wise*							
Choice Crisps) . .	110	8.0	13.0	3.0	0	320	3.0
honey Dijon (*Kettle*							
Chips)	150	2.0	16.0	8.0	0	150	1.0
hot:							
(*Lay's Flamin' Hot*)	160	2.0	15.0	10.0	0	330	1.0
(*Pringles* Fiery) . . .	160	2.0	15.0	10.0	0	135	1.0
(*Snyder's* Louisiana),							
1.5 oz.	220	3.0	30.0	10.0	0	440	n.a.
(*Wise* Mighty Hot)	150	1.0	15.0	10.0	0	320	1.0
Buffalo wing							
(*Snyder's*)	150	2.0	20.0	7.0	0	330	n.a.
jalapeño:							
(*Lay's* Kettle Cooked)	140	2.0	16.0	8.0	0	170	1.0
(*Miss Vickie's*), 1 pkg.	190	2.0	22.0	11.0	0	240	1.0
(*Snyder's*)	150	2.0	20.0	6.0	0	330	n.a.
cheddar (*Cape Cod*)	140	2.0	16.0	8.0	0	260	2.0
cheddar (*Kettle Chips*							
Krinkle Cut)	150	2.0	16.0	9.0	0	210	1.0
w/tequila and lime							
(*Kettle Chips*) . . .	150	2.0	16.0	9.0	0	160	2.0

Food and Measure	cal.	prot. (gms)	carbo. (gms)	fat (gms)	chol. (mgs)	sod. (mgs)	fiber (gms)
ketchup (*Herr's Heinz*)	150	2.0	15.0	10.0	0	300	1.0
lime (*Lay's* Limón) ...	150	2.0	15.0	10.0	0	370	1.0
malt vinegar (*Terra* Frites)	150	2.0	18.0	8.0	0	200	3.0
mustard and honey (*Kettle Chips* Low Fat)	110	3.0	22.0	1.5	0	160	2.0
onion, French (*Kettle Chips* Low Fat)	110	3.0	22.0	1.5	0	200	2.0
onion and garlic:							
(*Garden of Eatin'*) .	140	2.0	16.0	8.0	0	140	1.0
(*Terra* Yukon Gold) .	130	2.0	19.0	5.0	0	65	1.0
(*Wise*)	150	2.0	14.0	10.0	0	310	1.0
Parmesan garlic (*Garden of Eatin'*) .	140	2.0	16.0	8.0	0	160	1.0
pepper, cracked (*Snyder's*)	140	2.0	20.0	6.0	0	230	n.a.
pizza (*Pringles* Pizzalicious)	160	1.0	14.0	11.0	0	200	1.0
ranch:							
(*Lay's Hidden Valley Ranch* Wavy) ...	150	2.0	16.0	10.0	0	200	1.0
(*Pringles* Ranch-Rageous)	150	2.0	15.0	10.0	0	130	1.0
red pepper, roasted, w/goat cheese (*Kettle Chips*)	150	2.0	16.0	8.0	0	180	1.0
salsa w/mesquite (*Kettle Chips*)	140	2.0	15.0	8.0	0	160	1.0
salt and pepper:							
(*Terra* Yukon Gold) .	130	2.0	19.0	5.0	0	120	1.0
fresh ground (*Kettle Chips*) ...	140	2.0	16.0	9.0	0	170	2.0
fresh ground (*Kettle Chips* Krinkle Cut)	140	2.0	15.0	8.0	0	170	1.0
sea salt (*Kettle Chips* Organic)	150	2.0	16.0	9.0	0	210	2.0
sea salt (*Terra* Kettles)	140	2.0	18.0	6.0	0	65	<1.0
sea salt, cracked pepper (*Cape Cod* Nantucket Spice)	140	2.0	16.0	7.0	0	160	1.0
salt and vinegar:							
(*Garden of Eatin'*) .	150	2.0	16.0	9.0	0	210	1.0
(*Lay's*)	150	2.0	15.0	10.0	0	380	1.0
(*Pringles*)	160	1.0	15.0	11.0	0	200	1.0
(*Snyder's*)	140	2.0	19.0	6.0	0	250	1.0

Food and Measure	cal.	prot. (gms)	carbo. (gms)	fat (gms)	chol. (mgs)	sod. (mgs)	fiber (gms)
Potato chips/crisps, salt and vinegar *(cont.)*							
(*Terra* Yukon Gold) .	130	2.0	20.0	5.0	0	110	2.0
(*Wise*)	150	2.0	14.0	10.0	0	290	1.0
sea salt (*Cape Cod*)	150	2.0	17.0	8.0	0	130	1.0
sea salt (*Kettle Chips*)	150	2.0	15.0	8.0	0	180	1.0
sea salt (*Lay's* Kettle Cooked)	140	2.0	17.0	7.0	0	260	1.0
sea salt (*Miss Vicklie's*), 1 pkg. .	190	2.0	24.0	10.0	0	360	1.0
sea salt:							
(*Lay's* Natural)	150	2.0	15.0	10.0	0	150	1.0
(*Ruffles* Natural Reduced Fat) . . .	140	2.0	17.0	7.0	0	160	1.0
w/blue potato (*Terra* Kettles)	140	2.0	18.0	6.0	0	90	<1.0
w/sweet potato (*Terra* Kettles) . .	140	2.0	18.0	7.0	0	120	<1.0
seasoned salt (*Terra Frites*)	150	2.0	18.0	8.0	0	160	3.0
shoestring (*Jays*)	150	1.0	16.0	9.0	0	190	1.0
sour cream and onion:							
(*Kettle Chips*)	150	2.0	16.0	9.0	0	110	2.0
(*Lay's*)	160	2.0	12.0	11.0	<5	210	1.0
(*Lay's* Baked!)	120	2.0	21.0	3.0	0	210	2.0
(*Pringles*)	160	2.0	15.0	10.0	0	135	1.0
(*Pringles* Reduced Fat)	140	2.0	18.0	7.0	0	140	1.0
(*Ruffles*)	160	2.0	14.0	10.0	0	190	1.0
(*Snyder's*)	150	2.0	19.0	7.0	0	270	1.0
(*Wise* Ridgies)	150	2.0	14.0	10.0	0	210	1.0
sun-dried tomato and balsamic vinegar (*Terra Red Bliss*) . .	140	2.0	18.0	7.0	0	85	3.0
taco (*Snyder's* Fiesta)	150	2.0	20.0	7.0	0	270	1.0
tomato and onion (*Terra Frites* Américaine)	150	2.0	18.0	8.0	0	180	2.0
yogurt and green onion:							
(*Barbara's*)	150	2.0	15.0	9.0	0	240	1.0
(*Kettle Chips*)	150	2.0	15.0	8.0	0	170	1.0
(*Terra* Yukon Gold) .	130	2.0	19.0	5.0	0	75	1.0
Potato dish, can or pkg.:							
au gratin:							
(*Del Monte Savory Sides*), ½ cup . .	80	2.0	13.0	2.5	0	470	1.0

Food and Measure	cal.	prot. (gms)	carbo. (gms)	fat (gms)	chol. (mgs)	sod. (mgs)	fiber (gms)
w/ham (*Hormel Cure 81* Bowl), 10 oz. . .	310	12.0	32.0	15.0	35	960	1.0
w/chickpeas (*Tasty Bite* Bombay), ½ pkg. . . .	105	5.0	13.0	4.0	0	412	3.0
scalloped:							
(*Glory*), ½ cup	70	2.0	14.0	.5	0	590	1.0
and ham (*Dinty Moore* Cup),							
1 cont.	230	9.0	20.0	12.0	35	1000	2.0
smothered, ½ cup:							
beef gravy (*Glory*) . . .	50	2.0	11.0	0	0	600	<1.0
chicken gravy (*Glory*)	50	1.0	11.0	0	0	820	<1.0
herbs and garlic (*Glory*)	50	1.0	11.0	0	0	540	1.0
Potato dish, freeze-dried, 1 serving:							
and beef (*Mountain House*), ½ pouch . .	250	12.0	38.0	6.0	20	1040	3.0
and cheese:							
(*Mountain House*), ½ pouch	240	10.0	38.0	5.0	15	710	3.0
cheddar, w/chives (*AlpineAire*)	220	7.0	39.0	5.0	n.a.	550	3.0
hash browns (*Alpine-Aire* Red & Green) .	220	3.0	24.0	11.0	0	200	0
mashed:							
(*AlpineAire* Instant)	100	2.0	22.0	0	0	10	0
garlic (*AlpineAire*) .	25	1.0	5.0	1.0	0	130	0
Potato dish, frozen, 1 pkg., except as noted:							
au gratin:							
(*Stouffer's*), ½ cup	150	5.0	18.0	6.0	15	510	2.0
baked, twice, butter flavor (*Ore-Ida*), 5 oz.	170	4.0	26.0	6.0	0	350	2.0
cheddar:							
(*Lean Cuisine Everyday Favorites*), 10⅜ oz.	260	13.0	36.0	7.0	25	620	5.0
bake (*Stouffer's*), 10 oz.	240	7.0	19.0	15.0	20	460	1.0
cheddar broccoli:							
(*Healthy Choice*), 10.5 oz.	280	13.0	41.0	7.0	25	550	6.0

Food and Measure	cal.	prot. (gms)	carbo. (gms)	fat (gms)	chol. (mgs)	sod. (mgs)	fiber (gms)
Potato dish, frozen *(cont.)*							
pancakes, see "Potato pancakes"							
roasted, w/broccoli, cheese sauce:							
(*Birds Eye*), ⅔ cup	100	2.0	15.0	4.0	0	470	1.0
(*Green Giant*), ¾ cup	120	4.0	19.0	3.5	5	520	2.0
(*Lean Cuisine Everyday Favorites*), 10.25 oz.	230	11.0	35.0	5.0	15	660	5.0
(*Smart Ones*), 10 oz.	250	8.0	33.0	6.0	20	510	4.0
roasted, w/garlic and herbs (*Green Giant*), 1¼ cups	270	3.0	33.0	14.0	0	610	4.0
whipped, and gravy (*Stouffer's*), ½ of 10-oz. pkg.	170	2.0	17.0	10.0	15	490	2.0
Potato dish, mix:							
au gratin:							
(*Betty Crocker*), ⅔ cup*	150	3.0	22.0	6.0	<5	650	1.0
cheesy (*Velveeta*), 2.1 oz. mix	180	5.0	26.0	6.0	10	770	2.0
bacon and cheddar, twice baked (*Betty Crocker*), ¾ cup*	180	6.0	21.0	9.0	85	540	1.0
broccoli au gratin (*Betty Crocker*), ⅔ cup*	120	3.0	20.0	4.0	0	660	2.0
cheddar:							
au gratin, cheesy (*Betty Crocker Deluxe*), ½ cup*	180	3.0	22.0	9.0	5	660	1.0
and bacon (*Betty Crocker*), ⅔ cup*	130	3.0	21.0	4.5	<5	700	1.0
cheese, three (*Betty Crocker*), ⅔ cup*	130	3.0	21.0	4.0	<5	600	1.0
garlic, roasted (*Betty Crocker*), ½ cup*	120	2.0	19.0	4.0	0	530	1.0
hash browns (*Betty Crocker*), ½ cup*	160	2.0	26.0	5.0	0	320	2.0
julienne (*Betty Crocker*), ⅔ cup*	110	2.0	19.0	3.5	<5	650	1.0
mashed:							
(*Barbara's*), ⅓ cup	70	2.0	17.0	0	0	10	1.0

Food and Measure	cal.	prot. (gms)	carbo. (gms)	fat (gms)	chol. (mgs)	sod. (mgs)	fiber (gms)
w/beef gravy, hearty (*Betty Crocker* Homestyle), ¾ cup*	170	3.0	24.0	7.0	0	760	2.0
butter, creamy (*Betty Crocker* Homestyle), ½ cup*	160	3.0	21.0	7.0	5	430	1.0
butter and herb (*Betty Crocker*), ½ cup*	160	3.0	20.0	7.0	<5	460	1.0
cheddar and bacon (*Betty Crocker*), ½ cup*	150	3.0	20.0	7.0	5	390	1.0
cheese, four (*Betty Crocker*), ½ cup*	160	3.0	20.0	7.0	5	530	1.0
w/chicken gravy, roasted (*Betty Crocker* Homestyle), ¾ cup*	170	3.0	25.0	7.0	5	670	1.0
chicken and herb (*Betty Crocker*), ½ cup*	150	3.0	21.0	7.0	<5	510	1.0
garlic, roasted (*Betty Crocker*), ½ cup*	160	3.0	20.0	8.0	<5	400	1.0
garlic, roasted, and cheddar (*Betty Crocker*), ½ cup*	160	3.0	20.0	7.0	<5	490	1.0
sour cream and chive (*Betty Crocker*), ½ cup*	150	3.0	21.0	7.0	5	450	1.0
ranch (*Betty Crocker*), ⅔ cup*	130	3.0	23.0	3.5	<5	670	1.0
scalloped: (*Betty Crocker*), ½ cup*	130	3.0	22.0	4.0	<5	620	1.0
bacon, cheesy (*Velveeta*), 2.1 oz. mix	190	6.0	26.0	7.0	15	840	2.0
cheesy (*Betty Crocker*), ½ cup*	150	3.0	21.0	6.0	<5	620	2.0
creamy roasted garlic (*Betty Crocker* Deluxe), ⅔ cup*	160	3.0	25.0	5.0	10	700	1.0
sour cream and chive (*Betty Crocker*), ⅔ cup*	120	2.0	21.0	4.0	<5	690	1.0

Food and Measure	cal.	prot. (gms)	carbo. (gms)	fat (gms)	chol. (mgs)	sod. (mgs)	fiber (gms)
Potato entree, see "Potato dish"							
Potato flour:							
(*Shiloh Farms*), ¼ cup	100	2.0	23.0	0	0	10	2.0
1 cup	571	11.0	132.9	.5	0	88	9.4
Potato nuggets, frozen, w/cheese and dill, breaded (*Kineret*), 3½ pcs., 2.8 oz. . . .	180	6.0	19.0	9.0	10	440	5.0
Potato pancake, frozen:							
(*Dr. Praeger's*), 1.5-oz. pc.	75	2.0	10.0	3.0	15	150	1.0
(*Dr. Praeger's* Bombay), 1.45-oz. pc.	75	2.0	10.0	3.0	15	150	1.0
(*Kineret* Latkas), 1.5-oz. pc.	70	1.0	9.0	3.0	0	100	1.0
mini (*Kineret* Latkas), 11 pcs., 3 oz.	170	2.0	21.0	8.0	0	320	2.0
nuggets (*Dr. Praeger's*), 4 pcs. 1.4 oz.	60	2.0	7.0	2.5	15	95	<1.0
Potato pancake mix (*Carmel*), 3 tbsp. . . .	80	2.0	18.0	1.0	0	500	2.0
Potato salad, refrigerated:							
(*Blue Ridge Farm*), 4 oz.	180	2.0	22.0	10.0	10	550	1.0
(*Hellmann's* Classic), 4.9 oz.	290	2.0	27.0	19.0	10	650	3.0
(*Reser's* Homestyle), ½ cup	190	3.0	28.0	8.0	10	590	3.0
(*Reser's* Regular), ½ cup	230	3.0	28.0	12.0	10	490	3.0
bacon cheese (*Hellmann's*), 4.9 oz. . . .	300	3.0	24.0	22.0	15	660	2.0
w/egg (*Reser's*), ½ cup	240	3.0	29.0	13.0	15	560	3.0
Potato salad mix (*Suddenly Salad*), ¾ cup*	280	4.0	24.0	20	60	440	2.0
Potato salad seasoning (*Watkins*), ¼ tsp. . . .	0	0	0	0	0	135	0
Potato seasoning mix, dry:							
french fries (*Shake 'n Bake*), 1/12 pkg. . .	15	0	3.0	0	0	460	0

Food and Measure	cal.	prot. (gms)	carbo. (gms)	fat (gms)	chol. (mgs)	sod. (mgs)	fiber (gms)
roasted Italian herb (*Produce Partners*), 2 tsp.	30	0	2.0	1.5	0	430	0
topping (*Produce Partners* Potato Toppers), 1 tbsp.	35	1.0	4.0	1.0	0	190	0
Potato soy crisps, 1 oz.:							
barbecue (*GeniSoy*)	90	6.0	17.0	3.0	0	410	2.0
Parmesan garlic or ranch (*GeniSoy*)	90	6.0	16.0	3.0	0	440	2.0
sea salt and pepper (*GeniSoy*)	90	6.0	16.0	3.0	0	220	2.0
Potato starch (*Mani-schewitz*), 1 tbsp.	30	0	8.0	0	0	0	0
Potato sticks (see also "Potato chips/crisps"), shoestring, canned:							
(*Butterfield*), ⅔ cup	150	2.0	16.0	9.0	0	90	2.0
(*Butterfield* Single Serve), 1 cup	250	3.0	26.0	15.0	0	150	3.0
Poultry seasoning (see also "Chicken seasoning"):							
1 tsp.	5	.1	1.0	.1	0	tr.	.2
and game pepper rub (*Ducks Unlimited*), ¼ tsp.	0	0	0	0	0	110	0
Pout, ocean, meat only:							
raw, 4 oz.	90	18.9	0	1.0	59	69	0
baked, broiled, or microwaved, 4 oz.	116	24.2	0	1.3	76	88	0
Praline sauce (*Trader Vic's*), 2 tbsp.	120	1.0	21.0	5.0	0	50	0
Pretzel, 1 oz., except as noted:							
(*Cape Cod*)	130	3.0	27.0	1.0	0	410	<1.0
(*Goldfish*)	110	3.0	22.0	1.0	0	430	<1.0
(*Mr. Salty*), 1.1 oz.	120	3.0	25.0	1.0	0	370	0
(*Rold Gold* Thins)	110	2.0	23.0	1.0	0	560	1.0
(*Snyder's* Homestyle)	120	3.0	25.0	1.0	0	230	<1.0
(*Snyder's* Olde Tyme)	120	3.0	24.0	1.0	0	120	<1.0
(*Snyder's* Snack Mix)	150	3.0	16.0	3.5	0	310	<1.0
(*Snyder's* Snaps)	120	3.0	25.0	1.0	0	390	<1.0
(*Snyder's* Thins)	110	3.0	23.0	0	0	330	<1.0

Food and Measure	cal.	prot. (gms)	carbo. (gms)	fat (gms)	chol. (mgs)	sod. (mgs)	fiber (gms)
Pretzel *(cont.)*							
butter:							
(*Rold Gold* Checkers)	110	3.0	22.0	1.5	<5	300	1.0
(*Snyder's* Snaps) ..	120	3.0	25.0	1.0	0	270	<1.0
sticks, tiny (*Snyder's*)	120	3.0	25.0	0	0	360	<1.0
cheddar (*Rold Gold* Tiny							
Twists)	110	3.0	22.0	1.0	0	370	1.0
hard (*Snyder's* Unsalted)	100	3.0	22.0	0	0	90	<1.0
honey mustard (*Rold*							
Gold Tiny Twists) ..	110	3.0	23.0	1.0	0	430	1.0
honey wheat:							
sticks (*Snyder's*) ..	120	3.0	24.0	2.0	0	230	<1.0
sticks (*Snyder's*							
Organic)	130	3.0	24.0	2.0	0	210	<1.0
twists (*Rold Gold*							
Tiny)	110	2.0	22.0	1.0	0	410	1.0
mini:							
(*Quinlan* Low Fat),							
1.5 oz.	170	4.0	34.0	1.5	0	630	1.0
(*Snyder's*)	110	3.0	25.0	0	0	250	<1.0
(*Snyders* Organic							
Classic)	110	3.0	25.0	0	0	250	<1.0
(*Snyder's* Unsalted)	110	3.0	25.0	0	0	75	<1.0
multigrain, five, sticks							
(*Snyder's*)	120	3.0	23.0	2.0	0	160	1.0
mustard, deli-style							
(*Gardetto's* Mix),							
½ cup, 1.1 oz.	130	3.0	24.0	2.0	0	220	1.0
oat bran:							
(*Shiloh Farms*)	110	3.0	21.0	1.0	0	260	2.0
(*Shiloh Farms* No							
Salt)	110	3.0	21.0	1.0	0	60	2.0
sticks (*Snyder's*							
Organic)	120	3.0	25.0	0	0	320	1.0
pumpernickel onion:							
sticks (*Snyder's*) ..	120	3.0	23.0	2.0	0	280	1.0
sticks (*Snyder's*							
Organic)	120	3.0	24.0	1.5	0	225	1.0
rods:							
(*Rold Gold*)	110	3.0	22.0	1.0	0	610	1.0
(*Snyder's*)	120	3.0	24.0	1.0	0	400	<1.0
sourdough:							
(*Rold Gold* Specials)	110	3.0	23.0	.5	0	470	1.0

Food and Measure	cal.	prot. (gms)	carbo. (gms)	fat (gms)	chol. (mgs)	sod. (mgs)	fiber (gms)
(*Snyder's* Nibblers Fat Free)	120	3.0	25.0	0	0	200	<1.0
(*Snyder's* Nibblers Unsalted)	120	3.0	25.0	0	0	50	<1.0
hard (*Rold Gold*) ..	100	2.0	21.0	.5	0	500	1.0
hard (*Snyder's*) ...	100	3.0	22.0	0	0	240	1.0
sourdough, seasoned:							
(*Snyder's* Pieces New York Deli)	150	2.0	16.0	8.0	0	240	<1.0
buttermilk ranch (*Snyder's* Pieces)	140	2.0	19.0	6.0	0	230	1.0
cheddar (*Snyder's* Pieces)	130	2.0	18.0	6.0	0	260	<1.0
garlic bread (*Snyder's* Nibbers)	130	2.0	24.0	3.0	0	180	<1.0
honey barbecue (*Snyder's* Pieces)	130	4.0	17.0	5.0	0	150	<1.0
honey mustard onion (*Snyder's* Nibblers)	130	3.0	23.0	0	0	50	<1.0
honey mustard onion (*Snyder's* Pieces)	140	2.0	18.0	7.0	0	240	<1.0
jalapeño (*Snyder's* Pieces)	140	2.0	20.0	5.0	0	370	<1.0
spelt:							
(*Shiloh Farms* Big), .8-oz. pc.	90	3.0	18.0	1.0	0	410	2.0
(*Shiloh Farms* Big No Salt), .8-oz. pc. .	90	3.0	17.0	1.0	0	0	2.0
(*Shiloh Farms* Mini)	110	3.0	23.0	.5	0	350	3.0
(*Shiloh Farms* Mini No Salt)	110	3.0	23.0	.5	0	10	3.0
sticks:							
(*Rold Gold*)	100	2.0	23.0	0	0	460	1.0
(*Snyder's*)	110	3.0	25.0	1.0	0	250	<1.0
(*Snyder's* Dipping) .	110	3.0	23.0	1.0	0	300	<1.0
(*Snyder's* Old Fashioned)	120	3.0	23.0	1.5	0	200	<1.0
sesame (*Snyder's* Old Fashioned)	120	3.0	23.0	2.0	0	200	<1.0
twists:							
(*Rold Gold* Braided)	110	2.0	22.0	1.0	0	410	1.0
(*Rold Gold* Tiny) ..	110	2.0	23.0	1.0	0	580	1.0
(*Rold Gold* Tiny Fat Free)	100	3.0	23.0	0	0	420	1.0

Food and Measure	cal.	prot. (gms)	carbo. (gms)	fat (gms)	chol. (mgs)	sod. (mgs)	fiber (gms)
Pretzel *(cont.)*							
whole wheat:							
(*Shiloh Farms*)	90	2.0	20.0	.5	0	260	3.0
(*Shiloh Farms* No							
Salt)	90	2.0	18.0	0	0	30	3.0
Pretzel, soft, frozen:							
(*SuperPretzel*),							
2.25-oz. pc.:							
no salt added	180	6.0	36.0	1.0	0	140	2.0
w/salt added	180	6.0	36.0	1.0	0	930	2.0
(*SuperPretzel*),							
2.5-oz. pc.:							
no salt added	190	6.0	40.0	1.0	0	160	2.0
w/salt added	190	6.0	40.0	1.0	0	940	2.0
(*SuperPretzel Soft							
Pretzel Bites*), 5 pcs.,							
1.9 oz.:							
no salt added	140	5.0	29.0	.5	0	115	<1.0
w/salt added	140	5.0	29.0	.5	0	900	<1.0
filled, 2 pcs., 1.8 oz.:							
cheddar (*Super-*							
Pretzel Softstix) .	140	5.0	23.0	3.5	10	260	<1.0
onion veggie cream							
cheese (*Super-*							
Pretzel Pretzelfils)	140	4.0	22.0	4.0	10	150	1.0
pepperjack (*Super-*							
pretzel Pretzelfils)	140	5.0	22.0	3.5	5	370	1.0
pizza (*SuperPretzel							
Pretzelfils*)	130	4.0	23.0	2.5	<5	210	1.0
Pretzel dip, honey-							
mustard:							
(*Nance's*), 2 tbsp.	90	1.0	18.0	2.0	0	600	0
(*Snyder's*), 1 oz.	70	1.0	15.0	1.0	0	240	0
Pretzel sandwich, 1 oz.:							
cheddar (*Snyder's*) ...	150	3.0	16.0	8.0	<5	200	<1.0
peanut butter (*Snyder's*)	140	4.0	16.0	7.0	0	140	<1.0
Prickly pear:							
(*Andy Boy* Cactus Pear),							
1 large, trimmed,							
3.6 oz.	40	1.0	8.0	1.0	0	25	2.0
(*Frieda's* Cactus Pear),							
5 oz.	60	1.0	13.0	.5	0	5	5.0
4.8-oz. fruit, 3.6 oz.							
trimmed	42	.8	9.9	.5	0	5	3.7
1 cup	61	1.1	14.3	.8	0	7	5.4

Food and Measure	cal.	prot. (gms)	carbo. (gms)	fat (gms)	chol. (mgs)	sod. (mgs)	fiber (gms)
Prosciutto, 1 oz.:							
(*Boar's Head* Riserva Stradolce)	60	8.0	0	3.0	15	770	0
(*Fiorucci*)	80	7.0	0	6.0	30	690	0
Prune, see "Plum, dried"							
Prune juice, 8 fl. oz.:							
(*L&A*)	180	0	41.0	0	0	10	0
(*Langers* Plus)	180	0	41.0	0	0	10	1.0
(*R.W. Knudsen* Organic)	170	1.0	46.0	0	0	20	3.0
(*Sunsweet*)	170	1.0	42.0	0	0	35	3.0
(*S&W*)	180	2.0	41.0	0	0	10	1.0
(*Tree of Life* Pure Fruit)	180	1.0	43.0	0	0	0	2.0
canned	182	1.6	44.7	.1	0	10	2.6
Psyllium husk (*Shiloh Farms*), 2 tbsp. ...	30	0	8.0	0	0	5	8.0
Pudding (see also specific listings), 4-oz. cont., except as noted:							
banana:							
creamy (*Kozy Shack*)	130	3.0	22.0	3.0	15	150	0
creme pie (*Hunt's Dessert Favorites*), 3.5 oz.	140	1.0	20.0	6.0	0	150	0
butterscotch (*Hunt's Snack Packs*), 3.5 oz.	130	2.0	20.0	4.5	0	170	0
chocolate:							
(*Handi-Snacks* Mega Cup), 5.25 oz. ...	170	2.0	31.0	6.0	0	220	1.0
(*Hunt's Snack Packs*), 3.5 oz.	140	2.0	22.0	5.0	0	140	0
(*Jell-O*)	140	2.0	27.0	4.0	0	190	1.0
(*Jell-O*), 1/5 of 22-oz. cont.	190	3.0	33.0	5.0	0	230	1.0
(*Jell-O* Fat Free) ...	100	2.0	23.0	0	0	180	1.0
(*Jell-O* Sugar Free), 3.75 oz.	60	2.0	14.0	1.5	0	180	1.0
(*Kozy Shack* Real) .	140	4.0	24.0	3.5	15	140	<1.0
chocolate brownie (*Hunt's Dessert Favorites*), 3.5 oz. .	190	2.0	28.0	7.0	0	135	0
chocolate chip cookie (*Handi-Snacks* Doubles), 3.5 oz. ...	120	2.0	22.0	4.0	0	160	1.0

Food and Measure	cal.	prot. (gms)	carbo. (gms)	fat (gms)	chol. (mgs)	sod. (mgs)	fiber (gms)
Pudding (cont.)							
chocolate fudge:							
(*Hunt's Snack Packs*),							
3.5 oz.	150	2.0	23.0	5.0	0	160	0
sundae (*Jell-O*) . . .	140	2.0	25.0	3.5	0	170	0
chocolate marshmallow							
(*Hunt's Snack Packs*),							
3.5 oz.	130	2.0	21.0	5.0	0	140	0
chocolate mud pie							
(*Hunt's Dessert*							
Favorites), 3.5 oz. .	170	2.0	25.0	7.0	0	130	0
chocolate peanut butter							
pie (*Hunt's Dessert*							
Favorites), 3.5 oz. .	190	3.0	27.0	8.0	0	170	0
chocolate/vanilla:							
(*Handi-Snacks*),							
3.5 oz.	110	1.0	21.0	3.5	0	150	1.0
(*Handi-Snacks*							
Doubles), 3.5 oz.	120	1.0	22.0	3.5	0	150	0
chocolate/vanilla swirl:							
(*Jell-O*)	140	2.0	26.0	4.0	0	170	1.0
(*Jell-O* Fat Free) . . .	100	2.0	23.0	0	0	200	1.0
(*Jell-O* Sugar Free),							
3.75 oz.	60	2.0	13.0	1.5	0	190	1.0
cookie (*Jell-O Oreo*) . .	140	2.0	27.0	4.0	0	170	1.0
créme caramel flan							
(*Kozy Shack*)	140	4.0	23.0	4.0	45	105	<1.0
devil's food (*Jell-O* Fat							
Free)	100	2.0	22.0	0	0	190	1.0
dulce de leche:							
(*Hunt's Dessert*							
Favorites), 3.5 oz.	140	1.0	23.0	5.0	0	190	0
(*Kozy Shack*)	160	4.0	25.0	4.0	20	95	0
lemon (*Hunt's Snack*							
Packs), 3.5 oz.	120	0	23.0	3.0	0	60	0
orange or strawberry							
cream swirl (*Jell-O*							
Creme Savers)	130	2.0	25.0	3.0	10	85	0
tapioca:							
(*Hunt's Snack Packs*),							
3.5 oz.	130	2.0	20.0	4.5	0	135	0
(*Jell-O*)	130	1.0	25.0	3.0	0	150	0
(*Jell-O* Fat Free)	100	1.0	23.0	0	0	230	0

Food and Measure	cal.	prot. (gms)	carbo. (gms)	fat (gms)	chol. (mgs)	sod. (mgs)	fiber (gms)
(*Kozy Shack* Old Fashioned)	130	3.0	23.0	3.0	15	140	0
vanilla:							
(*Hunt's Snack Packs*), 3.5 oz.	130	1.0	21.0	4.5	0	140	0
(*Jell-O*)	130	1.0	24.0	3.5	0	160	0
(*Kozy Shack* Natural)	130	3.0	22.0	3.0	15	150	0
vanilla caramel sundae (*Jell-O* Fat Free) ...	100	1.0	23.0	0	0	230	0
vanilla/chocolate:							
(*Jell-O* Fat Free) ...	100	1.0	24.0	0	0	230	0
Pudding bar, frozen, all varieties (*Jell-O* Pops), 1.75-fl.-oz. bar	90	2.0	16.0	3.0	0	40	<1.0
Pudding and pie filling mix, dry mix, ¼ pkg. or 1 serving:							
banana cream:							
(*Jell-O* Cook & Serve)	80	0	20.0	0	0	180	0
(*Jell-O* Instant)	90	0	23.0	0	0	360	0
(*Jell-O* Sugar/Fat Free)	25	0	6.0	0	0	320	0
butter cream (*Jell-O* Instant)	90	0	23.0	0	0	360	0
butterscotch:							
(*Jell-O* Cook & Serve)	100	0	24.0	0	0	130	1.0
(*Jell-O* Instant)	90	0	23.0	0	0	390	0
cheesecake (*Jell-O* Instant)	100	0	24.0	0	0	360	0
chocolate:							
(*Jell-O* Cook & Serve)	90	1.0	22.0	0	0	110	1.0
(*Jell-O* Cook & Serve Sugar Free)	30	1.0	7.0	0	0	110	1.0
(*Jell-O* Instant)	100	0	25.0	0	0	420	1.0
(*Jell-O* Instant Sugar/ Fat Free)	35	1.0	8.0	0	0	300	1.0
milk (*Jell-O* Cook & Serve)	90	1.0	22.0	0	0	125	1.0
white (*Jell-O* Instant)	90	0	23.0	0	0	350	0
white (*Jell-O* Instant Sugar/Fat Free) .	25	0	6.0	0	0	320	0
chocolate cherry (*Jell-O* Instant)	100	1.0	25.0	0	0	420	1.0

Food and Measure	cal.	prot. (gms)	carbo. (gms)	fat (gms)	chol. (mgs)	sod. (mgs)	fiber (gms)
Pudding *(cont.)*							
chocolate fudge:							
(*Jell-O* Cook & Serve)	90	1.0	22.0	0	0	115	1.0
(*Jell-O* Instant)	100	1.0	25.0	0	0	380	1.0
(*Jell-O* Instant Sugar/							
Fat Free)	35	1.0	8.0	0	0	300	1.0
chocolate mint (*Jell-O*							
Instant)	100	1.0	25.0	0	0	380	1.0
coconut cream:							
(*Jell-O* Cook & Serve)	90	1.0	18.0	2.5	0	150	1.0
(*Jell-O* Instant)	.100	0	21.0	2.5	0	270	1.0
cookies and cream							
(*Jell-O Oreo* Instant)	120	0	28.0	1.0	0	390	0
devil's food (*Jell-O*							
Instant)	140	0	25.0	0	0	360	1.0
lemon:							
(*Jell-O* Cook & Serve)	50	0	12.0	0	0	70	0
(*Jell-O* Instant)	90	0	24.0	0	0	310	0
pistachio:							
(*Jell-O* Instant)	100	0	23.0	.5	0	360	0
(*Jell-O* Instant Sugar/							
Fat Free)	30	0	6.0	0	0	300	0
tapioca:							
(*Jell-O* Americana) .	90	0	22.0	0	0	115	0
vanilla:							
(*Jell-O* Cook & Serve)	80	0	20.0	0	0	135	0
(*Jell-O* Cook & Serve							
Sugar Free)	20	0.	5.0	0	0	115	0
(*Jell-O* Instant)	90	0	23.0	0	0	350	0
(*Jell-O* Instant Sugar/							
Fat Free)	25	0	6.0	0	0	300	0
French (*Jell-O* Instant)	90	0	23.0	0	0	350	0
Pudding, plum (*Crosse*							
& Blackwell), 1/3 pkg.	410	4.0	91.0	4.0	10	290	4.0
Puff pastry shell, see							
"Pastry, puff"							
Pummelo (see also							
"Melogold"):							
(*Frieda's*), 5 oz.	50	1.0	13.0	0	0	0	1.0
1 lb. 3 oz. fruit							
w/out rind	231	4.6	58.6	.2	0	6	6.1
sections, 1 cup	72	1.4	18.3	.1	0	2	1.9
Pumpkin, fresh:							
mini (*Frieda's* Orange/							
White), 3/4 cup, 3 oz.	20	1.0	6.0	0	0	0	1.0

Food and Measure	cal.	prot. (gms)	carbo. (gms)	fat (gms)	chol. (mgs)	sod. (mgs)	fiber (gms)
pulp, ½ cup:							
raw, 1" cubes	15	.6	3.8	.1	0	1	1.0
boiled, drained, mashed	24	.9	6.0	.1	0	2	1.0
Pumpkin, canned, ½ cup:							
(*Libby's* Pure)	40	2.0	9.0	.5	0	5	5.0
w/or w/out winter squash	41	1.3	9.9	.3	0	6	3.4
Pumpkin butter (*Lost Acres*), 1 tbsp.	45	0	11.0	0	0	25	0
Pumpkin flower:							
raw, ½ cup	3	.2	.5	<.1	0	1	<1.0
boiled, drained, ½ cup	10	.7	2.2	.1	0	4	.6
Pumpkin leaf:							
raw, ½ cup	4	.6	.5	.1	0	2	<1.0
boiled, drained, ½ cup	7	1.0	1.2	.1	0	3	.9
Pumpkin pie spice, 1 tsp.	6	.1	1.2	.2	0	1	.3
Pumpkin seeds:							
in shell, roasted:							
1 oz. or 85 seeds . .	127	5.3	15.3	5.5	0	5	n.a.
1 cup	285	11.9	34.4	12.4	0	12	n.a.
salted, 1 oz.	127	5.3	15.3	5.5	0	163	n.a.
shelled:							
(*Shiloh Farms*), ¼ cup	180	9.0	4.0	14.0	0	5	3.0
1 oz., 142 kernels .	154	7.0	5.1	13.0	0	5	n.a.
shelled, dry-roasted:							
(*Eden* Organic), ¼ cup	200	10.0	5.0	16.0	0	100	5.0
spicy, w/tamari (*Eden* Organic), ¼ cup .	200	10.0	5.0	16.0	0	75	5.0
shelled, roasted:							
(*Tree of Life* Salted), ¼ cup, 2 oz.	300	13.0	8.0	24.0	0	330	4.0
1 oz.	148	9.4	3.8	12.0	0	5	1.8
salted, 1 oz.	148	9.4	3.8	12.0	0	163	1.8
Purslane, ½ cup:							
raw	4	.3	.7	<.1	0	10	<1.0
boiled, drained	10	.9	2.1	.1	0	26	<1.0

Q

Food and Measure	cal.	prot. (gms)	carbo. (gms)	fat (gms)	chol. (mgs)	sod. (mgs)	fiber (gms)
Quail:							
raw, meat w/skin:							
1 quail, 3.8 oz.							
(4.3 oz. w/bone) .	210	21.4	0	13.1	83	58	0
1 oz.	54	5.6	0	3.4	22	15	0
raw, meat only:							
1 quail, 3.2 oz.							
(4.3 oz. w/bone							
and skin)	123	20.0	0	4.2	64	47	0
1 oz. . . . . , .	38	6.2	0	1.3	20	14	0
raw, breast meat only:							
1 breast, 2 oz.	69	12.7	0	1.8	32	31	0
1 oz.	35	6.4	0	.8	16	16	0
cooked, meat w/skin,							
1 oz.	66	7.1	0	4.0	25	15	0
Quesadilla, frozen:							
beef steak, shredded							
(*El Monterey* Carb							
Friendly), 3.5-oz. pc.	260	15.0	15.0	15.0	45	590	9.0
cheese, three:							
(*Cedarlane*), 3-oz. pc.	250	10.0	25.0	11.0	25	420	0
chicken (*Tyson* Meal Kit),							
3.9-oz. pc.*	250	15.0	26.0	10.0	35	430	3.0
chicken/cheese:							
(*El Monterey* Carb							
Friendly),							
3.5-oz. pc.	210	16.0	16.0	9.0	20	590	9.0
char-broiled (*El							
Monterey* Mexican							
Grill), 3.5-oz. pc.	230	15.0	20.0	10.0	40	650	1.0
chicken/cheese, three:							
(*El Monterey*),							
3.5-oz. pc.	260	13.0	20.0	14.0	35	420	1.0

Food and Measure	cal.	prot. (gms)	carbo. (gms)	fat (gms)	chol. (mgs)	sod. (mgs)	fiber (gms)
fried (*El Monterey Cruncheros*), 2 pcs., 6 oz.	450	19.0	34.0	26.0	55	840	1.0
Quiche, frozen, 6 oz.:							
broccoli cheddar (*Cedarlane Carb Buster*)	320	21.0	7.0	24.0	255	470	2.0
cheese, four (*Cedarlane Carb Buster*)	500	35.0	5.0	38.0	300	750	<1.0
spinach artichoke (*Cedarlane Carb Buster*)	330	22.0	7.0	25.0	260	700	2.0
Quince:							
(*Frieda's*), 5 oz.	80	1.0	21.0	0	0	5	3.0
1 medium, 5.3 oz.	53	.4	14.1	.1	0	4	1.7
peeled, seeded, 1 oz. .	16	.1	4.3	<.1	0	1	.5
Quinoa, dry, ¼ cup, except as noted:							
(*Arrowhead Mills*), ⅓ cup	160	6.0	30.0	2.5	0	10	3.0
(*Eden* Organic)	180	7.0	29.0	3.5	0	10	11.0
(*Shiloh Farms*)	150	5.0	28.0	2.0	0	0	4.0
red (*Shiloh Farms*) . . .	163	6.0	29.0	3.0	0	5	4.0
Quinoa flour (*Shiloh Farms*), ¼ cup	150	5.0	30.0	2.5	0	25	4.0
Quinoa seeds (*Arrowhead Mills*), ¼ cup .	140	5.0	25.0	2.0	0	0	4.0

R

Food and Measure	cal.	prot. (gms)	carbo. (gms)	fat (gms)	chol. (mgs)	sod. (mgs)	fiber (gms)
Rabbit, domesticated, meat only:							
roasted, 4 oz.	223	33.0	0	9.1	93	53	0
stewed, 4 oz.	234	34.5	0	9.6	98	42	0
stewed, diced, 1 cup .	288	42.5	0	11.8	120	52	0
Rabbit, wild, meat only, stewed:							
4 oz.	196	37.4	0	4.0	139	51	0
diced, 1 cup	242	46.2	0	4.9	172	63	0
Raccoon, meat only, roasted, 4 oz.	289	33.1	0	16.4	109	90	0
Radiatore pasta entree, frozen, Romano (*Smart Ones*), 10.4-oz. pkg.	280	12.0	40.0	8.0	15	510	4.0
Radiatore pasta mix, basil and herb:							
(*Near East*), 2 oz. . . .	200	8.0	39.0	2.0	5	380	3.0
(*Near East*), 1 cup*	240	8.0	41.0	6.0	5	380	3.0
and cheese (*Velveeta*), 4 oz. mix	360	14.0	46.0	13.0	30	1030	2.0
w/sun-dried tomato, basil sauce (*Annie's*), 1 cup*	350	12.0	52.0	11.0	30	500	1.0
Radicchio, fresh:							
(*Frieda's*), 2 cups, 3 oz.	20	1.0	4.0	0	0	20	1.0
3 oz.	20	1.2	3.8	.2	0	19	.8
1 medium leaf, .3 oz. . .	2	.1	.4	<.1	0	2	0
shredded, 1 cup	9	.6	1.8	.1	0	8	.4
Radish:							
(*Dole*), 3 oz.	15	1.0	3.0	0	0	25	0
10 medium, ¾–1" . . .	7	.3	1.6	.2	0	11	.7
sliced, ½ cup	12	.4	2.1	.3	0	14	.9

Food and Measure	cal.	prot. (gms)	carbo. (gms)	fat (gms)	chol. (mgs)	sod. (mgs)	fiber (gms)
Radish, black (*Frieda's*),							
¾ cup, 3 oz.	15	1.0	3.0	0	0	20	1.0
Radish, Oriental:							
(*Frieda's* Chinese Lo							
Bok), ⅔ cup, 3 oz. .	25	1.0	5.0	0	0	55	2.0
(*Frieda's* Daikon),							
½ cup, 1.1 oz.	15	1.0	1.0	1.0	0	0	0
(*Frieda's* Korean Moo),							
⅔ cup, 3 oz.	15	1.0	3.0	0	0	20	1.0
7" pc., 11.9 oz.	61	2.0	12.8	.3	0	71	5.4
sliced, ½ cup	8	.3	1.8	<.1	0	9	.7
boiled, drained, sliced,							
½ cup	12	.5	2.5	.2	0	10	1.2
Radish, Oriental, dried:							
daikon, shredded (*Eden*),							
2 tbsp.	45	1.0	9.0	0	0	20	3.0
½ cup, .5 oz.	157	4.6	36.8	.8	0	161	4.8
Radish, pickled, see							
"Daikon, picked"							
Radish, white-icicle:							
1 medium, .6 oz.	2	.2	.5	<.1	0	3	.2
sliced, ½ cup	7	.6	1.3	.1	0	8	.7
Radish sprouts							
(*Jonathan's*), 1 cup	57	3.0	3.0	2.0	0	5	2.0
Raisin sauce (*Reese*),							
¼ cup	150	0	36.0	0	0	55	0
Raisins, ¼ cup, except							
as noted:							
seeded, not packed . .	107	.9	28.5	.2	0	11	2.5
seedless:							
(*Dole*)	130	1.0	31.0	0	0	10	2.0
(*Shiloh Farms*),							
⅓ cup	126	1.0	31.0	0	0	8	2.0
(*Tree of Life*)	130	1.0	31.0	0	0	10	2.0
golden, not packed	110	1.3	28.9	.2	0	5	1.5
not packed	109	1.2	28.7	.2	0	5	1.5
vine-dried (*Frieda's*							
Raisins on the Vine),							
4 oz.	316	3.0	77.0	1.0	0	20	6.0
chocolate coated, see							
"Candy"							
cinnamon (*Dole Cinna-*							
Raisins)	130	1.0	32.0	.5	0	5	2.0

Food and Measure	cal.	prot. (gms)	carbo. (gms)	fat (gms)	chol. (mgs)	sod. (mgs)	fiber (gms)
Rambuten, canned, in syrup, ½ cup	62	.5	15.7	.2	0	17	1.4
Ranch dip, 2 tbsp:							
(*Cabot*)	50	1.0	1.0	5.0	15	160	0
(*Litehouse*)	120	1.0	2.0	13.0	10	210	0
(*Ott's* Dipping Sauce) .	150	0	1.0	16.0	10	250	0
(*Ruffles*)	60	1.0	1.0	5.0	<5	240	<1.0
creamy (*Kraft*)	60	1.0	3.0	4.5	0	190	0
creamy (*Reser's*)	110	1.0	1.0	11.0	15	190	0
salsa (*Litehouse*)	60	1.0	2.0	6.0	5	200	0
Ranch dip mix (*Mc-Cormick*), ¾ tsp. dry	5	0	0	0	0	300	0
Rapini, see "Broccoli rabe"							
Raspberry, fresh:							
(*Dole*), 1 cup	50	1.0	17.0	0	0	0	8.0
½ cup	31	.6	7.1	.3	0	<1	4.2
Raspberry, canned, in heavy syrup (*Oregon*), ½ cup	120	1.0	30.0	0	0	10	5.0
Raspberry, dried (*Frieda's*), ⅓ cup, 1.4 oz.	145	1.0	36.0	.5	0	0	1.0
Raspberry, frozen:							
(*Cascadian Farm*), 1¼ cup	70	1.0	15.0	0	0	0	7.0
(*C&W*), thawed, ¾ cup	70	2.0	7.0	0	0	0	7.0
(*Tree of Life*), ⅔ cup .	50	0	12.0	0	0	0	2.0
sweetened, ½ cup ...	129	.9	32.7	.2	0	1	5.5
Raspberry drink, 8 fl. oz.:							
(*Nantucket Nectars* Organic Very)	120	0	30.0	0	0	30	0
(*Newman's Own* Razz-Ma-Tazz)	120	0	28.0	0	0	5	0
(*Walnut Acres*)	130	0	32.0	0	0	15	0
Raspberry juice, frozen* (*Cascadian Farm*), 8 fl. oz.	120	0	29.0	0	0	10	0
Raspberry mist, blue, drink mixer (*Rose's* Cocktail Infusions), 1.5 fl. oz.	60	0	15.0	0	0	25	0

Food and Measure	cal.	prot. (gms)	carbo. (gms)	fat (gms)	chol. (mgs)	sod. (mgs)	fiber (gms)
Raspberry syrup, red (*Smucker's*), ¼ cup	210	0	52.0	0	0	0	0
Raspberry topping (*Smucker's Plate-Scapers*), 2 tbsp. . . .	100	0	25.0	0	0	5	0
Raspberry-peach drink (*Snapple*), 8 fl. oz. .	120	0	29.0	0	0	10	0
Raspberry-peach juice (*R.W. Knudsen*), 8 fl. oz.	150	<1.0	31.0	0	0	25	0
Raspberry-tamarind sauce, dipping (*Helen's Tropical Exotics*), 2 tbsp.	50	0	11.0	1.0	0	0	1.0
Ravioli, frozen or refrigerated, 1 cup, except as noted:							
artichoke lemon parsley (*Cafferata* Oki Doki)	158	6.0	31.0	1.0	0	320	2.0
cheese, five, and soy (*Cafferata* 10 Carb)	178	15.0	14.0	6.5	40	250	4.0
cheese, four, 1¼ cups:							
(*Buitoni*)	330	12.0	40.0	14.0	65	630	3.0
(*Buitoni* Light)	230	12.0	37.0	4.0	35	390	2.0
cheese, four, and chive (*Monterey Carb Smart*), 3.5 oz. . . .	260	18.0	18.0	13.0	110	410	5.0
cheese, three, mini (*Buitoni*)	270	12.0	43.0	6.0	35	330	2.0
cheese and sun-dried tomato (*Cafferata* Sunny)	152	6.0	22.0	4.0	35	230	0
chicken, 1¼ cups:							
Parmesan (*Buitoni*)	310	14.0	45.0	8.0	55	620	2.0
roasted garlic (*Buitoni*)	340	14.0	47.0	11.0	50	550	2.0
beef:							
(*Buitoni* Classic), 1¼ cups	340	15.0	48.0	10.0	60	530	2.0
mini (*Buitoni*)	300	12.0	46.0	7.0	35	370	2.0
butternut squash (*Cafferata* Squash By Gosh)	188	7.0	33.0	3.0	25	310	1.0

Food and Measure	cal.	prot. (gms)	carbo. (gms)	fat (gms)	chol. (mgs)	sod. (mgs)	fiber (gms)
Ravioli *(cont.)*							
edamame and roasted corn (*Cafferata* Soy Good 4 U)	158	6.0	31.0	1.0	0	170	1.0
lobster (*Andrea*), 3 pcs. cooked, 4.7 oz. ...	192	10.0	30.0	3.0	20	209	2.0
mozzerella herb (*Buitoni* Double Stuffed), 1½ cups .	340	16.0	43.0	12.0	55	620	3.0
mushroom (*Cafferata* Magical)	196	9.0	31.0	4.0	40	290	0
pesto (*Cafferata* Manifesto)	190	10.0	24.0	6.0	45	290	0
seafood (*Monterey Carb Smart*), 3.5 oz.	220	15.0	18.0	9.0	125	330	5.0
spinach and ricotta (*Monterey Carb Smart*), 3.5 oz. ...	240	16.0	18.0	11.0	105	440	5.0
spinach and roasted garlic (*Andrea*), 3 pcs. cooked, 4.7 oz.	200	9.0	27.0	5.0	20	190	1.0
vegetable, garden (*Buitoni*)	250	11.0	39.0	5.0	40	500	2.0
walnut and gorgonzola (*Cafferata* Nutty Gorgonzola)	222	10.0	25.0	9.0	45	340	2.0
whole wheat pasta: chicken, roasted, sun-dried tomato (*Monterey*)	230	15.0	34.0	5.0	40	180	4.0
tomato, basil, and mozzarella (*Monterey*)	250	12.0	34.0	7.0	35	250	4.0
vegetable and cheese (*Monterey*)	240	12.0	35.0	6.0	25	340	4.0
Ravioli entree, can or pkg., 1 cup:							
beef:							
meat sauce (*SpagghettiOs* Raviolios)	290	12.0	39.0	10.0	20	1160	3.0
meat sauce (*SpaghettiOs* Superior)	270	11.0	43.0	6.0	10	1060	5.0
mini (*Kid's Kitchen*)	240	10.0	35.0	7.0	20	1000	1.0

Food and Measure	cal.	prot. (gms)	carbo. (gms)	fat (gms)	chol. (mgs)	sod. (mgs)	fiber (gms)
cheese, tomato sauce (*Annie's* Organic Cheesy)	180	6.0	31.0	3.5	5	730	3.0
Ravioli entree, frozen, 1 pkg.:							
butternut squash (*Linda McCartney*), 10 oz.	450	12.0	49.0	17.0	35	580	3.0
cheese:							
(*Amy's*), 8 oz.	340	15.0	43.0	12.0	25	580	3.0
(*Contessa* Minute Meal Bowl), 9 oz.	310	17.0	33.0	13.0	35	710	6.0
(*Lean Cuisine Everyday Favorites*), 8.5 oz.	250	10.0	38.0	6.0	35	590	3.0
(*Stouffer's*), 10⅝ oz.	370	16.0	55.0	9.0	60	710	4.0
w/Alfredo broccoli sauce (*Michelina's* Authentico), 8 oz.	390	17.0	42.0	18.0	80	820	2.0
and rigatoni, Italian style (*Stouffer's*), 8.25 oz.	460	18.0	52.0	20.0	85	860	3.0
chicken, roasted, Italian style (*Stouffer's*), 8.25 oz.	370	20.0	42.0	14.0	80	1030	2.0
Florentine (*Smart Ones*), 8.5 oz.	220	9.0	34.0	5.0	20	510	3.0
meatless (*Hain Vegetarian Classics*), 10 oz.	220	14.0	40.0	3.0	0	200	8.0
Recaito (*Goya*), 1 tsp.	0	0	0	0	0	35	0
Red bean (see also "Kidney beans"), canned, ½ cup:							
(*Allens*)	100	6.0	19.0	.5	0	310	9.0
(*Bush's*)	110	6.0	19.0	.5	0	460	6.0
(*Eden* Organic Small) .	100	6.0	17.0	.5	0	65	5.0
(*Glory* New Orleans) .	130	9.0	22.0	0	0	680	7.0
(*S&W* Louisiana)	80	6.0	20.0	0	0	480	5.0
(*Westbrae Natural* Organic)	100	6.0	19.0	0	0	140	7.0
w/rice (*Glory*)	90	5.0	18.0	.5	0	680	3.0
Red bean dish, frozen, seasoned, and rice (*Glory* Savory Accents), ½ cup ..	90	4.0	17.0	.5	0	360	3.0

Food and Measure	cal.	prot. (gms)	carbo. (gms)	fat (gms)	chol. (mgs)	sod. (mgs)	fiber (gms)
Red kuri squash (*Frieda's*), ¾ cup, 3 oz.	30	1.0	7.0	0	0	0	1.0
Red snapper, see "Snapper"							
Redfish, see "Ocean perch"							
Refried beans, canned, ½ cup:							
(*Allens*)	150	7.0	24.0	2.5	0	360	11.0
(*Amy's* Traditional) . . .	140	7.0	21.0	3.0	0	390	6.0
(*Bush's*)	150	9.0	24.0	3.0	0	490	7.0
(*Bush's* Fat Free)	130	9.0	24.0	0	0	490	7.0
(*Las Palmas*)	150	8.0	23.0	3.0	0	540	9.0
(*Old El Paso* Fat Free)	100	6.0	18.0	0	0	580	6.0
(*Old El Paso* Traditional)	100	6.0	17.0	.5	0	570	6.0
(*Pace* Traditional)	80	5.0	16.0	0	0	590	5.0
(*Taco Bell* Fat Free) . .	110	7.0	21.0	0	0	460	6.0
(*Taco Bell* Vegetarian Blend)	140	5.0	23.0	3.0	0	530	7.0
(*Zapata*)	130	8.0	22.0	0	0	290	7.0
black beans:							
(*Allens* No Fat)	120	7.0	23.0	0	0	500	8.0
(*Amy's*)	140	7.0	20.0	3.0	0	440	6.0
(*Ducal*)	230	7.0	26.0	11.0	0	490	6.0
(*Eden* Organic)	110	6.0	18.0	1.5	0	180	7.0
(*Goya*)	150	9.0	25.0	2.5	0	460	8.0
(*Zapata*)	120	8.0	20.0	0	0	290	5.0
and black soybean (*Eden* Organic) . .	90	8.0	13.0	3.0	0	170	6.0
spicy (*Eden* Organic)	110	6.0	18.0	1.5	0	180	7.0
green chilis (*Amy's*) . .	130	7.0	20.0	3.0	0	440	6.0
kidney beans (*Eden* Organic)	80	7.0	15.0	1.0	0	180	6.0
pinto beans:							
(*Goya* Traditional) .	140	9.0	24.0	1.5	0	480	7.0
regular or spicy (*Eden* Organic) . .	90	6.0	19.0	1.0	0	180	7.0
red beans (*Ducal*) . . .	200	6.0	20.0	11.0	0	610	10.0
spicy:							
(*Old El Paso* Fat Free)	100	6.0	18.0	0	0	760	6.0
(*Pace*)	90	5.0	17.0	0	0	590	5.0
(*Zapata*)	130	8.0	24.0	0	0	370	8.0

Food and Measure	cal.	prot. (gms)	carbo. (gms)	fat (gms)	chol. (mgs)	sod. (mgs)	fiber (gms)
Refried beans, mix,							
instant (*Fantastic*),							
¼ cup	130	7.0	23.0	1.5	0	330	8.0
Relish, see "Pickle							
relish" and specific							
listings							
Relish, mixed, hot,							
Indian (*Patak's*),							
1 tbsp.	40	<1.0	<1.0	4.0	0	410	0
Rémoulade:							
dressing (*Louisiana*							
New Orleans), 1 tbsp.	80	0	2.0	7.0	0	100	0
sauce (*Zatarain's*),							
2 tbsp.	50	1.0	4.0	4.0	0	360	<1.0
Rennet (*Junket*),							
1 tablet	1	0	0	0	0	165	0
Rhubarb, fresh:							
1 stalk	11	.5	2.3	.1	0	2	.9
diced, ½ cup	13	.6	2.8	.1	0	2	1.1
Rhubarb, canned, in							
extra heavy syrup							
(*Oregon*), ½ cup . .	180	<1.0	44.0	0	0	15	3.0
Rhubard, frozen,							
sweetened, cooked,							
½ cup	139	.5	37.4	.1	0	2	2.4
Rice (see also "Wild							
rice"), dry, ¼ cup,							
except as noted:							
Arborio:							
(*Fantastic*)	160	3.0	36.0	0	0	0	<1.0
(*Goya*)	154	3.0	36.0	0	0	0	1.0
(*Lundberg Nutra-*							
Farmed)	160	4.0	35.0	1.0	0	0	1.0
(*S&W*)	150	3.0	35.0	0	0	0	<1.0
basmati, brown:							
(*Arrowhead Mills*) .	140	3.0	31.0	1.5	0	0	2.0
(*Lundberg* Organic)	160	4.0	34.0	1.5	0	0	2.0
(*Lundberg Nutra-*							
Farmed/Royal) . .	170	4.0	38.0	2.0	0	0	2.0
(*Shiloh Farms*)	150	3.0	33.0	1.0	0	0	2.0
basmati, white:							
(*Arrowhead Mills*) .	150	3.0	33.0	.5	0	0	<1.0
(*Fantastic*)	160	3.0	36.0	0	0	0	<1.0
(*Lundberg* Organic)	180	4.0	38.0	.5	0	0	1.0

Food and Measure	cal.	prot. (gms)	carbo. (gms)	fat (gms)	chol. (mgs)	sod. (mgs)	fiber (gms)
Rice, basmati, white *(cont.)*							
(*Lundberg* Nutra-Farmed)	180	4.0	41.0	.5	0	0	0
(*Mahatma* Indian) .	150	3.0	36.0	0	0	0	0
(*S&W* Indian)	160	3.0	36.0	0	0	0	0
blends:							
(*Lundberg Jubilee*)	170	4.0	39.0	1.5	0	0	3.0
(*Lundberg Wild Blend*)	150	4.0	35.0	1.5	0	0	3.0
basmati/wild (*Lundberg*)	150	4.0	34.0	1.5	0	0	2.0
basmati/wild (*Shiloh Farms*)	160	4.0	32.0	1.0	0	0	2.0
brown (*Lundberg Countrywild*) . . .	150	3.0	35.0	1.5	0	0	3.0
brown/wild (*Fanci Food*)	160	7.0	34.0	.5	0	0	1.0
brown/wild (*Gourmet House*)	160	7.0	34.0	.5	0	0	1.0
field rice (*Lundberg Black Japonica*) .	170	5.0	38.0	2.0	0	0	3.0
white/wild (*Gourmet House*)	170	4.0	35.0	0	0	0	1.0
white/wild (*S&W*) .	140	3.0	31.0	0	0	0	<1.0
wild rice garden (*Fanci Food*) . . .	190	5.0	40.0	.5	0	15	1.0
wild rice garden (*Gourmet House*)	190	5.0	40.0	.5	0	15	1.0
brown:							
(*Carolina*)	150	3.0	32.0	1.0	0	0	1.0
(*Lundberg Christmas*)	170	4.0	37.0	1.5	0	0	<3.0
(*Lundberg Wehani*)	170	3.0	38.0	1.5	0	0	3.0
(*Success* Boil-in-Bag), ½ cup	150	4.0	33.0	1.0	0	0	2.0
(*S&W*)	150	3.0	32.0	1.0	0	0	1.0
(*Uncle Ben's* Whole Grain Instant) . . .	170	4.0	34.0	1.5	0	10	2.0
(*Uncle Ben's* Whole Grain Original) . .	170	5.0	35.0	1.5	0	0	2.0
precooked (*Uncle Ben's Ready Rice*), 1 cup*	220	5.0	41.0	4.0	0	5	1.0
brown, long grain:							
(*Arrowhead Mills*) .	160	6.0	32.0	1.0	0	0	1.0
(*Lundberg* Organic)	170	4.0	38.0	1.5	0	0	3.0

Food and Measure	cal.	prot. (gms)	carbo. (gms)	fat (gms)	chol. (mgs)	sod. (mgs)	fiber (gms)
(*Lundberg Nutra-Farmed*)	170	3.0	37.0	2.0	0	0	3.0
(*Mahatma*)	150	3.0	32.0	1.0	0	0	1.0
(*River Maid*)	150	3.0	32.0	1.0	0	0	<1.0
brown, medium grain (*Lundberg* Organic Golden Rose)	160	3.0	34.0	1.0	0	0	1.0
brown, short grain: (*Arrowhead Mills*) .	180	4.0	38.0	1.0	0	0	2.0
(*Lundberg Nutra-Farmed*/Organic)	170	3.0	40.0	1.5	0	0	3.0
glutinous or sweet ...	171	3.2	37.8	.3	0	3	1.3
jasmine: (*Fantastic*)	160	3.0	36.0	0	0	0	<1.0
(*Mahatma* Thai) ...	150	3.0	36.0	0	0	0	0
(*A Taste of Thai* Soft)	160	3.0	36.0	0	0	0	0
(*Thai Kitchen*), 1 cup*	160	3.0	36.0	0	0	15	<1.0
(*Success* Boil-in-Bag), ½ cup	190	4.0	43.0	0	0	0	0
(*S&W* Thai)	150	3.0	36.0	0	0	0	0
white (*Lundberg Nuta-Farmed*/Organic)	160	3.0	36.0	.5	0	0	0
sushi (*Lundberg* Organic)	160	3.0	36.0	0	0	0	1.0
white: (*Success* Boil-in-Bag), ½ cup	190	4.0	43.0	0	0	0	0
(*Success* Boil-in-Bag 14 oz.), ½ cup ..	190	4.0	43.0	0	0	0	<1.0
white, long grain: (*Shiloh Farms*)	150	3.0	32.0	1.0	0	0	2.0
(*S&W*)	150	3.0	35.0	0	0	0	0
(*Uncle Ben's* Instant)	160	3.0	36.0	0	0	5	0
(*Uncle Ben's* Converted* Original) .	170	4.0	38.0	0	0	0	0
extra (*Carolina*) ...	150	3.0	35.0	0	0	0	0
extra (*Mahatma*) ..	150	3.0	35.0	0	0	0	0
parboiled (*Carolina* Gold)	150	3.0	32.0	1.0	0	0	1.0
parboiled (*Mahatma* Gold)	150	3.0	35.0	0	0	0	0
precooked (*Uncle Ben's* Boil-in-Bag), ⅓ cup	190	4.0	41.0	0	0	5	0

Food and Measure	cal.	prot. (gms)	carbo. (gms)	fat (gms)	chol. (mgs)	sod. (mgs)	fiber (gms)
Rice, white, long grain *(cont.)*							
precooked (*Uncle Ben's Ready Rice*), 1 cup*	230	4.0	44.0	3.5	0	0	1.0
white, medium grain (*Water Maid*)	160	3.0	37.0	0	0	0	<1.0
white, short grain:							
(*Goya* Valencia)	150	3.0	33.0	0	0	0	0
(*Mahatma* Valencia)	150	3.0	36.0	0	0	0	0
(*Shiloh Farms*)	170	4.0	36.0	1.0	0	0	2.0
Rice and beans, see "Rice dish, mix"							
Rice beverage (see also "Rice-soy beverage"), 8 fl. oz.:							
(*AmaZake* Gimme Green)	190	5.0	37.0	2.5	0	35	0
(*AmaZake* Oh So Original)	150	3.0	34.0	0	0	20	0
(*AmaZake* Rice Nog)	190	3.0	39.0	2.0	0	65	0
(*Lundberg Drink Rice* Original)	120	1.0	22.0	2.5	0	85	<1.0
(*Rice Dream/Rice Dream* Enriched	120	1.0	25.0	2.0	0	90	0
(*Rice Dream* Heartwise)	130	1.0	27.0	2.0	0	80	3.0
(*Westbrae*)	110	1.0	20.0	2.5	0	110	0
almond (*AmaZake* Shake)	200	4.0	36.0	4.0	0	20	0
banana (*AmaZake* Appeal)	160	3.0	35.0	0	0	20	0
carob (*Rice Dream*)	150	1.0	32.0	2.5	0	100	0
chai (*AmaZake* Tiger)	170	3.0	35.0	2.0	0	20	0
chocolate:							
(*AmaZake* Chimp)	190	9.0	35.0	2.0	0	20	0
(*Rice Dream* Enriched)	170	1.0	36.0	3.0	0	115	0
almond (*AmaZake*)	200	4.0	36.0	4.0	0	20	0
hazelnut (*AmaZake*)	200	4.0	36.0	4.0	0	20	0
mango (*AmaZake*)	170	2.0	35.0	0	0	40	0
mocha java (*AmaZake*)	180	3.0	37.0	2.0	0	20	0
vanilla:							
(*AmaZake* Gorilla)	190	9.0	35.0	2.0	0	20	0
(*Lundberg Drink Rice*)	120	1.0	22.0	2.5	0	85	<1.0
(*Rice Dream* Heartwise)	140	1.0	30.0	2.0	0	80	3.0
(*Rice Dream/Rice Dream* Enriched)	130	1.0	28.0	2.0	0	90	0

Food and Measure	cal.	prot. (gms)	carbo. (gms)	fat (gms)	chol. (mgs)	sod. (mgs)	fiber (gms)
(*Westbrae*)	110	1.0	20.0	2.5	0	110	0
vanilla pecan pie (*AmaZake*)	200	4.0	36.0	4.0	0	20	0
Rice bran (*Shiloh Farms*), ¼ cup	260	0	30.0	12.0	0	0	8.0
Rice cake (see also "Popcorn cake"), 1 pc., except as noted:							
apple cinnamon, buttery caramel, or honey nut (*Lundberg Nutra-Farmed*), .75 oz.	80	2.0	18.0	.5	0	0	<1.0
brown rice:							
(*Lundberg Nutra-Farmed/*Organic), .7 oz.	70	1.0	15.0	0	0	55	0
(*Lundberg Nutra-Farmed/*Organic Salt Free), .7 oz. .	70	1.0	16.0	0	0	0	0
koku seaweed (*Lundberg Organic*), .75 oz.	80	2.0	17.0	0	0	95	1.0
mochi (*Lundberg Nutra-Farmed/*Organic), .7 oz.	70	1.0	15.0	0	0	55	0
multigrain (*Lundberg Organic*), .7 oz. ...	80	1.0	16.0	0	0	65	<1.0
sesame:							
double (*Westbrae Natural*), 2 pcs., .5 oz.	50	1.0	10.0	0	0	85	0
garlic (*Westbrae Natural*), 2 pcs., .5 oz.	50	1.0	10.0	0	0	65	0
koku (*Lundberg Organic*), .75 oz.	80	2.0	17.0	0	0	35	2.0
tamari (*Lundberg Nutra-Farmed/*Organic), .7 oz. .	70	2.0	16.0	.5	0	120	2.0
teriyaki (*Westbrae Natural*), 2 pcs., .5 oz.	50	1.0	10.0	0	0	45	0

Food and Measure	cal.	prot. (gms)	carbo. (gms)	fat (gms)	chol. (mgs)	sod. (mgs)	fiber (gms)
Rice cake, sesame *(cont.)*							
toasted (*Lundberg Nutra-Farmed*),							
.7 oz.	70	2.0	14.0	0	0	65	1.0
tamari seaweed (*Lundberg* Organic), .7 oz.	70	1.0	15.0	0	0	125	0
wild rice (*Lundberg Nutra-Farmed/ Organic*), .7 oz. . . .	70	1.0	15.0	0	0	55	0
Rice chips/puffs, see "Rice snacks"							
Rice dish, canned,							
Spanish (*Zapata*), ⅔ cup	100	2.0	21.0	1.0	0	320	3.0
Rice dish, frozen, see "Rice entree, frozen"							
Rice dish, mix (see also "Grains, mixed, dish"):							
almond, toasted, pilaf:							
(*Near East*), 2 oz. . .	200	6.0	40.0	3.0	0	640	2.0
(*Near East*), 1 cup*	230	6.0	40.0	6.0	10	670	2.0
and beans:							
black (*Carolina*), 2 oz.	200	7.0	39.0	1.5	0	930	5.0
black (*Mahatma*), 2 oz.	180	4.0	42.0	.5	0	760	2.0
red (*Carolina/ Mahatma*), 2 oz. . .	190	7.0	40.0	1.0	0	790	6.0
red (*Goya*), ¼ cup .	160	5.0	35.0	0	0	610	3.0
red (*Success* Boil-in-Bag), 2 oz.	240	8.0	51.0	1.0	0	920	8.0
beef/beef favor:							
(*Mahatma*), 2 oz. . .	200	4.0	41.0	2.0	0	950	<1.0
(*Success* Boil-in-Bag), 2 oz.	190	5.0	43.0	.5	0	920	2.0
biryani (*Neera's*), 1 cup*	132	3.0	29.0	1.0	0	4	1.0
broccoli au gratin (*Uncle Ben's Country Inn*), 1 cup*	200	4.0	43.0	2.0	5	790	1.0
broccoli and cheese:							
(*Mahatma*), 2 oz. . .	200	5.0	41.0	1.5	5	620	2.0
(*Success* Boil-in-Bag), 2 oz.	210	5.0	40.0	4.5	5	840	1.0

Food and Measure	cal.	prot. (gms)	carbo. (gms)	fat (gms)	chol. (mgs)	sod. (mgs)	fiber (gms)
cheddar (*Annie's* Organic), 1 cup*	270	10.0	40.0	8.0	20	740	2.0
brown rice:							
(*Lundberg* Quick Hearty Harvest), 1 cup*	140	3.0	30.0	1.0	0	15	3.0
and wild (*Success* Boil-in-Bag), 2 oz.	190	6.0	41.0	1.0	0	790	3.0
wild and mushroom (*Lundberg* Quick), 1 cup*	260	6.0	53.0	3.0	0	800	4.0
picante Spanish (*Lundberg* Quick Fiesta), 1 cup*	260	6.0	53.0	2.5	0	670	5.0
pilaf (*Near East*), 2 oz.	180	5.0	41.0	1.0	0	670	3.0
pilaf (*Near East*), 1 cup*	210	5.0	41.0	4.0	10	700	3.0
roasted garlic pesto (*Lundberg* Quick), 1 cup*	260	6.0	52.0	3.5	0	830	5.0
vegetarian chicken (*Lundberg* Quick Savory), 1 cup*	260	6.0	53.0	2.5	0	910	5.0
butter/butter flavor:							
(*Uncle Ben's Ready Rice*), 1 cup*	190	4.0	47.0	4.5	0	850	1.0
herb pilaf (*Marrakesh Express*), 1 cup*	200	5.0	43.0	.5	0	840	0
Cantonese (*Health Valley* Cup), ½ cup	140	7.0	27.0	1.0	0	280	2.0
cheddar broccoli pilaf (*Marrakesh Express*), 1 cup*	200	5.0	40.0	2.0	0	790	0
cheese:							
(*Success* Boil-in-Bag), 2 oz.	220	5.0	39.0	4.5	5	960	1.0
four (*Uncle Ben's Flavorful Rice*), 1 cup*	190	5.0	43.0	1.0	5	550	1.0
nacho (*Mahatma*), 2.5 oz.	250	6.0	49.0	3.0	5	1260	<1.0
three (*Uncle Ben's Country Inn*), 1 cup*	200	6.0	40.0	1.0	5	800	1.0

Food and Measure	cal.	prot. (gms)	carbo. (gms)	fat (gms)	chol. (mgs)	sod. (mgs)	fiber (gms)
Rice dish, mix *(cont.)*							
chicken/chicken flavor:							
(*Carolina*), 2 oz. . . .	190	5.0	42.0	0	0	970	<1.0
(*Health Valley* Cup), ½ cup	140	7.0	26.0	1.0	0	280	3.0
(*Mahatma*), 2 oz. . .	190	5.0	41.0	.5	0	970	1.0
(*Success* Boil-in-Bag), 1.5 oz.	150	4.0	32.0	1.0	0	720	1.0
(*Uncle Ben's Country Inn*), 1 cup*	200	6.0	41.0	1.0	0	940	1.0
and herb (*Uncle Ben's Flavorful Rice*), 1 cup*	200	5.0	44.0	1.0	0	800	<1.0
pilaf (*Near East*), 2 oz.	190	5.0	43.0	.5	0	800	2.0
pilaf (*Near East*), 1 cup*	220	5.0	43.0	4.0	10	830	2.0
roasted (*Uncle Ben's Flavorful Rice*), 1 cup*	200	5.0	44.0	1.0	0	840	<1.0
roasted (*Uncle Ben's Ready Rice*), 1 cup*	230	5.0	44.0	4.0	0	960	1.0
roasted, and broccoli (*Success* Boil-in-Bag), 2 oz.	190	6.0	42.0	1.0	0	860	1.0
roasted, and garlic pilaf (*Near East*), 2 oz.	200	5.0	44.0	.5	0	570	2.0
roasted, and garlic pilaf (*Near East*), 1 cup*	220	5.0	44.0	3.0	5	600	2.0
chicken and broccoli (*Uncle Ben's Country Inn*), 1 cup*	190	5.0	42.0	1.0	0	910	1.0
chicken and vegetable (*Uncle Ben's Country Inn*), 1 cup*	200	5.0	41.0	1.5	0	720	1.0
chicken and wild rice (*Uncle Ben's Country Inn*), 1 cup*	200	5.0	42.0	1.0	0	800	1.0
chili, Thai, 1 cup*:							
green, and garlic (*Thai Kitchen* Jasmine)	200	3.0	39.0	2.0	0	510	<1.0
spicy (*Thai Kitchen* Jasmine)	210	4.0	43.0	2.5	0	520	0

Food and Measure	cal.	prot. (gms)	carbo. (gms)	fat (gms)	chol. (mgs)	sod. (mgs)	fiber (gms)
sweet, and onion (*Thai Kitchen* Jasmine)	210	4.0	42.0	3.0	0	530	0
coconut ginger:							
(*A Taste of Thai*), ¾ cup*	190	5.0	42.0	0	0	430	2.0
Thai (*Lundberg* Sensations), ½ cup .	114	3.0	22.0	2.0	0	137	2.0
curry:							
w/carrots, onion (*Goya*), ¼ cup ..	150	3.0	34.0	.5	0	530	3.0
w/lentils (*Lundberg* One-Step), 1 cup*	160	5.0	38.0	1.0	0	400	5.0
pilaf (*Near East*), 2 oz.	190	4.0	44.0	.5	0	600	2.0
pilaf (*Near East*), 1 cup*	220	4.0	44.0	3.5	10	640	2.0
yellow, Thai (*Thai Kitchen* Jasmine), 1 cup*	190	3.0	41.0	2.0	0	360	0
dirty rice, 1 cup*:							
(*Lipton Cajun Sides*)	280	8.0	50.0	5.5	5	860	2.0
(*Neera's* Jamaican)	175	3.0	28.0	6.0	0	5	2.0
fried, Oriental (*Uncle Ben's Country Inn*), 1 cup*	200	6.0	42.0	1.0	0	580	1.0
garlic, roasted:							
and chili (*Thai Kitchen* Jasmine), 1 cup*	190	3.0	42.0	.5	0	670	<1.0
herb (*Annie's* Organic), 1 cup*	280	6.0	43.0	8.0	20	670	1.0
garlic basil:							
(*A Taste of Thai*), ¾ cup*	160	5.0	35.0	0	0	370	0
w/lentils (*Lundberg* One-Step), 1 cup*	160	6.0	37.0	1.0	0	480	5.0
garlic butter, 1 cup*:							
(*Lipton Cajun Sides*)	300	7.0	48.0	8.0	10	790	1.0
(*Uncle Ben's Flavorful Rice*)	200	5.0	44.0	.5	0	750	<1.0
garlic and herb pilaf:							
(*Near East*), 2 oz...	190	5.0	44.0	.5	0	680	1.0
(*Near East*), 1 cup*	220	5.0	44.0	3.5	0	680	1.0

Food and Measure	cal.	prot. (gms)	carbo. (gms)	fat (gms)	chol. (mgs)	sod. (mgs)	fiber (gms)
Rice dish, mix *(cont.)*							
ginger miso (*Lundberg* Sensations), ½ cup	116	3.0	24.0	1.0	0	150	1.0
jambalaya (*Mahatma*), 1.5 oz.	140	4.0	32.0	0	0	840	<1.0
lemon herb (*Uncle Ben's Flavorful Rice*), 1 cup*	200	4.0	45.0	.5	0	740	<1.0
lemongrass and ginger (*Thai Kitchen* Jasmine), 1 cup*	200	3.0	42.0	2.5	0	550	0
long grain and wild:							
(*Carolina/Mahatma*), 2 oz.	190	5.0	41.0	.5	0	710	2.0
(*Success* Boil-in-Bag), 2 oz.	190	5.0	42.0	0	0	890	1.0
(*Uncle Ben's* Fast Cook Recipe), 1 cup*	200	6.0	43.0	1.0	0	690	1.0
(*Uncle Ben's* Original Recipe), 1 cup* .	200	6.0	42.0	0	0	670	1.0
(*Uncle Ben's Ready Rice*), 1 cup* . . .	240	5.0	44.0	3.5	0	500	1.0
butter and herb (*Uncle Ben's*), 1 cup*	190	5.0	40.0	1.0	0	810	1.0
garlic, roasted (*Uncle Ben's*), 1 cup* . .	200	5.0	42.0	1.0	0	750	1.0
garlic and herb (*Near East*), 2 oz.	190	5.0	43.0	.5	0	680	2.0
garlic and herb (*Near East*), 1 cup* . . .	220	5.0	43.0	4.0	10	720	2.0
mushroom (*Uncle Ben's*), 1 cup* . .	200	6.0	41.0	1.5	0	590	3.0
pilaf (*Near East*), 2 oz.	190	5.0	43.0	.5	0	800	2.0
pilaf (*Near East*), 1 cup*	220	5.0	43.0	4.0	10	830	2.0
vegetable, roasted, and chicken (*Near East*), 2 oz.	190	5.0	43.0	.5	0	730	2.0
vegetable, roasted, and chicken (*Near East*), 1 cup* . . .	220	5.0	43.0	4.0	10	770	2.0
vegetable and herb (*Uncle Ben's*), 1 cup*	200	5.0	42.0	1.5	0	800	1.0

Food and Measure	cal.	prot. (gms)	carbo. (gms)	fat (gms)	chol. (mgs)	sod. (mgs)	fiber (gms)
Mexican:							
(*Goya*), ¼ cup	160	3.0	37.0	0	0	520	0
(*Uncle Ben's Country Inn* Fiesta), 1 cup*	200	5.0	42.0	1.0	0	680	1.0
cheesy (*Old El Paso*), ⅓ pkg.	250	4.0	55.0	2.0	<5	780	2.0
cheesy (*Old El Paso*), ⅓ pkg.*	290	4.0	55.0	6.0	<5	820	2.0
mushroom:							
portobello, risotto (*Buitoni*), 1 serving	210	5.0	48.0	0	0	930	0
shiitake (*Health Valley* Cup), ½ cup	140	7.0	26.0	1.5	0	280	2.0
mushroom, wild:							
herb pilaf (*Near East*), 2 oz.	190	5.0	44.0	.5	0	530	2.0
herb pilaf (*Near East*), 1 cup*	220	5.0	44.0	3.5	10	570	2.0
risotto (*Marrakesh Express*), 1 cup*	200	5.0	42.0	1.0	0	610	1.0
Parmesan:							
and butter (*Uncle Ben's Flavorful Rice*), 1 cup* ...	200	5.0	44.0	1.0	0	860	<1.0
pilaf (*Marrakesh Express*), 1 cup*	200	5.0	42.0	1.0	0	870	1.0
pilaf (see also specific listings):							
(*Carolina/Mahatma* Classic), 2 oz. ..	190	5.0	43.0	0	0	810	1.0
(*Near East*), 2 oz. ..	190	5.0	44.0	0	0	780	1.0
(*Near East*), 1 cup*	220	5.0	44.0	3.5	10	820	1.0
(*Success* Boil-in-Bag), 2 oz.	200	5.0	44.0	0	0	630	2.0
(*Uncle Ben's Country Inn*), 1 cup*	200	5.0	43.0	1.0	0	640	1.0
(*Uncle Ben's Ready Rice*), 1 cup* ...	190	5.0	44.0	4.0	0	1110	1.0
Moroccan (*Lundberg* Sensations), ½ cup	100	2.0	22.0	.5	0	171	1.0
pilau (*Neera's* Shahi), 1 cup*	286	6.0	48.0	8.0	0	6	2.0

Food and Measure	cal.	prot. (gms)	carbo. (gms)	fat (gms)	chol. (mgs)	sod. (mgs)	fiber (gms)
Rice dish, mix *(cont.)*							
primavera:							
(*Goya*), ¼ cup	160	5.0	35.0	0	0	570	1.0
(*Health Valley* Cup), ½ cup	140	7.0	26.0	1.0	0	290	2.0
red pepper risotto (*Marrakesh Express*), 1 cup*	200	5.0	42.0	1.0	0	810	1.0
risotto, (see also specific listings):							
Alfredo (*Lundberg* Risotto), ¼ pkg. .	140	3.0	31.0	0	0	410	1.0
Florentine (*Lundberg* Risotto), ¼ pkg. ..	140	3.0	31.0	0	0	460	1.0
garlic primavera (*Lundberg* Risotto), ¼ pkg.	140	4.0	29.0	1.0	0	520	1.0
Italian herb (*Lundberg* Risotto), ¼ pkg.	140	4.0	28.0	1.0	0	530	1.0
Milano (*Lundberg* Risotto), ¼ pkg. .	140	2.0	34.0	0	0	675	1.0
Parmesan (*Marrakesh Express*), 1 cup*	200	5.0	42.0	1.0	0	870	1.0
Parmesan, creamy (*Lundberg Risotto*), ¼ pkg.	140	5.0	27.0	1.5	5	490	1.0
rosemary and potato (*Buitoni*), 1 serving	210	4.0	47.0	1.0	10	810	2.0
Tuscan (*Lundberg* Risotto), ¼ pkg. .	140	3.0	31.0	0	0	650	1.0
vegetable, garden (*Buitoni*), 1 serving	210	4.0	47.0	.5	0	930	0
saffron, see "yellow," below							
Southwestern, zesty (*Lundberg* Sensations), ½ cup	102	2.0	22.0	.5	0	171	1.0
Spanish:							
(*Carolina/Mahatma* Authentic), 2 oz. .	180	4.0	42.0	.5	0	760	2.0
(*Old El Paso*), ⅓ pkg.*	250	5.0	55.0	1.0	0	830	2.0
(*Old El Paso*), ⅓ pkg.*	280	4.0	55.0	4.5	0	870	2.0

Food and Measure	cal.	prot. (gms)	carbo. (gms)	fat (gms)	chol. (mgs)	sod. (mgs)	fiber (gms)
(*Success* Boil-in-Bag), 2 oz.	190	5.0	43.0	.5	0	780	1.0
(*Uncle Ben's Flavorful Rice*), 1 cup* . . .	200	4.0	45.0	.5	0	880	<1.0
(*Uncle Ben's Ready Rice*), 1 cup* . . .	240	5.0	44.0	3.5	0	500	1.0
pilaf (*Near East*), 2 oz.	240	5.0	54.0	.5	0	1010	2.0
pilaf (*Near East*), 1 cup*	310	5.0	54.0	8.0	20	1090	2.0
teriyaki:							
(*Lipton Asian Sides*), ½ cup	240	6.0	51.0	1.0	0	780	1.0
(*Uncle Ben's Ready Rice*), 1 cup* . . .	190	5.0	51.0	4.0	0	730	1.0
stir-fry (*Kraft*), ¼ pkg.	210	5.0	46.0	0	0	1020	2.0
Thai:							
(*Health Valley* Cup), ½ cup	140	7.0	27.0	1.0	0	280	2.0
seasoned (*A Taste of Thai* Golden), ¾ cup*	180	3.0	38.0	1.5	0	390	0
tomato, 1 cup*:							
herb (*Uncle Ben's Flavorful Rice*) . .	200	4.0	45.0	.5	0	850	<1.0
sun-dried, herb risotto (*Marrakesh Express*)	190	5.0	42.0	0	0	500	1.0
tomato basil:							
pilaf (*Marrakesh Express*), 1 cup*	190	6.0	41.0	0	0	570	0
risotto (*Buitoni*), 1 serving	210	4.0	46.0	.5	0	870	0
risotto (*Lundberg* Risotto), ¼ pkg. .	140	4.0	30.0	1.0	0	630	1.0
yellow:							
(*Carolina/Mahatma* Saffron), 2 oz. . .	190	4.0	43.0	0	0	970	<1.0
(*Carolina/Mahatma* Spicy), 2 oz.	180	4.0	41.0	.5	0	1150	<1.0
(*Goya*), 2 oz.	180	4.0	40.0	.5	0	560	0
(*Success* Boil-in-Bag), 1.5 oz.	150	3.0	33.0	0	0	670	<1.0
yellow, Spanish style:							
(*Goya*), ¼ cup	170	4.0	37.0	0	0	640	1.0

Food and Measure	cal.	prot. (gms)	carbo. (gms)	fat (gms)	chol. (mgs)	sod. (mgs)	fiber (gms)
Rice dish, mix, yellow, Spanish style *(cont.)*							
(*Vigo* Saffron), ⅓ cup	190	5.0	43.0	0	0	730	.5
Rice entree, freeze-dried, 1 serving:							
black beans and (*AlpineAire* Santa Fe)	340	11.0	69.0	2.0	0	770	10.0
Mexican, w/cheese (*AlpineAire*)	230	8.0	39.0	5.0	n.a.	580	3.0
mushroom pilaf, w/vegetables (*Alpine-Aire*)	330	13.0	66.0	2.0	0	840	4.0
wild rice pilaf:							
w/almonds (*Alpine-Aire*)	340	10.	58.0	7.0	0	900	7.0
mushroom (*Mountain House* Can), 1 cup	240	6.0	44.0	4.0	10	650	2.0
mushroom (*Mountain House* Double), ½ pouch	290	8.0	55.0	4.5	10	810	3.0
Rice entree, frozen, 1 pkg., except as noted:							
and beans, Santa Fe: (*Lean Cuisine Everyday Favorites*), 10⅜ oz.	290	11.0	50.0	5.0	15	580	5.0
(*Michelina's Lean Gourmet*), 9 oz. . .	350	9.0	56.0	9.0	25	950	3.0
(*Smart Ones*), 10 oz.	300	12.0	49.0	8.0	20	620	6.0
and beans, Southwest (*Linda McCartney*), 10 oz.	350	9.0	43.0	11.0	25	770	4.0
broccoli, cheese sauce:							
(*Birds Eye*), 10 oz. . .	300	6.0	49.0	9.0	5	1080	1.0
(*Green Giant* Cheesy), 10 oz.	300	8.0	56.0	5.0	5	970	2.0
brown, w/vegetables:							
(*Amy's* Bowls), 10 oz.	240	9.0	36.0	8.0	0	510	5.0
black-eyed peas (*Amy's* Bowls), 9 oz.	290	11.0	38.0	11.0	0	580	8.0
teriyaki (*Amy's* Bowls), 9.5 oz. . .	280	10.0	52.0	3.5	0	780	4.0

Food and Measure	cal.	prot. (gms)	carbo. (gms)	fat (gms)	chol. (mgs)	sod. (mgs)	fiber (gms)
chicken and, see "Chicken entree, frozen"							
fried rice:							
chicken (*Contessa*), 1¾ cups*	260	17.0	49.0	3.5	100	680	4.0
chicken (*Lean Cuisine* Café Classics Bowl), 10 oz.	310	17.0	45.0	7.0	50	690	3.0
chicken (*Tyson* Meal Kit), ½ of 28-oz. pkg.	440	27.0	69.0	6.0	30	1810	5.0
chicken (*Uncle Ben's* Rice Bowl), 12 oz.	410	24.0	65.0	7.0	85	1680	3.0
shrimp (*Ethnic Gourmet*), 11 oz.	460	13.0	63.0	17.0	50	870	4.0
shrimp (*Gorton's* Shrimp Bowl), 10.5 oz.	350	13.0	68.0	2.5	85	1100	1.0
shrimp (*Michelina's Yu Sing* Bowls), 11 oz.	430	13.0	76.0	7.0	115	1350	3.0
paella, w/chicken and seafood (*Contessa*), 1½ cups*	200	17.0	28.0	3.0	50	780	2.0
pilaf, w/vegetables: (*Green Giant*), 10 oz.	230	6.0	44.0	3.5	5	1250	3.0
herb butter sauce (*Birds Eye*), 1 cup	190	4.0	34.0	4.0	10	450	1.0
Thai stir-fry (*Amy's*), 9.5 oz.	310	8.0	45.0	11.0	0	420	5.0
and vegetables: (*Green Giant* Medley), 10 oz.	280	8.0	52.0	4.0	0	970	4.0
Creole (*Glory* Savory Accents), ½ cup	120	3.0	25.0	1.0	0	740	2.0
white/wild, green beans (*Green Giant*), 10 oz.	280	6.0	51.0	6.0	0	1350	3.0
Rice entree, pkg., 1 pkg or cont.:							
black beans and (*Hormel* Bowl Southwest), 10 oz.	190	5.0	34.0	4.5	0	1510	4.0
cheddar broccoli (*Bowl Appétit!*)	290	8.0	51.0	7.0	10	930	2.0

Food and Measure	cal.	prot. (gms)	carbo. (gms)	fat (gms)	chol. (mgs)	sod. (mgs)	fiber (gms)
Rice entree, pkg. *(cont.)*							
w/chicken, see "Chicken entree"							
herb roasted (*Hormel* Cup), 7.5 oz.	190	8.0	28.0	6.0	25	960	2.0
Masala beans, basmati (*Tasty Bite*), 12 oz. .	426	14.0	75.0	8.0	0	600	13.0
mushroom risotto, Tuscan (*Fantastic Fast Naurals*), 8 oz.	310	9.0	50.0	7.0	5	660	2.0
paella, Spanish (*Fantastic Fast Naturals*), 8 oz.	280	6.0	55.0	5.0	0	650	4.0
Southwestern:							
(*Bowl Appétit!*) . . .	260	8.0	52.0	3.0	5	920	3.0
(*Hormel* Cup), 7.5 oz.	150	4.0	25.0	3.5	0	1140	2.0
sweet and sour:							
(*Hormel* Bowl), 10 oz.	240	9.0	49.0	1.5	20	930	3.0
(*Hormel* Cup), 7.5 oz.	190	7.0	37.0	1.0	15	710	2.0
teriyaki:							
(*Hormel* Bowl), 10 oz.	240	10.0	47.0	2.0	20	1810	3.0
(*Hormel* Cup), 7.5 oz.	190	7.0	35.0	1.5	15	1370	2.0
Rice flour, ¼ cup, except as noted:							
brown:							
(*Arrowhead Mills*), ⅓ cup	130	3.0	27.0	1.0	0	0	2.0
(*Hodgson Mill*), <¼ cup	110	3.0	23.0	1.0	0	0	1.0
(*Lundberg* Organic)	110	2.0	22.0	1.5	0	0	2.0
(*Lundberg* Nutra-Farmed)	120	3.0	26.0	1.5	0	0	1.0
(*Shiloh Farms*)	130	2.0	27.0	1.0	0	0	2.0
1 cup	574	11.4	120.8	4.4	0	12	7.3
white:							
(*Arrowhead Mills*), ⅓ cup	120	2.0	28.0	0	0	0	<1.0
1 cup	578	9.4	126.6	2.2	0	1	3.9
Rice pasta, see "Pasta"							
Rice pudding, ready-to-eat, ½ cup, 4 oz., except as noted:							
(*Kozy Shack* European Style)	140	4.0	22.0	3.0	25	135	0

Food and Measure	cal.	prot. (gms)	carbo. (gms)	fat (gms)	chol. (mgs)	sod. (mgs)	fiber (gms)
(*Kozy Shack* Original) chocolate and vanilla	130	4.0	22.0	3.0	20	135	0
(*Handi-Snacks*), 3.5 oz.	140	0	19.0	6.0	0	130	0
cinnamon raisin (*Kozy Shack*)	140	4.0	24.0	3.0	20	130	0
Rice pudding mix, dry:							
(*Uncle Ben's*), ¼ pkg.	90	1.0	23.0	0	0	100	0
(*Watkins*), 1½ tsp.	50	1.0	12.0	0	0	190	0
cinnamon raisin:							
(*Lundberg* Elegant), ½ cup	70	0	16.0	0	0	0	1.0
(*Uncle Ben's*), ⅓ pkg.	160	2.0	37.0	1.0	0	180	0
coconut (*Lundberg* Elegant), ½ cup ...	70	0	13.0	2.0	0	0	1.0
honey almond (*Lundberg* Elegant), ½ cup	70	2.0	15.0	.5	0	0	1.0
vanilla, French (*Uncle Ben's*), ⅓ pkg.	120	2.0	28.0	0	0	90	1.0
Rice seasoning, Mexican (*Lawry's*), 1⅓ tbsp.	30	<1.0	6.0	0	0	620	0
Rice snacks (see also "Crackers" and "Rice cakes"):							
(*Grainaissance Mochi* Bake & Serve), 1.5 oz., ⅛ pkg.:							
cashew-date	110	2.0	24.0	2.0	0	35	0
chocolate brownie .	130	3.0	24.0	2.0	0	35	0
original or wheat-grass/mugwort ..	110	2.0	24.0	1.0	0	0	0
pizza	110	2.0	24.0	1.0	0	65	0
raisin-cinnamon ...	120	2.0	25.0	1.0	0	35	0
sesame-garlic	110	2.0	23.0	1.5	0	20	0
super seed	120	3.0	23.0	2.0	0	35	0
chips, brown rice (*Eden*), 1.1 oz.	150	2.0	19.0	7.0	0	100	0
puffs, five-flavor arare (*Eden*), 1.1 oz.	110	3.0	24.0	0	0	160	2.0
Rice syrup, brown (*Lundberg Sweet Dreams Nutra-Farmed*/ Organic), ¼ cup	170	0	42.0	0	0	5	0

Food and Measure	cal.	prot. (gms)	carbo. (gms)	fat (gms)	chol. (mgs)	sod. (mgs)	fiber (gms)
Rice-soy beverage:							
(*EdenBlend* Organic), 8 fl. oz.	120	7.0	18.0	3.0	0	85	0
(*EdenBlend* Organic), 8.45-oz. cont.	130	7.0	19.0	3.5	0	100	0
Rigatoni pasta dinner, frozen, jumbo, and meatballs (*Lean Cuisine Dinnertime Selections*), 15⅜-oz. pkg.	390	24.0	50.0	10.0	30	790	6.0
Rigatoni pasta entree, frozen, 1 pkg.:							
w/broccoli and chicken:							
(*Healthy Choice*), 9 oz.	280	19.0	34.0	7.0	30	600	3.0
creamy (*Smart Ones*), 9 oz.	240	16.0	39.0	3.5	25	780	4.0
w/chicken, white meat (*Stouffer's*), 8⅜ oz.	420	25.0	46.0	15.0	50	780	3.0
and ravioli, see "Ravioli entree, frozen"							
stuffed:							
cheese (*Michelina's* Authentico), 8.5 oz.	300	11.0	42.0	8.0	45	700	3.0
cheese (*Michelina's* Homestyle Bowls), 11 oz.	360	14.0	53.0	9.0	55	750	5.0
cheese (*Michelina's* Lean Gourmet), 8.5 oz.	260	10.0	37.0	7.0	35	700	3.0
cheese, three (*Lean Cuisine* Café Classics Bowl), 10 oz.	260	12.0	38.0	7.0	20	690	4.0
sausage, Italian style (*Stouffer's*), 9⅛ oz.	380	18.0	46.0	14.0	60	880	3.0
Risotto, see "Rice dish, mix"							
Rockfish, meat only:							
raw, 4 oz.	107	21.3	0	1.8	39	68	0
baked, broiled, or microwaved, 4 oz. .	137	27.3	0	2.3	50	87	0
Roe (see also "Caviar"), mixed species:							
raw, 1 oz., 2 tbsp. . . .	40	6.3	.4	1.8	106	26	0

Food and Measure	cal.	prot. (gms)	carbo. (gms)	fat (gms)	chol. (mgs)	sod. (mgs)	fiber (gms)
baked, broiled, or microwaved, 1 oz. . .	58	8.1	.5	2.3	135	33	0
Roll (see also "Biscuit"), 1 roll, except as noted:							
brown and serve or plain, 2 oz.	170	4.8	28.6	4.1	<1	295	1.7
club (*Pepperidge Farm Hot & Crusty*)	130	4.0	24.0	1.5	0	250	1.0
dinner:							
(*Pepperidge Farm Parker House*) . .	80	3.0	14.0	1.5	0	95	<1.0
soft (*Pepperidge Farm Country Style*)	90	3.0	17.0	1.5	0	150	1.0
egg, 2 oz.	174	5.4	29.5	3.6	28	309	2.1
French:							
(*Pepperidge Farm Hot & Crusty*) . . .	100	4.0	20.0	1.0	0	220	1.0
2 oz.	157	4.9	28.5	2.4	0	345	1.8
7-grain (*Pepperidge Farm Hot & Crusty*)	80	4.0	19.0	2.0	0	270	2.0
hamburger:							
(*Pepperidge Farm*) .	120	5.0	21.0	2.5	0	220	1.0
(*Pepperidge Farm Carb Style*)	110	7.0	17.0	1.0	<5	230	3.0
wheat (*Sara Lee Classic*)	200	7.0	38.0	3.5	0	390	3.0
wheat (*Sara Lee Classic Heart Healthy*)	190	7.0	37.0	2.5	0	370	3.0
2 oz.	162	4.8	28.5	2.9	0	318	1.5
hoagie, soft, w/sesame seeds (*Pepperidge Farm*)	200	7.0	33.0	5.0	0	320	2.0
hot dog:							
(*Pepperidge Farm*) .	140	5.0	24.0	2.5	0	270	<1.0
(*Pepperidge Farm Carb Style*)	120	8.0	20.0	1.0	<5	230	3.0
(*Sara Lee* Gourmet)	120	4.0	23.0	1.5	0	230	<1.0
2 oz.	162	4.8	28.5	2.9	0	318	1.5
mixed grain, 2 oz. . .	149	5.4	25.3	3.4	0	260	2.2
kaiser or hard:							
2 oz.	166	5.6	29.9	2.4	0	308	1.3

Food and Measure	cal.	prot. (gms)	carbo. (gms)	fat (gms)	chol. (mgs)	sod. (mgs)	fiber (gms)
Roll, kaiser or hard (cont.)							
oat bran, 2 oz.	134	5.4	22.8	2.6	0	234	2.3
party, round (*Pepperidge Farm*), 3 pcs.	130	5.0	26.0	2.0	0	190	1.0
rye, 2 oz.	162	5.8	30.1	1.9	0	506	2.8
sandwich bun:							
onion (*Anzio & Sons*)	190	6.0	34.0	3.0	10	360	1.0
onion, w/poppy seeds (*Pepperidge Farm*)	150	6.0	25.0	2.5	0	250	1.0
potato, golden (*Pepperidge Farm Farmhouse*)	220	8.0	36.0	4.5	0	360	<1.0
sesame seed (*Pepperidge Farm*)	130	5.0	22.0	3.0	0	220	1.0
sesame white (*Pepperidge Farm Farmhouse*)	230	8.0	36.0	6.0	<5	370	5.0
wheat (*Pepperidge Farm Farmhouse Country*)	210	8.0	36.0	4.0	0	370	1.0
white (*Pepperidge Farm Farmhouse Hearty*)	210	8.0	35.0	4.5	0	390	<1.0
sourdough (*Pepperidge Farm* Hot & Crusty)	100	4.0	19.0	1.0	0	240	1.0
wheat, 2 oz.	155	4.9	26.1	3.8	0	193	2.2
wheat, whole, 2 oz. . .	151	4.9	29.0	2.7	0	271	4.3
Roll, frozen or re-frigerated (see also "Biscuit, frozen or refrigerated"), ready-to-bake, 1 pc.:							
butter swirl:							
(*Rhodes Anytime!*)	100	2.0	16.0	3.5	5	240	0
w/frosting* (*Rhodes AnyTime!*)	140	2.0	21.0	6.0	12	163	0
crescent:							
(*Grands!*)	270	5.0	29.0	15.0	0	510	<1.0
(*Pillsbury* Big & Flaky)	180	3.0	18.0	10.0	0	380	<1.0
(*Pillsbury* Original/ Butter Flake)	110	2.0	11.0	6.0	0	220	0
(*Pillsbury* Reduced Fat)	100	2.0	12.0	4.5	0	230	0

Food and Measure	cal.	prot. (gms)	carbo. (gms)	fat (gms)	chol. (mgs)	sod. (mgs)	fiber (gms)
dinner:							
(*Pillsbury* Oven Baked Butter Flake)	160	4.0	20.0	7.0	0	370	0
(*Pillsbury Carb Monitor* Oven Baked)	70	6.0	11.0	2.0	0	190	4.0
French, crusty (*Pillsbury Home Baked Classics*)	110	4.0	19.0	1.5	0	220	0
sourdough, crusty (*Pillsbury Home Baked Classics*) .	100	4.0	18.0	1.5	0	200	<1.0
white (*Pillsbury*) ..	110	4.0	18.0	2.0	0	270	<1.0
white, soft (*Pillsbury Microwave*)	150	4.0	25.0	3.5	5	200	<1.0
white, soft (*Pillsbury* Oven Baked)	110	3.0	17.0	4.0	0	190	<1.0
whole wheat (*Pillsbury* Oven Baked)	90	4.0	17.0	1.0	0	170	2.0
egg twists (*Kineret* Chall-Ettes)	160	6.0	27.0	4.0	20	240	<1.0
wheat, cracked (*Rhodes*)	140	6.0	24.0	3.0	0	210	3.0
white:							
(*Rhodes* Fat Free) .	85	3.0	17.0	0	0	136	1.0
dinner (*Rhodes*) ...	95	3.0	17.0	2.0	0	140	0
Texas (*Rhodes*) ...	150	5.0	27.0	3.0	0	220	1.0
Roll, sweet, see "Bun, sweet"							
Romaine, see "Lettuce" and "Salad blend"							
Roman beans, canned (*Goya*), ½ cup	90	7.0	19.0	0	0	370	6.0
Roseapple, 1 oz.	7	.2	1.6	.1	0	<1	<1.0
Roselle, 1 oz., ½ cup	14	.3	3.2	.2	0	2	<1.0
Rosemary, fresh, 1 oz.	37	.9	5.9	1.7	0	7	4.0
Rosemary, dried, 1 tsp.	4	.1	.8	.2	0	1	.2
Rotelle pasta dish, frozen, and vegetables, herb butter sauce (*Birds Eye*), 1 cup .	160	5.0	26.0	4.0	0	240	1.0
Rotini pasta entree, three cheese (*Bowl Appétit!*), 1 pkg. ...	360	13.0	56.0	10.0	15	980	2.0
Rotini pasta mix: and cheese (*Velveeta*), ½ of 9.4-oz. pkg. ...	400	15.0	49.0	16.0	25	1220	2.0

Food and Measure	cal.	prot. (gms)	carbo. (gms)	fat (gms)	chol. (mgs)	sod. (mgs)	fiber (gms)
Rotini pasta mix *(cont.)*							
four cheese sauce							
(*Annie's*), 1 cup* ..	350	12.0	49.0	12.0	30	620	1.0
white cheddar sauce							
(*Annie's* Creamy							
Deluxe), 1 cup* ...	300	13.0	44.0	9.0	25	720	2.0
Roughy, orange, meat							
only:							
raw, 4 oz.	78	16.7	0	.8	23	72	0
baked, broiled, or							
microwaved, 4 oz. .	101	21.4	0	1.0	29	92	0
Rowal, ½ cup, 4 oz. .	127	2.6	27.2	2.0	0	5	7.1
Rum runner, drink							
mixer, frozen							
(*Bacardi*), 2 fl. oz. .	120	0	32.0	0	0	5	0
Rutabaga, fresh:							
1 large, 1.7 lbs.	278	9.3	62.8	1.5	0	154	19.3
cubed, ½ cup:							
raw	25	.8	5.7	.1	0	14	1.8
boiled, drained	33	1.1	7.4	.2	0	17	1.5
boiled, drained, mashed,							
½ cup	47	1.6	10.5	.3	0	25	2.2
Rutabaga, canned,							
diced (*Sunshine*),							
½ cup	30	<1.0	7.0	0	0	220	1.0
Rye, whole grain:							
(*Shiloh Farms*), ¼ cup	160	6.0	34.0	1.0	0	0	6.0
1 cup	567	25.0	117.9	4.2	0	10	24.7
Rye flour:							
(*Arrowhead Mills*),							
¼ cup	110	3.0	23.0	.5	0	0	4.0
(*Hodgson Mill/Hodgson*							
Mill Organic), <¼ cup	90	3.0	22.0	1.0	0	0	5.0
dark, 1 cup	415	18.0	88.0	3.4	0	2	28.9
light, 1 cup	374	8.6	81.8	1.4	0	2	14.9
medium, 1 cup	361	9.9	79.0	1.8	0	3	14.9
Rye malt, see "Malt							
syrup"							

S

Food and Measure	cal.	prot. (gms)	carbo. (gms)	fat (gms)	chol. (mgs)	sod. (mgs)	fiber (gms)
Sablefish, meat only:							
raw, 4 oz.	222	15.2	0	17.4	56	64	0
baked, broiled, or							
microwaved, 4 oz. . .	284	19.5	0	22.2	71	82	0
Sablefish, smoked:							
(*Acme*), 2 oz.	150	8.0	0	13.0	35	370	0
4 oz.	291	20.0	0	22.8	73	836	0
Safflower kernels,							
dried, 1 oz.	147	4.6	9.7	10.9	0	<1	1.0
Safflower meal,							
partially defatted,							
1 oz.	97	10.1	13.8	.7	0	n.a.	<3.0
Saffron, 1 tsp.	2	.1	.5	<.1	0	1	0
Sage, ground, 1 tsp. .	2	.1	.4	.1	0	<1	0
Sake, see "Wine"							
Salad blend (see also							
"Lettuce" and "Salad							
kit"), fresh, 3 oz.,							
except as noted:							
(*Dole* American)	15	1.0	3.0	0	0	10	1.0
(*Dole* European)	15	1.0	3.0	0	0	15	1.0
(*Dole* French)	15	1.0	4.0	0	0	20	2.0
(*Dole* Italian)	15	1.0	3.0	0	0	10	1.0
(*Dole* Mediterranean) .	15	1.0	3.0	0	0	20	2.0
(*Dole Very Veggie*) . . .	20	1.0	4.0	0	0	15	1.0
(*Fresh Express*							
American)	15	1.0	3.0	0	0	10	1.0
(*Fresh Express* Italian)	15	1.0	2.0	0	0	10	1.0
(*Fresh Express* Royal							
Blend)	20	1.0	5.0	0	0	30	2.0
(*Fresh Express Greener*							
European)	15	1.0	3.0	0	0	10	1.0
(*Fresh Express Rivera*)	10	1.0	2.0	0	0	5	1.0

Food and Measure	cal.	prot. (gms)	carbo. (gms)	fat (gms)	chol. (mgs)	sod. (mgs)	fiber (gms)
Salad blend (cont.)							
(Fresh Express Veggie Lover's)	20	1.0	4.0	0	0	15	1.0
(Ready Pac All American), 3 cups, 3.2 oz.	15	1.0	3.0	0	0	10	1.0
(Ready Pac Bordeaux), 5-oz. pkg.	35	2.0	5.0	0	0	20	2.0
(Ready Pac Continental)	20	1.0	4.0	0	0	15	2.0
(Ready Pac Costa Brava)	15	1.0	3.0	0	0	20	2.0
(Ready Pac Milano/ Monterey Organic) .	15	1.0	3.0	0	0	10	2.0
(Ready Pac Parisian) .	20	1.0	4.0	0	0	20	1.0
(Ready Pac Portofino), 5-oz. pkg.	25	3.0	4.0	0	0	125	2.0
(Ready Pac Santa Barbara)	15	1.0	3.0	0	0	20	<1.0
(Ready Pac Lafayette)	10	0	3.0	0	0	5	1.0
butter, leaf (Dole Butter Mix)	10	1.0	3.0	0	0	10	1.0
w/carrots, double (Fresh Express Green & Crisp)	20	1.0	4.0	0	0	15	1.0
coleslaw:							
(Dole Angel Hair) . .	25	1.0	5.0	0	0	20	2.0
(Dole Classic)	25	1.0	5.0	0	0	25	2.0
(Fresh Express Angel Hair), ⅓ of 10-oz. pkg.	20	1.0	5.0	0	0	15	2.0
(Fresh Express Old Fashioned), 3.2 oz.	25	1.0	5.0	0	0	15	2.0
3-color (Fresh Express), 3.2. oz.	20	1.0	5.0	0	0	15	2.0
field greens:							
(Dole)	15	1.0	4.0	0	0	30	2.0
(Fresh Express Fancy Field Greens) . . .	15	1.0	3.0	0	0	15	2.0
iceberg blend (Ready Pac Classic Crisp/ Hearty Green)	10	<1.0	2.0	0	0	5	<1.0
iceberg, carrots, red cabbage:							
(Dole Classic Iceberg)	15	1.0	4.0	0	0	15	1.0
(Fresh Express Iceberg Garden Salad Zip Bag)	15	1.0	3.0	0	0	10	4.0

Food and Measure	cal.	prot. (gms)	carbo. (gms)	fat (gms)	chol. (mgs)	sod. (mgs)	fiber (gms)
romaine (*Dole Greener Selection*)	15	1.0	3.0	0	0	10	1.0
w/iceberg and romaine (*Fresh Express* Green & Crisp), 3.4 oz.	15	1.0	3.0	0	0	10	1.0
leafy greens (*Ready Pac*)	15	2.0	2.0	0	0	100	2.0
mesclun blend (*Ready Pac* Organic), 4.5-oz. pkg.	35	3.0	7.0	0	0	40	3.0
romaine blend:							
carrots, red cabbage (*Dole* Classic)	15	1.0	4.0	0	0	10	1.0
iceberg (*Dole Just Lettuce*)	15	1.0	3.0	0	0	10	1.0
leaf (*Dole* Leafy)	15	1.0	3.0	0	0	15	1.0
spring mix (*Ready Pac*), 5-oz. pkg.	35	3.0	7.0	0	0	40	3.0
Salad bowl, w/dressing, fresh (*Ready Pac Bistro to Go*), 1 bowl:							
chef salad, 10 oz.	350	21.0	9.0	25.0	70	1060	2.0
Cobb salad, 8.75 oz.	410	20.0	7.0	32.0	165	1300	2.0
chicken Caesar, 7.8 oz.	380	26.0	8.0	27.0	75	1050	2.0
Greek salad, 10.2 oz.	400	6.0	5.0	35.0	20	910	3.0
spinach bacon, 5.9 oz.	300	17.0	22.0	17.0	155	980	1.0
veggie, spring mix, 6.5 oz.	330	12.0	18.0	23.0	15	1120	3.0
Salad kit, w/dressing, fresh, 3.5 oz., except as noted:							
Caesar:							
(*Dole*)	170	3.0	8.0	15.0	10	440	2.0
(*Dole* Light)	100	3.0	8.0	7.0	10	370	1.0
(*Fresh Express*)	160	3.0	9.0	14.0	10	410	1.0
(*Fresh Express* Light)	100	2.0	14.0	0	0	410	1.0
(*Fresh Express* Supreme)	150	3.0	8.0	13.0	10	390	1.0
creamy garlic (*Dole*)	180	3.0	8.0	15.0	5	420	1.0
coleslaw (*Fresh Express*), ⅓ of 11-oz. pkg.	120	1.0	12.0	8.0	5	135	2.0
Oriental (*Fresh Express*)	140	2.0	13.0	9.0	0	350	2.0

Food and Measure	cal.	prot. (gms)	carbo. (gms)	fat (gms)	chol. (mgs)	sod. (mgs)	fiber (gms)
Salad kit *(cont.)*							
ranch:							
(Fresh Express) ...	140	2.0	8.0	11.0	5	280	1.0
sunflower *(Dole)* ..	160	2.0	5.0	16.0	5	220	2.0
Romano *(Dole)*	150	3.0	9.0	16.0	5	220	2.0
taco *(Fresh Express Taco Fiesta)*	110	3.0	7.0	8.0	10	230	1.0
Salad dressing, 2 tbsp., except as noted:							
(Albert's Steakhouse) .	130	0	4.0	13.0	0	400	0
(Annie's Naturals Goddess)	130	1.0	2.0	13.0	0	320	0
(Ott's Famous)	80	0	8.0	5.0	0	200	0
(Ott's Famous Fat Free)	35	0	9.0	0	0	310	0
(Ott's Famous Reduced Calorie) ....,	50	0	8.0	2.5	0	330,	0
(Wish-Bone Western Fat Free)	45	0	12.0	0	0	260	0
(Wish-Bone Western Original Sweet & Smooth)	150	0	10.0	12.0	0	250	0
(Wish-Bone Western Just 2 Good!)	70	0	13.0	2.0	0	270	0
bacon *(Wish-Bone Western)*	150	0	10.0	12.0	0	250	0
basil:							
garlic vinaigrette *(Annie's Naturals)*	130	0	<1.0	14.0	0	120	0
Parmesan *(Bernstein's)*	100	1.0	2.0	10.0	5	400	0
balsamic vinaigrette:							
(Annie's Naturals) .	100	0	3.0	10	0	75	0
(Cains)	100	0	6.0	9.0	0	230	0
(Kraft Special Collection)	90	0	4.0	8.0	0	300	0
(Litehouse Natural)	80	0	4.0	7.0	0	150	0
(Litehouse Organic)	80	0	3.0	7.0	0	210	0
(Newman's Own) ..	90	0	3.0	9.0	0	350	0
(Newman's Own Lighten Up!)* ...	45	0	2.0	4.0	0	470	0
(Wish-Bone)	60	0	3.0	5.0	0	280	0
basil *(Ken's)*	110	0	12.0	0	0	290	0
Italian *(Wish-Bone)*	70	0	5.0	6.0	0	370	0
berry vinaigrette *(Wish-Bone)*	50	0	2.0	5.0	0	135	0

Food and Measure	cal.	prot. (gms)	carbo. (gms)	fat (gms)	chol. (mgs)	sod. (mgs)	fiber (gms)
blue/bleu cheese:							
(*Cains*)	120	0	2.0	12.0	10	270	0
(*Kraft Roka*)	130	1.0	2.0	13.0	5	310	0
(*Kraft Roka Carb Well*)	120	0	0	13.0	5	260	0
(*Kraft Roka Light Done Right*)	70	1.0	3.0	6.0	5	290	0
(*Litehouse Big Bleu*)	160	1.0	1.0	17.0	15	230	0
(*Litehouse Chunky/ Original*)	150	1.0	1.0	16.0	15	210	0
(*Litehouse Lite*) . . .	70	1.0	2.0	6.0	5	210	0
(*Litehouse Organic*)	100	<1.0	2.0	10.0	10	300	0
(*Litehouse One Carb Plus*)	150	1.0	1.0	16.0	15	210	0
(*Ott's*)	100	0	3.0	10.0	10	180	0
(*Wish-Bone Just 2 Good*)	45	<1.0	6.0	2.0	0	310	0
(*Wish-Bone Western*)	140	0	9.0	12.0	0	250	0
chunky (*Bernstein's*)	120	1.0	2.0	13.0	5	180	0
chunky (*Ken's*)	140	0	1.0	15.0	0	290	0
chunky (*Marie's*) . .	170	1.0	0	19.0	15	160	0
chunky (*Wish-Bone*)	160	0	2.0	17.0	0	260	0
chunky (*Wish-Bone Fat Free*)	35	<1.0	7.0	0	0	280	<1.0
vinaigrette (*La Martinique*)	160	2.0	0	17.0	5	450	0
vinaigrette (*Litehouse Natural*) . .	130	1.0	3.0	13.0	5	210	0
buttermilk (*Annie's Naturals Organic*) . .	70	<1.0	1.0	7.0	10	210	0
Caesar:							
(*Annie's Naturals*) .	120	1.0	1.0	12.0	<5	170	0
(*Cains Fat Free*) . . .	30	0	7.0	0	0	590	0
(*Cains Light*)	70	1.0	5.0	5.0	5	470	0
(*Kraft Carb Well*) . .	110	1.0	0	11.0	5	310	0
(*Litehouse*)	140	1.0	1.0	14.0	15	210	0
(*Litehouse Fat Free*)	15	1.0	2.0	0	0	290	0
(*Litehouse Organic*)	110	<1.0	1.0	12.0	10	230	0
(*Litehouse One Carb Plus*)	140	1.0	1.0	14.0	15	200	0
(*Marie's*)	170	1.0	1.0	19.0	15	150	0
(*Newman's Own*) . .	150	1.0	1.0	16.0	<5	420	0
(*Ott's*)	110	1.0	2.0	11.0	20	290	0
(*Wish-Bone Just 2 Good Classic*) . . .	45	<1.0	5.0	2.0	<5	310	0

Food and Measure	cal.	prot. (gms)	carbo. (gms)	fat (gms)	chol. (mgs)	sod. (mgs)	fiber (gms)
Salad dressing, Caesar *(cont.)*							
asiago, creamy (*Brianna's*)	140	1.0	1.0	15.0	20	280	0
cilantro pepita (*El Torito*)	140	1.0	2.0	14.0	10	260	0
creamy (*Bernstein's*)	120	0	1.0	13.0	15	200	0
creamy (*Cains*)	170	1.0	1.0	19.0	10	170	0
creamy (*Ken's*)	170	1.0	0	19.0	15	290	0
creamy (*Newman's Own*)	150	1.0	1.0	16.0	<5	450	0
creamy (*Wish-Bone*)	170	<1.0	1.0	18.0	10	300	0
creamy (*Wish-Bone Just 2 Good*) ...	50	<1.0	7.0	2.0	10	300	0
creamy garlic (*Litehouse* Natural) ..	150	1.0	1.0	16.0	10	115	0
Italian, w/oregano (*Kraft* Special Collection)	100	1.0	2.0	10.0	0	470	0
vinaigrette w/ Parmesan (*Kraft* Special Collection)	60	1.0	1.0	5.0	5	440	0
cheese (*Bernstein's* Fantastico)	100	1.0	2.0	10.0	5	400	0
cilantro lime vinaigrette (*Annie's Naturals*) .	100	0	2.0	10.0	0	90	0
citrus vinaigrette (*Wish-Bone Citrus Splash*)	90	0	7.0	7.0	0	290	0
coleslaw:							
(*Hidden Valley*) ...	150	0	5.0	15.0	10	170	0
(*Kraft* Coleslaw Maker)	110	0	7.0	9.0	10	230	0
(*Litehouse*)	90	0	7.0	7.0	5	95	0
(*Marie's*)	150	0	8.0	13.0	0	180	0
cranberry vinaigrette (*Litehouse* Natural/ Fat Free)	25	0	6.0	0	0	95	0
Dijon:							
honey (*Cains* Fat Free)	35	0	9.0	0	0	250	0
lime (*Newman's Own* Parisienne)	120	0	0	13.0	0	220	0
dill cucumber, creamy (*Cains* Fat Free) ...	35	0	8.0	0	0	380	0
feta, chunky (*Marie's*)	160	1.0	1.0	17.0	15	160	0

Food and Measure	cal.	prot. (gms)	carbo. (gms)	fat (gms)	chol. (mgs)	sod. (mgs)	fiber (gms)
French:							
(*Annie's Naturals*) .	90	0	3.0	9.0	0	170	0
(*Cains*)	120	0	7.0	11.0	0	170	0
(*Cains* Light)	50	1.0	5.0	3.5	0	410	0
(*Ken's* Country) . . .	150	0	10.0	12.0	0	220	0
(*Kraft Catalina*)	140	0	8.0	12.0	0	410	0
(*Kraft Catalina* Fat Free)	35	0	8.0	0	0	320	1.0
(*Wish-Bone* Deluxe)	50	0	8.0	2.0	0	250	<1.0
(*Wish-Bone Just 2 Good* Deluxe) . . .	50	0	8.0	2.0	0	250	<1.0
creamy (*Kraft*)	160	0	5.0	15.0	0	270	0
creamy (*Kraft Carb Well*)	100	1.0	0	11.0	5	360	0
creamy (*Kraft Light Done Right*)	80	0	9.0	4.5	0	280	0
creamy (*Wish-Bone Western*)	130	0	9.0	11.0	0	270	0
herb garden (*Bernstein's*)	130	0	8.0	11.0	0	260	0
sweet honey (*Kraft Catalina* Special Collection)	130	0	8.0	11.0	0	320	0
sweet red (*Litehouse*)	110	0	11.0	7.0	0	180	0
sweet and spicy (*Wish-Bone*) . . .	130	0	6.0	12.0	0	330	0
sweet and spicy (*Wish-Bone Just 2 Good*)	50	0	9.0	2.0	0	250	0
vinaigrette (*La Martinique* True)	170	0	0	19.0	0	430	0
garlic, green (*Annie's Naturals* Organic) . .	90	<1.0	2.0	9.0	0	140	0
garlic, roasted:							
creamy (*Bernstein's*)	150	1.0	3.0	15.0	5	280	0
vinaigrette (*Kraft* Special Collection)	50	0	3.0	4.0	0	280	0
vinaigrette (*Wish-Bone*)	70	0	3.0	6.0	0	290	0
garlic and herb vinaigrette (*Wish-Bone*)	70	0	5.0	5.0	0	430	0
ginger:							
(*Makoto*)	80	1.0	2.0	8.0	0	620	0

Food and Measure	cal.	prot. (gms)	carbo. (gms)	fat (gms)	chol. (mgs)	sod. (mgs)	fiber (gms)
Salad dressing, ginger *(cont.)*							
vinaigrette (*Annie's Naturals* Low Fat)	40	1.0	4.0	2.0	0	270	0
green goddess:							
(*Annie's Naturals Organic*)	130	<1.0	2.0	13.0	<5	380	0
(*Seven Seas*)	130	0	1.0	13.0	0	260	0
Greek:							
(*Cains*)	160	0	2.0	17.0	5	190	0
vinaigrette (*Kraft* Special Collection)	110	0	2.0	11.0	0	280	0
honey bacon (*Litehouse* Fat Free)	45	0	11.0	0	0	240	0
honey Dijon:							
(*Kraft*)	110	0	6.0	10.0	0	210	0
(*Kraft* Fat Free)	50	1.0	10.0	0	0	340	1.0
(*Litehouse* Fat Free)	40	0	9.0	0	0	115	0
(*Wish-Bone Just 2 Good*)	50	0	8.0	2.0	0	250	<1.0
vinaigrette (*Wish-Bone*)	80	0	6.0	6.0	0	360	0
honey mustard:							
(*Annie's Naturals* Low Fat)	45	0	6.0	2.0	0	200	0
(*Litehouse*)	130	0	3.0	14.0	10	160	0
(*Ott's*)	100	0	8.0	8.0	0	280	0
huckleberry vinaigrette (*Litehouse* Natural/ Fat Free)	20	0	4.0	0	0	95	0
Italian:							
(*Annie's Naturals* Tuscany)	80	0	5.0	7.0	0	240	0
(*Bernstein's* Dressing & Marinade)	110	0	1.0	12.0	0	330	0
(*Bernstein's* Restaurant Recipe)	120	1.0	1.0	12.0	5	360	0
(*Cains*)	80	0	3.0	8.0	0	470	0
(*Cains* Bellissimo) .	150	0	2.0	16.0	0	200	0
(*Cains* Fat Free) ...	15	0	4.0	0	0	490	0
(*Cains* Robust)	100	0	4.0	10.0	0	500	0
(*Ken's*)	150	0	1.0	17.0	0	460	0
(*Kraft* Fat Free)	15	0	4.0	0	0	430	0
(*Kraft* House)	70	0	3.0	6.0	<5	310	0
(*Kraft Carb Well*) ..	70	0	0	8.0	0	300	0

Food and Measure	cal.	prot. (gms)	carbo. (gms)	fat (gms)	chol. (mgs)	sod. (mgs)	fiber (gms)
(*Kraft Carb Well Light*)	20	0	0	1.5	0	490	0
(*Kraft Light Done Right* House) ...	40	0	3.0	3.0	0	270	0
(*Litehouse One Carb Plus*)	100	0	1.0	11.0	0	290	0
(*Newman's Own* Family Recipe) ..	120	1.0	1.0	13.0	0	400	0
(*Newman's Own Lighten Up!*) ...	60	0	0	6.0	0	260	0
(*Ott's Fat Free*)	20	0	5.0	0	0	280	0
(*Ott's St. Louis Style*)	120	0	6.0	10.0	0	360	0
(*Seven Seas Viva*) .	90	0	2.0	9.0	0	380	0
(*Seven Seas Viva* Fat Free)	15	0	2.0	0	0	480	0
(*Seven Seas Viva* Reduced Fat) ...	45	0	2.0	4.0	0	370	0
(*Seven Seas Viva* Robust)	90	0	2.0	9.0	0	380	0
(*Wish-Bone*)	80	0	3.0	8.0	0	490	0
(*Wish-Bone* Fat Free)	20	0	4.0	0	0	390	0
(*Wish-Bone* House)	100	0	3.0	10.0	5	260	0
(*Wish-Bone* Robusto)	80	0	3.0	8.0	0	530	0
(*Wish-Bone Just 2 Good*)	35	0	4.0	2.0	0	490	0
(*Wish-Bone Just 2 Good* Country) ..	30	0	3.0	2.0	0	300	0
balsamic (*Bernstein's*)	110	0	2.0	11.0	0	270	0
cheese, five (*Wish-Bone*)	120	<1.0	6.0	10.0	0	410	0
cheese, three (*Kraft*)	130	1.0	1.0	14.0	0	310	0
creamy (*Cains*)	120	0	4.0	12.0	0	290	0
creamy (*Kraft*)	110	0	2.0	11.0	0	250	0
creamy (*Litehouse*)	110	0	3.0	11.0	0	105	0
creamy (*Ott's*)	90	0	1.0	10.0	0	210	0
creamy (*Seven Seas*)	110	0	2.0	12.0	0	510	0
creamy (*Wish-Bone*)	110	<1.0	4.0	10.0	0	240	0
herb, sweet (*Bernstein's*)	130	0	8.0	11.0	0	380	0
herb and garlic (*Bernstein's*)	130	1.0	3.0	13.0	5	280	0
Parmesan basil (*Wish-Bone Just 2 Good*)	45	<1.0	7.0	1.5	<5	310	0

Food and Measure	cal.	prot. (gms)	carbo. (gms)	fat (gms)	chol. (mgs)	sod. (mgs)	fiber (gms)
Salad dressing, Italian *(cont.)*							
pesto (*Kraft* Special Collection)	70	1.0	5.0	5.0	0 –	270	0
red wine and garlic (*Bernstein's*)	110	0	2.0	11.0	0	250	0
roasted red pepper, w/Parmesan (*Kraft*)	35	0	4.0	2.0	0	340	0
w/Romano (*Ken's*) .	110	0	1.0	12.0	0	300	0
vinaigrette (*Kraft* Special Collection Classic)	50	0	4.0	4.0	0	420	0
vinegar and oil (*Ott's*)	100	0	1.0	11.0	0	300	0
zesty (*Kraft*)	110	0	2.0	11.0	0	530	0
zesty (*Kraft Light Done Right*)	25	0	2.0	1.5	0	470	0
lemon chive (*Annie's Naturals*)	150	0	1.0	16.0	0	150	0
olive oil:							
vinaigrette (*Wish-Bone*)	60	0	4.0	5.0	0	250	0
and vinegar (*Newman's Own*)	150	0	1.0	16.0	0	150	0
onion, Vidalia:							
(*Albert's/Ott's*)	110	0	7.0	9.0	0	115	0
honey mustard (*Albert's*)	130	0	13.0	9.0	0	390	0
sweet (*Ken's*)	110	0	9.0	9.0	0	120	0
papaya poppy seed (*Annie's Naturals* Organic)	120	0	4.00	11.0	0	200	0
Parmesan:							
(*Newman's Own* Parmesiano Italiano)	140	1.0	2.0	14.0	10	270	0
w/cracked peppercorns (*Ken's*) ...	170	1.0	2.0	18.0	10	300	0
garlic (*Litehouse*) ..	120	1.0	1.0	13.0	10	200	0
Italian, w/basil (*Kraft* Special Collection)	90	1.0	2.0	9.0	5	360	0
and roasted garlic (*Newman's Own*)	110	0	2.0	11.0	0	250	0
Parmesan Romano:							
(*Cains*)	170	1.0	3.0	17.0	5	220	0
(*Kraft* Special Collection)	140	1.0	1.0	14.0	10	310	0

Food and Measure	cal.	prot. (gms)	carbo. (gms)	fat (gms)	chol. (mgs)	sod. (mgs)	fiber (gms)
peanut, Thai (*Litehouse*)	100	1.0	4.0	9.0	0	200	0
peppercorn Parmesan							
(*Cains*)	150	1.0	2.0	16.0	5	330	0
poppy seed:							
(*Albert's/Ott's*)	150	0	7.0	14.0	0	130	0
(*Albert's* Lite)	80	0	7.0	5.0	0	210	0
(*La Martinique*) . . .	170	0	8.0	15.0	0	330	0
(*Litehouse*)	130	0	6.0	12.0	10	210	0
(*Marie's*)	150	0	8.0	13.0	10	180	0
(*Ott's* Fat Free)	45	0	12.0	0	0	210	0
creamy (*Kraft*							
Special Collection)	130	0	8.0	10.0	0	250	0
ranch:							
(*Annie's Naturals*							
Cowgirl)	120	1.0	3.0	11.0	10	260	0
(*Cains*)	180	0	1.0	19.0	5	270	0
(*Cains* Light)	80	1.0	6.0	6.0	10	320	0
(*Ken's*)	140	0	2.0	15.0	10	310	0
(*Kraft*)	170	0	2.0	18.0	10	280	0
(*Kraft* Fat Free)	50	0	11.0	0	0	350	0
(*Kraft Carb Well*) . .	110	0	0	11.0	5	310	0
(*Kraft Light Done*							
Right)	80	0	3.0	7.0	10	300	0
(*Litehouse*)	120	1.0	2.0	12.0	10	180	0
(*Litehouse* Country) ·	120	1.0	1.0	13.0	10	190	0
(*Litehouse* Fat Free)	15	0	2.0	0	0	210	0
(*Litehouse* Lite) . . .	60	1.0	2.0	6.0	5	200	0
(*Litehouse* Organic)	100	<1.0	2.0	10.0	10	300	0
(*Litehouse One Carb*							
Plus)	120	1.0	1.0	13.0	10	230	0
(*Hidden Valley*							
Original)	140	1.0	1.0	14.0	10	260	0
(*Newman's Own*) . .	140	0	2.0	15.0	10	250	0
(*Ott's*)	156	1.0	2.0	16.0	9	269	0
(*Ott's* Dipping Sauce)	150	0	1.0	16.0	10	250	0
(*Wish-Bone*)	160	<1.0	1.0	17.0	10	200	0
(*Wish-Bone* Fat Free)	30	0	7.0	0	0	280	<1.0
(*Wish-Bone Just 2*							
Good)	40	0	5.0	2.0	0	290	<1.0
(*Wish-Bone Ranch*							
Up! Classic)	140	0	2.0	15.0	10	230	0
(*Wish-Bone Ranch*							
Up! Zesty)	140	0	2.0	15.0	0	270	0
buttermilk (*Ken's*) .	180	0	1.0	20.0	5	280	0

Salad dressing, ranch *(cont.)*

Food and Measure	cal.	prot. (gms)	carbo. (gms)	fat (gms)	chol. (mgs)	sod. (mgs)	fiber (gms)
buttermilk (*Kraft*) ..	150	0	2.0	16.0	5	240	0
buttermilk (*Kraft Carb Well Light*) .	60	1.0	0	6.0	5	430	0
cheesy (*Wish-Bone Ranch Up!*)	150	0	2.0	16.0	0	260	0
chipotle (*Litehouse Natural*)	110	1.0	1.0	12.0	10	260	0
garlic (*Kraft*)	180	0	1.0	19.0	10	270	0
garlic (*Wish-Bone*) .	140	0	2.0	15.0	0	310	0
jalapeño (*Litehouse*)	120	1.0	1.0	12.0	10	200	0
jalapeño (*Marie's*) .	160	1.0	1.0	17.0	10	220	0
onion, spring (*Wish-Bone*)	130	0	2.0	14.0	0	310	0
Parmesan garlic (*Bernstein's*)	140	1.0	2.0	14.0	10	300	0
Parmesan peppercorn (*Wish-Bone Just 2 Good*) ...	50	0	7.0	2.0	0	270	<1.0
peppercorn (*Cains Fat Free*)	45	0	10.0	0	0	270	0
peppercorn (*Litehouse*)	100	1.0	2.0	10.0	10	190	0
salsa (*Litehouse Lite*)	50	0	2.0	4.5	5	190	0
serrano (*El Torito*) .	150	0	2.0	15.0	10	320	0
Southwest (*Litehouse One Carb Plus*) ..	120	1.0	1.0	13.0	10	210	0
raspberry vinaigrette:							
(*Albert's*)	120	0	8.0	10.0	0	250	0
(*Annie's Naturals Low Fat*)	35	0	5.0	1.5	0	75	0
(*Cains Fat Free*) ...	35	0	8.0	0	0	270	0
(*Cains Light*)	120	0	8.0	10.0	0	250	0
(*Kraft Light Done Right*)	60	0	5.0	4.0	0	270	0
(*Litehouse Fat Free*)	25	0	6.0	0	0	90	0
red (*Ott's*)	156	1.0	2.0	16.0	9	269	0
raspberry and walnut (*Newman's Own Lighten Up!*)	70	0	7.0	5.0	0	120	0
red pepper, roasted:							
(*Litehouse Natural*)	110	0	2.0	11.0	0	180	0
w/Parmesan (*Kraft*)	35	0	4.0	2.0	0	340	0
vinaigrette (*Annie's Naturals*)	70	0	3.0	6.0	0	240	0

Food and Measure	cal.	prot. (gms)	carbo. (gms)	fat (gms)	chol. (mgs)	sod. (mgs)	fiber (gms)
red wine vinaigrette:							
(*Seven Seas*)	90	0	2.0	9.0	0	480	0
(*Seven Seas* Fat Free)	15	0	3.0	0	0	400	0
(*Seven Seas* Reduced							
Fat)	45	0	3.0	4.0	0	320	0
(*Wish-Bone*)	80	0	9.0	5.0	0	240	0
(*Wish-Bone* Fat Free)	30	0	7.0	0	0	230	0
Chianti (*Cains*)	130	0	5.0	12.0	0	250	0
olive oil (*Annie's*							
Naturals)	160	0	1.0	17.0	0	120	0
red wine vinegar and							
oil (*Newman's Own*)	110	0	3.0	10.0	0	430	0
Russian:							
(*Wish-Bone*)	110	0	14.0	6.0	0	360	0
creamy (*Seven Seas*)	140	0	3.0	14.0	0	50	0
sea veggie and sesame							
vinaigrette (*Annie's*							
Naturals)	110	1.0	1.0	11.0	0	330	0
sesame, Asian:							
(*Annie's Naturals*) .	140	0	4.0	14.0	0	210	0
cilantro (*Annie*							
Chun's Noodle/							
Salad), 1 tbsp. . .	60	0	4.0	4.0	0	400	0
ginger (*Litehouse*							
Asian/Fat Free) . .	35	0	8.0	0	0	230	0
ginger vinaigrette							
(*Annie's Naturals*)	100	1.0	4.0	9.0	0	240	0
soy (*Trader Vic's*) . .	110	<1.0	3.0	11.0	0	200	0
shiitake sesame vinai-							
grette (*Annie's*							
Naturals)	120	0	1.0	13.0	0	250	0
sweet and sour (*Old*							
Dutch)	50	0	13.0	0	0	480	0
tamari:							
mustard (*San-J*) . .	25	1.0	5.0	0	0	240	0
peanut (*San-J*)	60	3.0	9.0	2.0	0	230	0
sesame (*San-J*) . . .	45	1.0	5.0	2.0	0	600	0
vinaigrette (*San-J*) .	45	1.0	4.0	3.0	0	670	0
Thousand Island:							
(*Annie's Naturals*							
Organic)	90	<1.0	5.0	7.0	<5	140	0
(*Ken's*)	140	0	4.0	13.0	15	300	0
(*Kraft*)	120	0	5.0	10.0	10	310	0
(*Kraft* Fat Free)	450	0	10.0	0	0	260	0

Food and Measure	cal.	prot. (gms)	carbo. (gms)	fat (gms)	chol. (mgs)	sod. (mgs)	fiber (gms)
Salad dressing, Thousand Island *(cont.)*							
(*Litehouse*)	120	0	3.0	13.0	10	250	0
(*Newman's Own* Two)	140	0	4.0	14.0	10	260	0
(*Ott's*)	100	0	6.0	8.0	10	190	0
(*Wish-Bone*)	130	0	6.0	12.0	10	330	0
(*Wish-Bone Just 2 Good*)	50	0	9.0	2.0	5	290	0
tomato, sun-dried (*Kraft* Special Collection)	60	0	4.0	5.0	0	340	0
tomato bacon, tangy (*Kraft* Special Collection)	130	1.0	8.0	10.0	0	410	0
tuna salad (*Kraft* Tuna Salad Maker), 1 tbsp.	35	0	2.0	2.5	5	135	0
vinaigrette (see also specific listings): (*Litehouse* Fat Free)	10	0	1.0	0	0	310	0
blush wine (*Cains* Fat Free)	40	0	9.0	0	0	500	0
blush wine (*Cains* Light)	70	0	8.0	4.5	0	480	0
Mediterranean (*Litehouse One Carb Plus*)	25	0	1.0	2.0	0	310	0
olive oil (*Bernstein's*)	90	0	3.0	9.0	0	280	0
vinegar free (*Annie's Naturals* Gardenstyle)	120	0	2.0	12.0	0	110	0
yogurt w/dill (*Annie's Naturals* Organic Nonfat)	20	1.0	3.0	0	0	320	0
Salad dressing mix, 1/8 pkt. mix, except as noted:							
Caesar, gourmet (*Good Seasons*)	15	0	2.0	0	0	300	0
cheese garlic (*Good Seasons*)	5	0	1.0	0	0	330	0
garlic herb (*Good Seasons*)	5	0	1.0	0	0	340	0
Italian: (*Good Seasons* Cruet Kit)	5	0	1.0	0	0	320	0
(*Good Seasons* Fat Free)	10	0	3.0	0	0	290	0

Food and Measure	cal.	prot. (gms)	carbo. (gms)	fat (gms)	chol. (mgs)	sod. (mgs)	fiber (gms)
mild (*Good Seasons*)	10	0	2.0	0	0	370	0
Parmesan (*Good Seasons*)	10	0	2.0	0	0	330	0
zesty (*Good Seasons*)	5	0	1.0	0	0	220	0
peanut (*A Taste of Thai*), 2 tbsp.*	40	1.0	7.0	1.5	0	340	1.0
sesame, Oriental (*Good Seasons*)	15	0	3.0	0	0	360	0
Salad dressing/topping kit, approx. 1/5 pkg.:							
balsamic Italian (*Linsey Et Tu Caesar*)	120	2.0	9.0	8.0	0	125	1.0
Caesar:							
(*Linsey Et Tu Caesar*)	140	2.0	8.0	12.0	10	280	<1.0
(*Linsey Et Tu Caesar Light*)	94	2.0	9.0	6.0	5	260	0
Greek (*Linsey Et Tu Caesar Authentic*) . .	120	1.0	6.0	9.0	0	210	0
Oriental (*Linsey Et Tu Caesar*)	80	1.0	14.0	1.5	0	140	<1.0
spinach (*Linsey Et Tu Caesar*)	110	1.0	8.0	8.0	5	220	0
Salad toppers (see also "Bacon bits" and "Croutons"):							
(*McCormick Salad Toppins*), 1⅓ tbsp.	35	1.0	2.0	1.5	0	90	0
(*Produce Partners Crunchies*), 1 tbsp.	30	1.0	2.0	1.5	0	110	0
garden vegetable (*McCormick Salad Toppins*), 1⅓ tbsp.	35	1.0	3.0	2.0	0	60	0
Salami, 2 oz., except as noted:							
(*Hatfield Deli Choice*) .	130	8.0	2.0	10.0	30	510	0
beef:							
(*Boar's Head*)	120	10.0	0	9.0	25	470	0
(*Hansel & Gretel*) . .	170	7.0	4.0	14.0	35	660	0
(*Hebrew National*) .	150	8.0	0	13.0	35	420	0
(*Hebrew National Chub*)	160	8.0	0	14.0	35	500	0
lean (*Hebrew National*)	90	9.0	1.0	5.0	25	480	0

Food and Measure	cal.	prot. (gms)	carbo. (gms)	fat (gms)	chol. (mgs)	sod. (mgs)	fiber (gms)
Salami *(cont.)*							
cooked:							
(*Boar's Head*)	130	8.0	0	11.0	40	550	0
(*Deli Delight*)	100	9.0	4.0	5.0	35	400	0
regular or hot							
(*Hansel & Gretel*)	160	7.0	4.0	12.0	40	770	0
cotto, 1 oz.:							
(*Oscar Mayer*)	70	3.0	1.0	5.0	25	280	0
(*Oscar Mayer* 50%							
Less Fat)	45	4.0	0	3.0	20	280	0
beef (*Oscar Mayer*)	60	4.0	1.0	4.5	20	360	0
dry, Italian (*Boar's Head*							
Bianco D'Oro), 1 oz.	110	7.0	1.0	8.0	25	470	0
Genoa:							
(*Boar's Head*)	180	12.0	1.0	14.0	55	970	0
(*Hansel & Gretel*) . .	220	11.0	3.0	18.0	50	980	0
(*Hormel Pillow Pack*)	210	12.0	0	18.0	50	940	0
(*Sara Lee* Sliced),							
4 slices, 1 oz. . . .	110	6.0	1.0	10.0	35	390	0
(*Tyson* Sliced),							
4 slices, 1 oz. . . .	110	6.0	1.0	9.0	25	440	0
hard:							
(*Boar's Head*), 1 oz.	110	6.0	<1.0	9.0	30	490	0
(*Hansel & Gretel*) . .	230	12.0	2.0	20.0	50	920	0
(*Oscar Mayer*), 1 oz.	100	7.0	1.0	8.0	25	510	0
(*Sara Lee* Sliced),							
4 slices, 1 oz. . . .	120	6.0	0	11.0	40	410	0
(*Tyson* Sliced),							
4 slices, 1 oz. . . .	110	6.0	1.0	3.0	25	460	0
"Salami," vegetarian:							
(*Worthington*), 3 slices,							
2 oz.	120	12.0	3.0	7.0	0	800	2.0
slices (*Yves*), 2.2 oz. .	90	17.0	5.0	0	0	390	1.0
Salisbury steak, see							
"Beef dinner" and							
"Beef entree"-							
Salmon, meat only:							
Atlantic, farmed, 4 oz.:							
raw	207	22.6	0	12.3	67	66	0
baked, broiled, or							
microwaved	234	25.0	0	14.0	71	69	0
Atlantic, wild, 4 oz.:							
raw	161	22.5	0	7.2	62	50	0
baked, broiled, or							
microwaved	206	28.8	0	9.2	81	64	0

Food and Measure	cal.	prot. (gms)	carbo. (gms)	fat (gms)	chol. (mgs)	sod. (mgs)	fiber (gms)
Chinook, 4 oz.:							
raw	204	22.8	0	11.9	75	53	0
baked, broiled, or							
microwaved	262	29.2	0	15.2	96	68	0
chum, 4 oz.:							
raw	136	22.8	0	4.3	84	112	0
baked, broiled, or							
microwaved	175	29.3	0	5.5	108	73	0
coho, farmed, 4 oz.:							
raw	182	24.1	0	8.7	58	53	0
baked, broiled, or							
microwaved	202	27.6	0	9.3	71	59	0
coho, wild, 4 oz.:							
raw	165	25.0	0	6.7	51	53	0
baked, broiled, or							
microwaved	158	26.6	0	4.9	62	66	0
boiled, poached, or							
steamed	209	31.0	0	8.5	65	60	0
pink, 4 oz.:							
raw	132	22.6	0	3.9	59	76	0
baked, broiled, or							
microwaved	169	29.0	0	5.0	76	98	0
sockeye, 4 oz.:							
raw	191	24.2	0	9.7	70	53	0
baked, broiled, or							
microwaved	245	31.0	0	12.4	99	75	0
Salmon, baked (*Acme*),							
2 oz.	130	11.0	1.0	9.0	30	420	0
Salmon, canned,							
¼ cup, except as							
noted:							
chum, drained, 4 oz. .	160	24.3	0	6.2	44	552	0
keta (*Bumble Bee*) . . .	90	13.0	0	4.0	40	270	0
pink:							
(*Bumble Bee*)	90	12.0	0	5.0	40	270	0
(*Crown Prince* Low							
Sodium)	90	12.0	0	5.0	60	60	0
wild Alaskan							
(*Miramonte*)	90	12.0	0	5.0	40	60	0
red:							
(*Bumble Bee/Bumble*							
bee Blueback) . .	110	13.0	0	7.0	40	270	0
blueback							
(*Rubinstein's*) . . .	110	13.0	0	7.0	40	270	0

Food and Measure	cal.	prot. (gms)	carbo. (gms)	fat (gms)	chol. (mgs)	sod. (mgs)	fiber (gms)
Salmon, canned, red *(cont.)*							
medium (*Bumble Bee*)	90	12.0	0	5.0	40	270	0
sockeye, drained, w/bone, 4 oz. . . .	174	23.2	0	8.3	50	611	0
Salmon, marinated (*Spence & Co. Gravlax*), 2 oz.	120	13.0	<1.0	7.0	30	910	<1.0
Salmon, smoked, 2 oz.							
(*Acme*)	70	13.0	0	2.5	30	790	0
(*Echo Falls*)	100	13.0	2.0	4.0	40	720	0
Atlantic:							
(*Ducktrap River Kendall Brook*) . .	130	11.0	0	9.0	10	690	0
(*Ducktrap River Spruce Point*) . .	110	12.0	0	7.0	35	680	0
(*Ducktrap River Winter Harbor*) . .	130	11.0	0	9.0	10	690	0
Chinook	66	10.4	0	2.4	13	445	0
keta (*SeaBear Beer Garden*)	86	11.2	4.7	2.7	13	448	1.9
king, wild, Nova style (*SeaBear*)	60	12.0	0	1.5	20	660	0
lox (*Vita*)	50	11.0	<1.0	1.0	20	800	0
Nova (*Vita*)	50	11.0	<1.0	1.0	20	580	0
pastrami style:							
(*Ducktrap River Spruce Point*) . .	130	11.0	0	9.0	10	690	0
(*Spence & Co.*) . . .	120	13.0	<1.0	7.0	30	910	<1.0
roasted (*Ducktrap River*)	100	13.0	0	6.0	10	430	0
sockeye, wild:							
(*SeaBear*)	110	14.0	0	6.0	80	340	0
Nova style (*SeaBear*)	60	12.0	1.0	5.0	15	850	0
Salmon, smoked, canned, in oil (*Bumble Bee*), 1 can drained, 3 oz.	150	16.0	0	9.0	55	400	0
Salmon, smoked, spread:							
(*Sau•Sea*), 2 tbsp. . . .	100	2.0	1.0	10.0	20	55	0
(*SeaBear*), 8 oz.	578	22.3	6.5	51.4	186	459	.5
Salmon burger, frozen (*Dr. Praeger's*), 2.75-oz. pc.	100	7.5	11.0	3.0	7	200	3.0

Food and Measure	cal.	prot. (gms)	carbo. (gms)	fat (gms)	chol. (mgs)	sod. (mgs)	fiber (gms)
Salmon cake, frozen (*Dr. Praeger's*), 2.9-oz. pc.	158	12.0	14.0	6.0	30	190	<1.0
Salmon entree, frozen:
w/basil (*Lean Cuisine Spa Cuisine*), 9.5-oz. pkg.	260	17.0	31.0	8.0	30	680	5.0
grilled:
(*Gorton's* Classic) 3.8-oz. pc.	100	15.0	1.0	3.5	20	310	0
lemon butter (*Gorton's*), 3.8-oz. pc.	100	17.0	1.0	3.0	60	250	0
lemon butter (*Mrs. Paul's* Meals), 11-oz. pkg.	280	22.0	35.0	5.0	70	520	3.0
stuffed, w/spinach and cheese (*Oven Poppers*), 5-oz. pc.	290	18.0	10.0	18.0	60	440	0
Salmon entree, pkg., poached sockeye (*SeaBear*), 2 oz.	90	14.0	0	4.5	65	45	0
Salmon frankfurter, see "Frankfurter"
Salmon gefilte fish, see "Gefilte fish, frozen"
Salmon oil, see "Oil"
Salmon pastrami (*A&B Famous*), 2 oz.	110	10.0	1.0	7.0	20	880	0
Salmon pâté:
(*Trois Petits Cochons*), 2 oz.	110	6.0	2.0	9.0	35	180	0
smoked (*Ducktrap River*), ¼ cup	150	7.0	1.0	14.0	35	410	0
Salmon salami (*A&B Famous*), 2 oz.	120	8.0	2.0	9.0	20	470	0
Salmon seasoning mix (*Old Bay* Classic), 1/5 pkg.	40	1.0	3.0	1.5	55	115	0
Salsa (see also "Picante sauce"), except as noted:
(*Cedar's* Boston)	10	<1.0	<1.0	0	0	125	0
(*D.L. Jardine's* Bobos)	15	1.0	3.0	0	0	200	<1.0

Food and Measure	cal.	prot. (gms)	carbo. (gms)	fat (gms)	chol. (mgs)	sod. (mgs)	fiber (gms)
Salsa *(cont.)*							
(*D.L. Jardine's* Texacante)	10	0	2.0	0	0	125	<1.0
(*El Torito* Original Restaurant)	10	0	2.0	0	0	180	0
(*Guiltless Gourmet* Southwestern Grill)	15	0	2.0	0	0	115	0
(*Herdez* Casera)	10	0	1.0	0	0	240	0
(*Herdez* Ranchera) ...	15	0	1.0	0	0	220	0
(*Herdez* Taquera)	10	0	2.0	0	0	280	0
(*Herdez* Verde)	10	0	1.0	0	0	310	0
(*La Victoria* Ranchera)	10	0	2.0	0	0	125	0
(*La Victoria* Salsa Victoria)	10	0	2.0	0	0	115	0
(*La Victoria* Suprema)	10	0	1.0	0	0	135	0
(*La Victoria* Thick 'n Chunky)	10	0	2.0	0	0	125	0
(*La Victoria* Verde) ...	10	0	2.0	0	0	140	0
(*Neera's* Caribbean), 1 tbsp.	25	0	7.0	0	0	60	0
(*Newman's Own* Bandito)	10	0	2.0	0	0	105	1.0
(*Pace* Chunky)	10	0	2.0	0	0	210	1.0
(*Pace* Dip)	10	0	2.0	0	0	240	<1.0
(*Tostitos* Restaurant Style)	15	<1.0	3.0	0	0	210	<1.0
artichoke:							
(*D.L. Jardine's* Cowpoke)	15	0	2.0	.5	0	230	0
(*Jose Goldstein*) ...	15	0	2.0	0	0	135	0
black bean and corn:							
(*Amy's*)	15	1.0	3.0	0	0	170	1.0
(*Fiesta*)	10	0	2.0	0	0	60	0
(*Frontier Traders*) ..	15	1.0	3.0	0	0	150	1.0
(*Muir Glen*)	15	0.	2.0	0	0	125	0
(*Walnut Acres* Midnight Sun) ..	15	1.0	3.0	0	0	125	1.0
cheese (con queso), see "Cheese dip"							
w/cheese (*Kaukauna*) .	15	0	3.0	0	0	170	0
cherry (*D.L. Jardine's* Cowboy)	25	0	6.0	0	0	75	0
chipotle:							
(*D.L. Jardine's* Ole)	10	0	2.0	0	0	105	<1.0

Food and Measure	cal.	prot. (gms)	carbo. (gms)	fat (gms)	chol. (mgs)	sod. (mgs)	fiber (gms)
(*Pace* Chunky)	10	0	2.0	0	0	230	1.0
cilantro:							
(*Pace* Chunky)	10	0	2.0	0	0	270	1.0
(*Walnut Acres* Fiesta)	10	0	2.0	0	0	135	0
olive (*D.L. Jardine's*)	10	1.0	2.0	0	0	230	<1.0
corn (*Garden of Eatin'*)	15	0	3.0	0	0	190	0
cranberry orange (*D.L. Jardine's*)	15	0	4.0	0	0	100	<1.0
fire-roasted tomato:							
(*Pace* Chunky)	10	0	2.0	0	0	230	1.0
(*Tostitos*)	15	<1.0	2.0	0	0	280	1.0
mild or medium (*El Torito*)	10	0	2.0	0	0	170	0
mild or medium (*Zapata* Verde) ..	10	0	2.0	0	0	100	0
mild, medium, or hot (*Zapata* Roja) ...	10	0	2.0	0	0	130	0
garlic:							
(*Jose Goldstein* XXX)	10	0	2.0	0	0	160	0
(*Garden of Eatin'*) .	10	0	2.0	0	0	180	0
(*Pace* Chunky Grande)	10	0	3.0	0	0	200	1.0
cactus (*Jose Goldstein*)	10	0	2.0	0	0	230	0
chipotle (*Jose Goldstein*)	5	0	2.0	0	0	140	0
chipotle or cilantro (*Muir Glen*)	10	0	2.0	0	0	125	0
garlic, roasted:							
(*Newman's Own*) ..	10	1.0	2.0	0	0	150	1.0
and olive (*Jose Goldstein*)	10	0	1.0	1.0	0	115	0
green chili (*Pace Territorial House*) ..	10	0	2.0	0	0	180	<1.0
habanero:							
(*D.L. Jardine's*) ...	10	0	2.0	0	0	220	0
(*Frontier Traders* Wild & Hot)	10	0	2.0	0	0	110	0
garlic (*Pain Is Good*)	15	0	2.0	0	0	160	0
hot:							
(*Chi-Chi's*)	10	0	2.0	0	0	220	0
(*Chi-Chi's* Fiesta) ..	10	0	2.0	0	0	210	0
(*Herdez*)	10	0	1.0	0	0	240	0
(*Old El Paso Gotta Have Hot* Thick N' Chunky)	10	0	3.0	0	0	230	0

Food and Measure	cal.	prot. (gms)	carbo. (gms)	fat (gms)	chol. (mgs)	sod. (mgs)	fiber (gms)
Salsa *(cont.)*							
jalapeño:							
green (*La Victoria*)	10	0	2.0	0	0	150	0
red (*La Victoria*)	10	0	2.0	0	0	95	0
smoked (*Fiesta*)	15	0	2.0	0	0	240	0
smoked (*Frontier Traders*)	10	0	2.0	0	0	240	0
lime cilantro (*D.L. Jardine's*)	10	0	3.0	0	0	210	0
lime and garlic (*Pace* Chunky)	15	0	3.0	0	0	210	1.0
mango (*D.L. Jardine's* Mariachi)	15	0	3.0	0	0	180	0
medium:							
(*Garden of Eatin'*)	20	1.0	4.0	0	0	190	0
(*Herdez*)	10	0	1.0	0	0	270	0
(*Litehouse*)	10	0	3.0	0	0	210	0
(*Muir Glen*)	10	0	2.0	0	0	125	0
(*Taco Bell* Thick 'n Chunky)	15	0	2.0	0	0	240	1.0
medium or mild :							
(*Amy's*)	10	0	2.0	0	0	190	0
(*Cape Cod*)	15	<1.0	3.0	0	0	210	1.0
(*Chi-Chi's*)	10	0	2.0	0	0	150	0
(*Chi-Chi's* All Natural)	10	0	2.0	0	0	140	0
(*Herdez* Casera)	10	0	1.0	0	0	270	0
(*Old El Paso* Salsa Verde)	10	0	2.0	0	0	95	0
(*Old El Paso* Thick N' Chunky)	10	0	3.0	0	0	230	0
(*Red Gold*)	10	0	2.0	0	0	120	1.0
(*Tostitos*)	15	<1.0	3.0	0	0	260	1.0
mild:							
(*Old El Paso* Wild for Mild* Thick n' Chunky)	10	0	2.0	0	0	230	0
(*Taco Bell* Thick 'n Chunky)	15	0	3.0	0	0	230	1.0
peach:							
(*D.L. Jardine's*)	20	0	5.0	0	0	95	0
(*Frontier Traders* Wild & Mild)	15	0	4.0	0	0	100	0
(*Newman's Own*)	25	0	6.0	0	0	90	1.0

Food and Measure	cal.	prot. (gms)	carbo. (gms)	fat (gms)	chol. (mgs)	sod. (mgs)	fiber (gms)
Southwest, sweet (*Walnut Acres*) ..	20	0	5.0	0	0	85	0
pepper:							
garden (*Old El Paso*)	10	0	2.0	0	0	240	<1.0
roasted, and garlic (*Pace* Chunky) ..	10	0	2.0	0	0	230	1.0
pineapple:							
(*D.L. Jardine's*) ...	15	0	4.0	0	0	85	0
(*Newman's Own*) ..	15	0	3.0	0	0	90	1.0
chipotle (*D.L. Jardine's*)	15	1.0	3.0	0	0	130	0
Jamaican (*Pain Is Good*)	15	0	3.0	0	0	110	0
raspberry:							
(*D.L. Jardine's*) ...	15	0	4.0	0	0	90	<1.0
(*Frontier Traders* Wild & Mild) ...	15	0	4.0	0	0	70	0
Chardonnay (*D.L. Jardine's*)	15	0	4.0	0	0	95	0
red pepper, roasted:							
(*Guiltless Gourmet*)	15	0	2.0	0	0	130	0
and garlic (*Pace* Chunky)	10	0	2.0	0	0	230	<1.0
Southwest Tex-Mex (*Frontier Traders*) ..	10	0	2.0	0	0	110	0
sweet (*Synder's* Garden Style)	20	0	5.0	0	0	95	0
tequila lime (*Chi-Chi's*)	15	0	3.0	0	0	160	0
tomatillo, fire-roasted (*Fiesta*)	60	3.0	12.0	.5	0	390	0
tomato, roasted (*Chi-Chi's*)	10	0	2.0	0	0	180	0
Salsa dip (see also "Cheese dip"), sour cream (*Cabot* Salsa Grande), 2 tbsp.	50	1.0	1.0	5.0	15	130	0
Salsa seasoning mix, fresh (*Lawry's*), ½ tsp.	5	0	1.0	0	0	90	0
Salsify:							
raw:							
(*Frieda's*), ¾ cup, 3 oz.	70	3.0	16.0	0	0	15	3.0
untrimmed, 1 lb. ..	325	13.0	73.4	.8	0	79	13.0
sliced, ½ cup	55	2.2	12.5	.1	0	13	2.2

Food and Measure	cal.	prot. (gms)	carbo. (gms)	fat (gms)	chol. (mgs)	sod. (mgs)	fiber (gms)
Salsify (cont.)							
boiled, drained, sliced,							
½ cup	46	1.9	10.5	.1	0	11	2.1
Salt, ¼ tsp.:							
(*Morton*)	0	0	0	0	0	590	0
popcorn, fine ground							
(*Fanci Food*)	0	0	0	0	0	640	0
sea:							
(*Hain*)	0	0	0	0	0	590	0
(*Shiloh Farms*)	0	0	0	0	0	420	0
French (*Eden*)	0	0	0	0	0	392	0
Portuguese (*Eden*) .	0	0	0	0	0	408	0
Salt, seasoned (see							
also specific listings),							
¼ tsp.:							
(*Lawry's*)	0	0	0	0	0	380	0
(*McCormick* Salt 'n							
Spice)............	0	0	0	0	0	250	0
(*McCormick Season-*							
All)	0	0	0	0	0	350	0
black pepper (*Lawry's*)	0	0	0	0	0	170	0
butter flavor							
(*McCormick*)	0	0	0	0	0	310	0
hickory smoked							
(*McCormick*)	0	0	0	0	0	455	0
peppered (*McCormick*							
Season-All)	0	0	0	0	0	110	0
red pepper (*Lawry's*) .	0	0	0	0	0	300	0
spicy (*McCormick*							
Season-All)	0	0	0	0	0	250	0
Salt, substitute:							
(*Morton*), ¼ tsp.	0	0	0	0	0	0	0
(*Nu-Salt*), ¼ tsp.	0	0	0	0	0	0	0
Salt pork, raw, 1 oz. .	212	1.4	0	22.8	25	404	0
Sandwich, see specific							
listings							
Sandwich sauce,							
canned, ¼ cup,							
except as noted:							
(*Hormel Not-So-*							
Sloppy-Joe)	60	1.0	13.0	0	0	640	1.0
sloppy Joe:							
(*Del Monte*)	50	1.0	11.0	0	0	620	0
(*Heinz*)	40	1.0	10.0	0	0	360	1.0
(*Manwich* Original)	30	1.0	6.0	0	0	380	1.0

Food and Measure	cal.	prot. (gms)	carbo. (gms)	fat (gms)	chol. (mgs)	sod. (mgs)	fiber (gms)
hickory smoke (*Del Monte*)	60	1.0	14.0	0	0	660	0
vegetarian (*Worthington*), ½ cup	140	9.0	23.0	1.0	0	580	3.0
Sandwich sauce seasoning mix, see "Sloppy Joe seasoning mix"							
Sandwich spread (see also "Meat spread," and specific listings):							
(*Black Bear*), 1 tbsp. .	50	0	3.0	4.0	<5	105	0
(*Cains*), 1 tbsp.	70	0	2.0	7.0	5	80	0
(*Hellmann's*), 1 tbsp. .	50	0	2.0	5.0	<5	200	0
burger (*Kraft*), 2 tbsp.	150	0	4.0	15.0	15	210	0
Sapodilla:							
(*Frieda's*), 3-oz. fruit .	70	0	17.0	1.0	0	10	5.0
1 medium, 3" x 2½" . .	140	.7	33.9	1.9	0	20	9.0
½ cup	100	.5	24.1	1.3	0	15	6.4
Sapote:							
(*Frieda's*), 5 oz.	190	3.0	47.0	1.0	0	15	4.0
11.2-oz. fruit, 7.9 oz. trimmed	301	4.8	76.0	1.4	0	23	5.9
trimmed, 1 oz.	38	.6	9.6	.2	0	3	.7
Sardine, fresh, see "Herring"							
Sardine, canned (see also "Herring, canned"):							
Atlantic, in oil:							
drained, 2 oz.	118	14.8	0	6.5	81	286	0
2 medium, 3" long .	50	5.9	0	2.8	34	121	0
in hot sauce:							
(*Beach Cliff/Brunswick* Louisiana), 3.75-oz. can	150	18.0	2.0	8.0	110	420	0
(*Bela*), ¼ cup	110	13.0	0	7.0	20	120	0
(*Bumble Bee*), 2 oz.	90	8.0	0	6.0	30	250	0
in lemon sauce:							
(*Bela*), ¼ cup	130	12.0	0	9.0	20	115	0
(*Goya*), ¼ cup	120	10.0	0	9.0	20	300	0
in mustard sauce:							
(*Beach Cliff/Brunswick*), 3.75-oz. can	150	20.0	2.0	8.0	110	460	0
(*Bumble Bee*), 2 oz.	70	8.0	1.0	3.5	20	260	1.0

Food and Measure	cal.	prot. (gms)	carbo. (gms)	fat (gms)	chol. (mgs)	sod. (mgs)	fiber (gms)
Sardine, canned, in mustard sauce *(cont.)*							
(*Crown Prince* Brisling),							
3.7-oz. can	170	17.0	2.0	10.0	105	820	2.0
(*Yankee Clipper*),							
¼ cup	90	10.0	1.0	5.0	35	260	0
in olive oil, drained:							
(*Beach Cliff* 3.75 oz.),							
3.4 oz.	200	20.0	0	14.0	105	270	0
(*Bela*), ¼ cup	120	13.0	0	7.0	20	130	0
(*Crown Prince* Brisling),							
2.9-oz. can	260	16.0	0	22.0	85	400	0
(*Goya*), ¼ cup	130	13.0	0	9.0	20	20	0
skin/boneless (*Crown Prince*),							
3.5-oz. can	230	24.0	0	15.0	40	300	<1.0
skin/boneless (*Granadaisa*),							
¼ cup	120	13.0	0	7.0	24	280	0
in soy oil, drained:							
(*Beach Cliff* Oval),							
2 oz.	100	12.0	0	6.0	50	80	0
(*Beach Cliff/Bruns- wick* 3.75 oz.),							
3.4 oz.	200	22.0	1.0	12.0	115	260	0
(*Bumble Bee*), 2 oz.	100	10.0	0	7.0	25	250	0
(*Yankee Clipper*),							
¼ cup	120	14.0	0	7.0	40	110	0
w/green chili (*Beach Cliff* 3.75 oz.),							
3.4 oz.	180	19.0	1.0	12.0	100	250	0
w/hot Tabasco pepper (*Bruns- wick* 3.75 oz.),							
3.3 oz.	190	21.0	0	12.0	110	280	0
spiced (*Goya*), ¼ cup	120	12.0	0	9.0	20	280	0
in tomato sauce:							
(*Beach Cliff*),							
3.75-oz. can	140	17.0	2.0	6.0	90	520	0
(*Beach Cliff* Oval),							
2 oz.	70	0	1.0	3.5	45	200	0
(*Brunswick*),							
3.75-oz. can	150	16.0	3.0	8.0	100	520	0
(*Goya*), ¼ cup	130	12.0	1.0	9.0	20	300	0

Food and Measure	cal.	prot. (gms)	carbo. (gms)	fat (gms)	chol. (mgs)	sod. (mgs)	fiber (gms)
(*Yankee Clipper*), ¼ cup	90	10.0	1.0	5.0	40	220	0
Pacific, 2 oz.	101	9.3	n.a.	6.8	35	235	<1.0
in water:							
(*Bumble Bee*), 2 oz.	90	10.0	0	6.0	25	250	0
(*Brunswick* 3.75 oz.), 3.3 oz.	150	19.0	0	8.0	115	240	0
(*Crown Prince* Brisling), 2.9-oz. can	220	15.0	3.0	16.0	50	115	0
skin/boneless (*Crown Prince*), 3.2-oz. can	130	22.0	0	5.0	35	360	0
Sardine oil, see "Oil"							
Satsuma, see "Tangerine"							
Sauce, see specific sauce listings							
Sauce, all purpose, 2 tbsp.:							
(*Ott's* Famous)	80	0	8.0	5.0	0	200	0
(*Silver Dollar City*) . . .	30	0	8.0	0	0	180	0
Sauerbraten season- ing mix (*Knorr Recipe Classics*), 1 tbsp.	35	<1.0	6.0	1.0	0	440	0
Sauerkraut, 2 tbsp., except as noted:							
(*Boar's Head*)	5	0	1.0	0	0	180	<1.0
(*Claussen*)	5	0	1.0	0	0	220	1.0
(*Del Monte*)	0	0	<1.0	0	0	180	<1.0
(*Eden* Organic), ½ cup	25	2.0	4.0	0	0	580	3.0
(*Hebrew National*) . . .	5	0	1.0	0	0	180	1.0
(*S&W*)	0	0	1.0	0	0	180	<1.0
Bavarian style:							
(*Bush's*)	15	0	3.0	0	0	105	1.0
(*Del Monte*)	15	0	4.0	0	0	180	0
chopped or shredded (*Bush's*)	5	0	1.0	0	0	180	1.0
Sausage (see also specific listings), cooked, except as noted:							
beef, smoked, 1 link: (*Arnold's*), 1.8 oz. . .	200	8.0	1.0	18.0	75	610	0

Food and Measure	cal.	prot. (gms)	carbo. (gms)	fat (gms)	chol. (mgs)	sod. (mgs)	fiber (gms)
Sausage, beef, smoked *(cont.)*							
hot (*Arnold's*), 1.8 oz.	210	8.0	1.0	19.0	75	610	0
spicy (*Johnsonville* Hot Links), 2.7 oz.	230	9.0	2.0	20.0	40	620	0
chicken, 1 link, 2-oz., except as noted:							
Andouille, Cajun (*Bilinski*)	80	9.0	1.0	4.0	60	300	0
apple, smoked (*Aidells*), 3.5 oz. .	210	16.0	1.0	16.0	90	730	0
apple, smoked, minis (*Aidells*), 5 links, 2 oz.	100	16.0	1.0	8.0	50	370	0
apple Chardonnay (*Bilinski*)	70	10.0	2.5	5.5	60	350	0
cilantro (*Bilinski*) . .	70	9.0	1.0	3.5	40	270	1.0
garlic, roasted (*Bell & Evans*), 2.25 oz.	80	9.0	2.0	4.0	45	320	0
Italian, mild, w/pepper and onion (*Bilinski*) .	70	9.0	1.0	3.5	60	270	0
Italian, sweet (*Bell & Evans*), 2.25 oz. .	80	9.0	2.0	4.5	50	330	0
jalapeño (*Bilinski*) .	70	9.0	0	4.0	55	270	0
lemon, smoked (*Aidell's*), 3.5 oz.	210	15.0	1.0	16.0	90	700	0
mango (*Aidell's*), 3.5 oz.	210	17.0	6.0	13.0	65	740	0
mango, breakfast (*Aidells*), 2 links, 2 oz.	170	9.0	3.0	7.0	40	420	0
maple apple (*Bell & Evans*), 2.25 oz. .	110	9.0	8.0	6.0	45	550	0
pesto (*Bilinski*) . . .	90	10.0	0	5.0	40	320	0
spinach (*Bilinski*) . .	70	9.0	1.0	3.5	40	270	1.0
sun-dried tomato (*Bilinski*)	70	10.0	2.0	3.5	40	280	0
sun-dried tomato and basil (*Bell & Evans*), 2.25 oz. .	80	9.0	2.0	4.5	45	350	0
chicken, raw, Italian (*Organic Valley*), 3 oz.	140	14.0	0	9.0	80	580	0
chicken/turkey, see "turkey/chicken," below							

Food and Measure	cal.	prot. (gms)	carbo. (gms)	fat (gms)	chol. (mgs)	sod. (mgs)	fiber (gms)
duck, smoked (*Aidells*), 3.5-oz. link	220	17.0	1.0	16.0	60	700	0
garlic:							
(*Johnsonville* Irish O' Garlic), 3-oz. link	290	14.0	1.0	25.0	65	800	0
(*Trois Petits Cochons* Saucisson a l'Ail), 2 oz.	80	11.0	1.0	3.5	35	430	0
Italian:							
(*Johnsonville* Heat & Serve), 2.7-oz. link	260	12.0	3.0	23.0	50	920	0
hot (*Hatfield* Burgers), 3-oz. patty	210	16.0	3.0	14.0	45	650	0
hot (*Hatfield* Rope), 2 oz.	140	10.0	2.0	9.0	30	430	0
hot or mild, ground, (*Johnsonville*), 2-oz. patty	160	8.0	1.0	13.0	35	390	0
hot or sweet (*Hatfield* Grillers), 2-oz. link	160	10.0	2.0	13.0	35	510	0
hot, sweet, or mild, fresh (*Johnsonville*), 3-oz. link .	290	14.0	1.0	25.0	65	800	0
mild, precooked (*Johnsonville*), 2.7-oz. link	240	9.0	2.0	22.0	50	760	0
sweet (*Hatfield* Burgers), 3-oz. patty	210	16.0	2.0	14.0	50	780	0
sweet (*Hatfield* Rope), 2 oz.	140	10.0	1.0	9.0	30	520	0
Italian, raw (*Organic Valley*), 3-oz. link . .	240	12.0	<1.0	21.0	60	650	0
Polish, 1 link:							
fresh, grilled (*Johnsonville*), 3 oz. . .	290	14.0	1.0	25.0	65	800	0
precooked (*Johnsonville*), 2.7 oz.	240	9.0	2.0	21.0	60	640	0
pork, chub (*Jimmy Dean*), 2 oz.	220	7.0	0	21.0	40	280	0
pork, fresh:							
ground, grilled (*Johnsonville*), 2 oz.	160	8.0	1.0	13.0	35	390	0

Food and Measure	cal.	prot. (gms)	carbo. (gms)	fat (gms)	chol. (mgs)	sod. (mgs)	fiber (gms)
Sausage, pork, fresh *(cont.)*							
link, raw, 1 oz.	118	3.3	.3	11.4	19	189	0
link, cooked, .5 oz.							
(1 oz. raw)	105	5.6	.3	8.8	24	367	0
patty, raw, 2 oz. . . .	286	6.6	.6	22.8	39	378	0
pork, link, 3 links,							
except as noted:							
(*Johnsonville* Break-							
fast Original) . . .	190	10.0	1.0	16.0	40	610	0
(*Little Sizzlers*)	200	8.0	0	19.0	40	580	0
(*Patrick Cudahy* Pre-							
cooked), 2 links .	260	8.0	<1.0	25.0	55	400	0
brown sugar honey							
(*Johnsonville*							
Breakfast Links) .	190	7.0	5.0	15.0	35	460	0
hickory smoke							
(*Johnsonville*) . .	200	10.0	2.0	17.0	40	590	0
hot and spicy (*Little*							
Sizzlers)	170	8.0	0	19.0	40	670	0
maple (*Johnsonville*							
Vermont Breakfast							
Links)	200	10.0	1.0	18.0	40	600	0
maple (*Little Sizzlers*)	200	8.0	2.0	19.0	40	580	0
mild (*Jones Dairy*							
Farm Golden							
Brown Precooked),							
2 links	100	7.0	1.0	8.0	35	300	0
pepper and onion,							
pan fried (*Hatfield*							
Grillers), 1 link . .	180	13.0	3.0	11.0	40	700	0
pork, patty, 2 pcs.,							
except as noted:							
(*Johnsonville* Break-							
fast Patties)	180	11.0	1.0	15.0	40	580	0
(*Jones Dairy Farm*							
Golden Brown Pre-							
cooked), 1 pc. . .	150	5.0	1.0	14.0	30	240	0
(*Little Sizzlers*)	200	8.0	0	19.0	40	580	0
(*Patrick Cudahy* Pre-							
cooked)	230	8.0	<1.0	22.0	50	390	0
(*Swift Premium*							
Brown 'N Serve							
Original)	180	6.0	2.0	16.0	40	420	0

Food and Measure	cal.	prot. (gms)	carbo. (gms)	fat (gms)	chol. (mgs)	sod. (mgs)	fiber (gms)
pork, raw:							
(*Organic Valley* Breakfast), 2 links	130	9.0	0	10.0	40	420	0
chub, raw (*Organic Valley*), 4 oz. ...	250	18.0	<1.0	19.0	75	840	0
pork/beef, fresh, .5-oz. link	112	3.9	.8	10.3	20	228	0
pork/turkey (*Healthy Choice* Breakfast), 3 links or 3 patties .	70	8.0	3.0	3.0	25	480	0
smoked, 1 link, except as noted:							
(*Boar's Head* Natural Casing), 4 oz. ...	310	15.0	2.0	27.0	65	920	0
(*Healthy Choice*), 2 oz.	80	7.0	6.0	2.5	25	480	0
(*Johnsonville*), 2.7 oz.	240	9.0	2.0	21.0	60	640	0
(*Johnsonville* Little Smokies), 6 links, 2 oz.	180	6.0	1.0	16.0	35	480	0
(*Oscar Mayer* Little Smokies), 6 links, 2 oz.	170	7.0	1.0	15.0	35	570	0
Andouille (*Aidells* Cajun), 3.5 oz. ..	220	16.0	1.0	17.0	55	770	0
Andouille (*Johnson-ville* New Orleans), 2.7 oz.	230	9.0	2.0	20.0	40	630	0
cheese (*Johnsonville* Bedder with Cheddar/Swiss-wurst), 2.7 oz. ..	240	9.0	2.0	21.0	60	640	0
cheese (*Oscar Mayer* Little Smokies), 6 links, 2 oz. ...	180	6.0	2.0	16.0	30	590	0
hot (*Boar's Head*), 3.2 oz.	250	6.0	<1.0	22.0	55	740	0
turkey:							
raw (*Louis Rich* Chub), 2.5 oz. ..	120	12.0	1.0	8.0	55	430	0
raw (*Shady Brook Farms* Breakfast), 2.3 oz.	80	10.0	0	4.0	35	480	0

Food and Measure	cal.	prot. (gms)	carbo. (gms)	fat (gms)	chol. (mgs)	sod. (mgs)	fiber (gms)
Sausage, turkey *(cont.)*							
raw (*Wampler* Break-							
fast), 4 oz.	230	17.0	1.0	7.0	100	880	0
smoked (*Louis Rich*),							
2-oz. link	90	8.0	2.0	5.0	35	520	0
turkey, Italian, 1 link:							
hot (*Perdue*), 2.9 oz.	150	16.0	1.0	9.0	60	470	0
sweet (*Perdue*),							
2.4 oz.	150	16.0	1.0	9.0	60	490	0
turkey, Italian, raw:							
hot (*Perdue*), 3.2 oz.	150	16.0	1.0	9.0	60	500	0
hot (*Shady Brook*							
Farms 92% Fat							
Free), 3 oz.	110	13.0	1.0	7.0	50	600	0
sweet (*Perdue*),							
2.7 oz.	150	16.0	1.0	9.0	60	510	0
sweet (*Shady Brook*							
Farms 92% Fat							
Free), 3 oz.	110	13.0	1.0	7.0	50	570	0
turkey/chicken,							
3.5-oz. link, except							
as noted:							
Andouille, Cajun,							
minis (*Aidells*),							
5 links, 2 oz. . . .	80	11.0	1.0	3.0	45	490	0
artichoke and garlic,							
smoked (*Aidells*)	160	16.0	3.0	10.0	90	650	0
black bean, Cuban							
(*Aidells*)	180	15.0	6.0	11.0	90	850	0
curry, Burmese,							
smoked (*Aidells*)	220	18.0	3.0	15.0	95	730	0
habanero green chili,							
smoked (*Aidells*)	170	16.0	2.0	11.0	55	600	0
New Mexico, smoked							
(*Aidells*)	210	15.0	2.0	16.0	80	600	0
pesto, smoked							
(*Aidells*)	220	18.0	2.0	16.0	75	780	0
portobello mushroom							
(*Aidells*)	160	15.0	3.0	9.0	85	700	0
roasted red pepper							
w/corn (*Aidells*) .	120	18.0	2.0	4.0	70	800	0
sun-dried tomato,							
smoked (*Aidells*)	210	19.0	1.0	14.0	80	730	0

Food and Measure	cal.	prot. (gms)	carbo. (gms)	fat (gms)	chol. (mgs)	sod. (mgs)	fiber (gms)
sun-dried tomato, smoked, minis (*Aidells*), 5 links, 2 oz.	110	11.0	1.0	7.0	45	370	0
Sausage, canned:							
pickled, regular or hot (*Hormel*), 6 links, 2 oz.	130	8.0	1.0	10.0	40	420	0
Vienna:							
(*Armour*), 3 links . .	150	5.0	0	14.0	50	430	0
(*Goya*), 3 links	130	5.0	1.0	12.0	45	330	0
(*Hormel*), 2 oz. . . .	150	5.0	0	14.0	50	420	0
chicken (*Hormel*), 2 oz.	100	6.0	0	7.0	50	480	0
Sausage, freeze-dried, pork (*Mountain House*), 2 patties . .	220	25.0	2.0	13.0	90	1050	0
"Sausage," vegetarian, canned (see also specific listings):							
(*Loma Linda* Linkettes), 1.2-oz. link	70	7.0	1.0	4.0	0	160	1.0
(*Loma Linda* Little Links), 2 links, 1.6 oz.	90	8.0	3.0	5.0	0	250	2.0
(*Loma Linda* Veja-Links), 1.1-oz. link	45	5.0	3.0	1.5	0	220	0
(*Worthington* Saucettes), 1.3-oz. link	90	6.0	1.0	6.0	0	200	1.0
(*Worthington* Super-Links), 1.7-oz. link .	110	7.0	2.0	8.0	0	350	1.0
"Sausage," vegetarian, frozen (see also specific listings):							
crumbles (*Morningstar Farms*), ⅔ cup	90	11.0	5.0	2.5	0	440	1.0
links:							
(*Boca* Breakfast), 2 links, 1.6 oz. . .	70	8.0	5.0	3.0	0	330	2.0
(*Morningstar Farms*), 2 links, 1.6 oz. . .	80	9.0	3.0	3.0	0	320	2.0
(*Quorn*), 2 links, 1.6 oz.	70	8.0	2.0	3.0	0	210	1.0
(*Worthington* Prosage), 2 links, 1.6 oz.	80	9.0	3.0	3.0	0	320	2.0

Food and Measure	cal.	prot. (gms)	carbo. (gms)	fat (gms)	chol. (mgs)	sod. (mgs)	fiber (gms)
"Sausage," vegetarian, frozen, links *(cont.)*							
(*Yves*), 2 oz.	70	11.0	3.0	2.0	0	440	2.0
.9-oz. link	64	4.6	2.5	4.5	0	222	.7
Italian (*Boca*),							
2.5-oz. link	130	13.0	6.0	6.0	0	650	1.0
smoked (*Boca*),							
2.5-oz. link	130	14.0	6.0	6.0	0	680	1.0
patties:							
(*Boca* Breakfast),							
1.3-oz. pc.	60	7.0	5.0	2.0	0	280	2.0
(*Morningstar Farms*),							
1.3-oz. pc.	80	10.0	3.0	3.0	0	270	2.0
(*Worthington Prosage*),							
1.4-oz, pc.	80	10.0	3.0	3.0	0	300	2.0
(*Yves*), 1.7-oz. pc. .	80	11.0	4.0	2.0	0	350	2.0
1.3-oz. pc.	97	7.0	3.7	6.9	0	337	1.1
Sausage seasoning							
(*Tone's*), 1 tsp.	12	.4	2.7	.3	0	1	.7
Sausage stick (see also "Beef jerky"), beef or spicy (*Johnsonville* Snack Stix), 1 oz. . .	120	5.0	0	11.0	25	400	0
Sausage sub, frozen, Italian, and peppers (*Michelina's Hot Subs*), 2.1-oz. pc. .	310	11.0	39.0	12.0	15	810	2.0
Savory, ground, 1 tsp.	4	.1	1.0	.1	0	<1	<1.0
Sbarro, 1 slice or serving:							
pizza:							
cheese	460	24.0	60.0	13.0	30	1080	3.0
chicken vegetable . .	530	24.0	69.0	17.0	45	1260	5.0
mushroom	460	19.0	62.0	14.0	20	1310	4.0
pepperoni	730	35.0	61.0	37.0	75	2200	3.0
sausage	670	35.0	60.0	31.0	80	1810	3.0
supreme	630	31.0	63.0	27.0	60	1720	3.0
tomato, fresh	450	20.0	60.0	14.0	25	1040	3.0
white	570	30.0	59.0	23.0	55	1150	2.0
pizza, gourmet:							
broccoli spinach . . .	720	29.0	88.0	28.0	30	1540	6.0
cheese	660	30.0	84.0	21.0	40	1460	4.0
ham, pineapple, and bacon	680	33.0	88.0	21.0	45	1820	4.0

Food and Measure	cal.	prot. (gms)	carbo. (gms)	fat (gms)	chol. (mgs)	sod. (mgs)	fiber (gms)
meat delight	780	41.0	84.0	29.0	80	2250	4.0
mushroom	610	22.0	85.0	20.0	20	1600	5.0
mushroom, spinach	710	29.0	87.0	27.0	30	1680	6.0
spinach, yellow							
pepper	670	28.0	86.0	24.0	30	1470	5.0
tomato basil	700	28.0	87.0	25.0	40	1650	5.0
pizza, low carb:							
cheese	310	34.0	18.0	14.0	25	640	n.a.
pepperoni	420	36.0	18.0	14.0	60	940	n.a.
sausage/pepperoni .	560	44.0	18.0	35.0	95	1300	n.a.
pizza, stuffed:							
pepperoni	960	52.0	89.0	34.0	50	1610	4.0
Philly cheesesteak .	830	38.0	94.0	33.0	70	2090	5.0
spinach broccoli ...	790	32.0	89.0	34.0	50	1610	5.0
calzone, cheese ...	770	39.0	87.0	28.0	90	1410	3.0
stromboli:							
pepperoni	890	39.0	82.0	44.0	80	2470	3.0
spinach, tomato,							
broccoli	680	29.0	84.0	24.0	35	1420	5.0
salads:							
Caesar	80	2.0	6.0	5.0	5	200	1.0
cucumber tomato ..	130	1.0	9.0	11.0	0	85	2.0
fruit	130	2.0	32.0	1.0	0	15	3.0
Greek	60	2.0	3.0	5.0	10	130	<1.0
mixed garden	35	2.0	7.0	0	0	15	3.0
pasta primavera ...	190	4.0	21.0	10.0	0	1180	2.0
stringbean tomato .	100	1.0	9.0	7.0	0	80	2.0
dinner plates:							
baked ziti w/sauce .	700	39.0	43.0	41.0	135	1220	4.0
chicken Francese ..	640	63.0	8.0	38.0	175	590	2.0
chicken Parmesan .	520	64.0	16.0	22.0	175	750	2.0
chicken Portofino ..	730	63.0	7.0	48.0	225	790	1.0
chicken Vesuvio ...	690	63.0	8.0	43.0	225	810	1.0
eggplant rollatini							
w/cheese	580	21.0	40.0	38.0	50	900	4.0
garlic rolls	170	5.0	28.0	4.5	0	370	<1.0
lasagna, meat	650	41.0	36.0	37.0	130	1130	3.0
meatballs	140	8.0	10.0	9.0	30	880	1.0
pasta Milano	640	45.0	41.0	32.0	175	740	6.0
pasta rustica	600	10.0	39.0	47.0	70	2288	5.0
penne w/sausage,							
peppers	710	35.0	33.0	49.0	130	1690	4.0
penne alla vodka ..	640	23.0	67.0	28.0	120	1000	5.0
sausage and peppers	410	17.0	19.0	30.0	55	1340	4.0

Food and Measure	cal.	prot. (gms)	carbo. (gms)	fat (gms)	chol. (mgs)	sod. (mgs)	fiber (gms)
Sbarro, dinner plates *(cont.)*							
spaghetti w/:							
chicken Parmesan	930	75.0	75.0	36.0	175	950	6.0
chicken Vesuvio .	850	50.0	64.0	41.0	145	1100	4.0
meatballs	680	19.0	96.0	25.0	15	1720	9.0
sauce	820	20.0	120.0	28.0	0	890	10.0
vegetables, mixed .	190	3.0	14.0	15.0	0	330	4.0
dessert, cake:							
Black Forest	480	3.0	59.0	24.0	50	340	1.0
carrot	540	5.0	64.0	29.0	65	400	1.0
cheesecake	560	9.0	42.0	40.0	170	450	1.0
milk chocolate	490	4.0	59.0	25.0	30	310	1.0
Scallion, see "Onion, green"							
Scallop, meat only:							
raw, 4 oz.	100	19.0	2.7	.9	38	183	0
raw, 2 large or 5 small, 1.1 oz.	26	5.0	.7	.2	10	48	0
steamed, 4 oz.	127	26.3	0	1.6	60	301	0
Scallop, frozen (*Contessa*), 4 oz. ..	80	19.0	<1.0	0	<5	430	0
"Scallop," imitation:							
(*Louis Kemp Scallop Delights* Bay Style), ½ cup, 3 oz.	80	8.0	12.0	0	10	385	0
from surimi, 4 oz. ...	112	14.5	12.1	.5	25	902	0
Scallop, smoked (*Ducktrap River*), ¼ cup	60	10.0	0	1.0	60	260	0
"Scallop," vegetarian, canned (*Worthington Skallops*), ½ cup, 3 oz.	90	17.0	4.0	1.0	0	390	3.0
Scallop dish, frozen:							
breaded, fried (*Mrs. Paul's*), 3.5 oz., 13 pcs.	220	12.0	27.0	7.0	25	440	1.0
cakes (*Yankee Trader*), 3-oz. cake	180	10.0	10.0	9.0	30	420	1.0
caviche, (*Sau•Sea*), ½ cup	70	6.0	5.0	3.0	45	310	1.0
Scallop squash (see also "Sunburst Squash"), ½ cup:							
raw, sliced	12	.8	2.5	.1	0	1	1.2

Food and Measure	cal.	prot. (gms)	carbo. (gms)	fat (gms)	chol. (mgs)	sod. (mgs)	fiber (gms)
boiled, drained, sliced	14	.9	3.0	.2	0	1	1.1
boiled, drained, mashed	19	1.2	4.0	.2	0	1	1.4
Scampi sauce, cooking (*Golden Dipt*), 2 tbsp.	210	0	4.0	25.0	0	140	0
Scarlet runner bean, canned (*Westbrae Natural* Organic Heirloom Beans), ½ cup	100	6.0	20.0	0	0	140	7.0
Schlotzsky's Deli, 1 serving:							
sandwich, on sourdough bun, except as noted:							
BLT:							
regular	578	21.0	70.0	24.0	41	1548	3.0
small	379	13.0	47.0	15.0	26	1010	2.0
chicken, Dijon, wheat:							
regular	496	38.0	74.0	6.0	68	2202	6.0
small	329	25.0	49.0	4.0	46	1456	4.0
chicken, fiesta, jalapeño cheese:							
regular	839	50.0	79.0	36.0	n.a.	2947	4.0
small	577	34.0	53.0	25.0	n.a.	1995	3.0
chicken, pesto:							
regular	512	37.0	73.0	9.0	71	1927	4.0
small	346	25.0	49.0	6.0	48	1297	2.0
chicken, Santa Fe:							
regular, jalapeño cheese	605	42.0	81.0	14.0	n.a.	2448	5.0
small, jalapeño cheese	404	28.0	54.0	9.0	n.a.	1654	3.0
chicken breast:							
regular	499	36.0	80.0	4.0	n.a.	2338	4.0
small	337	24.0	54.0	3.0	n.a.	1588	3.0
chicken club:							
regular	686	44.0	75.0	23.0	106	2403	4.0
small	458	29.0	50.0	15.0	71	1591	3.0
corned beef, dark rye:							
regular	593	43.0	78.0	12.0	n.a.	2929	4.0
small	393	29.0	52.0	8.0	n.a.	1924	3.0
pastrami/Swiss, dark rye:							
regular	882	60.0	81.0	36.0	n.a.	3977	4.0
small	586	40.0	54.0	24.0	n.a.	2622	3.0

Food and Measure	cal.	prot. (gms)	carbo. (gms)	fat (gms)	chol. (mgs)	sod. (mgs)	fiber (gms)
Schlotzsky's Deli, sandwich *(cont.)*					—		
The Philly:							
regular	840	57.0	86.0	29.0	n.a.	3103	4.0
small	571	39.0	57.0	21.0	n.a.	2064	2.0
Reuben, dark rye:							
corned beef,							
regular	838	54.0	82.0	33.0	n.a.	3955	4.0
corned beef, small	534	34.0	55.0	20.0	n.a.	2568	3.0
pastrami, regular	944	59.0	83.0	41.0	n.a.	4183	4.0
pastrami, small ..	635	40.0	56.0	28.0	n.a.	2857	3.0
turkey, regular ..	823	50.0	80.0	34.0	n.a.	3925	4.0
turkey, small ...	554	34.0	54.0	23.0	n.a.	2684	3.0
roast beef:							
regular	623	43.0	78.0	15.0	n.a.	2418	3.0
small	418	29.0	52.0	10.0	n.a.	1622	2.0
roast beef/cheese:							
regular	855	57.0	83.0	32.0	n.a.	3021	4.0
small	586	39.0	56.0	23.0	n.a.	2040	3.0
Texas Schlotsky's,							
jalapeño cheese:							
regular	776	43.0	76.0	32.0	n.a.	3388	3.0
small	537	30.0	51.0	23.0	n.a.	2288	2.0
tuna, wheat:							
regular	496	30.0	77.0	10.0	n.a.	1801	5.0
small	334	20.0	52.0	7.0	n.a.	1230	3.0
tuna melt, wheat:							
regular	740	44.0	83.0	29.0	n.a.	2459	6.0
small	509	30.0	56.0	21.0	n.a.	1677	4.0
turkey, smoked:							
regular	498	34.0	75.0	7.0	60	2123	3.0
small	335	23.0	50.0	5.0	40	1426	2.0
turkey/bacon club,							
wheat:							
regular	834	52.0	79.0	35.0	n.a.	3040	5.0
small	571	35.0	53.0	24.0	n.a.	2038	3.0
turkey guacamole:							
regular	643	36.0	84.0	19.0	n.a.	2711	3.0
small	423	24.0	56.0	12.0	n.a.	1789	2.0
vegetable club:							
regular	541	19.0	76.0	18.0	n.a.	1567	5.0
small	367	13.0	50.0	13.0	n.a.	1036	3.0
The Vegetarian,							
wheat:							
regular	482	18.0	79.0	11.0	n.a.	1475	5.0
small	324	12.0	53.0	7.0	n.a.	996	4.0

Food and Measure	cal.	prot. (gms)	carbo. (gms)	fat (gms)	chol. (mgs)	sod. (mgs)	fiber (gms)
Western vegetarian:							
regular	611	18.0	76.0	28.0	n.a.	1193	4.0
small	425	12.0	51.0	20.0	n.a.	816	3.0
sandwich, *The Original:*							
large, family size	1390	65.0	152.0	58.0	n.a.	4592	7.0
regular	738	34.0	79.0	31.0	n.a.	2560	4.0
small	525	24.0	53.0	24.0	n.a.	1781	3.0
deluxe:							
regular	930	53.0	84.0	42.0	n.a.	4296	4.0
deluxe, small ...	693	39.0	57.0	34.0	n.a.	3155	3.0
ham and cheese:							
regular	749	44.0	82.0	27.0	n.a.	3459	4.0
small	512	30.0	55.0	19.0	n.a.	2323	3.0
turkey, original:							
regular	822	51.0	81.0	32.0	n.a.	3127	4.0
small	583	36.0	54.0	24.0	n.a.	2161	3.0
wraps:							
chicken:							
Asian almond ...	459	24.0	72.0	7.0	n.a.	2391	4.0
Caesar	511	26.0	40.0	27.0	n.a.	1536	3.0
salsa, w/cheddar	460	27.0	44.0	17.0	n.a.	1419	3.0
tuna, zesty albacore	311	18.0	45.0	7.0	n.a.	1226	3.0
soup, 8-oz. cup:							
black bean, Monterey	240	11.0	42.0	4.0	n.a.	1010	17.0
broccoli cheese ...	252	7.0	23.0	17.0	17	1104	1.0
cheese, Wisconsin .	319	4.0	26.0	25.0	22	1104	1.0
chicken gumbo ...	110	4.0	13.0	5.0	20	1114	2.0
chicken noodle	122	8.0	18.0	2.0	39	1104	1.0
chicken tortilla ...	150	10.0	13.0	6.0	n.a.	1470	1.0
chicken w/wild rice	360	8.0	36.0	19.0	n.a.	1090	0
chili, Timberline ...	210	14.0	24.0	7.0	32	814	7.0
clam chowder, Boston	233	5.0	24.0	15.0	10	1062	1.0
corn chowder	284	2.0	38.0	17.0	6	1010	1.0
minestrone	89	3.0	17.0	1.0	0	1048	3.0
potato w/bacon ...	226	2.0	31.0	13.0	5	1209	2.0
ravioli tomato	111	6.0	21.0	2.0	17	1115	1.0
red beans and rice .	167	8.0	32.0	1.0	0	934	4.0
tomato basil, Tuscan	320	4.0	13.0	29.0	n.a.	1010	3.0
vegetable beef,							
gourmet	120	7.0	14.0	4.0	n.a.	1090	2.0
vegetarian vegetable	138	3.0	20.0	6.0	n.a.	1536	6.0
salad, deli, small:							
chicken..........	286	25.0	6.0	17.0	n.a.	736	2.0
coleslaw	188	1.0	24.0	10.0	6	275	3.0

Food and Measure	cal.	prot. (gms)	carbo. (gms)	fat (gms)	chol. (mgs)	sod. (mgs)	fiber (gms)
Schlotzsky's Deli, salad, deli, small *(cont.)*							
fresh fruit	86	1.0	21.0	1.0	0	22	3.0
macaroni	275	4.0	23.0	19.0	13	642	2.0
pasta, California ...	58	0	10.0	3.0	0	250	1.0
pasta, chicken pesto	326	18.0	40.0	11.0	n.a.	580	3.0
potato	288	4.0	35.0	15.0	13	600	4.0
potato, mustard ...	250	4.0	31.0	13.0	6	1050	4.0
tuna, albacore	136	20.0	2.0	9.0	n.a.	632	0
salad, leaf, no dressing, croutons, noodles:							
Caesar	30	3.0	3.0	1.0	0	89	2.0
chef, ham/turkey ..	202	18.0	13.0	11.0	n.a.	1122	3.0
chef, smoked turkey	199	19.0	13.0	10.0	n.a.	1010	3.0
chicken, Caesar ...	111	16.0	4.0	3.0	n.a.	433	2.0
chicken, Chinese ..	127	16.0	10.0	3.0	n.a.	360	2.0
garden	48	3.0	7.0	1.0	0	119	3.0
garden, small	23	1.0	3.0	1.0	0	58	2.0
Greek	127	9.0	10.0	11.0	n.a.	652	4.0
salad dressing, 1 pkt.:							
balsamic vinaigrette, Greek	170	0	2.0	17.0	0	330	0
Caesar	260	2.0	1.0	27.0	25	250	0
Italian, light	90	0	3.0	8.0	0	690	0
ranch	270	0	1.0	29.0	5	370	0
ranch, spicy	230	1.0	2.0	25.0	15	310	0
ranch, spicy, light ..	140	1.0	9.0	11.0	15	350	0
sesame ginger vinaigrette	170	1.0	8.0	15.0	0	370	0
Thousand Island ..	220	0	6.0	21.0	30	360	0
salad extras, 1 pkt.:							
chow mein noodles	74	2.0	1.0	4.0	0	111	1.0
garlic cheese croutons	46	1.0	5.0	2.0	0	142	0
pizza, 8" sourdough:							
bacon, tomato, and mushroom	611	27.0	78.0	22.0	n.a.	1966	4.0
cheese, double	580	26.0	76.0	19.0	n.a.	1791	4.0
cheese, double, and pepperoni	721	33.0	77.0	32.0	n.a.	2220	4.0
chicken, barbecue .	683	37.0	93.0	15.0	n.a.	2533	2.0
chicken, kung pao .	718	43.0	92.0	20.0	n.a.	2426	5.0
chicken, Thai	663	40.0	89.0	17.0	n.a.	2297	5.0
chicken and pesto .	649	40.0	78.0	19.0	74	2187	4.0

Food and Measure	cal.	prot. (gms)	carbo. (gms)	fat (gms)	chol. (mgs)	sod. (mgs)	fiber (gms)
combination, the							
original	625	26.0	79.0	23.0	n.a.	2068	5.0
herb, Tuscan	541	22.0	80.0	15.0	n.a.	2003	5.0
meat, three	805	37.0	74.0	39.0	n.a.	2797	3.0
Mediterranean	524	21.0	72.0	18.0	32	1879	3.0
smoked turkey and							
jalapeño	624	39.0	80.0	17.0	n.a.	2610	4.0
tomato and pesto ..	539	23.0	76.0	16.0	27	1670	4.0
vegetarian special .	551	24.0	76.0	17.0	27	1812	4.0
buns:							
dark rye, regular ..	327	10.0	68.0	2.0	0	819	3.0
dark rye, small	218	7.0	45.0	1.0	0	546	2.0
jalapeño cheese:							
regular	353	12.0	66.0	4.0	6	945	2.0
small	235	8.0	44.0	3.0	4	630	2.0
sourdough:							
large	667	22.0	136.0	4.0	0	1725	5.0
regular	333	11.0	68.0	2.0	0	863	2.0
small	225	7.0	46.0	1.0	0	582	2.0
wheat, regular	336	12.0	66.0	3.0	0	864	4.0
wheat, small	226	8.0	45.0	2.0	0	583	2.0
desserts, 1 pc.:							
cheesecake:							
cookies and crème	330	6.0	36.0	18.0	35	320	1.0
New York	310	7.0	31.0	18.0	60	230	0
strawberry swirl .	300	6.0	30.0	17.0	55	230	0
cookie:							
chocolate chip ..	160	2.0	23.0	7.0	10	150	0
fudge chocolate							
chip	170	2.0	22.0	8.0	10	170	1.0
oatmeal raisin ..	150	1.0	24.0	5.0	10	140	1.0
peanut butter ...	170	2.0	21.0	8.0	10	190	1.0
sugar	160	2.0	23.0	6.0	15	180	0
white chocolate							
macadamia ...	170	2.0	22.0	8.0	10	140	0
fudge brownie cake	410	5.0	46.0	25.0	35	135	3.0
Schnitzel, vegetarian,							
frozen (*Garden*							
Gourmet), 2.9-oz. pc.	100	10.0	5.0	4.0	0	500	6.0
Scone, all fruit varieties							
(*Health Valley*),							
2.1-oz. pc.	180	4.0	43.0	0	0	190	5.0
Scorpion drink mixer							
(*Trader Vic's*), 4 fl. oz.	80	0	21.0	0	0	20	0

Food and Measure	cal.	prot. (gms)	carbo. (gms)	fat (gms)	chol. (mgs)	sod. (mgs)	fiber (gms)
Scrapple, 2 oz.:							
(*Dietz & Watson*)	150	5.0	7.0	9.0	35	300	0
(*Hatfield*)	90	5.0	5.0	6.0	35	350	0
beef (*Hatfield*)	90	4.0	6.0	5.0	15	350	0
Scrod, fresh, see "Cod, Atlantic"							
Scup, meat only:							
raw, 4 oz.	119	21.4	0	3.1	59	48	0
baked, broiled, or microwaved, 4 oz. .	153	27.5	0	4.0	76	61	0
Sea bass, meat only:							
raw, 4 oz.	110	20.9	0	2.3	47	77	0
baked, broiled, or microwaved, 4 oz. .	141	26.8	0	2.9	60	99	0
Sea trout, meat only:							
raw, 4 oz.	118	19.0	0	4.1	94	66	0
baked, broiled, or microwaved, 4 oz. .	151	24.3	0	5.3	120	84	0
Sea vegetables, see "Seaweed"							
Seafood, see specific listings							
Seafood coating mix (see also "Batter and breading mix" and "Fish coating mix):							
Cajun (*Luzianne*), 2 tbsp.	100	2.0	22.0	1.0	0	1200	1.0
fry mix (*Golden Dipt* Fry Easy), 1⅔ tbsp.	50	0	9.0	0	0	490	0
shrimp and seafood (*Golden Dipt Oven Easy*), 2 tbsp.	70	1.0	8.0	2.0	0	230	0
Seafood salad kit, w/crab, crackers, 1 pkg.:							
(*Bumble Bee*):							
2.75-oz. can salad .	90	4.0	15.0	1.0	10	550	1.0
6 crackers, .6 oz. . .	90	2.0	12.0	4.5	0	180	0
Seafood sauce (see also specific listings), cocktail, ¼ cup, except as noted:							
(*Crosse & Blackwell*) .	100	1.0	23.0	0	0	710	0
(*Del Monte*)	100	1.0	24.0	0	0	910	0

Food and Measure	cal.	prot. (gms)	carbo. (gms)	fat (gms)	chol. (mgs)	sod. (mgs)	fiber (gms)
(*Heinz*)	60	1.0	15.0	0	0	690	1.0
(*Kraft*)	60	1.0	13.0	.5	0	800	1.0
(*Litehouse*), 2 tbsp. . .	25	0	5.0	0	0	220	0
(*Old Bay*)	110	0	18.0	.5	0	960	0
(*Red Gold*)	70	0	17.0	0	0	480	1.0
(*S&W*), 1 tbsp.	20	0	5.0	0	0	220	0
hot and spicy (*Kraft*) .	60	1.0	11.0	.5	0	900	1.0
Seafood seasoning (see also "Seafood coating mix" and specific listings):							
(*Old Bay*), ¼ tsp.	0	0	0	0	0	160	0
w/garlic and herb (*Old Bay*), ¼ tsp.	0	0	0	0	0	100	0
w/lemon and herb (*Old Bay*), ¼ tsp.	0	0	0	0	0	150	0
Seasoning (see also specific listings), ¼ tsp., except as noted:							
(*Ac'cent*), ⅛ tsp.	0	0	0	0	0	160	0
(*Sa-son* con Cilantro) .	0	0	0	0	0	170	0
(*Sa-son Ac'cent*)	0	0	0	0	0	150	0
(*Sazon Goya* con Achiote)	0	0	0	0	0	160	0
(*Sazon Goya* con Azafran)	0	0	0	0	0	150	0
blend, all varieties (*Mrs. Dash*)	0	0	0	0	0	0	0
Seaweed:							
agar:							
raw, 2 tbsp.	3	.5	.7	0	0	1	<.1
dried, 1 oz.	87	1.8	22.9	.1	0	29	2.2
freeze-dried, bar or flakes (*Eden* Agar Agar), .5 oz.	10	0	2.0	0	0	10	2.0
arame (*Eden*), ½ cup, .4 oz.	30	1.0	7.0	0	0	120	7.0
dulse flakes (*Maine Coast Sea Vegetables*), 1 tbsp.	13	1.0	2.0	0	0	87	2.0
hiziki (*Eden*), ½ cup . .	30	0	6.0	0	0	160	6.0
Irish moss, raw, 1 oz.	14	.4	3.5	<.1	0	19	.4
kelp, raw, 1 oz.	12	.5	2.7	.2	0	66	.4

Food and Measure	cal.	prot. (gms)	carbo. (gms)	fat (gms)	chol. (mgs)	sod. (mgs)	fiber (gms)
Seaweed, *(cont.)*							
kombu (*Eden*), ½ of							
7" pc.	10	0	2.0	0	0	90	1.0
laver, raw, 1 oz.	10	1.6	1.4	.1	0	1	4.1
nori, 1 sheet:							
(*Eden/Eden Sushi*) . . .	10	1.0	1.0	0	0	5	1.0
(*Sushi Chef*)	10	1.0	2.0	0	0	20	1.0
spirulina, 1 oz.:							
raw	8	1.7	.7	.1	0	28	n.a.
dried	82	16.3	6.8	2.2	0	297	1.0
wakame:							
(*Eden*), ½ cup	25	2.0	4.0	0	0	660	4.0
raw, 1 oz.	13	.9	2.6	.2	0	247	.1
flakes, instant (*Eden*),							
1 tsp.	3	0	0	0	0	72	0
Seaweed chips (*Eden*							
Sea Vegetable),							
1.1 oz.	140	1.0	23.0	5.0	0	220	0
Seitan:							
(*White Wave* Traditional),							
3 oz.	140	31.0	3.0	1.0	0	440	1.0
chicken style:							
(*White Wave* Box),							
3 oz.	130	24.0	9.0	0	0	170	3.0
(*White Wave* Water							
Pack), 1 pc.							
w/broth, 5 oz.	130	20.0	12.0	0	0	470	10.0
strips, stir-fry (*White*							
Wave), 3 oz.	100	22.0	2.0	1.0	0	200	0
Semolina, whole grain,							
1 cup	601	21.2	121.6	1.8	0	2	6.5
Semolina flour (*Hodg-*							
son Mill Pasta Flour),							
<¼ cup	110	4.0	22.0	.5	0	0	2.0
Sesame butter (*Kettle*							
Roaster Fresh							
Unsalted), 1 oz. . . .	168	5.0	6.0	15.0	0	3	0
Sesame flour, 1 oz.:							
high fat	149	8.7	7.6	10.5	0	12	1.8
partially defatted	108	11.4	10.0	3.4	0	12	1.7
low fat	95	14.2	10.1	.5	0	11	1.4
Sesame meal, partially							
defatted, 1 oz.	161	4.8	7.4	13.6	0	11	1.1

Food and Measure	cal.	prot. (gms)	carbo. (gms)	fat (gms)	chol. (mgs)	sod. (mgs)	fiber (gms)
Sesame nut mix (*Planters*), 1 oz. ...	160	5.0	9.0	13.0	0	240	2.0
Sesame paste (see also "Tahini"), from whole seeds, 1 tbsp.	95	2.9	4.1	8.1	0	2	.9
Sesame salt, regular or garlic (*Eden Organic Seaweed Gomasio*), ½ tsp. ...	10	0	0	.5	0	35	0
Sesame seed condiment (*Eden Shake*), ½ tsp.	5	0	1.0	0	0	25	1.0
Sesame seeds:							
black (*Shiloh Farms*), ¼ cup	160	5.0	6.0	14.0	0	3	3.1
whole:							
(*Arrowhead Mills*), ¼ cup	190	6.0	8.0	17.0	0	0	4.0
(*Shiloh Farms*), ¼ cup	200	7.0	8.0	20.0	0	20	5.0
dried, 1 tbsp.	52	1.6	2.1	4.5	0	1	1.1
roasted, toasted, 1 oz.	160	4.8	7.3	13.6	0	3	4.0
kernels:							
(*Arrowhead Mills*), ¼ cup	210	9.0	3.0	19.0	0	15	1.0
(*Shiloh Farms*), ¼ cup	210	7.0	5.0	20.0	0	10	5.0
dried, 1 tsp.	16	.7	.3	1.5	0	1	<1.0
toasted, 1 oz.	161	4.8	7.4	13.6	0	11	4.8
Sesame spread, see "Sesame butter"							
Sesame stick snack, 1.1 oz.:							
cheddar (*Shiloh Farms*)	160	5.0	15.0	9.0	0	160	3.0
garlic (*Shiloh Farms*) .	170	5.0	13.0	11.0	0	230	3.0
oat bran (*Shiloh Farms*)	160	5.0	15.0	9.0	0	160	5.0
poppy onion (*Shiloh Farms*)	170	5.0	12.0	11.0	0	250	3.0
spelt (*Shiloh Farms*) .	170	5.0	13.0	11.0	0	170	5.0
Sesbania flower:							
raw, 1 cup	5	.3	1.4	<.1	0	3	n.a.
steamed, ½ cup	11	.6	2.7	<.1	0	6	n.a.
Shad, meat only:							
raw, 4 oz.	223	19.2	0	15.6	85	58	0

Food and Measure	cal.	prot. (gms)	carbo. (gms)	fat (gms)	chol. (mgs)	sod. (mgs)	fiber (gms)
Shad *(cont.)*							
baked, broiled, or							
microwaved, 4 oz. . .	286	24.6	0	20.0	109	74	0
Shallot, fresh:							
(*Frieda's*), 1.1 oz.	20	1.0	5.0	0	0	0	0
peeled, 1 oz.	20	.7	4.8	<.1	0	3	<1.0
chopped, 1 tbsp.	7	.3	1.7	<.1	0	1	<1.0
Shallot, freeze-dried,							
1 tbsp.	3	.1	.7	tr.	0	1	<1.0
Shark, meat only, raw,							
4 oz.	148	23.8	0	5.1	58	90	0
Sheepshead, meat only:							
raw, 4 oz.	123	22.9	0	2.7	56	81	0
baked, broiled, or							
microwaved, 4 oz. .	143	29.5	0	1.8	73	83	0
Shellie beans, canned							
w/liquid, ½ cup . . .	37	2.1	7.6	.2	0	408	4.1
Shells, pasta, entree,							
frozen, 1 pkg.:							
and cheese (*Michelina's*							
Zap'ems), 8 oz. . . .	350	14.0	46.0	11.0	20	570	2.0
stuffed:							
(*Amy's* Bowls), 10 oz.	300	19.0	30.0	12.0	30	740	5.0
(*Healthy Choice*),							
11.15 oz.	290	17.0	40.0	6.0	20	470	5.0
vegetables and, garlic							
butter sauce (*Birds*							
Eye), 9 oz.	270	6.0	32.0	13.0	15	430	3.0
Shells, pasta, mix:							
Alfredo, 1 cup*							
(*Annie's* Natural) . .	360	11.0	49.0	13.0	35	640	1.0
(*Annie's* Organic) . .	370	12.0	47.0	16.0	40	700	1.0
cheddar, 1 cup*:							
Mexican (*Annie's*							
Organic)	280	11.0	49.0	4.0	10	540	1.0
white (*Annie's* Natu-							
ral Family)	360	11.0	49.0	13.0	35	650	1.0
white (*Annie's*							
Organic)	370	12.0	48.0	15.0	40	640	1.0
white (*Annie's*							
Organic Family) .	280	13.0	47.0	5.0	10	580	2.0
white or Wisconsin							
(*Annie's* Natural)	290	11.0	49.0	5.0	15	580	1.0
whole wheat shells							
(*Annie's* Organic)	360	12.0	47.0	15.0	40	640	5.0

Food and Measure	cal.	prot. (gms)	carbo. (gms)	fat (gms)	chol. (mgs)	sod. (mgs)	fiber (gms)
Wisconsin (*Annie's* Creamy Deluxe) .	320	14.0	46.0	10.0	25	760	2.0
Wisconsin (*Annie's* Organic)	370	11.0	49.0	15.0	40	650	1.0
cheese, 4 oz. mix:							
(*Velveeta* Light) . . .	320	15.0	53.0	5.0	20	1130	2.0
(*Velveeta* Original 12 oz.)	360	14.0	48.0	12.0	20	950	2.0
(*Velveeta* Original Family Size)	360	15.0	46.0	13.0	30	960	2.0
bacon (*Velveeta*) . .	400	18.0	47.0	16.0	50	1230	2.0
cheese, salsa (*Velveeta*), ½ of 10.85-oz. pkg.	380	17.0	47.0	14.0	40	1180	2.0
"cheese," nondairy (*Road's End Organics Shells & Chreese*), ¾ cup mix	320	14.0	62.0	1.0	0	390	7.0
Shepherd's pie, see "Beef entree, frozen"							
Shepherd's pie, meatless, frozen (*Amy's*), 8-oz. pkg.	160	5.0	27.0	4.0	0	490	5.0
Sherbet (see also "Sorbet"), ½ cup, except as noted:							
berry rainbow (*Dreyer's/ Edy's*)	130	1.0	29.0	1.0	5	35	0
cherry amaretto (*Turkey Hill* Orchard)	120	1.0	28.0	1.0	5	15	0
cherry chip (*Darigold*)	130	1.0	28.0	2.0	5	35	<1.0
lime (*Dreyer's/Edy's*) .	130	1.0	28.0	1.5	5	35	0
lime, orange, lemon (*Hood Fruit Scoops*)	120	1.0	26.0	1.0	<5	35	0
orange:							
(*Breyer's*)	130	1.0	28.0	1.5	5	25	0
(*Darigold*)	120	1.0	26.0	1.0	5	35	0
(*Hood Fruit Scoops*)	120	1.0	26.0	1.0	<5	35	0
(*Turkey Hill* Grove) .	120	1.0	26.0	1.0	5	20	0
Swiss (*Dreyer's/Edy's*)	150	1.0	30.0	3.0	5	40	0
orange, and ice cream:							
(*Breyer's* Take Two)	130	2.0	21.0	4.5	15	35	0
(*Breyer's* Creamsicle)	130	2.0	20.0	5.0	15	35	0
(*Darigold* Float) . . .	120	2.0	21.0	4.0	15	40	0
(*Dreyer's/Edy's*) . . .	120	2.0	23.0	2.0	10	40	0

Food and Measure	cal.	prot. (gms)	carbo. (gms)	fat (gms)	chol. (mgs)	sod. (mgs)	fiber (gms)
Sherbet, orange, and ice cream *(cont.)*							
(*Peak Pleasures*) ..	130	1.0	19.0	5.0	20	40	0
swirl (*Turkey Hill*) .	140	2.0	20.0	6.0	25	40	0
rainbow, fruit:							
(*Breyer's*)	130	1.0	27.0	1.5	5	25	0
(*Darigold*)	120	1.0	26.0	1.0	5	30	0
(*Turkey Hill*)	120	1.0	26.0	1.0	5	20	0
swirl (*Hood Fruit*							
Scoops)	120	1.0	26.0	1.0	<5	30	0
raspberry:							
(*Darigold*)	120	1.0	26.0	1.0	5	30	0
(*Dreyer's/Edy's*) ...	130	1.0	28.0	1.0	5	35	0
raspberry orange lime							
(*Hood Fruit Scoops*)	120	1.0	26.0	1.0	<5	30	0
tropical rainbow							
(*Dreyer's/Edy's*) ...	130	1.0	29.0	1.0	5	35	0
Sherbet bar, see "Iced confection bar"							
Shiso leaf powder							
(*Eden*), 1 tsp.	0	0	0	0	0	200	2.0
Shortening, 1 tbsp.:							
all varieties (*Crisco*) ..	110	0	0	12.0	0	0	0
soy and cottonseed ..	113	0	0	12.8	0	0	0
Shrimp, meat only:							
raw, 4 oz.	120	23.0	1.0	2.0	173	168	0
raw, 4 large, 1 oz. ...	30	5.7	.3	.5	43	42	0
boiled or steamed:							
4 oz.	112	23.7	0	1.2	221	254	0
4 large, .8 oz.	22	4.6	0	.2	43	49	0
Shrimp, canned, drained:							
all varieties (*Bumble Bee/Orleans*), 2 oz.,							
¼ cup	40	10.0	0	0	115	650	0
small (*Crown Prince*),							
½ can	120	26.0	2.0	.5	250	810	1.0
1 cup	154	29.6	1.3	2.5	222	216	0
Shrimp, frozen, cleaned, tail-on:							
raw, 4 oz.:							
(*Contessa*)	70	18.0	0	0	135	550	0
all sizes (*Chicken of The Sea*)	120	23.0	1.0	2.0	170	170	0

Food and Measure	cal.	prot. (gms)	carbo. (gms)	fat (gms)	chol. (mgs)	sod. (mgs)	fiber (gms)
cooked, 3 oz.:							
(*Chicken of the Sea*)	80	18.0	0	1.0	165	190	0
(*Contessa*), 3 oz. . .	60	14.0	0	0	130	360	0
"Shrimp," imitation,							
from surimi, 4 oz. .	115	14.1	10.4	1.7	41	800	0
Shrimp, smoked							
(*Ducktrap River*),							
¼ cup	60	10.0	0	2.0	120	440	0
Shrimp appetizer,							
frozen/refrigerated:							
caviche (*Sau•Sea*),							
½ cup	70	6.0	5.0	3.0	45	310	1.0
cocktail (*Margaritaville*							
Paradise), ½ pkg.:							
shrimp, 3 oz.	60	12.0	0	0	130	340	0
sauce, 2 tbsp.	26	6.0	0	0	0	391	0
w/cocktail sauce:							
(*Contessa* Party							
Platter), 4 oz. . . .	90	14.0	6.0	0	140	610	0
(*Sau•Sea*), 4-oz. jar	110	8.0	20.0	0	85	710	3.0
(*Sau•Sea*), 6-oz. jar	170	11.0	30.0	0	120	850	4.0
coconut (*Margaritaville*							
Calypso), ½ pkg.:							
shrimp, 4 oz.	300	12.0	25.0	17.0	70	530	0
sauce, 2 tbsp.	50	0	14.0	0	0	160	0
Shrimp coating mix,							
see "Seafood coating							
mix"							
Shrimp cocktail, see							
"Shrimp appetizer"							
Shrimp dinner, frozen,							
creamy garlic							
(*Healthy Choice*							
Dinners), 11.5 oz. .	270	19.0	35.0	6.0	75	600	6.0
Shrimp entree, freeze-							
dried, 1 serving:							
Alfredo (*AlpineAire*) . .	330	17.0	44.0	9.0	25	710	2.0
Newburg (*AlpineAire*)	320	14.0	50.0	7.0	15	510	2.0
Shrimp entree, frozen,							
1 pkg., except as							
noted:							
Alfredo:							
(*Gorton's* Shrimp							
Bowl), 10.5 oz. . . .	250	13.0	39.0	5.0	75	1230	4.0

Food and Measure	cal.	prot. (gms)	carbo. (gms)	fat (gms)	chol. (mgs)	sod. (mgs)	fiber (gms)
Shrimp entree, frozen, Alfredo *(cont.)*							
(*Michelina's* Home-style Bowls), 10 oz.	370	17.0	42.0	16.0	110	650	2.0
(*Michelina's Signature*), 8 oz.	290	15.0	31.0	13.0	100	540	2.0
and vegetables (*Michelina's* Home-style Bowls), 11 oz.	370	17.0	53.0	9.0	65	840	3.0
and angel hair pasta (*Lean Cuisine* Café Classics), 10 oz.	240	14.0	35.0	5.0	50	640	2.0
arrabiata (*Contessa* Minute Meal Bowl), 10.5 oz.	250	14.0	36.0	6.0	85	1380	5.0
fajita (*Contessa*), 2 pcs., 8 oz.	180	9.0	29.0	3.5	45	710	4.0
fried rice, see "Rice entree, frozen"							
garlic (*Birds Eye Voila!*), 1 cup*	220	9.0	27.0	8.0	10	510	2.0
garlic butter (*Gorton's* Shrimp Bowl), 10.5 oz.	260	13.0	38.0	6.0	65	910	2.0
jerk (*Margaritaville* Jammin'), ½ of 8-oz. pkg.	140	16.0	4.0	7.0	145	1040	0
kung pao (*Contessa*), 1¾ cups*	200	10.0	30.0	3.5	45	760	3.0
lime (*Margaritaville* Island), ½ of 8-oz. pkg.	130	16.0	2.0	7.0	155	720	0
marinara, w/linguine (*Smart Ones*), 9 oz.	180	8.0	28.0	2.0	35	650	4.0
Mediterranean (*Contessa*), 8 oz. . .	180	11.0	27.0	3.0	50	920	3.0
pad Thai (*Ethnic Gourmet*), 10 oz. . .	350	9.0	64.0	7.0	55	650	3.0
Parmesan penne (*Uncle Ben's* Pasta Bowl), 12 oz.	380	24.0	58.0	7.0	100	1430	2.0
w/pasta, vegetables (*Michelina's Lean Gourmet*), 8 oz.	260	13.0	37.0	6.0	55	590	2.0

Food and Measure	cal.	prot. (gms)	carbo. (gms)	fat (gms)	chol. (mgs)	sod. (mgs)	fiber (gms)
penne (*Contessa* Minute Meal Bowl), 10 oz. .	370	14.0	33.0	20.0	125	1270	4.0
primavera:							
(*Contessa*), 1½ cups*	350	11.0	30.0	21.0	60	780	2.0
(*Gorton's* Shrimp Bowl), 10.5 oz. . . .	270	13.0	41.0	6.0	55	1250	1.0
Santa Fe (*Contessa*), 1½ cups*	200	10.0	30.0	3.5	45	760	3.0
scampi:							
(*Contessa*), 4 oz. . .	340	10.0	5.0	30.0	85	690	0
(*Margaritaville* Sunset), ½ pkg.	270	12.0	10.0	20.0	130	460	0
(*SeaPak* Traditional), ⅓ of 12-oz. pkg.	350	13.0	4.0	32.0	95	600	0
Parmesan sauce (*SeaPak*), ⅓ of 12-oz. pkg.	350	14.0	2.0	33.0	115	490	0
soy ginger (*Contessa* Minute Meal Bowl), 11 oz.	270	14.0	53.0	3.5	55	910	4.0
stir-fry (*Contessa*), 1¾ cups*	140	9.0	26.0	.5	55	1250	4.0
sweet and sour (*Contessa*), 1½ cups*	180	9.0	40.0	0	50	430	3.0
teriyaki (*Gorton's* Shrimp Bowl), 10.5 oz.	320	10.0	57.0	6.0	45	1250	2.0
Shrimp sauce (*Crosse & Blackwell*), ¼ cup	110	1.0	25.0	0	0	790	0
Shrimp spread, w/roasted garlic (*Sau•Sea*), 2 tbsp. .	70	3.0	1.0	8.0	35	75	0
Sloppy Joe sauce, see "Sandwich sauce"							
Sloppy Joe seasoning:							
(*Fantastic*), ¼ cup . . .	70	10.0	11.0	.5	0	450	3.0
(*Lawry's*), 2 tsp.	20	0	5.0	0	0	520	0
(*McCormick*), 1 tsp. . .	20	0	3.0	0	0	300	0
Smelt, rainbow, meat only:							
raw, 4 oz.	110	20.0	0	2.8	80	68	0
baked, broiled, or microwaved, 4 oz. .	141	25.6	0	3.5	102	87	0

Food and Measure	cal.	prot. (gms)	carbo. (gms)	fat (gms)	chol. (mgs)	sod. (mgs)	fiber (gms)
Smoothie mix, 1⅔ tbsp.:							
banana frost or pineapple (*Produce Partners*)	80	0	18.0	0	0	0	0
chocolate banana (*Produce Partners*)	80	0	18.0	0	0	15	0
orange (*Produce Partners*)	60	0	14.0	0	0	0	0
strawberry (*Produce Partners*)	80	0	19.0	0	0	0	0
Smoothie snack, all fruit flavors (*Jell-O Snacks*), 4 oz.	100	1.0	18.0	2.5	10	40	0
Snack chips (see also "Snack mix" and specific grain and vegetable listings):							
(*Ritz* Original), 1.1 oz.	140	2.0	23.0	5.0	0	400	1.0
cheddar (*Ritz*), 1.1 oz.	150	2.0	20.0	6.0	5	320	1.0
pepper, three (*Guiltless Carbs*), 1 oz.	110	14.0	9.0	3.0	0	390	3.0
ranch (*Guiltless Carbs* Southwest), 1 oz.	110	14.0	9.0	3.0	0	420	3.0
salsa verde (*Guiltless Carbs*), 1 oz.	110	14.0	9.0	3.0	0	460	3.0
sour cream and onion (*Ritz*), 1.1 oz.	150	2.0	20.0	6.0	0	350	1.0
Snack mix (see also "Trail mix"):							
(*Cheez-It* Party Mix), ½ cup	130	3.0	19.0	4.5	0	340	1.0
(*Chex* Bold Party Blend), ½ cup	140	3.0	20.0	6.0	0	390	<1.0
(*Chex* Traditional), ⅔ cup	130	2.0	22.0	4.0	0	380	1.0
(*Gardetto's* Original), ½ cup	170	4.0	20.0	7.0	0	330	1.0
(*Gardetto's* Reduced Fat), ½ cup	130	3.0	20.0	5.0	0	320	1.0
(*Munchies* Mini Mix), 1 oz., 1 cup	140	2.0	18.0	6.0	0	230	<1.0
(*Munchies* Flamin' Hot), 1 oz., ¾ cup	140	2.0	17.0	6.0	0	190	<1.0

Food and Measure	cal.	prot. (gms)	carbo. (gms)	fat (gms)	chol. (mgs)	sod. (mgs)	fiber (gms)
(*Nabisco Mixers*), 1.1 oz.	140	2.0	21.0	5.0	0	350	1.0
cheese:							
cheddar (*Chex*), ⅔ cup	130	2.0	22.0	4.0	0	370	<1.0
cheddar (*Nabisco Mixers*), 1 oz.	140	2.0	17.0	6.0	0	360	1.0
blend, Italian (*Gardetto's*), ½ cup	140	3.0	20.0	5.0	0	350	<1.0
honey nut (*Chex*), ½ cup	130	2.0	23.0	4.0	0	250	1.0
hot and spicy (*Chex*), ⅔ cup	130	2.0	22.0	4.0	0	420	1.0
Italian recipe (*Gardetto's*), ½ cup	150	3.0	20.0	6.0	0	310	1.0
Oriental (*New England Naturals* Party Mix), ⅓ cup	170	6.0	14.0	10.0	0	125	2.0
peanut lovers (*Chex*), ½ cup	140	3.0	19.0	6.0	0	340	1.0
sweet and salt (*Chex Trail Mix*), ½ cup ..	140	2.0	22.0	4.5	0	230	1.0
Tex-Mex (*New England Naturals*), ⅓ cup ..	160	5.0	13.0	10.0	0	190	3.0
Snail, fresh, raw, 1 oz.	26	4.6	<.1	.4	14	20	0
Snail, canned (*Fanci Food* Very Large), 6 pcs.	25	5.0	0	.5	65	85	0
Snail, sea, see "Whelk"							
Snap bean (see also "Green bean"), fresh, all varieties (*Frieda's*), ⅔ cup, 3 oz.	25	2.0	6.0	0	0	5	3.0
Snapper, meat only:							
raw, 4 oz.	113	23.3	0	1.5	42	73	0
baked, broiled, or microwaved, 4 oz. ..	145	30.0	0	2.0	53	65	0
Snow pea, see "Peas, edible-podded"							
Snow pea sprouts (*Jonathan's*), 1 cup	40	3.0	8.0	0	0	0	3.0

Food and Measure	cal.	prot. (gms)	carbo. (gms)	fat (gms)	chol. (mgs)	sod. (mgs)	fiber (gms)
Soft drinks, carbonated, 12 fl. oz., except as noted:							
all flavors:							
(*Clearly Canadian*), 8 fl. oz.	45	0	10.0	0	0	10	0
(*Ocean Spray Juice Spritzers*), 11.75 fl. oz.	160	0	40.0	0	0	50	0
birch beer (*Pennsylvania Dutch*), 8 fl. oz.	110	0	28.0	0	0	30	0
blackberry (*Nantucket Nectars NectarFizz*), 8 fl. oz.	80	0	21.0	0	0	35	0
boysenberry (*R.W. Knudsen* Spritzer) .	160	<1.0	40.0	0	0	25	0
cherries and cream (*Stewart's*)	190	0	49.0	0	0	55	0
cherry:							
(*Santa Cruz Organic* Spritzer)	140	0	34.0	0	0	20	0
black (*R.W. Knudsen* Spritzer)	170	<1.0	42.0	0	0	20	0
sparkling (*R.W. Knudsen* Spritzer)	110	<1.0	28.0	0	0	15	0
coconut (*Goya*)	200	0	45.0	0	0	65	0
cola:							
(*Coca-Cola* Classic)	140	0	39.0	0	0	50	0
(*Coca-Cola* Classic), 8 fl. oz.	100	0	27.0	0	0	35	0
(*Goya* Champagne)	200	0	47.0	0	0	60	0
(*Pepsi/Pepsi* Free) .	150	0	41.0	0	0	35	0
(*Pepsi/Pepsi* Free), 8 fl. oz.	100	0	27.0	0	0	25	0
(*Pepsi Edge*), 8 fl. oz.	50	0	13.0	0	0	25	0
(*RC*), 8 fl. oz.	110	0	29.0	0	0	30	0
cherry (*Dr Pepper*)	150	0	40.0	0	0	55	0
cherry (*R.W. Knudsen* Spritzer)	170	<1.0	42.0	0	0	20	0
cherry, wild (*Pepsi*), 8 fl. oz.	100	0	28.0	0	0	20	0
lemon (*Pepsi Twist*), 8 fl. oz.	100	0	28.0	0	0	35	0
lime (*Coca-Cola*) . .	140	0	39.0	0	0	35	0

Food and Measure	cal.	prot. (gms)	carbo. (gms)	fat (gms)	chol. (mgs)	sod. (mgs)	fiber (gms)
vanilla (*Pepsi*), 8 fl. oz.	110	0	28.0	0	0	25	0
citrus, 8 fl. oz.:							
(*Mountain Dew*) . . .	110	0	31.0	0	0	50	0
(*Mountain Dew Code Red*)	110	0	31.0	0	0	110	0
(*Mountain Dew Livewire*)	110	0	31.0	0	0	45	0
(*7Up*)	100	0	26.0	0	0	50	0
(*7Up Plus*)	10	0	2.0	0	0	50	0
Collins mixer (*Canada Dry*), 8 fl. oz.	80	0	22.0	0	0	35	0
cranberry:							
(*Nantucket Nectars NectarFizz*), 8 fl. oz.	90	0	23.0	0	0	35	0
(*R.W. Knudsen Spritzer*)	190	1.0	45.0	0	0	65	0
sparkling (*R.W. Knudsen Spritzer*)	130	<1.0	30.0	0	0	45	0
cream:							
(*A&W*), 8 fl. oz. . . .	120	0	31.0	0	0	30	0
(*Mug*), 8 fl. oz.	120	0	32.0	0	0	45	0
(*Stewart's*)	180	0	45.0	0	0	50	0
vanilla (*R.W. Knudsen* Spritzer)	160	<1.0	35.0	0	0	20	0
vanilla (*Santa Cruz Organic* Spritzer)	160	0	40.0	0	0	10	0
fruit punch (*Goya*) . . .	190	0	49.0	0	0	40	0
ginger ale:							
(*Canada Dry*)	120	0	33.0	0	0	40	0
(*Canada Dry*), 8 fl. oz.	90	0	25.0	0	0	35	0
(*Health Valley*)	160	0	40.0	0	0	0	0
(*R.W. Knudsen* Spritzer)	160	1.0	40.0	0	0	25	0
(*Santa Cruz Organic* Spritzer)	150	0	37.0	0	0	0	0
(*Schweppes*)	120	0	34.0	0	0	60	0
(*Schweppes*), 8 fl. oz.	80	0	23.0	0	0	40	0
(*Seagrams's*), 8 fl. oz.	90	0	24.0	0	0	30	0
(*White Rock*), 8 fl. oz.	80	0	21.0	0	0	20	0
grape (*Schweppes*), 8 fl. oz.	100	0	26.0	0	0	40	0

Food and Measure	cal.	prot. (gms)	carbo. (gms)	fat (gms)	chol. (mgs)	sod. (mgs)	fiber (gms)
Soft drinks *(cont.)*							
ginger beer:							
(*Goya*)	190	0	43.0	0	0	30	0
(*Old Tyme*), 10 fl. oz.	140	0	34.0	0	0	25	0
(*Reed's* Jamaican							
Brew Premium/							
Extra Ginger) . . .	145	0	37.4	0	0	5	0
(*Stewart's*)	200	0	50.0	0	0	50	0
grape:							
(*Goya*)	230	0	59.0	0	0	5	0
(*R.W. Knudsen*							
Spritzer)	170	<1.0	41.0	0	0	30	0
(*Stewart's*)	190	0	48.0	0	0	50	0
(*Welch's*)	190	0	51.0	0	0	55	0
Concord (*Santa Cruz*							
Organic Spritzer)	150	0	36.0	0	0	15	0
grapefruit, pink (*Nan-*							
tucket Nectars							
NectarFizz), 8 fl. oz.	90	0	24.0	0	0	35	0
kiwi lime (*R.W.*							
Knudsen Spritzer) .	130	<1.0	32.0	0	0	25	0
lemon ginger (*Trè*							
Limone), 8 fl. oz. . .	90	0	22.0	0	0	30	0
lemon lime:							
(*Goya*)	170	0	42.0	0	0	35	0
(*R.W. Knudsen*							
Spritzer)	170	1.0	42.0	0	0	25	0
(*Santa Cruz Organic*							
Spritzer)	130	0	33.0	0	0	10	0
(*Sierra Mist*), 8 fl. oz.	100	0	26.0	0	0	25	0
(*Sprite/Sprite Remix*)	140	0	38.0	0	0	70	0
(*Sprite/Sprite Remix*),							
8 fl. oz.	100	0	26.0	0	0	45	0
lemonade (see also							
"Lemonade"):							
(*Nantucket Nectars*							
NectarFizz), 8 fl. oz.	90	0	24.0	0	0	35	0
(*Santa Cruz Organic*							
Spritzer)	100	0	26.0	0	0	0	0
Jamaican (*R.W.*							
Knudsen Spritzer)	170	<1.0	41.0	0	0	25	0
raspberry (*Santa*							
Cruz Organic							
Spritzer)	120	0	29.0	0	0	0	0

Food and Measure	cal.	prot. (gms)	carbo. (gms)	fat (gms)	chol. (mgs)	sod. (mgs)	fiber (gms)
lime, mandarin (*R.W. Knudsen* Spritzer) .	170	1.0	42.0	0	0	25	0
mango (*R.W. Knudsen* Spritzer Fandango) .	190	1.0	45.0	0	0	30	0
orange:							
(*Fanta*), 8 fl. oz. . . .	110	0	30.0	0	0	35	0
(*Slice*)	190	0	50.0	0	0	55	0
(*Sunkist*), 8 fl. oz. .	130	0	35.0	0	0	30	0
mandarin (*Goya*) . .	170	0	44.0	0	0	35	0
orange and cream (*Stewart's*)	190	0	48.0	0	0	65	0
orange mango:							
(*Nantucket Nectars NectarFizz*), 8 fl. oz.	90	0	24.0	0	0	35	0
(*Santa Cruz Organic* Spritzer)	130	0	33.0	0	0	0	0
orange passion fruit (*R.W. Knudsen* Spritzer)	160	1.0	40.0	0	0	25	0
peach (*R.W. Knudsen* Spritzer)	160	2.0	37.0	0	0	35	0
pineapple (*Goya*)	170	0	43.0	0	0	40	0
raspberry, red (*R.W. Knudsen* Spritzer) .	170	<1.0	38.0	0	0	25	0
raspberry lime (*Nantucket Nectars NectarFizz*), 8 fl. oz.	90	0	24.0	0	0	35	0
root beer:							
(*A&W*), 8 fl. oz. . . .	120	0	31.0	0	0	30	0
(*Barq's*), 8 fl. oz. . .	110	0	30.0	0	0	50	0
(*Mug*), 8 fl. oz.	100	0	29.0	0	0	45	0
(*Santa Cruz Organic* Spritzer)	150	0	36.0	0	0	0	0
old-fashioned or sarsaparilla (*Health Valley*) . .	160	0	40.0	0	0	0	0
sangria (*Goya*)	170	0	43.0	0	0	5	0
strawberry:							
(*Fanta*), 8 fl. oz. . . .	120	0	33.0	0	0	30	0
(*Goya*)	200	0	48.0	0	0	5	0
(*R.W. Knudsen* Spritzer)	170	<1.0	42.0	0	0	25	0
tangerine (*R.W. Knudsen* Spritzer) .	170	2.0	40.0	0	0	35	0

Food and Measure	cal.	prot. (gms)	carbo. (gms)	fat (gms)	chol. (mgs)	sod. (mgs)	fiber (gms)
Soft drinks (cont.)							
tonic:							
(Canada Dry), 8 fl. oz.	90	0	24.0	0	0	35	0
(Schweppes)	130	0	35.0	0	0	55	0
(Schweppes), 8 fl. oz.	90	0	23.0	0	0	35	0
(Seagram's), 8 fl. oz.	80	0	22.0	0	0	30	0
vanilla cream, see "cream," above							
Sofrito (Goya Jar), 1 tsp.	0	0	0	0	0	45	0
Sole, see "Flatfish"							
Sole entree, frozen, 5-oz. pc., except as noted:							
w/garlic, shrimp, almonds (Oven Poppers)	260	16.0	16.0	14.0	40	380	0
w/shrimp, lobster in Newberg sauce:							
(Oven Poppers) ...	150	20.0	7.0	5.0	80	430	0
(Oven Poppers), 6-oz. pc.	165	23.0	4.0	6.0	108	528	<1.0
w/spinach, cheese (Oven Poppers) ...	210	15.0	13.0	10.0	55	270	0
stuffed:							
w/broccoli, cheese (Oven Poppers) .	150	20.0	4.0	6.0	55	330	1.0
w/crab (Oven Poppers)	240	17.0	15.0	13.0	35	400	0
w/crab, miniature (Oven Poppers), 2-oz. pc.	120	6.0	8.0	7.0	25	140	0
w/lump crabmeat (Oven Poppers) .	200	18.0	9.0	10.0	80	430	0
Sonic, 1 serving:							
breakfast:							
burrito	731	195.0	29.0	47.0	167	1535	2.0
pancake on a stick, w/sausage	240	7.0	22.0	14.0	30	520	n.a.
Toaster, egg/cheese:							
bacon	500	96.0	28.0	29.0	156	1698	3.0
ham	436	60.0	33.0	19.0	174	2079	3.0
sausage	570	123.0	24.0	36.0	126	1038	3.0

Food and Measure	cal.	prot. (gms)	carbo. (gms)	fat (gms)	chol. (mgs)	sod. (mgs)	fiber (gms)
burgers:							
cheeseburger:							
bacon	727	23.0	44.0	49.0	67	1433	2.0
Sonic No. 1	647	18.0	44.0	42.0	52	1103	2.0
Sonic No. 2	551	18.0	44.0	31.0	44	1111	2.0
Jr. burger	353	14.0	27.0	21.0	45	1294	1.0
Sonic No. 1	577	14.0	43.0	36.0	37	753	2.0
Sonic No. 2	481	14.0	43.0	25.0	29	761	2.0
SuperSonic No. 1 ..	929	28.0	45.0	66.0	96	1476	2.0
SuperSonic No. 2 ..	839	28.0	46.0	55.0	88	1571	3.0
Toaster sandwich:							
bacon cheddar							
burger	675	26.0	60.0	38.0	59	1786	4.0
BLT	581	19.0	42.0	41.0	47	1307	3.0
chicken club	675	39.0	75.0	29.0	85	1458	3.0
grilled cheese	282	12.0	39.0	12.0	15	830	2.0
sandwiches:							
chicken, breaded ..	582	28.0	66.0	23.0	53	427	2.0
chicken, grilled	343	27.0	31.0	13.0	70	829	2.0
steak, country fried	748	24.0	56.0	47.0	60	804	2.0
chicken:							
Jumbo Popcorn Chicken:							
family	2083	116.0	142.0	117.0	264	7595	7.0
large	521	29.0	36.0	29.0	66	1899	2.0
snack	347	19.0	24.0	20.0	44	1266	1.0
Wacky Pack	260	15.0	18.0	15.0	33	949	1.0
strip, dinner	749	32.0	86.0	32.0	47	1973	5.0
strip, snack	272	19.0	22.0	13.0	35	760	0
coneys:							
plain	262	8.0	22.0	16.0	30	657	1.0
plain, extra long ...	483	14.0	44.0	27.0	50	1162	1.0
cheese	366	13.0	24.0	24.0	52	962	1.0
cheese, extra long .	666	23.0	47.0	42.0	87	1648	2.0
corn dog	262	6.0	23.0	17.0	15	480	1.0
wraps:							
chicken, grilled	539	29.0	40.0	27.0	70	1035	2.0
w/out dressing ..	393	2.0	38.0	12.0	65	820	2.0
chicken strip	574	20.0	55.0	29.0	28	1071	2.0
w/out dressing ..	428	20.0	53.0	13.0	23	856	2.0
Fritos chili cheese .	743	23.0	68.0	42.0	52	1172	5.0
salad, no dressing:							
chicken, grilled	355	33.0	20.0	17.0	95	807	3.0
chicken, Santa Fe ..	426	36.0	33.0	18.0	95	882	6.0

Food and Measure	cal.	prot. (gms)	carbo. (gms)	fat (gms)	chol. (mgs)	sod. (mgs)	fiber (gms)
Sonic, salad, no dressing *(cont.)*							
Jumbo Popcorn							
Chicken	475	26.0	38.0	26.0	63	1286	4.0
salad dressing, 2 oz.:							
honey mustard	240	1.0	14.0	21.0	15	300	0
ranch	260	0	0	28.0	20	490	0
ranch, light	120	1.0	14.0	7.0	15	740	0
Faves & Craves:							
Ched 'R' Peppers . .	256	8.0	29.0	12.0	28	1056	4.0
fries:							
large	252	3.0	30.0	13.0	0	758	5.0
regular	195	2.0	22.0	11.0	0	648	4.0
SuperSonic	358	5.0	44.0	18.0	0	963	7.0
fries, cheese:							
large	322	7.0	31.0	19.0	15	1108	5.0
regular	265	6.0	23.0	17.0	15	998	4.0
chili, large	357	8.0	32.0	22.0	22	1062	5.0
chili, regular	299	8.0	24.0	19.0	22	952	4.0
Fritos chili pie	611	18.0	36.0	44.0	53	816	3.0
mozzarella sticks . .	382	20.0	35.0	19.0	50	1300	0
onion rings:							
large	507	12.0	102.0	7.0	0	486	10.0
regular	331	8.0	66.0	5.0	0	311	7.0
SuperSonic	706	16.0	141.0	10.0	1	788	11.0
tater tots:							
large	365	0	40.0	21.0	0	1358	4.0
regular	259	0	27.0	16.0	0	1046	3.0
SuperSonic	485	6.0	53.0	28.0	0	1670	5.0
tater tots, cheese:							
large	435	4.0	41.0	27.0	15	1708	4.0
regular	329	4.0	28.0	22.0	15	1396	3.0
chili, large	547	9.0	43.0	36.0	37	1844	5.0
chili, regular	363	5.0	28.0	25.0	22	1350	3.0
add-ons:							
add bacon	80	5.0	0	7.0	15	330	0
add cheese	70	4.0	1.0	6.0	15	350	0
cheddar, shredded .	104	6.0	1.0	9.0	28	491	0
dressing, 1 oz.:							
honey mustard . .	110	0	9.0	9.0	10	300	0
ranch dressing . .	147	0	2.0	16.0	5	215	0
1000 Island	150	0	3.0	15.0	10	170	0
jalapeños-nacho . . .	5	0	1.0	0	0	302	1.0
marinara sauce . . .	15	0	3.0	0	0	260	0

Food and Measure	cal.	prot. (gms)	carbo. (gms)	fat (gms)	chol. (mgs)	sod. (mgs)	fiber (gms)
pickle relish	40	0	11.0	0	0	248	0
slaw, .9 oz.	45	0	4.0	3.0	0	45	1.0
Sonic chili	52	2.0	1.0	4.0	8	59	0
Sonic green chilies .	10	0	3.0	0	0	24	0
Sonic hickory							
barbecue sauce .	41	0	10.0	0	0	429	0
Sopressata, hot or							
sweet (*Boar's Head*),							
1 oz.	100	8.0	<1.0	8.0	15	540	0
Sorbet (see also							
"Sherbet"), ½ cup:							
apple cinnamon							
(*Whole Fruit*)	140	0	34.0	0	0	30	1.0
berry, mixed (*Sharon's*)	90	0	23.0	0	0	11	1.0
blueberry (*Whole Fruit*)	130	0	32.0	0	0	15	1.0
boysenberry (*Whole*							
Fruit)	150	0	37.0	0	0	20	1.0
chocolate:							
(*Häagen-Dazs*)	130	2.0	28.0	.5	0	70	2.0
(*Sharon's*)	130	1.0	22.0	5.0	0	5	1.0
Belgian dark (*Godiva*)	130	1.0	32.0	.5	0	30	2.0
raspberry swirl							
(*Godiva*)	140	1.0	36.0	.5	0	40	2.0
coconut:							
(*Sharon's*)	160	1.0	22.0	8.0	0	8	1.0
(*Whole Fruit*)	140	1.0	28.0	3.0	5	20	0
grapefruit, pink							
(*Whole Fruit*) ...	130	0	32.0	0	0	10	0
lemon:							
(*Häagen-Dazs* Zesty)	110	0	25.0	0	0	25	<1.0
(*Sharon's*)	75	0	19.0	0	0	8	0
(*Whole Fruit*)	140	0	35.0	0	0	20	0
(*Whole Fruit* No							
Sugar)	60	0	23.0	0	0	10	7.0
mango:							
(*Häagen-Dazs*)	120	0	37.0	0	0	10	0
(*Sharon's*)	80	0	20.0	0	0	0	1.0
(*Whole Fruit*)	130	0	33.0	0	0	0	0
orange (*Whole Fruit*							
Mandarin)	120	0	31.0	0	0	25	0
passion fruit (*Sharon's*)	80	1.0	20.0	0	0	8	0
peach:							
(*Häagen-Dazs*)	130	0	33.0	0	0	0	<1.0

Food and Measure	cal.	prot. (gms)	carbo. (gms)	fat (gms)	chol. (mgs)	sod. (mgs)	fiber (gms)
Sorbet, peach *(cont.)*							
(*Whole Fruit*)	130	0	32.0	0	0	10	1.0
(*Whole Fruit* No							
Sugar)	60	0	23.0	0	0	0	7.0
raspberry:							
(*Häagen-Dazs*)	120	0	30.0	0	0	0	2.0
(*Sharon's*)	80	0	20.0	0	0	8	2.0
(*Whole Fruit*)	130	0	33.0	0	0	15	1.0
(*Whole Fruit* No							
Sugar)	60	0	23.0	0	0	0	7.0
strawberry:							
(*Häagen-Dazs*)	120	0	30.0	0	0	10	<1.0
(*Whole Fruit*)	120	0	31.0	0	0	10	0
(*Whole Fruit* No							
Sugar)	60	0	22.0	0	0	0	6.0
strawberry banana							
(*Whole Fruit*)	120	0	31.0	0	0	5	<1.0
tropical:							
(*Häagen-Dazs*)	150	0	38.0	0	0	25	0
(*Whole Fruit*)	150	0	38.0	0	0	15	0
Sorbet bar (see also							
"Fruit bar"), 1 bar:							
marshmallow swirl							
(*Cool Cotton Candy*)	100	1.0	20.0	1.0	10	20	0
mocha fudge (*Healthy*							
Choice)	90	2.0	17.0	1.5	5	50	1.0
orange, w/vanilla ice							
cream:							
(*Tropicana* Light) ..	80	1.0	12.0	3.0	10	30	0
(*Tropicana* Real Fruit)	80	1.0	14.0	2.5	10	20	0
chocolate dipped							
(*Tropicana*)	120	2.0	19.0	5.0	5	35	0
orange or raspberry,							
vanilla ice cream:							
(*Tropicana* Swirls) .	80	1.0	12.0	3.0	10	30	0
(*Tropicana* Swirls No							
Sugar)	60	2.0	11.0	2.0	10	30	0
(*Tropicana* Swirls							
Single)	130	2.0	20.0	5.0	20	45	0
raspberry orange swirl							
(*Healthy Choice*) ..	90	1.0	18.0	1.0	5	35	1.0
raspberry w/vanilla							
yogurt (*Häagen-Dazs*)	90	2.0	21.0	0	0	12	<1.0

Food and Measure	cal.	prot. (gms)	carbo. (gms)	fat (gms)	chol. (mgs)	sod. (mgs)	fiber (gms)
strawberry:							
w/banana yogurt							
(*Häagen-Dazs*) ..	90	2.0	20.0	0	0	20	0
w/strawberry sorbet							
(*Healthy Choice*)	80	3.0	13.0	1.5	5	60	0
w/vanilla ice cream							
(*Tropicana* Light)	80	1.0	12.0	3.0	10	30	0
Sorghum, whole grain,							
1 cup	650	21.7	143.3	6.3	0	12	n.a.
Sorghum syrup:							
½ cup	479	0	123.7	0	0	13	0
1 tbsp.	61	0	15.7	0	0	2	0
Sorrel, see "Dock"							
Soup, ready-to-serve,							
1 cup, except as							
noted:							
alphabet (*Amy's*)	80	3.0	16.0	.5	0	580	2.0
bean:							
(*Westbrae Natural*							
Great Plains							
Savory)	120	8.0	23.0	0	0	540	7.0
(*Westbrae Natural*							
Louisiana Stew) .	130	8.0	25.0	0	0	550	7.0
five, vegetable							
(*Health Valley*) ..	140	10.0	32.0	0	0	250	10.0
w/bacon (*Campbell's*							
Kitchen Classics)	180	9.0	28.0	4.0	5	820	8.0
and ham (*Campbell's*							
Chunky Hearty) .	180	11.0	30.0	2.0	10	800	8.0
and ham (*Campbell's*							
Select)	170	9.0	30.0	1.0	5	680	7.0
and ham (*Healthy*							
Choice)	170	11.0	29.0	2.5	10	480	6.0
bean, black:							
(*Health Valley*)	130	7.0	25.0	1.0	0	380	5.0
(*Health Valley* No							
Salt)	130	7.0	25.0	1.0	0	25	5.0
(*Progresso* Hearty)	170	8.0	30.0	1.5	<5	730	10.0
(*Walnut Acres* Cuban)	150	7.0	30.0	1.0	0	630	8.0
(*Westbrae Natural*							
Alabama Gumbo)	140	8.0	26.0	0	0	530	6.0
vegetable (*Amy's*) .	130	6.0	25.0	1.5	0	580	5.0
vegetable (*Health*							
Valley)	110	11.0	24.0	0	0	280	9.0

Food and Measure	cal.	prot. (gms)	carbo. (gms)	fat (gms)	chol. (mgs)	sod. (mgs)	fiber (gms)
Soup *(cont.)*							
beef:							
barley (*Progresso* 97% Fat Free) ..	130	9.0	20.0	2.0	10	710	4.0
barley (*Progresso* Steak Soup)	140	9.0	16.0	4.5	10	670	3.0
barley, roasted (*Campbell's Select*)	150	9.0	24.0	1.5	15	860	4.0
mushroom (*Progresso* Steak Soup)	100	7.0	14.0	1.5	10	1030	1.0
mushroom medley (*Campbell's Carb Request* Savory)	70	7.0	7.0	2.0	10	870	1.0
w/portobello, rice (*Campbell's Select*)	110	8.0	15.0	1.5	10	860	2.0
w/portobello, rice (*Campbell's Select* Micro Cup)	90	8.0	13.0	1.0	15	780	2.0
and potato, baked (*Progresso* Steak Soup)	100	6.0	15.0	2.0	10	860	1.0
and potato, chunky (*Healthy Choice*)	110	8.0	19.0	1.0	10	480	2.0
w/rice, white/wild (*Campbell's Chunky*)	150	9.0	24.0	2.5	10	960	2.0
slow roasted, w/mushrooms (*Campbell's Chunky*)	120	8.0	18.0	1.5	15	830	3.0
vegetable (*Progresso* Steak Soup)	130	10.0	16.0	2.5	20	850	2.0
w/vegetables, country (*Campbell's Chunky*)	160	11.0	22.0	3.0	15	910	4.0
w/vegetables, country (*Campbell's Chunky* Micro Bowl)	190	10.0	18.0	9.0	40	890	3.0
beef broth:							
(*College Inn*)	25	4.0	0	1.0	0	900	0

Food and Measure	cal.	prot. (gms)	carbo. (gms)	fat (gms)	chol. (mgs)	sod. (mgs)	fiber (gms)
(*College Inn* Fat Free Lower Sodium)	15	4.0	0	0	0	450	0
(*Kitchen Basics* Stock)	20	4.0	0	0	0	480	0
(*Swanson* Clear) . .	15	2.0	0	.5	0	890	0
(*Swanson* Lower Sodium)	15	2.0	1.0	0	<5	440	0
(*Tyson*)	15	2.0	1.0	.5	0	860	0
w/onion (*Swanson*)	20	2.0	2.0	.5	0	830	0
beef flavor broth:							
(*Health Valley*)	10	2.0	0	0	0	390	0
(*Health Valley* No Salt)	10	1.0	0	0	0	120	0
(*Health Valley* Organic)	15	2.0	2.0	0	0	390	0
broccoli:							
carotene (*Health Valley* Super) . . .	70	6.0	16.0	0	0	240	7.0
cream of (*Campbell's Soup at Hand*), 1 cont.	160	4.0	16.0	8.0	5	910	3.0
creamy (*Imagine*) .	70	3.0	10.0	1.5	0	370	2.0
butternut squash:							
(*Amy's*)	100	2.0	20.0	2.5	0	580	2.0
(*Amy's* Light Sodium)	100	2.0	20.0	2.5	0	290	2.0
creamy (*Imagine*) .	120	2.0	23.0	2.0	0	370	2.0
cheddar chicken chowder (*Progresso*)	210	6.0	25.0	9.0	10	890	2.0
chicken:							
(*Healthy Choice* Hearty)	120	8.0	20.0	2.0	20	480	3.0
(*Progresso* Home-style White Meat)	90	7.0	11.0	1.5	15	900	<1.0
Alfredo (*Campbell's Select*)	210	11.0	15.0	12.0	30	930	2.0
barley (*Progresso* White Meat)	100	7.0	15.0	1.5	15	890	3.0
creamy (*Campbell's Soup at Hand*), 1 cont.	150	4.0	15.0	8.0	10	970	2.0
and dumplings (*Campbell's Chunky*)	190	10.0	17.0	9.0	25	890	2.0

Food and Measure	cal.	prot. (gms)	carbo. (gms)	fat (gms)	chol. (mgs)	sod. (mgs)	fiber (gms)
Soup, chicken *(cont.)*							
and dumplings (*Campbell's Chunky* Micro Bowl)	190	10.0	18.0	9.0	40	890	3.0
and dumplings (*Healthy Choice*)	140	11.0	19.0	3.0	35	480	4.0
w/meatball (*Progresso* Chickarina)	130	8.0	12.0	5.0	20	1010	<1.0
pasta, w/roasted garlic (*Campbell's Select*)	100	8.0	18.0	1.0	15	820	2.0
rosemary, w/roasted potatoes (*Campbell's Select*) ...	110	7.0	17.0	1.0	10	890	2.0
rotini, hearty (*Progresso* White Meat)	90	8.0	12.0	1.5	15	970	<1.0
and stars (*Campbell's Soup at Hand*), 1 cont.	70	3.0	11.0	1.5	5	960	2.0
tortilla, Mexican style (*Campbell's Select*)	150	8.0	22.0	3.0	10	890	4.0
chicken, grilled:							
(*Progresso* Italiano White Meat)	110	9.0	14.0	2.5	20	1090	1.0
sausage gumbo (*Campbell's Chunky*)	140	9.0	21.0	2.5	15	890	3.0
w/sun-dried tomatoes, mushrooms (*Campbell's Select*)	110	8.0	18.0	.5	15	790	2.0
w/vegetables, pasta (*Campbell's Chunky*)	110	8.0	15.0	1.5	15	890	2.0
w/vegetables, pasta (*Campbell's Chunky* Micro Bowl)	100	8.0	13.0	2.0	15	850	2.0
chicken, roasted:							
(*Healthy Choice* Italian)	120	9.0	19.0	2.5	15	480	4.0
(*Progresso* Italiano White Meat)	80	6.0	10.0	1.5	15	1020	<1.0

Food and Measure	cal.	prot. (gms)	carbo. (gms)	fat (gms)	chol. (mgs)	sod. (mgs)	fiber (gms)
w/garlic (*Healthy Choice*)	120	8.0	21.0	2.0	5	480	2.0
herb, garden (*Progresso* White Meat)	70	6.0	9.0	1.5	15	920	1.0
herb, w/potatoes and garlic (*Campbell's Chunky*)	110	8.0	17.0	1.5	15	870	3.0
honey, w/potato (*Campbell's Select*)	110	7.0	19.0	1.0	15	860	3.0
w/penne, garden vegetables (*Campbell's Carb Request*)	70	9.0	7.0	1.0	15	890	2.0
and rotini (*Progresso* White Meat)	80	6.0	11.0	1.5	15	870	<1.0
w/rotini and penne pasta (*Campbell's Select*)	100	8.0	16.0	.5	10	860	2.0
w/white/wild rice (*Campbell's Select*)	100	7.0	18.0	.5	15	870	2.0
w/wild rice (*Progresso* 97% Fat Free)	90	6.0	12.0	1.5	10	700	<1.0
chicken broccoli cheese: (*Campbell's Carb Request*)	130	9.0	8.0	7.0	10	820	5.0
and potato (*Campbell's Chunky*) ..	190	7.0	14.0	12.0	20	960	1.0
chicken broth:							
(*Allens*)	10	1.0	0	0	0	620	0
(*Campbell's* Low Sodium), 1 can .	25	4.0	1.0	.5	5	140	0
(*College Inn*)	15	2.0	0	.5	0	910	0
(*Health Valley* Fat Free)	20	5.0	0	0	0	390	0
(*Health Valley* Low Fat)	35	5.0	0	1.5	25	390	0
(*Health Valley* No Salt)	35	5.0	0	1.5	25	130	0
(*Health Valley* Organic)	25	2.0	2.0	1.0	0	440	0
(*Imagine* Free Range)	20	1.0	2.0	.5	0	570	<1.0

Food and Measure	cal.	prot. (gms)	carbo. (gms)	fat (gms)	chol. (mgs)	sod. (mgs)	fiber (gms)
Soup, chicken broth *(cont.)*							
(*Kitchen Basics* Stock)	20	3.0	1.0	0	0	480	0
(*Pacific* Free Range)	10	1.0	1.0	0	0	570	0
(*Swanson*)	15	1.0	1.0	.5	<5	960	0
(*Swanson Natural Goodness*)	15	3.0	1.0	0	0	570	0
(*Tyson*)	15	1.0	2.0	.5	0	980	0
(*Tyson* Reduced Sodium)	15	1.0	2.0	.5	0	570	0
w/ginger (*Annie Chun's*)	30	4.0	3.0	0	0	730	0
w/Italian herbs (*Swanson*)	20	1.0	3.0	1.0	<5	840	0
roasted (*Tyson*) ...	15	1.0	2.0	.5	0	970	0
w/roasted garlic (*College Inn*) ...	20	1.0	3.0	0	0	1000	0
w/roasted garlic (*Swanson*)	20	1.0	2.0	1.0	<5	950	0
chicken flavor broth (*Imagine* No-Chicken)	20	1.0	4.0	.5	0	460	<1.0
chicken gumbo (*Healthy Choice* Zesty)	100	6.0	16.0	2.0	20	480	3.0
chicken noodle:							
(*Campbell's* Low Sodium), 1 can .	170	12.0	17.0	6.0	30	140	2.0
(*Campbell's Chunky* Classic)	100	9.0	16.0	2.5	20	860	2.0
(*Campbell's Chunky* Classic Micro Bowl)	110	8.0	15.0	2.0	25	860	1.0
(*Campbell's Kitchen Classics*)	90	6.0	13.0	1.0	10	870	1.0
(*Health Valley* 99% Fat Free	130	9.0	20.0	2.0	15	390	2.0
(*Health Valley* Rich & Hearty)	100	7.0	13.0	2.5	15	580	2.0
(*Healthy Choice* Old Fashioned)	110	7.0	16.0	2.0	20	480	3.0
(*Progresso* 97% Fat Free)	90	7.0	13.0	1.5	20	950	<1.0
(*Progresso* White Meat)	90	0	9.0	2.0	25	950	<1.0

Food and Measure	cal.	prot. (gms)	carbo. (gms)	fat (gms)	chol. (mgs)	sod. (mgs)	fiber (gms)
egg noodles (*Campbell's Select*) ...	110	9.0	14.0	1.5	15	990	1.0
egg noodles (*Campbell's Select* Micro Cup)	90	8.0	12.0	1.5	20	960	2.0
mini noodles (*Campbell's Soup at Hand*), 1 cont. ...	80	4.0	12.0	1.5	10	980	2.0
chicken rice:							
(*Campbell's Select*)	100	7.0	18.0	.5	15	920	2.0
(*Healthy Choice*) ..	90	7.0	12.0	3.0	15	480	2.0
(*Healthy Choice* Fiesta)	100	6.0	17.0	2.0	5	480	3.0
white/wild (*Campbell's Kitchen Classics*)	100	5.0	18.0	1.0	10	800	2.0
white/wild, savory (*Campbell's Chunky*)	120	8.0	19.0	1.5	15	840	2.0
wild (*Progresso* White Meat)	100	7.0	15.0	1.5	15	850	1.0
w/vegetables (*Progresso* White Meat)	90	6.0	13.0	2.0	10	890	1.0
chicken vegetable:							
(*Campbell's Select*)	110	7.0	19.0	.5	10	870	3.0
(*Progresso* White Meat)	90	7.0	13.0	1.5	15	820	2.0
hearty (*Campbell's Chunky*)	100	7.0	14.0	1.5	15	790	2.0
herbed, roasted vegetables (*Campbell's Select*) ...	100	8.0	15.0	.5	15	890	2.0
clam chowder, Manhattan:							
(*Campbell's Chunky*)	130	5.0	19.0	3.5	5	880	2.0
(*Progresso*)	110	6.0	17.0	2.0	10	880	2.0
clam chowder, New England:							
(*Campbell's Chunky*)	240	7.0	21.0	14.0	10	890	2.0
(*Campbell's Kitchen Classics*)	240	5.0	20.0	16.0	10	720	3.0
(*Campbell's Select*)	220	6.0	16.0	14.0	10	870	2.0
(*Campbell's Select* 98% Fat Free) ..	110	6.0	18.0	1.5	10	840	2.0

Soup, clam chowder, New England *(cont.)*

Food and Measure	cal.	prot. (gms)	carbo. (gms)	fat (gms)	chol. (mgs)	sod. (mgs)	fiber (gms)
(*Campbell's Select* 98% Fat Free Micro Bowl)	100	6.0	16.0	1.5	10	890	3.0
(*Campbell's Soup at Hand*), 1 cont. ..	110	3.0	12.0	6.0	5	980	4.0
(*Healthy Choice*) ..	110	4.0	21.0	1.5	15	480	3.0
(*Progresso*)	230	6.0	23.0	13.0	25	790	1.0
(*Progresso* 97% Fat Free)	110	5.0	18.0	1.5	5	610	2.0
coconut ginger (*Thai Kitchen*), 7 oz.	187	3.0	11.0	15.0	0	800	1.0
consommé, madrilène:							
clear (*Dominique's*)	30	8.0	<1.0	0	0	890	0
red (*Dominique's*) .	35	7.0	2.0	0	0	900	<1.0
corn:							
creamy (*Imagine*) .	100	5.0	15.0	3.0	0	340	1.0
vegetable (*Health Valley*)	70	5.0	17.0	0	0	135	7.0
corn chowder:							
(*Walnut Acres*)	150	4.0	28.0	3.0	10	690	2.0
chicken (*Campbell's Chunky*)	230	9.0	19.0	13.0	20	850	2.0
Southwestern (*Progresso*)	200	4.0	29.0	7.0	5	780	3.0
escarole in chicken broth (*Progresso*) .	25	1.0	3.0	1.0	<5	930	1.0
ginger carrot (*Walnut Acres*)	100	2.0	22.0	1.0	0	550	3.0
ham, honey roasted w/potatoes (*Campbell's Chunky*)	130	8.0	20.0	2.5	15	810	3.0
hot and sour (*Thai Kitchen*), 7 oz.	40	2.0	7.0	.5	0	800	1.5
Italian style wedding:							
(*Campbell's Select*)	110	8.0	16.0	2.5	10	840	2.0
(*Campbell's Select* Micro Cup)	110	7.0	15.0	2.0	15	770	2.0
lentil:							
(*Amy's*)	150	8.0	19.0	4.5	0	590	9.0
(*Campbell's Kitchen Classics*)	120	7.0	23.0	.5	5	750	5.0
(*Campbell's Select* Savory)	140	8.0	27.0	.5	5	860	6.0

Food and Measure	cal.	prot. (gms)	carbo. (gms)	fat (gms)	chol. (mgs)	sod. (mgs)	fiber (gms)
(*Campbell's Select* Savory Micro Cup)	130	8.0	24.0	.5	5	860	5.0
(*Health Valley* Organic)	100	8.0	21.0	1.0	0	380	8.0
(*Health Valley* Organic No Salt)	100	8.0	21.0	1.0	0	25	8.0
(*Progresso*)	140	9.0	22.0	2.0	0	750	7.0
(*Progresso* Vegetable Classics 99% Fat Free)	130	8.0	20.0	.5	0	440	6.0
(*Walnut Acres* Mediterranean) . .	130	7.0	26.0	0	0	620	8.0
(*Westbrae Natural* Mediterranean) . .	140	10.0	24.0	0	0	540	10.0
carrot (*Health Valley*)	100	10.0	25.0	0	0	220	7.0
vegetable (*Amy's*) .	150	8.0	23.0	4.0	0	680	9.0
vegetable (*Amy's* Light Sodium) . .	150	7.0	23.0	4.0	0	340	6.0
macaroni and bean (*Progresso*)	160	7.0	23.0	4.0	<5	800	6.0
meatball, Mediterranean (*Campbell's Carb Request*)	90	8.0	5.0	4.5	20	890	2.0
Mexican style (*Campbell's Soup at Hand Fiesta*), 1 cont.	130	7.0	22.0	3.0	15	930	3.0
minestrone:							
(*Amy's*)	90	3.0	17.0	1.5	0	540	3.0
(*Campbell's Kitchen Classics*)	110	4.0	22.0	.5	0	840	3.0
(*Campbell's Select*)	100	5.0	20.0	0	0	790	4.0
(*Campbell's Select* Micro Cup)	100	4.0	19.0	.5	5	900	4.0
(*Health Valley* Italian)	90	8.0	21.0	0	0	210	8.0
(*Health Valley* Organic)	110	3.0	17.0	0	0	380	3.0
(*Health Valley* Organic No Salt)	70	3.0	17.0	0	0	45	3.0
(*Progresso*)	120	5.0	21.0	2.0	0	960	5.0
(*Progresso* 97% Fat Free)	110	5.0	19.0	1.0	0	630	4.0
(*Walnut Acres*)	100	3.0	22.0	0	0	650	3.0
(*Westbrae Natural* Hearty Milano) . .	120	7.0	24.0	0	0	570	6.0

Food and Measure	cal.	prot. (gms)	carbo. (gms)	fat (gms)	chol. (mgs)	sod. (mgs)	fiber (gms)
Soup, minestrone *(cont.)*							
herb and shell (*Progresso*)	120	5.0	22.0	1.5	0	1050	4.0
miso broth (*Annie Chun's*)	35	2.0	5.0	1.0	0	870	1.0
mushroom:							
barley (*Health Valley*)	70	2.0	17.0	0	0	380	3.0
barley (*Health Valley No Salt*)	70	2.0	17.0	0	0	25	3.0
portobello, creamy (*Imagine*)	80	4.0	10.0	3.0	0	310	2.0
mushroom, cream of:							
(*Amy's*)	140	3.0	13.0	9.0	5	590	2.0
(*Campbell's* Low Sodium), 1 can .	200	3.0	19.0	12.0	10	90	3.0
creamy (*Campbell's Soup at Hand*), 1 cont.	120	2.0	8.0	8.0	5	890	2.0
creamy (*Progresso*)	180	2.0	12.0	14.0	30	930	<1.0
mushroom broth:							
(*Health Valley*)	10	0	2.0	0	0	390	0
shiitake (*Annie Chun's*)	25	2.0	3.0	0	0	900	0
penne, in chicken broth (*Progresso*)	80	4.0	14.0	1.0	0	1020	<1.0
noodle:							
(*Amy's No Chicken*)	90	5.0	12.0	3.0	0	540	2.0
(*Westbrae Natural* New York Un-Chicken)	60	2.0	10.0	1.0	10	820	<1.0
onion, French (*Progresso*)	50	<1.0	9.0	1.5	<5	900	1.0
pasta:							
cacciatore (*Health Valley*)	100	4.0	20.0	0	0	290	4.0
Romano (*Health Valley*)	100	4.0	20.0	0	0	290	4.0
pasta and bean:							
(*Health Valley* Fagioli)	120	6.0	25.0	0	0	290	4.0
3-bean (*Amy's*) ...	130	5.0	19.0	5.0	0	680	4.0
pea, split:							
(*Amy's*)	100	7.0	19.0	0	0	570	4.0
(*Campbell's* Low Sodium), 1 can .	240	12.0	38.0	4.0	5	50	6.0

Food and Measure	cal.	prot. (gms)	carbo. (gms)	fat (gms)	chol. (mgs)	sod. (mgs)	fiber (gms)
(*Health Valley*)	110	10.0	23.0	0	0	160	8.0
(*Health Valley* No Salt)	110	10.0	23.0	0	0	115	8.0
(*Westbrae Natural* Old World)	150	10.0	28.0	0	0	590	6.0
carrot (*Health Valley*)	110	8.0	17.0	0	0	230	4.0
green (*Progresso*) .	170	10.0	25.0	3.0	5	870	5.0
w/ham (*Campbell's Chunky*)	170	12.0	27.0	2.5	10	780	4.0
w/ham (*Campbell's Select*)	160	10.0	29.0	1.0	5	860	5.0
w/ham (*Healthy Choice*)	170	11.0	30.0	2.5	5	480	4.0
w/ham (*Progresso*)	150	9.0	20.0	4.0	15	830	5.0
pepper steak (*Campbell's Chunky*)	120	9.0	18.0	1.5	15	740	3.0
pizza (*Campbell's Soup at Hand*), 1 cont. ...	130	5.0	27.0	.5	5	850	2.0
potato:							
(*Campbell's Soup at Hand* Velvety), 1 cont.	150	2.0	21.0	6.0	5	860	4.0
cheddar, white (*Progresso* 97% Fat Free)	100	2.0	20.0	1.5	<5	680	2.0
cream of (*Campbell's Kitchen Classics*)	160	2.0	20.0	8.0	5	780	2.0
creamy, w/roasted garlic (*Campbell's Select*)	180	3.0	20.0	10.0	10	770	2.0
potato, baked:							
w/bacon bits, chives (*Campbell's Chunky*)	160	6.0	21.0	5.0	15	940	1.0
w/cheddar, bacon bits (*Campbell's Chunky*)	180	5.0	23.0	8.0	15	970	2.0
w/steak, cheese (*Campbell's Chunky*)	210	10.0	21.0	9.0	25	970	3.0
potato chowder:							
w/broccoli and cheese (*Progresso*)	160	5.0	21.0	6.0	<5	960	1.0

Food and Measure	cal.	prot. (gms)	carbo. (gms)	fat (gms)	chol. (mgs)	sod. (mgs)	fiber (gms)
Soup, potato chowder *(cont.)*							
w/ham (*Campbell's Chunky* Old Fashioned)	190	6.0	17.0	11.0	15	800	2.0
w/ham and cheese (*Progresso*)	170	6.0	21.0	7.0	10	860	1.0
roasted garlic (*Progresso*)	180	2.0	23.0	9.0	10	900	2.0
potato leek:							
(*Health Valley*)	70	4.0	15.0	0	0	230	3.0
(*Health Valley* No Salt)	70	4.0	15.0	0	0	20	3.0
creamy (*Imagine*) .	90	3.0	14.0	2.5	0	380	2.0
pumpkin potato (*Walnut Acres* Autumn Harvest)	100	3.0	19.0	2.0	5	620	2.0
ravioli, w/vegetables:							
three cheese (*Campbell's Select*) . . .	140	5.0	20.0	4.0	20	820	4.0
tomato cheese (*Campbell's Chunky*)	150	4.0	27.0	3.5	5	930	4.0
rib roast, seasoned, w/potatoes, herbs (*Campbell's Chunky*)	110	8.0	17.0	1.0	10	890	3.0
Salisbury steak, mushrooms, onions (*Campbell's Chunky*)	150	9.0	18.0	4.5	20	890	2.0
sausage w/chicken, spicy (*Campbell's Carb Request*)	100	8.0	7.0	4.0	15	840	2.0
seafood stock (*Kitchen Basics*)	10	3.0	0	0	0	420	0
sirloin burger, w/country vegetables:							
(*Campbell's Chunky*)	180	10.0	17.0	8.0	20	890	3.0
(*Campbell's Chunky* Micro Bowl)	160	10.0	18.0	5.0	15	890	3.0
sirloin steak, grilled, w/hearty vegetables:							
(*Campbell's Chunky*)	130	8.0	19.0	2.0	10	920	4.0
(*Campbell's Chunky* Micro Bowl)	130	9.0	18.0	2.0	15	920	3.0

Food and Measure	cal.	prot. (gms)	carbo. (gms)	fat (gms)	chol. (mgs)	sod. (mgs)	fiber (gms)
steak, grilled (*Progresso* Steak Soup)	120	10.0	13.0	3.5	20	1030	1.0
steak and potato (*Campbell's Chunky*)	130	10.0	18.0	2.0	15	920	2.0
tomato:							
(*Campbell's 32 oz.*)	100	2.0	21.0	.5	5	760	2.0
(*Campbell's Kitchen Classics*)	100	2.0	24.0	0	0	760	1.0
(*Campbell's Soup at Hand* Classic), 1 cont.	120	3.0	27.0	0	0	970	2.0
(*Health Valley*)	80	3.0	18.0	0	0	380	1.0
(*Health Valley* No Salt)	80	3.0	18.0	0	0	35	1.0
(*Progresso* Hearty)	110	2.0	23.0	1.0	0	1110	2.0
basil (*Progresso*) ..	160	3.0	29.0	3.0	0	1060	2.0
chunky (*Health Valley*)	80	3.0	18.0	0	0	380	2.0
chunky (*Health Valley* No Salt)	80	3.0	18.0	0	0	70	2.0
garden (*Campbell's Select*)	100	3.0	21.0	.5	5	700	3.0
w/roasted garlic, herbs (*Campbell's 32 oz.*)	120	2.0	28.0	.5	0	770	2.0
rotini (*Progresso*) .	140	4.0	30.0	.5	0	1000	2.0
savory (*Walnut Acres*)	120	4.0	23.0	2.0	5	580	2.0
w/tomato pieces (*Campbell's* Low Sodium), 1 can .	160	4.0	25.0	5.0	10	90	4.0
vegetable (*Health Valley*)	80	6.0	17.0	0	0	240	5.0
tomato, cream of:							
(*Amy's*)	100	2.0	17.0	2.0	10	690	4.0
(*Amy's* Sodium Light)	100	2.0	17.0	2.0	10	340	3.0
creamy (*Campbell's 32 oz.*)	130	3.0	26.0	1.5	5	760	2.0
creamy (*Campbell's Kitchen Classics*)	140	3.0	24.0	3.5	10	730	2.0
creamy (*Campbell's Soup at Hand*), 1 cont.	190	4.0	34.0	4.0	5	940	4.0
creamy (*Healthy Choice*)	100	3.0	22.0	1.5	0	480	2.0

Food and Measure	cal.	prot. (gms)	carbo. (gms)	fat (gms)	chol. (mgs)	sod. (mgs)	fiber (gms)
Soup, tomato, cream of *(cont.)*							
creamy (*Imagine*)	90	2.0	17.0	1.5	0	520	2.0
creamy (*Progresso*)	190	4.0	30.0	6.0	15	900	1.0
tomato bisque (*Amy's*)	120	2.0	21.0	3.5	10	680	2.0
tortellini, cheese:							
w/chicken, vegetables							
(*Campbell's*							
Chunky)	110	5.0	18.0	2.0	10	890	2.0
herb (*Progresso*) ..	140	4.0	23.0	3.0	<5	700	2.0
turkey:							
chili, w/beans							
(*Campbell's*							
Chunky)	190	15.0	27.0	2.0	20	880	6.0
noodle (*Progresso*							
White Meat)	90	7.0	11.0	1.5	20	1060	<1.0
pot pie (*Campbell's*							
Chunky)	180	9.0	18.0	8.0	20	870	3.0
rice, w/vegetables							
(*Progresso* White							
Meat)	110	7.0	18.0	1.0	15	910	1.0
vegetable:							
(*Campbell's Chunky*)	110	3.0	22.0	1.0	0	770	4.0
(*Campbell's Kitchen*							
Classics)	100	3.0	22.0	.5	0	820	3.0
(*Campbell's Select*)	100	3.0	21.0	.5	0	900	3.0
(*Campbell's Select*							
Fiesta)	120	4.0	24.0	.5	15	790	2.0
(*Health Valley*)	80	3.0	18.0	0	0	380	4.0
(*Health Valley* No							
Salt)	80	3.0	18.0	0	0	40	4.0
(*Healthy Choice*							
Country)	100	4.0	22.0	.5	0	480	4.0
(*Progresso*)	90	3.0	17.0	1.0	0	930	2.0
(*Progresso* Italiano)	90	3.0	15.0	2.0	0	990	4.0
(*Westbrae Natural*							
Santa Fe)	160	9.0	31.0	0	0	380	8.0
(*Westbrae Natural*							
Spicy Southwest)	130	7.0	35.0	0	0	540	6.0
barley (*Amy's*)	70	2.0	13.0	1.0	0	580	3.0
barley (*Health Valley*)	90	6.0	19.0	0	0	210	4.0
blended medley							
(*Campbell's Soup*							
at Hand), 1 cont.	110	3.0	21.0	2.0	10	970	3.0

Food and Measure	cal.	prot. (gms)	carbo. (gms)	fat (gms)	chol. (mgs)	sod. (mgs)	fiber (gms)
14, garden (*Health Valley*)	80	6.0	17.0	0	0	250	4.0
garden (*Healthy Choice*)	120	6.0	25.0	1.0	0	480	4.0
herb and rotini (*Progresso*)	100	4.0	19.0	1.0	0	1100	5.0
w/pasta (*Campbell's Chunky*)	130	4.0	23.0	2.0	<5	930	3.0
vegetarian (*Progresso*)	100	4.0	20.0	.5	0	990	4.0
vegetable beef:							
(*Campbell's Chunky Old Fashioned*) . .	130	9.0	18.0	2.5	15	910	6.0
(*Campbell's Select*)	110	8.0	16.0	2.0	15	910	3.0
(*Campbell's Soup at Hand*), 1 cont. . .	60	3.0	10.0	1.0	5	830	2.0
(*Healthy Choice*) . .	130	9.0	24.0	1.0	10	480	4.0
chunky (*Campbell's Low Sodium*), 1 can	160	14.0	17.0	4.0	40	90	6.0
vegetable broth:							
(*College Inn* Garden)	25	0	6.0	0	0	590	0
(*Health Valley*)	20	0	5.0	0	0	330	0
(*Health Valley Organic*)	15	0	4.0	0	0	390	0
(*Imagine*)	30	1.0	5.0	.5	0	460	1.0
(*Kitchen Basics Stock*)	20	0	0	0	0	330	0
(*Pacific* Stock)	15	0	3.0	0	0	530	0
(*Swanson*)	15	0	3.0	0	0	940	0
Soup, condensed, undiluted, ½ cup:							
asparagus, cream of (*Campbell's*)	100	2.0	10.0	7.0	5	870	1.0
bean, w/bacon (*Campbell's*)	170	8.0	25.0	4.0	5	860	8.0
bean, black (*Campbell's*)	110	5.0	19.0	2.0	0	900	5.0
beef, w/vegetables and barley (*Campbell's*)	90	5.0	15.0	1.5	10	890	3.0
beef broth (*Campbell's*)	15	3.0	1.0	0	0	860	0
beef consommé (*Campbell's*)	20	4.0	1.0	0	0	810	0
beef noodle (*Campbell's*)	70	4.0	9.0	2.5	15	870	<1.0

Food and Measure	cal.	prot. (gms)	carbo. (gms)	fat (gms)	chol. (mgs)	sod. (mgs)	fiber (gms)
Soup, condensed *(cont.)*							
broccoli cream of:							
(*Campbell's*)	90	2.0	12.0	3.5	5	750	1.0
(*Campbell's* 98% Fat Free)	60	2.0	12.0	1.0	5	700	2.0
broccoli cheese:							
(*Campbell's*)	100	2.0	12.0	4.5	5	820	0
(*Campbell's* 98% Fat Free)	70	3.0	12.0	1.5	5	790	1.0
celery, cream of:							
(*Campbell's*)	100	1.0	10.0	6.0	5	860	1.0
(*Campbell's* 98% Fat Free)	60	1.0	8.0	3.0	<5	780	1.0
(*Campbell's Healthy Request*)	70	1.0	11.0	2.0	<5	430	0
cheddar cheese (*Campbell's*)	100	3.0	12.0	4.5	10	950	1.0
cheese, nacho (*Campbell's* Fiesta)	120	3.0	10.0	8.0	10	800	1.0
chicken:							
alphabet (*Campbell's*)	70	4.0	11.0	1.5	10	880	1.0
dumplings (*Campbell's*)	80	4.0	10.0	3.0	15	960	1.0
gumbo (*Campbell's*)	60	2.0	10.0	1.0	5	870	1.0
and stars (*Campbell's*)	70	3.0	12.0	2.0	5	860	1.0
vegetable (*Campbell's*)	80	3.0	15.0	1.0	5	890	2.0
vegetable, creamy (*Campbell's* Southwest Style)	110	5.0	21.0	1.0	5	830	4.0
won ton (*Campbell's*)	45	3.0	6.0	1.0	10	870	0
chicken, cream of:							
(*Campbell's*)	120	3.0	11.0	7.0	10	870	1.0
(*Campbell's* 98% Fat Free)	70	3.0	10.0	2.0	10	890	<1.0
(*Campbell's Healthy Request*)	70	2.0	12.0	2.5	10	450	1.0
w/herbs (*Campbell's*)	90	3.0	10.0	4.0	10	890	1.0
and mushrooms (*Campbell's*)	120	3.0	9.0	8.0	10	900	1.0
chicken broth (*Campbell's*)	20	1.0	1.0	1.0	<5	770	0

Food and Measure	cal.	prot. (gms)	carbo. (gms)	fat (gms)	chol. (mgs)	sod. (mgs)	fiber (gms)
chicken noodle:							
(*Campbell's*)	60	3.0	8.0	1.5	15	890	<1.0
(*Campbell's* 26 oz.)	60	3.0	8.0	2.0	10	890	<1.0
(*Campbell's* Home-style)	70	4.0	8.0	2.0	10	940	1.0
(*Campbell's Healthy Request*)	60	3.0	8.0	2.0	10	450	1.0
(*Campbell's Noodle O's*)	80	4.0	12.0	2.5	10	930	1.0
creamy (*Campbell's*)	120	4.0	13.0	7.0	15	870	0
chicken w/rice:							
(*Campbell's*)	80	2.0	14.0	1.5	5	820	1.0
(*Campbell's Healthy Request*)	80	2.0	13.0	2.0	5	420	1.0
white/wild (*Campbell's*)	70	3.0	12.0	1.5	5	820	1.0
white/wild, hearty (*Campbell's Healthy Request*)	110	5.0	17.0	2.0	10	360	2.0
chili beef (*Campbell's* Fiesta)	170	7.0	25.0	5.0	10	770	8.0
clam bisque (*Chincoteague*) . . .	100	8.0	13.0	2.0	15	990	1.0
clam chowder, Manhattan:							
(*Campbell's*)	70	2.0	12.0	.5	<5	880	2.0
(*Chincoteague*) . . .	100	8.0	13.0	2.0	15	990	1.0
clam chowder, New England:							
(*Campbell's*)	90	4.0	13.0	2.5	5	880	1.0
(*Campbell's* 98% Fat Free)	80	3.0	13.0	2.0	<5	940	1.0
(*Chincoteague*) . . .	80	5.0	10.0	2.5	10	590	<1.0
(*Chincoteague* 99% Fat Free)	70	2.0	12.0	1.0	5	610	<1.0
corn chowder (*Chincoteague*) . . .	100	2.0	16.0	3.5	0	890	1.0
crab:							
(*Chincoteague* She)	70	4.0	7.0	3.0	20	770	0
and cheddar (*Chincoteague*) .	90	4.0	10.0	3.5	20	590	0
cream of (*Chincoteague*) .	200	11.0	23.0	6.0	35	830	0

Food and Measure	cal.	prot. (gms)	carbo. (gms)	fat (gms)	chol. (mgs)	sod. (mgs)	fiber (gms)
Soup, condensed, crab *(cont.)*							
red, vegetable (*Chincoteague*) .	90	5.0	12.0	2.5	15	880	2.0
lobster bisque:							
(*Chincoteague*) . . .	90	4.0	10.0	4.0	15	650	0
cheddar (*Chincoteague*) .	110	4.0	10.0	6.0	20	610	0
minestrone:							
(*Campbell's*)	90	4.0	17.0	1.0	<5	960	3.0
(*Campbell's Healthy Request*)	80	3.0	15.0	.5	5	460	3.0
mushroom:							
beefy (*Campbell's*) .	50	3.0	6.0	2.0	10	890	0
golden (*Campbell's*)	80	2.0	10.0	3.5	5	890	1.0
mushroom, cream of:							
(*Campbell's*)	100	1.0	9.0	7.0	5	790	1.0
(*Campbell's 98% Fat Free*)	70	1.0	9.0	3.0	5	900	2.0
(*Campbell's Healthy Request*)	70	1.0	10.0	2.5	<5	460	1.0
w/roasted garlic (*Campbell's*)	70	2.0	11.0	2.0	5	790	1.0
noodle:							
(*Campbell's Fun Shapes*)	80	4.0	12.0	1.5	5	780	2.0
curly (*Campbell's*) .	80	4.0	11.0	2.0	15	840	1.0
double, in chicken broth (*Campbell's*)	100	4.0	17.0	1.5	10	830	2.0
mega, in chicken broth (*Campbell's*)	90	4.0	14.0	2.0	15	800	2.0
onion:							
cream of (*Campbell's*)	100	2.0	12.0	5.0	10	880	1.0
French (*Campbell's*)	45	2.0	6.0	1.5	<5	900	1.0
oyster stew:							
(*Campbell's*)	80	2.0	5.0	6.0	20	910	0
(*Chincoteague*) . . .	80	3.0	11.0	3.5	25	680	0
pasta:							
(*Campbell's Goldfish*)	130	3.0	28.0	.5	0	720	1.0
w/chicken, chicken broth (*Campbell's Goldfish*)	70	3.0	11.0	1.5	10	800	1.0
pea, green (*Campbell's*)	180	9.0	28.0	3.0	5	870	4.0
pea, split, w/ham and bacon (*Campbell's*)	180	10.0	27.0	3.5	5	850	5.0

Food and Measure	cal.	prot. (gms)	carbo. (gms)	fat (gms)	chol. (mgs)	sod. (mgs)	fiber (gms)
pepper pot (*Campbell's*)	90	4.0	9.0	4.0	20	940	1.0
potato, cream of (*Campbell's*)	100	2.0	15.0	3.0	10	880	1.0
Scotch broth (*Campbell's*)	70	3.0	9.0	2.0	5	880	2.0
shrimp, cream of (*Campbell's*)	90	1.0	8.0	6.0	15	880	1.0
shrimp bisque (*Chincoteague*) ...	80	2.0	10.0	3.0	20	590	0
tomato:							
(*Campbell's*)	90	2.0	20.0	0	0	710	1.0
(*Campbell's Healthy Request*)	90	2.0	18.0	1.5	0	450	1.0
bisque (*Campbell's*)	130	2.0	23.0	3.5	5	880	1.0
noodle (*Campbell's*)	120	3.0	25.0	.5	5	660	2.0
rice (*Campbell's Old Fashioned*)	110	1.0	23.0	2.0	<5	770	1.0
turkey noodle (*Campbell's*)	70	3.0	9.0	2.0	10	890	1.0
vegetable:							
(*Campbell's*)	100	4.0	20.0	.5	5	890	3.0
(*Campbell's California Style*) .	70	3.0	13.0	.5	5	810	2.0
(*Campbell's Old Fashioned*)	80	3.0	14.0	1.5	5	940	2.0
(*Campbell's Healthy Request*)	100	4.0	20.0	1.0	<5	480	3.0
beef (*Campbell's*) ..	80	5.0	15.0	1.0	5	890	3.0
beef (*Campbell's Healthy Request*)	90	5.0	15.0	1.0	5	480	3.0
w/pasta, hearty (*Campbell's*)	90	3.0	19.0	.5	0	890	2.0
vegetarian (*Campbell's*)	90	3.0	18.0	.5	0	790	2.0
Soup, semi-condensed, undiluted:							
broth, vegetarian (*Westbrae Natural California Un-Chicken*), ¾ cup ...	15	1.0	2.0	.5	0	890	0
clam chowder, Manhattan (*Bookbinder's*), ½ cup	60	4.0	10.0	0	5	800	<1.0

Food and Measure	cal.	prot. (gms)	carbo. (gms)	fat (gms)	chol. (mgs)	sod. (mgs)	fiber (gms)
Soup, semi-condensed *(cont.)*							
lobster bisque (*Bookbinder's*), ½ cup	100	5.0	10.0	4.0	20	850	0
mushroom, creamy (Westbrae Natural Monte Carlo), ¾ cup	70	1.0	10.0	3.0	10	680	0
pepperpot, seafood (*Bookbinder's*), ½ cup	140	7.0	23.0	2.0	10	1120	1.0
seafood bisque (*Bookbinder's*), ½ cup	130	8.0	9.0	7.0	35	930	0
shrimp bisque (*Bookbinder's*), ½ cup	100	4.0	10.0	4.0	25	850	0
snapper (*Bookbinder's*), ½ cup	110	3.0	12.0	5.0	0	530	<1.0
tomato (*Westbrae Natural* Tuscany), ¾ cup	70	2.0	16.0	0	0	710	0
Soup, freeze-dried, 1 serving:							
bean, multi (*AlpineAire*)	170	10.0	28.0	2.0	0	570	8.0
broccoli, cream of (*AlpineAire*)	130	5.0	21.0	3.0	15	1090	2.0
corn chowder (*AlpineAire* Kernel's)	210	14.0	36.0	1.0	0	490	9.0
minestrone (*AlpineAire* Alpine)	180	7.0	34.0	2.0	0	510	6.0
potato cheddar, creamy (*AlpineAire*)	210	7.0	36.0	4.0	20	1290	3.0
seafood chowder (*Mountain House*)	270	19.0	19.0	12.0	90	910	1.0
split pea (*AlpineAire* Soup-er)	200	14.0	34.0	1.0	0	620	9.0
Soup, frozen, 1 cup:							
asparagus, creamy (*Impromptu Gourmet*)	240	6.0	14.0	18.0	45	970	1.0
bean, white, and vegetable (*Moosewood* Tuscan)	130	6.0	24.0	2.0	0	760	5.0
broccoli and cheese, creamy (*Moosewood*)	160	5.0	7.0	6.0	20	800	3.0
chicken noodle (*Organic Classics*)	110	7.0	15.0	3.0	15	760	2.0

Food and Measure	cal.	prot. (gms)	carbo. (gms)	fat (gms)	chol. (mgs)	sod. (mgs)	fiber (gms)
clam chowder, New England (*Boston Chowda*)	280	11.0	20.0	17.0	60	900	1.0
crab, Charleston (*Boston Chowda She-Crab*)	320	11.0	16.0	23.0	90	550	<1.0
lobster bisque:							
(*Boston Chowda Rockport*)	260	9.0	12.0	19.0	40	1400	1.0
(*Impromptu Gourmet*)	210	10.0	10.0	14.0	80	1230	0
mushroom barley (*Moosewood* Hearty)	90	3.0	14.0	2.0	0	720	3.0
potato and corn chowder (*Moosewood*) .	160	5.0	26.0	5.0	15	390	3.0
salmon, smoked, chowder (*Impromptu Gourmet*)	260	10.0	21.0	15.0	50	750	1.0
seafood chowder (*Organic Classics*) .	160	11.0	17.0	6.0	50	800	1.0
shrimp and sausage gumbo (*Boston Chowda*)	420	14.0	38.0	23.0	70	490	2.0
tomato and rice (*Moosewood* Mediterranean)	100	3.0	16.0	3.0	0	510	2.0
Soup, mix, dry, 1 cont. or pkg., except as noted:							
bean:							
3-bean (*Bean Cuisine* Bouillabaisse), 1 cup*	220	6.0	17.0	0	0	0	5.0
5-bean (*Fantastic Big Soup*), ½ cont...	180	10.0	33.0	1.5	0	470	9.0
and ham (*Hormel Micro Cup*)	190	9.0	29.0	4.0	15	790	2.0
bean, black:							
(*Bean Cuisine* Island), 1 cup*	210	6.0	17.0	0	0	0	7.0
(*Fantastic Big Soup* Jumpin'), ½ cont.	230	13.0	41.0	1.5	0	690	19.0
w/couscous, spicy (*Health Valley* Cup), ⅓ cup	130	6.0	29.0	0	0	290	5.0

Food and Measure	cal.	prot. (gms)	carbo. (gms)	fat (gms)	chol. (mgs)	sod. (mgs)	fiber (gms)
Soup, mix, bean, black *(cont.)*							
w/rice (*Health Valley* Cup Zesty), ⅓ cup	100	5.0	22.0	0	0	240	4.0
and rice (*Uncle Ben's* Hearty), ⅓ pkg. .	150	7.0	28.0	1.5	0	720	7.0
bean, white (*Bean Cuisine* Provencal), 1 cup*	250	10.0	32.0	1.0	0	15	11.0
beef, vegetarian:							
barley (*Fantastic Carb 'Tastic*)	90	4.0	14.0	1.0	5	750	6.0
noodle (*Fantastic Big Soup* Noodle Bowl), ½ cont.	100	5.0	21.0	0	0	580	2.0
beef stew, hearty (*Wyler's Soup Starter*), 1 cup* w/water	90	2.0	19.0	0	0	810	2.0
beef vegetable:							
(*Hormel* Micro Cup)	90	6.0	15.0	1.0	10	790	1.0
beefy (*Instant Gourmet*)	100	9.0	6.0	4.0	30	960	1.0
broccoli:							
cheddar (*Fantastic Carb'Tastic*)	110	7.0	13.0	3.0	5	560	7.0
cheddar (*Instant Gourmet*)	140	6.0	6.0	10.0	35	740	2.0
cheddar (*Produce Partners*), 2 tbsp.	70	1.0	5.0	3.0	10	720	0
cheddar (*Wyler's Soup Starter*), 1 cup*	110	3.0	19.0	3.0	5	710	2.0
cheddar, creamy (*Fantastic Big Soup*), ½ cont...	130	5.0	21.0	2.5	10	490	2.0
cheese (*Cup-a-Soup*)	90	2.0	17.0	1.5	5	840	0
cheese and rice (*Uncle Ben's* Hearty), ⅓ pkg. .	110	3.0	19.0	2.0	5	680	1.0
cream of (*Produce Partners*), 1⅓ tbsp.	35	0	4.0	0	0	700	0
ginger, Asian (*Fantastic Carb 'Tastic*)	80	7.0	11.0	1.5	0	680	9.0

Food and Measure	cal.	prot. (gms)	carbo. (gms)	fat (gms)	chol. (mgs)	sod. (mgs)	fiber (gms)
Mandarin (*Fantiasic Big Soup* Noodle Bowl), ½ cont. . .	110	5.0	20.0	0	0	630	2.0
cheese (*Watkins* Soup and Sauce Base), 2½ tbsp.	80	1.0	14.0	2.0	5	440	0
chicken:							
w/asparagus (*Instant Gourmet*) .	130	8.0	5.0	9.0	35	610	1.0
cream of (*Cup-a-Soup*)	70	1.0	14.0	1.5	0	730	0
spicy Thai (*Cup-a-Soup*)	60	1.0	12.0	1.0	0	890	0
"chicken," vegetarian:							
gumbo (*Fantastic Carb 'Tastic*)	90	9.0	9.0	1.5	0	470	4.0
Mandarin (*Fantastic Carb 'Tastic*)	90	9.0	13.0	1.0	0	660	10.0
chicken noodle:							
(*Fantastic Big Soup* Noodle Bowl), ½ cont.	90	4.0	19.0	.5	0	590	1.0
(*Fantastic* Simmer), ⅓ cup	120	6.0	22.0	.5	0	690	2.0
(*Hormel* Micro Cup)	100	7.0	12.0	2.5	35	790	0
(*Wyler's Soup Starter*), 1 cup* w/water	70	3.0	13.0	1.0	10	910	1.0
chicken rice (*Hormel* Micro Cup)	110	4.0	18.0	3.0	15	950	1.0
chili (*Fantastic Big Soup* Cha Cha), ½ cont.	220	14.0	37.0	2.0	0	440	11.0
clam chowder, New England (*Hormel* Micro Cup)	140	5.0	18.0	5.0	20	800	1.0
corn chowder:							
bean (*Bean Cuisine* Santa Fe), 1 cup*	160	6.0	18.0	0	0	10	6.0
and potato (*Fantastic Big Soup*), ½ cont.	130	5.0	26.0	1.0	5	340	2.0
w/tomatoes (*Health Valley* Cup), ½ cup	100	5.0	21.0	0	0	270	3.0

Food and Measure	cal.	prot. (gms)	carbo. (gms)	fat (gms)	chol. (mgs)	sod. (mgs)	fiber (gms)
Soup, mix *(cont.)*							
couscous w/lentils *(Fantastic Big Soup)*, ½ cont.	170	9.0	35.0	1.0	0	460	5.0
cream *(Watkins* Soup Base), 2½ tbsp.	90	1.0	4.0	8.0	15	1150	0
garlic herb *(Fantastic Soup/Dip)*, 2¼ tsp.	20	0	5.0	0	0	540	0
hot and sour:							
(Fantastic Big Soup Noodle Bowl), ½ cont.	130	4.0	22.0	2.0	0	710	1.0
(Fantastic Carb 'Tastic)	70	6.0	7.0	2.5	0	410	1.0
lentil:							
(Bean Cuisine Lots of Lentils), 1 cup*	230	6.0	17.0	0	0	5	5.0
(Fantastic Big Soup Country), ½ cont.	180	12.0	32.0	1.5	0	220	9.0
w/couscous *(Health Valley* Cup), ⅓ cup	130	7.0	28.0	0	0	270	5.0
minestrone *(Fantastic Big Soup)*, ½ cont.	140	7.0	27.0	1.5	0	470	4.0
miso:							
dark *(San-J)*	40	3.0	3.0	1.5	0	1200	1.0
mild *(San-J)*	45	3.0	5.0	1.5	0	1340	1.0
red *(Westbrae Natural* Instant)	35	2.0	3.0	1.5	0	750	0
w/tofu *(Fantastic Big Soup* Noodle Bowl), ½ cont.	100	4.0	19.0	1.0	0	580	<1.0
sesame *(Fantastic Big Soup* Noodle Bowl), ½ cont.	90	3.0	17.0	1.0	0	550	<1.0
white *(San-J)*	40	3.0	3.0	1.5	0	830	0
white *(Westbrae Natural* Instant)	35	2.0	3.0	1.5	0	780	0
mushroom:							
(Watkins Soup and Sauce Base), 2 tbsp.	60	2.0	9.0	2.0	5	540	0
shiitake *(Fantastic Carb 'Tastic)*	80	6.0	9.0	2.0	0	610	7.0

Food and Measure	cal.	prot. (gms)	carbo. (gms)	fat (gms)	chol. (mgs)	sod. (mgs)	fiber (gms)
and chicken w/garlic (*Instant Gourmet*)	100	7.0	8.0	4.0	15	960	2.0
noodle:							
beef flavor (*Cup-a-Soup* Asian)	70	2.0	14.0	1.0	0	680	0
chicken flavor (*Cup-a-Soup*)	80	2.0	17.0	.5	<5	920	0
chicken flavor, w/vegetables (*Health Valley* Cup), ½ cup	110	5.0	24.0	0	0	270	3.0
thin cut (*Azumaya* Asian), 1 cup ...	120	6.0	24.0	0	0	820	<1.0
wide cut (*Azumaya* Asian), 1 cup ...	120	5.0	24.0	0	0	600	<1.0
noodle, ramen:							
buckwheat or brown rice (*Westbrae Natural*), ½ pkg.	140	5.0	30.0	1.0	0	750	2.0
chicken free, vegetarian (*Fantastic Big Soup*), ½ cont.	100	7.0	19.0	.5	0	420	2.0
curry (*Westbrae Natural*), ½ pkg.	140	5.0	30.0	1.0	0	720	3.0
5 spice (*Westbrae Natural*), ½ pkg.	140	5.0	30.0	1.0	0	700	3.0
miso (*Westbrae Natural*), ½ pkg.	140	5.0	29.0	1.0	0	750	4.0
mushroom (*Westbrae Natural*), ½ pkg.	140	5.0	30.0	.5	0	710	3.0
seaweed (*Westbrae Natural*), ½ pkg.	140	5.0	30.0	.5	0	690	3.0
spinach (*Westbrae Natural*), ½ pkg.	140	5.0	29.0	.5	0	760	3.0
vegetable curry (*Fantastic Big Soup*), ½ cont...	110	5.0	20.0	1.0	0	490	2.0
vegetable miso (*Fantastic Big Soup*), ½ cont...	100	5.0	19.0	1.0	0	430	1.0
onion:							
(*Fantastic* Soup/Dip), 2½ tsp.	25	1.0	6.0	0	0	480	1.0

Food and Measure	cal.	prot. (gms)	carbo. (gms)	fat (gms)	chol. (mgs)	sod. (mgs)	fiber (gms)
Soup, mix, onion *(cont.)*							
mushroom (*Fantastic* Soup and Dip), 1½ tbsp.	25	0	6.0	0	0	480	<1.0
pasta:							
(*Health Valley* Cup Italiano), ½ cup .	140	5.0	31.0	0	0	270	3.0
marinara, Mediterranean, or Parmesan (*Health Valley* Cup), ½ cup	100	5.0	20.0	0	0	290	1.0
pea, split:							
(*Fantastic* Simmer), ¼ cup	125	8.0	2.0	1.0	0	580	6.0
(*Fantastic Big Soup*), ½ cont.	160	11.0	7.0	1.0	0	410	7.0
garden, w/carrots (*Health Valley* Cup), ⅓ cup	110	7.0	22.0	0	0	270	2.0
potato:							
cream of (*Produce Partners*), 1 tbsp.	25	0	3.0	0	0	710	0
creamy (*Fantastic* Simmer), ¼ cup .	130	4.0	22.0	3.0	10	680	1.0
potato broccoli, creamy (*Health Valley* Cup), ⅓ cup	80	4.0	17.0	0	0	290	3.0
rice noodles, 1 cup*:							
curry (*Thai Kitchen*)	140	2.0	28.0	2.0	0	875	0
curry (*Thai Kitchen* Bangkok Instant*)	90	1.0	16.0	3.0	0	510	0
garlic, roasted (*Thai Kitchen* Soup Bowls)	120	2.2	25.0	1.5	0	756	0
garlic and vegetables (*Thai Kitchen* Instant)	80	1.0	17.0	1.5	0	470	0
ginger (*Thai Kitchen* Instant)	80	1.0	16.0	2.0	0	510	0
ginger (*Thai Kitchen* Soup Bowls) ...	120	2.2	24.0	1.8	0	690	0
hot and sour (*Thai Kitchen*)	130	2.0	30.0	.5	0	830	0

Food and Measure	cal.	prot. (gms)	carbo. (gms)	fat (gms)	chol. (mgs)	sod. (mgs)	fiber (gms)
hot and sour (*Thai Kitchen* Soup Bowls)	115	2.0	24.0	1.5	0	700	0
lemongrass and chili (*Thai Kitchen*) ..	285	4.0	60.0	3.0	0	530	0
lemongrass and chili (*Thai Kitchen* Instant)	80	1.0	17.0	1.5	0	520	0
mushroom (*Thai Kitchen* Soup Bowls)	120	3.9	25.0	1.5	0	881	0
onion, spring (*Thai Kitchen* Instant) .	90	1.0	16.0	1.5	0	430	0
onion, spring (*Thai Kitchen* Soup Bowls)	120	2.0	25.0	1.5	0	627	0
shrimp bisque (*Instant Gourmet* Bay Shrimp)	150	6.0	7.0	11.0	35	720	1.0
Thai:							
w/mushrooms (*Tasty Bite* Tom Yum), ½ pkg.	80	2.0	5.0	6.0	0	630	<1.0
spicy (*Fantastic Big Soup* Noodle Bowl), ½ cont.	110	3.0	22.0	1.0	0	460	1.0
w/vegetables (*Tasty Bite* Gang Pha), ½ pkg.	25	<1.0	4.0	0	0	620	1.0
tomato:							
w/croutons (*Cup-a-Soup*)	90	1.0	16.0	2.5	0	870	<1.0
noodle, Italian (*Fantasic Big Soup* Noodle Bowl), ½ cont.	130	5.0	26.0	1.0	0	480	2.0
sun-dried, basil (*Fantastic Carb 'Tastic*)	70	5.0	10.0	1.0	0	440	7.0
tortilla (*Chi-Chi's* Fiesta), 1/5 pkg.	80	3.0	13.0	1.5	0	800	1.9
vegetable:							
(*Fantastic* Soup and Dip), 1½ tsp.	25	1.0	5.0	0	0	480	<1.0

Food and Measure	cal.	prot. (gms)	carbo. (gms)	fat (gms)	chol. (mgs)	sod. (mgs)	fiber (gms)
Soup, mix, vegetable *(cont.)*							
barley (*Fantastic Simmer*), ¼ cup .	120	4.0	26.0	0	0	690	3.0
barley (*Fantastic Big Soup*), ½ cont. . .	120	4.0	27.0	.5	0	420	5.0
spring (*Cup-a-Soup*)	50	1.0	11.0	.5	0	720	<1.0
spring (*Fantastic Big Soup* Noodle Bowl), ½ cont.	90	4.0	19.0	0	0	590	<1.0
wakame (*San-J*)	50	0	12.0	0	0	910	0
Sour cream, see "Cream, sour"							
Soursop, ½ cup	75	1.1	18.9	.3	0	16	3.7
Soy, cultured, see "Yogurt," soy							
Soy bean, see "Soybean"							
Soy beverage, 8 fl. oz., except as noted:							
(*Edensoy* Extra Organic Original)	130	11.0	13.0	4.0	0	100	3.0
(*Edensoy* Extra Organic Original), 8.45 fl. oz.	135	11.0	14.0	4.0	0	105	3.0
(*Edensoy* Light Organic Original)	100	5.0	14.0	2.0	0	85	0
(*Edensoy* Light Organic Original), 8.45 fl. oz.	100	5.0	15.0	2.0	0	90	0
(*Edensoy* Organic Original)	140	11.0	14.0	5.0	0	105	2.0
(*Edensoy* Organic Original), 8.45 fl. oz.	145	11.0	14.0	5.0	0	110	2.0
(*Edensoy* Organic Unsweetened)	120	12.0	5.0	6.0	0	5	2.0
(*8th Continent*)	90	7.0	11.0	3.0	0	170	0
(*Organic Valley* Original)	100	7.0	11.0	3.0	0	95	3.0
(*Pearl* Organic Original)	110	7.0	12.0	3.5	0	110	1.0
(*Power Dream*), 11 fl. oz.	260	10.0	48.0	5.0	0	180	2.0
(*Silk*)	100	7.0	8.0	4.0	0	120	1.0
(*Silk*), 11 fl. oz.	140	10.0	11.0	6.0	0	170	1.0
(*Silk* Enhanced)	110	7.0	8.0	5.0	0	120	1.0
(*Silk* Light)	70	6.0	8.0	2.0	0	120	1.0
(*Silk* Unsweetened) . .	90	7.0	5.0	4.0	0	85	1.0

Food and Measure	cal.	prot. (gms)	carbo. (gms)	fat (gms)	chol. (mgs)	sod. (mgs)	fiber (gms)
(*Silk* Unsweetened Aseptic)	90	7.0	5.0	4.0	0	120	1.0
(*Soy Dream* Original) .	130	7.0	17.0	.5	0	140	n.a.
(*WestSoy* Lite)	90	4.0	15.0	1.5	0	90	2.0
(*WestSoy* Low Fat) ..	90	4.0	14.0	1.5	0	90	2.0
(*WestSoy* Non Fat) ...	70	6.0	10.0	0	0	105	<1.0
(*WestSoy* Organic Original)	130	8.0	18.0	3.5	0	125	3.0
(*WestSoy* Organic Unsweetened)	90	9.0	5.0	4.5	0	30	4.0
(*WestSoy* Plus)	130	7.0	17.0	3.0	0	125	3.0
(*WestSoy* Smart Plus)	180	11.0	22.0	5.0	0	85	5.0
banana berry (*WestSoy* Smoothie)	140	3.0	28.0	1.5	0	15	2.0
cappucino (*WestSoy* Soy Slender)	70	7.0	4.0	3.0	0	125	3.0
carob:							
(*Edensoy* Organic) .	170	7.0	27.0	4.0	0	95	0
(*Edensoy* Organic), 8.45 fl. oz.	170	7.0	28.0	4.0	0	100	0
(*Soy Dream*)	210	7.0	36.0	4.0	0	160	1.0
chai:							
(*Power Dream* Sky High), 11 fl. oz. .	250	10.0	42.0	5.0	0	70	<1.0
(*Silk*)	140	6.0	19.0	4.0	0	100	0
(*WestSoy* Original) .	130	2.0	25.0	3.0	0	65	<1.0
chocolate:							
(*Edensoy* Organic) .	175	8.0	28.0	4.0	0	105	1.0
(*Edensoy* Organic), 8.45 fl. oz.	180	8.0	29.0	4.0	0	110	1.0
(*8th Continent*) ...	140	7.0	23.0	3.0	0	190	1.0
(*8th Continent* Light)	90	7.0	11.0	1.5	0	190	<1.0
(*Organic Valley*) ...	120	5.0	19.0	2.5	0	140	3.0
(*Silk*)	140	5.0	23.0	3.5	0	100	2.0
(*Silk*); 6.5 fl. oz. ...	120	4.0	19.0	3.0	0	80	2.0
(*Silk*), 11 fl. oz. ...	190	7.0	32.0	5.0	0	140	2.0
(*Soy Dream* Enriched)	210	7.0	37.0	3.5	0	160	1.0
(*WestSoy* Lite)	130	4.0	25.0	1.5	0	55	2.0
(*WestSoy* Low Fat)	150	6.0	24.0	3.0	0	25	3.0
(*WestSoy* Organic Unsweetened) ..	100	9.0	6.0	4.5	0	30	5.0
(*WestSoy* Shake) ..	170	7.0	30.0	3.5	0	130	4.0
(*WestSoy* Soy Slender)	70	7.0	5.0	3.0	0	125	4.0

Food and Measure	cal.	prot. (gms)	carbo. (gms)	fat (gms)	chol. (mgs)	sod. (mgs)	fiber (gms)
Soy beverage, chocolate *(cont.)*							
(*WestSoy VigorAid*),							
1 cont.	260	12.0	42.0	5.0	0	100	6.0
coffee:							
(*Power Dream* Java							
Jolt), 11 fl. oz. . .	240	10.0	42.0	4.5	0	70	2.0
(*Silk* Soylatte)	170	5.0	25.0	3.5	0	100	1.0
(*Silk* Soylatte),							
11 fl. oz.	200	7.0	34.0	4.5	0	140	1.0
green tea (*Pearl*							
Organic)	110	7.0	13.0	3.5	0	95	1.0
kefir blend, all flavors							
(*Lifeway Soy Treat*)	160	7.0	23.0	4.0	0	2	0
mango:							
(*Power Dream*							
Passion), 11 fl. oz.	320	8.0	65.0	4.5	0	100	1.0
(*Silk Live!*), 10 fl. oz.	230	7.0	41.0	4.0	0	120	4.0
mocha (*Silk*)	140	5.0	22.0	3.5	0	100	0
peach (*Soy Live!*),							
10 fl. oz.	220	7.0	38.0	4.0	0	120	4.0
raspberry (*Silk Live!*),							
10 fl. oz.	200	7.0	40.0	4.0	0	120	4.0
spice (*Silk* Soylatte),							
11 fl. oz.	190	8.0	27.0	5.0	0	160	1.0
strawberry:							
(*Silk*), 6.5 fl. oz. . . .	130	5.0	21.0	3.0	0	95	1.0
(*Silk Live!*), 10 fl. oz.	220	7.0	40.0	4.0	0	120	4.0
tropical:							
(*Pearl* Organic							
Delight)	110	7.0	14.0	3.5	0	70	0
(*WestSoy* Smoothie							
Whip)	140	3.0	28.0	1.5	0	20	2.0
vanilla:							
(*Edensoy* Organic) .	150	7.0	24.0	3.0	0	85	1.0
(*Edensoy* Organic),							
8.45 fl. oz.	155	7.0	25.0	3.0	0	90	1.0
(*Edensoy* Extra							
Organic)	150	7.0	23.0	3.0	0	90	1.0
(*Edensoy* Extra Or-							
ganic), 8.45 fl. oz.	150	7.0	24.0	3.0	0	95	1.0
(*Edensoy* Light							
Organic)	120	4.0	20.0	2.0	0	85	0
(*Edensoy* Light Or-							
ganic), 8.45 fl. oz.	120	4.0	22.0	2.0	0	90	0

Food and Measure	cal.	prot. (gms)	carbo. (gms)	fat (gms)	chol. (mgs)	sod. (mgs)	fiber (gms)
(8th Continent) ...	90	7.0	11.0	3.0	0	170	0
(8th Continent Light)	60	7.0	4.0	1.0	0	190	0
(Organic Valley) ...	110	6.0	14.0	3.0	0	90	3.0
(Pearl Organic Creamy)	110	7.0	11.0	3.5	0	90	0
(Power Dream Blast), 11 fl. oz.	240	10.0	39.0	5.0	0	170	2.0
(Silk)	100	6.0	10.0	3.5	0	95	1.0
(Silk), 6.5 fl. oz. ...	100	5.0	14.0	3.0	0	80	1.0
(Silk), 11 fl. oz. ...	140	8.0	14.0	5.0	0	130	1.0
(Silk Light)	80	6.0	10.0	2.0	0	95	1.0
(Silk Very)	130	6.0	19.0	3.5	0	140	1.0
(Soy Dream)	150	7.0	22.0	4.0	0	140	0
(Soy Dream Enriched)	150	7.0	22.0	4.0	0	140	0
(WestSoy Lite)	110	4.0	19.0	1.5	0	65	2.0
(WestSoy Low Fat)	120	4.0	21.0	1.5	0	90	2.0
(WestSoy Non Fat) .	80	6.0	12.0	0	0	105	<1.0
(WestSoy Organic Unsweetened) ..	100	9.0	5.0	4.5	0	30	4.0
(WestSoy Shake) ..	170	7.0	28.0	3.0	0	125	3.0
(WestSoy Soy Slender)	70	6.0	4.0	3.0	0	125	3.0
(WestSoy Plus) ...	130	7.0	19.0	3.0	0	125	3.0
(WestSoy Smart Plus)	190	11.0	25.0	5.0	0	85	5.0
(WestSoy VigorAid), 1 cont.	230	11.0	37.0	5.0	0	90	5.0
chai tea (Bolthouse Farms Perfectly Protein)	160	10.0	25.0	3.0	0	60	0
Soy butter, see "Soy spread"							
Soy chips/crisps (see also "Potato-soy crisps"), 1 oz., except as noted:							
apple cinnamon (Geni-Soy Crisps)	120	7.0	17.0	2.0	0	160	2.0
barbecue (GeniSoy Crisps Zesty)	110	7.0	17.0	2.0	0	160	2.0
caramel (Hain Pure-Snax Munchies), 7 pcs., .5 oz.	40	2.0	8.0	0	0	10	<1.0
cheddar, white (Hain PureSnax Munchies), 9 pcs., .5 oz.	60	3.0	6.0	2.5	0	240	1.0

Food and Measure	cal.	prot. (gms)	carbo. (gms)	fat (gms)	chol. (mgs)	sod. (mgs)	fiber (gms)
Soy chips/crisps *(cont.)*							
cheese:							
nacho (*GeniSoy* Crisps)	110	7.0	15.0	2.0	0	170	2.0
rich (*GeniSoy* Crisps)	100	7.0	14.0	2.0	0	320	2.0
garlic, roasted, onion (*GeniSoy* Crisps) ..	100	7.0	14.0	2.0	0	320	2.0
Parmesan, garlic, olive oil (*Synder's* Crisps)	160	8.0	11.0	9.0	0	340	1.0
ranch:							
(*GeniSoy* Crisps) ..	110	7.0	15.0	2.0	0	330	2.0
(*Hain PureSnax* Munchies), 9 pcs., .5 oz.	60	3.0	8.0	2.0	0	150	1.0
salt and vinegar (*Geni-Soy* Crisps)	100	7.0	14.0	2.0	0	290	2.0
sea salted (*GeniSoy* Crisps)	100	7.0	14.0	2.0	0	260	2.0
tomato, Romano, olive oil (*Snyder's* Crisps)	160	8.0	12.0	9.0	0	360	n.a.
Soy flour, see "Soy-bean flour"							
Soy meal, defatted, raw, 1 cup	414	54.8	49.0	2.9	0	3	14.0
Soy milk, see "Soy beverage"							
Soy nuts, roasted:							
(*Frieda's*), ⅓ cup, 1.1 oz.	140	11.0	9.0	7.0	0	0	1.0
(*Frieda's* Salted), ⅓ cup, 1.1 oz.	140	11.0	9.0	7.0	0	50	1.0
(*GeniSoy* Unsalted), 1 oz.	120	12.0	9.0	4.0	0	10	5.0
(*Tree of Life*), 1.1 oz. .	150	12.0	9.0	7.0	0	10	3.0
(*Tree of Life* Salted), 1.3 oz.	150	12.0	9.0	7.0	0	80	3.0
barbecue (*GeniSoy* Zesty), 1 oz.	120	12.0	9.0	4.0	0	420	5.0
barbecue, honey, or wasabi (*Frieda's*), ¼ cup	140	10.0	11.0	7.0	0	110	5.0
hickory smoked (*Geni-Soy*), 1 oz.	120	12.0	9.0	4.0	0	90	5.0
sea salted (*GeniSoy*), 1 oz.	120	12.0	9.0	4.0	0	150	2.0

Food and Measure	cal.	prot. (gms)	carbo. (gms)	fat (gms)	chol. (mgs)	sod. (mgs)	fiber (gms)
toasted:							
1 oz. or 95 kernels .	129	10.5	8.7	6.8	0	1	1.0
whole, 1 cup	490	40.0	33.0	25.9	0	4	3.9
Soy protein, concentrate, 1 oz.:							
w/alcohol	94	16.5	8.8	.1	0	1	<2.0
acid/water wash	94	16.5	8.8	.1	0	255	<2.0
Soy sauce, 1 tbsp.:							
(*House of Tsang* Low Sodium)	5	0	0	0	0	300	0
(*House of Tsang* Mandarin Marinade)	25	6.0	0	0	0	680	0
(*Kikkoman*)	10	2.0	0	0	0	920	0
(*Kikkoman* Lite)	10	1.0	1.0	0	0	575	0
(*World Harbors* Angostura)	10	1.0	1.0	0	0	670	0
(*World Harbors Angostura* All Natural) ..	15	1.0	2.0	0	0	440	0
ginger flavor:							
(*House of Tsang*) ..	20	0	4.0	0	0	760	0
(*House of Tsang* Low Sodium) ...	10	0	2.0	0	0	320	0
shoyu:							
(*Eden* Imported) ...	15	2.0	2.0	0	0	1010	0
(*Eden* Organic)	15	2.0	2.0	0	0	1040	0
(*Eden* Organic Imported Reduced Sodium)	10	2.0	2.0	0	0	500	0
(*San-J* Organic) ...	20	2.0	1.0	0	0	960	0
(*Tree of Life* Wheat Free Organic) ...	15	2.0	0	0	0	960	0
tamari:							
(*Eden* Organic)	15	2.0	2.0	0	0	860	0
(*Eden* Organic Imported)	10	2.0	2.0	0	0	990	0
(*San-J*)	15	2.0	1.0	0	0	960	0
(*San-J* Reduced Sodium)	20	2.0	1.0	0	0	700	0
(*San-J* Wheat Free Organic)	15	2.0	1.0	0	0	940	0
(*Tree of Life* Wheat Free Organic) ...	15	2.0	0	0	0	940	0
Soy spread, creamy or crunchy (*Soy Wonder*), 2 tbsp. ..	170	8.0	10.0	11.0	0	170	1.0

Food and Measure	cal.	prot. (gms)	carbo. (gms)	fat (gms)	chol. (mgs)	sod. (mgs)	fiber (gms)
Soybean, fresh (see also "Edamame"):							
raw, shelled, ½ cup ..	188	16.6	14.1	8.7	0	19	5.4
boiled, drained, ½ cup	127	11.1	10.0	5.8	0	13	3.8
Soybean, canned, ½ cup:							
(*Westbrae Natural* Organic)	150	13.0	11.0	7.0	0	140	3.0
black (*Eden* Organic) .	120	11.0	8.0	6.0	0	30	7.0
Soybean, dried:							
dry, ¼ cup:							
(*Arrowhead Mills*) .	160	14.0	11.0	8.0	0	0	4.0
black or yellow (*Shiloh Farms*) ..	170	15.0	14.0	8.0	0	0	10.0
dry-roasted	194	17.0	14.1	9.3	0	1	3.5
roasted	202	15.2	14.5	10.9	0	70	3.5
boiled, ½ cup	149	14.3	8.5	7.7	0	1	5.2
Soybean, frozen:							
in pod, see "Edamame"							
shelled (*C&W* Sweet), ½ cup	100	9.0	16.0	1.0	0	5	10.0
Soybean curd or cake, see "Tofu"							
Soybean flakes (*Shiloh Farms*), ½ cup	250	20.0	18.0	11.0	0	3	0
Soybean flour, ¼ cup:							
(*Arrowhead Mills*) ...	100	7.0	9.0	4.5	0	0	4.0
(*Hodgson Mill*), <¼ cup	80	15.0	9.0	0	0	10	6.0
(*Hodgson Mill* Organic), <¼ cup	110	9.0	9.0	5.0	0	0	4.0
(*Shiloh Farms*)	100	10.0	7.0	5.0	0	1	3.5
stirred:							
full fat, raw	93	7.4	7.5	4.4	0	3	2.1
defatted	82	11.8	9.6	.3	0	5	4.4
lowfat	72	10.2	8.4	.6	0	4	2.3
Soybean grits, roasted (*Shiloh Farms*), ¼ cup	100	10.0	7.0	5.0	0	1	3.5
Soybean kernels, roasted, see "Soy nuts"							
Soybean sprouts,							
(*Jonathan's*), 1 cup	100	11.0	8.0	6.0	0	10	2.0
steamed, ½ cup	38	4.0	3.1	2.1	0	5	.4

Food and Measure	cal.	prot. (gms)	carbo. (gms)	fat (gms)	chol. (mgs)	sod. (mgs)	fiber (gms)
Spaghetti, see "Pasta"							
Spaghetti entree, can or pkg., 1 cup, except as noted:							
(*SpaghettiOs*)	180	6.0	37.0	1.0	5	850	3.0
(*SpaghettiOs* A to Z's)	180	6.0	36.0	1.0	<5	880	3.0
(*SpaghettiOs* Fun Shapes Smilers) ...	170	6.0	33.0	1.0	5	850	3.0
(*SpaghettiOs* Plus Calcium)	170	6.0	35.0	1.0	5	620	3.0
(*SpaghettiOs* Spaghetti)	200	7.0	40.0	1.5	5	950	3.0
w/franks:							
(*SpaghettiOs*)	230	9.0	27.0	10.0	20	930	5.0
(*SpaghettiOs* A to Z's)	230	9.0	33.0	7.0	15	990	2.0
rings (*Kid's Kitchen*)	240	9.0	32.0	9.0	25	840	1.0
meat sauce:							
(*Hormel* Bowl), 10 oz.	270	12.0	41.0	7.0	15	980	4.0
(*Hormel* Meal), 1 cont.	220	10.0	31.0	7.0	20	790	2.0
(*SpaghettiOs*)	170	8.0	31.0	2.0	10	890	3.0
w/meatballs:							
(*Kid's Kitchen*)	230	10.0	28.0	8.0	20	800	2.0
(*SpaghettiOs*)	240	11.0	32.0	8.0	25	890	3.0
(*SpaghettiOs* A to Z's)	260	11.0	33.0	9.0	20	990	3.0
(*SpaghettiOs* Fun Shapes Smilers) .	240	11.0	32.0	8.0	25	890	3.0
rings (*Kid's Kitchen*)	230	11.0	31.0	7.0	25	1190	1.0
tomato cheese sauce (*SpaghettiOs*)	200	7.0	40.0	1.5	5	950	2.0
Spaghetti entree, dried, 1 serving:							
marinara, w/mushrooms (*AlpineAire*)	320	17.0	53.0	5.0	0	550	6.0
meat and sauce:							
(*Mountain House* Can/Four), 1 cup	230	12.0	32.0	7.0	20	680	2.0
(*Mountain House* Double), ½ pouch	270	14.0	37.0	8.0	20	790	2.0
(*Mountain House* Single)	340	17.0	46.0	10.0	25	990	3.0
Spaghetti entree, frozen, 1 pkg.:							
Bolognese (*Smart Ones*), 11.5 oz.	280	17.0	43.0	5.0	15	670	5.0

Food and Measure	cal.	prot. (gms)	carbo. (gms)	fat (gms)	chol. (mgs)	sod. (mgs)	fiber (gms)
Spaghetti entree, frozen *(cont.)*							
cheese bake (*Stouffer's*),							
12 oz.	500	23.0	45.0	25.0	130	1250	4.0
marinara:							
(*Michelina's* Zap'ems),							
8 oz.	230	8.0	46.0	2.0	0	380	4.0
(*Smart Ones*), 9 oz.	280	9.0	46.0	7.0	5	690	4.0
w/meat sauce:							
(*Healthy Choice*),							
10 oz.	280	14.0	36.0	8.0	20	600	5.0
(*Lean Cuisine Every-*							
day Favorites),							
9.5 oz.	280	13.0	48.0	4.0	15	580	3.0
(*Michelina's* Authen-							
tico), 8.5 oz.	250	11.0	45.0	4.0	15	670	4.0
(*Michelina's Lean*							
Gourmet), 9 oz. .	280	13.0	45.0	5.0	15	530	4.0
(*Stouffer's*), 12 oz. .	400	24.0	51.0	11.0	30	830	4.0
w/meatballs:							
(*Lean Cuisine Every-*							
day Favorites),							
9.5 oz.	270	17.0	38.0	5.0	25	590	3.0
(*Michelina's* Authen-							
tico), 9 oz.	300	15.0	44.0	8.0	20	810	4.0
(*Michelina's* Zap'ems),							
8 oz.	260	13.0	38.0	7.0	15	720	4.0
(*Stouffer's*), 12⅝ oz.	460	21.0	58.0	16.0	40	880	4.0
tomato basil sauce							
(*Michelina's* Zap'ems),							
8 oz.	240	9.0	47.0	3.0	5	410	4.0
Spaghetti sauce, see							
"Pasta sauce"							
Spaghetti squash:							
raw (*Frieda's*), ¾ cup,							
3 oz.	30	1.0	6.0	0	0	15	1.0
baked or boiled, drained,							
½ cup	23	.5	5.0	.2	0	14	1.1
Spanikopita, see							
"Spinach entrée,							
frozen" and "Spinach							
snack rolls/nuggets"							
Spareribs, see "Pork"							
and "Pork, frozen or							
refrigerated"							

Food and Measure	cal.	prot. (gms)	carbo. (gms)	fat (gms)	chol. (mgs)	sod. (mgs)	fiber (gms)
Spelt, grain, ¼ cup:							
(*Purity Foods* Berries)	130	7.0	32.0	1.0	0	0	8.0
(*Shiloh Farms*)	130	7.0	32.0	1.0	0	0	8.0
Spelt chips (*VitaSpelt* Flatchips), 1 oz. ...	70	2.0	15.0	.5	0	110	.5
Spelt flakes, see "Cereal, ready-to-eat"							
Spelt flour:							
(*Arrowhead Mills*), ⅓ cup	130	4.0	25.0	1.0	0	0	4.0
(*Hodgson Mill* Organic), <¼ cup	85	5.0	21.0	1.0	0	0	5.0
(*Shiloh Farms*), ¼ cup	110	5.0	23.0	1.0	0	0	2.0
white (*Shiloh Farms*), ¼ cup	100	4.0	21.0	.5	0	0	1.0
Spinach, fresh:							
raw:							
(*Dole/Dole* Baby), 3 oz.	20	2.0	3.0	0	0	65	2.0
baby (*Dole* Organic), 3 oz.	35	2.0	9.0	0	0	135	4.0
baby (*Fresh Express*), 1½ cups, 3 oz. ...	20	2.0	3.0	0	0	65	2.0
baby (*Ready Pac*), 4 cups, 3 oz.	40	2.0	10.0	0	0	160	5.0
flat leaf (*Fresh Express*), 1½ cups, 3 oz.	40	2.0	10.0	0	0	160	5.0
cooked, ½ cup:							
(*Ready Pac*)	20	2.0	3.0	0	0	60	<1.0
boiled, drained	21	2.7	3.4	.2	0	63	2.2
Spinach, canned, ½ cup:							
leaf:							
(*Popeye* No Salt) ..	40	4.0	5.0	.5	0	30	2.0
(*S&W*)	30	2.0	4.0	0	0	360	2.0
cut (*Freshlike*)	45	5.0	5.0	1.0	0	200	3.0
leaf or chopped:							
(*Del Monte*)	30	2.0	4.0	0	0	360	2.0
(*Del Monte* No Salt)	30	2.0	4.0	0	0	85	2.0
(*Popeye*)	30	3.0	4.0	0	0	190	2.0
seasoned (*Glory*)	30	4.0	3.0	0	0	430	2.0
drained	25	3.0	3.6	.5	0	29	2.6

Food and Measure	cal.	prot. (gms)	carbo. (gms)	fat (gms)	chol. (mgs)	sod. (mgs)	fiber (gms)
Spinach, frozen (see also "Spinach dish"):							
leaf:							
(*Birds Eye*), ⅓ cup .	30	2.0	3.0	0	0	125	1.0
(*C&W*), ⅓ cup	20	2.0	2.0	0	0	115	2.0
cut leaf:							
(*Birds Eye*), 1 cup .	30	2.0	3.0	0	0	120	1.0
(*Cascadian Farm* Bag), ⅓ cup	20	2.0	3.0	0	0	130	3.0
(*Cascadian Farm* Box), ⅓ cup	25	2.0	3.0	0	0	160	1.0
(*Green Giant*), ⅓ cup cooked	15	2.0	2.0	0	0	100	2.0
(*Tree of Life*), 1 cup	20	2.0	2.0	1.0	0	110	2.0
cut leaf, in butter sauce (*Green Giant*), ½ cup	35	2.0	4.0	1.0	<5	310	2.0
cut leaf or chopped (*Seabrook Farms*), ⅓ cup	20	2.0	2.0	0	0	115	2.0
chopped:							
(*Birds Eye*), ⅓ cup .	30	2.0	3.0	0	0	125	1.0
(*C&W*), ⅓ cup	20	2.0	2.0	0	0	115	2.0
(*Green Giant*), ½ cup	25	3.0	3.0	0	0	200	2.0
chopped or leaf, drained, ½ cup	27	3.0	5.1	.2	0	82	2.6
Spinach, malabar, cooked, 1 cup	10	1.3	1.2	.4	0	24	.9
Spinach, New Zealand, chopped:							
raw, 1 oz. or ½ cup . .	4	.4	.7	.1	0	37	n.a.
boiled, drained, ½ cup	11	1.2	2.0	.2	0	97	n.a.
Spinach dip, frozen, w/cheese and arti- choke (*T.G.I. Friday's*), 2 tbsp.	50	2.0	2.0	3.5	10	150	0
Spinach dip mix, dry (*McCormick*), 1 tsp.	10	0	1.0	0	0	100	0
Spinach dish, frozen, ½ cup, except as noted:							
creamed:							
(*Birds Eye*)	100	3.0	7.0	7.0	35	630	1.0
(*Boston Market*) . .	180	6.0	7.0	13.0	20	550	3.0
(*C&W*)	110	3.0	5.0	8.0	30	410	2.0

Food and Measure	cal.	prot. (gms)	carbo. (gms)	fat (gms)	chol. (mgs)	sod. (mgs)	fiber (gms)
(*Green Giant*)	80	3.0	9.0	3.0	0	510	1.0
(*Seabrook Farms*) .	120	4.0	10.0	6.0	15	450	3.0
(*Stouffer's*), ½ of 9-oz. pkg.	200	4.0	10.0	16.0	25	510	2.0
pancake:							
(*Dr. Praeger's*), 1.3-oz. pc.	40	1.0	5.0	2.0	0	135	<1.0
(*Dr. Praeger's* Bombay), 1.3-oz. pc. .	70	2.0	8.5	3.0	15	155	1.0
nuggets (*Dr. Praeger's*), 4 pcs., 1.4 oz.	45	2.0	5.0	2.0	0	140	1.0
soufflé (*Stouffer's*), ⅓ of 12-oz. pkg.	130	6.0	9.0	8.0	90	450	1.0
Spinach entree, frozen, 1 pkg., except as noted:							
w/cheese, palak paneer: (*Amy's*), 10 oz.	240	8.0	38.0	6.0	5	580	5.0
(*Deep*), ½ of 10-oz. pkg.	230	8.0	7.0	19.0	25	690	4.0
(*Ethnic Gourmet*), 12 oz.	420	18.0	42.0	20.0	15	790	7.0
feta pie (*Cedarlane* Spanakopita), ½ of 10-oz. pkg.	260	12.0	38.0	8.0	20	650	2.0
Spinach entree, pkg.:							
w/cheese and rice: (*Tamarind Tree* Palak Paneer), 9.25-oz. pkg.	380	14.0	46.0	15.0	35	640	6.0
(*Tasty Bite* Kashmir), ½ of 10-oz. pkg.	117	6.0	8.0	8.0	0	693	3.0
dal, w/rice (*Tasty Bite*), 12-oz. pkg.	372	12.0	62.0	9.0	0	649	8.0
w/garbanzos, rice (*Tamarind Tree* Saag Chole), 9.25-oz. pkg.	370	14.0	55.0	10.0	0	800	13.0
Spinach snack rolls/ nuggets, frozen: (*Health is Wealth* Muchees*), 2 pcs., 1 oz.	60	2.0	9.0	2.5	0	105	1.0

Food and Measure	cal.	prot. (gms)	carbo. (gms)	fat (gms)	chol. (mgs)	sod. (mgs)	fiber (gms)
Spinach snack rolls/nuggets *(cont.)*							
w/cheese, breaded (*Kineret*), 3½ pcs., 2.8 oz.	180	8.0	19.0	8.0	5	620	6.0
w/feta cheese:							
(*Amy's*), 5-6 pcs. . .	170	7.0	24.0	6.0	15	430	2.0
(*Athens/Apollo* Spanikopita), 2 pcs., 2 oz.	170	4.0	17.0	10.0	20	200	<1.0
(*Health is Wealth Muchees*), 2 pcs., 1 oz.	70	2.0	9.0	3.0	5	115	1.0
Spinach-feta pocket, frozen (*Amy's*), 4.5-oz. pc.	250	11.0	34.0	9.0	20	590	3.0
Spiny lobster, meat only:							
raw, 4 oz.	127	23.4	2.8	1.7	80	201	0
boiled or steamed:							
2 lbs. in shell	233	43.1	5.1	3.2	146	370	0
4 oz.	138	29.9	3.5	2.2	102	257	0
Spleen, braised:							
beef, 4 oz.	164	28.5	0	4.8	394	65	0
lamb, 4 oz.	177	30.0	0	5.4	437	66	0
pork, 4 oz.	169	32.0	0	3.6	572	121	0
veal, 4 oz.	146	27.3	0	3.3	507	66	0
Split peas:							
dry, ¼ cup:							
green (*Arrowhead Mills*)	160	12.0	24.0	1.0	0	10	4.0
green (*Goya*)	110	11.0	27.0	0	0	25	11.0
green or yellow (*Shiloh Farms*) . .	110	11.0	27.0	0	0	25	11.0
yellow (*Goya*)	110	10.0	28.0	0	0	20	12.0
boiled, ½ cup	116	8.2	20.7	.4	0	2	8.1
Sports bar, see "Granola/cereal bar"							
Spring roll, frozen, 2 pcs., 1.6 oz.:							
(*Health is Wealth*) . . .	70	2.0	10.0	2.0	0	200	5.0
hot and spicy (*Health is Wealth*)	90	4.0	16.0	1.5	0	310	1.0
Thai (*Health is Wealth*)	90	4.0	15.0	1.5	0	280	1.0

Food and Measure	cal.	prot. (gms)	carbo. (gms)	fat (gms)	chol. (mgs)	sod. (mgs)	fiber (gms)
SpriteMelon (*Frieda's*), 10.6-oz. melon	115	0	29.0	0	0	190	2.0
Sports drink, all flavors, 8 fl. oz.:							
(*Gatorade*)	50	0	14.0	0	0	110	0
(*Recharge*)	70	<1.0	18.0	0	0	25	0
Spot, meat only:							
raw, 4 oz.	140	21.0	0	5.6	68	33	0
baked, broiled, or microwaved, 4 oz. .	179	26.9	0	7.1	87	42	0
Sprouts, see "Bean sprouts" and specific listings							
Sprouts, mixed, 1 cup:							
(*Jonathan's*)	100	7.0	21.0	0	0	10	4.0
(*Jonathan's* Gourmet)	20	3.0	3.0	0	0	10	2.0
hot and spicy (*Jonathan's*)	25	3.0	4.0	0	0	15	2.0
salad (*Jonathan's*) . . .	80	4.0	10.0	0	0	15	4.0
Squab, fresh, raw:							
meat w/skin, 4 oz. . . .	333	20.9	0	27.0	108	61	0
breast meat only, 4 oz.	161	19.8	0	8.5	102	62	0
Squid, fresh, meat only, raw, 4 oz.	104	17.7	3.5	1.6	265	50	0
Squirrel, meat only, roasted, 4 oz.	196	34.9	0	5.3	137	135	0
Star fruit, see "Carambola"							
Star spangled squash (*Frieda's*), ⅔ cup, 3 oz.	20	2.0	3.0	0	0	0	1.0
Starbucks:							
Chantico, 6 fl. oz.	390	11.0	51.0	21.0	25	105	6.0
Classics, no cream/ topping, 12 fl. oz.:							
caramel apple cider	230	0	55.0	0	0	15	0
chocolate milk, whole	270	12.0	33.0	12.0	40	150	1.0
chocolate milk, nonfat	190	13.0	35.0	1.5	5.0	170	1.0
hot chocolate, whole	270	12.0	33.0	12.0	40	150	1.0
hot chocolate, nonfat	190	13.0	35.0	1.5	5	170	1.0
pumpkin spice créme, whole . . .	290	12.0	38.0	10.0	40	210	0

Food and Measure	cal.	prot. (gms)	carbo. (gms)	fat (gms)	chol. (mgs)	sod. (mgs)	fiber (gms)
Starbucks, Classics *(cont.)*							
toffee nut créme, whole	260	11.0	31.0	11.0	45	270	0
vanilla créme, whole	250	10.0	29.0	10.0	30	135	0
white hot chocolate, whole	370	13.0	49.0	15.0	45	240	0
coffee, brewed, 12 fl. oz. :							
coffee of week	5	0	1.0	0	0	0	0
iced, shaken	60	0	15.0	0	0	0	0
espresso, hot, whole milk, no cream/ topping, 12 fl. oz.:							
caffé Americano ...	10	1.0	2.0	0	0	0	0
caffé latte	200	11.0	16.0	11.0	45	160	0
caffé misto/café au lait	110	6.0	8.0	6.0	25	85	0
caffé mocha	240	10.0	31.0	10.0	35	125	.0
cappuccino	120	7.0	10.0	6.0	25	95	0
caramel macchiato .	240	10.0	28.0	10.0	30	135	0
caramel mocha ...	290	9.0	46.0	9.0	25	100	1.0
cinnamon spice mocha	240	10.0	30.0	10.0	35	135	0
pumpkin spice latte	280	11.0	38.0	9.0	35	190	0
syrup latte	240	9.0	29.0	9.0	30	120	0
toffee nut latte	250	10.0	30.0	10.0	40	260	0
vanilla latte	240	9.0	29.0	9.0	30	120	0
white chocolate mocha	320	11.0	43.0	12.0	35	200	0
espresso, iced, whole milk, no cream/ topping, 12 fl. oz.:							
caffé Americano ...	10	1.0	2.0	0	0	0	0
caffé latte	120	11.0	6.0	10.0	25	95	0
caffé mocha	170	7.0	26.0	6.0	20	75	1.0
caramel macchiato .	190	7.0	24.0	8.0	30	110	0
caramel mocha ...	230	6.0	42.0	6.0	15	55	0
syrup or vanilla latte	160	6.0	23.0	5.0	15	75	0
white chocolate mocha	270	8.0	42.0	9.0	20	160	0
Frappuccino coffee blend, no cream/ topping, 12 fl. oz.:							
caffé vanilla	240	4.0	51.0	2.5	10	190	0

Food and Measure	cal.	prot. (gms)	carbo. (gms)	fat (gms)	chol. (mgs)	sod. (mgs)	fiber (gms)
caramel	210	4.0	43.0	2.5	10	180	0
caramel mocha ...	260	5.0	52.0	3.5	10	190	0
coffee	190	4.0	38.0	2.5	10	180	0
espresso	160	4.0	33.0	2.0	10	160	0
java chip	270	5.0	51.0	7.0	10	220	1.0
mocha	220	5.0	44.0	3.0	10	180	0
pumpkin spice	230	5.0	47.0	2.5	10	210	0
toffee nut	210	4.0	43.0	2.5	10	220	0
white chocolate mocha	240	5.0	48.0	3.5	10	210	0
Frappuccino créme blend, no cream/ topping, 12 fl. oz.:							
caramel chocolate .	330	11.0	62.0	5.0	<5	260	<1.0
double chocolate chip	330	12.0	57.0	8.0	<5	300	2.0
strawberries/créme	330	10.0	65.0	3.5	<5	270	0
Tazo chai créme ...	280	10.0	52.0	3.5	<5	270	0
toffee nut	260	11.0	48.0	3.5	<5	260	0
vanilla bean	270	10.0	51.0	3.5	<5	370	0
Tazo tea, whole milk, 12 fl. oz.:							
chai latte	210	6.0	36.0	5.0	20	85	0
chai latte, iced	200	5.0	36.0	5.0	20	80	0
Tazo tea, iced	60	0	16.0	0	0	5	0
Tazo tea lemonade ...	90	0	23.0	0	0	15	0
drink extras:							
syrup, 1 pump:							
flavored	20	0	5.0	0	0	0	0
mocha	25	1.0	6.0	.5	0	0	0
toppings:							
chocolate	5	0	1.0	0	0	0	0
caramel	15	0	2.0	.5	0	5	0
sprinkles	0	0	<1.0	0	0	0	0
whipped cream:							
cold drinks	90	0	2.0	9.0	35	5	0
hot drinks	80	0	1.0	8.0	30	5	0
bagels, 5 oz.:							
plain	430	15.0	92.0	1.0	0	660	3.0
cinnamon raisin ...	440	13.0	96.0	1.0	0	570	3.0
sesame	440	16.0	92.0	3.0	0	630	6.0
bars:							
caramel apple	310	3.0	38.0	16.0	40	150	2.0
caramel brownie ..	580	5.0	60.0	36.0	100	230	2.0
carrot cake	420	4.0	46.0	25.0	85	440	<1.0

Food and Measure	cal.	prot. (gms)	carbo. (gms)	fat (gms)	chol. (mgs)	sod. (mgs)	fiber (gms)
Starbucks, bars *(cont.)*							
chocolate marsh-							
mallow	510	5.0	61.0	27.0	60	230	2.0
chocolate peanut							
butter stack	670	9.0	67.0	42.0	45	350	4.0
cranberry bliss	320	3.0	38.0	18.0	30	160	<1.0
espresso brownie ..	370	4.0	43.0	21.0	85	115	2.0
espresso brownie,							
enrobed or fudge	430	5.0	48.0	25.0	75	140	3.0
lemon	310	4.0	44.0	14.0	140	130	0
milk chocolate pea-							
nut butter brownie	460	6.0	45.0	29.0	50	170	2.0
oatmeal cranberry							
mountain	430	7.0	49.0	24.0	60	320	3.0
Oreo dream bar ...	420	5.0	33.0	30.0	65	200	2.0
pecan almond	490	4.0	38.0	37.0	40	170	2.0
peppermint brownie	440	4.0	48.0	27.0	55	135	2.0
raspberry sammy ..	300	3.0	41.0	14.0	35	115	1.0
seven layer	600	8.0	63.0	37.0	10	270	4.0
toffee cream cheese							
chew	440	5.0	38.0	31.0	65	400	2.0
toffee crunch	430	4.0	56.0	21.0	50	420	1.0
biscotti:							
chocolate hazelnut .	110	2.0	15.0	5.0	25	80	1.0
vanilla almond	110	2.0	15.0	5.0	25	75	1.0
cakes:							
apple harvest torte .	350	3.0	53.0	15.0	0	140	4.0
bundt:							
chocolate big baby	330	5.0	45.0	15.0	25	380	4.0
lemon yogurt ...	350	4.0	56.0	13.0	55	250	<1.0
coffee cake:							
apple walnut	320	4.0	41.0	17.0	55	330	1.0
blueberry walnut	340	4.0	43.0	18.0	60	360	1.0
cinnamon walnut	360	4.0	46.0	18.0	65	390	1.0
classic	570	7.0	75.0	28.0	75	310	2.0
crumble berry ..	520	6.0	69.0	26.0	75	350	2.0
hazelnut	630	9.0	74.0	35.0	125	460	2.0
sour cream	420	5.0	43.0	25.0	95	260	1.0
crumb cake	670	8.0	89.0	32.0	115	360	1.0
gingerbread, holiday	480	5.0	81.0	16.0	100	410	1.0
key lime crumb ...	550	8.0	71.0	27.0	190	370	1.0
pound cake:							
banana	360	4.0	47.0	18.0	100	380	1.0
cranberry walnut	390	6.0	45.0	21.0	110	310	1.0

Food and Measure	cal.	prot. (gms)	carbo. (gms)	fat (gms)	chol. (mgs)	sod. (mgs)	fiber (gms)
carrot, iced	540	5.0	101.0	13.0	35.0	320	3.0
lemon, iced	500	6.0	69.0	23.0	145	390	<1.0
marble	400	6.0	49.0	21.0	130	370	<1.0
orange poppy							
cheese	490	8.0	55.0	27.0	140	380	2.0
pumpkin	310	5.0	47.0	12.0	65	360	2.0
zucchini	370	5.0	47.0	19.0	55	250	2.0
pullman:							
banana	400	5.0	57.0	17.0	65	320	2.0
chocolate	380	5.0	54.0	17.0	55	270	2.0
cranberry walnut	360	5.0	53.0	15.0	25	240	2.0
lemon glazed . . .	370	5.0	55.0	15.0	90	180	<1.0
marble chocolate							
chip	440	6.0	61.0	20.0	95	250	1.0
orange poppy							
cheese	450	7.0	55.0	22.0	110	290	1.0
pumpkin	370	4.0	51.0	17.0	60	340	2.0
cookies:							
black and white . . .	430	4.0	68.0	17.0	50	210	2.0
cinnamon twist . . .	60	0	9.0	2.0	0	25	0
graham, dark or milk							
chocolate	140	2.0	17.0	8.0	<5	60	<1.0
double chocolate							
chunk	430	5.0	58.0	21.0	15	350	3.0
oatmeal raisin	390	6.0	65.0	15.0	15	340	3.0
Madeline	80	1.0	11.0	3.5	25	30	0
shortbread	100	1.0	12.0	6.0	15	65	0
white chocolate							
macadamia	470	6.0	54.0	27.0	15	350	2.0
croissants:							
almond filled	330	6.0	39.0	18.0	30	230	2.0
butter, apricot glaze	320	5.0	37.0	17.0	25	280	1.0
chocolate filled	350	5.0	43.0	19.0	30	210	2.0
raspberry cream							
cheese filled	260	4.0	34.0	12.0	30	270	1.0
muffins:							
blueberry	380	5.0	49.0	19.0	70	380	1.0
chocolate cream							
cheese	450	5.0	53.0	24.0	80	420	1.0
cranberry orange . .	410	5.0	53.0	20.0	70	400	2.0
morning sunrise . . .	330	5.0	54.0	12.0	35	550	2.0
scones:							
apricot currant	450	7.0	67.0	17.0	60	360	3.0
blueberry	460	5.0	68.0	18.0	50	400	3.0

Food and Measure	cal.	prot. (gms)	carbo. (gms)	fat (gms)	chol. (mgs)	sod. (mgs)	fiber (gms)
***Starbucks,* scones** *(cont.)*							
butterscotch pecan	520	7.0	64.0	27.0	50	390	2.0
cinnamon chip, iced	510	6.0	71.0	23.0	50	480	2.0
maple oat, iced . . .	490	7.0	69.0	22.0	45	430	2.0
raspberry	440	7.0	65.0	18.0	50	360	2.0
sweet rolls:							
caramel pecan sticky	730	10.0	75.0	40.0	40	860	7.0
cinnamon	620	9.0	80.0	29.0	45	740	3.0
cinnamon twist . . .	320	5.0	37.0	17.0	25	280	1.0
Danish, mocha swirl:							
apple	370	5.0	44.0	19.0	25	330	2.0
cheese	460	7.0	44.0	28.0	50	400	1.0
raspberry	370	5.0	45.0	19.0	25	380	1.0
Steak sauce, 1 tbsp.:							
(*A.1.*)	15	0	3.0	0	0	280	0
(*A.1.* Bold and Spicy							
w/*Tabasco*)	20	0	5.0	0	0	260	0
(*A.1.* Carb Well)	5	0	1.0	0	0	230	0
(*Crosse & Blackwell*) .	30	0	7.0	0	0	95	0
(*Heinz 57*)	20	0	4.0	0	0	190	0
(*HP*)	15	0	3.0	0	0	150	0
(*Kikkoman*)	20	0	5.0	0	0	290	0
(*Lawry's*)	15	0	3.0	0	0	260	0
(*Newman's Own*)	20	0	4.0	.5	0	85	0
(*Peter Luger*)	30	0	7.0	0	0	125	0
(*Pickapeppa*)	18	0	4.0	0	0	95	0
(*San-J* Japanese)	13	2.0	2.0	0	0	930	0
(*Watkins*)	20	0	4.0	0	0	200	0
and burger (*TryMe*							
Bullfighter)	15	0	4.0	0	0	220	0
garlic, roasted (*A.1.*) .	20	0	5.0	0	0	300	0
teriyaki (*A.1.*)	20	0	5.0	0	0	30	0
Steak sauce, cooking,							
see "Grilling sauce"							
Steak seasoning:							
(*D.L. Jardine's*), 1 tbsp.	25	1.0	4.0	.5	0	3920	<1.0
broiled (*McCormick*),							
¼ tsp.	0	0	0	0	0	230	0
Stir-fry sauce (see also							
"Marinade," and							
specific listings),							
1 tbsp., except as							
noted:							
(*House of Tsang* Classic)	25	0	4.0	1.0	0	570	0

Food and Measure	cal.	prot. (gms)	carbo. (gms)	fat (gms)	chol. (mgs)	sod. (mgs)	fiber (gms)
(*House of Tsang Bangkok Padang*) ..	45	1.0	4.0	2.5	0	250	0
(*House of Tsang Saigon Sizzle*)	45	0	7.0	2.0	0	380	0
(*Kikkoman*)	20	<1.0	4.0	0	0	520	0
(*Litehouse*), 2 tbsp. ...	45	1.0	10.0	0	0	430	0
citrus (*House of Tsang Imperial*)	25	0	5.0	0	0	170	0
garlic, and rib sauce (*Mikee*)	30	0	10.0	0	0	550	0
oyster flavored (*House of Tsang*)	30	0	7.0	0	0	600	0
teriyaki (*House of Tsang Korean*)	35	0	5.0	1.5	0	460	0
sweet and sour (*House of Tsang*)	36	0	8.0	0	0	50	0
Szechuan, spicy (*House of Tsang*)	25	0	4.0	1.0	0	500	0
Stir-fry seasoning mix (*Produce Partners*), 2 tsp. dry	30	0	2.0	1.5	0	430	0
Stomach, pork, raw, 1 oz.	44	4.7	0	2.7	55	15	0
Strawberry, fresh:							
(*Del Monte*), 8 medium, 5.2 oz.	45	1.0	12.0	0	0	0	4.0
(*Dole*), 8 medium ...	45	1.0	12.0	0	0	0	4.0
halves, ½ cup	23	.5	5.3	.3	0	1	1.8
pureed, ½ cup	35	.7	8.1	.4	0	1	2.7
Strawberry, canned, in heavy syrup, ½ cup	117	.7	29.9	.3	0	5	2.2
Strawberry, dried (*Frieda's*), ½ cup, 1.4 oz.	150	1.0	34.0	0	0	0	3.0
Strawberry, frozen:							
whole:							
(*Cascadian Farm*), 1 cup	45	<1.0	13.0	0	0	0	3.0
(*C&W*), ⅔ cup	50	0	12.0	0	0	0	2.0
(*Tree of Life*), ¾ cup	50	0	13.0	0	0	0	2.0
unsweetened, ½ cup .	39	.5	10.1	.1	0	2	2.3
Strawberry drink, 8 fl. oz., except as noted:							
(*Capri Sun*), 6.75 fl. oz.	90	0	25.0	0	0	15	0

Food and Measure	cal.	prot. (gms)	carbo. (gms)	fat (gms)	chol. (mgs)	sod. (mgs)	fiber (gms)
Strawberry drink *(cont.)*							
(*Hi-C Blast*)	120	0	32.0	0	0	140	0
(*Yoo-hoo*)	130	3.0	29.0	.5	0	110	0
sparkling (*R.W. Knudsen*)	110	<1.0	28.0	0	0	15	0
Strawberry drink blend, 8 fl. oz., except as noted:							
all varieties (*Langers*)	120	0	30.0	0	0	10	0
banana: (*Snapple-a-Day*),							
11.5 fl. oz.	210	7.0	43.0	0	0	110	5.0
(*V8 Splash*)	110	0	27.0	0	0	40	0
(*V8 Splash* Smoothies)	130	3.0	30.0	0	0	60	1.0
daiquiri (*Sobe Lizard Lava*)	120	0	32.0	0	0	20	0
kiwi: (*Capri Sun*),							
6.75 fl. oz.	100	0	26.0	0	0	15	0
(*Hi-C Blast*)	120	0	31.0	0	0	140	0
(*V8 Splash*)	110	0	27.0	0	0	35	0
passion fruit: (*Minute Maid*)	120	0	31.0	0	0	75	0
(*Minute Maid*), 12-fl.-oz. can ...	170	0	46.0	0	0	120	0
raspberry (*Minute Maid*)	120	0	33.0	0	0	20	0
Strawberry glaze:							
(*Great Expectations*), ⅓ cup	150	0	38.0	0	0	20	0
(*Litehouse*), 3 tbsp. ...	100	0	26.0	0	0	70	0
(*Litehouse* Sugar Free), 3 tbsp.	35	0	8.0	0	0	40	0
Strawberry juice (*Ceres*), 8 fl. oz. ...	115	0	28.0	0	0	35	1.0
Strawberry milk, see "Milk, flavored"							
Strawberry milk drink mix (*Nesquik*), 2 tbsp.	90	0	21.0	0	0	0	0
Strawberry syrup:							
(*Hershey's*), 2 tbsp. ...	100	0	26.0	0	0	10	0
(*Nesquik*), 2 tbsp.	110	0	27.0	0	0	0	0

Food and Measure	cal.	prot. (gms)	carbo. (gms)	fat (gms)	chol. (mgs)	sod. (mgs)	fiber (gms)
(*Smucker's*), ¼ cup ..	210	0	52.0	0	0	0	0
(*Smucker's Sundae Syrup*), 2 tbsp.	110	0	26.0	0	0	5	0
Strawberry topping (*Smucker's*), 2 tbsp.	100	0	24.0	0	0	0	0
Strawberry-banana juice, 8 fl. oz.:							
(*Bolthouse Farms*) ...	124	1.0	29.0	0	0	10	<1.0
(*Juicy Juice*)	120	0	30.0	0	0	20	0
String bean, see "Green bean"							
Stuffing, ¾ cup:							
corn bread (*Pepperidge Farm*)	170	4.0	33.0	2.0	0	480	2.0
cube (*Pepperidge Farm Country Style*)	140	5.0	27.0	1.5	0	380	2.0
herb (*Pepperidge Farm*)	170	5.0	33.0	1.5	0	600	3.0
sage and onion (*Pepperidge Farm*) .	140	5.0	26.0	1.0	0	540	3.0
Stuffing, frozen, corn-bread (*Glory* Savory Accents Dressing), ½ cup	240	4.0	33.0	10.0	0	430	1.0
Stuffing mix, dry:							
chicken:							
(*Pepperidge Farm One-Step*), ½ cup	110	2.0	12.0	6.0	<5	300	<1.0
(*Stove Top*), 1/6 of 6-oz. pkg.......	110	4.0	20.0	1.0	0	430	1.0
(*Stove Top*), 1/8 of 8-oz. cont.	120	3.0	19.0	3.0	0	460	1.0
(*Stove Top* Lower Sodium), 1/6 of 6-oz. pkg.......	110	4.0	21.0	1.0	0	260	1.0
corn bread:							
(*Mrs. Cubbison's*), ¾ cup	120	4.0	24.0	1.0	0	340	2.0
(*Pepperidge Farm One-Step*), ½ cup	170	3.0	26.0	6.0	0	300	2.0
(*Stove Top*), 1/6 of 6-oz. pkg.......	110	4.0	21.0	1.0	0	490	1.0
(*Stove Top*), 1/8 of 8-oz. cont.	120	3.0	19.0	3.0	0	530	1.0

Food and Measure	cal.	prot. (gms)	carbo. (gms)	fat (gms)	chol. (mgs)	sod. (mgs)	fiber (gms)
Stuffing mix *(cont.)*							
herb:							
(*Stove Top* Home-style), ⅛ of 8-oz. cont.	120	3.0	19.0	2.5	0	440	1.0
garden (*Pepperidge Farm* One-Step), ½ cup	90	3.0	14.0	3.0	<5	280	<1.0
herb seasoned cube (*Mrs. Cubbison's*), ¾ cup	120	3.0	24.0	1.0	0	340	1.0
pork (*Stove Top*), 1/6 of 6-oz. pkg. . .	110	3.0	20.0	1.0	0	450	1.0
seasoned (*Mrs. Cubbison's* Dressing), ¾ cup	120	4.0	24.0	1.0	0	340	2.0
turkey:							
(*Pepperidge Farm* One-Step), ½ cup	90	3.0	14.0	3.0	<5	350	<1.0
(*Stove Top*), 1/6 of 6-oz. pkg.	110	3.0	20.0	1.0	0	450	1.0
Sturgeon, meat only:							
raw, 4 oz.	120	18.3	0	4.6	68	61	0
baked, broiled, or microwaved, 4 oz. .	153	23.5	0	5.9	87	78	0
smoked, 4 oz.	196	35.4	0	5.0	91	838	0
Subway, 1 serving:							
breakfast, French toast, w/syrup	350	2.0	57.0	8.0	280	350	2.0
breakfast, omelette:							
bacon	240	20.0	2.0	17.0	570	350	0
cheese	240	19.0	2.0	17.0	570	370	0
ham	230	21.0	2.0	14.0	575	550	0
steak	250	24.0	3.0	15.0	580	390	1.0
vegetable	210	17.0	4.0	14.0	560	250	1.0
Western	220	19.0	4.0	14.0	565	360	1.0
breakfast sandwich:							
on deli round:							
bacon/egg	320	15.0	34.0	15.0	190	520	3.0
cheese/egg	320	14.0	34.0	15.0	190	550	3.0
ham/egg	310	16.0	35.0	13.0	190	720	3.0
steak/egg	330	19.0	35.0	14.0	190	570	3.0
vegetable/egg . . .	290	12.0	36.0	12.0	180	410	3.0
Western/egg	300	14.0	36.0	12.0	180	530	3.0

Food and Measure	cal.	prot. (gms)	carbo. (gms)	fat (gms)	chol. (mgs)	sod. (mgs)	fiber (gms)
on 6" white/wheat:							
bacon/egg	360	17.0	42.0	15.0	190	600	3.0
cheese/egg	360	16.0	42.0	15.0	190	620	3.0
ham/egg	350	18.0	43.0	13.0	190	790	3.0
steak/egg	370	22.0	43.0	14.0	190	640	4.0
vegetable/egg ...	330	14.0	44.0	12.0	180	480	4.0
Western/egg	340	16.0	44.0	12.0	180	610	4.0
6" sub, cold:							
cold cut combo ...	410	21.0	47.0	17.0	60	1550	4.0
Subway seafood ...	450	16.0	51.0	22.0	25	1150	5.0
tuna, classic	530	22.0	45.0	31.0	45	1030	4.0
6" sub, toasted:							
cheese steak	360	24.0	47.0	10.0	35	1090	5.0
cheese steak, chipotle South- west	450	24.0	48.0	20.0	45	1310	6.0
chicken/bacon ranch	530	36.0	47.0	25.0	90	1400	5.0
Italian BMT	450	23.0	47.0	21.0	55	1790	4.0
meatball marinara .	560	24.0	63.0	24.0	45	1610	7.0
turkey/ham/bacon melt	380	25.0	48.0	12.0	45	1610	4.0
6" sub, 6 grams fat or less:							
chicken breast, roasted	330	24.0	47.0	5.0	45	1020	4.0
chicken teriyaki ...	370	26.0	59.0	5.0	50	1220	4.0
ham, honey mustard	320	18.0	53.0	5.0	25	1420	4.0
roast beef	290	19.0	45.0	5.0	20	920	4.0
Subway Club	320	24.0	47.0	6.0	35	1310	4.0
turkey breast	280	18.0	46.0	4.5	20	1020	4.0
turkey breast/ham .	290	20.0	47.0	5.0	25	1230	4.0
Veggie Delite	230	9.0	44.0	3.0	0	520	4.0
6" double meat (DM):							
cheese steak	450	37.0	50.0	14.0	60	1470	6.0
cheese steak, chipotle South- west	540	37.0	51.0	24.0	70	1680	7.0
chicken, roasted ...	430	39.0	50.0	8.0	90	1520	4.0
chicken teriyaki ...	490	43.0	68.0	7.0	100	1630	4.0
cold cut combo ...	550	31.0	49.0	28.0	110	2380	4.0
ham	380	28.0	57.0	7.0	50	2180	4.0
Italian BMT	630	34.0	49.0	35.0	100	2890	4.0
meatball marinara .	960	37.0	82.0	42.0	85	2490	10.0
roast beef	360	29.0	46.0	7.0	40	1320	4.0

Food and Measure	cal.	prot. (gms)	carbo. (gms)	fat (gms)	chol. (mgs)	sod. (mgs)	fiber (gms)
Subway, 6" double meat *(cont.)*							
Subway Club	420	39.0	50.0	8.0	65	2100	4.0
Subway seafood ...	640	20.0	58.0	38.0	40	1580	5.0
tuna, classic	790	32.0	45.0	55.0	80	1340	4.0
turkey breast	340	28.0	48.0	6.0	40	1520	4.0
turkey breast/ham .	360	31.0	50.0	7.0	50	1950	4.0
turkey breast/ham/							
bacon melt	450	36.0	51.0	14.0	70	2330	4.0
deli-style sandwich:							
ham	210	11.0	36.0	4.0	10	770	3.0
roast beef	220	13.0	35.0	4.5	15	660	3.0
tuna, classic	350	14.0	35.0	18.0	30	750	3.0
turkey breast	210	13.0	36.0	3.5	15	730	3.0
wraps:							
chicken/bacon ranch							
w/cheese	440	41.0	18.0	27.0	90	1670	9.0
tuna, w/cheese	440	27.0	16.0	32.0	45	1310	9.0
turkey breast	190	24.0	18.0	6.0	20	1290	9.0
turkey/bacon melt							
w/cheese	440	34.0	20.0	28.0	65	1870	9.0
condiments/extras:							
bacon, 2 slices	45	3.0	0	3.5	10	180	0
chipotle sauce	100	0	1.0	10.0	8	220	0
honey mustard sauce	30	0	7.0	0	0	140	0
mayo, 1 tbsp.	110	0	0	12.0	10	80	0
mayo, light, 1 tbsp.	45	0	1.0	5.0	10	100	0
mustard, 2 tsp.	5	0	1.0	0	0	115	0
olive oil blend, 1 tsp.	45	0	0	5.0	0	0	0
onion sauce, sweet	40	0	9.0	0	0	100	0
ranch dressing	70	0	0	8.0	0	205	0
red wine vinaigrette	30	0	6.0	0	0	340	0
salad, no dressing:							
chicken, grilled, baby							
spinach	140	20.0	11.0	3.0	50	450	4.0
Subway Club	160	18.0	15.0	4.0	35	880	4.0
tuna, w/cheese	360	16.0	12.0	29.0	45	600	4.0
Veggie Delite	60	3.0	12.0	1.0	0	90	4.0
salad dressing, 2 oz.:							
Greek vinaigrette ...	200	1.0	3.0	21.0	0	590	0
honey mustard	200	1.0	1.0	22.0	0	510	0
Italian, fat free	35	1.0	7.0	0	0	720	0
ranch	200	1.0	1.0	22.0	10	550	.5
soup, 1 cup:							
broccoli, cream of .	130	5.0	15.0	6.0	10	860	2.0

Food and Measure	cal.	prot. (gms)	carbo. (gms)	fat (gms)	chol. (mgs)	sod. (mgs)	fiber (gms)
broccoli cheese ...	180	5.0	16.0	11.0	15	1120	2.0
brown/wild rice, w/chicken	190	6.0	17.0	11.0	20	990	2.0
cheese w/ham/bacon	240	8.0	17.0	15.0	20	1160	1.0
chicken dumpling ..	130	7.0	16.0	4.5	30	1030	1.0
chicken noodle	60	6.0	7.0	1.5	10	940	1.0
chicken rice, Spanish	90	5.0	13.0	2.0	5	800	1.0
chili con carne	240	15.0	23.0	10.0	15	860	8.0
clam chowder	110	5.0	16.0	3.5	10	990	1.0
minestrone	90	7.0	7.0	4.0	20	1180	1.0
potato, w/bacon ...	200	4.0	21.0	11.0	15	840	2.0
tomato vegetable rotini	100	3.0	20.0	.5	0	2340	2.0
vegetable beef	90	5.0	15.0	1.0	5	1050	3.0
Fruzie Express, small:							
berry lishus	110	1.0	28.0	0	0	30	1.0
berry lishus, banana	140	1.0	35.0	0	0	30	2.0
pineapple delight ..	130	1.0	33.0	0	0	25	1.0
peach pizzazz	100	0	26.0	0	0	25	0
pineapple delight, banana	160	1.0	40.0	0	0	25	2.0
sunrise refresher ..	120	1.0	29.0	0	0	20	1.0
cookies/dessert:							
apple pie	245	0	37.0	10.0	0	290	1.0
chocolate chip	210	2.0	30.0	10.0	15	160	1.0
chocolate chunk ...	220	2.0	30.0	10.0	10	105	1.0
double chocolate chip	210	2.0	30.0	10.0	15	170	1.0
fruit roll, 1 pc.	50	0	12.0	1.0	0	55	0
M&M's	210	2.0	30.0	10.0	15	105	1.0
oatmeal raisin	200	4.0	26.0	8.0	15	170	2.0
peanut butter	220	4.0	26.0	12.0	10	200	1.0
sugar	230	2.0	28.0	12.0	15	135	0
white chip macadamia	220	0	37.0	10.0	0	290	1.0
Succotash, canned:							
(*Glory*), ½ cup	80	3.0	17.0	0	0	580	3.0
cream-style, ½ cup ..	103	3.5	23.4	.7	0	325	4.0
Succotash, frozen boiled, drained, ½ cup	79	3.7	17.0	.8	0	38	4.6
Sucker, white, meat only: raw, 4 oz.	105	19.0	0	2.6	47	45	0

Food and Measure	cal.	prot. (gms)	carbo. (gms)	fat (gms)	chol. (mgs)	sod. (mgs)	fiber (gms)
Sucker *(cont.)*							
baked, broiled, or							
microwaved, 4 oz. .	135	24.4	0	3.4	60	58	0
Sugar, beet or cane:							
brown:							
(*Hain* Organic), 1 tsp.	15	0	4.0	0	0	0	0
1 oz.	107	0	27.6	0	0	11	0
1 cup, not packed .	546	0	141.0	0	0	57	0
1 cup, packed	828	0	214.0	0	0	86	0
granulated:							
(*Hain* Organic), 1 tsp.	10	0	3.0	0	0	0	0
1 oz.	110	0	28.3	0	0	<1	0
1 cup	773	0	199.8	0	0	<1	0
1 tbsp.	46	0	12.0	0	0	<1	0
1 tsp.	15	0	4.0	0	0	<1	0
powdered/confectioner's:							
(*Hain* Organic),							
¼ cup	140	0	37.0	0	0	0	0
1 cup, sifted	389	0	99.5	0	0	1	0
1 tbsp., unsifted . . .	31	0	8.0	0	0	<1	0
Sugar, date (*Shiloh*							
Farms), 1½ tsp. . . .	15	0	3.0	0	0	0	0
Sugar, maple, 1 oz. . .	99	0	25.5	0	0	4	0
Sugar, substitute (see							
also "Fructose"):							
(*Equal*), 1 pkt.	4	0	<1.0	0	0	0	0
(*NutraSweet*), 1 tsp. .	2	0	<1.0	0	0	0	0
(*Splenda*), 1 pkt.	0	0	<1.0	0	0	0	0
(*Sugar Twin*), 1 pkt. . .	0	0	<1.0	0	0	0	0
(*Sweet 'n Low*), 1 pkt. .	4	0	1.0	0	0	0	0
white or brown (*Sugar*							
Twin), 1 tsp.	0	0	0	0	0	0	0
Sugar, turbinado:							
(*Hain*), 1 tsp.	15	0	4.0	0	0	0	0
(*Tree of Life*), 1 tsp. . .	15	0	4.0	0	0	0	0
Sugar apple:							
1 medium, 9.9 oz. . . .	146	3.2	36.6	.5	0	15	6.8
½ cup	118	2.6	29.6	.4	0	12	5.5
Sugar cane juice drink							
(*Foco*), 11.8-fl.-oz.							
can	150	1.0	37.0	0	0	70	0
Sugar snap peas, see							
"Peas, edible-podded"							

Food and Measure	cal.	prot. (gms)	carbo. (gms)	fat (gms)	chol. (mgs)	sod. (mgs)	fiber (gms)
Summer sausage, 2 oz.:							
(*Johnsonville* Old World)	190	10.0	1.0	16.0	40	680	0
(*Johnsonville* Original/							
Beef)	180	10.0	1.0	15.0	40	680	0
(*Old Smokehouse*) . . .	200	8.0	2.0	18.0	55	970	0
beef:							
(*Hickory Farms Beef*							
Stick Original) . .	190	9.0	1.0	16.0	40	750	0
smoked (*Hickory*							
Farms Beef Stick)	190	9.0	1.0	16.0	45	790	0
garlic (*Johnsonville*) .	180	10.0	1.0	15.0	40	680	0
Summer squash (see							
also specific listings),							
all varieties, 1 cup:							
raw, sliced	23	1.3	4.9	.2	0	2	2.2
boiled, drained, sliced	36	1.6	7.8	.6	0	2	2.5
Sun choke, see							
"Jerasalem artichoke"							
Sunburst squash, baby							
(*Frieda's*), ⅔ cup,							
3 oz.	15	1.0	3.0	0	0	0	1.0
Sunfish, pumpkinseed,							
meat only:							
raw, 4 oz.	101	22.0	0	.8	76	91	0
baked, broiled, or							
microwaved, 4 oz. .	129	28.2	0	1.0	98	117	0
Sunflower butter:							
(*Kettle Roaster Fresh*							
Unsalted), 1 oz. . . .	160	6.0	5.0	14.0	0	1	0
1 tbsp.	93	3.2	4.4	7.6	0	1	.8
Sunflower seed,							
shelled:							
(*Arrowhead Mills*),							
¼ cup	170	7.0	6.0	15.0	0	0	3.0
(*Frito Lay*), 3 tbsp., 1 oz.	180	7.0	5.0	15.0	0	160	2.0
(*Shiloh Farms*), ¼ cup	180	8.0	6.0	14.0	0	10	2.0
unsalted, 1 oz.:							
dry-roasted	165	5.5	6.8	14.1	0	1	3.2
oil-roasted	174	6.1	4.2	16.3	0	1	4.2
toasted	176	4.9	5.8	16.1	0	1	3.3
roasted, salted:							
(*Planters*), 1 oz. . . .	180	7.0	5.0	15.0	0	120	2.0
(*Planters*), ½ of							
3-oz. pkg.	280	10.0	8.0	23.0	0	180	4.0

Food and Measure	cal.	prot. (gms)	carbo. (gms)	fat (gms)	chol. (mgs)	sod. (mgs)	fiber (gms)
Sunflower seed *(cont.)*							
tamari (*New England Naturals*), ¼ cup, 1.2 oz.	190	8.0	7.0	15.0	0	115	5.0
Sunflower seed flour, partially defatted, 1 cup	261	38.5	28.7	1.3	0	2	4.2
Sunflower sprouts, (*Jonathan's*), 1 cup	45	2.0	2.0	4.0	0	0	1.0
Surimi, pollock, 4 oz.	112	17.2	7.8	1.0	34	162	0
Sushi, supermarket (*Southern Tsunami Sushi Bar*), rolls, except as noted:							
California, 9 pcs.	290	7.0	54.0	5.0	<5	380	3.0
carrot/cucumber, 12 pc.	232	4.9	51.5	.6	0	179	2.3
combo rolls:							
fullmoon, 6 pcs.	307	11.2	50.1	6.9	37	471	2.2
marina, 6 pcs.	426	22.4	73.4	4.8	86	402	.6
meteor special, 11 pcs.	371	18.9	66.7	3.2	65	350	2.1
shoreline, 10 pcs. .	473	21.5	84.0	5.7	70	468	2.4
crab, ocean, 9 pcs. ..	344	14.2	53.6	8.2	24	433	3.9
"crab"/cucumber, 12 pcs.	239	6.6	51.6	.6	3	314	1.6
cream cheese, 9 pcs. .	569	23.1	53.1	29.4	105	386	2.4
cucumber, 12 pcs.	225	4.8	50.0	.6	0	172	1.8
dragon, 9 pcs.	643	21.9	62.9	33.7	111	671	7.3
eel, 9 pcs.	467	20.4	55.5	18.1	111	661	2.2
eel/carrot, 12 pcs.	315	11.2	51.6	7.0	48	309	2.1
inari, 4 pcs.	260	8.0	46.0	5.0	0	400	1.0
orange, 9 pcs.	394	16.2	65.0	7.8	7	764	3.9
rainbow, 9 pcs.	480	14.0	92.0	10.0	40	700	4.0
salads:							
calamari, 4 oz.	182	20.2	20.2	2.3	304	1013	0
edamame, plain, 4 oz.	171	14.0	12.5	7.3	0	16	4.8
edamame mixed, 4 oz.	60	3.4	4.5	3.1	0	176	.6
harusame, 2 oz.	59	.7	13.2	.4	0	560	0
seaweed, seabreeze, 2 oz.	56	0	11.3	1.3	0	805	0
salmon, 9 pcs.:							
grilled	348	18.4	54.4	6.4	34	208	3.3
spicy	362	18.3	52.4	8.8	36	250	2.4

Food and Measure	cal.	prot. (gms)	carbo. (gms)	fat (gms)	chol. (mgs)	sod. (mgs)	fiber (gms)
shrimp, 9 pcs.:							
crunchy	650	36.8	83.0	19.0	130	1247	4.0
spicy	334	18.9	52.4	5.5	126	365	2.4
shrimp/avocado, 12 pcs.	280	10.4	50.4	4.2	50	230	2.5
tempura, 9 pcs.	603	28.6	92.6	13.2	29	1296	4.4
tofu, 9 pcs.........	250	8.0	48.0	3.0	0	440	3.0
tsunami, 9 pcs.	480	22.0	63.2	15.5	29	273	2.7
tuna, spicy, 9 pcs. ...	290	14.0	45.0	6.0	15	290	3.0
tuna/cucumber, 12 pcs.	247	10.6	49.4	.8	12	181	1.7
vegetable combo, 9 pcs.	240	4.0	45.0	4.0	0	390	1.0
Swamp cabbage:							
raw, .6-oz. shoot	2	.3	.4	<.1	0	15	.3
boiled, drained, chopped,							
½ cup	10	1.0	1.8	.1	0	60	.9
Sweet dumpling							
squash (*Frieda's*),							
¾ cup, 3 oz.	30	1.0	7.0	0	0	0	1.0
Sweet peas, see "Peas,							
green"							
Sweet potato:							
raw:							
5" x 2" potato	136	2.1	31.6	.4	0	17	3.9
cut (*Glory*), 4.9 oz.	140	2.0	36.0	0	0	50	4.0
baked in skin:							
5" x 2" potato	118	2.0	27.7	.1	0	12	3.4
mashed, ½ cup ...	103	1.7	24.3	.1	0	10	3.0
boiled w/out skin:							
4 oz.	86	1.6	20.1	.2	0	31	2.8
mashed, ½ cup ...	125	2.5	31.7	.3	0	48	4.5
Sweet potato, canned,							
½ cup, except as							
noted:							
candied:							
(*Glory*)	210	1.0	52.0	0	0	240	1.0
(*Royal Prince*)	210	1.0	50.0	0	0	30	2.0
(*S&W*)	170	2.0	46.0	0	0	360	4.0
cut (*Princella/Sugary							
Sam*), ⅔ cup	160	0	39.0	0	0	35	3.0
mashed:							
(*Glory* Casserole) ..	180	2.0	43.0	0	0	250	2.0
(*Princella/Sugary							
Sam*), ⅔ cup ...	120	1.0	28.0	0	0	30	3.0
in syrup:							
(*Sylvia's* Yams) ...	120	0	30.0	0	0	30	2.0

Food and Measure	cal.	prot. (gms)	carbo. (gms)	fat (gms)	chol. (mgs)	sod. (mgs)	fiber (gms)
Sweet potato, canned, in syrup *(cont.)*							
light syrup (*Glory*) .	120	0	30.0	0	0	30	2.0
whole (*Royal Prince/ Trappey's*), 3 pcs.	200	1.0	48.0	0	0	40	4.0
w/liquid	101	1.1	23.9	.2	0	50	2.8
drained	106	1.3	24.9	.3	0	38	2.9
orange pineapple (*Royal Prince*)	210	1.0	50.0	0	0	30	3.0
Sweet potato, frozen:							
baked, cubed, ½ cup .	88	1.5	20.6	.1	0	7	2.6
candied (*Green Giant*), ¾ cup	240	2.0	41.0	7.0	0	430	3.0
casserole (*Glory* Savory Accents), ½ cup . .	170	1.0	37.0	2.0	0	210	0
fries:							
(*Ian's* Natural), 2.5 oz.	70	1.0	13.0	2.5	0	25	1.0
straight cut (*McCain Premium Golden Crisp*), 3 oz.	120	1.0	22.0	3.0	0	180	2.0
Sweet potato chips, 1 oz.:							
(*Terra*)	140	1.0	18.0	7.0	0	10	1.0
jalapeño (*Terra*)	140	1.0	18.0	7.0	0	65	1.0
Southern recipe (*Terra Frites*)	160	1.0	15.0	10.0	0	80	2.0
spiced (*Terra*)	140	1.0	16.0	7.0	0	105	3.0
Sweet potato leaf:							
raw, chopped, ½ cup .	6	.7	1.1	.1	0	2	<1.0
steamed, ½ cup	11	.7	2.3	.1	0	4	.6
Sweet and sour drink mixer (*Angostura*), 2 fl. oz.	70	0	17.0	0	0	25	0
Sweet and sour sauce, 2 tbsp., except as noted:							
(*Contadina*), 1 tbsp. . . .	40	0	8.0	1.0	0	115	0
(*Kikkoman*)	35	0	9.0	0	0	190	0
(*Kraft*)	60	0	13.0	0	0	125	0
(*Port Arthur*)	50	0	13.0	0	0	140	0
(*Sagawa's* Sweet & Sour/Sassy)	50	0	11.0	0	0	250	0
(*San-J* Sweet & Tangy)	50	1.0	13.0	0	0	320	0
(*World Harbors* Sweet & Sour)	60	0	14.0	0	0	250	0

Food and Measure	cal.	prot. (gms)	carbo. (gms)	fat (gms)	chol. (mgs)	sod. (mgs)	fiber (gms)
(*World Harbors* Sweet & Tangy)	60	0	14.0	0	0	220	0
barbecue, see "Barbecue sauce"							
duck sauce:							
(*Ka•Me*)	60	0	15.0	0	0	180	0
(*La Choy*)	60	0	15.0	0	0	120	0
(*Mee Tu*)	80	0	19.0	0	0	260	1.0
(*Mikee*), 1 tbsp. . . .	25	0	6.0	0	0	120	0
w/ginger (*Ka•Me*)	50	0	13.0	0	0	60	0
Sweetbreads, see "Pancreas" and "Thymus"							
Swiss chard, fresh:							
raw:							
(*Frieda's*), 1 cup, 3 oz.	15	2.0	3.0	0	0	180	1.0
chopped, ½ cup . . .	3	.3	.7	<.1	0	38	.3
boiled, drained, chopped, ½ cup . . .	18	1.7	3.6	.1	0	158	1.8
Swiss chard, frozen (*C&W*), ½ cup	20	1.0	3.0	0	0	260	2.0
Swordfish, fresh, meat only:							
raw, 4 oz.	137	22.5	0	4.6	45	102	0
baked, broiled, or microwaved, 4 oz. .	176	28.8	0	5.8	57	130	0
Syrup, see specific syrup listings							
Szechuan sauce (see also "Stir-fry sauce"):							
(*Ka•Me*), 1 tbsp.	25	1.0	2.0	1.5	0	390	0
(*San-J*), 1 tsp.	5	0	1.0	0	0	180	0

T

Food and Measure	cal.	prot. (gms)	carbo. (gms)	fat (gms)	chol. (mgs)	sod. (mgs)	fiber (gms)
Tabouli salad:							
(*Cedar's*), 2 tbsp.	30	1.0	3.0	1.0	0	63	1.0
(*Joseph's*), 2 tbsp. . . .	30	1.0	5.0	1.0	0	40	1.0
Tabouli salad mix:							
(*Fantastic*), 2 tbsp. . . .	70	2.0	15.0	0	0	280	4.0
(*Near East*), 1 oz.	80	3.0	21.0	0	0	270	5.0
(*Near East*), ⅔ cup* .	110	4.0	23.0	3.0	0	270	5.0
Taco, frozen, 1 pc., except as noted:							
beef, mini (*El Monterey* Fiesta Minis), 4 pcs., 4 oz.	260	9.0	27.0	12.0	15	250	3.0
beef/cheese:							
(*El Monterey* Soft Taco), 5.5 oz.	440	18.0	42.0	22.0	40	930	3.0
spicy (*El Monterey* Soft Taco), 5.5 oz.	420	19.0	40.0	22.0	40	800	2.0
chicken/cheese, spicy (*El Monterey* Soft Taco), 5.5 oz.	340	15.0	44.0	11.0	20	730	4.0
Taco, breakfast, sausage, egg, cheese (*El Monterey* Soft), 4.5-oz. pc.	370	12.0	29.0	23.0	60	790	1.0
Taco entree kit, pkg.:							
(*Old El Paso* Dinner Kit), 1/6 pkg.	130	2.0	18.0	5.0	0	750	1.0
w/chicken breast* .	260	22.0	19.0	11.0	55	850	1.0
w/lean beef*	300	19.0	19.0	16.0	60	840	1.0
(*Old El Paso* Hard & Soft Dinner Kit):							
hard, ⅓ pkg.	130	2.0	19.0	5.0	0	760	2.0
hard, w/lean beef, 2 pcs.*	310	18.0	19.0	18.0	55	880	2.0

Food and Measure	cal.	prot. (gms)	carbo. (gms)	fat (gms)	chol. (mgs)	sod. (mgs)	fiber (gms)
soft, ⅓ pkg.	190	4.0	32.0	5.0	0	1030	1.0
soft, w/lean beef,							
2 pcs.*	360	19.0	32.0	17.0	55	1110	1.0
(*Old El Paso* Soft							
Dinner Kit), 1/5 pkg.	190	4.0	32.0	5.0	0	1170	2.0
w/chicken breast* .	350	28.0	32.0	12.0	70	1230	2.0
w/lean ground beef*	390	22.0	33.0	19.0	70	1270	2.0
(*Taco Bell* Dinner),							
1/6 pkg. mix	130	3.0	19.0	4.5	0	540	2.0
cheesy, 1/6 pkg. mix:							
(*Taco Bell* Dinner							
Double Decker) .	230	5.0	29.0	10.0	5	1020	2.0
w/shells, sauce							
(*Taco Bell* Dinner)	180	4.0	20.0	10.0	5	790	1.0
Taco filling, vegetarian							
(*SoyTaco*), 1 oz. . . .	50	4.0	3.0	3.0	0	180	2.0
Taco filling mix							
(*Fantastic*), ¼ cup .	80	11.0	10.0	1.0	0	430	4.0
Taco Bell, 1 serving:							
Big Bell Value Menu:							
burrito:							
bean especial . . .	600	21.0	82.0	21.0	15	1760	12.0
beef combo	470	22.0	52.0	19.0	45	1620	5.0
beef/potato	530	15.0	65.0	24.0	40	1670	4.0
chicken, spicy . .	430	14.0	50.0	19.0	30	1160	4.0
caramel apple							
empanada	290	3.0	37.0	15.0	<5	290	1.0
cheesy potatoes . . .	280	4.0	27.0	18.0	20	800	2.0
taco:							
chicken, spicy . .	180	10.0	21.0	7.0	20	580	2.0
Double Decker . .	340	14.0	39.0	14.0	25	810	5.0
Double Decker							
Supreme	380	15.0	41.0	18.0	40	820	5.0
soft, grande	450	19.0	44.0	21.0	45	1410	2.0
burritos:							
bean	370	14.0	55.0	10.0	10	1200	8.0
beef, fiesta	390	14.0	50.0	15.0	25	1160	3.0
beef, grilled *Stuft* . .	720	27.0	79.0	33.0	55	2090	7.0
beef, *Supreme*	440	17.0	52.0	18.0	40	1330	5.0
chicken, fiesta	370	18.0	48.0	12.0	30	1090	3.0
chicken, grilled *Stuft*	680	35.0	76.0	26.0	70	1950	7.0
chicken *Supreme* . .	410	21.0	50.0	14.0	45	1270	5.0
chili cheese	390	16.0	40.0	18.0	40	1080	3.0

Food and Measure	cal.	prot. (gms)	carbo. (gms)	fat (gms)	chol. (mgs)	sod. (mgs)	fiber (gms)
Taco Bell, burritos (cont.)							
steak, fiesta	370	16.0	48.0	13.0	25	1080	4.0
steak, grilled *Stuft* .	680	31.0	76.0	28.0	55	1940	8.0
steak, *Supreme* ...	420	19.0	50.0	16.0	35	1260	6.0
7-layer	530	18.0	66.0	21.0	25	1350	10.0
chalupas:							
beef, *Baja*	430	13.0	32.0	27.0	30	760	2.0
beef, nacho	380	12.0	33.0	22.0	20	740	1.0
beef, *Supreme*	390	14.0	31.0	24.0	35	600	1.0
chicken, *Baja*	400	17.0	30.0	24.0	40	690	2.0
chicken, nacho	350	16.0	31.0	18.0	25	670	1.0
chicken, *Supreme* .	370	17.0	30.0	20.0	45	530	1.0
steak, *Baja*	400	15.0	30.0	25.0	30	680	2.0
steak, nacho	350	14.0	31.0	19.0	20	670	2.0
steak, *Supreme* ...	370	15.0	29.0	22.0	35	520	2.0
gorditas:							
beef, *Baja*	350	13.0	31.0	19.0	30	760	2.0
beef, nacho	300	12.0	32.0	13.0	20	740	2.0
beef, *Supreme*	310	14.0	30.0	16.0	35	600	2.0
chicken, *Baja*	320	17.0	29.0	15.0	40	690	2.0
chicken, nacho	270	16.0	30.0	10.0	25	670	2.0
chicken, *Supreme* .	290	17.0	28.0	12.0	45	530	2.0
steak, *Baja*	320	15.0	29.0	16.0	30	680	2.0
steak, nacho	270	14.0	30.0	11.0	20	670	2.0
steak, *Supreme* ...	290	16.0	28.0	13.0	35	520	2.0
taco:							
regular	170	8.0	13.0	10.0	25	350	<1.0
Supreme	220	9.0	14.0	14.0	35	360	1.0
taco, soft:							
beef	210	10.0	21.0	10.0	25	620	<1.0
beef, *Supreme*	260	11.0	23.0	14.0	35	640	1.0
chicken, Ranchero .	270	14.0	21.0	14.0	35	710	2.0
steak, grilled	280	12.0	21.0	17.0	30	650	1.0
specialties:							
Border Bowl, chicken	730	23.0	65.0	42.0	45	1640	12.0
Border Bowl, chicken,							
no dressing	500	22.0	60.0	19.0	30	1400	12.0
Enchirito, beef	380	19.0	35.0	18.0	45	1430	5.0
Enchirito, chicken .	350	23.0	33.0	14.0	55	1360	5.0
Enchirito, steak ...	360	21.0	33.0	16.0	45	1350	5.0
express taco salad .	630	26.0	58.0	33.0	65	1390	10.0
express taco salad,							
no chips	410	23.0	32.0	21.0	65	1300	8.0

Food and Measure	cal.	prot. (gms)	carbo. (gms)	fat (gms)	chol. (mgs)	sod. (mgs)	fiber (gms)
Fiesta Taco Salad	870	31.0	80.0	47.0	65	1780	12.0
no shell	500	24.0	42.0	27.0	65	1520	10.0
no shell/strips	420	24.0	34.0	21.0	65	1480	9.0
Mexican pizza	550	21.0	47.0	31.0	45	1040	5.0
MexiMelt	290	10.0	23.0	16.0	40	880	2.0
quesadilla, cheese	490	19.0	39.0	28.0	55	1150	3.0
quesadilla, chicken	540	28.0	40.0	30.0	80	1380	3.0
quesadilla, steak	540	26.0	40.0	31.0	75	1370	3.0
Southwest steak bowl	700	30.0	73.0	32.0	55	2050	13.0
tostada	250	00.0	29.0	10.0	15	710	7.0
nachos/sides:							
cinnamon twists	160	<1.0	28.0	5.0	0	150	0
Mexican rice	210	6.0	23.0	10.0	15	740	3.0
nachos	320	5.0	33.0	19.0	<5	530	2.0
nachos *BellGrande*	780	20.0	80.0	43.0	35	1300	11.0
nachos supreme	450	13.0	42.0	26.0	35	810	5.0
pintos 'n cheese	180	10.0	20.0	7.0	15	700	6.0
Taco John's, 1 serving:							
burritos:							
bean	380	15.0	53.0	12.0	15	830	10.0
beef, grilled	590	27.0	49.0	32.0	75	1240	9.0
beefy	430	22.0	41.0	20.0	55	870	8.0
chicken, grilled	590	33.0	47.0	30.0	95	1790	8.0
chicken/potato	460	18.0	54.0	19.0	35	1470	8.0
chicken/potato, crunchy	590	20.0	62.0	29.0	35	1420	8.0
combination	400	18.0	47.0	16.0	35	850	9.0
meat/potato	490	15.0	55.0	23.0	30	1190	9.0
super	450	19.0	49.0	20.0	40	920	10.0
quesadilla:							
cheese	480	20.0	39.0	28.0	50	960	6.0
chicken	540	29.0	41.0	29.0	75	1430	7.0
tacos:							
chicken, softshell	190	14.0	19.0	6.0	30	760	4.0
crispy	180	9.0	13.0	10.0	25	270	3.0
softshell	220	11.0	21.0	10.0	25	470	4.0
Taco Bravo	340	15.0	39.0	14.0	25.0	650	8.0
taco burger	280	14.0	28.0	12.0	35	600	3.0
local favorites:							
Beefy Cheesy Taco Bravo	410	18.0	35.0	22.0	50	850	6.0
burrito:							
chicken fajita	340	22.0	39.0	11.0	50	1120	7.0

Food and Measure	cal.	prot. (gms)	carbo. (gms)	fat (gms)	chol. (mgs)	sod. (mgs)	fiber (gms)
***Taco John's,* local favorites, burrito** *(cont.)*							
chicken festiva ..	530	21.0	58.0	24.0	50	1300	8.0
el grande	720	32.0	67.0	36.0	90	1640	10.0
el grande, chicken	660	39.0	64.0	28.0	100	2210	9.0
platter, smothered	830	33.0	102.0	33.0	55	2230	16.0
ranch, beef	420	17.0	41.0	22.0	45	860	8.0
ranch, chicken ..	390	20.0	40.0	18.0	50	1140	7.0
smothered	500	23.0	56.0	21.0	50	1330	11.0
enchilada:							
chili	740	31.0	71.0	38.0	75	1470	8.0
double	720	37.0	54.0	40.0	105	2090	11.0
platter, beef	780	32.0	80.0	37.0	70	2460	11.0
platter, chicken ..	700	30.0	73.0	32.0	65	2460	9.0
cheese crisp	210	10.0	11.0	14.0	35	260	1.0
chilito	430	20.0	38.0	22.0	60	1040	7.0
chili *Potato Olés* ...	610	13.0	59.0	36.0	25	2290	7.0
chimi platter, beef/							
bean	760	27.0	88.0	34.0	50	1930	9.0
Mexi Rolls	480	20.0	33.0	30.0	50	1270	3.0
Mexi Rolls, no nacho							
cheese	370	16.0	29.0	21.0	40	530	3.0
taco, el grande	510	24.0	32.0	32.0	75	820	4.0
tostada	180	9.0	14.0	10.0	25	270	3.0
tostada, bean	160	6.0	19.0	6.0	5	250	3.0
salad, no dressing:							
chicken festiva	580	29.0	60.0	24.0	65	1190	11.0
no tortilla	380	24.0	25.0	20.0	65	820	5.0
chicken festiva,							
crunchy	750	33.0	71.0	37.0	60	1140	10.0
no tortilla	550	27.0	36.0	33.0	60	770	4.0
chicken taco	530	27.0	45.0	27.0	70	1330	3.0
side salad	80	3.0	6.0	5.0	5	50	1.0
taco	580	23.0	46.0	32.0	60	960	4.0
nachos/sides:							
chicken, crunchy ..	450	29.0	24.0	27.0	60	1040	0
chili, Texas style ...	270	15.0	26.0	12.0	35	1400	4.0
Mexican rice	240	4.0	36.0	8.0	0	1100	1.0
nachos	380	6.0	38.0	23.0	10	970	<1.0
super	830	22.0	73.0	51.0	60	1730	5.0
super chicken ...	780	31.0	62.0	45.0	90	2250	3.0
Potato Olés:							
large	790	7.0	86.0	47.0	0	2290	8.0
medium	620	5.0	67.0	36.0	0	1780	6.0
small	440	4.0	48.0	26.0	0	1270	5.0

Food and Measure	cal.	prot. (gms)	carbo. (gms)	fat (gms)	chol. (mgs)	sod. (mgs)	fiber (gms)
super	980	22.0	82.0	62.0	60	2950	10.0
w/nacho cheese .	550	7.0	52.0	35.0	10	2000	5.0
refried beans	400	18.0	50.0	14.0	15	1110	11.0
condiments, 2 oz.,							
except as noted:							
barbecue sauce ...	70	0	15.0	0	0	490	0
chipotle cream sauce	300	0	4.0	30.0	20	380	0
dressing:							
Italian, creamy ..	180	0	4.0	20.0	0	430	0
house	90	0	3.0	10.0	0	360	0
ranch	190	2.0	4.0	21.0	30	470	0
ranch, bacon ...	170	1.0	14.0	13.0	15	490	0
guacamole	90	0	6.0	9.0	0	360	0
jalapeños	15	1.0	3.0	0	0	950	1.0
pico de gallo	15	1.0	4.0	0	0	160	<1.0
sauce, 1 oz.:							
hot	5	0	1.0	0	0	135	0
mild	5	0	1.0	0	0	140	0
super hot	10	0	2.0	0	0	25	<1.0
sour cream	120	2.0	2.0	12.0	25	30	0
desserts:							
apple grande	240	5.0	36.0	9.0	5	220	0
choco taco	300	4.0	38.0	15.0	15	110	1.0
churro	230	2.0	31.0	11.0	10	120	1.0
Taco sauce, 1 tbsp.,							
except as noted:							
(*Chi-Chi's* Fiesta							
Squeezable)	10	0	1.0	0	0	75	0
(*La Victoria* Salsa Brava)	0	0	0	0	0	25	0
(*Pace* Taco Topper) ..	10	0	2.0	0	0	130	0
(*Pace* Mexican							
Creations), 2 tbsp. .	15	0	3.0	0	0	390	0
green:							
(*Pace* Taco Topper)	5	0	1.0	0	0	100	0
(*La Victoria*)	0	0	<1.0	0·	0	70	0
hot or medium (*Old El*							
Paso)	5	0	1.0	0	0	90	0
medium (*Taco Bell*),							
2 tbsp.	10	0	2.0	0	0	170	1.0
mild:							
(*Old El Paso*)	5	0	1.0	0	0	85	0
(*Taco Bell*), 2 tbsp.	15	0	3.0	0	0	160	1.0
hot (*La Victoria*)	5	0	1.0	0	0	90	0

Food and Measure	cal.	prot. (gms)	carbo. (gms)	fat (gms)	chol. (mgs)	sod. (mgs)	fiber (gms)
Taco seasoning mix, 2 tsp., except as noted:							
(*Chi-Chi's* Fiesta), 1/5 pkg.	25	0	4.0	0	0	400	1.0
(*Ducks Unlimited*) . . .	15	0	3.0	0	0	340	0
(*Lawry's*)	15	0	3.0	0	0	340	<1.0
(*Lawry's* Family Pack)	15	0	3.0	0	0	330	<1.0
(*McCormick*)	20	0	3.0	0	0	430	0
(*McCormick* 30% Less Sodium)	20	0	3.0	0	0	300	0
(*Old El Paso*)	15	0	4.0	0	0	560	0
(*Old El Paso* 40% Less Sodium)	15	0	4.0	0	0	330	0
(*Taco Bell*)	20	1.0	3.0	0	0	410	1.0
(*Wick Fowler's*)	20	0	3.0	1.0	0	510	0
chicken:							
(*Lawry's*)	20	0	5.0	0	0	440	<1.0
(*McCormick*)	25	0	4.0	0	0	450	0
hot:							
(*Lawry's*)	15	0	3.0	0	0	370	<1.0
(*McCormick*)	20	0	3.0	0	0	430	0
mild:							
(*McCormick*)	20	1.0	4.0	0	0	460	0
(*Old El Paso*)	15	0	4.0	0	0	360	0
Taco shell (see also "Tostada shell"):							
(*Old El Paso*), 3 pcs. . .	150	2.0	20.0	7.0	0	135	1.0
(*Old El Paso* Super Stuffer), 2 pcs.	170	2.0	23.0	8.0	0	160	2.0
(*Taco Bell*), 1.1-oz. pc.	150	2.0	21.0	6.0	0	5	2.0
(*Zapata*), 2 pcs.	110	2.0	14.0	5.0	0	5	1.0
corn, blue or yellow (*Garden of Eatin'*), 2 pcs.	140	2.0	17.0	7.0	0	5	1.0
corn, white (*Old El Paso*), 3 pcs.	150	2.0	20.0	7.0	0	140	1.0
mini (*Old El Paso* Fun Shells), 7 pcs.	150	2.0	19.0	7.0	0	130	1.0
salad shell (*Old El Paso*), .8-oz. pc.	110	1.0	14.0	6.0	0	5	<1.0
soft, see "Tortilla"							
Taco snack, frozen (*Michelina's* Zap'ems Rockin'), 5.5-oz. pkg.	350	12.0	34.0	18.0	50	520	2.0

Food and Measure	cal.	prot. (gms)	carbo. (gms)	fat (gms)	chol. (mgs)	sod. (mgs)	fiber (gms)
TacoTime, 1 serving:							
burritos:							
bean, crisp	427	15.0	53.0	18.0	12	453	9.0
bean, soft	380	16.0	58.0	10.0	15	715	13.0
beef, Big Juan	640	34.0	71.0	25.0	60	1120	15.0
beef/bean/cheese . .	617	39.0	66.0	23.0	63	1343	18.0
Casita Burrito	647	40.0	54.0	31.0	89	1233	16.0
chicken, Big Juan . .	620	34.0	69.0	24.0	65	1230	12.0
chicken, crisp	422	17.0	32.0	25.0	54	795	2.0
chicken/black bean .	400	19.0	45.0	18.0	35	580	5.0
chicken BLT	580	23.0	38.0	39.0	50	1020	5.0
meat, crisp	552	34.0	39.0	30.0	58	1000	7.0
meat, soft	491	31.0	48.0	21.0	56	1197	12.0
veggie	491	21.0	70.0	16.0	24	643	10.0
tacos:							
crisp	295	22.0	16.0	17.0	48	609	5.0
soft	316	24.0	23.0	15.0	48	599	5.0
soft, ½ lb.	512	33.0	46.0	23.0	63	1111	12.0
soft, chicken, ½ lb.	387	21.0	41.0	16.0	48	933	7.0
soft, super	510	29.0	50.0	23.0	60	590	11.0
salads:							
chicken	370	19.0	27.0	21.0	48	861	3.0
chicken fiesta	390	20.0	35.0	19.0	45	840	4.0
taco, regular	479	30.0	30.0	28.0	63	895	7.0
tostada	628	36.0	48.0	33.0	82	1004	13.0
nachos, etc.:							
cheddar melt	205	11.0	17.0	11.0	30	255	1.0
Mexi-rice	159	3.0	30.0	2.0	0	530	1.0
nachos	680	26.0	61.0	38.0	78	1250	11.0
nachos deluxe	1048	46.0	91.0	57.0	109	2252	17.0
Refritos	326	18.0	44.0	10.0	22	525	13.0
taco cheeseburger .	633	31.0	48.0	36.0	66	1291	7.0
fries:							
cheddar, large	704	16.0	54.0	48.0	0	1862	0
cheddar, medium . .	505	11.0	40.0	35.0	0	1346	0
cheddar, small	352	8.0	27.0	24.0	0	931	0
Mexi-fries, large . . .	532	6.0	54.0	34.0	0	1598	0
Mexi-fries, medium	390	4.0	40.0	25.0	0	1170	0
Mexi-fries, small . .	266	3.0	27.0	17.0	0	799	0
stuffed, large	990	16.0	88.0	73.0	35	2580	6.0
stuffed, medium . . .	640	12.0	50.0	44.0	25	1740	5.0
stuffed, small	490	8.0	34.0	37.0	20	1400	3.0
sauces/dressings:							
green sauce	5	0	2.0	0	0	115	<1.0

Food and Measure	cal.	prot. (gms)	carbo. (gms)	fat (gms)	chol. (mgs)	sod. (mgs)	fiber (gms)
TacoTime, sauces/dressings *(cont.)*							
hot sauce	10	0	2.0	0	0	120	0
salsa Fresca	65	0	16.0	0	0	350	0
Thousand Island ...	120	0	3.0	12.0	5	120	0
dessert:							
Crustos, cinnamon .	373	9.0	47.0	15.0	0	86	0
fruit empanada	250	5.0	37.0	9.0	0	46	0
Tahini, sesame:							
(Alma), ¼ cup	340	10.0	12.0	31.0	0	70	1.0
(Arrowhead Mills), 2 tbsp.	190	8.0	3.0	18.0	0	10	<1.0
(Joyva), 2 tbsp.	200	5.0	3.0	18.0	0	75	1.0
(Peloponnese), 1 tbsp.	100	4.0	2.0	8.0	0	20	1.0
(Sesame King), 2 tbsp.	210	6.0	5.0	19.0	0	5	3.0
(Tree of Life), 2 tbsp. .	180	5.0	8.0	15.0	0	10	5.0
Tamale, canned, 2 pcs., except as noted:							
beef:							
(Hormel), 7.5-oz. can	200	6.0	22.0	10.0	25	1060	3.0
(Hormel Jumbo) ..	190	6.0	21.0	10.0	25	980	3.0
regular or hot-spicy *(Hormel)*	140	4.0	15.0	7.0	15	710	2.0
chicken *(Hormel)*	130	3.0	15.0	7.0	30	660	1.0
Tamale, frozen, 1 pc.:							
beef:							
(El Monterey Quick Classics), 4.5 oz.	300	9.0	26.0	18.0	25	670	3.0
shredded *(El Monterey Quick Classics),* 4 oz. ..	200	7.0	24.0	9.0	20	660	2.0
chicken *(El Monterey Quick Classics),* 4.5 oz.	260	10.0	28.0	12.0	20	770	2.0
pork *(Goya)*	240	6.0	31.0	10.0	15	390	2.0
Tamale pie, frozen, meatless *(Amy's* Mexican), 8 oz. ...	150	5.0	27.0	3.0	0	590	4.0
Tamari, see "Soy sauce"							
Tamarillo, red or gold *(Frieda's),* 2 pcs., 4.2 oz.	40	2.0	9.0	0	0	0	4.0
Tamarind:							
1 fruit, 3" x 1"	5	.1	1.3	<.1	0	1	.1
pulp, ½ cup	144	1.7	37.5	.4	0	17	3.1

Food and Measure	cal.	prot. (gms)	carbo. (gms)	fat (gms)	chol. (mgs)	sod. (mgs)	fiber (gms)
Tamarind drink:							
(*Foco*), 11.8 fl. oz. . . .	230	0	55.0	0	0	55	0
nectar (*Goya*), 12 fl. oz.	240	1.0	59.0	0	0	20	1.0
Tamarind sauce:							
(*Neera's* Asian), 2 tsp.	61	0	16.0	0	0	110	0
dipping (*Neera's*), 1 tsp.	15	0	3.0	0	0	98	0
Tamarindo (*Frieda's*),							
1.1-oz. pod	70	1.0	19.0	0	0	10	2.0
Tandoori paste, see							
"Curry paste"							
Tangerine, fresh:							
(*Chiquita*), 3.8-oz. fruit	50	1.0	15.0	.5	0	0	3.0
(*Del Monte* Satsuma),							
3.8-oz. fruit	50	1.0	15.0	0	0	0	3.0
(*Dole* Tangerine/							
Mandarin/Tangelo),							
1 medium	50	1.0	15.0	.5	0	0	3.0
(*Frieda's* Delite/Pixie							
Mandarin), 1 cup,							
5 oz.	60	0	16.0	0	0	0	3.0
(*Frieda's* Page							
Mandarin), 1 cup,							
5 oz.	60	0	12.0	0	0	0	3.0
(*Frieda's* Satsuma							
Mandarin), 1 cup,							
5 oz.	60	1.0	16.0	0	0	0	3.0
(*Sunkist*), 3.8-oz. fruit	50	1.0	15.0	.5	0	0	3.0
1 large 2½" diam.,							
3.5 oz.	43	.6	11.0	.2	0	1	2.3
sections, 1 cup	86	1.2	21.8	.4	0	2	4.5
Tangerine, can or jar							
(mandarin orange):							
in juice, ½ cup:							
w/liquid	46	.8	11.9	<.1	0	6	.9
lightly sweetened							
(*S&W* Natural							
Style)	60	1.0	14.0	0	0	10	1.0
in light syrup:							
(*Del Monte*), ½ cup	80	0	19.0	0	0	10	<1.0
(*Del Monte*),							
4-oz. can	70	0	17.0	0	0	10	<1.0
(*Del Monte Fruit Cup*),							
4.5 oz.	70	0	17.0	0	0	10	<1.0

Food and Measure	cal.	prot. (gms)	carbo. (gms)	fat (gms)	chol. (mgs)	sod. (mgs)	fiber (gms)
Tangerine, can or jar, in light syrup *(cont.)*							
(*Del Monte Sunfresh*),							
½ cup	80	0	19.0	0	0	15	<1.0
(*Dole*), ½ cup	80	0	19.0	0	0	10	1.0
(*Fanci Food*), ⅓ cup	80	1.0	19.0	0	0	15	1.0
(*S&W*), ½ cup	80	0	19.0	0	0	10	<1.0
w/liquid, ½ cup . . .	77	.6	20.4	.1	0	8	.9
in orange gelatin (*Del Monte* Lite), 4.5-oz.							
cup	60	0	14.0	0	0	40	0
Tangerine drink (*Ocean Spray* Mandarin							
Magic), 8 fl. oz. . . .	120	0	31.0	0	0	60	0
Tangerine juice, 8 fl. oz.:							
(*Noble* Express)	125	1.0	30.0	0	0	0	0
fresh	106	1.2	25.0	1.2	0	2	.5
canned, sweetened . .	125	1.3	29.9	.5	0	2	.5
frozen*	111	1.0	26.7	.3	0	2	.5
Tannier, see "Malanga"							
Tapenade, see "Olive spread"							
Tapioca:							
(*Minute*), 1½ tsp. . . .	20	0	5.0	0	0	0	0
(*Reese* Pearls), 1 tbsp.	35	0	9.0	0	0	0	0
Tapioca pudding, see "Pudding"and "Pudding and pie filling mix"							
Tapioca flour (*Shiloh Farms*), 1½ tbsp. . .	45	0	11.0	0	0	0	tr.
Taquito, frozen, 3 pcs., 4.5 oz., except as noted:							
corn:							
beef (*El Monterey Quick Classics*),							
5 pcs., 5 oz.	260	10.0	31.0	10.0	30	420	2.0
chicken (*El Monterey*)	270	12.0	31.0	10.0	30	600	2.0
chicken (*El Monterey Quick Classics*),							
5 pcs., 5 oz.	300	13.0	37.0	10.0	25	340	1.0
steak, shredded (*El Monterey*)	280	11.0	31.0	11.0	40	490	2.0

Food and Measure	cal.	prot. (gms)	carbo. (gms)	fat (gms)	chol. (mgs)	sod. (mgs)	fiber (gms)
flour:							
beef/cheese, shredded (*El Monterey*)	390	12.0	37.0	20.0	35	700	1.0
beef/cheese, shredded (*El Monterey* Fiesta Pack)	330	12.0	36.0	15.0	30	430	1.0
chicken breast, charbroiled (*El Monterey* Mexican Grill), 3 pcs., 5 oz.	380	15.0	36.0	19.0	35	670	1.0
chicken/cheese (*El Monterey*)	370	11.0	38.0	18.0	20	650	2.0
chicken/cheese (*El Monterey* Fiesta Pack)	310	11.0	36.0	13.0	20	540	1.0
chicken, cheese, zesty (*El Monterey* Fiesta Minis), 3 pcs., 4 oz.	380	9.0	41.0	20.0	15	1490	1.0
flour, batter-dipped, 4 pcs., 5.6 oz.:							
beef/cheese, taco (*El Monterey Crucheros*)	420	13.0	40.0	24.0	40	1080	2.0
chicken, Southwest (*El Monterey Crucheros*)	400	14.0	52.0	17.0	25	880	2.0
chicken/cheese (*El Monterey Crucheros*)	360	14.0	41.0	15.0	30	900	2.0
Taquito, breakfast, egg, cheese, bacon (*El Monterey*), 3 pcs., 4.5 oz.	300	12.0	38.0	12.0	110	730	1.0
Taramosalata (*Krinos*), 1 tbsp.	90	1.0	0	10.0	15	115	0
Taro, fresh:							
raw:							
(*Frieda's* Taro Root), ²⁄₃ cup, 3 oz. ...	90	1.0	22.0	0	0	10	3.0
sliced, ½ cup	56	.8	13.8	.1	0	6	2.1
cooked, sliced, ½ cup	94	.3	22.8	.1	0	10	3.4

Food and Measure	cal.	prot. (gms)	carbo. (gms)	fat (gms)	chol. (mgs)	sod. (mgs)	fiber (gms)
Taro *(cont.)*							
Tahitian, ½ cup:							
raw, sliced	25	1.7	4.3	.6	0	31	n.a.
cooked, sliced	30	2.8	4.7	.5	0	37	n.a.
Taro chips/crisps (see also "Vegetable chips/crisps"):							
(*Terra* Chips), 1 oz. . . .	140	1.0	19.0	6.0	0	110	4.0
1 oz...............	141	.7	19.3	7.1	0	97	n.a.
½ cup	57	.3	8.1	3.1	0	44	n.a.
spiced (*Terra* Chips), 1 oz............	130	1.0	20.0	5.0	0	170	2.0
Taro leaf:							
raw, ½ cup	6	.7	.9	.1	0	1	.5
steamed, ½ cup	17	2.0	2.9	.3	0	1	1.5
Taro shoots, ½ cup:							
raw, sliced	5	.4	1.0	<.1	0	<1	n.a.
cooked, sliced	10	.5	2.2	.1	0	1	n.a.
Tarragon, ground, 1 tsp.	5	.4	.8	.1	0	1	.1
Tart shell, see "Pastry shell"							
Tartar sauce, 2 tbsp.:							
(*Cains*)	150	0	2.0	16.0	15	115	0
(*Kraft*)	70	0	4.0	6.0	5	230	0
(*Kraft* Fat Free)	25	0	5.0	0	0	200	0
(*Litehouse*)	140	0	2.0	15.0	15	250	0
(*Old Bay*)	130	0	3.0	12.0	15	210	0
hot and spicy (*Kraft*) .	70	0	4.0	6.0	5	240	0
lemon herb (*Kraft*) ...	150	0	1.0	16.0	15	170	0
TCBY, ½ cup, except as noted:							
ice cream, hand dip:							
butter pecan	260	3.0	17.0	20.0	45	130	<1.0
chocolate chocolate chocolate chunk	210	4.0	21.0	13.0	50	50	0
cookie dough ...	200	3.0	18.0	14.0	50	50	0
chocolate fudge ...	260	4.0	27.0	16.0	45	65	<1.0
lemon meringue pie	230	3.0	29.0	12.0	55	65	0
mint chocolate	230	3.0	23.0	15.0	50	45	<1.0
oatmeal raisin	220	3.0	25.0	12.0	45	90	0
pralines & cream ..	210	3.0	22.0	13.0	45	65	0
strawberry, very berry	180	3.0	19.0	11.0	40	45	0
vanilla bean	210	3.0	17.0	13.0	55	45	0

Food and Measure	cal.	prot. (gms)	carbo. (gms)	fat (gms)	chol. (mgs)	sod. (mgs)	fiber (gms)
white chunk macadamia	250	3.0	23.0	16.0	45	75	0
Fruithead Smoothie, w/yogurt, 20 oz.:							
Berry Slim	410	5.0	95.0	3.0	10	50	2.0
Healthy Balance . . .	410	5.0	95.0	3.0	10	50	2.0
Holy-Cal	470	4.0	114.0	3.0	10	65	3.0
A Lotta Colada	550	6.0	99.0	17.0	0	95	3.0
Peachy Lean	470	4.0	116.0	3.0	10	70	<1.0
Raspberry DeLite . .	360	4.0	85.0	3.0	10	50	4.0
Raspberry Revitalizer	370	5.0	84.0	3.0	10	50	3.0
Tropical Replenisher	370	4.0	87.0	3.0	10	50	1.0
Workout Whey	460	4.0	112.0	3.0	10	85	1.0
Fruithead Smoothie, w/out yogurt, 20 oz.:							
Berry Slim	300	1.0	75.0	0	0	5	2.0
Healthy Balance . . .	300	1.0	75.0	0	0	5	2.0
Holy-Cal	360	1.0	94.0	0	0	25	3.0
A Lotta Colada	380	2.0	69.0	12.0	0	20	3.0
Peachy Lean	360	1.0	96.0	0	0	30	<1.0
Raspberry DeLite . .	240	2.0	59.0	0	0	15	3.0
Raspberry Revitalizer	300	2.0	79.0	0	0	0	6.0
Tropical Replenisher	240	1.0	61.0	0	0	20	2.0
Workout Whey	340	1.0	92.0	0	0	25	1.0
sorbet, all flavors	100	0	24.0	0	0	30	0
yogurt, soft serve, all flavors:							
96% fat free	140	4.0	23.0	3.0	15	60	0
nonfat	110	4.0	23.0	0	<5	60	0
nonfat no sugar . . .	90	4.0	20.0	0	<5	35	0
Tea (see also "Tea, iced"), plain, regular or instant, all varieties, 1 bag or tsp. .	0	0	0	0	0	0	0
Tea, iced, 8 fl. oz., except as noted:							
(*Hood*)	100	0	25.0	0	0	10	0
(*Sobe Dragon*)	110	0	30.0	0	0	15	0
(*Sobe Zen Tea 3G*) . . .	100	0	26.0	0	0	10	0
(*Turkey Hill*)	90	0	22.0	0	0	15	0
(*Turkey Hill* Decaf) . . .	80	0	20.0	0	0	15	0
all fruit varieties (*Ocean Spray*)	100	0	24.0	0	0	35	0

Food and Measure	cal.	prot. (gms)	carbo. (gms)	fat (gms)	chol. (mgs)	sod. (mgs)	fiber (gms)
Tea, iced *(cont.)*							
black tea:							
(*AriZona* Botanical)	70	0	18.0	0	0	10	0
(*AriZona* Sweet) . . .	90	0	23.0	0	0	20	0
w/ginseng, herbs							
(*Sobe*)	100	0	27.0	0	0	15	0
w/milk (*Thai Kitchen*),							
11.5-oz. can	130	4.0	24.0	2.0	5	55	0
cherry (*Snapple* Very							
Cherry)	100	0	25.0	0	0	10	0
ginseng (*AriZona*) . . .	70	0	18.0	0	0	20	0
green tea:							
(*AriZona* Botanical)	60	0	16.0	0	0	10	0
(*AriZona* Sweet) . . .	70	0	18.0	0	0	20	0
(*Turkey Hill*)	70	0	17.0	0	0	20	0
w/enchinacea, herbs							
(*Sobe*)	90	0	24.0	0	0	10	0
lime (*Snapple*)	100	0	25.0	0	0	10	0
herbal:							
(*AriZona* Rx Energy)	120	0	31.0	0	0	25	0
(*AriZona* Rx Health)	70	0	19.0	0	0	20	0
(*AriZona* Rx Memory)	80	0	20.0	0	0	20	0
(*AriZona* Rx Stress)	70	0	16.0	0	0	20	0
kiwi (*Snapple* Teawi) .	100	0	26.0	0	0	10	0
lemon:							
(*AriZona*)	90	0	25.0	0	0	20	0
(*Nantucket Nectars*							
Squeezed)	90	0	23.0	0	0	0	0
(*Nestea*)	80	0	22.0	0	0	70	0
(*Newman's Own*							
Lemon-Aided) . .	110	0	27.0	0	0	40	0
(*Snapple*)	100	0	25.0	0	0	10	0
(*Turkey Hill*)	100	0	24.0	0	0	10	0
lemonade:							
(*Minute Maid*)	110	0	29.0	0	0	20	0
(*Nantucket Nectars*							
Squeezed Half and							
Half	100	0	26.0	0	0	0	0
(*Snapple*)	110	0	28.0	0	0	10	0
frozen* (*Minute Maid*)	100	0	28.0	0	0	0	0
lime (*Turkey Hill*)	100	0	25.0	0	0	10	0
mint:							
(*Snapple*)	110	0	27.0	0	0	10	0
(*Turkey Hill*)	90	0	21.0	0	0	10	0

Food and Measure	cal.	prot. (gms)	carbo. (gms)	fat (gms)	chol. (mgs)	sod. (mgs)	fiber (gms)
oolong:							
(*Turkey Hill*)	100	0	25.0	0	0	10	0
blueberry (*Turkey Hill*)	100	0	24.0	0	0	10	0
w/ginseng, herbs (*Sobe*)	90	0	25.0	0	0	15	0
orange:							
(*Turkey Hill*)	100	0	25.0	0	0	10	0
mandarin (*AriZona*)	70	0	19.0	0	0	20	0
peach:							
(*AriZona*)	70	0	18.0	0	0	20	0
(*Snapple*)	100	0	26.0	0	0	10	0
(*Turkey Hill*)	110	0	28.0	0	0	10	0
plum, Asian (*AriZona*)	70	0	18.0	0	0	20	0
raspberry:							
(*AriZona*)	90	0	25.0	0	0	20	0
(*Snapple*)	100	0	26.0	0	0	10	0
(*Turkey Hill*)	110	0	28.0	0	0	10	0
red tea (*AriZona Botanical*)	60	0	16.0	0	0	10	0
Tea, iced, mix, chai latte (*General Foods International Coffee*), 2 tbsp.	110	0	20.0	4.0	0	95	0
Teff, grain (*Shiloh Farms*), ¼ cup	160	5.0	32.0	1.0	0	5	6.0
Teff flour:							
(*Arrowhead Mills*), 2 oz.	200	7.0	41.0	1.0	0	6	7.7
(*Shiloh Farms*), ¼ cup	160	5.0	32.0	1.0	0	5	6.0
Teff seeds (*Arrowhead Mills*), 2 oz.	200	7.0	41.0	1.0	0	6	7.7
Tekka (*Eden*), 1 tsp. ...	5	.4	.5	0	0	70	0
Tempeh:							
(*White Wave* Original), ⅓ block	180	16.0	12.0	8.0	0	10	8.0
five grain (*White Wave*), ⅓ block	180	12.0	17.0	7.0	0	10	8.0
sea veggie (*White Wave*), ⅓ block ...	180	12.0	14.0	8.0	0	240	12.0
soy rice (*White Wave*), ⅓ block	180	12.0	17.0	7.0	0	10	5.0
1 oz.	55	5.3	2.7	3.1	0	3	n.a.
½ cup	160	15.4	7.8	9.0	0	7	n.a.

Food and Measure	cal.	prot. (gms)	carbo. (gms)	fat (gms)	chol. (mgs)	sod. (mgs)	fiber (gms)
Temptation melon (*Frieda's*), 1/10 melon, 4.7 oz.	55	1.0	14.0	0	0	45	1.0
Tempura batter mix (*Golden Dipt* Fry Easy), ¼ cup	100	1.0	20.0	0	0	150	0
Tenderizer, see "Meat tenderizer"							
Teriyaki sauce (see also "Marinade"):							
(*Annie Chun's*), 1 tbsp.	25	1.0	5.0	0	0	350	0
(*Sagawa's*), 1 tbsp. ..	30	1.0	6.0	0	0	380	0
(*San-J*), 1 tbsp.	10	1.0	3.0	0	0	450	0
baste/glaze, 2 tbsp.:							
(*Kikkoman*)	50	1.0	11.0	0	0	810	0
w/honey, pineapple (*Kikkoman*)	80	1.0	18.0	0	0	770	0
Texas toast, see "Bread, frozen"							
Tex-Mex seasoning (*McCormick 1 Step*), 2 tsp.	25	0	3.0	1.0	0	590	0
Thai entree, pkg., see "Noodle entree, pkg."							
Thai sauce (see also "Peanut sauce" and specific listings):							
(*Neera's*), 1 tsp.	29	0	8.0	1.0	0	164	0
(*World Harbors*), 2 tbsp.	40	0	8.0	0	0	350	0
barbecue, spicy (*Thai Kitchen*), 1 tbsp. ..	10	2.0	<1.0	0	0	690	0
chili:							
(*Kikkoman*), 2 tbsp.	70	0	15.0	1.0	0	240	1.0
sweet red (*A Taste of Thai*), 1 tsp. ...	10	0	2.0	0	0	40	0
garlic pepper (*A Taste of Thai*), 1 tsp.	10	2.0	2.0	0	0	230	0
spicy (*Thai Kitchen*), 1 tbsp.	15	0	4.0	0	0	195	0
sweet red (*Thai Kitchen*), 1 tbsp.	30	0	8.0	0	0	202	0

Food and Measure	cal.	prot. (gms)	carbo. (gms)	fat (gms)	chol. (mgs)	sod. (mgs)	fiber (gms)
chili paste, roasted red (*Thai Kitchen*), 1 tbsp.	26	0	2.0	2.0	0	280	0
fish, 1 tbsp.:							
(*A Taste of Thai Seasoning*)	15	2.0	1.0	0	0	1730	0
(*Thai Kitchen*)	10	2.0	<1.0	0	0	1190	0
pad Thai, 2 tbsp.:							
(*A Taste of Thai*) . .	90	1.0	20.0	1.0	0	790	1.0
(*Thai Kitchen*)	90	0	22.0	0	0	469	0
Thai snack nuggets, frozen (*Health is Wealth Munchees*), 3 oz.	180	5.0	27.0	5.0	0	420	3.0
Thyme, ground, 1 tsp.	4	.1	.9	.1	0	1	.3
Thymus, 4 oz.:							
beef, braised	362	24.8	0	28.3	333	132	0
veal, braised	197	35.8	0	4.9	532	75	0
Tilapia, fresh, baked or broiled, 3 oz. . . .	110	22.0	0	2.5	75	30	0
Tilapia entree, frozen, stuffed w/sun-dried tomato, shrimp, lobster (*Oven Poppers*), ½ of 10-oz. pkg.	180	19.0	8.0	8.0	80	320	0
Tilefish, meat only:							
raw, 4 oz.	109	19.9	0	2.6	57	60	0
baked, broiled, or microwaved, 4 oz. . .	167	27.8	0	5.3	73	67	0
T. J. Cinnamons:							
Cinnachips, 10-oz. bag	1130	14.0	157.0	50.0	42	700	3.0
cinnamon twist	260	3.0	33.0	13.0	5	190	10.0
The Original Gourmet Cinnamon Roll:							
no icing	500	8.0	81.0	17.0	30	370	0
w/cream cheese icing	651	8.0	103.0	37.0	40	420	0
pecan sticky roll	690	14.0	97.0	28.0	32	400	0
mocha chill, 12 oz.:							
no whipped cream .	260	10.0	48.0	3.5	15	190	10.0
w/whipped cream . .	310	10.0	49.0	6.0	25	190	10.0
mocha chill, 18 oz.:							
no whipped cream .	390	15.0	72.0	5.0	20	280	15.0
w/whipped cream . .	440	15.0	73.0	8.0	35	280	15.0

Food and Measure	cal.	prot. (gms)	carbo. (gms)	fat (gms)	chol. (mgs)	sod. (mgs)	fiber (gms)
Tiramisu, see "Cake, frozen"							
Toaster pastry and muffin (see also "Breakfast pocket/ sandwich"), 1 pc.:							
apple:							
(*Amy's* Toaster Pops)	140	4.0	26.0	3.0	0	130	<1.0
(*Toaster Strudel*) . .	190	2.0	26.0	9.0	5	180	0
iced (*Hot Pockets*) .	240	3.0	39.0	9.0	15	160	2.0
apple cinnamon (*Pop• Tarts*)	210	2.0	37.0	6.0	0	180	<1.0
berry, mixed (*Pop• Tarts* Wild!Berry) . .	210	2.0	39.0	5.0	0	170	<1.0
blueberry:							
(*Pop•Tarts*)	200	2.0	37.0	5.0	0	190	1.0
(*Toaster Strudel*) . .	190	2.0	26.0	9.0	5	190	0
frosted (*Pop•Tarts*)	200	2.0	37.0	5.0	0	170	1.0
muffin (*Organic Toaster Classics*)	170	3.0	27.0	5.0	25	270	<1.0
yogurt (*Pop•Tarts Yogurt Blasts*) . .	210	2.0	37.0	6.0	0	190	<1.0
brown sugar cinnamon:							
(*Pop•Tarts*)	210	3.0	35.0	6.0	0	190	1.0
(*Toaster Strudel*) . .	200	2.0	28.0	9.0	5	190	<1.0
frosted (*Pop•Tarts*)	210	3.0	34.0	7.0	0	180	1.0
frosted (*Pop•Tarts* Low Fat)	190	2.0	39.0	3.0	0	230	1.0
carrot spice muffin (*Organic Toaster Classics*)	180	3.0	29.0	6.0	20	230	<1.0
cherry:							
(*Toaster Strudel*) . .	190	3.0	26.0	9.0	5	190	<1.0
frosted (*Pop•Tarts*)	200	2.0	38.0	5.0	0	170	1.0
chocolate chip:							
(*Pop•Tarts*)	220	3.0	35.0	7.0	0	240	<1.0
cookie dough (*Pop• Tarts*)	200	2.0	35.0	5.0	0	190	<1.0
chocolate fudge:							
(*Toaster Strudel*) . .	200	2.0	25.0	10.0	5	180	0
frosted (*Pop•Tarts* Low Fat)	190	3.0	39.0	3.0	0	270	2.0

Food and Measure	cal.	prot. (gms)	carbo. (gms)	fat (gms)	chol. (mgs)	sod. (mgs)	fiber (gms)
or vanilla crème, frosted (*Pop•Tarts*)	200	3.0	37.0	5.0	0	220	1.0
corn (*Awrey's* Toastums)	180	2.0	22.0	9.0	30	125	0
cranberry corn muffin (*Organic Toaster Classics*)	170	3.0	26.0	6.0	25	260	1.0
cream cheese: (*Toaster Strudel* Danish Style) ...	200	3.0	23.0	11.0	10	220	0
raspberry (*Toaster Strudel*)	200	3.0	24.0	10.0	10	200	0
strawberry (*Amy's* Toaster Pops) ...	160	4.0	24.0	6.0	10	125	<1.0
strawberry (*Toaster Strudel*)	200	3.0	24.0	10.0	10	210	0
strawberry, iced (*Hot Pockets*)	240	3.0	34.0	10.0	20	200	2.0
grape, frosted (*Pop•Tarts*)	200	2.0	37.0	5.0	0	170	<1.0
hot fudge sundae (*Pop•Tarts*)	200	2.0	37.0	5.0	0	220	<1.0
maple oat muffin (*Organic Toaster Classics*)	190	4.0	29.0	6.0	30	210	2.0
raspberry: (*Toaster Strudel*) ..	190	2.0	26.0	9.0	5	190	0
frosted (*Pop•Tarts*)	210	2.0	37.0	5.0	0	170	<1.0
S'mores: (*Pop•Tarts*)	200	3.0	36.0	6.0	0	200	1.0
(*Toaster Strudel*) ..	200	3.0	27.0	9.0	5	190	<1.0
strawberry: (*Pop•Tarts*)	200	2.0	37.0	5.0	0	190	1.0
(*Toaster Strudel*) ..	200	2.0	25.0	9.0	5	190	<1.0
iced (*Hot Pockets*) .	240	3.0	39.0	8.0	15	170	2.0
frosted (*Pop•Tarts*)	200	2.0	38.0	5.0	0	170	1.0
frosted (*Pop•Tarts* Low Fat)	190	2.0	39.0	3.0	0	210	1.0
yogurt (*Pop•Tarts Yogurt Blasts*) ..	210	2.0	37.0	6.0	0	190	<1.0
wild berry (*Toaster Strudel*)	190	2.0	26.0	9.0	5	190	<1.0
Toffee, see "Candy"							

Food and Measure	cal.	prot. (gms)	carbo. (gms)	fat (gms)	chol. (mgs)	sod. (mgs)	fiber (gms)
Toffee baking chips,							
1 tbsp., .5 oz.:							
(*Hershey's Bake*							
Shoppe Heath Bits)	80	<1.0	9.0	4.5	<5	60	0
(*Hershey's Bake*							
Shoppe Heath Bits							
'O Brickle Bits)	80	<1.0	9.0	5.0	5	80	0
Toffee syrup (*Heath*							
Sundae), 2 tbsp. . .	100	0	24.0	0	0	130	0
Toffee topping (*Heath*							
Shell), 2 tbsp.	230	<1.0	17.0	17.0	0	40	<1.0
Tofu (see also "Seitan"							
and Tempeh"):							
(*White Wave* Reduced							
Fat), 1/5 of 1-lb. pkg.	90	10.0	1.0	4.0	0	5	2.0
fresh, ½ cup	94	10.0	2.3	5.9	0	9	1.5
fresh, extra firm:							
(*Azumaya*), 2.8 oz. . .	70	7.0	2.0	4.0	0	0	1.0
(*Azumaya* Lite),							
2.8 oz.	60	7.0	3.0	2.0	0	30	1.0
(*Frieda's*), 3 oz. . . .	90	10.0	1.0	5.0	0	10	0
(*Frieda's* Organic),							
3 oz.	70	7.0	2.0	4.0	0	10	0
(*White Wave*), 3 oz.	110	11.0	4.0	6.0	0	5	2.0
fresh, firm:							
(*Azumaya*), 2.8 oz. . .	70	7.0	2.0	4.0	0	0	<1.0
(*Frieda's*), 3 oz. . . .	60	6.0	2.0	3.0	0	10	0
(*Frieda's* Organic),							
3 oz.	70	7.0	1.0	4.0	0	10	0
(*Tree of Life*), 3.2 oz.	110	11.0	4.0	5.0	0	5	2.0
(*Tree of Life* Reduced							
Fat), 3.2 oz.	90	10.0	4.0	4.0	0	5	2.0
(*Tree of Life* Water							
Pack), 3.2 oz. . . .	100	9.0	2.0	5.0	0	5	0
(*White Wave* Box),							
1/5 of 1-lb. box .	90	10.0	1.0	6.0	0	10	1.0
(*White Wave* Water							
Pack), 1/5 of							
1-lb. pkg.	110	11.0	4.0	6.0	0	5	2.0
1 oz.	41	4.5	1.2	2.5	0	4	.7
½ cup	183	19.9	5.4	11.0	0	17	2.9
fresh, silken:							
(*Azumaya*), 3.2 oz. .	40	4.0	1.0	2.0	0	0	<1.0

Food and Measure	cal.	prot. (gms)	carbo. (gms)	fat (gms)	chol. (mgs)	sod. (mgs)	fiber (gms)
(*Azumaya* Lite),							
3.2 oz.	40	5.0	3.0	1.0	0	45	0
fresh, soft:							
(*Frieda's*), 3 oz. ...	45	5.0	1.0	2.5	0	15	0
(*Frieda's* Organic),							
3 oz.	50	5.0	2.0	2.5	0	10	0
(*White Wave* Water Pack), 1/5 of							
1-lb. pkg.	110	11.0	4.0	6.0	0	5	2.0
baked:							
(*Tree of Life*), 2.7 oz.	130	15.0	3.0	7.0	0	310	0
barbecue, hickory (*White Wave*),							
2 oz., ¼ pkg. ...	90	9.0	2.0	5.0	0	220	2.0
garlic herb (*Frieda's*),							
3 oz.	120	10.0	8.0	6.0	0	240	1.0
garlic herb Italian (*White Wave*),							
2 oz., ¼ pkg. ...	90	9.0	2.0	5.0	0	280	2.0
ginger teriyaki (*Frieda's*), 3 oz. .	150	10.0	13.0	6.0	0	520	1.0
lemon pepper (*White Wave* Zesty), 2 oz.,							
¼ pkg.	90	9.0	2.0	5.0	0	380	2.0
savory (*Tree of Life*),							
2.7 oz.	130	15.0	3.0	7.0	0	320	0
sesame garlic (*Frieda's*), 3 oz. .	130	10.0	10.0	6.0	0	210	1.0
teriyaki (*White Wave* Oriental), 2 oz.,							
¼ pkg.	90	9.0	2.0	5.0	0	400	2.0
Thai style (*White Wave*), 2 oz.,							
¼ pkg.	90	9.0	2.0	5.0	0	280	2.0
tomato basil (*White Wave* Roma), 2 oz.,							
¼ pkg.	90	9.0	2.0	5.0	0	280	2.0
dried (*Eden*), .4 oz. ..	50	5.0	0	2.5	0	0	2.0
salted and fermented (fuyu), 1 oz.	33	2.3	1.5	2.3	0	814	<1.0
seasoned, 3 oz.:							
garlic onion (*Azumaya* Zesty)	90	8.0	3.0	5.0	0	250	1.0

Food and Measure	cal.	prot. (gms)	carbo. (gms)	fat (gms)	chol. (mgs)	sod. (mgs)	fiber (gms)
Tofu, seasoned *(cont.)*							
Oriental spice (*Azumaya*)	90	8.0	3.0	5.0	0	220	1.0
smoked, all varieties (*Tree of Life*), 3 oz.	120	18.0	3.0	5.0	0	120	0
tenders, 4.5 oz.:							
black bean (*Tofu-Town Tofu Tenders Havana*)	200	16.0	15.0	8.0	0	930	2.0
*sesame ginger teriyaki (*TofuTown Tofu Tenders*) . . .	220	16.0	18.0	9.0	0	930	3.0
tahini (*TofuTown Tofu Tenders Mediterranean*) . .	240	16.0	11.0	14.0	0	790	2.0
tamari (*TofuTown Tofu Tenders*) . . .	150	15.0	5.0	8.0	0	310	2.0
Tofu, ground, frozen, plain or savory garlic (*Tree of Life* Ready Ground), ⅓ of 10-oz. pkg.	60	7.0	2.0	4.0	0	10	0
Tofu breakfast, frozen, 9-oz. pkg.:							
Rancheros (*Amy's* Meal)	360	18.0	37.0	17.0	15	580	7.0
scramble (*Amy's* Meal)	320	19.0	19.0	19.0	0	580	4.0
Tofu dessert, 3 oz.:							
almond (*Frieda's*)	60	2.0	9.0	1.0	0	0	0
peach mango (*Frieda's*)	60	2.0	9.0	1.5	0	0	0
Tofu pudding, see "Pudding, nondairy"							
Tofu salad, plain or sun-dried tomato (*Tree of Life* Egg Less Salad), 3 oz. . .	90	8.0	2.0	5.0	0	130	<1.0
Tofu scrambler mix (*Fantastic*), 1 tbsp. . .	35	1.0	7.0	0	0	260	1.0
Tofu seasoning mix (*TofuMate*), ¼ pkg.:							
breakfast scramble . . .	15	1.0	3.0	0	0	350	0
eggless salad	15	0	4.0	0	0	310	0
mandarin stir-fry	25	1.0	6.0	0	0	310	0
Mediterranean herb . .	15	1.0	3.0	0	0	330	0

Food and Measure	cal.	prot. (gms)	carbo. (gms)	fat (gms)	chol. (mgs)	sod. (mgs)	fiber (gms)
Szechuan stir-fry	25	1.0	4.0	0	0	280	0
Texas taco	15	1.0	3.0	0	0	360	0
Tom Collins drink mixer (*Holland House*), 4 fl. oz.	210	0	49.0	0	0	115	0
Tom and Jerry drink batter (*Trader Vic's*), 1 tbsp.	116	2.0	23.0	2.0	35	240	0
Tomatillo, fresh:							
(*Frieda's*), ⅔ cup, 3 oz.	25	1.0	5.0	1.0	0	0	2.0
1 medium, 1⅝" diam.	11	.3	2.0	.4	0	tr.	.6
chopped, ½ cup	21	.6	3.8	.7	0	1	1.3
Tomatillo, can or jar:							
whole:							
(*Embasa*), 3 pcs., 2.1 oz.	15	0	3.0	0	0	15	2.0
(*La Costeña*), 4 pcs., 4.3 oz.	40	1.0	4.0	2.5	0	260	4.0
(*La Victoria* Entero), 5 pcs., 4.5 oz. ...	40	1.0	7.0	1.0	0	410	5.0
crushed:							
(*Embasa*), ¼ cup ..	10	0	2.0	0	0	290	2.0
(*La Victoria*), 4.5 oz.	45	2.0	8.0	.5	0	400	7.0
(*Las Palmas*), ½ cup	45	1.0	7.0	1.5	0	n.a.	2.0
Tomato, fresh, ripe:							
raw:							
(*Del Monte*), 1 medium, 5.2 oz.	35	1.0	7.0	.5	0	0	1.0
(*Chiquita*), 1 medium, 5.2 oz.	35	1.0	7.0	.5	0	5	1.0
(*Frieda's* Baby Roma/ Teardrop), ⅔ cup, 3 oz.	20	1.0	4.0	0	0	10	1.0
2⅜" tomato	26	1.0	5.7	.4	0	11	1.4
chopped, 1 cup ...	38	1.5	8.4	.6	0	16	2.0
boiled:							
2 medium, 8.8 oz. ..	66	2.6	14.3	1.0	0	27	2.5
1 cup	65	2.6	14.0	1.0	0	27	2.4
orange:							
3.9-oz. tomato	18	1.3	3.5	.2	0	47	1.0
chopped, 1 cup ...	25	1.8	5.0	.3	0	66	1.4
yellow:							
7.8-oz. tomato	32	2.1	6.3	.6	0	49	1.5
chopped, 1 cup ...	21	1.4	4.1	.4	0	32	1.0

Food and Measure	cal.	prot. (gms)	carbo. (gms)	fat (gms)	chol. (mgs)	sod. (mgs)	fiber (gms)
Tomato, canned (see also "Tomato paste," "Tomato puree" and "Tomato sauce"), ½ cup, except as noted:							
whole, peeled:							
(*Del Monte*)	25	1.0	6.0	0	0	160	2.0
(*Eden* Organic)	30	1.0	4.0	0	0	10	1.0
(*Hunt's*)	20	1.0	4.0	0	0	190	1.0
(*Hunt's* No Salt) . . .	20	<1.0	4.0	0	0	15	1.0
(*Muir Glen* 14.5 oz.)	30	1.0	5.0	0	0	260	1.0
(*Muir Glen* 28 oz.) .	35	1.0	9.0	0	0	260	1.0
(*Progresso* Italian Style)	30	1.0	5.0	0	0	35	1.0
(*Red Gold/Red Pack*)	25	1.0	5.0	0	0	220	1.0
(*Red Pack* Plum) . .	30	1.0	5.0	0	0	180	2.0
(*S&W*)	30	1.0	7.0	0	0	380	2.0
(*Tuttorosso* Pear) . .	30	1.0	5.0	0	0	220	2.0
w/basil (*Eden* Organic)	30	1.0	4.0	0	0	10	1.0
w/basil (*Muir Glen*)	35	1.0	9.0	0	0	260	1.0
w/basil (*Tuttorosso*)	25	1.0	5.0	0	0	220	1.0
w/basil (*Tuttorosso* Pear)	30	1.0	5.0	0	0	220	2.0
fire-roasted (*Muir Glen*)	30	1.0	6.0	0	0	350	1.0
wedges (*Del Monte*) .	35	1.0	9.0	0	0	380	2.0
chunky, in puree (*Red Pack*)	30	1.0	6.0	0	0	270	1.0
diced:							
(*Contadina* Recipe Ready)	30	<1.0	6.0	0	0	200	1.0
(*Del Monte/Del Monte* Petite) . . .	25	1.0	6.0	0	0	250	2.0
(*Del Monte* No Salt)	25	1.0	6.0	0	0	50	2.0
(*Eden* Organic)	30	1.0	6.0	0	0	5	2.0
(*Hunt's* Original) . . .	20	1.0	5.0	0	0	380	<1.0
(*Hunt's* Petite)	20	1.0	5.0	0	0	330	1.0
(*Muir Glen* 14.5 oz.)	25	1.0	5.0	0	0	290	1.0
(*Muir Glen* 28 oz.) .	25	1.0	4.0	0	0	290	1.0
(*Muir Glen* No Salt)	25	1.0	6.0	0	0	45	1.0
(*Red Gold* Chili Ready)	35	1.0	8.0	0	0	220	1.0

Food and Measure	cal.	prot. (gms)	carbo. (gms)	fat (gms)	chol. (mgs)	sod. (mgs)	fiber (gms)
(*Red Gold/Red Pack*)	25	1.0	5.0	0	0	220	1.0
(*S&W Petite-Cut* Rich Juice)	25	1.0	6.0	0	0	250	2.0
(*S&W Ready-Cut* No Salt)	25	1.0	6.0	0	0	50	2.0
chunky, chili style (*Del Monte*)	30	1.0	8.0	0	0	670	2.0
chunky, pasta style (*Del Monte*)	45	1.0	11.0	0	0	560	2.0
w/balsamic vinegar/ basil/oil (*Hunt's*) .	60	1.0	8.0	0	0	460	1.0
w/basil/garlic, garlic/ onion, or Italian herbs (*Muir Glen*)	25	1.0	5.0	0	0	290	1.0
w/basil/garlic/ oregano (*Del Monte*)	50	2.0	11.0	0	0	650	<1.0
w/basil/garlic/ oregano (*Hunt's*)	25	1.0	6.0	0	0	530	1.0
w/basil/garlic/ oregano (*Red Pack*)	50	1.0	7.0	0	0	270	1.0
fire-roasted (*Muir Glen*)	30	1.0	6.0	0	0	290	1.0
fire-roasted, w/green chili (*Muir Glen*) .	30	1.0	6.0	0	0	420	1.0
w/garlic, roasted (*Contadina* Recipe Ready)	45	1.0	10.0	0	0	560	<1.0
w/garlic, roasted (*Hunt's*)	30	1.0	6.0	0	0	480	1.0
w/garlic, roasted (*S&W Ready-Cut*)	30	2.0	5.0	.5	0	240	<1.0
w/garlic, roasted, and onion (*Red Gold/ Red Pack*)	25	1.0	5.0	0	0	500	1.0
w/garlic and olive oil (*Del Monte* Petite)	45	1.0	10.0	.5	0	620	1.0
w/garlic and olive oil (*Red Gold/Red Pack* Petite)	45	1.0	9.0	1.0	0	490	1.0
w/garlic/onion (*Del Monte*)	40	2.0	8.0	.5	0	610	<1.0

Food and Measure	cal.	prot. (gms)	carbo. (gms)	fat (gms)	chol. (mgs)	sod. (mgs)	fiber (gms)
Tomato, canned, diced (cont.)							
w/green chili (Eden Organic)	30	2.0	5.0	0	0	35	2.0
w/green chili (Red Gold Petite)	20	1.0	4.0	0	0	380	1.0
w/green chili (Red Pack Petite)	25	1.0	5.0	0	0	340	1.0
w/green chili (S&W Ready-Cut)	30	1.0	6.0	0	0	500	1.0
w/green chili, mild (Del Monte)	30	1.0	6.0	0	0	500	1.0
w/green chili, mild (Hunt's Petite) . .	30	2.0	6.0	0	0	360	2.0
w/green pepper/ celery/onions (Hunt's)	45	1.0	10.0	0	0	340	1.0
w/green pepper/ onion (Del Monte)	40	1.0	9.0	0	0	480	2.0
Italian (Red Gold) .	50	1.0	7.0	2.0	0	270	1.0
Italian (S&W Ready-Cut)	25	1.0	4.0	0	0	190	1.0
Italian herbs (Contadina Recipe Ready)	45	1.0	10.0	0	0	470	<1.0
w/jalapeño (Del Monte Petite Cut)	30	1.0	6.0	0	0	500	1.0
w/jalapeño (S&W Petite-Cut)	30	1.0	7.0	0	0	380	2.0
marinara (Contadina Recipe Ready) . .	70	1.0	13.0	1.5	0	600	2.0
Mexican (Red Gold Fiesta Petite) . . .	25	1.0	5.0	0	0	250	1.0
w/mushrooms (Hunt's Petite) . .	40	1.0	6.0	1.0	0	380	<1.0
w/mushrooms/garlic (Del Monte)	45	1.0	10.0	0	0	590	1.0
w/onion (Red Gold Chili Ready)	35	1.0	8.0	0	0	220	1.0
w/onion, sweet (Hunt's)	45	1.0	10.0	0	0	460	<1.0
w/onion, sweet (Red Gold/Red Pack) .	45	1.0	10.0	0	0	490	1.0
w/onion/green pepper (S&W Ready-Cut)	40	1.0	9.0	0	0	480	2.0

Food and Measure	cal.	prot. (gms)	carbo. (gms)	fat (gms)	chol. (mgs)	sod. (mgs)	fiber (gms)
w/onion/roasted garlic (*S&W Petite-Cut*)	45	1.0	10.0	0	0	550	1.0
primavera (*Contadina* Recipe Ready)	60	1.0	13.0	0	0	560	2.0
w/red pepper, roasted (*Contadina* Recipe Ready)	60	1.0	13.0	0	0	550	2.0
in sauce (*Hunt's*) ..	30	<1.0	7.0	0	0	430	1.0
w/smoked chipotle (*Red Gold* Petite)	40	1.0	8.0	0	0	490	1.0
crushed, ¼ cup:							
(*Contadina* Recipe Ready)	20	<1.0	4.0	0	0	150	1.0
(*Hunt's*)	30	2.0	7.0	0	0	350	2.0
(*Progresso* Recipe Ready)	20	<1.0	3.0	0	0	95	0
(*Eden* Organic)	20	1.0	3.0	0	0	0	1.0
(*Red Gold*)	25	1.0	5.0	0	0	170	1.0
(*Red Pack* All Purpose)	30	1.0	6.0	0	0	180	1.0
(*Red Pack* Puree) ..	20	0	4.0	0	0	120	1.0
w/basil (*Muir Glen*)	25	1.0	5.0	0	0	85	1.0
w/basil (*Tuttorosso*)	10	0	4.0	0	0	210	1.0
w/basil, garlic, oregano (*Red Pack*)	20	1.0	4.0	0	0	90	1.0
w/basil, in heavy puree (*Tuttorosso*)	10	0	4.0	0	0	120	1.0
fire-roasted (*Muir Glen*)	20	1.0	5.0	0	0	160	1.0
w/garlic, roasted (*Contadina* Recipe Ready)	20	<1.0	3.0	0	0	150	1.0
w/green pepper, mushroom (*Red Gold*)	25	1.0	5.0	0	0	250	0
Italian (*S&W*)	20	1.0	4.0	0	0	95	1.0
Italian herbs (*Contadina* Recipe Ready)	20	<1.0	3.0	0	0	150	<1.0
in puree (*S&W*) ...	20	1.0	4.0	0	0	125	1.0

Food and Measure	cal.	prot. (gms)	carbo. (gms)	fat (gms)	chol. (mgs)	sod. (mgs)	fiber (gms)
Tomato, canned *(cont.)*							
ground, peeled, ¼ cup:							
(*Muir Glen*)	10	<1.0	3.0	0	0	100	1.0
(*Red Pack*)	30	1.0	6.0	0	0	180	1.0
stewed:							
(*Contadina*)	35	1.0	9.0	0	0	220	1.0
(*Del Monte*)	35	1.0	9.0	0	0	360	2.0
(*Del Monte* No Salt)	35	1.0	9.0	0	0	50	2.0
(*Hunt's*)	35	1.0	8.0	0	0	390	1.0
(*Hunt's* No Salt) . . .	40	2.0	9.0	0	0	30	1.0
(*Muir Glen*)	30	1.0	7.0	0	0	290	<1.0
(*Red Gold/Red Pack*)	35	1.0	8.0	0	0	270	1.0
(*S&W*)	35	1.0	7.0	0	0	270	2.0
(*S&W* No Salt)	35	1.0	9.0	0	0	50	2.0
w/basil and oregano (*Red Pack*)	35	1.0	8.0	0	0	270	1.0
Cajun (*Del Monte*) .	35	1.0	9.0	0	0	460	2.0
Cajun, Italian or Mexican (*S&W*) .	35	1.0	7.0	0	0	270	2.0
Italian (*Contadina*) .	35	1.0	8.0	0	0	260	1.0
Italian (*Del Monte*) .	30	1.0	8.0	0	0	420	2.0
Italian (*Red Gold*) .	35	1.0	8.0	0	0	270	1.0
Mexican (*Del Monte*)	35	1.0	9.0	0	0	400	2.0
Tomato, dried:							
1 oz.	73	4.0	15.8	.8	0	594	3.5
1 pc., 32 pcs. per cup	5	.3	1.1	.1	0	42	.3
½ cup	70	3.8	15.3	.8	0	566	3.3
chopped or halves (*Frieda's*), ⅓ cup, 1.1 oz.	100	2.0	19.0	1.0	0	10	2.0
yellow, chopped or halves (*Frieda's*), ½ cup, 3 oz.	220	12.0	47.0	2.5	0	1780	10.0
marinated, in oil:							
julienne or halves (*Frieda's*), 1 tbsp., .4 oz.	35	1.0	4.0	2.0	0	60	1.0
drained, ½ cup . . .	117	2.8	12.8	7.7	0	146	3.2
Tomato, dried, blend, seasoned (*Frieda's* Tomato Toss*), ½ cup, 1.1 oz.	100	6.0	19.0	0	0	105	4.0

Food and Measure	cal.	prot. (gms)	carbo. (gms)	fat (gms)	chol. (mgs)	sod. (mgs)	fiber (gms)
Tomato, freeze-dried:							
flakes (*AlpineAire*), ½ oz.	50	2.0	10.0	0	0	20	1.0
powder (*AlpineAire*), ⅔ oz.	70	3.0	13.0	0	0	25	0
Tomato, green, raw, 1 large, 6.4 oz.	44	2.2	9.3	.4	0	24	2.0
Tomato, pickled:							
(*Ba-Tampte*), ½ pc., 1.5 oz.	5	0	1.0	0	0	310	0
halves (*Claussen*), 1 oz.	5	0	1.0	0	0	320	0
Tomato, sun-dried, see "Tomato, dried"							
Tomato juice, 8 fl. oz., except as noted:							
(*Campbell's*)	50	2.0	10.0	0	0	750	2.0
(*Campbell's*), 5.5-fl.-oz. can	30	1.0	6.0	0	0	520	1.0
(*Campbell's* Low Sodium)	50	2.0	10.0	0	0	140	1.0
(*Campbell's Healthy Request*)	50	1.0	12.0	0	0	480	1.0
(*Del Monte*)	50	2.0	10.0	0	0	760	1.0
(*Red Gold*)	45	1.0	10.0	0	0	750	2.0
(*Red Gold* No Salt)	45	1.0	10.0	0	0	25	2.0
(*R.W. Knudsen* Organic)	60	2.0	14.0	0	0	390	0
(*Sacramento*)	45	1.0	10.0	0	0	750	2.0
(*S&W*)	50	2.0	10.0	0	0	760	1.0
(*S&W*), 6 fl. oz.	30	1.0	7.0	0	0	500	<1.0
(*Tree of Life Pure Fruit*)	50	1.0	10.0	0	0	480	0
Tomato paste, 2 tbsp.:							
(*Contadina*)	30	2.0	6.0	0	0	20	1.0
(*Del Monte*)	30	1.0	7.0	0	0	25	2.0
(*Hunt's*)	25	1.0	6.0	0	0	90	2.0
(*Hunt's* No Salt)	30	1.0	6.0	0	0	15	2.0
(*Muir Glen*)	30	2.0	6.0	0	0	20	1.0
(*Red Gold/Red Pack*)	30	2.0	6.0	0	0	20	1.0
(*S&W*)	30	2.0	6.0	0	0	20	1.0
w/basil, garlic, and oregano (*Hunt's*)	25	1.0	6.0	0	0	260	2.0
w/Italian seasoning (*Contadina*)	35	1.0	7.0	.5	0	290	1.0
w/pesto (*Contadina*)	35	1.0	5.0	.5	0	300	<1.0

Food and Measure	cal.	prot. (gms)	carbo. (gms)	fat (gms)	chol. (mgs)	sod. (mgs)	fiber (gms)
Tomato paste *(cont.)*							
w/roasted garlic							
(*Contadina*)	35	1.0	6.0	.5	0	300	1.0
Tomato puree, ¼ cup:							
(*Contadina*)	20	<1.0	4.0	0	0	15	<1.0
(*Hunt's*)	30	1.0	7.0	0	0	450	2.0
(*Muir Glen*)	20	1.0	5.0	0	0	20	1.0
(*Progresso*)	25	3.0	5.0	0	0	15	1.0
(*Red Gold/Red Pack*) .	25	1.0	5.0	0	0	10	1.0
(*S&W*)	30	1.0	6.0	0	0	15	2.0
(*Tuttorosso*)	25	1.0	5.0	0	0	10	1.0
w/basil (*Tuttorosso*) . .	25	1.0	5.0	0	0	10	1.0
Tomato relish, 1 tbsp.,							
except as noted:							
(*Heinz* Piccalilli)	15	0	4.0	0	0	75	0
hot (*Mrs. Renfro's*) . .	10	0	3.0	0	0	40	0
medium, Indian							
(*Patak's*)	10	0	2.0	.5	0	70	0
mild (*Mrs. Renfro's*) .	10	0	3.0	0	0	45	0
salsa (*Vlasic* Relish							
Mixers)	10	0	2.0	0	0	55	0
Tomato sauce, can or							
jar (see also "Pasta							
sauce" and "Tomato,							
canned"), ¼ cup:							
(*Contadina*)	15	<1.0	3.0	0	0	280	<1.0
(*Contadina* Extra Thick							
& Zesty)	20	1.0	3.0	0	0	340	1.0
(*Del Monte*)	20	<1.0	4.0	0	0	340	<1.0
(*Del Monte* No Salt) . .	20	0	4.0	0	0	20	<1.0
(*Goya*)	20	1.0	4.0	0	0	280	1.0
(*Hunt's*)	15	<1.0	3.0	0	0	360	<1.0
(*Hunt's* No Salt)	30	1.0	6.0	0	0	15	2.0
(*Muir Glen*)	20	<1.0	5.0	0	0	310	1.0
(*Muir Glen* Chunky) . .	20	<1.0	4.0	0	0	160	1.0
(*Muir Glen* No Salt) . .	20	<1.0	5.0	0	0	30	1.0
(*Red Gold/Red Pack*) .	20	0	5.0	0	0	280	1.0
(*Red Pack* No Salt) . .	20	0	5.0	0	0	15	1.0
(*S&W* Homestyle) . . .	20	1.0	4.0	0	0	260	1.0
(*Tuttorosso*)	20	0	5.0	0	0	280	1.0
w/basil, garlic, and							
oregano (*Hunt's*) . .	15	<1.0	3.0	0	0	350	<1.0
for chili (*Hunt's* Family							
Favorites)	25	1.0	5.0	0	0	400	1.0

Food and Measure	cal.	prot. (gms)	carbo. (gms)	fat (gms)	chol. (mgs)	sod. (mgs)	fiber (gms)
w/garlic, roasted (*Hunt's*)	15	<1.0	3.0	0	0	380	<1.0
w/garlic and onion (*Contadina*)	20	<1.0	4.0	0	0	270	<1.0
w/herbs and cheese ..	36	1.3	6.2	1.2	0	331	1.3
Italian style (*Contadina*)	15	<1.0	4.0	0	0	320	1.0
for lasagna (*Hunt's Family Favorites*) ..	30	1.0	6.0	0	0	330	1.0
for meat loaf (*Hunt's Family Favorites*) ..	30	1.0	7.0	0	0	390	2.0
w/onion	26	1.0	6.1	.1	0	338	1.1
w/onion, green pepper, and celery	26	.6	5.5	.5	0	341	.9
for pizza, see "Pizza sauce"							
w/tomato tidbits, no salt added	20	.8	4.3	.1	0	9	.9
Tomato-beef drink (*Beefamato*), 8 fl. oz.	50	0	11.0	0	0	830	0
Tomato-chile cocktail:							
(*Snap-E-Tom*), 6 fl. oz.	40	2.0	8.0	0	0	500	1.0
(*Snap-E-Tom*), 8 fl. oz.	60	3.0	13.0	0	0	840	2.0
Tomato-clam drink:							
(*Clamato*), 8 fl. oz. ...	60	1.0	11.0	0	0	830	0
cocktail (*Chincoteague*), 5 fl. oz.	70	9.0	10.0	0	0	460	0
Tongue, braised:							
beef, 4 oz.	321	25.1	.4	23.5	121	68	0
lamb, 4 oz.	312	24.5	0	23.0	214	76	0
pork, 4 oz.	307	27.3	0	21.1	166	124	0
veal (calves), 4 oz. ...	229	29.3	0	11.5	270	73	0
Tongue lunch meat, beef (*Hebrew National*), 2 oz. ...	12.0	10.0	0	9.0	50	330	0
Topping, dessert (see also specific listings), 2 tbsp.:							
(*Smucker's Magic Shell Turtle Delight*)	210	1.0	17.0	16.0	0	20	1.0
(*Smucker's Magic Shell Twix*)	210	1.0	18.0	15.0	0	35	1.0
(*Smucker's Milky Way*)	130	1.0	23.0	4.0	5	50	1.0
(*Smucker's Sunday Syrup 3 Musketeers*)	110	1.0	23.0	2.0	0	60	0

Food and Measure	cal.	prot. (gms)	carbo. (gms)	fat (gms)	chol. (mgs)	sod. (mgs)	fiber (gms)
Tortellini (see also "Tortelloni"), frozen or refrigerated, 1 cup, except as noted:							
cheese:							
mixed (*Buitoni*) ...	320	15.0	50.0	7.0	50	500	3.0
three (*Buitoni*)	320	15.0	50.0	7.0	40	480	3.0
three (*DiGiorno*), ⅓ of 9-oz. pkg. .	250	10.0	41.0	5.0	25	320	2.0
whole wheat pasta (*Moneterey*)	290	13.0	48.0	6.0	35	290	5.0
herb chicken (*Buitoni*)	340	13.0	52.0	9.0	40	410	2.0
olive, Sicilian, lemon (*Cafferata* Olota) ...	218	7.0	43.0	2.0	0	320	1.0
spinach and cheese (*Buitoni*)	330	15.0	49.0	8.0	55	510	3.0
Tortellini, pkg. (see also "Tortelloni"), ⅔ cup:							
cheese, 3 (*Barilla*) ...	230	8.0	33.0	8.0	40	480	3.0
cheese and spinach (*Barilla*)	230	8.0	32.0	7.0	35	340	3.0
Tortellini entree, frozen, pesto (*Amy's* Bowls), 9.5-oz. pkg.	470	18.0	58.0	19.0	40	640	3.0
Tortellini entree, pkg., cheese (*Hormel* Pasta Cup), 1 cont.	170	7.0	23.0	6.0	10	720	2.0
Tortelloni, frozen or refrigerated (see also "Tortellini"), 1 cup, except as noted							
cheese/roasted garlic (*Buitoni*)	270	12.0	37.0	8.0	35	360	2.0
chicken/proscuitto (*Buitoni*)	330	14.0	47.0	9.0	45	630	2.0
mozzarella/herb (*Buitoni*)	330	14.0	46.0	10.0	45	450	2.0
mozzarella/pepperoni (*Buitoni*)	330	15.0	45.0	10.0	45	440	2.0
portobello/cheese (*Buitoni*)	270	9.0	46.0	6.0	25	400	3.0

Food and Measure	cal.	prot. (gms)	carbo. (gms)	fat (gms)	chol. (mgs)	sod. (mgs)	fiber (gms)
sausage, sweet Italian (*Buitoni*)	330	13.0	48.0	9.0	35	280	3.0
spinach/cheese (*Monterey Carb Smart*), 3.5 oz. ...	230	16.0	21.0	9.0	115	500	6.0
tomato, sun-dried (*Buitoni*)	310	12.0	46.0	9.0	25	340	3.0
Tortelloni, pkg. (see also "Tortellini"), ¾ cup:							
cheese/garlic (*Barilla*)	230	8.0	31.0	8.0	60	450	4.0
porcini mushroom (*Barilla*)	240	8.0	32.0	8.0	60	350	5.0
ricotta/asparagus (*Barilla*)	240	7.0	32.0	8.0	55	450	4.0
ricotta/spinach (*Barilla*)	230	8.0	32.0	8.0	60	340	4.0
Tortilla (see also "Wraps"):							
corn, 2 pcs., 1.7 oz.:							
(*Garden of Eatin' Corntillas*)	120	3.0	29.0	1.5	0	0	5.0
blue (*Garden of Eatin'*)	110	3.0	22.0	1.5	0	0	2.0
flour:							
for burritos (*Old El Paso*), 1.4-oz. pc.	130	3.0	21.0	4.0	0	310	0
for soft tacos (*Old El Paso*), 1.8-oz. pc.	160	3.0	26.0	4.5	0	370	0
for soft tacos (*Taco Bell*), 2 pcs., 2.1 oz.	200	4.0	32.0	5.0	0	450	1.0
whole wheat (*Garden of Eatin'*), 1.7 oz.	140	4.0	22.0	3.0	0	170	2.0
Tortilla chips, see "Corn chips/crisps"							
Tostada shell (see also "Taco shell"):							
(*Old El Paso*), 3 pcs. .	150	2.0	20.0	7.0	0	135	1.0
(*Zapata*), 2 pcs.	110	2.0	14.0	5.0	0	5	1.0
Triple sec (*Angostura*), 1 tsp.	15	0	0	0	0	390	0
Trail mix:							
(*California Trail Mix*), ¼ cup, 1 oz.	110	1.0	18.0	4.5	0	0	2.0

Food and Measure	cal.	prot. (gms)	carbo. (gms)	fat (gms)	chol. (mgs)	sod. (mgs)	fiber (gms)
Trail mix *(cont.)*							
(*Cape Cod Cranberry Trail Mix*), ¼ cup, 1.1 oz.	130	2.0	17.0	7.0	0	15	2.0
(*Eden* All Mixed Up), 3 tbsp.	160	8.0	7.0	12.0	0	70	4.0
(*Eden* All Mixed Up Too), 3 tbsp.	140	5.0	10.0	11.0	0	15	4.0
(*GeniSoy* Happy Trails), 1 oz.	130	4.0	17.0	6.0	0	50	2.0
(*GeniSoy* Mountain Medley), 1 oz.	130	4.0	16.0	6.0	0	120	2.0
(*GeniSoy* Tropical Paradise), 1 oz. ...	119	3.0	18.0	4.0	0	90	2.0
(*Happy Trails Mix*), ¼ cup, 1.2 oz.	150	4.0	16.0	9.0	0	20	3.0
(*Kettle* Camping Mix), 1 oz.	140	4.0	11.0	10.0	0	0	2.0
(*Kettle* Chocolate Lovers Mix), 1 oz. .	130	3.0	16.0	7.0	0	10	2.0
(*Kettle* Deluxe Mix), 1 oz.	170	5.0	6.0	16.0	0	65	2.0
(*Kettle* Honey Cranberry Mix), 1 oz. ..	120	3.0	16.0	6.0	0	20	2.0
(*Kettle* Honey Roast Harvest Mix), 1 oz.	130	3.0	15.0	7.0	0	20	2.0
(*Kettle* Honey Roast Nuts & Fruit), 1 oz.	120	3.0	16.0	6.0	0	55	2.0
(*Kettle* Natural Chocolate Lovers Mix), 1 oz.	120	3.0	15.0	6.0	0	0	2.0
(*Kettle* Raw Hikers Mix), 1 oz.	120	3.0	15.0	6.0	0	0	2.0
(*Kettle* Southwest BBQ Mix), 1 oz.	150	6.0	11.0	10.0	0	200	2.0
(*Kettle* Sporting Mix), 1 oz.	150	5.0	10.0	11.0	0	0	2.0
(*Kettle* Truffle Trail Mix), 1 oz.	120	3.0	17.0	6.0	0	5	2.0
(*Kettle* X-Treme Trail Mix), 1 oz.	150	5.0	9.0	12.0	0	0	2.0
(*New England Naturals* Freedom Trail Mix), 3 tbsp., .9 oz.	130	4.0	10.0	9.0	0	0	1.0

Food and Measure	cal.	prot. (gms)	carbo. (gms)	fat (gms)	chol. (mgs)	sod. (mgs)	fiber (gms)
(*Organic Chocolate Trail Mix*), 3 tbsp., 1 oz.	140	4.0	14.0	9.0	0	20	2.0
(*Organic Harvest Trail Mix*), ¼ cup, 1.1 oz.	120	2.0	16.0	6.0	0	5	2.0
(*Planters* Fruit & Nut), 1 oz.	130	3.0	14.0	7.0	0	10	1.0
(*Planters Cheese Nips/ Mini Ritz*), 1 oz. . . .	160	5.0	9.0	12.0	0	95	2.0
(*Save the Forest* Fruit & Nut), ¼ cup, 1.1 oz.	130	2.0	19.0	8.0	0	0	2.0
(*Shiloh Farms* Path Finders), ¼ cup . . .	120	2.0	16.0	6.0	0	5	2.0
(*Tree of Life* Everyday), 1.1 oz.	150	4.0	14.0	10.0	0	120	2.0
(*Tree of Life* Organic), ¼ cup	130	4.0	14.0	8.0	0	0	2.0
(*Vanilla Passion Mix*), ¼ cup, 1.1 oz.	150	3.0	19.0	8.0	0	10	1.0
chocolate mix (*Save the Forest*), ¼ cup, 1.2 oz.	160	3.0	18.0	10.0	0	0	2.0
honey nut and caramel (*Planters*), 1.1 oz. .	160	4.0	17.0	9.0	0	160	1.0
macadamia/fruit (*Mauna Loa* Tropical), 1 oz., ¼ cup	180	3.0	23.0	8.0	0	50	2.0
nut and chocolate (*Planters*), 1.2 oz. .	170	11.0	16.0	11.0	0	20	2.0
nuts: seeds, raisins (*Planters*), 1 oz. . .	160	5.0	11.0	12.0	0	15	3.0
spicy, and Cajun sticks (*Planters*), 1 oz.	150	4.0	13.0	10.0	0	250	2.0
soy/mango (*Kettle* Organic Sunrise), 1 oz.	120	5.0	13.0	6.0	0	35	3.0
tropical (*New England Naturals* Delight), 3 tbsp., 1 oz.	120	3.0	16.0	6.0	0	0	2.0
Tree fern, cooked, chopped, ½ cup . . .	28	.2	7.8	.1	0	3	2.6
Triticale, whole grain, 1 cup	646	25.1	138.5	4.0	0	10	34.8

Food and Measure	cal.	prot. (gms)	carbo. (gms)	fat (gms)	chol. (mgs)	sod. (mgs)	fiber (gms)
Triticale flour, whole grain, 1 cup	440	17.1	95.1	2.4	0	3	19.0
Tropical punch, see "Fruit punch"							
Trout, meat only:							
mixed species:							
raw, 4 oz.	168	23.6	0	7.5	66	59	0
baked, broiled, or microwaved, 4 oz.	215	30.2	0	9.6	84	76	0
rainbow, farmed:							
raw, 4 oz.	156	23.7	0	6.1	67	40	0
baked, broiled, or microwaved, 4 oz.	192	27.5	0	8.2	77	48	0
rainbow, wild:							
raw, 4 oz.	135	23.2	0	3.9	67	35	0
baked, broiled, or microwaved, 4 oz.	170	26.0	0	6.6	78	64	0
sea, see "Sea trout"							
Trout, smoked, 2 oz.:							
peppered, rainbow (*Spence & Co.*) ...	100	14.0	0	5.0	30	430	0
rainbow (*Ducktrap River*)	110	14.0	0	6.0	15	590	0
Trout, smoked, spread:							
(*Alaska Smokehouse*), .75 oz.	107	5.0	0	9.0	21	248	0
pâté, ¼ cup:							
(*Ducktrap River*) ..	130	9.0	1.0	10.0	25	380	0
(*Ducktrap River* Lowfat)	70	10.0	1.0	3.0	5	280	0
Trout bean, canned (*Westbrae Natural Organic Heirloom Beans*), ½ cup	100	7.0	18.0	0	0	140	6.0
Tuna, meat only:							
bluefin:							
raw, 4 oz.	163	26.5	0	5.6	43	44	0
baked, broiled, or microwaved, 4 oz.	209	33.9	0	7.1	56	57	0
skipjack:							
raw, 4 oz.	117	25.0	0	1.2	53	42	0
baked, broiled, or microwaved, 4 oz.	150	32.0	0	1.5	68	53	0

Food and Measure	cal.	prot. (gms)	carbo. (gms)	fat (gms)	chol. (mgs)	sod. (mgs)	fiber (gms)
yellowfin:							
raw, 4 oz.	123	26.5	0	1.1	51	42	0
baked, broiled, or							
microwaved, 4 oz.	158	34.0	0	1.4	66	53	0
Tuna, canned, drained,							
2 oz. or ¼ cup,							
except as noted:							
chunk light, in oil:							
(*Bumble Bee*)	110	13.0	0	6.0	30	250	0
(*Bumble Bee/Coral*							
3 oz.), 2.6 oz. . . .	140	15.0	0	8.0	40	350	0
(*Coral*)	110	13.0	0	6.0	30	290	0
chunk light, in water:							
(*Bumble Bee*)	60	13.0	0	.5	30	250	0
(*Bumble Bee* 3 oz.),							
2.6 oz.	70	15.0	0	1.0	40	350	0
(*Bumble Bee* Pouch)	60	13.0	0	.5	30	250	0
(*Bumble Bee "Touch*							
of Lemon")	60	13.0	0	.5	30	250	0
(*Coral*)	60	13.0	0	.5	30	290	0
(*Crown Prince*							
Tongol)	60	14.0	0	0	35	140	0
(*Crown Prince*							
Tongol Low							
Sodium)	60	14.0	0	0	35	50	0
(*StarKist*)	60	13.0	0	.5	30	250	0
(*StarKist* Low							
Sodium)	60	13.0	0	.5	25	100	0
(*StarKist* Pouch) . .	90	19.0	0	1.0	45	380	0
(*StarKist Select/*							
Gourmet's Choice							
Fillet)	60	13.0	0	1.0	30	250	0
wild (*Tree of Life*							
Tongol)	50	12.0	0	0	45	140	0
wild (*Tree of Life*							
Tongol No Salt) .	50	12.0	0	0	45	50	0
chunk white, in oil:							
(*Bumble Bee*							
Albacore)	100	13.0	0	5.0	25	250	0
(*Bumble Bee*							
Albacore 3 oz.),							
2.6 oz.	140	16.0	0	8.0	35	350	0
chunk white, in water:							
(*Bumble Bee*							
Albacore)	60	13.0	0	1.0	25	250	0

Food and Measure	cal.	prot. (gms)	carbo. (gms)	fat (gms)	chol. (mgs)	sod. (mgs)	fiber (gms)
Tuna, canned, chunk white, in water *(cont.)*							
(*Bumble Bee* Albacore 3 oz.), 2.6 oz.	70	16.0	0	1.0	35	350	0
(*Bumble Bee* Albacore Very Low Sodium) . . .	70	15.0	0	1.0	25	35	0
(*Chicken of the Sea*)	60	13.0	0	1.0	25	250	0
hickory smoked (*Star-Kist Tuna Creations* Pouch)	60	13.0	0	1.0	20	280	0
solid light, in olive oil:							
(*Bumble Bee* Tonno)	120	15.0	0	6.0	35	250	0
(*Genova* Tonno) . . .	130	14.0	0	8.0	30	250	0
(*Progresso*)	160	13.0	0	12.0	30	250	0
solid white, Albacore, in oil:							
(*Bumble Bee* Albacore)	90	14.0	0	3.0	25	250	0
(*Bumble Bee* Albacore 3 oz.), 2.7 oz.	130	19.0	0	5.0	35	350	0
solid white, Albacore, in water:							
(*Bumble Bee* 3 oz.), 2.7 oz.	90	20.0	0	1.0	35	350	0
(*Bumble Bee* Pouch)	60	13.0	0	1.0	25	250	0
(*Bumble Bee/Bumble Bee Prime Fillet*)	70	15.0	0	1.0	25	250	0
(*Chicken of the Sea*)	70	15.0	0	1.0	25	250	0
(*Chicken of the Sea* Pouch)	60	13.0	0	1.0	25	250	0
(*Chicken of the Sea*), 3-oz. pouch	100	20.0	0	1.5	40	380	0
(*Crown Prince*) . . .	65	15.0	0	.5	30	150	0
(*Crown Prince* Low Sodium)	65	15.0	0	0	30	80	0
(*StarKist*)	70	15.0	0	1.0	25	250	0
Tuna, freeze-dried, albacore (*AlpineAire*), 1 oz.	110	26.0	0	.5	0	0	0
Tuna, smoked (*Acme*), 2 oz.	70	13.0	2.0	1.0	20	1	0
"Tuna," vegetarian, frozen (*Worthington Tuno*), ½ cup	90	7.0	3.0	6.0	0	300	2.0

Food and Measure	cal.	prot. (gms)	carbo. (gms)	fat (gms)	chol. (mgs)	sod. (mgs)	fiber (gms)
Tuna entree, freeze-dried, w/noodles and cheese (*Alpine-Aire*), 1½ cups	330	17.0	41.0	10.0	20	840	3.0
Tuna entree, frozen, 1 pkg.:							
casserole (*Healthy Choice*), 9 oz.	250	16.0	30.0	7.0	20	600	5.0
noodle:							
casserole (*Stouffer's*), 10 oz.	370	18.0	35.0	17.0	60	1060	2.0
gratin (*Smart Ones*), 9.5 oz.	270	14.0	38.0	7.0	40	640	3.0
Tuna entree, pkg.., albacore steak, 4 oz.:							
ginger and soy (*Bumble Bee*)	170	34.0	3.0	2.5	40	1030	0
lemon cracked pepper (*Bumble Bee*)	160	36.0	0	1.0	50	370	0
mesquite grilled (*Bumble Bee*)	150	35.0	0	1.5	40	370	0
Tuna entree, mix, 1 cup*:							
au gratin (*Tuna Helper*)	310	13.0	38.0	12.0	20	920	1.0
broccoli:							
cheesy (*Tuna Helper*)	300	16.0	38.0	10.0	20	870	1.0
creamy (*Tuna Helper*)	300	13.0	33.0	13.0	15	840	1.0
casserole (*Tuna Helper Oven Favorites Classic*)	290	11.0	37.0	11.0	15	1230	1.0
cheddar, garden (*Tuna Helper*)	290	13.0	36.0	11.0	20	990	1.0
fettuccine Alfredo (*Tuna Helper*)	300	12.0	32.0	14.0	15	900	1.0
melt (*Tuna Helper*) ...	300	12.0	34.0	13.0	20	920	0
Parmesan, creamy (*Tuna Helper*)	260	13.0	32.0	9.0	20	900	0
pasta:							
cheesy (*Tuna Helper*)	270	12.0	31.0	11.0	20	870	1.0
creamy (*Tuna Helper*)	290	12.0	32.0	13.0	15	880	2.0
spirals, creamy (*Annie's Organic Skillet Meal*)	260	18.0	30.0	7.0	80	650	1.0
tetrazzini (*Tuna Helper*)	280	14.0	31.0	12.0	20	900	1.0

Food and Measure	cal.	prot. (gms)	carbo. (gms)	fat (gms)	chol. (mgs)	sod. (mgs)	fiber (gms)
Tuna salad, ⅓ cup:							
(*Wampler*)	180	7.0	9.0	12.0	20	450	1.0
chunky, w/pickle relish							
(*Wampler*)	180	8.0	8.0	13.0	20	380	1.0
Tuna salad kit, w/out crackers, 5 oz.:							
w/mayo/onion (*Chicken of the Sea* Single!) .	380	22.0	18.0	24.0	55	640	1.0
w/salad dressing/sweet relish (*Chicken of the Sea* Single!)	320	22.0	19.0	17.0	50	700	1.0
Tuna salad lunch kit, w/crackers, 1 pkg.:							
(*Bumble Bee*):							
2.9-oz can salad . . .	190	8.0	6.0	16.0	15	270	1.0
6 crackers, .6 oz. . .	90	2.0	12.0	4.5	0	180	0
(*Bumble Bee* Fat Free):							
2.9-oz can salad . . .	70	7.0	10.0	0	20	450	0
6 crackers, .6 oz. . .	80	2.0	14.0	1.5	0	310	1.0
(*Bumble Bee*), w/mayo:							
2.9-oz can tuna . . .	70	15.0	0	1.0	40	358	0
6 crackers, .6 oz. . .	90	2.0	12.0	4.5	0	180	0
mayo, 3.7-oz. pkt. .	260	17.0	12.0	17.0	45	610	0
(*StarKist Lunch To-Go*), 4.5 oz.	210	20.0	27.0	9.0	40	720	1.5
Turban squash (*Frieda's*), ¾ cup, 3 oz.	30	1.0	7.0	0	0	0	1.0
Turbot, European, meat only:							
raw, 4 oz.	108	18.2	0	3.4	54	170	0
baked, broiled, or microwaved, 4 oz. . .	138	23.3	0	4.3	70	218	0
Turkey (see also "Turkey, frozen and refrigerated"), fresh, all classes, roasted:							
meat w/skin, 4 oz. . . .	236	31.9	0	11.0	93	77	0
meat only:							
4 oz.	193	3.2	0	5.6	86	79	0
diced, 1 cup	238	41.0	0	7.0	107	99	0
skin only, 1 oz.	125	5.6	0	11.2	32	15	0
dark meat:							
w/skin, 4 oz.	251	31.2	0	13.1	101	86	0

Food and Measure	cal.	prot. (gms)	carbo. (gms)	fat (gms)	chol. (mgs)	sod. (mgs)	fiber (gms)
meat only, 4 oz. . . .	212	32.4	0	8.2	96	90	0
meat only, diced, 1 cup	262	40.0	0	10.1	119	110	0
light meat:							
w/skin, 4 oz.	223	32.4	0	9.4	86	71	0
meat only, 4 oz. . . .	178	33.9	0	3.7	78	73	0
meat only, diced, 1 cup	219	41.9	0	4.5	97	89	0
breast, meat w/skin:							
½ breast, 1.9 lb., (4.2 lbs. raw w/bone)	1637	248.1	0	64.1	643	541	0
4 oz.	214	32.6	0	8.4	84	71	0
ground, see "Turkey ground"							
leg, meat w/skin:							
1.2 lb. (1.5 lbs. raw w/bone)	1133	152.2	0	53.6	466	420	0
4 oz.	236	31.6	0	11.1	96	87	0
wing, meat w/skin:							
6.6 oz. (9.9 oz. raw w/bone)	426	50.9	0	23.1	150	114	0
4 oz.	260	31.0	0	14.1	92	69	0
Turkey, canned, chunk, 2 oz.:							
(*Hormel*)	60	9.0	0	2.5	35	300	0
white (*Hormel*)	50	9.0	0	1.5	25	250	0
Turkey, freeze-dried, cooked, diced							
(*AlpineAire*), ½ oz. .	60	12.0	0	1.0	45	25	0
Turkey, frozen or re-frigerated, raw, 4 oz., except as noted:							
whole:							
(*Organic Valley*) . . .	190	23.0	0	10.0	70	70	0
(*Shady Brook Farms* Natural)	180	23.0	0	9.0	85	75	0
breast, bone-in:							
(*Shady Brook Farms* Natural)	190	24.0	0	9.0	70	60	0
(*Shady Brook Farms* Natural Hotel Style)	180	24.0	0	9.0	85	65	0

Food and Measure	cal.	prot. (gms)	carbo. (gms)	fat (gms)	chol. (mgs)	sod. (mgs)	fiber (gms)
Turkey, frozen or refrigerated, raw, breast, bone-in *(cont.)*							
split (*Shady Brook Farms* Natural) ..	190	24.0	0	9.0	70	60	0
breast, boneless, skinless:							
(*Organic Valley*) ...	120	28.0	0	.5	70	55	0
chops (*Shady Brook Farms*)	110	25.0	0	.5	65	250	0
cutlets, thin sliced (*Perdue/Perdue Fit & Easy*), 3.3 oz.	100	23.0	0	1.0	50	45	0
cutlets or scallopini cuts (*Shady Brook Farms*)	110	25.0	0	.5	60	240	0
London broil (*Perdue Fit & Easy*)	120	27.0	0	1.0	60	55	0
London broil (*Shady Brook Farms*) ...	130	28.0	0	.5	70	55	0
breast, marinated, rotisserie (*Perdue*) .	170	20.0	2.0	9.0	55	390	0
ground, see "Turkey, ground"							
necks (*Shady Brook Farms*)	150	23.0	0	6.0	90	105	0
tenderloin:							
(*Perdue Fit & Easy*)	120	27.0	0	1.0	60	55	0
(*Shady Brook Farms*)	130	28.0	0	.5	70	55	0
tenderloin, marinated:							
(*Shady Brook Farms Homestyle*)	130	21.0	0	3.5	55	500	0
honey mustard (*Always Tender*) .	120	21.0	4.0	2.0	50	510	0
rotisserie flavor (*Shady Brook Farms*)	130	21.0	0	3.5	50	730	0
teriyaki (*Always Tender*)	130	21.0	6.0	2.0	50	700	0
thighs (*Shady Brook Farms*)	145	20.0	0	7.0	75	0	0
wing portions (*Shady Brook Farms*)	240	23.0	0	16.0	75	60	0
wings (*Shady Brook Farms*)	210	24.0	0	12.0	110	70	0

Food and Measure	cal.	prot. (gms)	carbo. (gms)	fat (gms)	chol. (mgs)	sod. (mgs)	fiber (gms)
Turkey, frozen or re-frigerated, cooked, 3 oz., except as noted:							
whole, unseasoned:							
hen, dark (*Perdue*) .	180	20.0	0	11.0	85	65	0
hen, white (*Perdue*)	150	22.0	0	7.0	65	45	0
tom, dark (*Perdue*)	160	21.0	0	9.0	90	55	0
tom, white (*Perdue*)	140	23.0	0	5.0	65	50	0
whole:							
Cajun style fried (*Shady Brook Farms*)	160	19.0	2.0	7.0	65	880	0
oven roasted (*Shady Brook Farms*) ...	160	19.0	1.0	8.0	65	620	0
whole, smoked (*Shady Brook Farms*)	160	19.0	2.0	8.0	65	930	0
breast, unseasoned:							
whole (*Perdue*) ...	150	22.0	0	7.0	60	40	0
half (*Perdue*)	150	23.0	0	6.0	75	40	0
boneless, skinless (*Perdue Fit & Easy*)	110	26.0	0	.5	60	40	0
cutlet (*Perdue Fit & Easy*), 2.4-oz. pc.	90	20.0	0	.5	45	30	0
breast, in gravy (*Tyson*), 5 oz.	110	20.0	5.0	1.5	35	550	0
breast, marinated, rotisserie (*Perdue*) .	130	18.0	1.0	6.0	55	320	0
breast, oven roasted, bone-in (*Shady Brook Farms*)	160	20.0	1.0	7.0	60	610	0
breast, roasted, carved (*Perdue Short Cuts*), ½ cup, 2.5 oz.	80	16.0	4.0	0	40	570	0
breast, smoked, bone-in (*Shady Brook Farms*)	160	20.0	2.0	7.0	60	900	0
drumettes, roasted, unseasoned (*Perdue*), 3.3-oz. pc.	180	24.0	0	9.0	95	70	0
and gravy (*Hormel*), 5.7 oz.	130	21.0	4.0	3.0	45	1010	4.0
wings, unseasoned (*Perdue*)	160	22.0	0	8.0	90	65	0

Food and Measure	cal.	prot. (gms)	carbo. (gms)	fat (gms)	chol. (mgs)	sod. (mgs)	fiber (gms)
Turkey, ground:							
raw, 4 oz.:							
(*Louis Rich* Pure) . .	190	20.0	0	12.0	90	140	0
(*Shady Brook Farms* 15% Fat)	220	21.0	1.0	15.0	75	75	0
(*Shady Brook Farms* 7% Fat)	160	22.0	0	8.0	80	85	0
(*Wampler* 100%) . .	210	18.0	0	15.0	100	30	0
breast (*Perdue*) . . .	120	27.0	0	1.5	65	60	0
breast (*Shady Brook Farms* 99% Fat Free)	120	28.0	0	.5	70	55	0
lean or burger (*Perdue*)	170	21.0	0	9.0	90	120	0
patties (*Shady Brook Farms*)	170	20.0	0	9.0	90	105	0
patties (*Wampler* 100%)	210	18.0	0	15.0	100	30	0
patties, barbecue flavor (*Wampler*)	220	18.0	3.0	15.0	100	280	0
patties, seasoned (*Wampler*)	180	21.0	1.0	11.0	75	400	0
white (*Shady Brook Farms* 98% Fat Free)	130	26.0	0	2.0	65	70	0
cooked:							
breast (*Perdue*), 3 oz.	110	25.0	0	1.0	50	40	0
burger (*Perdue*), 4 oz.	160	20.0	0	2.5	85	85	0
lean (*Perdue*), 3 oz.	150	20.0	0	9.0	85	85	0
"Turkey," vegetarian:							
canned (*Worthington* Turkee Slices), 3 slices, 3.3 oz. . . .	110	14.0	5.0	12.0	0	530	0
frozen:							
roast (*Quorn*), 1/5 pc.	90	15.0	8.0	2.5	5	360	6.0
slices (*Yves*), 2.2 oz.	90	15.0	4.0	2.0	0	410	2.0
smoked (*Worthington*), 3 slices, 2 oz. . . .	140	10.0	4.0	9.0	0	450	0
Turkey bacon (*Louis Rich*), .5 oz.	35	2.0	0	2.5	15	180	0
Turkey bologna (*Louis Rich/Oscar Mayer* 50% Less Fat), 1 oz.	50	3.0	1.0	4.0	20	270	0

Food and Measure	cal.	prot. (gms)	carbo. (gms)	fat (gms)	chol. (mgs)	sod. (mgs)	fiber (gms)
Turkey burger, see "Turkey, ground"							
Turkey dinner, frozen, breast, 1 pkg.:							
grilled (*Healthy Choice* Dinners), 10 oz. . . .	250	18.0	31.0	5.0	35	600	5.0
roasted:							
(*Healthy Choice* Dinners Traditional), 10.5 oz.	330	21.0	50.0	5.0	35	600	4.0
(*Lean Cuisine Dinner-time Selections*), 14 oz.	340	20.0	50.0	7.0	30	840	6.0
(*Stouffer's* Homestyle Dinners), 16 oz.	450	23.0	60.0	13.0	40	1660	6.0
Turkey entree, can or pkg.:							
and dressing (*Hormel* Bowl), 10 oz.	290	22.0	33.0	8.0	45	1120	3.0
stew (*Dinty Moore* Can), 1 cup	140	10.0	19.0	3.0	20	910	2.0
Turkey entree, freeze-dried, 1 serving:							
(*AlpineAire* Wild Tyme)	370	21.0	47.0	11.0	55	610	7.0
mashed potato and gravy (*AlpineAire*) .	300	13.0	56.0	2.0	35	640	4.0
Romanoff (*AlpineAire*)	340	24.0	35.0	11.0	70	670	2.0
teriyaki (*AlpineAire*) . .	290	16.0	50.0	3.0	40	590	2.0
tetrazzini:							
(*Mountain House* Can), 1 cup	250	14.0	24.0	10.0	35	800	2.0
(*Mountain House* Double), ½ pouch	280	16.0	30.0	10.0	30	930	1.0
(*Mountain House* Single)	350	20.0	37.0	13.0	35	1170	2.0
Turkey entree, frozen, 1 pkg., except as noted:							
glazed tenderloins (*Lean Cuisine* Café Classics), 9 oz.	260	14.0	40.0	5.0	20	660	4.0
medallions, w/mushroom gravy (*Smart Ones* Higher Protein), 9 oz.	200	21.0	10.0	10.0	45	730	3.0

Food and Measure	cal.	prot. (gms)	carbo. (gms)	fat (gms)	chol. (mgs)	sod. (mgs)	fiber (gms)
Turkey entree, frozen *(cont.)*							
pie/pot pie:							
(*Boston Market*),							
1 cup	590	13.0	34.0	39.0	55	1110	2.0
(*Stouffer's*), 10 oz. .	740	25.0	52.0	48.0	60	1260	4.0
(*Stouffer's*), ½ of							
16-oz. pkg.	600	20.0	42.0	39.0	50	1020	3.0
(*Swanson*), 7 oz. . . .	320	9.0	31.0	17.0	30	780	5.0
roasted (*Pepperidge*							
Farm), 1 cup . . .	500	13.0	38.0	33.0	30	890	2.0
roasted:							
(*Lean Cuisine Skillet*							
Sensations 24 oz.),							
6.9 oz.	130	7.0	23.0	1.5	10	450	3.0
breast (*Healthy*							
Choice), 8.5 oz. .	230	18.0	25.0	6.0	35	580	4.0
breast (*Lean Cuisine*							
Café Classics),							
9.75 oz.	270	12.0	51.0	2.5	20	690	3.0
breast (*Stouffer's*							
Homestyle),							
9⅝ oz.	290	16.0	30.0	12.0	45	970	2.0
w/gravy, potato							
(*Michelina's* Au-							
thentico), 8 oz. . .	250	10.0	32.0	9.0	35	980	2.0
medallions (*Smart*							
Ones), 9 oz.	200	12.0	33.0	2.0	20	550	2.0
slow (*Smart Ones*							
Bistro Selections),							
10 oz.	220	18.0	18.0	8.0	50	720	2.0
slow, breast and							
mashed potato							
(*Healthy Choice*),							
8.5 oz.	200	18.0	19.0	5.0	40	600	4.0
and vegetables (*Lean*							
Cuisine Café							
Classics), 8 oz. . .	150	15.0	12.0	5.0	25	650	3.0
stuffed (*Smart Ones*							
Bistro Selections),							
10 oz.	270	13.0	37.0	7.0	30	720	5.0
w/stuffing, gravy:							
(*Glory* Savory							
Singles), 11 oz. .	440	18.0	49.0	18.0	30	1380	2.0

Food and Measure	cal.	prot. (gms)	carbo. (gms)	fat (gms)	chol. (mgs)	sod. (mgs)	fiber (gms)
potato (*Stouffer's Family Style Recipes Thanksgiving Tonight*), ¼ of 37-oz. pkg.	270	14.0	34.0	9.0	45	1020	2.0
stuffing baked (*Swanson*), 13.5 oz.	360	19.0	43.0	12.0	50	1210	3.0
tetrazzini (*Stouffer's*), 10 oz.	370	20.0	33.0	18.0	55	1040	2.0
Turkey fat, 1 tbsp.	115	0	0	12.8	13	0	0
Turkey frankfurter, see "Frankfurter"							
Turkey giblets:							
simmered, 4 oz.	189	30.1	2.4	5.8	474	67	0
simmered, diced, 1 cup	243	38.5	3.0	7.4	606	85	0
Turkey gravy, can or jar, ¼ cup:							
(*Campbell's*)	25	1.0	3.0	1.0	0	270	0
(*Campbell's Fat Free*) .	20	1.0	4.0	0	<5	290	0
(*Pacific Foods*)	25	1.0	4.0	.5	0	230	0
roast, slow:							
(*Franco-American*) .	20	1.0	4.0	.5	<5	320	0
(*Franco-American* Fat Free)	20	1.0	4.0	0	<5	320	0
roasted:							
(*Boston Market*) . .	25	1.0	2.0	1.0	<5	330	0
(*Heinz* Home Style)	20	0	3.0	.5	0	270	0
Turkey gravy mix, ¼ cup*:							
(*Lawry's*)	25	<1.0	4.0	1.0	0	320	0
(*McCormick*)	20-	0	3.0	0	0	350	0
Turkey ham, 2 oz., except as noted:							
(*Healthy Deli*)	80	10.0	2.0	2.5	30	470	0
(*Louis Rich/Oscar Mayer* 50% Less Fat), 1 oz.	35	5.0	1.0	1.5	20	350	0
(*Shady Brook Farms*) .	60	9.0	0	2.0	30	590	0
Black Forest (*Shady Brook Farms*)	70	10.0	3.0	2.5	30	470	0
honey roasted (*Sara Lee*)	70	9.0	2.0	3.0	40	700	0
smoked (*Louis Rich/ Oscar Mayer* 50% Less Fat), 1 oz. . . .	35	5.0	1.0	1.5	20	350	0

Food and Measure	cal.	prot. (gms)	carbo. (gms)	fat (gms)	chol. (mgs)	sod. (mgs)	fiber (gms)
Turkey ham salad (*Wampler*), ⅓ cup .	150	7.0	9.0	10.0	30	500	1.0
Turkey kielbasa, see "Kielbasa"							
Turkey lunch meat (see also "Turkey ham," etc.), breast, 2 oz., except as noted:							
(*Alpine Lace* Fat Free)	50	11.0	1.0	0	25	500	0
(*Boar's Head* Premium 47% Lower Sodium Skin-on)	60	12.0	0	1.5	25	320	0
(*Boar's Head* Premium 47% Lower Sodium Skinless)	60	12.0	0	.5	20	340	0
(*Dietz & Watson* Banquet Cater Style)	60	11.0	1.0	1.0	20	320	0
(*Dietz & Watson* Cater Ready)	50	12.0	1.0	1.0	20	200	0
(*Dietz & Watson* Gourmet/Golden Brown/Homestyle) .	60	11.0	1.0	1.0	20	430	0
(*Dietz & Watson* Gourmet Lite)	50	10.0	0	1.0	20	240	0
(*Dietz & Watson* Gourmet Lite No Salt)	60	14.0	1.0	.5	30	55	0
(*Dietz & Watson* No Salt)	50	13.0	0	.5	30	55	0
(*Dietz & Watson* Santa Fe)	60	12.0	1.0	.5	20	460	0
(*Hansel & Gretel*)	50	7.0	3.0	1.0	15	550	0
(*Hatfield Deli Choice* Premium)	90	18.0	1.0	.5	55	530	0
(*Louis Rich* 98% Fat Free), 1 oz.	30	5.0	1.0	.5	10	320	0
(*Wampler 5 Diamond*)	50	13.0	0	0	30	240	0
(*Wampler 5 Diamond* Skin-on)	70	12.0	0	2.5	35	240	0
(*Wampler 4 Diamond* Skinless)	60	11.0	0	1.5	20	400	0
(*Wampler 4 Diamond* Skinless No Salt) . .	60	12.0	0	0	30	25	0
(*Wampler 3 Diamond* Fat Free)	45	9.0	1.0	0	20	440	0

Food and Measure	cal.	prot. (gms)	carbo. (gms)	fat (gms)	chol. (mgs)	sod. (mgs)	fiber (gms)
braised:							
(*Dietz & Watson* Cater Ready) ...	50	12.0	1.0	1.0	20	200	0
(*Dietz & Watson* Homestyle)	55	11.0	1.0	.5	20	430	0
bacon flavor (*Dietz & Watson* Bacon Lovers)	70	12.0	1.0	2.5	30	430	0
Black Forest:							
(*Boar's Head*)	60	13.0	0	.5	25	360	0
(*Dietz & Watson*) ..	60	11.0	1.0	1.0	20	400	0
(*Wampler Deli Roast Collection*)	60	10.0	2.0	1.5	25	650	0
browned, w/broth (*Healthy Choice*) ..	50	10.0	1.0	1.0	20	400	0
Buffalo style:							
(*Dietz & Watson*) ..	70	11.0	1.0	2.0	30	420	0
(*Williams*)	60	12.0	<1.0	0	30	650	0
Cajun style:							
(*Perdue Carving*) ..	50	9.0	1.0	1.0	20	800	0
oven roasted, smoked (*Boar's Head*)	60	13.0	1.0	.5	25	750	0
garlic herb (*Williams*)	60	11.0	2.0	1.0	40	540	0
honey:							
(*Dietz & Watson*) ..	70	11.0	3.0	1.0	20	400	0
(*Healthy Deli*)	60	10.0	3.0	.5	20	480	0
(*Perdue Carving*) ..	50	10.0	1.0	1.0	20	390	0
barbecue (*Dietz & Watson*)	70	11.0	1.0	2.0	30	400	0
maple (*Dietz & Watson*)	70	11.0	3.0	1.0	20	400	0
maple (*Williams*) ..	60	11.0	1.0	1.0	40	540	0
honey roasted:							
(*Hatfield Deli Choice*)	70	13.0	3.0	0	30	380	0
(*Louis Rich* Fat Free)	60	11.0	3.0	0	20	660	0
(*Sara Lee*)	60	11.0	1.0	.5	20	500	0
(*Sara Lee* Sliced), 2 slices, 1.6 oz. .	50	10.0	1.0	.5	20	410	0
(*Tyson* Box), 5 slices, 1.8 oz.	50	8.0	4.0	1.0	15	590	0
w/cracked pepper (*Shady Brook Farms*)	60	11.0	4.0	0	25	470	0

Food and Measure	cal.	prot. (gms)	carbo. (gms)	fat (gms)	chol. (mgs)	sod. (mgs)	fiber (gms)
Turkey lunch meat *(cont.)*							
Italian style (*Dietz & Watson*)	60	11.0	1.0	1.0	20	430	0
London broil (*Dietz & Watson*)	60	11.0	0	1.0	20	460	0
maple glazed (*Boar's Head Honey Coat*) .	70	14.0	2.0	.5	30	440	0
oil browned:							
(*Wampler 4 Diamond*)	60	10.0	1.0	1.5	25	490	0
(*Wampler 3 Diamond*)	50	12.0	1.0	1.5	20	360	0
skin on (*Wampler 5 Diamond*)	70	11.0	3.0	1.0	15	390	0
skinless (*Wampler 5 Diamond*)	45	9.0	1.0	.5	20	530	0
skinless (*Wampler 3 Diamond*)	45	9.0	1.0	.5	20	530	0
oven browned (*Wampler 4 Diamond*)	50	9.0	1.0	1.0	20	540	0
oven roasted:							
(*Boar's Head* Golden Catering Style) . .	60	13.0	0	1.0	25	170	0
(*Boar's Head Oven-gold* Skin-on) . . .	60	12.0	1.0	1.5	35	360	0
(*Boar's Head Oven-gold* Skinless) . .	60	13.0	0	1.0	20	350	0
(*Dietz & Watson* Oven Classic) . . .	60	11.0	1.0	1.0	20	430	0
(*Healthy Choice* Hearty Slices), 1 oz.	30	5.0	1.0	1.0	15	240	0
(*Healthy Choice* Tub), 5 slices, 1.9 oz. . .	60	9.0	2.0	1.5	25	450	0
(*Healthy Choice Deli Thin*), 4 slices, 1.8 oz.	60	9.0	2.0	1.5	25	450	0
(*Hebrew National* Fat Free)	50	11.0	1.0	.5	20	430	0
(*Louis Rich* Fat Free)	50	11.0	1.0	0	20	660	0
(*Louis Rich Carving Board* 98% Fat Free), 2.3 oz. . . .	70	11.0	3.0	1.5	25	730	0
(*Louis Rich/Oscar Mayer* Fat Free), 1 oz.	25	4.0	1.0	0	10	340	0

Food and Measure	cal.	prot. (gms)	carbo. (gms)	fat (gms)	chol. (mgs)	sod. (mgs)	fiber (gms)
(*Louis Rich/Oscar Mayer* 98% Fat Free), 1 oz.	30	5.0	1.0	.5	10	310	0
(*Oscar Mayer* Deli Style Shaved), 1.8 oz.	50	8.0	2.0	1.0	20	570	0
(*Oscar Mayer* Deli Style Thin Sliced)	60	9.0	2.0	1.0	20	630	0
(*Perdue*)	50	10.0	1.0	1.0	20	420	0
(*Perdue Carving*) . .	70	12.0	1.0	2.0	25	510	0
(*Perdue Healthsense*)	60	10.0	3.0	0	20	290	0
(*Sara Lee*)	60	12.0	0	1.5	25	500	0
(*Sara Lee* Sliced), 2 slices, 1.6 oz. .	45	9.0	2.0	.5	20	470	0
(*Shady Brook Farms* Homestyle)	60	12.0	1.0	0	20	400	0
(*Tyson* Bag), 2 slices, 1.6 oz.	40	8.0	1.0	.5	15	560	0
(*Tyson* Box), 5 slices, 1.8 oz.	50	9.0	1.0	1.0	20	590	0
(*Wampler 3 Diamond*)	50	9.0	1.0	1.0	15	390	0
(*Wampler 2 Diamond*)	50	8.0	1.0	1.5	10	430	0
(*Wampler 1 Diamond*)	50	7.0	1.0	2.0	20	400	0
oil-braised (*Williams*)	70	14.0	0	1.5	35	440	0
rotisserie (*Sara Lee*)	70	11.0	1.0	2.0	25	450	0
skinless (*Healthy Choice* Golden) .	50	10.0	1.0	1.0	20	430	0
white (*Oscar Mayer* 95% Fat Free), 1 oz.	30	4.0	1.0	1.0	10	300	0
pan roasted:							
(*Perdue Carving Classic*)	70	14.0	0	2.0	30	390	0
(*Wampler Deli Roast Collection*)	50	12.0	0	1.0	25	250	0
braised homestyle (*Perdue Carving Classics*)	70	13.0	1.0	2.0	45	360	0
w/broth (*Wampler Deli Roast Collection*)	50	12.0	1.0	0	20	400	0
cracked pepper (*Perdue Carving Classics*)	50	10.0	2.0	0	20	470	0

Food and Measure	cal.	prot. (gms)	carbo. (gms)	fat (gms)	chol. (mgs)	sod. (mgs)	fiber (gms)
Turkey lunch meat, pan roasted *(cont.)*							
skinless (*Perdue Carving Classics*)	60	13.0	0	.5	30	390	0
pepper and garlic (*Dietz & Watson*)	60	11.0	1.0	.5	20	460	0
pepper/peppered:							
(*Sara Lee*)	50	10.0	2.0	0	20	420	0
(*Wampler Del Roast Collection*)	40	8.0	1.0	0	20	520	0
cracked (*Sara Lee*) .	50	11.0	2.0	.5	15	480	0
cracked (*Sara Lee* Sliced), 2 slices, 1.6 oz.	45	9.0	2.0	0	20	380	0
cracked black (*Dietz & Watson*)	60	11.0	1.0	1.0	20	430	0
cracked pepper (*Williams*)	60	12.0	1.0	0	20	450	0
roasted:							
(*Boar's Head Salsalito*)	60	13.0	1.0	.5	25	480	0
(*Hormel*)	50	11.0	0	1.0	25	680	0
(*Sara Lee* Golden) .	50	11.0	0	.5	20	530	0
golden (*Tyson* Bag), 2 slices, 2.25 oz.	70	13.0	2.0	0	35	880	0
rotisserie style (*Wampler Deli Roast Collection*)	50	9.0	1.0	1.5	20	500	0
spiced (*Wampler Deli Roast Collection*) . .	70	16.0	1.0	.5	25	380	0
smoked:							
(*Boar's Head Cracked Pepper Mill*)	60	13.0	0	.5	30	460	0
(*Dietz & Watson* Chef Carved)	60	11.0	1.0	1.0	20	400	0
(*Healthy Choice Deli Thin*), 4 slices, 1.8 oz.	60	9.0	2.0	1.5	25	450	0
(*Healthy Deli* Zero Carb Brick Oven)	50	11.0	0	.5	20	470	0
(*Hormel*)	60	11.0	1.0	1.0	25	700	0
(*Louis Rich Carving Board* 98% Fat Free), 2.3 oz. . . .	70	11.0	3.0	1.5	25	730	0
(*Wampler 4 Diamond*)	60	11.0	2.0	2.0	20	450	0

Food and Measure	cal.	prot. (gms)	carbo. (gms)	fat (gms)	chol. (mgs)	sod. (mgs)	fiber (gms)
(*Wampler 3 Diamond*)	45	8.0	1.0	1.0	15	430	0
(*Wampler 2 Diamond*)	60	8.0	2.0	2.5	20	380	0
(*Wampler 1 Diamond*)	50	8.0	1.0	1.5	20	520	0
hardwood (*Sara Lee*)	60	12.0	1.0	.5	20	550	0
hardwood (*Sara Lee* Sliced), 2 slices, 1.6 oz.	45	9.0	1.0	.5	20	440	0
hickory (*Louis Rich* Fat Free)	50	11.0	1.0	0	25	720	0
hickory (*Louis Rich/ Oscar Mayer* Fat Free), 1 oz.	25	4.0	1.0	0	10	300	0
hickory (*Louis Rich/ Oscar Mayer* 98% Fat Free), 1 oz. ...	30	5.0	1.0	.5	10	260	0
hickory (*Perdue*) ..	60	9.0	1.0	2.5	40	770	0
hickory (*Shady Brook Farms*)	50	10.0	1.0	0	25	470	0
hickory (*Tyson*), 2 slices, 2.25 oz.	70	13.0	1.0	0	90	940	0
hickory, pan roasted (*Perdue Carving Classics*)	70	12.0	1.0	2.5	30	540	0
honey (*Healthy Choice* Heart Slices), 1 oz. ...	35	5.0	1.0	1.0	15	240	0
honey (*Healthy Choice Deli Thin*), 4 slices, 1.8 oz. .	60	9.0	4.0	1.5	25	450	0
honey (*Hormel*) ...	70	11.0	3.0	1.0	25	680	0
honey (*Oscar Mayer* Deli Style Thin Sliced)	60	10.0	2.0	1.0	25	610	0
honey (*Perdue Carving*)	50	10.0	2.0	0	20	510	0
honey (*Tyson*), 2 slices, 2.25 oz.	70	13.0	5.0	0	35	880	0
honey (*Wampler 4 Diamond*)	70	9.0	4.0	2.0	25	560	0
honey (*Wampler 4 Diamond* Petite) .	50	9.0	4.0	0	25	380	0
honey, white lean (*Oscar Mayer*), 1 oz.	35	3.0	2.0	1.5	10	320	0

Food and Measure	cal.	prot. (gms)	carbo. (gms)	fat (gms)	chol. (mgs)	sod. (mgs)	fiber (gms)
Turkey lunch meat, smoked *(cont.)*							
mesquite (*Boar's Head Mesquite Wood Smoked*) .	60	13.0	1.0	.5	25	440	0
mesquite (*Dietz & Watson*)	50	11.0	0	.5	20	390	0
mesquite (*Healthy Choice*)	60	10.0	2.0	1.0	20	360	0
mesquite (*Healthy Choice Deli Thin*), 4 slices, 1.8 oz. . .	60	9.0	2.0	1.5	25	450	0
mesquite (*Oscar Mayer* Deli Style Thin Sliced)	60	10.0	2.0	1.0	25	690	0
mesquite (*Perdue Carving*)	50	10.0	0	1.0	25	510	0
mesquite (*Sara Lee*)	60	12.0	1.0	.5	20	560	0
mesquite, honey (*Wampler 4 Diamond*)	50	8.0	4.0	0	25	380	0
peppercorn (*Dietz & Watson*)	50	12.0	0	.5	20	320	0
skin on (*Wampler 5 Diamond*)	70	12.0	0	2.5	20	420	0
skinless (*Healthy Choice*)	50	10.0	1.0	1.0	20	430	0
white (*Louis Rich* 95% Fat Free), 1 oz.	35	5.0	1.0	1.5	15	280	0
white (*Oscar Mayer* 95% Fat Free), 1 oz.	30	4.0	1.0	1.0	10	320	0
Southwest grilled (*Healthy Choice*) . .	60	11.0	2.0	1.0	20	400	0
Turkey pastrami, 2 oz.:							
(*Boar's Head*)	60	13.0	1.0	.5	25	440	0
(*Dietz & Watson*)	60	12.0	1.0	.5	20	460	0
(*Healthy Deli*)	70	10.0	2.0	2.5	30	480	0
dark (*Perdue*)	70	9.0	2.0	3.0	40	670	0
Turkey pepperoni (*Hormel Pillow Pack*), 17 slices, 1.1 oz. . .	80	9.0	0	4.0	40	600	0
Turkey pie, see "Turkey entree"							

Food and Measure	cal.	prot. (gms)	carbo. (gms)	fat (gms)	chol. (mgs)	sod. (mgs)	fiber (gms)
Turkey pocket, frozen, 4.5-oz. pc.:							
(*Pot Pie Express*)	340	10.0	45.0	18.0	15	840	3.0
bacon club (*Croissant Pockets*)	320	14.0	30.0	15.0	20	750	3.0
broccoli and cheese (*Lean Pockets*)	270	13.0	39.0	7.0	25	530	3.0
and ham w/cheddar (*Lean Pockets*)	280	13.0	43.0	7.0	30	710	3.0
Turkey salami, 1 oz.:							
cooked	56	4.6	.2	3.9	23	285	0
cotto (*Louis Rich 50% Less Fat*)	40	4.0	0	2.5	20	280	0
Turkey sausage, see "Sausage"							
Turkey strips, smoked, 1 oz.:							
peppered (*Pemmican Premium Cut*)	70	10.0	5.0	1.0	25	670	1.0
sweet (*Pemmican Premium Cut*)	70	10.0	5.0	1.0	25	700	0
Turmeric, 1 tsp.	8	.2	1.4	.2	0	1	.5
Turnip:							
raw:							
1 large 6.5 oz.	51	1.7	11.8	.2	0	123	3.3
cubed, ½ cup	18	.6	4.1	.1	0	44	1.2
boiled, drained:							
cubed, ½ cup	16	.6	3.8	.6	0	39	1.6
mashed, ½ cup ...	24	.8	5.6	.9	0	58	2.3
Turnip, frozen, boiled, drained, ½ cup ...	18	1.2	3.4	.2	0	28	1.6
Turnip greens, fresh:							
raw, untrimmed, 1 lb.	85	4.8	18.2	1.0	0	126	7.6
raw, chopped:							
(*Del Monte*), 2 cups	25	1.0	5.0	0	0	30	1.0
(*Glory*), 2 cups ...	20	1.0	5.0	0	0	30	3.0
chopped, ½ cup ...	7	.4	1.6	.1	0	11	.7
boiled, chopped, ½ cup	15	.8	3.1	.2	0	21	2.2
Turnip greens, canned, ½ cup:							
(*Allens* No Salt)	25	2.0	3.0	.5	0	15	2.0
(*Bush's*)	25	2.0	3.0	0	0	300	2.0
w/diced turnip:							
(*Allens* No Salt) ...	30	1.0	5.0	.5	0	20	3.0

Food and Measure	cal.	prot. (gms)	carbo. (gms)	fat (gms)	chol. (mgs)	sod. (mgs)	fiber (gms)
Turnip greens, canned, w/diced turnip							
(*Bush's*)	30	1.0	5.0	0	0	380	2.0
seasoned (*Allens/ Sunshine*)	35	4.0	5.0	.5	0	860	2.0
seasoned (*Glory*) ..	35	2.0	6.0	0	0	430	2.0
seasoned:							
(*Allens/Sunshine*) .	35	4.0	5.0	.5	0	860	2.0
(*Glory*)	45	3.0	6.0	.5	0	630	2.0
(*Sylvia's*)	40	1.0	8.0	0	0	490	3.0
turkey flavor (*Glory*) .	35	3.0	5.0	0	0	540	2.0
Turnip greens, frozen:							
boiled, drained, 1 cup	28	3.4	4.7	.3	0	24	2.9
seasoned (*Glory* Savory Accents), ½ cup ..	45	2.0	8.0	0	0	600	2.0
Turnover, frozen, 1 pc.:							
apple:							
(*Pepperidge Farm*) .	290	4.0	36.0	15.0	0	230	2.0
(*Pillsbury*)	180	2.0	24.0	8.0	0	260	0
blueberry (*Pepperidge Farm*)	280	4.0	33.0	15.0	0	230	1.0
cherry:							
(*Pepperidge Farm*) .	280	4.0	34.0	15.0	0	250	1.0
(*Pillsbury*)	180	2.0	24.0	8.0	0	250	0
peach (*Pepperidge Farm*)	290	4.0	35.0	15.0	0	230	1.0
raspberry (*Pepperidge Farm*)	290	4.0	35.0	15.0	0	230	2.0
Turtle, green, raw, meat only, 4 oz. ...	101	22.5	0	.6	57	68	0

U-V

Food and Measure	cal.	prot. (gms)	carbo. (gms)	fat (gms)	chol. (mgs)	sod. (mgs)	fiber (gms)
Umeboshi plum, (*Eden*), .3-oz. pc.	5	0	1.0	0	0	710	0
Umeboshi plum paste (*Eden*), 1 tsp.	5	0	0	0	0	340	0
Uzbek melon (*Frieda's*), 1 cup, 1.4 oz.	35	1.0	9.0	0	0	15	1.0
Vanilla chai tea, see "Soy beverage"							
Vanilla drink mix (*Nesquik*), 2 tbsp. . .	90	0	21.0	0	0	0	0
Vanilla extract, imitation, 1 tbsp.:							
w/alcohol	31	0	.3	0	0	<1	0
w/out alcohol	7	0	1.8	0	0	<1	0
Vanilla syrup (*Ferrara*), 2 oz.	130	0	32.0	0	0	12	0
Vanilla topping (*Smucker's Plate-Scapers*), 2 tbsp. . . .	110	1.0	24.0	1.0	0	0	0
Veal, meat only, 4 oz.: cubed, lean only,							
braised or stewed .	213	39.6	0	4.9	164	105	0
ground, broiled	195	27.6	0	8.6	117	94	0
leg:							
braised, lean w/fat .	239	41.0	0	7.2	152	76	0
braised, lean only . .	230	41.6	0	5.8	159	76	0
roasted, lean w/fat .	181	31.4	0	5.3	117	77	0
roasted, lean only .	170	31.8	0	3.8	117	77	0
loin:							
braised, lean w/fat .	322	34.2	0	19.5	134	91	0
braised, lean only . .	256	38.1	0	10.4	142	95	0
roasted, lean w/fat .	246	28.1	0	14.0	117	105	0
roasted, lean only .	198	29.8	0	7.9	120	109	0

Food and Measure	cal.	prot. (gms)	carbo. (gms)	fat (gms)	chol. (mgs)	sod. (mgs)	fiber (gms)
Veal (cont.)							
rib:							
braised, lean w/fat .	285	36.8	0	14.2	158	108	0
braised, lean only . .	247	39.1	0	8.9	163	112	0
roasted, lean w/fat .	259	27.2	0	15.8	125	104	0
roasted, lean only .	201	29.2	0	8.4	130	110	0
shank, braised:							
lean w/fat	217	35.8	0	7.0	141	105	0
lean only	201	35.4	0	4.9	143	107	0
shoulder, whole:							
braised, lean w/fat .	259	36.4	0	11.5	143	108	0
braised, lean only . .	226	38.2	0	6.9	147	110	0
roasted, lean w/fat .	209	28.7	0	9.5	128	109	0
roasted, lean only .	193	29.3	0	7.5	129	110	0
shoulder, arm:							
braised, lean w/fat .	268	38.1	0	11.6	168	99	0
braised, lean only . .	228	40.5	0	6.0	176	102	0
roasted, lean w/fat .	208	28.9	0	9.4	122	102	0
roasted, lean only .	186	29.6	0	6.6	124	103	0
shoulder, blade:							
braised, lean w/fat .	255	35.4	0	11.4	174	111	0
braised, lean only . .	224	37.0	0	7.3	179	115	0
roasted, lean w/fat .	211	28.5	0	9.8	133	113	0
roasted, lean only .	194	29.1	0	7.8	135	116	0
sirloin:							
braised, lean w/fat .	286	35.4	0	14.9	122	90	0
braised, lean only . .	231	38.5	0	7.4	128	92	0
roasted, lean w/fat .	229	28.5	0	11.9	116	94	0
roasted, lean only .	191	29.8	0	7.1	118	96	0
Veal dinner, frozen, parmigiana (*Stouffer's* Homestyle Dinners), 17.5-oz. pkg.	490	23.0	62.0	17.0	65	1050	7.0
Veal entree, frozen, parmigiana (*Stouffer's* Homestyle), 11⅝-oz. pkg.	420	22.0	46.0	16.0	60	1050	5.0
Vegetable burger, see "Burger, vegetarian"							
Vegetable chips/crisps (see also specific listings), 1 oz., except as noted:							

Food and Measure	cal.	prot. (gms)	carbo. (gms)	fat (gms)	chol. (mgs)	sod. (mgs)	fiber (gms)
(*Eden/Eden* Wasabi Chips), 1.1 oz.	130	1.0	24.0	4.0	0	260	0
(*Synder's* Crisps)	140	1.0	18.0	7.0	0	290	n.a.
(*Terra* Chips Original) .	140	1.0	18.0	7.0	0	70	3.0
(*Terra Stix*)	150	1.0	16.0	9.0	0	110	3.0
(*Terra* Chips Mediterranean)	140	1.0	18.0	7.0	0	280	4.0
cheddar jalapeño (*Synder's* Crisps) ..	130	1.0	18.0	7.0	0	430	n.a.
mushroom, wild (*Terra Stix* Medley)	150	1.0	16.0	9.0	0	140	3.0
tomato, sun-dried, pesto (*Synder's* Crisps)	130	1.0	18.0	7.0	0	390	n.a.
tomato, zesty (*Terra* Chips)	140	1.0	18.0	7.0	0	230	4.0
twirls: (*Hain PureSnax* Crudités)	120	<1.0	22.0	4.0	0	210	1.0
sour cream and onion (*Hain Pure-Snax* Crudités) ..	120	<1.0	21.0	4.0	0	250	1.0
Vegetable dip (*Cabot Veggie*), 2 tbsp.	50	1.0	2.0	5.0	15	125	0
Vegetable dip mix: (*Fantastic* Soup/Dip), 1½ tsp.	25	1.0	5.0	0	0	480	<1.0
(*McCormick*), ½ tsp. .	5	0	0	0	0	130	0
Vegetable dish, frozen (see also "Vegetable entree, frozen," "Vegetables, mixed, frozen" and specific listings):							
crepes (*Kineret*), 2.2-oz. pc.	100	2.0	13.0	5.0	45	440	1.0
Southern casserole (*Glory* Savory Accents), ½ cup ..	140	2.0	20.0	5.0	15	480	2.0
tomato, okra, corn casserole (*Glory* Savory Accents), ½ cup	110	4.0	14.0	4.5	5	460	2.0

Food and Measure	cal.	prot. (gms)	carbo. (gms)	fat (gms)	chol. (mgs)	sod. (mgs)	fiber (gms)
Vegetable entree, frozen (see also "Vegetable entree mix, frozen," "Vegetarian entree, frozen" and specific listings), 1 pkg., except as noted:							
korma (*Ethnic Gourmet*), 12 oz.	330	8.0	52.0	9.0	0	710	7.0
pie/pot pie:							
(*Amy's*), 7.5 oz. . . .	429	9.0	54.0	19.0	50	590	4.0
(*Amy's* Country), 7.5 oz.	370	12.0	47.0	16.0	40	580	4.0
nondairy (*Amy's*), 7.5 oz.	360	10.0	50.0	13.0	0	590	4.0
stir-fry:							
(*Shanghai* Gourmet), 1 cup	90	3.0	12.0	3.0	0	340	4.0
w/rice (*Michelina's* Zap'ems), 8 oz. .	240	5.0	43.0	4.5	0	1090	3.0
teriyaki, w/rice (*Uncle Ben's* Rice Bowl), 12 oz. . . .	360	8.0	74.0	3.0	0	1350	4.0
wraps, see "Wraps, filled"							
Vegetable entree mix, frozen:							
beefy noodle (*Green Giant Create A Meal!*), 1¼ cups* w/ground beef	350	26.0	31.0	14.0	70	1130	3.0
cheesy pasta vegetable (*Green Giant Create A Meal!*), 1¼ cups* w/ground beef and milk	420	29.0	29.0	21.0	95	1350	2.0
chicken Alfredo (*Green Giant Create A Meal!*), 1¼ cups* w/chicken and milk	400	35.0	36.0	13.0	75	1100	3.0
garlic ginger stir-fry (*Green Giant Create A Meal!*), 1½ cups* w/chicken, oil, and water	270	27.0	25.0	7.0	55	1130	4.0

Food and Measure	cal.	prot. (gms)	carbo. (gms)	fat (gms)	chol. (mgs)	sod. (mgs)	fiber (gms)
garlic herb chicken (*Green Giant Create A Meal!*), 1¼ cups* w/chicken, oil, and water	380	32.0	30.0	15.0	80	870	3.0
lasagna, skillet (*Green Giant Create A Meal!*), 1¼ cups* w/ground beef and water	340	25.0	31.0	13.0	70	830	3.0
lemon pepper chicken (*Green Giant Create A Meal!*), 1⅔ cups* w/chicken and oil ..	310	29.0	30.0	8.0	65	1400	5.0
lo mein stir-fry (*Green Giant Create A Meal!*), 1¾ cups* w/chicken and oil	320	30.0	33.0	7.0	60	920	3.0
Parmesan herb chicken (*Green Giant Create A Meal!*), 1¾ cups* w/chicken and oil ..	340	31.0	29.0	11.0	70	1050	5.0
stew, homestyle (*Green Giant Create A Meal!*), 1 cup* w/ground beef and water	340	24.0	24.0	16.0	70	1370	3.0
sweet and sour (*Green Giant Create A Meal!*), 1¼ cups* w/chicken and oil	340	25.0	43.0	7.0	60	620	3.0
Szechuan stir-fry (*Green Giant Create A Meal!*), 1¼ cups* w/chicken and oil ..	310	26.0	20.0	14.0	60	1390	4.0
teriyaki stir-fry (*Green Giant Create A Meal!*), 1¼ cups* w/chicken and oil	230	27.0	18.0	6.0	55	920	4.0
Vegetable juice, 8 fl. oz., except as noted:							
(*Bolthouse Farms* Vedge)	60	3.0	11.0	0	0	440	2.0
(*Hain* Veggie)	45	2.0	11.0	.5	0	550	0

Food and Measure	cal.	prot. (gms)	carbo. (gms)	fat (gms)	chol. (mgs)	sod. (mgs)	fiber (gms)
Vegetable juice *(cont.)*							
(*Herdez* Original),							
12 fl. oz.	80	2.0	17.0	0	0	1040	2.0
(*Herdez* Picante Limon),							
12 fl. oz.	90	2.0	17.0	0	0	1040	2.0
(*Red Gold*)	50	1.0	11.0	0	0	650	2.0
(*R.W. Knudsen Very*							
Veggie Low Sodium)	50	1.0	11.0	0	0	35	0
(*R.W. Knudsen Very*							
Veggie Original/							
Organic/Spicy)	50	2.0	11.0	0	0	480	2.0
(*Sacramento*)	50	1.0	11.0	0	0	850	2.0
(*V8*)	50	2.0	10.0	0	0	590	2.0
(*V8* Calcium Enriched)	50	2.0	11.0	0	0	460	2.0
(*V8* Essential Anti-							
oxidants)	50	2.0	10.0	0	0	460	2.0
(*V8* Low Sodium)	50	2.0	10.0	0	0	140	2.0
(*Walnut Acres*)	50	2.0	12.0	0	0	580	1.0
cocktail	46	1.5-	11.0	.2	0	653	1.9
lemon twist (*V8*)	50	2.0	10.0	0	0	590	2.0
picante (*V8*)	50	2.0	10.0	.5	0	670	2.0
spicy hot (*V8*)	50	2.0	10.0	0	0	710	2.0
Vegetable oyster, see							
"Salsify"							
Vegetable pie, see							
"Vegetable entree,							
frozen"							
Vegetable pocket/							
sandwich (see also							
specific listings),							
4.5-oz. pc.:							
(*Amy's* Pie)	300	8.0	45.0	9.0	0	490	3.0
and mozzarella (*Smart*							
Ones Smartwich) . .	270	14.0	38.0	7.0	25	600	3.0
roasted (*Amy's*)	220	6.0	35.0	8.0	0	480	4.0
Vegetable protein:							
(*AlpineAire*), 2 oz. . . .	200	30.0	17.0	1.5	0	10	10.0
texturized (*Tree of Life*),							
2.8 oz.	216	41.0	24.0	1.0	0	8	14.0
Vegetable snack rolls							
(see also specific list-							
ings), frozen (*Health*							
is Wealth Munchees),							
2 pcs., 1 oz.	50	2.0	9.0	1.0	0	170	1.0

Food and Measure	cal.	prot. (gms)	carbo. (gms)	fat (gms)	chol. (mgs)	sod. (mgs)	fiber (gms)
Vegetables, see specific listings							
Vegetables, mixed, can or jar, ½ cup, except as noted:							
(*Del Monte*)	40	2.0	8.0	0	0	360	2.0
(*Del Monte* No Salt) . .	40	2.0	8.0	0	0	25	2.0
(*Del Monte Savory Sides* Homestyle Medley)	70	1.0	11.0	2.0	0	380	2.0
(*Freshlike*)	45	1.0	8.0	.5	0	410	2.0
(*Green Giant* Garden Medley)	40	1.0	9.0	0	0	370	1.0
(*S&W*)	45	2.0	10.0	0	0	360	2.0
(*Veg-All* Homestyle Large Cut)	40	1.0	8.0	0	0	350	2.0
(*Veg-All* Original)	40	1.0	8.0	0	0	290	2.0
(*Veg-All* Original No Salt)	40	1.0	8.0	0	0	25	2.0
Cajun (*Veg-All*)	50	2.0	10.0	0	0	410	3.0
w/potato (*Del Monte*) .	45	2.0	10.0	0	0	360	2.0
spiced (*Veg-All* Hot 'n Spicy)	40	1.0	8.0	0	0	370	2.0
stir-fry (*Port Arthur*), ⅓ cup	25	1.0	3.0	.5	0	170	0
Vegetables, mixed, freeze-dried, 1 serving:							
(*AlpineAire*)	30	1.0	6.0	0	0	50	1.0
garden (*AlpineAire*) . .	80	3.0	15.0	1.0	0	55	3.0
Vegetables, mixed, frozen (see also "Vegetable dishes, frozen" and specific vegetable listings):							
(*Birds Eye* Classic), ⅔ cup	60	2.0	12.0	0	0	20	2.0
(*Cascadian Farm*), ⅔ cup	50	2.0	12.0	0	0	50	2.0
(*Cascadian Farm* Gardener's Blend), ¾ cup	50	2.0	11.0	0	0	35	3.0
(*C&W* Fancy Organic), ¾ cup	60	2.0	11.0	0	0	15	2.0

Food and Measure	cal.	prot. (gms)	carbo. (gms)	fat (gms)	chol. (mgs)	sod. (mgs)	fiber (gms)
Vegetables, mixed, frozen *(cont.)*							
(*C&W Farmer's Harvest Fancy*), ¾ cup	60	3.0	11.0	0	0	45	2.0
(*C&W Farmer's Harvest Healthy Garden*), ¾ cup	25	1.0	4.0	0	0	30	2.0
(*C&W Ultimate Petite Mixed Vegetables*), ¾ cup	60	3.0	11.0	0	0	45	2.0
(*C&W The Ultimate Southwest Blend*), ⅔ cup	90	5.0	15.0	1.0	0	25	6.0
(*C&W The Ultimate Stir Fry*), ¾ cup	30	1.0	6.0	0	0	14	1.0
(*Dr. Praeger's*), ⅔ cup	60	3.0	12.0	0	0	85	3.0
(*Green Giant*), ¾ cup	50	2.0	10.0	0	0	40	2.0
(*McKenzie's* Garden Fresh), ⅔ cup	25	2.0	4.0	0	0	25	2.0
(*Tree of Life*), ½ cup .	65	3.0	13.0	0	0	60	3.0
Alfredo, in sauce:							
(*Green Giant*), 1 cup	70	4.0	8.0	2.0	5	360	2.0
(*Green Giant* Boil-in-Bag), ¾ cup	70	4.0	9.0	2.5	5	440	3.0
Asian, in sesame ginger sauce (*Birds Eye*), 1 cup	60	2.0	12.0	1.0	0	630	2.0
California blend (*Cascadian Farm*), ⅔ cup	25	2.0	5.0	0	0	25	2.0
in cheese sauce:							
cheddar, California blend (*Birds Eye*), ½ cup	80	2.0	8.0	4.0	5	390	1.0
winter blend (*Birds Eye*), 1⅓ cups ..	50	3.0	6.0	2.0	0	150	3.0
Chinese stir-fry (*Cascadian Farm*), 1 cup	25	2.0	6.0	0	0	15	2.0
gumbo mix (*McKenzie's*), ⅔ cup	35	1.0	8.0	0	0	30	2.0
Italian style, in oil, garlic (*Green Giant*), 1 cup	90	3.0	6.0	6.0	0	380	2.0

Food and Measure	cal.	prot. (gms)	carbo. (gms)	fat (gms)	chol. (mgs)	sod. (mgs)	fiber (gms)
soup mix, ⅔ cup:							
(*Birds Eye*)	50	1.0	9.0	0	0	60	2.0
(*McKenzie's*)	40	2.0	9.0	0	0	40	2.0
stir-fry, 7 vegetable							
(*Birds Eye*), 1 cup .	30	1.0	5.0	0	0	35	2.0
Szechuan, in sauce:							
(*Green Giant*), ⅔ cup	50	2.0	9.0	.5	0	410	2.0
sesame sauce (*Birds Eye*), 1 cup	60	1.0	9.0	2.0	0	460	2.0
teriyaki (*Green Giant*), 1¼ cups	80	2.0	6.0	5.0	0	490	2.0
Thai stir-fry (*Cascadian Farm*), ¾ cup	35	2.0	7.0	0	0	15	3.0
Tuscan, in herb tomato sauce (*Birds Eye*), 1 cup	50	1.0	7.0	2.0	0	180	2.0
Vegetables, mixed, pickled:							
(*Fanci Food* Giardiniera), ⅓ cup	5	0	1.0	0	0	500	0
(*Krinos*), 3 oz.	0	0	0	0	0	900	2.0
(*Zorba*), ½ cup	20	<1.0	2.0	1.0	0	850	0
hot (*Fanci Food* Medley), ⅓ cup	5	0	1.0	0	0	500	0
Vegetarian dish (see also "Vegetarian entree" and specific listings):							
canned:							
(*Loma Linda* Dinner Cuts), 2 slices, 3.3 oz.	90	18.0	4.0	1.0	0	500	2.0
(*Loma Linda* Tender Bits), 6 pcs., 3 oz.	120	13.0	7.0	4.0	0	440	3.0
(*Loma Linda* Tender Rounds), 6 pcs., 2.8 oz.	120	13.0	6.0	4.5	0	340	1.0
(*Worthington* Choplets), 2 slices, 3.3 oz.	90	18.0	4.0	1.0	0	500	2.0
(*Worthington* Savory Slices), 3 slices, 3 oz.	140	12.0	7.0	8.0	0	420	0

Food and Measure	cal.	prot. (gms)	carbo. (gms)	fat (gms)	chol. (mgs)	sod. (mgs)	fiber (gms)
Vegetarian dish, canned *(cont.)*							
cutlets, multi-grain (*Worthington*), 2 slices, 3.2 oz. . .	100	17.0	5.0	1.0	0	350	3.0
frozen:							
(*Worthington* Dinner Roast), ¾" slice, 3 oz.	180	14.0	6.0	11.0	0	580	3.0
(*Worthington* Fillets), 2 pcs., 3 oz.	180	16.0	8.0	9.0	0	650	4.0
croquettes (*Worthington* Golden), 4 pcs., 3 oz.	210	15.0	14.0	11.0	0	530	2.0
patties (*Worthington* FriPats), 2.3-oz. pc.	130	15.0	5.0	6.0	0	320	3.0
Vegetarian entree, frozen (see also "Vegetable entree, frozen," and specific listings), 1 pkg.:							
nuggets, Hawaiian (*Hain Vegetarian Classics*), 10 oz. . . .	310	13.0	55.0	5.0	0	495	6.0
portobello mushroom barley pilau (*Linda McCartney*), 10 oz.	250	7.0	33.0	6.0	10	920	8.0
teriyaki (*Ethnic Gourmet*), 12 oz. . .	330	7.0	71.0	2.5	0	870	4.0
Vegetarian entree, pkg. (see also specific listings), 1 pkg., except as noted:							
cacciatore (*Linsey Just Add Veggies!*), ¼ pkg.	240	15.0	40.0	2.5	0	320	5.0
curried garbanzos, potatoes, w/rice (*Tamarind Tree* Alu Chole), 9.25 oz. . . .	350	12.0	63.0	6.0	0	620	9.0
peas and cheese, w/rice (*Tasty Bite*), 12 oz. . .	427	18.0	54.0	15.0	13	491	11.0
peas and greens (*Tasty Bite*), ½ of 10-oz pkg.	138	4.0	9.0	10.0	3	417	4.0

Food and Measure	cal.	prot. (gms)	carbo. (gms)	fat (gms)	chol. (mgs)	sod. (mgs)	fiber (gms)
peas, mushrooms, w/rice (*Tamarind Tree* Dhingri Mutter), 9.25 oz.	290	8.0	53.0	5.0	0	680	7.0
pepper steak style (*Linsey Just Add Veggies!*), ¼ pkg. ..	320	15.0	24.0	4.0	0	930	4.0
sprouts curry, w/rice (*Tasty Bite*), 12 oz. ..	363	14.0	63.0	6.0	0	543	12.0
stir-fry, ¼ pkg.:							
Oriental (*Linsey Add Veggies!*) ..	330	15.0	60.0	2.5	0	890	3.0
teriyaki (*Linsey Just Add Veggies!*) ..	340	15.0	66.0	1.0	0	890	3.0
vegetables (*Tasty Bite* Jaipur), ½ of 10-oz. pkg.	169	7.0	10.0	11.0	3	372	4.0
vegetables, w/noodles:							
curry, green (*Tasty Bite*), ⅓ pkg.	150	3.0	30.0	1.5	0	210	0
curry, red (*Tasty Bite*), ⅓ pkg.	160	3.0	31.0	2.5	0	330	<1.0
curry, yellow (*Tasty Bite*), ⅓ pkg. ...	170	3.0	33.0	3.0	0	200	<1.0
vegetables, w/rice:							
(*Tasty Bite* Supreme), 12 oz.	317	11.0	55.0	6.0	4	410	11.0
creamy (*Tamarind Tree* Navratan Korma), 9.25 oz. .	430	12.0	60.0	16.0	5	700	7.0
spicy (*Tamarind Tree* Vegetable Jalfrazi), 9.25 oz.	310	8.0	57.0	6.0	0	600	7.0
Venison, meat only, 4 oz.:							
roasted	179	34.3	0	3.6	127	61	0
ground, pan-broiled ..	212	30.0	0	9.3	111	88	0
Vermicelli entree mix, garlic and olive oil:							
(*Near East*), 2 oz.	250	10.0	48.0	3.0	5	510	3.0
(*Near East*), 1 cup* ..	310	10.0	48.0	9.0	<5	510	3.0
Vienna sausage, see "Sausage, canned"							

Food and Measure	cal.	prot. (gms)	carbo. (gms)	fat (gms)	chol. (mgs)	sod. (mgs)	fiber (gms)
Vine spinach, raw, untrimmed, 1 lb. ..	86	8.2	15.4	1.4	0	109	4.0
Vinegar, 1 tbsp.:							
all varieties:							
(*S&W*)	0	0	0	0	0	0	0
except balsamic							
(*Progresso*)	0	0	0	0	0	0	0
apple cider:							
(*Tree of Life*)	0	0	1.0	0	0	0	0
or red wine (*Eden*) .	0	0	0	0	0	0	0
balsamic:							
(*Hain*)	10	0	2.0	0	0	5	0
(*Pompeian*)	5	0	2.0	0	0	0	0
(*Progresso*)	10	0	2.0	0	0	0	0
(*Regina*)	5	0	2.0	0	0	5	0
(*Zabar's*)	5	0	1.0	0	0	5	0
malt or tarragon (*Fanci Food*)	0	0	0	0	0	0	0
red wine:							
(*Pompeian*)	2	0	0	0	0	0	0
(*Regina*)	0	0	<1.0	0	0	0	0
red or white wine:							
(*Fanci Food*)	0	0	0	0	0	0	0
(*Hain*)	0	0	0	0	0	0	0
rice:							
brown (*Eden*)	2	0	0	0	0	0	0
seasoned (*Marukan*)	25	0	6.0	0	0	520	0
sushi (*Sushi Chef*) . . .	20	0	6.0	0	0	570	0
ume plum (*Eden*), 1 tsp.	2	0	0	0	0	1050	0
white wine:							
(*Regina*)	0	0	<1.0	0	0	0	0
raspberry (*Fanci Food*)	6	0	2.0	0	0	0	0

W

Food and Measure	cal.	prot. (gms)	carbo. (gms)	fat (gms)	chol. (mgs)	sod. (mgs)	fiber (gms)
Waffle, frozen, 2 pcs., except as noted:							
(*Aunt Jemima* Home-style)	190	4.0	32.0	5.0	0	420	1.0
(*Aunt Jemima* Low Fat)	160	4.0	30.0	2.5	<5	420	1.0
(*Eggo* Homestyle) ...	190	5.0	29.0	6.0	20	440	1.0
(*Eggo* Homestyle Minis), 3 sets of 4 pcs. ...	250	7.0	38.0	8.0	30	600	1.0
(*Eggo Froot Loops*) ..	200	4.0	30.0	7.0	15	390	1.0
(*Eggo Special K* 99% Fat Free)	190	8.0	37.0	1.0	0	400	1.0
(*Eggo Special K* Low Carb)	190	15.0	15.0	11.0	0	350	7.0
(*GoLean* Original)	170	8.0	33.0	3.0	0	330	6.0
(*Pillsbury* Homestyle)	170	3.0	29.0	5.0	0	540	<1.0
(*Belgian Chef*)	170	4.0	34.0	2.0	0	420	2.0
apple cinnamon (*Eggo*)	190	4.0	30.0	6.0	15	370	1.0
banana bread (*Eggo*) .	190	5.0	30.0	6.0	0	280	2.0
blueberry:							
(*Aunt Jemima*)	190	4.0	32.0	5.0	5	450	<1.0
(*Eggo*)	190	4.0	30.0	6.0	15	370	1.0
(*GoLean*)	170	8.0	33.0	3.0	0	320	6.0
(*Hungry Jack*)	210	3.0	33.0	7.0	0	540	<1.0
buttermilk:							
(*Aunt Jemima*)	200	5.0	33.0	5.0	5	470	1.0
(*Eggo*)	180	5.0	26.0	6.0	15	420	1.0
(*Pillsbury*)	170	4.0	28.0	5.0	0	480	<1.0
chocolate chip (*Eggo*)	200	4.0	32.0	6.0	15	380	1.0
cinnamon toast (*Eggo*), 3 sets of 4 pcs. ...	270	5.0	46.0	8.0	20	480	1.0
honey oat (*Heart to Heart*)	160	6.0	31.0	3.0	0	370	3.0
strawberry (*Eggo*) ...	190	4.0	32.0	6.0	15	400	1.0

Food and Measure	cal.	prot. (gms)	carbo. (gms)	fat (gms)	chol. (mgs)	sod. (mgs)	fiber (gms)
Waffle *(cont.)*							
whole wheat:							
(*Eggo Nutri-Grain*) .	170	5.0	28.0	5.0	0	420	3.0
(*Eggo Nutri-Grain* Low Fat)	140	5.0	28.0	2.5	0	430	3.0
Waffle, filled, 1 pc.:							
apple cinnamon (*Eggo Waf-fulls*)	150	2.0	25.0	5.0	10	310	<1.0
blueberry or strawberry (*Eggo Waf-fulls*) . . .	150	3.0	25.0	4.5	10	300	<1.0
Waffle mix, see "Pancake mix"							
Waffle sticks, 6 pcs. w/syrup:							
(*Pillsbury* Homestyle)	310	4.0	60.0	6.0	0	650	1.0
blueberry (*Pillsbury*) .	340	4.0	64.0	7.0	0	650	<1.0
chocolate chip (*Pillsbury*)	350	4.0	68.0	7.0	0	630	1.0
cinnamon (*Pillsbury*) .	320	4.0	62.0	6.0	0	620	1.0
Walnut, dried:							
(*Fisher*), 1 oz.	200	5.0	3.0	20.0	0	0	3.0
(*Planters*), 1.2 oz. . . .	210	5.0	6.0	20.0	0	0	2.0
black:							
(*Planters*), 2-oz. pkg.	340	14.0	8.0	31.0	0	0	3.0
shelled, 1 oz.	172	6.9	3.4	16.1	0	<1	1.4
chopped, 1 cup . . .	759	30.4	15.1	70.7	0	2	6.3
English or Persian:							
shelled, 1 oz.	182	4.1	5.2	17.6	0	3	1.4
pcs., 1 cup	770	17.2	22.0	74.2	0	12	5.8
halves, 1 cup	642	14.3	18.3	61.9	0	10	4.8
glazed, see "Candy"							
pieces (*Planters*), 1 oz.	190	4.0	5.0	18.0	0	0	1.0
Walnut topping, in syrup (*Smucker's*), 2 tbsp.	170	2.0	20.0	9.0	0	0	1.0
Wasabi, root, fresh, sliced, ½ cup	71	3.1	15.3	.4	0	11	5.0
Wasabi chips, see "Vegetable chips/ crisps"							
Wasabi powder (*Eden*), 1 tsp.	10	0	1.0	0	0	0	.5
Wasabi sauce, 1 tsp.:							
(*S&B* Tube)	15	0	3.0	.5	0	100	0

Food and Measure	cal.	prot. (gms)	carbo. (gms)	fat (gms)	chol. (mgs)	sod. (mgs)	fiber (gms)
w/ginger (*Gold's*)	15	0	1.0	1.5	5	15	0
Water chestnut, fresh:							
(*Frieda's*), 1 tbsp.,							
1.1 oz.	30	0	7.0	0	0	0	1.0
4 medium, 1.3 oz. ...	35	.5	8.6	<.1	0	5	1.1
sliced, ½ cup	60	.9	14.8	.1	0	9	1.9
Water chestnut, can							
or jar:							
whole:							
(*Port Arthur*), ½ cup	40	1.0	9.0	0	0	25	1.0
4 pcs., 1 oz.	14	.3	3.5	<.1	0	2	.7
sliced, ½ cup:							
w/liquid	35	.5	8.7	<.1	0	6	1.8
Watercress:							
(*Frieda's*), 1 cup, 3 oz.	10	2.0	1.0	0	0	35	2.0
10 sprigs, 11¼" 3	.6	.3	<.1	0	10	.6	
chopped, ½ cup	2	.4	.2	<.1	0	7	.4
Watermelon, fresh:							
1" slice, 10" diam. ...	152	3.0	34.6	2.0	0	10	2.4
diced (*Del Monte*),							
2 cups, 9.9 oz.	80	1.0	27.0	0	0	10	2.0
diced, ½ cup	25	.5	5.7	.3	0	2	.4
yellow seedless							
(*Frieda's*), ½ cup,							
3 oz.	25	1.0	6.0	0	0	0	0
Watermelon drink							
blend, 8 fl. oz.:							
(*AriZona*)	110	0	27.0	0	0	25	0
(*Snapple* What-a-Melon)	90	0	25.0	0	0	40	0
strawberry (*Nantucket*							
Nectars)	120	0	30.0	0	0	5	0
Watermelon juice							
blend (*Juicy Juice*),							
8 fl. oz.	120	0	31.0	0	0	20	0
Watermelon rind,							
pickled, sweet:							
(*Old South*), 2 cubes,							
1 oz.	70	0	17.0	0	0	40	0
(*Reese*), 2 cubes	70	0	17.0	0	0	40	0
Watermelon seeds,							
dried, 1 oz.	158	8.1	4.4	13.5	0	28	n.a.
Wax beans, fresh, see							
"Green bean"							

Food and Measure	cal.	prot. (gms)	carbo. (gms)	fat (gms)	chol. (mgs)	sod. (mgs)	fiber (gms)
Wax beans, canned, golden (*Del Monte*), ½ cup	20	1.0	4.0	0	0	360	2.0
Wax gourd, 1 cup:							
raw, cubed	17	.5	4.0	.3	0	147	3.8
boiled, drained, cubed	23	.7	5.3	.4	0	187	1.8
Welsh rarebit, frozen (*Stouffer's*), ¼ cup .	120	6.0	6.0	8.0	20	280	1.0
Wendy's, 1 serving:							
chicken:							
nuggets, 4 pcs. . . .	180	8.0	10.0	11.0	25	390	0
nuggets, 5 pcs. . . .	220	10.0	13.0	14.0	35	490	0
barbecue sauce .	40	1.0	11.0	0	0	160	0
honey mustard . .	130	0	6.0	12.0	10	220	0
sweet and sour .	45	0	12.0	0	0	120	0
strips, 3 pcs.	410	28.0	33.0	18.0	60	1470	0
chipotle sauce . .	140	0	4.0	13.0	20	170	0
honey mustard . .	170	1.0	6.0	16.0	15	210	0
ranch sauce	200	0	1.0	21.0	20	280	0
sandwiches:							
Big Bacon Classic .	580	35.0	46.0	29.0	95	1300	3.0
cheeseburger, Jr. . .	320	17.0	34.0	13.0	40	810	1.0
w/bacon	380	20.0	34.0	18.0	55	810	2.0
deluxe	360	18.0	37.0	16.0	45	880	2.0
cheeseburger, kids' meal	320	17.0	34.0	13.0	40	810	1.0
chicken fillet:							
homestyle	540	29.0	57.0	22.0	55	1320	2.0
spicy	510	29.0	57.0	19.0	55	1480	2.0
ultimate grill	360	31.0	44.0	7.0	75	1090	2.0
hamburger, Jr.	280	15.0	34.0	9.0	30	600	1.0
hamburger, kids' meal	270	15.0	33.0	9.0	30	600	1.0
Classic Single w/everything . . .	430	25.0	37.0	20.0	65	890	2.0
salad, *Garden Sensations:*							
chicken BLT	330	35.0	10.0	18.0	105	840	4.0
garlic croutons . .	70	2.0	9.0	3.0	0	125	2.0
honey mustard dressing	280	1.0	11.0	26.0	25	350	1.0
chicken strips	440	29.0	33.0	22.0	70	1180	5.0
ranch dressing . .	230	1.0	5.0	23.0	15	580	0
fresh fruit bowl . . .	130	2.0	33.0	0	0	35	3.0

Food and Measure	cal.	prot. (gms)	carbo. (gms)	fat (gms)	chol. (mgs)	sod. (mgs)	fiber (gms)
strawberry yogurt	90	4.0	16.0	1.0	5	50	0
Mandarin Chicken .	170	23.0	17.0	2.0	60	480	4.0
almonds	130	5.0	4.0	11.0	0	70	2.0
noodles	60	1.0	10.0	2.0	0	170	0
sesame dressing	250	1.0	19.0	19.0	0	560	0
spring mix	180	11.0	11.0	11.0	30	220	5.0
honey pecans . . .	130	2.0	5.0	13.0	0	65	2.0
vinaigrette	190	0	8.0	18.0	0	750	0
taco supreme	380	27.0	31.0	17.0	65	1000	9.0
salsa	30	1.0	6.0	0	0	440	0
sour cream	60	1.0	2.0	5.0	20	20	0
taco chips	210	3.0	29.0	9.0	0	240	2.0
salad dressing, light:							
French, fat free	80	0	19.0	0	0	210	0
honey mustard, low							
fat	110	0	21.0	3.0	0	340	0
ranch, reduced fat .	100	1.0	6.0	8.0	15	550	1.0
sides:							
chili, large	330	25.0	35.0	9.0	55	1170	8.0
chili, small	220	17.0	23.0	6.0	35	780	5.0
add cheddar	70	4.0	1.0	6.0	15	110	0
add hot season-							
ing	5	0	2.0	0	0	270	0
add saltines, 2 . .	25	1.0	5.0	.5	0	70	0
fries:							
Biggie	490	5.0	65.0	24.0	0	480	6.0
Great Biggie	590	6.0	77.0	29.0	0	570	7.0
kids meal	280	3.0	37.0	14.0	0	270	3.0
medium	440	5.0	58.0	21.0	0	430	5.0
fruit cup	80	1.0	20.0	0	0	20	2.0
mandarin orange							
cup	80	1.0	20.0	0	0	15	1.0
potato, baked, plain	270	7.0	61.0	0	0	0	7.0
Country Crock							
spread pkt. . . .	60	0	0	7.0	0	115	0
potato, baked, w/:							
bacon/cheese . . .	560	16.0	69.0	25.0	40	850	8.0
broccoli/cheese .	440	10.0	69.0	15.0	10	540	9.0
sour cream/chive	340	8.0	62.0	6.0	10	40	7.0
side salad	35	2.0	7.0	0	0	20	3.0
side salad, Caesar .	70	6.0	3.0	4.5	15	150	2.0
garlic croutons . .	70	2.0	9.0	3.0	0	125	0
Caesar dressing .	150	1.0	1.0	16.0	20	240	0

Food and Measure	cal.	prot. (gms)	carbo. (gms)	fat (gms)	chol. (mgs)	sod. (mgs)	fiber (gms)
Wendy's *(cont.)*							
Frosty cup:							
junior, 6 oz.	160	4.0	28.0	4.0	15	75	0
medium, 16 oz. ...	430	10.0	74.0	11.0	45	200	0
small. 12 oz.	330	8.0	56.0	8.0	35	150	0
Wheat, whole grain:							
(*Arrowhead Mills*),							
¼ cup	150	7.0	31.0	1.0	0	0	5.0
durum, 1 cup	651	26.3	136.6	4.7	0	3	n.a.
hard red:							
(*Shiloh Farms*),							
¼ cup	160	6.0	34.0	1.0	0	0	7.0
spring, 1 cup	632	29.6	130.6	3.7	0	4	24.2
winter, 1 cup	628	24.2	136.7	3.0	0	4	24.2
hard white:							
1 cup	657	21.7	145.7	3.3	0	4	n.a.
spring (*Shiloh*							
Farms), ¼ cup ..	160	5.0	33.0	1.0	0	4	11.0
soft red winter, 1 cup .	556	17.4	124.7	2.6	0	4	21.0
soft white, 1 cup	571	18.0	126.6	3.3	0	3	21.3
Wheat, parboiled, see							
"Bulgur"							
Wheat, sprouted, 1 cup	214	8.1	45.9	1.4	0	18	1.2
Wheat berries, see							
"Wheat kernels"							
Wheat bran (see also							
"Cereal"):							
coarse (*Shiloh Farms*),							
¼ cup	30	2.0	10.0	0	0	0	6.0
crude:							
(*Hodgson Mill*							
Unprocessed),							
¼ cup	30	2.0	10.0	0	0	0	7.0
2 tbsp.	15	1.1	4.5	.3	0	<1	3.0
fine (*Shiloh Farms*),							
¼ cup	30	3.0	7.0	.5	0	0	6.0
toasted (*Kretschmer*),							
¼ cup	30	3.0	10.0	1.0	0	0	7.0
untoasted (*Hodgson*							
Mill), 2 tbsp.	55	4.0	7.0	1.0	0	0	4.0
Wheat flakes, ⅓ cup:							
(*Shiloh Farms*)	110	4.0	24.0	.5	0	0	5.0
rolled (*Arrowhead Mills*)	110	4.0	24.0	.5	0	0	5.0

Food and Measure	cal.	prot. (gms)	carbo. (gms)	fat (gms)	chol. (mgs)	sod. (mgs)	fiber (gms)
Wheat flour (see also specific listings), ¼ cup, except as noted:							
(*Hodgson Mill* 50/50), <¼ cup	100	4.0	21.0	1.0	0	0	2.0
biscuit (*Gold Medal Baker's Blend*)	110	3.0	23.0	0	0	0	1.0
bread:							
(*Gold Medal Baker's Blend*)	120	4.0	25.0	0	0	0	1.0
(*Gold Medal Better for Bread*)	100	4.0	22.0	0	0	0	<1.0
(*Hodgson Mill* Best for Bread)	100	4.0	22.0	0	0	5	1.0
wheat (*Gold Medal Better for Bread*)	100	4.0	21.0	.5	0	0	1.0
cake:							
(*Swans Down*)	100	2.0	22.0	0	0	0	0
1 cup	395	8.9	85.1	.9	0	2	1.8
self-rising (*Presto*) .	90	3.0	20.0	0	0	310	1.0
cookie (*Gold Medal Baker's Blend*)	120	3.0	25.0	0	0	0	1.0
gluten, see "Wheat gluten"							
graham, whole wheat (*Hodgson Mill*), <¼ cup	100	3.0	22.0	1.0	0	0	3.0
pasta, see "Semolina flour"							
pastry:							
(*Arrowhead Mills*), ⅓ cup	110	4.0	23.0	.5	0	0	3.0
whole wheat (*Hodgson Mill*), <¼ cup	110	3.0	22.0	.5	0	0	3.0
seasoned (*Kentucky Kernel*), 4 tsp.	36	1.0	8.0	0	0	544	0
self-rising:							
(*Gold Medal*)	100	3.0	22.0	0	0	400	<1.0
1 cup	442	12.4	92.8	1.2	0	1587	4.0
tortilla mix, 1 cup	449	10.7	74.5	11.8	0	751	n.a.
white, all-purpose:							
(*Gold Medal/Gold Medal* Organic) .	100	3.0	22.0	0	0	0	<1.0

Food and Measure	cal.	prot. (gms)	carbo. (gms)	fat (gms)	chol. (mgs)	sod. (mgs)	fiber (gms)
Wheat flour, white, all-purpose *(cont.)*							
1 cup	455	12.9	95.4	1.2	0	2	3.4
presifted (*Wondra*) .	100	3.0	23.0	0	0	0	<1.0
white, unbleached:							
(*Arrowhead Mills*) .	120	3.0	26.0	.5	0	0	<1.0
(*Hodgson Mill*),							
<¼ cup	100	3.0	23.0	0	0	0	1.0
(*Hodgson Mill*							
Organic)	100	3.0	23.0	0	0	0	1.0
(*Shiloh Farms*),							
⅓ cup	160	5.0	33.0	.5	0	0	0
white, whole wheat							
(*Hodgson Mill*) ...	100	4.0	21.0	.5	0	0	3.0
whole grain, 1 cup ...	407	16.4	87.1	2.2	0	1	15.1
whole wheat:							
(*Arrowhead Mills*) .	130	5.0	26.0	1.0	0	0	4.0
(*Gold Medal*)	90	4.0	21.0	.5	0	0	3.0
(*Shiloh Farms*)	130	5.0	25.0	.5	0	0	4.0
Wheat germ:							
(*Hodgson Mill* Un-							
toasted), 2 tbsp....	55	4.0	7.0	1.0	0	0	4.0
(*Kretschmer*), 2 tbsp.	50	4.0	6.0	1.0	0	0	2.0
crude, 1 oz.	102	6.6	14.7	2.8	0	3	3.7
raw or flake (*Shiloh							
Farms*), 3 tbsp. ...	50	2.0	10.0	.5	0	0	2.0
honey crunch (*Kret-							
schmer*), 1⅔ tbsp.	50	4.0	8.0	1.0	0	0	1.0
toasted:							
(*Shiloh Farms* Glass),							
3 tbsp.	100	9.0	12.0	3.0	0	0	3.0
(*Tree of Life*), 3 tbsp.	100	9.0	12.0	3.0	0	0	3.0
1 oz.	108	8.3	14.1	3.0	0	1	3.7
Wheat gluten, vital:							
(*Hodgson Mill*), 4 tsp.	40	8.0	3.0	0	0	0	1.0
(*Shiloh Farms*), 3 tsp.	36	6.0	1.0	.5	0	11	0
Wheat kernels, ¼ cup:							
(*Purity Foods* Berries)	160	6.0	34.0	1.0	0	0	7.0
(*Shiloh Farms* Soft) ..	160	6.0	35.0	.5	0	0	7.0
Wheat malt syrup, see							
"Malt syrup"							
Wheat pilaf mix:							
(*Near East*), 2 oz.....	170	7.0	40.0	1.0	0	640	9.0
(*Near East*), 1 cup* ..	220	7.0	40.0	4.0	10	690	9.0

Food and Measure	cal.	prot. (gms)	carbo. (gms)	fat (gms)	chol. (mgs)	sod. (mgs)	fiber (gms)
Wheat salad, cracked							
(*Cedar's*), 3.5 oz. ...	150	5.0	26.0	3.0	0	220	2.0
Whelk, meat only:							
raw, 4 oz.	156	27.0	8.8	.5	74	234	0
boiled, steamed, or							
poached, 4 oz.	312	54.1	17.6	.9	147	467	0
Whey, fluid:							
acid, 1 cup	59	1.9	12.6	.2	0	118	0
sweet, 1 cup	66	2.1	12.6	.9	5	132	0
Whipped topping, see							
"Cream topping"							
Whiskey, see "Liquor"							
White bean, mature:							
boiled, ½ cup	125	8.6	22.6	.3	0	6	5.7
small:							
dry (*Jack Rabbit*),							
¼ cup	70	8.0	22.0	0	0	15	14.0
boiled, ½ cup	124	8.7	22.5	.3	0	5	5.6
White bean, canned:							
(*S&W*), ½ cup	80	7.0	19.0	.5	0	440	6.0
w/liquid, ½ cup	153	9.5	28.7	.4	0	595	6.3
Spanish style (*Goya*),							
7.5 oz.	130	13.0	29.0	1.0	0	990	12.0
White Castle, 1 serving:							
breakfast sandwich ..	340	14.0	17.0	25.0	130	900	0
burgers:							
cheeseburger	160	7.0	13.0	9.0	20	360	<1.0
bacon	200	10.0	13.0	12.0	30	500	<1.0
bacon, double ..	360	18.0	20.0	23.0	60	930	1.0
double	290	14.0	19.0	18.0	45	650	1.0
jalapeño	170	8.0	13.0	10.0	25	410	<1.0
hamburger	250	6.0	13.0	7.0	15	240	<1.0
double	250	11.0	19.0	14.0	30	400	1.0
chicken sandwich:							
breast, w/cheese ..	210	13.0	21.0	8.0	25	710	<1.0
ring, w/cheese	190	9.0	17.0	10.0	30	490	<1.0
fish sandwich, w/cheese	180	10.0	18.0	8.0	25	150	<1.0
sides:							
cheese sticks, 5 ...	420	17.0	37.0	23.0	40	1250	2.0
fries	300	4.0	37.0	14.0	0	235	4.0
onion rings, 8	210	2.0	28.0	10.0	0	220	1.0
White sauce mix:							
(*Knorr*), 2 tsp.	25	0	4.0	1.0	0	220	0
(*McCormick*), 2 tsp. .	20	0	3.0	.5	0	300	0

Food and Measure	cal.	prot. (gms)	carbo. (gms)	fat (gms)	chol. (mgs)	sod. (mgs)	fiber (gms)
Whitefish, meat only:							
raw, 4 oz.	153	21.7	0	6.7	68	58	0
baked, broiled, or							
microwaved, 4 oz. .	195	27.7	0	8.5	87	74	0
Whitefish, smoked:							
(*Acme*), 2 oz.	120	10.0	0	9.0	30	340	0
(*Ducktrap River*), 2 oz.	70	12.0	0	2.0	5	730	0
4 oz.	122	26.5	0	1.1	37	1156	0
chubs (*Acme*), 2 oz. .	80	9.0	0	4.5	25	380	0
Whitefish salad,							
smoked (*Acme*),							
4 tbsp.	170	7.0	3.0	14.0	37	345	1.0
Whiting, meat only:							
raw, 4 oz.	102	20.8	0	1.5	76	82	0
baked, broiled, or							
microwaved, 4 oz. .	130	26.6	0	1.9	95	150	0
Wiener, see							
"Frankfurter"							
Wild rice:							
raw, ¼ cup:							
(*Fanci Food*)	170	6.0	35.0	.5	0	0	2.0
(*Lundberg* Organic)	160	6.0	34.0	.5	0	0	3.0
(*Shiloh Farms*)	160	7.0	34.0	0	0	0	3.0
cracked (*Gourmet*							
House)	170	6.0	35.0	0	0	0	2.0
raw, quick, ½ cup:							
(*Fanci Food*)	170	6.0	25.0	0	0	0	2.0
(*Gourmet House*) . .	170	6.0	25.0	0	0	0	2.0
cooked, 1 cup	166	6.5	35.0	.6	0	6	1.5
Wild rice blends, see							
"Rice"							
Wild rice dishes, see							
"Rice dishes"							
Wine, 3.5 fl. oz., except							
as noted:							
dessert or apertif[1] . . .	158	.2	12.2	0	0	9	0
dry or table[2]:							
red	74	.2	1.8	0	0	5	0
rose	73	.2	1.4	0	0	5	0

1. Includes fortified wines containing more than 15% alcohol, such as port, sherry, vermouth, etc.
2. Includes wines containing less than 15% alcohol, such as burgundy, Chablis, champagne, etc.

Food and Measure	cal.	prot. (gms)	carbo. (gms)	fat (gms)	chol. (mgs)	sod. (mgs)	fiber (gms)
white	70	.1	.8	0	0	5	0
sake, 1 fl. oz.	39	.1	.1	0	0	<1	0
Wine, cooking, 2 tbsp., except as noted:							
Burgundy:							
(*Regina*)	25	0	3.0	0	0	190	0
or Chablis (*Fanci Food*)	20	0	0	0	0	150	0
Marsala (*Holland House*)	45	0	4.0	0	0	190	0
red (*Holland House*) .	20	0	1.0	0	0	190	0
rice, 1 tbsp.:							
(*Eden* Marin)	25	0	7.0	0	0	130	0
(*Sun Luck* Mirin) ..	20	0	5.0	0	0	55	0
Sauterne (*Regina*) ...	20	0	3.0	0	0	190	0
sherry:							
(*Fanci Food*)	40	0	2.0	0	0	160	0
(*Holland House*) ...	45	0	5.0	0	0	190	0
(*Regina*)	35	0	5.0	0	0	190	0
white, plain or w/lemon (*Holland House*) ...	20	0	0	0	0	190	0
Wine cooler (*Bartles & Jaymes*), 12 fl. oz.:							
berry, exotic	220	0	34.0	0	0	0	0
blackberry, luscious ..	240	0	40.0	0	0	0	0
blue Hawaiian	240	0	31.0	0	0	0	0
classic original	200	0	29.0	0	0	0	0
fuzzy navel	250	0	43.0	0	0	0	0
kiwi strawberry	230	0	37.0	0	0	0	0
lemonade, hard	240	0	38.0	0	0	0	0
raspberry lemonade, hard	230	0	37.0	0	0	0	0
strawberry daiquiri ...	230	0	38.0	0	0	0	0
tropical burst	240	0	39.0	0	0	0	0
Wing sauce (*Ott's*), 2 tbsp.	15	0	0	1.5	0	400	0
Winged bean, fresh:							
raw, sliced, ½ cup ...	11	1.5	1.0	.2	0	1	n.a.
boiled, drained, ½ cup	12	1.6	1.0	.2	0	1	n.a.
Winged bean, mature:							
dry, ½ cup	372	27.0	38.0	14.9	0	35	14.1
boiled, ½ cup	126	9.1	12.8	5.0	0	11	n.a.
Winged bean leaves, trimmed, 1 oz.	21	1.7	4.0	.3	0	3.	n.a.

Food and Measure	cal.	prot. (gms)	carbo. (gms)	fat (gms)	chol. (mgs)	sod. (mgs)	fiber (gms)
Winged bean tuber, trimmed, 1 oz.	45	3.3	8.0	.3	0	10	n.a.
Winter squash (see also specific listings), all varieties, 1 cup:							
raw, cubed	43	1.7	10.2	.3	0	5	1.7
boiled, drained, cubed	80	1.8	17.9	1.3	0	2	5.7
Winter squash, frozen, ½ cup:							
(*Cascadian Farm*)	70	2.0	19.0	0	0	0	2.0
cooked (*Birds Eye*) . .	45	0	11.0	0	0	0	2.0
Witloof, see "Chicory, witloof"							
Wolf fish, Atlantic, meat only:							
raw, 4 oz.	109	19.9	0	2.7	52	97	0
baked, broiled, or microwaved, 4 oz. .	139	25.4	0	3.5	67	124	0
Wonton wrapper (see also "Wrappers"): (*Frieda's* Fiesta), 4 pcs., 1 oz.	80	3.0	17.0	0	0	160	1.0
Worcestershire sauce: (*Annie's Naturals* Organic), 2 tbsp. . .	20	<1.0	5.0	0	0	460	0
(*Lea & Perrins*), 1 tsp.	5	0	1.0	0	0	65	0
(*World Harbors Angostura*), 1 tbsp.	5	0	1.0	0	0	20	0
white wine (*Lea & Perrins*), 1 tsp.	3	0	.7	0	0	50	0
Wrappers (see also "Egg roll wrapper" and "Wonton wrapper"):							
round (*Azumaya*), 10 pcs.	160	6.0	31.0	.5	10	370	1.0
square (*Azumaya*), 8 pcs.	160	6.0	31.0	.5	10	370	1.0
square, large (*Azumaya*), 3 pcs.	160	6.0	31.0	.5	10	370	1.0
Wraps (see also "Tortilla"), unfilled, 1 pc.:							
(*Cedar's* Low Carb), 1.5 oz.	70	6.0	14.0	1.5	0	320	9.0

Food and Measure	cal.	prot. (gms)	carbo. (gms)	fat (gms)	chol. (mgs)	sod. (mgs)	fiber (gms)
garlic pesto (*Aladdin Gourmet*), 3.5 oz. . . .	310	9.0	53.0	9.0	0	790	5.0
roasted red pepper (*Aladdin* Gourmet), 3.5 oz.	310	9.0	52.0	9.0	0	920	5.0
spinach (*Cedar's*), 2.5 oz.	180	6.0	34.0	3.0	0	380	3.0
wheat:							
(*Cedar's*), 2.5 oz. . .	220	6.0	38.0	4.5	0	460	3.0
(*Sahara*), 2.1 oz. . .	170	5.0	27.0	4.5	0	320	4.0
white:							
(*Cedar's*), 2.5 oz. . .	160	6.0	27.0	3.5	0	380	1.0
(*Sahara*), 2.1 oz. . .	170	5.0	29.0	4.5	0	320	<1.0
Wraps, filled (see also "Breakfast pocket/ sandwich"), frozen, 1 pc.:							
chicken tikka (*Ethnic Gourmet*), 8 oz. . . .	370	23.0	45.0	12.0	25	860	3.0
couscous vegetable (*Cedarlane Veggie Wraps*), 6 oz.	220	14.0	36.0	3.0	0	580	3.0
Indian samosa vege- table (*Amy's*), 5 oz. .	240	8.0	38.0	6.0	0	680	4.0
kung pao tofu (*Ethnic Gourmet*), 8 oz. . . .	410	16.0	48.0	17.0	0	970	4.0
peanut satay, vegetarian (*Ethnic Gourmet*), 8 oz.	420	17.0	49.0	17.0	0	990	6.0
pizza veggie (*Cedarlane Veggie Wraps*), 6 oz.	220	17.0	32.0	3.0	0	520	2.0
vegetable paneer (*Ethnic Gourmet*), 8 oz.	360	14.0	42.0	15.0	5	1060	4.0
vegetable/rice teriyaki (*Cedarlane*), 6 oz. .	320	10.0	56.0	6.0	0	480	2.0
veggie "ham" and cheese (*Cedarlane Veggie Wraps*), 6 oz.	350	29.0	36.0	10.0	15	660	1.0

Y

Food and Measure	cal.	prot. (gms)	carbo. (gms)	fat (gms)	chol. (mgs)	sod. (mgs)	fiber (gms)
Yachtwurst, w/pistachios, cooked, 2 oz.	150	8.3	.8	12.7	36	524	0
Yam (see also "Name yam"), cubed, ½ cup:							
raw	89	1.2	20.9	.1	0	7	3.1
baked or boiled	79	1.0	18.8	.1	0	6	2.7
Yam, canned or frozen, see "Sweet potato"							
Yam, mountain, Hawaiian, ½ cup:							
raw, cubed	46	.9	11.1	.1	0	9	n.a.
steamed, cubed	59	1.2	14.4	.1	0	9	n.a.
Yam bean, tuber:							
raw:							
(*Frieda's* Jicama), ¾ cup, 3 oz.	35	1.0	7.0	0	0	5	1.0
sliced, ½ cup	23	.4	5.3	.1	0	3	2.9
boiled, drained, 4 oz. .	43	.8	10.0	.1	0	5	n.a.
Yard-long bean, fresh:							
raw (*Frieda's* Dow Gok), ¾ cup, 3 oz. .	40	2.0	7.0	0	0	0	0
boiled, drained, sliced, ½ cup	25	1.3	4.8	.1	0	2	n.a.
Yard-long bean, mature:							
dry, ½ cup	292	20.4	52.0	1.1	0	14	4.0
boiled, ½ cup	102	7.1	18.1	.4	0	4	1.4
Yautia root, see "Malanga"							
Yeast, baker's:							
active, dry:							
(*Hodgson Mill*), 5/16 oz.	30	4.0	3.0	0	0	0	1.0
1 tbsp.	35	3.4	4.6	.6	0	6	.3

Food and Measure	cal.	prot. (gms)	carbo. (gms)	fat (gms)	chol. (mgs)	sod. (mgs)	fiber (gms)
compressed, .6-oz. . . .	6	<.1	1.1	0	0	2	<.1
fast rise (*Hodgson Mill*), 5/16 oz.	25	3.0	4.0	0	0	0	1.0
Yellow beans, dried, boiled, ½ cup	127	8.1	22.2	1.0	0	4	9.2
Yellow squash, fresh, see "Crookneck squash"							
Yellow squash, canned sliced (*Sunshine*), ½ cup	25	0	5.0	0	0	160	2.0
Yellowtail, meat only:							
raw, 4 oz.	166	26.3	0	6.0	62	44	0
baked, broiled, or microwaved, 4 oz. . .	212	33.6	0	7.6	81	57	0
Yogurt, 8 oz., except as noted:							
plain:							
(*Cabot* Nonfat)	100	10.0	19.0	0	5	135	0
(*Dannon* Lowfat) . .	160	9.0	14.0	8.0	35	150	0
(*Dannon* Lowfat), 6 oz.	110	9.0	14.0	2.5	15	140	0
(*Dannon* Nonfat), 6 oz.	90	9.0	14.0	0	<5	140	0
(*Darigold* Lowfat) . .	160	14.0	21.0	2.5	15	190	0
(*Stonyfield* Lowfat)	120	10.0	17.0	2.0	10	140	3.0
(*Stonyfield* Lowfat), 6 oz.	90	7.0	13.0	1.5	5	110	2.0
(*Stonyfield* Nonfat) .	110	10.0	18.0	0	0	150	3.0
(*Stonyfield* Nonfat), 6 oz.	80	8.0	14.0	0	0	115	2.0
(*Yoplait* Grande! Nonfat)	130	15.0	19.0	0	5	220	0
all flavors:							
(*Dannon* Natural Flavors), 6 oz. . .	150	7.0	26.0	2.5	10	115	0
(*Dannon* Light'n Fit Carb Control), 4 oz.	60	5.0	3.0	3.0	10	30	0
(*Dannon* Sprinkl'ins), 4.1 oz.	120	4.0	22.0	1.5	5	65	0
(*Trix*), 4 oz.	120	4.0	23.0	1.5	5	55	0
(*Yoplait* Thick & Creamy), 6 oz. . .	190	7.0	32.0	3.5	15	100	0

Food and Measure	cal.	prot. (gms)	carbo. (gms)	fat (gms)	chol. (mgs)	sod. (mgs)	fiber (gms)
Yogurt, all flavors *(cont.)*							
except banana/ Boston/lemon cream pie, and vanilla (*Yoplait* Light), 6 oz.	100	5.0	19.0	0	<5	85	0
except coconut crème pie, lemon, and piña colada (*Yoplait*), 6 oz. ...	170	5.0	33.0	1.5	10	80	0
except raspberry and key lime (*Dannon Light 'n Fit* Creamy), 6 oz.	100	8.0	16.0	0	<5	125	0
all fruit flavors:							
(*Danimals XL*), 5.75 oz.	170	7.0	29.0	3.0	15	105	0
(*Dannon Light 'n Fit* with Fiber), 4 oz.	70	4.0	13.0	0	<5	55	3.0
(*Go-Gurt*), 2.25 oz.	80	2.0	13.0	2.0	5	40	0
(*Yoplait* Light 6-Pack), 4 oz.	70	4.0	13.0	0	0	60	0
(*Yoplait* 99% Fat Free 6-Pack), 4 oz.	110	4.0	22.0	1.0	5	55	0
(*Yoplait Ultra*), 6 oz.	90	8.0	8.0	2.5	15	45	0
(*Yoplait Whips*), 4 oz.	140	5.0	25.0	2.5	10	75	0
(*Yumsters*), 4 oz. ...	120	5.0	21.0	2.0	10	60	0
except berry-banana (*Cabot* Nonfat) ..	130	8.0	24.0	0	5	115	0
except strawberry banana/cheesecake and raspberries and cream (*Breyers* Light Nonfat)	120	8.0	22.0	0	10	105	0
apple cinnamon (*Dannon* Fruit on the Bottom), 6 oz.	160	6.0	31.0	1.5	10	170	<1.0
apple cobbler (*Breyers* Smooth & Creamy)	230	7.0	46.0	2.0	20	120	0
apricot-mango:							
(*Darigold* Lowfat) ..	240	10.0	45.0	2.5	15	130	0

Food and Measure	cal.	prot. (gms)	carbo. (gms)	fat (gms)	chol. (mgs)	sod. (mgs)	fiber (gms)
(*Stonyfield* Nonfat), 6 oz.	130	6.0	26.0	0	0	100	2.0
banana cream:							
(*la Crème*), 4 oz. . .	150	5.0	21.0	5.0	20	80	0
pie (*Yoplait* Light), 6 oz.	110	6.0	20.0	0	<5	90	0
banana vanilla (*Stony-field* Lowfat Banilla)	200	8.0	38.0	2.5	10	130	4.0
berry:							
(*Stonyfield* Nonfat Bash), 6 oz.	130	6.0	25.0	0	0	115	2.0
mixed (*Breyers* Fruit on the Bottom) . .	240	9.0	46.0	2.0	20	130	0
mixed (*Dannon* Fruit on the Bottom), 6 oz.	150	6.0	28.0	1.5	10	135	0
berry-banana (*Cabot* Nonfat)	130	8.0	24.0	0	10	120	0
blackberry, 6 oz.:							
(*Stonyfield* Nonfat) .	140	7.0	29.0	0	0	120	2.0
pie (*Dannon* Light 'n Fit)	90	6.0	16.0	0	<5	95	0
blueberries and cream (*Breyers* Creme Savers*)	240	7.0	45.0	3.0	25	110	0
blueberry:							
(*Breyers* Fruit on the Bottom)	230	9.0	44.0	2.0	20	130	0
(*Dannon* Fruit on the Bottom), 6 oz. . .	150	6.0	29.0	1.5	10	105	0
(*Dannon* Creamy Fruit Blends), 6 oz.	170	6.0	33.0	2.0	10	105	0
(*Dannon* Light 'n Fit), 6 oz.	90	6.0	17.0	0	<5	95	0
(*Darigold* Lowfat) . .	240	10.0	45.0	2.5	15	150	0
(*Hood Carb Count-down*), 6 oz.	80	12.0	4.0	1.5	10	80	0
(*Stonyfield* Lowfat), 6 oz.	130	6.0	25.0	1.5	5	95	2.0
(*Stonyfield* Nonfat), 6 oz.	130	6.0	26.0	0	0	100	2.0
Boston crème pie (*Yoplait* Light), 6 oz.	110	6.0	20.0	0	<5	90	0

Food and Measure	cal.	prot. (gms)	carbo. (gms)	fat (gms)	chol. (mgs)	sod. (mgs)	fiber (gms)
Yogurt *(cont.)*							
boysenberry:							
(*Dannon* Fruit on the							
Bottom), 6 oz. ..	150	6.0	28.0	1.5	10	120	0
(*Darigold* Lowfat) ..	240	10.0	45.0	2.5	15	170	0
caramel (*Stonyfield*							
Lowfat), 6 oz.	190	6.0	38.0	1.5	5	140	2.0
cherry:							
(*Dannon* Fruit on the							
Bottom), 6 oz. ..	150	6.0	29.0	1.5	10	150	<1.0
(*Dannon* Creamy							
Fruit Blends), 6 oz.	170	6.0	31.0	2.0	10	115	0
(*Darigold* Lowfat) ..	240	10.0	44.0	2.5	15	150	0
black (*Breyers* Fruit							
on the Bottom) ..	240	9.0	46.0	2.0	20	130	0
black (*Stonyfield*							
Nonfat), 6 oz.	130	6.0	26.0	0	0	105	2.0
cherry parfait, black:							
(*Breyers* Smooth &							
Creamy Classic) .	230	7.0	46.0	2.0	20	110	0
(*Breyers* Smooth &							
Creamy Classic),							
4 oz.	110	4.0	23.0	1.0	10	55	0
cherry vanilla (*Dannon*							
Light 'n Fit), 6 oz. .	90	6.0	17.0	0	<5	95	0
chocolate (*Stonyfield*							
Nonfat Underground),							
6 oz.	180	7.0	29.0	0	0	105	2.0
chocolate, white,							
raspberry (*Dannon*							
Light 'n Fit), 6 oz. .	90	6.0	16.0	0	<5	95	0
coconut crème pie							
(*Yoplait*), 6 oz.	170	5.0	34.0	3.0	10	85	0
coffee (*Dannon* Natural),							
6 oz.	150	7.0	26.0	2.5	10	115	0
lemon:							
(*Stonyfield* Low Fat							
Luscious), 6 oz. . .	140	6.0	25.0	1.5	5	120	3.0
(*Stonyfield* Nonfat							
Lotsa), 6 oz.	140	7.0	28.0	0	0	115	2.0
(*Yoplait* Burst), 6 oz.	180	5.0	36.0	1.5	10	80	0
chiffon (*Dannon*							
Light 'n Fit), 6 oz.	90	6.0	16.0	0	<5	95	0

Food and Measure	cal.	prot. (gms)	carbo. (gms)	fat (gms)	chol. (mgs)	sod. (mgs)	fiber (gms)
creme pie (*Yoplait* Light), 6 oz.	110	6.0	20.0	0	<5	90	0
lime, key, 6 oz.:							
(*Dannon Light 'n Fit* Creamy)	100	8.0	16.0	0	<5	140	0
(*Stonyfield* Nonfat) .	140	7.0	29.0	0	0	120	2.0
maple vanilla (*Stonyfield* Lowfat), 6 oz. .	130	7.0	23.0	1.5	5	100	2.0
mocha latte (*Stonyfield* Lowfat), 6 oz.	140	7.0	25.0	1.5	5	105	2.0
orange:							
(*la Crème* Mousse), 2.6 oz.	120	3.0	15.0	5.0	20	60	0
and cream (*Breyers* Creme Savers) . .	240	7.0	45.0	3.0	25	230	0
orange mango (*Dannon Light 'n Fit*), 6 oz. .	90	6.0	16.0	0	<5	95	0
peach:							
(*Breyers* Fruit on the Bottom)	230	9.0	45.0	2.0	20	130	0
(*la Crème*), 4 oz. . .	150	5.0	21.0	5.0	20	80	0
(*Dannon* Fruit on the Bottom), 6 oz. . .	150	6.0	29.0	1.5	10	100	0
(*Dannon Creamy Fruit Blends*), 6 oz.	170	6.0	33.0	2.0	10	130	0
(*Dannon Light 'n Fit*), 6 oz.	90	6.0	16.0	0	<5	95	0
(*Darigold* Lowfat) . .	240	10.0	45.0	2.5	15	150	0
(*Stonyfield* Lowfat), 6 oz.	130	6.0	25.0	1.5	5	95	2.0
(*Stonyfield* Nonfat), 6 oz.	120	6.0	25.0	0	0	120	2.0
peaches and cream:							
(*Breyers* Smooth & Creamy Classic) .	240	7.0	48.0	2.0	20	105	0
(*Breyers* Smooth & Creamy Classic), 4 oz.	120	3.0	24.0	1.0	10	55	0
(*Breyers* Creme Savers)	240	7.0	45.0	3.0	25	110	0
piña colada (*Yoplait*), 6 oz.	170	5.0	33.0	2.0	10	95	0
pineapple (*Breyers* Fruit on the Bottom)	230	9.0	46.0	2.0	20	130	0

Yogurt *(cont.)*

Food and Measure	cal.	prot. (gms)	carbo. (gms)	fat (gms)	chol. (mgs)	sod. (mgs)	fiber (gms)
raspberries and cream:							
(*Breyers* Light Nonfat)	120	8.0	22.0	0	10	120	0
(*Breyers* Smooth & Creamy Classic) .	240	7.0	48.0	2.0	20	115	0
(*Breyers* Smooth & Creamy Classic), 4 oz.	120	3.0	24.0	1.0	10	55	0
(*Breyers* Creme Savers)	240	7.0	45.0	3.0	25	240	0
raspberry:							
(*Breyers* Fruit on the Bottom)	240	9.0	46.0	2.0	20	130	0
(*la Crème*), 4 oz. . .	140	5.0	20.0	5.0	20	85	0
(*Dannon* Fruit on the Bottom), 6 oz. . .	150	6.0	29.0	1.5	10	130	0
(*Dannon Creamy Fruit Blends*), 6 oz.	170	6.0	32.0	2.0	10	110	<1.0
(*Dannon Light 'n Fit*), 6 oz.	90	6.0	16.0	0	<5	140	0
(*Dannon Light 'n Fit Creamy*), 6 oz. . .	100	8.0	17.0	0	<5	130	0
(*Darigold* Lowfat) . .	240	10.0	44.0	2.5	15	150	0
(*Hood Carb Countdown*), 6 oz.	90	12.0	4.0	1.5	10	80	0
(*Stonyfield* Lowfat), 6 oz.	130	6.0	25.0	1.5	5	105	3.0
(*Stonyfield* Nonfat), 6 oz.	130	6.0	25.0	0	0	100	2.0
raspberry lemon (*Darigold* Lowfat) . .	240	10.0	45.0	2.5	15	130	0
strawberries and cream:							
(*Breyers* Smooth & Creamy Classic), 4 oz.	120	3.0	24.0	1.0	10	50	0
(*Breyers* Creme Savers)	240	7.0	45.0	3.0	25	240	0
strawberry:							
(*Breyers* Fruit on the Bottom)	240	9.0	46.0	2.0	20	130	0
(*Breyers* Smooth & Creamy Classic) .	230	7.0	46.0	2.0	20	105	0
(*Breyers* Smooth & Creamy Classic), 4 oz.	115	4.0	23.0	1.0	10	50	0

Food and Measure	cal.	prot. (gms)	carbo. (gms)	fat (gms)	chol. (mgs)	sod. (mgs)	fiber (gms)
(*la Crème*), 4 oz. ..	140	5.0	20.0	5.0	20	75	0
(*la Crème* Mousse), 2.6 oz.	120	3.0	15.0	5.0	20	55	0
(*Dannon* Fruit on the Bottom), 6 oz. ..	160	6.0	30.0	1.5	10	130	0
(*Dannon Creamy Fruit Blends*), 6 oz.	170	6.0	31.0	2.0	10	115	0
(*Dannon Light 'n Fit*), 6 oz.	90	6.0	17.0	0	<5	120	0
(*Darigold* Lowfat) ..	240	10.0	45.0	2.5	15	150	0
(*Hood Carb Countdown*), 6 oz.	80	12.0	4.0	1.5	10	80	0
(*Stonyfield* Lowfat)	120	10.0	17.0	2.0	10	140	3.0
(*Stonyfield* Lowfat), 6 oz.	130	6.0	25.0	1.5	5	95	2.0
(*Stonyfield* Nonfat) .	180	9.0	36.0	0	0	150	3.0
(*Stonyfield* Nonfat), 6 oz.	130	6.0	26.0	0	0	130	2.0
(*Yoplait* Grande! 99% Fat Free)	250	9.0	48.0	2.5	15	130	0
strawberry banana:							
(*Breyers* Fruit on the Bottom)	240	9.0	46.0	2.0	20	130	0
(*Breyers* Light Nonfat)	120	8.0	22.0	0	10	115	0
(*Breyers* Smooth & Creamy Classic) .	240	7.0	49.0	2.0	20	100	0
(*Breyers* Smooth & Creamy Classic), 4 oz.	120	3.0	24.0	1.0	10	50	0
(*Dannon* Fruit on the Bottom), 6 oz. ..	160	6.0	30.0	1.5	10	105	0
(*Dannon Creamy Fruit Blends*), 6 oz.	170	6.0	32.0	2.0	10	100	0
(*Dannon Light 'n Fit*), 6 oz.	90	6.0	17.0	0	<5	105	0
(*Darigold* Lowfat) ..	240	10.0	46.0	2.5	15	130	0
(*Hood Carb Countdown*), 6 oz.	80	12.0	4.0	1.5	10	80	0
strawberry cheesecake:							
(*Breyers* Light Nonfat)	120	8.0	22.0	0	10	115	0
(*Breyers* Smooth & Creamy)	230	7.0	47.0	2.0	20	105	0

Food and Measure	cal.	prot. (gms)	carbo. (gms)	fat (gms)	chol. (mgs)	sod. (mgs)	fiber (gms)
Yogurt, strawberry cheesecake *(cont.)*							
(*Stonyfield* Nonfat), 6 oz.	140	7.0	29.0	0	0	120	2.0
strawberry kiwi:							
(*Dannon Light 'n Fit*), 6 oz.	90	6.0	17.0	0	<5	105	0
(*Darigold* Lowfat)	240	10.0	45.0	2.5	15	150	0
vanilla:							
(*Breyers* Smooth & Creamy)	240	7.0	47.0	2.0	20	105	0
(*Cabot* Nonfat)	130	8.0	24.0	0	10	115	0
(*la Crème*), 4 oz. . .	140	5.0	20.0	5.0	20	75	0
(*Dannon Light 'n Fit*), 6 oz.	90	6.0	16.0	0	<5	95	0
(*Darigold* Lowfat) . .	240	10.0	45.0	2.5	15	150	0
(*Stonyfield* Lowfat)	190	9.0	34.0	2.0	10	135	3.0
(*Stonyfield* Lowfat), 6 oz.	140	7.0	25.0	1.5	5	100	2.0
(*Yoplait* Grande! 99% Fat Free)	250	9.0	48.0	2.5	15	130	0
(*Yoplait* Light Very), 6 oz.	110	6.0	20.0	0	<5	90	0
vanilla, French:							
(*la Crème* Mousse), 2.6 oz.	120	3.0	15.0	5.0	20	50	0
(*Hood Carb Count-down*), 6 oz.	80	12.0	3.0	1.5	10	90	0
(*Stonyfield* Nonfat) .	180	9.0	36.0	0	0	140	3.0
(*Stonyfield* Nonfat), 6 oz.	140	7.0	28.0	0	0	110	2.0
Yogurt, frozen, ½ cup:							
(*Ben & Jerry's Half Baked*)	190	5.0	35.0	3.0	20	100	<1.0
black cherry vanilla swirl (*Dreyer's/Edy's* Nonfat)	90	3.0	20.0	0	0	45	0
blueberry (*Turkey Hill Muffin*)	120	3.0	23.0	3.0	10	80	2.0
caramel brownie sundae (*Hood* Nonfat)	120	3.0	28.0	0	0	60	0
caramel praline swirl (*Dreyer's/Edy's* Nonfat)	100	3.0	23.0	0	0	60	0

Food and Measure	cal.	prot. (gms)	carbo. (gms)	fat (gms)	chol. (mgs)	sod. (mgs)	fiber (gms)
cherry chocolate chip (*Ben & Jerry's Cherry Garcia*)	170	4.0	32.0	3.0	20	65	<1.0
chocolate (*Stonyfield* Nonfat)	100	4.0	19.0	0	0	55	<1.0
chocolate almond praline (*Hood*)	140	3.0	24.0	3.0	10	60	0
chocolate cherry cordial (*Turkey Hill* Nonfat)	110	3.0	23.0	0	0	80	1.0
chocolate chip cookie dough (*Turkey Hill*)	120	3.0	22.0	3.5	10	90	3.0
chocolate fudge brownie:							
(*Ben & Jerry's*)	190	5.0	35.0	2.5	15	100	1.0
(*Häagen-Dazs*)	200	9.0	35.0	2.5	35	140	2.0
chocolate marshmallow: (*Turkey Hill* Nonfat)	120	3.0	25.0	0	0	110	1.0
caramel (*Ben & Jerry's Phish Food*)	220	4.0	41.0	4.5	15	95	1.0
chocolate mint chip (*Stonyfield* Lowfat)	130	4.0	22.0	3.0	0	50	<1.0
coffee:							
(*Häagen-Dazs*)	200	8.0	31.0	4.5	65	50	0
(*Stonyfield* Nonfat Decaf)	90	4.0	19.0	0	<5	65	0
cookies and cream:							
(*Dreyer's/Edy's*) ...	120	2.0	19.0	3.5	10	45	0
(*Hood*)	140	3.0	25.0	3.5	10	75	0
crème caramel (*Stonyfield* Lowfat)	120	4.0	23.0	1.5	<5	90	0
dulce de leche (*Häagen-Dazs*)	190	6.0	35.0	2.5	5	75	0
graham, w/peanut butter (*Turkey Hill* Graham Canyon) ..	160	3.0	23.0	7.0	5	105	3.0
lemon (*Turkey Hill* Nonfat Southern Pie)	120	3.0	25.0	0	0	115	0
mint cookies and cream (*Turkey Hill*)	110	4.0	22.0	1.5	0	80	1.0
mocha fudge: (*Hood* Nonfat)	110	3.0	27.0	0	0	55	0
almond (*Stonyfield* Lowfat)	130	5.0	23.0	2.5	0	60	1.0

Food and Measure	cal.	prot. (gms)	carbo. (gms)	fat (gms)	chol. (mgs)	sod. (mgs)	fiber (gms)
Yogurt, frozen *(cont.)*							
Neapolitan (*Turkey Hill* Nonfat)	90	3.0	19.0	0	0	60	1.0
peach:							
(*Green's* Lowfat) . .	120	2.0	22.0	2.0	10	60	0
(*Green's* Nonfat) . . .	110	3.0	23.0	0	0	70	0
peanut butter marsh- mallow (*Turkey Hill*)	140	3.0	25.0	4.0	5	130	2.0
raspberry:							
(*Stonyfield* Nonfat) .	100	3.0	21.0	0	0	55	0
double (*Hood* Nonfat)	120	2.0	26.0	0	0	55	0
raspberry vanilla							
(*Dreyer's/Edy's*) . . .	90	2.0	16.0	2.5	10	25	0
strawberry:							
(*Häagen-Dazs*)	140	5.0	31.0	0	<5	40	0
(*Hood* Nonfat)	100	2.0	23.0	0	0	50	0
coffee crunch (*Dreyer's/ Edy's Heath*)	120	2.0	18.0	4.0	10	45	0
vanilla:							
(*Dreyer's/Edy's*) . . .	100	2.0	17.0	2.5	10	30	0
(*Dreyer's/Edy's* Nonfat)	90	3.0	19.0	0	0	45	0
(*Green's* Lowfat) . .	120	3.0	20.0	2.5	10	65	0
(*Green's* Nonfat) . . .	110	3.0	22.0	0	0	75	0
(*Hood* Nonfat)	110	3.0	24.0	0	0	55	0
(*Stonyfield* Nonfat) .	90	4.0	19.0	0	<5	65	0
bean (*Turkey Hill*) .	100	3.0	19.0	2.0	10	55	3.0
vanilla chocolate swirl (*Dreyer's/Edy's* Nonfat)	90	3.0	19.0	0	0	45	0
vanilla, chocolate, strawberry (*Hood Classic Trio*)	120	3.0	22.0	2.5	10	50	0
vanilla fudge swirl:							
(*Green's* Nonfat) . . .	120	3.0	25.0	0	0	70	0
(*Stonyfield* Nonfat) .	110	4.0	23.0	0	0	60	0
(*Turkey Hill* Nonfat Fudge Ripple) . . .	100	3.0	22.0	0	0	90	0
vanilla Swiss almond (*Hood*)	150	3.0	25.0	4.0	10	60	0
"Yogurt," soy, 6 oz., except as noted:							
plain (*Silk*), 8 oz.	140	5.0	22.0	3.0	0	30	1.0
apricot mango (*Silk*) .	160	4.0	30.0	2.0	0	20	1.0

Food and Measure	cal.	prot. (gms)	carbo. (gms)	fat (gms)	chol. (mgs)	sod. (mgs)	fiber (gms)
banana strawberry (*Silk*)	160	4.0	29.0	2.0	0	20	1.0
blueberry (*Silk*)	150	4.0	29.0	2.0	0	20	1.0
cherry, black (*Silk*) ..	160	4.0	29.0	2.0	0	20	1.0
lemon (*Silk*)	160	4.0	31.0	2.0	0	20	1.0
lime, key (*Silk*)	160	4.0	30.0	2.0	0	20	1.0
peach (*Silk*)	150	4.0	32.0	2.0	0	20	1.0
raspberry (*Silk*)	160	4.0	30.0	2.0	0	20	1.0
strawberry (*Silk*)	160	4.0	31.0	2.0	0	20	1.0
vanilla (*Silk*)	130	4.0	25.0	2.0	0	20	1.0
Yogurt bar, frozen, 1 pc.:							
all flavors:							
chocolate coated (*Yoplait* Triple Dipped)	110	2.0	11.0	6.0	<5	35	0
fruit, w/fruit pieces (*Yoplait* Double Smoothies)	45	1.0	11.0	0	0	35	0
sorbet and, see "Sorbet bar"							
strawberry w/cereal (*Yoplait* Breakfast) .	120	4.0	23.0	1.5	5	115	<1.0
vanilla w/cereal (*Yoplait* Breakfast) .	120	4.0	24.0	1.5	5	115	<1.0
Yogurt drink (see also "Kefir"):							
(*DanActive* Original), 3.3 fl. oz.	90	3.0	16.0	1.5	10	50	0
all varieties:							
(*Breyers Creme Savers* Smoothie), 10 fl. oz.	190	8.0	32.0	3.0	20	280	0
(*Danimals*), 3.1 fl. oz.	90	4.0	16.0	1.5	5	55	0
(*Dannon Light 'n Fit Carb Control* Smoothie), 7 fl. oz.	70	6.0	4.0	3.0	10	35	0
(*Yoplait Nouriche* Breakfast Smoothie), 11 fl. oz.	290	10.0	60.0	0	5	290	6.0
(*Yoplait Nouriche* Breakfast Smoothie Light), 11 fl. oz.	170	10.0	33.0	0	10	250	5.0

Food and Measure	cal.	prot. (gms)	carbo. (gms)	fat (gms)	chol. (mgs)	sod. (mgs)	fiber (gms)
Yogurt drink, all varieties *(cont.)*							
except strawberry (*Hood Carb Count-down* Smoothie), 10 fl. oz.	100	13.0	4.0	3.0	10	45	0
banana berry (*Dannon Fusion*), 10 fl. oz. ...	270	8.0	52.0	3.5	15	130	0
berry:							
mixed (*Dannon Light 'n Fit* Smoothie), 7 fl. oz.	80	5.0	15.0	0	0	85	0
wild (*Dannon Fusion*), 10 fl. oz.	280	8.0	53.0	3.5	15	170	0
cherry berry (*Dannon Fusion*), 10 fl. oz. ...	280	8.0	53.0	3.5	15	160	<1.0
orange (*DanActive*), 3.3 fl. oz.	100	3.0	18.0	1.5	5	45	5
peach passion fruit:							
(*Dannon Fusion*), 10 fl. oz.	270	8.0	51.0	3.5	15	180	0
(*Dannon Light 'n Fit* Smoothie), 7 fl. oz	80	5.0	15.0	0	0	85	0
raspberry (*Dannon Light 'n Fit* Smoothie), 7 fl. oz.	80	5.0	15.0	0	0	95	<1.0
strawberry:							
(*DanActive*), 3.3 fl. oz.	100	3.0	18.0	1.5	5	50	0
(*Dannon Light 'n Fit* Smoothie), 7 fl. oz.	80	5.0	14.0	0	0	85	0
(*Hood Carb Count-down* Smoothie), 10 fl. oz.	100	13.0	4.0	3.0	10	50	0
strawberry banana (*Dannon Light 'n Fit* Smoothie), 7 fl. oz.	80	5.0	15.0	0	0	85	0
strawberry kiwi (*Dannon Fusion*), 10 fl. oz.	270	8.0	52.0	3.5	15	160	0
tropical fruit: (*Dannon Fusion*), 10 fl. oz.	270	8.0	52.0	3.5	15	130	0

Food and Measure	cal.	prot. (gms)	carbo. (gms)	fat (gms)	chol. (mgs)	sod. (mgs)	fiber (gms)
(*Dannon Light 'n Fit* Smoothie), 7 fl. oz.	80	5.0	15.0	0	0	85	0
vanilla (*DanActive*), 3.3 fl. oz.	100	3.0	18.0	1.5	5	50	0
Yogurt sandwich, frozen, 1 pc.:							
orange vanilla, w/cereal waffles (*Yoplait* Breakfast)	180	4.0	33.0	4.5	0	130	0
vanilla (*Turkey Hill*) ..	160	4.0	30.0	3.5	5	180	3.0
Yogurt seasoning (*Neera's*), 1 tsp.	6	0	2.0	0	0	2	0
Yogurt smoothie, see "Yogurt drink"							
Youngberry juice, (*Ceres*), 8 fl. oz. ...	120	0	30.0	0	0	10	0
Yu choy sum (*Frieda's*), 1 cup, 3 oz.	20	2.0	3.0	0	0	20	0
Yuca root (*Frieda's*), ⅔ cup, 3 oz.	100	3.0	23.0	0	0	5	1.0

Z

Food and Measure	cal.	prot. (gms)	carbo. (gms)	fat (gms)	chol. (mgs)	sod. (mgs)	fiber (gms)
Ziti pasta entree, frozen, three cheese (*Smart Ones*), 10-oz. pkg.	290	11.0	47.0	7.0	5	600	5.0
Zucchini, fresh, w/skin, ½ cup, except as noted:							
raw:							
chopped	9	.7	1.8	.1	0	2	.7
sliced	8	.7	1.6	.1	0	2	.7
baby (*Frieda's*), ⅔ cup, 3 oz. . . .	20	2.0	3.0	0	0	0	0
baby, 1 large, 3⅛" .	3	.4	.5	<.1	0	tr.	<.1
boiled, drained:							
sliced	14	.6	3.5	<.1	0	2	1.3
mashed	19	.8	4.7	.1	0	3	1.7
Zucchini, canned, Italian style, ½ cup:							
(*Del Monte*)	30	1.0	7.0	0	0	490	1.0
w/tomato juice	33	1.2	7.8	.1	0	424	1.0
Zucchini, frozen:							
w/skin, boiled, drained, 1 cup	38	2.6	7.9	.3	0	5	2.9
yellow and green (*C&W*), ⅔ cup	15	1.0	2.0	0	0	15	1.0
Zucchini, breaded, frozen (*Empire Kosher*), 7 pcs., 3 oz.	100	5.0	18.0	.5	0	280	1.0
Zucchini, marinated, sun-dried, in jars (*Antica Italia*), 1 oz.	160	0	2.0	17.0	0	15	1.0